MODERN COLPOSCOPY

Textbook and Atlas,
Second Edition

Daron G. Ferris, MD
J. Thomas Cox, MD
Dennis M. O'Connor, MD
V. Cecil Wright, MD
John Foerster, MFA, CMI

American Society for Colposcopy and Cervical Pathology

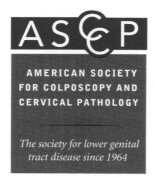

ASCP

AMERICAN SOCIETY
FOR COLPOSCOPY AND
CERVICAL PATHOLOGY

*The society for lower genital
tract disease since 1964*

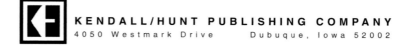

KENDALL/HUNT PUBLISHING COMPANY
4050 Westmark Drive   Dubuque, Iowa 52002

ISBN 0-7872-6467-9

Kendal/Hunt Publishing Company has the exclusive rights to reproduce this work,
to prepare derivative works from this work, to publicly distribute this work,
to publicly perform this work and to publicly display this work.

Printed in the United States of America
10 9 8 7 6 5 4 3 2

Dedication

This book is dedicated to a select group of understanding individuals:

To my partner in life, Deborah, and to our children, Jonathan and Jamie. For all the love, support, and the many missed walks on the beach. And to my two mentors, Mark Schiffman, MD and Tom Wright, MD: brothers in science and in friendship.
J. Thomas Cox, MD

To my loving wife, Pamella, and supportive parents, Herschel and Georga; their presence, compassion, and guidance are truly appreciated.
Daron G. Ferris, MD

To my wife, Louise, and children (David, Rick, Sarah, and Elizabeth), for their continued patience when husband and dad had to work on "Those Book Chapters," and to the members of the ASCCP, for providing the focus to produce a quality product worthy of their acceptance.
Dennis M. O'Connor, MD

I dedicate my work in this volume to three giants of gynecology and gynecologic oncology that I had the good fortune to train under: the late Clyde Randall, the late John B. Graham and the late Stanley Way.
V. Cecil Wright, MD

Acknowledgments

Many wonderful individuals and entities contributed to the production of this textbook, in addition to the authors. We thank Welch Allyn, Inc. (Skaneateles Falls, NY) for their very generous financial support of our project. We sincerely appreciate Drs. Vesna Kesic, Kenneth L. Noller, Gordon D. Davis, V. Cecil Wright, Richard Reid, Teresa M. Darragh, Joel Palefsky, Duane E. Townsend, Kenneth D. Hatch, and Burton A. Krumholz providing additional colposcopic images. We are particularly grateful to Drs. L. Stewart Massad, Hope K. Haefner, Burton A. Krumholz, E. J. Mayeaux, Jr., Alan Waxman, and Mark Schiffman for their critical but helpful CME review. Dr. Thomas C. Wright should be recognized for having co-authored the original *Contemporary Colposcopy* videotape and for his valuable contributions in planning, organizing and reviewing in the initial phase of development of the book. We also thank Melody Collins and Karen Shipp for their careful editorial review of the textbook. Kelly Smith contributed significantly by digitally scanning the colposcopic images and Tecia German, Deborah Cox, and Mary Ann Riopelle should be recognized for coordination and transcription of the textbook. John Foerster, Robert Finkbeiner, and Andrew Rekito have created a remarkable new standard for medical illustrations in a colposcopy textbook. Kathy Poole is also thanked for her patience, support and central coordination of this effort.

Contents

Authors

Daron G. Ferris, MD
Professor
Departments of Family Medicine and
Obstetrics and Gynecology
Medical College of Georgia
Augusta, Georgia

J. Thomas Cox, MD
Director
Gynecology and Colposcopic Clinic
Student Health Services
University of California, Santa Barbara
Santa Barbara, California

Dennis M. O'Connor, MD
Clinical Pathology Associates
Louisville, Kentucky
Clinical Associate Professor
Department of Obstetrics/Gynecology
and Pathology
University of Louisville School of Medicine
Louisville, Kentucky

V. Cecil Wright, MD
Professor Emeritus
Department of Obstetrics/Gynecology
University of Western Ontario
London, Ontario, Canada

John Foerster, MFA, CMI
Augusta, Georgia

Medical Illustrators

John Foerster, MFA, CMI
Augusta, Georgia

Robert Finkbeiner, MS
Pittsburgh, Pennsylvania

Andrew Rekito, MS
Augusta, Georgia

Reviewers

Hope K. Haefner, MD
Director
The University of Michigan Center for Vulvar Diseases
Associate Professor of Obstetrics and Gynecology
The University of Michigan Hospitals
Ann Arbor, Michigan

Burton A. Krumholz, MD
Professor of Gynecology, Obstetrics, and Women's
  Health
Albert Einstein College of Medicine
Chief of Colposcopy and Laser Surgery
Department of Obstetrics and Gynecology
Long Island Jewish Medical Center
North Shore-LIJ Health System
New Hyde Park, New York

L. Stewart Massad, MD
Associate Professor
Division of Gynecologic Oncology
Department of Obstetrics and Gynecology
Southern Illinois University School of Medicine
Springfield, Illinois

Edward J. Mayeaux, Jr, MD
Professor of Family Medicine
Professor of Obstetrics and Gynecology
Louisiana State University Health Sciences Center
Shreveport, Louisiana

Alan G. Waxman, MD
Associate Professor
Department of Obstetrics and Gynecology
University of New Mexico School of Medicine
Albuquerque, New Mexico

CME Credits

Is This Educational Activity Right for Me?

The *Modern Colposcopy, Textbook and Atlas, Second Edition* teaching kit is intended for both the beginning and advanced colposcopist (e.g., obstetrician-gynecologist, family physician, resident, nurse practitioner, physician's assistant, pathologist, etc.). The participant should be a licensed physician or advanced practice clinician who has completed advanced clinical training from an accredited institution.

Educational Objectives

Upon completion of this activity you should be able to:

- Describe the anatomy, cytology, histology, and colposcopic findings of the normal and abnormal cervix, vagina, and vulva;
- Elicit and document an appropriate history including risk factors for lower genital tract neoplasia;
- Understand the pathophysiology of lower genital tract neoplasia including the role of oncogenic HPV in preinvasive and invasive diseases of the cervix, vagina, and vulva;
- Describe the various screening technologies to detect cervicovaginal abnormalities and the strengths and limitations of each;
- Discuss the challenges of colposcopy for selected patient populations, such as adolescents, underserved women, and pregnant women;
- Perform appropriate cytologic sampling, colposcopic evaluation and biopsies (including endocervical sampling), and become familiar with instrumentation and necessary supplies;
- Understand the normal operation and function of a surgical pathology and cytopathology laboratory;
- Recognize the diagnostic characteristics of cervical abnormalities (low-grade and high-grade cervical lesions as well as cervical cancer) on cytologic, colposcopic, and histologic exam;
- Interpret and correlate cytologic, colposcopic, and histologic results;
- Formulate a plan of care for the management of women with Pap test abnormalities according to the 2001 ASCCP Consensus Guidelines, the ASCUS/LSIL Triage Study (ALTS), and other evidence-based guidelines;
- Implement treatment options to include cryosurgery and electrosurgical loop excision;
- Understand new treatments for vulvar and vaginal pain;
- Provide appropriate patient education and support; and,
- Perform quality assurance measures.

Educational Components

Textbook: A leading reference for the physician, resident, or advanced practice clinician who wishes to bridge the gap between the obvious need for increased early detection of cervical, vaginal, and vulvar disease, and the intensive education required for colposcopy. *Modern Colposcopy, Textbook and Atlas, Second Edition* is organized into twenty chapters, providing practical, evidence-based knowledge on cervical cancer screening, colposcopy equipment and supplies, lower genital tract disease triage and management, the natural history and epidemiology of human papillomavirus, the challenges of colposcopy for special patient populations, and the new evidence-based guidelines for cervical cytological abnormalities and cervical cancer precursors. The textbook contains 750 pages, with over 1200 color plates, illustrations, and tables throughout the text.

    CD-ROM: 20 case studies on cervical and vulvar disease that require the user to diagnose and develop a management plan based on patient history, findings on physical examination, and biopsy test results. All cases reflect the new Bethesda 2001 nomenclature and the ASCCP Consensus Guidelines for the Management of Women with Cervical Cytological Abnormalities and Cervical Intraepithclial Neoplasia. This CD-ROM will help users do the following: a) make appropriate diagnoses of a variety of colposcopic lesions considering patient history, presenting signs and symptoms, and clinical evaluation; b) identify select physical characteristics demonstrated by a variety of colposcopic lesions; c) identify appropriate management options and describe a plan of care for a variety of patients presenting with select colposcopic diagnoses; and, d) apply components of grading criteria to develop a consistent system for grading colposcopic lesions. The CD-ROM also contains the CME unit pages such as the self-exam CME post-test, the Program Evaluation Form, the CME coupon for additional program users, etc.

DVD: Formerly the ASCCP's *Contemporary Colposcopy* videotape, this live, 42-minute DVD depicts the instruments, procedural knowledge, and techniques used when performing colposcopy. The video features normal cervices, atypical cervices, low-grade and high-grade CIN, and cancer. Colposcopy of the vagina and vulva are also featured.

ACCME accreditation

The American Society for Colposcopy and Cervical Pathology is accredited by the Accreditation Council for Continuing Medical Education (ACCME) to provide continuing medical education for physicians.

Continuing medical education credits

ASCCP—The American Society for Colposcopy and Cervical Pathology designates this educational activity for a maximum of 28.5 Category 1 credits toward the the Society's program for continuing Professional Development Physician's Recognition Award of the AMA. Each physician should claim only those credits that he/she actually spent in the activity. The *Modern Colposcopy, Textbook and Atlas, Second Edition* teaching kit was planned and produced in accordance with ACCME's *Essential Areas and Elements*.

Instructions for obtaining continuing medical education credit

To complete this program successfully and receive credit and certificate of attendance, participants must follow these steps:

- Read the educational objectives;
- Read the textbook (20 CME hours Category 1);
- View the CD-ROM Case Studies (8 CME hours Category 1);
- View the DVD program (0.5 CME hour Category 1);
- Read, complete and submit CME Exam answers, to the ASCCP national office (form located on the CD-ROM); and,
- Read, complete and submit the Program Evaluation Form to the ASCCP national office (form located on the CD-ROM).

To earn your CME credits, please complete and submit the CME Exam and Program Evaluation Form with the CME coupon found on the CD-ROM. From the Main Menu, select the CME button to access the form that may be completed electronically or downloaded and physically sent to the ASCCP National Office. Should others wish to obtain CME credit for the program, they may submit the completed Program Evaluation Form, CME Exam form, and CME Coupon, and mail, along with a check for $100.00 to: ASCCP National Office, 20 West Washington Street, Suite 1, Hagerstown, MD 21740.

This program was originally released in 2004. Continuing medical education credits will be available from ASCCP through December 31, 2007. After 2007, ASCCP will review the program for affirmation of credit.

Disclaimer

The *Modern Colposcopy, Textbook and Atlas, Second Edition* is an educational resource and as such does not define a standard of care, nor is it intended to dictate an exclusive course of treatment or procedure to be followed. It presents methods and techniques of clinical practice that are acceptable and used by recognized authorities, for consideration by licensed physicians and healthcare providers to incorporate into their practice. Variations of practice, taking into account the needs of the individual patient, resources, and limitation unique to the institution or type of practice, may be appropriate.

The statements and opinions expressed within this educational program are those of the authors and are not necessarily those of the American Society for Colposcopy and Cervical Pathology (ASCCP). ASCCP disclaims any responsibility and/or liability for such information.

Disclosure of Interest

Current guidelines state that the participants in CME activities should be made aware of any affiliation, financial interest, or potential conflict of interest within the past twelve months that may affect the author's presentation(s). Each author and reviewer has been requested to complete a disclosure of interest statement. Those reporting an affiliation are listed below. All remaining authors and reviewers declare that neither they nor any business associate or any member of their immediate family have financial interests or other relationships with the manufacturer(s) of any products or provider(s) of any of the services discussed in this program. Any discussion of off-label use of products is noted as appropriate.

The following codes identify the relationship to industry: Advisor (A); Advisory Board (AB), Clinical Trial Support, (CTC) Consultant (C), Educational Grant (EG), Equipment Support (E), General Support (G), Honorarium (H), Invention (I), Research Support (R), Speaker's Bureau (S), and/or Speaker's Bureau Advisor (SA), Stockholder (SH).

J. Thomas Cox, MD
3M Pharmaceuticals (S)
Cytyc Corporation (S)
Digene Corporation (S)

Daron G. Ferris, MD
3M Pharmaceuticals (C), (R), (S), (H)
Cytyc Corporation (S), (R-Past), (H)
Digene Corporation (S), (R-past)
GlaxoSmithKline Worldwide (R), (C), (H)
Merck Pharmaceuticals (C), (R), (S)

Wallach Surgical Corporation (I)
Welch Allyn Inc, (C), (EG), (R- past)
SpectRx, Inc (R)
Medispectra (R- past)
Polartechnics (R- past)

Edward J. Mayeaux, Jr, MD
3M Pharmaceuticals (S)

Hope K. Haefner, MD
Ortho McNeil (S)

Educational Grant/Equipment Sponsor Disclosure
ASCCP received an unrestricted educational grant from Welch Allyn Inc. to produce and publish the *Modern Colposcopy, Textbook and Atlas, Second Edition* program.

ASCCP annually offers educational grant (E) and equipment sponsorship (ES) opportunities to exhibitors and manufacturing companies to help defray the costs of presenting postgraduate courses in colposcopy education. At the time of this printing (May 2004), the following corporations participated in the 2004 Friends program:

- Cooper Surgical (ES)
- Cytyc Corporation (E)
- Elsevier Science/Saunders/Mosby (E)
- Wallach Surgical (ES)
- Welch Allyn (ES)
- Lippincott Williams, and Wilkins (E)

The Challenge of Colposcopy Today
Historical Perspective

Table of Contents

1.1 Inventing the Colposcope

The study of the cervix *in vivo* began only after Recamier's invention of the modern speculum in 1818. By the early 1900s, a few reports of white lesions on the cervix, termed *leukoplakia* (Figure 1.1), had appeared in the literature, several of which had been observed to progress to invasive cancer.[1,2] A Viennese investigator, von Franque, assigned his assistant, Hans Hinselmann, to study leukoplakia (Table 1.1). Hinselmann's conclusion was that leukoplakia was always a sign of either a precancerous or a cancerous condition.[3] Concerned with the limitations of palpation and *naked-eye* examinations in the diagnosis of early cervical cancer, he set out to devise an instrument that would illuminate and magnify the cervix.[4] He mounted a Leitz binocular dissecting microscope with an attached light source to a stand. Using 3.5x to 30x magnification, Hinselmann was able to do more than his original intention of detecting the smallest possible invasive cancer. With the colposcope, he began to describe the characteristics of intraepithelial carcinomas (carcinoma in situ and lesser grades of cervical intraepithelial neoplasia [CIN]). While evaluating the effect of dilute acetic acid in removing mucus, he discovered the colposcopic sign of acetowhitening.

These discoveries followed closely on the footsteps of the histologic descriptions of lesions noted to be only in the surface epithelium. Carcinoma in situ, both in the absence of invasive carcinoma and at the periphery of such lesions, had been studied histologically by von Franque,[5] Schaeunstein,[6] and Schottlander and Kermauer.[7] Cullen provided similar observations during his research at Johns Hopkins University. By stripping away the leukoplakia and

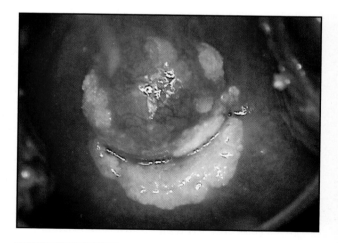

FIGURE 1.1 The earliest changes noted on the cervix with the naked eye were white lesions, termed leukoplakia. Although it is currently known that most areas of leukoplakia are not associated with cervical neoplasia, the initial reports of this finding concluded that it was always secondary to a precancerous or a cancerous process. This photomicrograph demonstrates an area of leukoplakia associated with a low-grade intraepithelial lesion.

Table 1.1 The Birth of Colposcopy

1901	von Franque and others describe the earliest histologic changes of cervical cancer as *surface carcinoma* or *intraepithelial carcinoma*.
1924	Hinselmann collaborates with Leitz to produce a binocular microscope with an attached light source on a movable stand.
1931	Emmert (USA) introduces colposcopy to the United States in an article in the *Journal of the American Medical Association*.[15]
1932–39	Colposcopy clinics are established in Switzerland (Mestwerdt and Wespi), England (Shaw), Spain (Usandizaga), Brazil (de Morales), Germany (Hinselmann), and Argentina (Jakob).[28]
1939	Kraatz (Germany) describes the use of colored filters.[28]

evaluating the underlying epithelium with the colposcope, it was possible to describe the fine detail of the morphologic changes.[8] Through meticulous comparison of the visual findings with the histologic detail, the colposcopic appearance of the *ground leukoplakia or Leukoplakiegrund* (now termed *punctation*) and the *Mosaic leukoplakia or Felderung* (now known as *mosaic*) were determined to be disturbances of epithelial architecture.[9,10] Early investigators tried to explain all such *atypical* colposcopic patterns as part of the same process leading to cervical cancer. But some atypical patterns represent only benign disorders. This misperception resulted in the grouping of benign disorders of maturation, characterized only by wide bands of typical-appearing prickle cells, with CIN, characterized by similar bulky epithelial pegs of mostly atypical undifferentiated cells. These abnormal areas, recognized as involving primarily the transformation zone,[4,11] were labeled the *matrix area of carcinoma*.[12]

Areas of "disordered maturation", which would now be called atypical or reactive metaplasia, were originally characterized as *simple atypical*, and what is now termed CIN was called *marked atypical*. Not until the 1950s did pathologists define these as two distinct entities. Glatthar subdivided marked atypical epithelium into categories that have more recently been termed histologically as CIN grades 1, 2, and 3, or cytologically as low-grade and high-grade squamous intraepithelial lesions (LSIL and HSIL, respectively).[13] Subsequently, Dietel reported on the long-term follow-up of 390 women originally diagnosed as having simple atypical cells within the matrix area of the cervix.[14] Over a period of up to 23 years, he did not find a single malignant transformation of such acanthotic epithelium.

These observations began to explain why many matrix areas, which we now call the *atypical transformation zone*, failed to consistently indicate a premalignant state. Instead, histological sections often revealed only florid metaplasia, often with underlying stromal inflammation, or disorders of maturation, such as that found in the congenital transformation zone (See Chapter 2). The colposcopic differentiation of metaplasia and benign disorders of maturation from CIN continues to be a perplexing problem. When colposcopy is used as a tool only in response to abnormal cervical cytology, the impression is that virtually all atypical transformation zones will contain corresponding abnormal histology. When the colposcope is used for routine screening, however, it becomes readily apparent that the relationship between abnormal colposcopic appearances and cervical pathology is not so simple.[14] Despite these problems, colposcopy quickly became the primary cervical screening method in much of Europe and remained so long after the introduction of cervical cytologic screening. Emmert introduced the colposcope to the United States with an article in the *Journal of the American Medical Association* in 1931, however in contrast to the European experience, colposcopy never became established as a primary screening test in North America.[15]

1.2 Developing Methods for Cervical Screening

In 1926 at the Colthea Hospital in Romania, Aurel Babes introduced cytologic sampling as a means for detecting cervical cancer (Table 1.2). During this same period at Cornell University in the United States, George Papanicolaou (Figure 1.2), while researching hormonal effects on vaginal cells, discovered that the presence of abnormal cells in the vaginal pool is a feature of early cervical cancer. In 1928, Babes published his methods in the French literature[16] during the same year that Papanicolaou first presented his data on vaginal smears.[17] It was not until 1943, however, that publication of Papanicolaou and Traut's *Diagno-*

Table 1.2   Developing Methods for Cervical Screening

1926	Babes (Rumania) precedes Papanicolaou by several months in describing cervical/vaginal cytology in the detection of cervical carcinoma.
1927	Fischer-Wasels reports on the particular importance of metaplasia in the process of cervical carcinogenesis.
1928	Papanicolaou presents his observations on association of abnormal cells in the vaginal pool with cervical carcinoma. Schiller (Germany) reports that an iodine stain is useful in screening for cervical cancer. Schiller's test is subsequently used as an additional colposcopic aid.
1930s–40s	Low-cost primary screening for cervical neoplasia with Schiller's solution is established in North America. Colposcopy becomes the primary screening method for cervical neoplasia in Europe.
1941	Papanicolaou and Traut (USA) publish early findings on cervical cytology.
1943	Papanicolaou and Traut publish the first book on the diagnosis of cervical neoplasia by vaginal pool smears. Colposcopists in Switzerland and in Austria use cervical cytology to identify women who need colposcopy.
1944	Cytologic screening is introduced to Europe.
1947	Ayre (Canada) introduces a wooden spatula for cytologic sampling of the cervix.[28]
1949–54	Cervical screening with the Papanicolaou (Pap) smear begins to gain acceptance in the United States.
1950	Glatthar subdivides *markedly atypical* epithelium into categories that more closely resembled the subsequent histologic designations of cervical intraepithelial neoplasia (CIN) grades 1, 2, and 3.
1954–55	Dietel documents that not all acetowhite *matrix areas* have a premalignant potential. Koss describes the *koilocyte*.

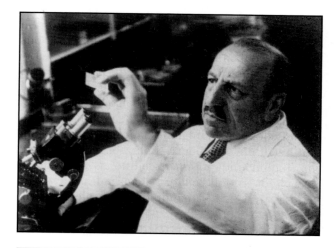

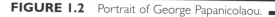

FIGURE 1.2   Portrait of George Papanicolaou.

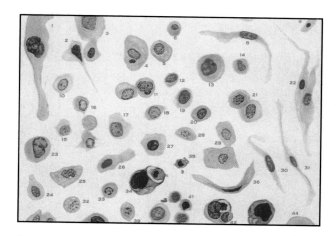

FIGURE 1.3   Drawings from Papanicolaou's early work on cervical cytology in the vaginal pool illustrate cells ranging from normal to cancer.

sis of Uterine Cancer by the Vaginal Smear[18] led the way to using cervical exfoliative cytology as a method of screening for cervical disease in the U.S. (Figure 1.3). Papanicolaou's pioneering work in cervical cytology occurred virtually simultaneously with the development of the colposcope.[4] Since colposcopy and cytology both were initially intended to detect only early invasive cervical cancer, the primary focus in the early days of both procedures was on the diagnosis of invasive cervical cancer in its earliest stages. Documentation by investigators of the many colposcopic appearances in both the healthy and the diseased cervix, and correlation of these findings with histology, subsequently showed that the most important role of colposcopy was its capacity to detect pre-invasive cervical disease. Similar conclusions about the role of cervical cytology were being developed concurrently.

At about the same time that Babes and Papanicolaou were developing cervical cytology as a screen for cervical cancer, Walter Schiller at the II Universitäts Frauenklinik in Vienna proposed the application of an iodine solution to the cervix as an inexpensive alternative cervical screen.[19] Schiller based his iodine test on Warberg's observation that "carcinomatous tissue uses up much more glycogen than normal tissue. While normal squamous epithelium, especially when honeycomb cells are well developed, stains mahogany brown with iodine solution, carcinomatous tissue remains unstained".[20] Schiller also noted that columnar epithelium did not stain, nor did poorly estrogenized squamous epithelium, whereas neoplastic lesions, whether cervical or vaginal, stained mustard-yellow color (Figure 1.4). Investigators subsequently began to experiment with the use of Schiller's stain during the colposcopic examination. In 1932, Schiller immigrated to Boston and brought with him the concept of cervical screening with iodine solution. However, the Schiller's iodine test was soon found to be too non-specific for primary screening of the cervix since many non-neoplastic conditions, including immature metaplasia and normal repair, also resulted in non-staining areas. Therefore, the advent of Papanicolaou testing during the 1940s quickly supplanted Schiller's testing in primary cervical screening. Today, the Schiller's test is rarely used except as part of a colposcopic evaluation in the follow-up of abnormal cytology.

1.3 Growth and Acceptance of Colposcopy

In the United States acceptance of colposcopy came about slowly, but in Europe it flourished under the guidance of the further pioneering work of Coupez,[21] Ganse,[22] Kolstad,[23] Limburg,[24] Mestwerdt,[25] Navratil,[26] and Wespi.[27] (Table 1.3) Use of colposcopy outside Germany and the German-speaking areas of Austria, Switzerland, and South America, however, was rare until the 1950s, as colposcopy was only introduced in the early years in areas with considerable German influence. Improved equipment with better optics and illumination and the advent of colpophotography led to more precise descriptions of the capillary vascular bed of both normal and neoplastic cervical epithelium. These improvements eventually led to wider acceptance of colposcopy and establishment of colposcopy departments in Japan by Ando and Masubuchi (1950), in France by Palmer (1952), and in England by Stallworthy (1955).[28] Resistance to colposcopy continued to be intense in the United States. As late as 1952, Novak, in his obstetrical and gynecologic textbook, stated that any discussion of colposcopic technique and terminology would "scarcely be profitable."[29] In 1953 the arrival of the German colposcopist Bolten in Philadelphia paved the way for eventual acceptance of colposcopy in the United States.[30] Bolten immediately established a colposcopy clinic at Jefferson Medical College and trained Lang.[31] Bolten then moved to New Orleans to establish another colposcopy clinic at Louisiana State University Medical School in 1954, where he trained a nucleus of disciples—Bise, Dampier, Schneider, Torres, Ward and Weese. These individuals would eventually be very important in establishing the role of colposcopy in the United States.[28]

By the 1960s, some of the earlier barriers to the acceptance of colposcopy in the United States began to fall, as an increasing understanding of the natural history of cervical carcinogenesis and improvements in colposcopic terminology eroded skepticism. The early descriptive terminology was in German and was not readily understood in English-speaking countries. More meaningful terminology for cytologic and

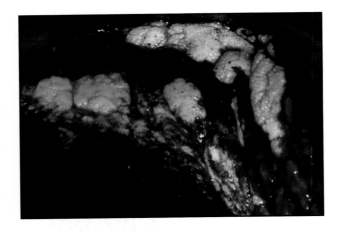

FIGURE 1.4 Schiller's iodine stains normal glycogen containing cells, but does not fully stain columnar, metaplastic or neoplastic cells. Both metaplastic and neoplastic cells take on a yellow mustard stain, whereas columnar cells completely reject the iodine uptake. Both maturing metaplasia and low-grade human papillomavirus associated changes often stain in a variegated or "tortoise shell" effect. Here can be seen multiple yellow mustard staining HPV lesions on the vaginal wall.

histologic features of tumor progression was eventually developed. Wider acceptance followed a better understanding of the morphologic changes underlying colposcopic images and English-language colposcopic terminology developed by Adolph Stafl and Malcolm Coppleson. [32,33]

Vence came to Miami in 1962 from Columbia, South America, and trained Scott in colposcopy. Scott, together with the small nucleus of colposcopists trained by Bolten, set up the American Society for Colposcopy and Colpomicroscopy in 1964.[28] Cervical cytology gained a foothold in cancer detection in the early 1950s but continued to compete with rather than complement colposcopy. This competition continued to limit colposcopy to only a minor following until the early work of Coppleson,[33,34,35] Stafl,[36] Burke,[37] Richart,[38,39] and Townsend[40] began to break down the perception that cytology and colposcopy were competing disciplines.

Coppleson, Pixley, and Reid[33] were particularly instrumental in changing the ponderous Germanic terminology to one more descriptive and communicative for modern colposcopists. Tireless teaching by these contemporary colposcopists helped to rapidly expand the cadre of colposcopic enthusiasts. By the late 1970s, colposcopy had become widely recognized in the United States as a complementary and necessary response to abnormal cervical cytology.

In other countries, however, the role of colposcopy continues to be viewed differently. In Germany and in much of Latin America, colposcopy has been incorporated into the routine gynecologic examination and continues to be used as a primary screen for cervical disease. In many other European countries and in North America, colposcopy is considered a diagnostic tool reserved for women with abnormal Papanicolaou (Pap) tests rather than a screening procedure.

Table 1.3 Growth and Acceptance of Colposcopy

1933–50	The conflict in Europe ends the development of colposcopy in the United States, as war interrupts the dialogue between European colposcopy pioneers and North American clinicians. Despite the war, advances in colposcopy continue to be made in Europe and South America.
1942	Triete (Germany) produces the first colpophotographs.[28]
1944	De la Riva (Spain) describes the value of colposcopy in the detection and treatment of cervical precancerous changes in the prevention of cervical carcinoma. Europeans begin screening with cervical cytology.[28]
1949	Hinselmann visits South America, giving stimulus to the burgeoning practice of colposcopy in Argentina, Brazil, and other countries.
1950	Ando and Masubichi introduce colposcopy to Japan. Primary mass screening with the colposcope becomes standard in Hungary 10 years before cervical cytology is used for the same purpose. Navratil establishes colposcopy as a routine technique in Austria.[28]
1953–54	Mestwerdt produces the first atlas on colposcopy. Bolten moves from Germany to the United States and establishes the first U.S. colposcopy clinics in Philadelphia and New Orleans. A small nucleus of U.S. enthusiasts is trained (i.e., Lang, Weese, Torres, Ward, Schneider, Dampier, Bise, and Hull).
1954	Stallworthy (England) sets up the first colposcopy department at Oxford in the United Kingdom. Colposcopy begins to flourish under advocates such as Anderson (1962), Jordan (1969), and Singer (1973).[28]
1961	Matew-Aragones and Usandizagas (Spain) describe colposcopic findings in pregnancy.[28]
1962	Vence comes from Colombia to Miami where he trains Scott and establishes the third center for colposcopy in the United States.
1963	Koller advocates a saline wash with colposcopic evaluation prior to the application of acetic acid and iodine stain, noting that the angioarchitecture is more easily identified prior to the application of these stains. Kolstad (Norway) develops photographic techniques to document fine angioarchitecture and describes the relationship between intercapillary distance and the degree of histologic abnormality.
1964	Disciples of Bolten and Vence establish the American Society for Colposcopy and Colpomicroscopy.

1.4 Development of Colposcopy-Based Management Algorithms for Abnormal Papanicolaou Test Results

1.4.1 Management before the introduction of colposcopy

The wide acceptance of colposcopy in the 1970s as a method for localizing lesions on the cervix brought a more rational approach to the management of women with abnormal Papanicolaou tests. Prior to this time, the response to an abnormal Pap test depended entirely upon the grade of the cytologic abnormality (Table 1.4). The response to *minor* cytologic abnormalities was to simply repeat the Pap test in 6 to 12 months. This was because minor cytologic abnormalities were thought to be rarely associated with HSIL (CIN 2,3) or invasive cancer. It was not until the 1980s that published studies demonstrated a high rate (10% to 30%) of high-grade disease and occasional invasive cervical cancer in women with minor cytologic abnormalities.[41] Cancer was occasionally missed by the failure of some women to return for proscribed follow-up Pap tests. For other women, the *standard of care* (two normal follow-up Pap tests) did not always detect disease.[42]

Somewhat paradoxically, using the grade of a cytologic abnormality alone to govern clinical responses also resulted in overtreatment of many women with high-grade disease. High-grade Pap test results, including those suspicious for cancer, were managed aggressively by cervical conization because blind four-quadrant biopsy was known to miss significant lesions. If dysplasia of any grade was found in the conization specimen, the patient was usually considered cured. Diagnosis of *carcinoma in situ*, however, usually required a hysterectomy, even for very young patients who desired to maintain their fertility. This approach to high-grade cytologic abnormalities had many drawbacks. Conization was expensive, as it required anesthesia and operating room time and had the potential for significant complications (e.g., bleeding, infection, cervical stenosis, and the risk of cervical incompetence).

Therefore, prior to the widespread use of colposcopy, management of women with cytologic abnormalities resulted in both underevaluation and overtreatment. Only those lesions correctly diagnosed by means of cytology as high-grade were actually triaged to confirmatory diagnostic and therapeutic procedures while many significant lesions remained undetected because of inadequate evaluation of lower-grade cytology. Moreover, considerable harm was caused by the widespread use of conization and hysterectomy to manage preinvasive lesions.

1.4.2 Management after the introduction of colposcopy
1.4.2.1 Management before The Bethesda System

The introduction of colposcopy and colposcopically directed biopsy dramatically changed the management of high-grade cytologic abnormalities and the treatment of proven cervical neoplasia. Colposcopy allowed the clinician to diagnose all grades of preinvasive disease and invasive cancer. Moreover, colposcopists were able to delineate the location of neoplasia on the cervix or in the vagina. As a result, more conservative (e.g., less radical) treatment methods, such as cryotherapy, laser ablation, and loop electrosurgical excision, largely supplanted cold-knife conization excision for the treatment of preinvasive disease.[43–46] Additionally, during the late 1960s through the 1980s, significant advances were made in understanding the pathogenesis of invasive cervical cancer. In 1967, Richart and Barron[47] published their work on the natural history of

Table 1.4. Management of Various Papanicolaou (Pap) Classifications before the Introduction of Colposcopy

Class I	Annual Pap test
Class IIA	Vaginal sulfa cream daily for 7 days followed by repeat Pap test in 6 to 12 months
IIB	Repeat Pap test in 3 to 6 months
Class III	Conization (some just repeated the Pap)
Class IV	Conization
Class V	Conization

cervical carcinogenesis as a continuum of disease from mild dysplasia to cervical cancer (Table 1.5). This work began to change the concept that dysplasia and carcinoma in situ require different treatments. Meisels and Fortin first established HPV as the etiologic agent in koilocytotic atypia in 1976.[48] Subsequently, the ability to document the presence of HPV within cervical neoplastic lesions, which began with the development of HPV DNA probes during the early 1980s, led to the establishment of HPV as the etiologic agent in most cervical cancers. The management of cervical preinvasive disease changed dramatically as these breakthroughs increased understanding of the disease process, and as colposcopy and conservative outpatient treatment methods became widely available.[49]

Until the late 1980s, only women with *dysplastic* cervical cytology were referred for colposcopy. However, more minor cervical cytologic abnormalities, including those with cellular changes secondary to HPV but without evidence of dysplasia, were still managed by means of repeat cervical cytology. This restrictive approach had the benefit of keeping the volume of women referred for colposcopy within a manageable range. Outpatient therapy was employed to effectively eradicate all but invasive disease and preinvasive disease not amenable to such treatment. However, the series of events that follow led to an expanding role for colposcopy.

1.4.2.2 Management after The Bethesda System

In 1988, a public outcry followed the revelation of problems inherent in cervical cytologic screening.[50] The U.S. government responded by changing regulations for cytology laboratories, and the National Cancer Institute convened a conference in Bethesda, Maryland, for the purpose of revising cervical cytologic terminology (Table 1.6). The resultant Bethesda System (TBS) dramatically changed cervical cytologic classification and reporting,[51] with similar impact on modern colposcopic practice. Not only was koilocytotic atypia now included with dysplasia in a single category of abnormality called LSIL, but even atypia that could not be reliably designated as *within normal limits* was placed in an abnormal category termed atypical squamous cells of undetermined significance

---

Table 1.5   The Role of Colposcopy in Conservative Management of Cervical Neoplasia before the Introduction of The Bethesda System

1967	Richart and Barron publish their work on the natural history of cervical carcinogenesis as a continuum of disease from mild dysplasia to cervical cancer, breaking down the concept that dysplasia and carcinoma in situ must be treated differently. Publications begin to promote more conservative approaches to treating cervical intraepithelial neoplasia (CIN 1,2,and 3 or mild, moderate, and severe dysplasia). Coppleson and Reid popularize colposcopy in Australia.
1970s	Colposcopy with directed cervical biopsy is reported to reduce the need for cone biopsy in the majority of women with abnormal Pap smear results. Cryotherapy becomes the dominant outpatient treatment modality for CIN. Canadian gynecologists establish colposcopy clinics.
1971	Coppleson, Pixley and Reid publish the first edition of their colposcopy text and further the understanding of the transformation zone in the development of cervical intraepithelial neoplasia (CIN).
1972	Argentina hosts The First World Congress of Colposcopy and Uterine Cervical Pathology, following which the International Federation of Cervical Pathology and Colposcopy (IFCPC) is founded to provide a worldwide organization of colposcopy societies.
1974	The CO_2 laser is introduced for the ablation of cervical intraepithelial neoplasia. The IFCPC standardizes colposcopic terminology and publishes its International Nomenclature of Colposcopic Findings.
1975	Zur Hausen (Germany) suggests that cervical neoplasia may be associated with human papillomavirus (HPV).
1980s	CO_2 laser begins to dominate outpatient treatment of CIN.
1983	Cartier describes electrodiathermy loop excision of cervical lesions.
1985	Ueki (Japan) publishes the first book on cervical adenocarcinoma.[28]

Table 1.6   The Role of Colposcopy and Outpatient Procedures in the Conservative Management of Cervical Neoplasia after the Introduction of The Bethesda System

1988	The first Bethesda System for reporting cervical cytology is published in the *Journal of the American Medical Association*. The colposcopic pool is greatly expanded to women with lesser degrees of cytologic atypia.
1989	Prendiville (UK) introduces large loop electrosurgical excision of the transformation zone (LLETZ).
1990s	Loop electrosurgical excision procedure (LEEP) using smaller size loops is adopted in the United States and widely criticized for overuse. A balance between use of LEEP for major, and cryotherapy for minor, lesions is accepted. Laser treatment of cervical intraepithelial neoplasia (CIN) falls out of favor due to higher cost and greater need for expertise.
1991	The Second Bethesda Conference refines The Bethesda System for reporting cervical cytology.
1995	The International Agency for Research on Cancer (IARC) confirms that human papillomavirus (HPV) is necessary in the etiology of most cervical cancers.
1996	Several new cervical screening technologies are introduced, including liquid-based cervical cytology and automated computer-based rescreening of Pap smears.
Late 1990s	Intense efforts to evaluate low-cost cervical screening modalities for resource-poor countries begin. Computer-based digital imaging systems, improved molecular probes for HPV, and computer analysis of differences in electromagnetic wavelengths of light and electrical stimulation emitted by normal and neoplastic tissues undergo intense study.
2001	The 2001 Bethesda Workshop further refines TBS cervical cytology terminology of 1988 and 1991.[66] The American Society for Colposcopy and Cervical Pathology hosts the ASCCP Consensus Conference for the Management of Abnormal Cervical Cytology and Cervical Cancer Precursors in Bethesda, MD.[67,68] Comprehensive evidence-based management guidelines for abnormal cytology and histology are developed for the first time by a consensus process involving 29 major national and international organizations with interest in cervical cancer screening.
2002	First data documenting efficacy of a prophylactic HPV vaccine are published in the *New England Journal of Medicine*.[71]

(ASCUS). The inclusion of these minor cellular changes in abnormal Pap test classifications, along with increased insecurity regarding the potential for false-negative repeat Pap tests, changed the traditional colposcopic triage guidelines.[41,52–56] The result was the referral of up to three times more women to colposcopy than would have been referred when the threshold for colposcopic referral began with dysplasia/CIN 1[57] (Figure 1.5). Although some women with high-grade lesions and invasive cervical cancer that might have been missed otherwise were now referred for colposcopic evaluation and treatment, so were many normal women and women with transient low-grade lesions induced by human papillomavirus (HPV) that had little clinical significance. Biopsy of trivial colposcopic changes may result in histologic overcall, since differentiation between variants of the normal metaplastic process and cervical neoplasia is

often quite difficult.[58–60] Improved sensitivity came at the price of subsequent overdiagnosis that has led to unnecessary treatment with high financial and psychological costs. Additionally, initial enthusiasm for in-office easy excision of the abnormal transformation zone led many to proceed directly to loop electrosurgical excision procedure (LEEP) of the transformation zone as the initial follow-up to high-grade cytology, rather than proceeding first to colposcopy-directed biopsy. Such "see and treat" LEEP procedures resulted in overtreatment of many women for disease that they did not have and subsequently has been discredited except when cytology and colposcopy both are interpreted as high-grade and the patient is deemed unreliable for follow-up.

As a consequence of this lowered threshold for referral, modern colposcopists have a much more difficult task than did their predecessors, who had to

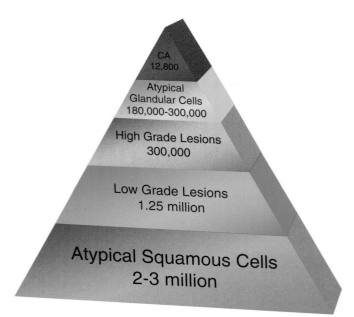

CA
12,800

Atypical
Glandular Cells
180,000-300,000

High Grade Lesions
300,000

Low Grade Lesions
1.25 million

Atypical Squamous Cells
2-3 million

FIGURE 1.5 Many have argued that The Bethesda System more than doubled the number of women considered to have abnormal Pap smear results by including atypical cells in the epithelial abnormality category. This expanded the potential colposcopic pool by at least 2,000,000 Pap findings of atypical squamous cells of undetermined significance (ASCUS), which was previously part of the Papanicolaou Class IIA category. Additionally, another 500,000 Pap findings of koilocytotic atypia, originally part of Papanicolaou Class IIB, were included with CIN 1 in the category LSIL, increasing the concern for this Pap interpretation as well. Since most protocols considered the Pap result of ASCUS to be only atypical and not abnormal, the general recommendation was to repeat these Pap smear tests and to colposcopically examine only those women with repeat abnormalities on Pap testing. HSIL denotes high-grade squamous intraepithelial lesions; LSIL, low-grade squamous intraepithelial lesions.

respond only to markedly abnormal cervical cytology that carried a high probability of finding high-grade disease at colposcopy. Only a well-trained colposcopist can capably minimize both the risks of failed detection of cervical neoplasia and the risk of overcall inherent in the colposcopic examination of normal women.

1.5 New Colposcopic Challenges

Several new challenges for the modern colposcopist have developed. First, in the past two decades, the colposcopist has been called upon to provide increasing expertise in the evaluation of areas of the female lower genital tract other than the cervix (e.g., vagina, vulva and anus). Many colposcopists have been unprepared to evaluate non-cervical areas because of a lack of experience with both normal and abnormal findings in these areas. Inexperience has led to biopsy of normal anatomic variants that have often been overcalled histologically.

Second, colposcopy was once the almost-exclusive domain of gynecologists and gynecologic oncologists who had more opportunity to see invasive cervical cancers. For physician colposcopists, residency training has provided at least a baseline familiarity with colposcopic principles, and for some, a substantial basis of excellence. However, often missing from colposcopy training is the provision of an adequate understanding of the histologic and cytologic basis of disease, an imperative for the practice of expert colposcopy. During the 1990s, the almost exclusive domain of gynecologists as colposcopists

has expanded to include generalists and nurse practitioners. As the base of colposcopic practitioners has expanded, while cervical cancer rates have fallen, the opportunity to see cervical and other lower genital tract cancers has diminished to the point that most colposcopists see very few, if any, invasive cervical cancers during their careers. Despite this, cancer prevention remains the purpose of cervical cytologic screening and colposcopic triage, so colposcopists must obtain adequate exposure to the colposcopic findings of early invasive cervical and other lower genital tract cancers by other means. To ensure this level of exposure, several organizations have developed multimedia continuing education programs in the field of colposcopy, assisted by self-study of colposcopic atlases and other teaching aids.

Third, contemporary colposcopists confront the dilemma of an apparently increasing incidence of adenocarcinomas-in-situ and invasive adenocarcinoma of the cervix, [61-63] two entities extremely difficult to diagnose by means of colposcopy. Colposcopy has long been considered to be less reliable in the evaluation of glandular intraepithelial neoplasia than in similar squamous preinvasive disease, as its presence in the canal and its subtle colposcopic appearance make it difficult to detect and to interpret.[64,65] Recognition of coexisting squamous intraepithelial neoplasia, often located just distal to glandular abnormalities, becomes even more imperative if colposcopists are to diagnosis glandular disease. In the future, advances in microcolposcopy may improve access to the endocervical canal.

One of the adverse consequences of managed health care has been the financial pressure exerted on many clinicians who have not had residency training in colposcopy to provide comprehensive expertise in the diagnosis and treatment of women with abnormal Pap test findings. Competence in colposcopy requires an understanding of the pathogenesis and natural history of the diseases of the lower genital tract as well as the procedure and instruments required for colposcopy. Proper triage and evaluation of women with abnormal Pap test results depends on a clear understanding of these principles. Inexperience in recognizing colposcopic patterns associated with the abnormal transformation zone, failure to biopsy the most abnormal area, and failure to take a sufficient number of biopsies from a large abnormal transformation zone are common errors for the inexperienced healthcare provider.[64] Mastery of complex skills and precepts are required to attain and to retain adequate expertise for competence. Some measure of legal protection is afforded by the proficiency thus attained.

Expanding colposcopic expertise to all clinicians who care for women provides an opportunity for a more cost-effective and accessible response to abnormal cervical cytology. However, it may be difficult to expand the base of clinicians who provide this service while ensuring they acquire and maintain adequate expertise in performing colposcopy and interpreting the findings. To facilitate this process, all colposcopists who have attained a degree of excellence should carry on the tradition of sharing their experience and expertise in the training of others.

1.6 Role of Colposcopy in This New Century

The acceptance of colposcopy in the United States and the development of outpatient treatment modalities for CIN have occurred rather slowly. As we move into this new century, however, dramatic changes are occurring rapidly in all aspects of medicine, including diagnosis and management of cervical disease. In order to provide good patient care, it is essential that the practicing colposcopist recognize these changes and modify clinical practices accordingly. Dramatic advances are occurring in the understanding of the pathogenesis of cervical cancer and its precursors. New insights into the role of HPV and the molecular events leading to cervical cancer are occurring almost monthly. In this age of molecular medicine, it is essential that the modern colposcopist keep abreast of these advances, recently translated into clinical practice in the form of new cytologic terminology[66] and new cervical screening and management guidelines [discussed in Chapters 18 and 19].[67,68] In addition to advances in the fields of molecular biology and molecular pathology, technical advances in optics, electromagnetic imaging, and image analysis will provide new tools for the colposcopist.[69,70] Although colposcopes used by clinicians today are considerably improved compared with the original colposcopes, they are probably more similar to the first colposcopes than they will be to the devices that will be used to evaluate the cervix in this new century. Although it is not known exactly how colposcopes and other diagnostic instruments will evolve in the future, it appears unlikely that colposcopic evaluation of the cervix will be limited to use of visible light, acetic acid, and magnification. Digital imaging computer systems, use of molecular biologic tests for HPV or its protein products, and computer analysis of different wavelengths of light and electrical stimulation reflected by normal, cancerous, and precancerous tissues are but a few of the new technologies likely to play a significant role in cervical screening in the near future. Additionally, successful HPV vaccines, discussed in Chapter 5, are likely to be available within a few years.[71]

It is our aim to provide a scientific and clinical foundation that will enable novice as well as experienced colposcopists to move confidently into this new century and become ever-evolving "modern colposcopists."

References

1. von Franque O. Leukoplakia und carcinoma vaginae et uteri. *Z Geburtshilfe* 1907;60:237–9.

2. Hinselmann H. Zur kenntnis der pracancerosen veranderungen der portio. *Zentralbl Gynakol* 1927;51:901–2.

3. Hinselmann H. Die atiologie, symptomatologie und diagnostik des uteruscarcinoms. In: Veit J, Stockel W, eds. *Handbuch der Gynekologie* Munich: Bergmann,1930:854–6: Vol 6:1.

4. Hinselmann H. Verbessrung der inspektionsmoglichkeiten von vulva, vagina und portio. *Munchner Med Wochenschr* 1925;72:1733–6.

5. von Franque O. Das beginnende portiokankroid und die ausbreitungswege des gebarmutterhalskrebses. *Z Geburtshilfe* 1901;44:173–7.

6. Schauenstein W. Histologie untersuchungen uber atypisches plattenepithel an der portio und an der innenflache der cervix uteri. *Arch Gynakol* 1908;85:576–9.

7. Schottlander J, Kermauner F. *Zur Kenntnis des Uteruskarzinoms* Berlin: Karger, 1912.

8. Hinselmann H. Ausgewahlte gesichtspunlte zur beurteilung des zusammenhanges der "matrixbezirke" und des karzinomsder sichtbaren abschnitte des weiblichen genitaltrakes. *Z Geburtshilfe* 1933;104:228–30.

9. Hinselmann H. Die Kolposkopie. In: *Klinische Fortbildung. Neue Deutsche Klinik* 1936; (suppl).4:717.

10. Hinselmann H. *Einfurung in die Kolposkopie.* Hamburg: Hartung, 1933.

11. Hinselmann H. Der begriff der umwandlungszone der portio. *Arch Gynakol* 1927;131:422–4.

12. Hinselmann H. Die linische und mikroskopische fruhdiagnose des portiokarzinoms. *Arch Gynakol* 1934:156:239–40.

13. Glatthaar E. Studien Uber die Morphogenese des Plattenepithelkarzinoms der Portio Vaginalis Uteri. Basle: Karger, 1950.

14. Dietel H, Focken A. Das schicksal des atypischen epithels an der portio. *Geburtshilfe Frauenheilkd* 1955;15:593–5.

15. Emmert F. The recognition of cancer of the uterus in its earliest stages. *JAMA* 1931;97:1684.

16. Babes A. Diagnostic du cancer du col uterine par les frottis. *La Presse Medicale.* 1928;36:451. Reprinted in English *Acta Cytol* 1967;11:217.

17. Papanicolaou G N. New cancer diagnosis. Proceedings Third Race Betterment Conference, Battle Creek, Michigan. Race Betterment Foundation, 1928.

18. Papanicolaou G N, Traut H F. *Diagnosis of Uterine Cancer by the Vaginal Smear.* New York: Commonwealth Fund, 1943.

19. Schiller J. Jodpinselung und abschabung des portioepithels. *Zentralbl Gynakol* 1929;53:1056.

20. Bolten K. Introduction to Colposcopy. *A Diagnostic Aid in Benign and Preclinical Cancerous Lesions of the Cervix Uteri,* Chapter 3. Grune & Stratton, 1960, New York.

21. Coupez F. Dysplasia of the cervix uteri. *Rev Franc Gynec Obstet.* 1965;60:579.

22. Ganse R. The influence of indirect metaplasia on the formation of carcinoma in situ of the portio. *Acta Un Int Cancer* 1963;19:1375–8.

23. Kolstad P. Carcinoma of the cervix. Stage 0. Diagnosis and treatment. *Am J Obstet Gynecol* 1966;96:1098–103.

24. Limburg H. Die *Fruhdiagnose des iteruscarcinoms.* Stuttgart: Theime, 1956.

25. Mestwerdt G. *Atlas der Kolposkopie.* Jena: Fischer, 1953.

26. Navratil E. Colposcopy. In: Gray L A, ed. *Dysplasia, carcinoma in situ and microinvasive carcinoma of the cervix uteri.* Springfield, Il: Thomas 1964:228–83.

27. Wespi H. *Early Carcinoma of the Uterine Cervix: Pathogenesis and Detection.* New York: Grune and Stratton, 1949.

28. Torres J E, Riopelle M A. History of colposcopy in the United States. In: Wright V C, Ed., *Contemporary Colposcopy.* Philadelphia: Obstet Gynecol Clin N Am 1993;20:1–12.

29. Novak E. *Gynecologic and Obstetric Pathology.* Philadelphia: W. B. Saunders, 1952.

30. Scheffery L C, Bolten K A, Lang W R. Colposcopy. *Obstet Gynecol* 1955;5:294.

31. Bise J R. In memorium Karl August Bolten. *The Colposcopist* 1972;1:1.

32. Stafl A. Colposcopy in diagnosis of cervical neoplasia. *Am J Obstet Gynecol* 1973;115(2):286–7.

33. Coppleson M, Pixley E, Reid B. Colposcopy. *A Scientific and Practical Approach to the Cervix in Health and Disease.* Springfield, Il: Charles C. Thomas, 1971.

34. Coppleson M, Reid B. The colposcopic study of the cervix during pregnancy and the puerperium. *J Obstet Gynaecol Br Commonw* 1966;73:375.

35. Coppleson M., Reid B L. *Pre-clinical Carcinoma of the Cervix Uteri; Its Origin, Nature and Management.* Pergamon Press, Oxford. 1967.

36. Stafl A. The clinical diagnosis of early cervical cancer. *Obstet Gynec Surv* 1969;24:976–82.

37. Burke L, Mathews B. *Colposcopy in Clinical Practice.* Philadelphia: FA Davis, 1977.

38. Richart R M. A clinical staining test for the in vivo delineation of dysplasia and carcinoma in situ. *Am J Obstet Gynecol* 1963;86:703–4.

39. Richart R M. Observations on the biology of cervical dysplasia. *Bull Sloane Hosp Women* 1964;10:170–4.

40. Townsend D E, Ostergard D, Mishell D. Abnormal Papanicolaou smears: evaluation by colposcopy, biopsies, and endocervical curettage. *Am J Obstet Gynecol* 1970;108:429–36.

41. Jones D E D, Creaseman W T, Dombroski R A, Lentz S S, Waeltz J L. Evaluation of the atypical Pap smear. *Am J Obstet Gynecol* 1987;157:544–9.

42. Mayeaux E J, Harper M B, Abreo F, et al. A comparison of the reliability of repeat cervical smears and colposcopy in patients with abnormal cervical cytology. *J Fam Pract* 1995;40:57–62.

43. Richart R M, Sciarra J J. Treatment of cervical dysplasia by outpatient electrocauterization. *Am J Obstet Gynecol* 1968;101:200–3.

44. Creasman W T, Weed J C, Curry S L, et al. Efficacy of cryosurgical treatment of severe cervical intraepithelial neoplasia. *Obstet Gynecol* 1972;41:501–5.

45. Wright V C, Davies E, Riopelle M A. Laser surgery for cervical intraepithelial neoplasia: principles and results. *Am J Obstet Gynecol* 1983;145–81.

46. Prendiville W, Cullimore J, Norman S. Large loop excision of the transformation zone (LLETZ): A new method of management for women with intraepithelial neoplasia. *Br J Obstet Gynecol* 1989;96:1054–60.

47. Richart R M, Barron B A. A follow-up study of patients with cervical dysplasia. *Am J Obstet Gynecol* 1969;105:386–93.

48. Meisels A, Fortin R. Condylomatous lesions of the cervix and vagina. I. Cytologic patterns. *Acta Cytol* 1976;20:505–9.

49. Shafti M I, Luesley D M. Management of low grade lesions: follow-up or treat? Cervical intraepithelial neoplasia. In: Jones H W, ed. *Bailliere's Clinical Obstetrics and Gynecology* London: Bailliere Tindall. 1995;9:121–33.

50. Bogdanich W. Wall Street Journal 1987.

51. National Cancer Institute Workshop. The 1988 Bethesda System for reporting cervical/vaginal cytologic diagnosis. *JAMA* 1989;262:931–4.

52. Yobs A R, Swanson R A, Lamotte L C. Laboratory reliability of the Papanicolaou smear. *Obstet Gynecol* 1985;65:235–43.

53. Davey D D, Naryshkin S, Nielsen M L, Kline T S. Atypical squamous cells of undetermined significance: interlaboratory comparisons and quality assurance monitors. *Diagn Cytopathol* 1994;11:390–6.

54. Van der Graaf Y, Vooijs G P, Gailland H L J, Go D M D S. Screening errors in cervical cytologic screening. *Acta Cytol* 1987;31:434–8.

55. Lindheim S R, Smith-Nguyen G. Aggressive evaluation for atypical squamous cells in Papanicolaou smears. *J Reprod Med* 1990;35:971–3.

56. Slawson D C, Bennett J H, Herman J M. Follow-up Papanicolaou smear for cervical atypia. Are we missing significant disease? *J Fam Pract* 1993;36:289–93.

57. Gordon P, Hatch K. Survey of colposcopy practices by obstetrician gynecologists. *J Reprod Med* 1992;37:861–3.

58. Robertson A J, Anderson J M, Swanson Beck J, et al. Observer variability in histopathological reporting of cervical biopsy specimens. *J Clin Pathol* 1989;42:231–8.

59. Ishmail S M, Colcough A B, Dinnen J S, et al. Observer variation in histopathological diagnosis and grading of cervical intraepithelial neoplasia. *BMJ* 1989;298:707–10.

60. Ishmail S M, Colclough A B, Dennen J S, et al. Reporting cervical intraepithelial neoplasia (CIN): intra- and interpathologist variation and factors associated with disagreement. *Histol Pathol* 1990;16:371–6.

61. Peters R K, Mack T M, Thomas D, et al. Increased frequency of adenocarcinoma of the uterine cervix in young women in Los Angeles County. *J Natl Cancer Inst* 1986;76:423–8.

62. Schwartz S M, Weiss N S. Increased incidence of adenocarcinoma of the cervix in young women in the United States. *Am J Epidemiol* 1986;124:1045–7.

63. Vesterinen E, Forss M, Nieminen U. Increase in cervical adenocarcinoma: a report of 520 cases of cervical carcinoma including 112 tumors with glandular elements. *Obstet Gynecol* 1989;33:49–53.

64. Luesley D M, Jordan J A, Woodman C B J, et al. A retrospective review of adenocarcinoma in situ and glandular atypia of the uterine cervix. *Br J Obstet Gynecol* 1987;94:699–703.

65. Anderson E S, Arrfmann E. Adenocarcinoma in situ of the uterine cervix; a clinicopathologic study of 36 cases. *Gynecol Oncol* 1989;35:1–7.

66. Solomon D, Davey D, Kurman R, et al. for the Forum Group Members and the Bethesda 2001 Workshop. The 2001 Bethesda System: terminology for reporting results of cervical cytology. *JAMA*. 2002;287:2114–9.

67. Wright T C, Jr., Cox J T, Massad L S, Twiggs L B, Wilkinson E J, for the 2001 ASCCP-Sponsored Consensus Conference. 2001 consensus guidelines for the management of women with cervical cytological abnormalities. *JAMA* 2002 Apr;287(16):2120–9.

68. Wright T C Jr, Cox J T, Massad L S, Carlson J, Twiggs L B, Wilkinson E J; American Society for Colposcopy and Cervical Pathology. 2001 consensus guidelines for the management of women with cervical intraepithelial neoplasia. *Am J Obstet Gynecol* 2003 Jul;189(1):295–304.

69. Coppleson M, Reid B L, Skladnev V, et al. An electronic approach to the detection of pre-cancer and cancer of the uterine cervix: a preliminary evaluation of Polarprobe. *Int J Gynecol Cancer* 1994;4:79.

70. Mitchell M F, Cantor S B, Ramanujam N et al. Fluorescence spectroscopy for diagnosis of squamous intraepithelial lesions of the cervix. *Obstet Gynecol* 1999;93:462.

71. Koutsky L A, Ault K A, Wheeler C M, et al. A controlled trial of a human papillomavirus type 16 vaccine. *N Engl J Med* 2002;347:1645–51.

Anatomy and Histology of the Normal Female Lower Genital Tract

Table of Contents

2.1 Introduction

The female lower genital tract includes the cervix, vagina and vulva and is unique in that these sites are readily accessible for evaluation. A medical subspecialty (cytopathology) and a procedure (colposcopy) are devoted to the screening, diagnosis, and management of these sites. To better understand the significance of female lower genital tract abnormalities and the basis for colposcopy, one must have an understanding of the normal anatomy, histology, and cytology of this region.

2.2 The Cervix
2.2.1 Embryology

The development of the female genital tract begins approximately 4 weeks after conception. At that time, a lack of testicular development results in an absence of Müllerian-inhibiting substance. The Müllerian ducts form as invaginations from the urogenital folds. These ducts extend caudally through the mesenchyme lateral to the mesonephros. By week seven, they turn medial and anterior to the mesonephros, meeting at the midline. Continued caudal growth results in the fused ducts eventually joining the urogenital sinus. The solid tip enlarges at the urogenital sinus and becomes the Müllerian tubercle. The midline septum within the ducts is lost, forming a single uterovaginal canal, which is lined by columnar epithelium. By the 11th week of gestation, stratified squamous cells partially replace the columnar cells, and by the 16th week of gestation, a rudimentary cervix is recognizable (Figure 2.1).[1,2]

The point at which the columnar and squamous cells meet is known as the *original* or *native squamocolumnar junction (SCJ).*[1,3] The location of the original SCJ varies throughout fetal life. In the second to early third trimester of gestation, the junction is located within the endocervical canal. After 32 weeks' gestation, it extends toward the vagina but by term regresses back into the canal.[4] In some individuals, however, it remains on the outer cervix and can be located on the vaginal surface at the time of delivery.[1,4]

It is unclear why squamous cells partially replace the Müllerian columnar cells in the fetal cervix. The squamous cells may originate from a cranial extension of the urogenital sinus or from the mesonephros. The degree of squamous replacement probably is also influenced by the adjacent vaginal stroma and further modulated by the presence or absence of sex

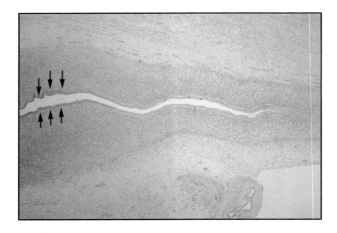

FIGURE 2.1 Junction of the embryonic lower uterine segment and cervix in a fetus at 4- to 5-months' gestation. The arrows point to the area of transition from columnar to squamous epithelium. The fused vagina is toward the right. A cross section of an embryonic fallopian tube is present in the lower portion of the photograph (hematoxylin and eosin, low power magnification).

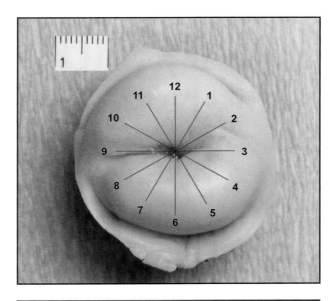

FIGURE 2.2 Gross photograph of an adult parous cervix. Lateral scars are indicative of prior vaginal deliveries. By convention, identification of a lesion site is by the nearest clock-face number.

steroid hormones, particularly estrogen. Increased estrogen is known to cause delayed caudal extension of the Müllerian duct and disruption of squamous cell development.[5]

2.2.2 Anatomy

The cervix, which is derived from the Latin word for *neck*, is the inferior extension of the uterus and is divided into two portions. The lower portion (*portio*, or vaginal cervix) extends into the vagina and is the structure that can be visualized after speculum placement. The upper or supravaginal cervix extends from the vaginal attachment to the lower uterine segment. The cervix is oriented obliquely in the vagina. Consequently, the posterior cervix represents the majority of the portio and comprises one half of the total cervix volume.[3,6,7] When examined through the opened speculum, the cervix appears as a raised oval to circular structure. Accordingly, topographic areas on the cervical surface are conventionally identified using the numbers on a clock face (Figure 2.2). In the nulliparous patient, the cylindrical cervix comprises approximately 50 percent of the total uterine size.[7,8] It is approximately 3 cm in length and approximately 2 cm in diameter. The centrally located external cervical os or beginning of the endocervical canal is round and measures 3 mm to 5 mm in diameter. During pregnancy, the cervix enlarges because of vascular congestion and proliferation of elastic fibers and smooth muscle cells. After vaginal delivery, the external os broadens into a horizontal slit with stellate lines attributable to scarring from cervical lacerations.[6-8] The cervical canal is approximately 3 cm in length and extends from the external os to the lower uterine segment or isthmus. The canal has a fusiform shape and the diameter varies, being approximately 8 mm at its widest point. At the cervicouterine junction, the canal narrows and becomes rounded. This portion is known as the *internal cervical os*. The cervical canal contains ridges known as *plicae palmatae* or *arbor vitae uterina*. These small ridges are no longer apparent after vaginal delivery (Figure 2.3).[3,6]

The cervix is supported by the parametrial soft tissue, the uterosacral ligaments, and the cardinal ligaments of Mackenrodt. The latter provide the major source of cervical support and extend from the lateral cervix through the broad ligament base to the levator ani muscle.[6,7]

The cervix is perfused by the descending cervicovaginal branches of the uterine artery, which enter the cervix laterally through the parametrial soft tissues. Venous drainage parallels the arterial supply and likewise courses laterally through the parametria into the uterine and hypogastric veins.[8] The lymphatic drainage of the cervix originates from the superficial stromal lymphatic spaces and extends into the parametrial tissues. These efferent channels continue to the paracervical, obturator, hypogastric, iliac, and eventually to the para-aortic lymph nodes.[9] Sensory nerves from the cervix and lower vagina arise

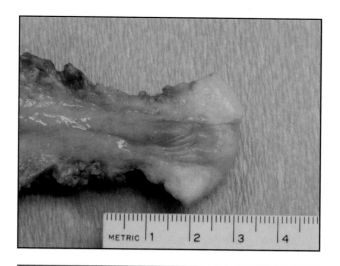

FIGURE 2.3 Gross photograph of a lower uterine segment and endocervix. The parallel plicae palmatae ridges are best seen near the external os. The remaining canal is covered by glistening, clear mucus.

from the deep stroma and endocervical canal. They then proceed through the paracervical and uterosacral plexes (Frankenhäuser's ganglion) and the pelvic nerves to the second, third and fourth sacral nerve roots.[6-8] The relative lack of ectocervical surface innervation may account for the minimal discomfort noted with an ectocervical biopsy or cryotherapy, compared with the significant cramping that can result from an endocervical curettage or loop excision. (Figure 2.4)

2.2.3 Histology
2.2.3.1 Squamous epithelium
The majority of the cervix portio is covered by stratified squamous epithelium. This area is also known as the *ecto-* or *exocervix*. As the squamous cells mature, they enlarge and increase in overall volume while the amount of nuclear material decreases. The overall effect is a characteristic basket-weave pattern.[3]

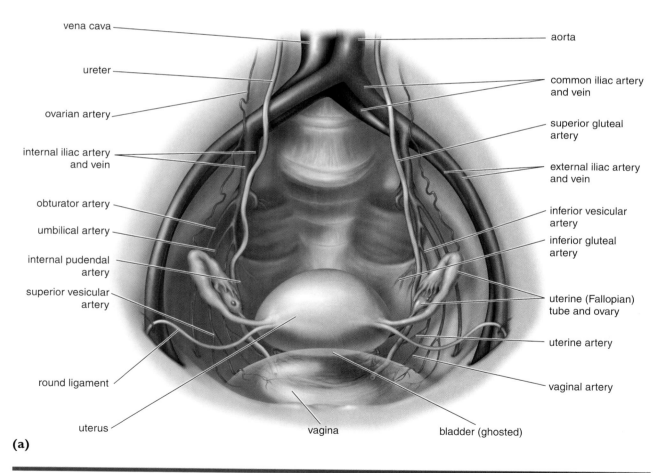

vena cava

ureter

ovarian artery

internal iliac artery and vein

obturator artery

umbilical artery

internal pudendal artery

superior vesicular artery

round ligament

uterus

vagina

aorta

common iliac artery and vein

superior gluteal artery

external iliac artery and vein

inferior vesicular artery

inferior gluteal artery

uterine (Fallopian) tube and ovary

uterine artery

vaginal artery

bladder (ghosted)

(a)

FIGURES 2.4a–c Vascular supply, support, and lymphatic drainage of the cervix. **(a)** Vascular supply: Blood flow is primarily through the descending branches of the uterine arteries, which arise from the hypogastric arteries.

(continued)

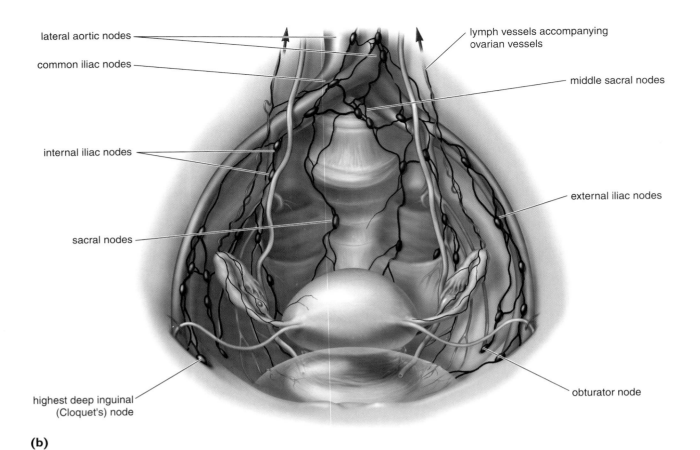

lateral aortic nodes

common iliac nodes

internal iliac nodes

sacral nodes

highest deep inguinal (Cloquet's) node

lymph vessels accompanying ovarian vessels

middle sacral nodes

external iliac nodes

obturator node

(b)

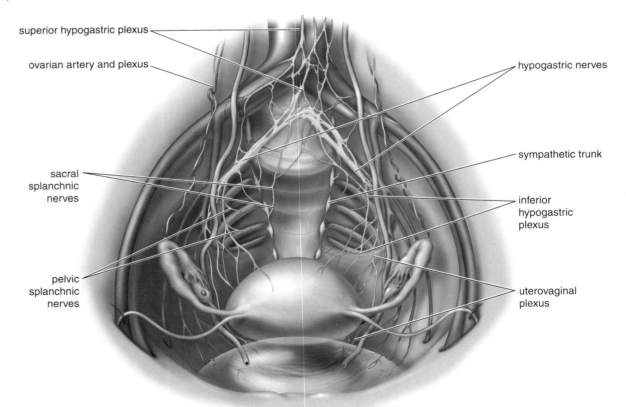

superior hypogastric plexus

ovarian artery and plexus

sacral splanchnic nerves

pelvic splanchnic nerves

hypogastric nerves

sympathetic trunk

inferior hypogastric plexus

uterovaginal plexus

(c)

FIGURES 2.4a–c (continued) **(b)** The lymphatic drainage flows through the adjacent parametrial nodes into the hypogastric and iliac nodes, which eventually drain into the para-aortic nodes. **(c)** Innervation of the pelvis and female genital tract.

Cervical squamous cells have been arbitrarily divided into four distinct layers (Figure 2.5).[3,10] The basal or germinal cell layer is composed of one to two layers of small cuboidal cells that contain large darkly staining round- to oval-shaped nuclei. Mitotic figures are occasionally seen. The parabasal or prickle-cell layer is composed of irregular polyhedral cells with large, dark, oval nuclei. Nucleoli can be seen in the majority of these cells. On electron microscopy, tonofilaments are present, indicating a squamous differentiation. Numerous desmosomes (cell adhesion sites) are also seen. The intermediate or navicular cells, which are flattened cells with glycogen rich clear cytoplasm, comprise the majority of the squamous cells. The nuclei are small, dark, and round, and nucleoli are no longer seen. The superficial or stratum corneum layer is composed of flat, elongated cells with small pyknotic nuclei. Collagen is present in the more superficial cells. Scanning electron microscopy of these squamous cells indicates numerous small ridges on the cell surface, which may suggest the presence of keratin filaments.[3] Since maturation of squamous cells varies considerably, only the basal and superficial cells can be consistently identified.[3,6,10] Langerhans cells and rare melanocytes are interspersed among the squamous cells.[3,6]

Maturation of squamous cells, which is estrogen dependent, can take as little as 4 days. In the pre- and postmenopausal state, the less mature squamous cells (basal and parabasal) predominate (Figure 2.6).[3,11] These cells contain numerous epidermal growth factor and estrogen receptors. Epidermal growth factor stimulates mitotic activity, induces keratinization, and promotes squamous cell differentiation. Estrogen stimulates DNA synthesis and shortens the cell cycle.[12]

The cytoskeleton of a cell consists of three types of filaments: microtubules, intermediate filaments, and microfilaments. The intermediate filaments, which are insoluble proteins with unique biochemical properties, make up the majority of the cytoskeleton matrix. The cytokeratins are intermediate filament proteins unique to epithelial cells. Excluding hair keratins, there are at least 20 different polypeptides. These cytokeratins maintain their integrity during cell transformation, including malignant change. Nevertheless, they may vary depending on epithelial cell type. Cytokeratins 1, 4, 5, 6, 10, 13, 14, 15, 16, 19, and 20 are expressed in the ectocervical squamous cells.[10,13–15] Some investigators suggest that alterations of cytokeratins contribute to the contrast effect of acetic acid, which is used during colposcopic examination.[14]

The basement membrane lies beneath the basal cells. On electron microscopy it usually measures three microns in thickness and consists of a *lamina densa* that borders the underlying cervical stroma and a *lamina lucida* that borders the basal cell. The basal cells contain foot processes that anchor the cell into the basement membrane.[11]

2.2.3.2 Columnar epithelium

A single layer of tall columnar cells lines the endocervical canal. Some pathologists may refer to these cells as glandular cells. The nuclei in these cells are round to oval in shape and basal in position (Figure 2.7). The majority of these columnar cells secrete mucus using

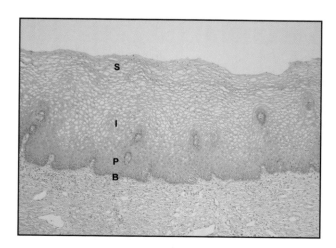

FIGURE 2.5 Normal ectocervix. The stratified squamous cells are divided into four more or less distinct layers. **B:** Basal cell layer. **P:** Parabasal cell layer. **I:** Intermediate cell layer. **S:** Superficial cell layer. The latter two layers have clear cytoplasm, consistent with glycogenation (hematoxylin and eosin, medium power magnification). ▬▬▬

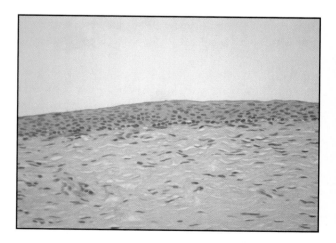

FIGURE 2.6 Atrophic ectocervix. The number of squamous cell layers is decreased and parabasal cells predominate (hematoxylin and eosin, high power magnification). ▬

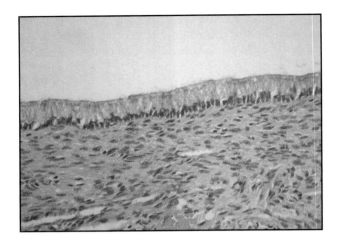

FIGURE 2.7 Normal endocervix. A single layer of columnar cells with basal nuclei covers the surface (hematoxylin and eosin, high power magnification). ▬▬

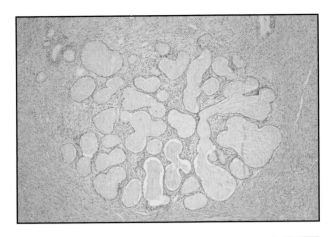

FIGURE 2.9 Tunnel clusters. Closely packed endocervical glands with compressed surface epithelium are present (hematoxylin and eosin, medium power magnification). ▬

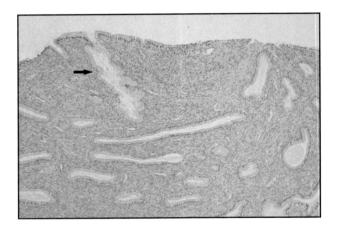

FIGURE 2.8 Endocervical glands. Although they are called glands because of their appearance in cross section, the structures should be considered crypts (arrow) (hematoxylin and eosin, medium power magnification). ▬▬

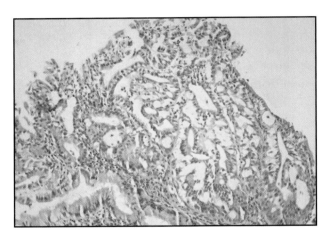

FIGURE 2.10 Microglandular hyperplasia. Numerous small glands are present. The nuclei are uniform and no mitoses are seen (hematoxylin and eosin, medium power).

apocrine and merocrine processes but a few columnar cells are ciliated and may participate in sperm transport.[3,6] Transmission electron microscopy demonstrates the presence of cilia, mucin droplets, and secretory granules of varying sizes.[11] Endocervical columnar cells consistently express cytokeratins 7, 8, 16, 18 and 19.[10,15]

Endocervical cells invaginate into the cervical stroma to a depth of approximately 5 mm to 8 mm (Figure 2.8). Since there are no ductal and acinar structures, this process technically represents crypt formation, but, by convention, they are called endocervical glands because of their rounded shape seen on cross section.[3] Compression of a group of arborizing glands

can result in the formation of *tunnel clusters,* which can be mistaken for atypical glandular hyperplasia because of a superficial architectural complexity (Figure 2.9). However, the columnar cells are benign. *Microglandular hyperplasia* is another form of benign gland proliferation that results in sheets of endocervical cells that coalesce to form individual cell spaces and small gland-like structures. The benign nature of this condition is reflected again by the lack of mitoses and benign nuclear features (Figure 2.10). Microglandular hyperplasia is often seen in young women using hormonal contraception or who are pregnant.[3,6]

The area where the stratified squamous and columnar cells meet is known as the *squamocolumnar*

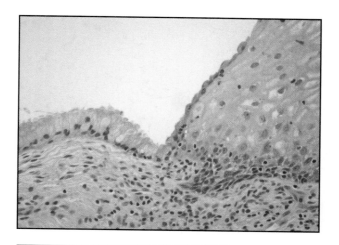

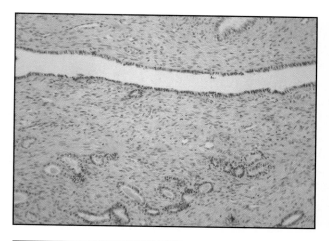

FIGURE 2.11   The squamocolumnar junction. A single layer of columnar cells (left) abruptly meets multiple layers of stratified squamous cells. A few degenerated columnar cells are present on the immediately adjacent squamous cells (hematoxylin and eosin, high power magnification). ▬

FIGURE 2.12   Müllerian remnants. A large duct is surrounded by smaller cyst-like spaces, many of which contain eosinophilic material. All structures are lined by cuboidal cells (hematoxylin and eosin, medium power magnification).

junction (SCJ) (Figure 2.11). This junction is abrupt in about one third of examined specimens. The remainder have evidence of a gradual transformation from one cell type to the other (see 2.4.1 *The transformation zone*).[3,7]

The cervical stroma is composed of fibrous connective tissue, with lesser amounts of smooth muscle and elastic fibers. In approximately 1 percent of cervices, small rounded structures lined by flattened cuboidal cells can be seen deep within the stroma at the 3 o'clock and at the 9 o'clock regions. These represent embryologic mesonephric or Wolffian remnants (Figure 2.12).[3] Capillary arcades are located in the superficial stroma. Straight vessel loops branch from these arcades and extend into the basal and parabasal layers of the squamous epithelium. In the endocervix, the small capillary loops are located directly beneath the columnar cells.

2.2.4 The transformation zone

2.2.4.1 Formation of squamous metaplasia

Metaplasia is defined as a transformation from one mature cell type to a different type of mature cell. The process usually involves conversion from a columnar cell to a stratified squamous cell, although conversion from one glandular cell type to another also occurs. Metaplasia occurs in different body sites, such as the bronchi, stomach, bladder, and salivary gland. However, metaplasia in the uterine cervix has always generated enormous interest because of its neoplastic potential.[13]

Historically, areas of cervical squamous metaplasia were originally misidentified either as early-differentiated carcinomas or as folds in the upper squamous epithelium.[16] German pathologists eventually described the process of metaplasia using terms such as epidermidalization or epidermoidalization to identify these areas. Later, it was variously reclassified as reserve cell hyperplasia, squamocolumnar prosoplasia, or metaplasia.[17]

Factors that induce squamous metaplasia in the cervix are still poorly understood but may include environmental conditions, mechanical irritation, chronic inflammation, pH changes, or changes in sex steroid hormone balance. Metaplasia probably begins when the original SCJ moves onto the portio and exposes the delicate columnar cells to an acidic bacteria-laden vaginal environment (Figure 2.13). Gradually, immature and then mature metaplastic squamous cells replace the columnar cells. These metaplastic cells eventually convert into stratified squamous cells, which normally exist in this milieu.[3,6,7,18] During a woman's lifetime, the SCJ returns to the endocervical canal, which has the more neutral pH of cervical mucus. As stated earlier, the position of the SCJ at birth is known as the original or native SCJ. Following metaplasia-induced migration, it is known as the new SCJ or, simply, the SCJ. The transformation zone, then, is technically defined as the area bordered by the original or native SCJ and the new SCJ.[19]

For decades, it was unclear how this transformation took place. The mechanism of squamous metaplasia has been described as proliferation of subcolumnar

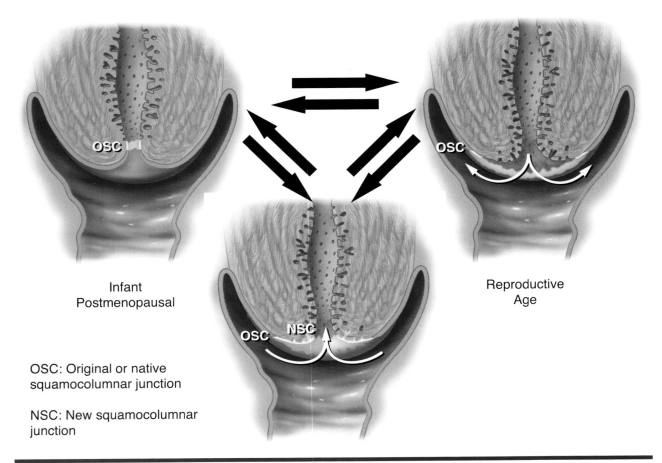

Infant
Postmenopausal

Reproductive
Age

OSC: Original or native
squamocolumnar junction

NSC: New squamocolumnar
junction

FIGURE 2.13   The physiology of squamous metaplasia. In infants and postmenopausal women, the original or native squamocolumnar junction is located in the endocervical canal. In reproductive-age women, this junction moves out on the portio, exposing the delicate columnar surface to the acidic vagina. Over time, the columnar cells are replaced by squamous cells (metaplasia), which create a new squamocolumnar junction that moves back into the canal. The area between the original squamocolumnar junction and the newly formed squamocolumnar junction after metaplasia is complete is known as the transformation zone (Modified with permission from Wright and Ferenczy.[6]) ▬

nests of squamous basal cells or development from undifferentiated embryonic rests within the superficial cervical stroma.[20,21] The evolution of the transformation zone may require several mechanisms. The two most commonly accepted involve the continued epithelialization with new squamous cells derived from previously formed squamous epithelium and development of metaplasia from the subcolumnar reserve cells. The origin of reserve cells remains obscure. Suggested parent cells include embryonal urogenital crest cells, fetal squamous cells, and stromal fibroblasts.[20] Presently, investigators believe that these reserve cells probably arise from the dedifferentiation of overlying columnar cells.[13,19] The presence of cytokeratins 5, 6, 8, 13, 14, 15, 16, 17, 18, and 19 in variable amounts indicates an epithelial origin of these cells.[10,22]

Initially, reserve cells appear as a single cell layer directly beneath the columnar cells to be replaced. Over time, these flattened cuboidal cells proliferate into multiple layers of immature squamoid metaplastic cells and push the columnar cells away from their underlying capillary vascular supply. These cells eventually degenerate and slough off the underlying immature metaplasia. As the reserve cells proliferate and differentiate into immature squamous cells cytokeratins 8 and 18 (unique to reserve and columnar cells) are lost and cytokeratin 19 predominates throughout the entire epithelial thickness.[13,22] As the immature metaplastic cells mature into squamous cells, cytokeratins 15 and 19 become limited to the basal and parabasal cells, while the surface cells begin to express other cytokeratins (4, 10, 13 and 14) commonly seen in intermediate and superficial squa-

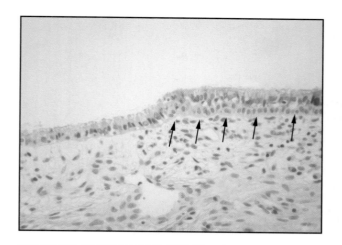

FIGURE 2.14 Reserve cells. A second layer of round cells has formed under the columnar endocervical cells (arrows). This is alternately known as *reserve cell hyperplasia* (hematoxylin and eosin, high power magnification).

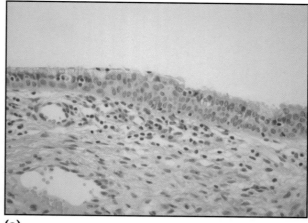

(a)

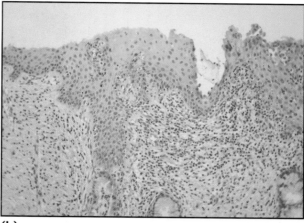

(b)

FIGURES 2.15a,b Development of squamous metaplasia. **(a)** Proliferation of reserve cells leads to the presence of immature squamous cells directly underneath the remaining columnar cells (hematoxylin and eosin, high power). **(b)** As metaplasia progresses, the immature cells acquire more cytoplasm and develop squamous cell characteristics. The remaining columnar cells degenerate and are lost. Chronic inflammatory cells are present in the superficial stroma (hematoxylin and eosin, medium power magnification).

mous cells. In contrast, cytokeratins 6 and 16 predominate in metaplastic cells that have the potential to become dysplastic.[13,20,22] Other predictors of dysplastic potential in squamous metaplasia include the degree of metaplastic proliferation and rate of metaplastic change.[7,23,24]

2.2.4.2 The histology of squamous metaplasia

Sixty percent of cervices will have a gradual transformation from columnar to mature squamous epithelium. Metaplasia is most commonly seen in the lower third of the endocervical canal.[7] The first evidence of squamous metaplasia is the identification of a single layer of subcolumnar reserve cells, known histologically as reserve cell hyperplasia (Figure 2.14). The reserve cells are cuboidal with scant cytoplasm and large round to oval nuclei. They can be seen beneath the surface columnar cells and the endocervix glands. As the reserve cells proliferate, the amount of cytoplasm increases. The nuclei decrease somewhat in size, develop sharp nuclear membranes, and acquire prominent nucleoli. As the process continues, the cells flatten toward the surface and acquire cytoplasmic glycogen; the nuclei become small and round with uniform chromatin and lose their nucleoli.[3,6,25,26] The remaining surface columnar cells degenerate and slough (Figure 2.15). As the metaplasia evolves within the endocervix glands, there is squamous bridging across the lumens, resulting in smaller gland structures. In the past, this has been called adenomatous hyperplasia or mucoid degeneration (Figure 2.16).[3] Lastly, the endocervical glands undergo

ing metaplasia become solid round structures that converge into the surface squamous cells.

The process of metaplasia is highly variable and it is common to see islands of well-developed metaplasia interspersed by non-metaplastic columnar epithelium (Figure 2.17). Other areas can show well-developed mature squamous epithelium overlying endocervical glands with little or no metaplastic proliferation.[3,6]

As metaplasia is a process brought about by irritation or inflammation, it is common to see plasma

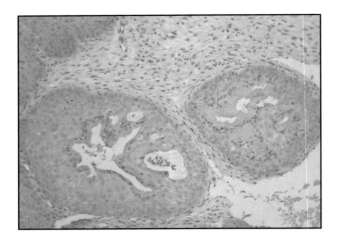

FIGURE 2.16 Partial replacement of glandular epithelium by immature squamous cells. The small spaces give the glands an adenomatous appearance (hematoxylin and eosin, medium power magnification). ■

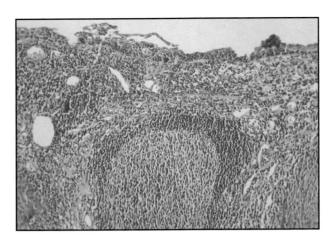

FIGURE 2.18 Follicular cervicitis. A central germinal follicle is surrounded by numerous chronic inflammatory cells. Reactive squamous metaplastic cells cover the surface (hematoxylin and eosin, medium power magnification). ■

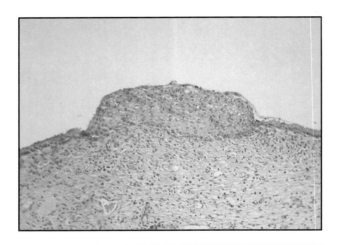

FIGURE 2.17 Focal squamous metaplasia. The area of squamous metaplasia is bordered on each side by a single layer of columnar cells (hematoxylin and eosin, high power magnification). ■

epithelium. Smaller biopsy specimens usually lack evidence of all the features common to metaplasia, such as the presence of reserve cells, immature metaplastic cell proliferation, and maturation. Nevertheless, the pathologist can establish the presence of the transformation zone by noting the presence of columnar cells beneath or adjacent to squamous epithelium (Figure 2.19).

2.2.5 Cytology

Papanicolaou (Pap) test sampling of the cervix involves scraping of the ectocervical surface and a portion of the nonvisualized endocervical canal using various sampling devices. Stratified squamous cells are markedly cohesive. As maturation continues, however, functional desmosomes diminish and individual squamous cells separate from each other. Therefore, the ectocervical cells removed for cytologic examination are those that have exfoliated from the surface and appear as individual cells under the microscope in Pap test specimens. On the other hand, endocervical cells are not stratified and generally do not exfoliate. When scraped, endocervical cells are usually removed in clumps that appear as cell clusters on microscopic examination.

In a background of abundant estrogen, the cytologic specimen will contain mostly superficial and intermediate cells (Figure 2.20). These cells are navicular in shape with a diameter of approximately 40 μm. The cytoplasm is abundant and usually eosinophilic (pink after Papanicolaou staining). When glycogenated, they show a perinuclear yellow color. The nucleus of the superficial cell is centrally located, small (5 μm), round,

cells and lymphocytes. Occasionally, acute inflammatory cells are present in the underlying stroma and the surface metaplastic cells. Extensive chronic inflammation can result in the formation of small lymphoid follicles within the superficial stroma (Figure 2.18). This is known as *chronic follicular cervicitis;* investigators have noted this change in women with *Chlamydia trachomatis* infections of the cervix.[27]

Pathologists usually observe a continual blending of all the metaplastic processes when examining large cervical specimens from conization procedures and hysterectomies, although occasionally, there is an abrupt transition from columnar to squamous

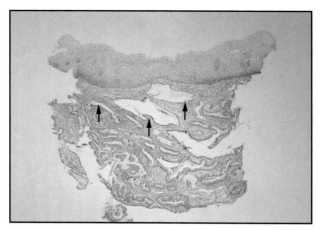

(a)

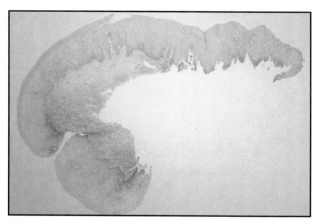

(b)

FIGURES 2.19a,b   Cervical biopsies. **(a)** The presence of endocervical glands (arrows) beneath squamous epithelial cells signifies the transformation zone (hematoxylin and eosin, low power). **(b)** A lack of endocervical glands signifies the microscopic absence of the transformation zone (hematoxylin and eosin, low power magnification).

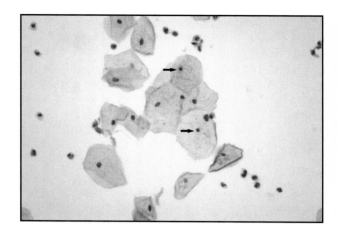

FIGURE 2.20   Superficial and intermediate cells. Although the squamous cells all have the same polygonal shape, there is a difference in nuclear sizes. The cells with the smaller pyknotic nuclei (arrows) are the superficial cells. Also present are scattered neutrophils (liquid preparation, Papanicolaou stain, high power magnification).

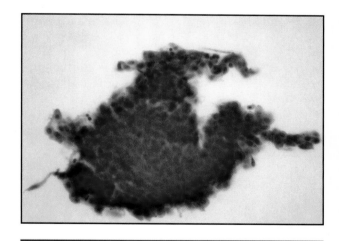

FIGURE 2.21   Atrophic smear. A sheet of uniformly round parabasal cells (best seen in the periphery) in an otherwise clean background (liquid preparation, Papanicolaou stain, high power magnification).

and dark. An intermediate cell nucleus is slightly larger (8 μm to 10 μm) and contains fine, evenly distributed chromatin. The amount of cell exfoliation varies with the menstrual cycle.[10] During the proliferative phase, there is an increased exfoliation of well-glycogenated superficial cells. However, intermediate cells predominate in the progesterone enhanced secretory phase, and there is less glycogen.[28]

Parabasal cells and rare intermediate cells are more common in the cytologic specimens of postmenopausal women (Figure 2.21). Parabasal cells do not exfoliate as readily as do more mature squamous cells, and, like columnar cells, they are often removed in groups. These cells are smaller and more

rounded with large centrally located nuclei. The nuclear membranes in these cells are smooth and the nuclear chromatin is usually granular or finely stippled. Air-drying is more commonly seen in conventional specimens from postmenopausal women, as there is little background mucus present. Consequently, the nuclei tend to smudge and the cytoplasm is eosinophilic.[6,10]

When present, the columnar cells are either linear in arrangement or grouped in a honeycomb pattern (Figure 2.22). The nuclei are basal, relatively large and round, and contain one to two micronucleoli. The chromatin is uniform and finely granular. Occasionally multinucleation occurs, and cilia are infrequently seen.[10]

Although basal cells are almost never present on a cytologic specimen, reserve cells can be seen. They are usually found within a mucoid background in linear sheets. They are commonly seen adjacent to columnar cells, which attest to their subcolumnar origin. Reserve cells are round to oval with irregular cell borders and finely vacuolated cytoplasm. The small nuclei are round to bean shaped and have prominent chromatin. Because of their arrangement and size, these cells can be difficult to discriminate from a high-grade squamous dysplasia (Figure 2.23). However, squamous dysplastic cells will have irregularly shaped nuclei and lack smooth nuclear membranes.

The presence of metaplastic cells is considered minimal cytologic evidence that a specimen contains transformation zone elements. The cells are typically seen in small individual cell groups or sheets (Figure 2.24). They have cyanophilic (blue-green) cytoplasm and are smaller in size than the mature squamous epithelial cells. The nuclei are slightly larger than intermediate cell nuclei. The nuclear membranes are smooth and round and the chromatin is granular to finely stippled. Micronucleoli may be present.[6,22]

The appearance of metaplastic cells can be cytologically similar to that of parabasal cells. Because of this, it is difficult to differentiate metaplastic cells from parabasal cells in a postmenopausal woman; however, parabasal cells tend to be more cohesive and eosinophilic, and they are rarely seen in a woman of reproductive age. Therefore, the presence of small oval to polyhedral cells with cyanophilic cytoplasm and slightly enlarged nuclei in a background of mature squamous cells represents evidence of squamous metaplasia.

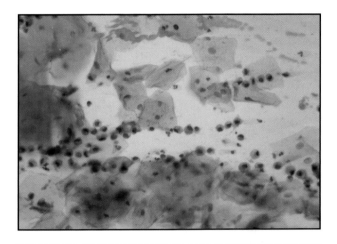

FIGURE 2.23   Reserve cells. The small round to oval cells are linear in arrangement. Note the small basophilic nuclei and the finely vacuolated cytoplasm (conventional preparation, Papanicolaou stain, high power magnification).

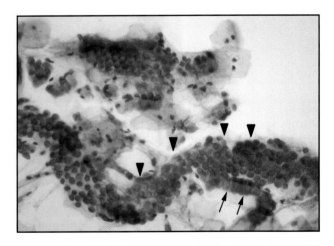

FIGURE 2.22   Endocervical cells. Although some cells demonstrate the typical "picket fence" tall, columnar architecture (small arrows), the majority are seen on-end in a "honeycomb" arrangement (arrowheads). The nuclei are slightly larger than the normal intermediate cell nucleus (liquid preparation, Papanicolaou stain, high power magnification). ▬

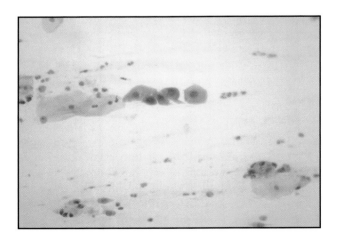

FIGURE 2.24   Metaplastic cells. The cyanophilic cells (center) are smaller than the mature squamous cell (lower right corner) and have a more rounded shape. The nuclei are slightly larger than an intermediate cell nucleus (conventional preparation, Papanicolaou stain, high power magnification). ▬

2.3 The Vagina

2.3.1 Embryology

By the seventh week postconception, the solid tip of the Müllerian duct reaches the dorsal wall of the urogenital sinus. As the tip enlarges to form the Müllerian tubercle, sinus cells proliferate medial to the mesonephric ducts and just lateral to the tubercle. This sinus-cell proliferation becomes the sinovaginal bulbs. Both the tubercle and the sinovaginal bulbs continue to enlarge and cavitate, forming the rudimentary vagina by the 10th week of gestation. Although originally lined by columnar epithelium, replacement by squamous cells begins at around 11 weeks, coincidental to the appearance of estrogen receptors along the vaginal wall. The replacement begins at the urogenital sinus, probably the site of origin, and progresses upward to the external cervical os. Proliferation and stratification of the squamous cells leads to secondary occlusion of the vaginal lumen. By the 16th week of gestation, under continued estrogen modulation, the vaginal squamous cells mature, glycogenate, and begin to exfoliate. This exfoliative process results in secondary cavitation of the essentially solid vaginal plate (Figure 2.25). Vaginal development is practically complete by the fifth month of pregnancy.[5,29]

The process by which squamous cells partially replace the original columnar cells lining the rudimentary uterovaginal canal and the extent to which this occurs is not completely understood[5] (see also

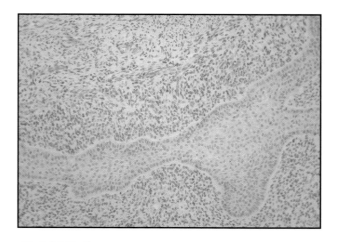

FIGURE 2.25   Vaginal plate, fetus of 18 to 20 weeks' gestation. Cavitation has not occurred yet, although the original columnar cells have been replaced by immature squamous cells. Immature mesenchyme borders the squamous cells laterally (hematoxylin and eosin, medium power magnification). ▬

Section 1.1). Nevertheless, evolution of the terminal Müllerian ducts and urogenital sinus into the cervix and vagina becomes hormonally dependent after completion of gonadal differentiation. Specifically, the reaction of these ducts to estrogen depends on the intensity and timing of the exposure. Exposure to large pharmacologic levels of estrogen during vaginal development in mice has resulted in delayed vaginal growth and retarded squamous replacement of the original columnar cells. In the human, exposure to exogenous estrogen early in the second trimester can result in persistent glandular epithelium, known as adenosis, and other anomalies, such as transverse vaginal ridges, and cobblestone mucosal surfaces.

Persistence of the adjacent mesonephric ducts may lead to formation of cysts in the vaginal stroma, known as Gartner's duct cysts. These cysts can grow to considerable size, compressing the vaginal lumen and extending into the broad ligament (Figure 2.26).

2.3.2 Anatomy

The vagina, which is Latin for *sheath*, is a mucosa-lined tube that extends from the vulva to the cervix. It separates the bladder neck and urethra from the rectum and anus. Normally, the anterior and posterior walls of the vagina lie in close approximation centrally while being more lax peripherally. This results in the non-distended vagina having an "H" shape on cross section. The vagina is extremely pliable and can stretch considerably during intercourse and childbirth.[5,8]

The vagina is positioned perpendicular to the uterus and is offset approximately 60° from the vestibule. The uterus is attached to the upper vagina at the recessed vaginal fornices. Because of the angle of attachment, the posterior fornix is usually longer than the anterior fornix. Accordingly, the anterior vaginal wall is shorter than the posterior wall, the former measuring 6 cm to 8 cm and the latter measuring 7 cm to 10 cm in length (Figure 2.27). In nulliparous women, small transverse ridges known as *rugae* cover the surface. These mucosal folds are not apparent after childbirth and during the postmenopausal period. In the nonpregnant state, the mucosal surface is kept moist by cervical secretions. The amount of vaginal secretions increases considerably during sexual arousal and excitement, probably through direct passage of fluids through the mucosa. A mixture of cervical mucus and exfoliated surface epithelial cells can result in a thin-layered milky discharge known as a leukorrhea. During pregnancy, under the influence of increased estrogen levels, the amount of physiologic discharge can increase considerably. In an adult woman, the vagina is

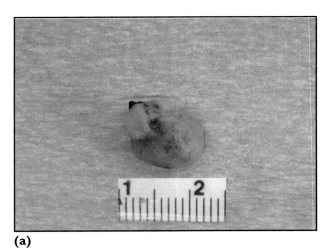

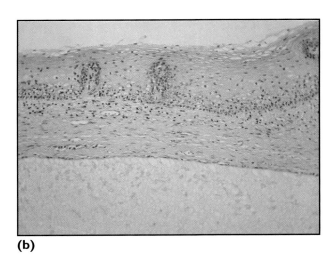

(a)

(b)

FIGURES 2.26a,b   Gartner's duct cyst. **(a)** Grossly, the cyst is unilocular and smooth walled. A small amount of elliptical vaginal mucosa is attached to the outer surface. **(b)** Microscopically, the cyst is lined by a single layer of cuboidal cells (hematoxylin and eosin, medium power magnification).

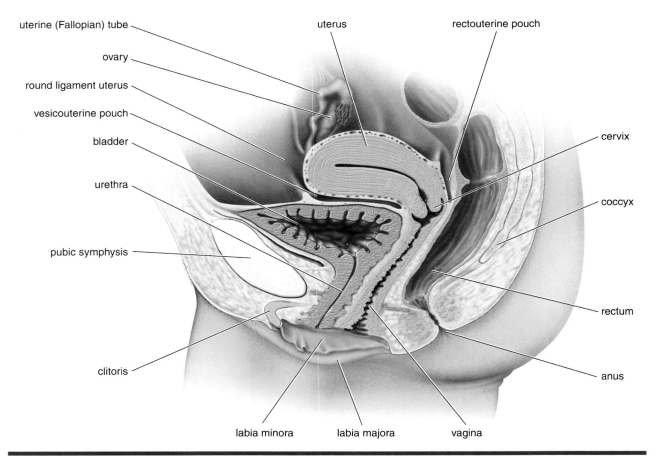

FIGURE 2.27   Sagittal section of the female pelvis, showing the relationship of the vagina to the cervix and adjacent pelvic organs (bladder and rectum).

normally acidic at a pH between 3.5 and 4.5. This acidic environment is derived through the breakdown of surface epithelial cell glycogen into lactic acid by lactobacilli. Estrogen also has some minor direct influence on the pH of the vagina, which is lowest during midcycle and highest just before menses.[5,8]

The vagina is surrounded by an ill-defined muscular coat, which is divided into an outer layer composed of longitudinal fibers and an inner coat that contains circular fibers. Most of the mid- and lower-vaginal support comes from the pubovaginalis and iliococcygeus portion of the levator ani muscle and the transverse perineal muscles. The cardinal and uterosacral ligaments provide support the upper vagina as well as the cervix.[5]

The vascular supply of the vagina is complex and has contributions from the arteries that supply the cervix (descending cervicovaginal arteries), bladder (inferior vesical arteries), and vulva (middle hemorrhoidal and internal pudendal arteries). The venous drainage starts in plexes that are found in the vaginal stroma and progresses parallel to the arterial system to enter the hypogastric veins. Lymphatic drainage of the vagina is also site dependent: the upper vagina drains into the paracervical and hypogastric nodes while the lower vagina drains into the superficial iliac and deep pelvic nodes, in a route similar to that of the vulva. The anterior midvagina drains into the paravesical nodes and the posterior midvagina drains into the pararectal nodes.[9]

Innervation of the vagina is through the sacral plexes, particularly S 2–5. The vagina is devoid of specialized receptors seen in the vulva; however, free nerve endings, which register pain, are occasionally found, primarily in the lower third of the vagina. The vagina is devoid of the ability to sense temperature.[8]

2.3.3 Histology

The histology of the vagina recapitulates the cervix, in that stratified squamous epithelial cells cover the surface (Figure 2.28). As in the cervix, the cells are divided into different layers that reflect the various degrees of squamous cell maturity. The basal cells are small oval cells with large nuclei arranged in a palisade against the basement membrane. The parabasal cells are slightly larger and make up an additional two to three layers above the basal cells. The intermediate cells correspond to the similar layer in the cervix. As they mature, the cytoplasm acquires abundant glycogen, and their orientation is more parallel to the basement membrane and surface. The superficial squamous cells are glycogenated flattened cells with small pyknotic nuclei. Other cell types found in

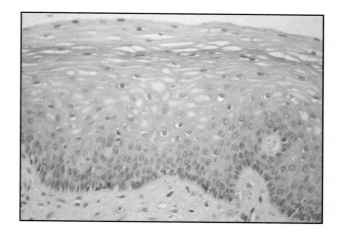

FIGURE 2.28   Vaginal squamous mucosa. The surface epithelial cells are similar in appearance to the cervix (hematoxylin and eosin, medium power magnification). ▬

the vagina include rare melanocytes at the base and Langerhans cells throughout the epithelial surface. Epithelial cells are arranged in layers that average 26 to 28 rows. The majority of epithelial cells are in the superficial and intermediate layers, each averaging about 10 rows.[5] The thickness of the vaginal epithelium is hormonally dependent; during the non-ovulatory portion of the menstrual cycle, it averages 24 cell layers, and during ovulation, 29.[30] A lack of estrogen results in epithelial cell atrophy. The surface cell layers are thinned; basal and parabasal cells predominate. As such, the amount of glycogen present in the epithelium is greatly diminished. Langerhans cell numbers, which reflect the immune status of the vagina, do not change with cyclic alterations in levels of estrogen or progesterone.

Cytokeratin expression in the vagina is similar to that in the cervix and reflects squamous cell maturity. Cells in the basal and adjacent suprabasal layers show early differentiation and express cytokeratin 13. The intermediate cells express a combination of cytokeratin 13 and 10, while the superficial cells express cytokeratin 10 exclusively.[31]

The vaginal stroma is composed of a mixture of elastic tissue and abundant lymph-vascular spaces. Occasionally, a thin layer of slightly enlarged fibroblastic cells is found directly beneath the epithelial surface. The nuclei of these stromal cells can also be mildly atypical and it is important that the pathologist not confuse this layer with a vaginal sarcoma.[9]

Theoretically, the vagina is devoid of glandular elements or columnar cells. Nevertheless, mesonephric or Wolffian remnants can occasionally be found in the lateral vaginal walls. As with mesonephric remnants in the cervix, these vestiges are usually composed of a

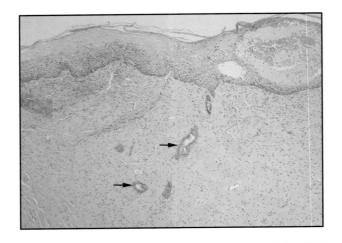

FIGURE 2.29 Vaginal adenosis. Small gland-like structures (arrows) directly lined by endocervical-type cells are present beneath the squamous mucosa. (hematoxylin and eosin, medium power magnification).

central duct surrounded by small gland-like structures. The lining is composed of flattened bland cells with round nuclei; the lumens are commonly filled with inspissated proteinaceous material. Occasionally, endocervical-type glandular cells are also seen in the vagina, a finding known as *adenosis* (Figure 2.29).[3] During embryogenesis, the müllerian lining of the original tubo-uterovaginal canal is composed of columnar type cells that have the potential to differentiate into the various cells that line the adult tube, endometrium, and endocervix. Accordingly, the columnar cells found in adenosis can recapitulate these same glandular structures. However about 70% of adenosis is an endocervical cell type.[3] Adenosis acquired considerable notoriety from its association with in-utero diethylstilbestrol (DES) exposure from its potential to develop into clear cell adenocarcinoma (for more information, see Chapters 13 and 14).[29] Nevertheless, it can also be seen in normal vaginas, particularly during the healing process after ablative or erosive therapy (5-fluorouracil cream). As in the cervix, the glandular cells of adenosis eventually are replaced by squamous epithelium through the process of squamous metaplasia.

2.3.4 Cytology

Exfoliated squamous cells in the vagina are morphologically identical to those seen in the ectocervix. In well-estrogenized women, superficial and intermediate cells predominate; in postmenopausal women, primarily parabasal cells are seen. Historically, prior to the development of direct estrogen assays, a matu-

ration index was calculated to infer estrogen levels by quantifying the degree of hormonal influence on the vagina. One hundred vaginal squamous cells would be counted and characterized as ratios of superficial, intermediate, and parabasal cells. This indirect assessment of estrogen levels can be inaccurate because of contamination by cervical metaplastic cells and is rarely used today.

The presence of glandular cells on a vaginal cytologic specimen is consistent with adenosis. It is therefore important that colposcopists identify the correct source of a cytologic specimen and provide appropriate history, particularly regarding surgical removal of the uterus or cervix. Since vaginal metaplasia can occur only in the presence of adenosis, pathologists must be careful not to misinterpret small parabasal-type cells, more commonly seen in postmenopausal women, as metaplastic cells.

2.4 The Vulva
2.4.1 Embryology

The mesoderm along the anterior cloaca proliferates and creates a mound beneath the overlying ectoderm around the fourth week after conception. At the same time, small folds develop lateral to the central cloacal membrane of the urogenital sinus. By the sixth week of gestation, the rudimentary external genitalia are recognizable and consist of a urogenital membrane, a genital tubercle, two urogenital folds, and two labial scrotal swellings. The urogenital and labioscrotal folds fuse anteriorly to form the mons pubis by the seventh week. Posterior fusion separates the urogenital membrane from the anal membrane and results in formation of the posterior fourchette and perineum. By the end of the seventh week of gestation, the urogenital membrane disappears, exteriorizing the urogenital sinus. At eight to nine weeks, if testes are present, Leydig cells begin producing testosterone. If the target cells in the external genitalia contain the enzyme 5 alpha reductase, testosterone is converted into dehydrotestosterone and, by 10 weeks' gestation, male structures develop. If no testosterone is produced or the reductase enzyme is not found in the epithelial cells, a vulva develops. Specifically, the genital tubercle folds posteriorly and becomes the clitoris, the urogenital sinus becomes a portion of the vestibule that includes the introitus and hymeneal membrane, the urogenital folds become the remaining vestibule and labia minora, and the labial scrotal swellings become the labia majora. The entire conversion to

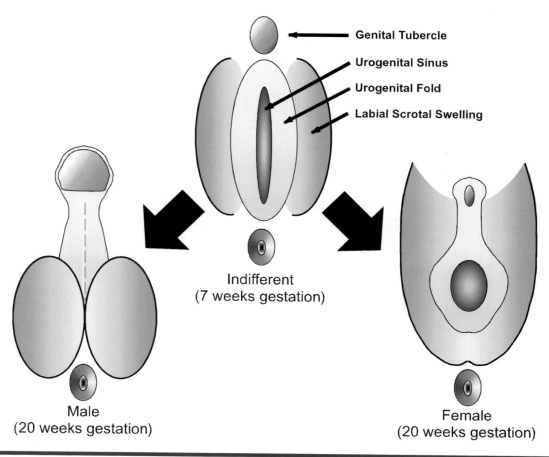

FIGURE 2.30 Development of the external genitalia. In the female, the urogenital sinus and urogenital folds remain open, forming the labia minora, vestibule, and introitus.

female structures is completed by 20 weeks' gestational age (Figure 2.30).[2,32]

The vulva represents the fusion of ectodermal elements (the surface epithelia of the labia majora and minora) and endodermal elements (the epithelia of the vestibule and vagina). Ectodermal squamous epithelium is keratinized while endodermal epithelium is not. The point where these two types of epithelia meet is known as *Hart's line*. Although this line represents a transition from one surface type to another, it does not have the same degree of significance as the transformation zone in the cervix, as the transformation on the vulva is from one squamous cell type to another and overall cell proliferation is minimal and has no neoplastic potential. In addition, ectodermal glandular structures are more representative of skin adnexa while the vestibular glands are derived from endoderm. Table 2.1 describes the male homologues of the different female vestibular glands.

As described previously, the period between 10 and 20 weeks' gestation is critical to the develop-

Table 2.1 Male and Female External Genitalia Homologous Glandular Structures

Female	Male
Skene's Glands	Prostrate
Minor Vestibular Glands	Penile Glands of Littre
Bartholin's Glands	Cowper's Glands

ment of the vulva. Epithelial contact with androgens at this time results in a variable androgenic influence on the external genitalia. Reasons for androgen exposure may include drug or exogenous hormone intake, placental aromatase deficiency, maternal androgenic tumors, and congenital adrenal hyperplasia. The end result is a female pseudohermaphrodite with ambiguous genital development characterized by clitoral hypertrophy, hypospadias, and scrotalization of nonfused labia (Figure 2.31).[32]

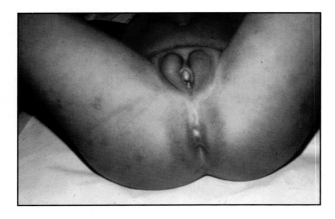

FIGURE 2.31 Ambiguous genitalia. There is enlargement of the labia majora and clitoralmegaly, with enlargement of the clitoral hood.

2.4.2 Anatomy

The vulva, which is the Latin word for *covering*, is the area of the female external genital tract that extends from the symphysis pubis anteriorly to the anus posteriorly and lateral to the inguinal-gluteal folds. The area includes the mons pubis, the labia minora, and labia majora, the clitoris, the vestibule and associated structures, the posterior fourchette, and the perineum. The *vestibule* represents that portion of the vulva medial to the labia minora that extends from the clitoral region anteriorly to the area of labia fusion beneath the introitus (the *posterior fourchette*). The urethral meatus and the introitus lie within the vestibule. The *pilosebaceous line* is the border separating the lateral skin covered by pubic hairs from the medial non hair-bearing skin. (Figure 2.32).[33]

The labia majora are lateral skin folds that vary in size depending on the amount of underlying adipose tissue. After childbearing, they decrease in size and become almost completely absent in postmenopausal

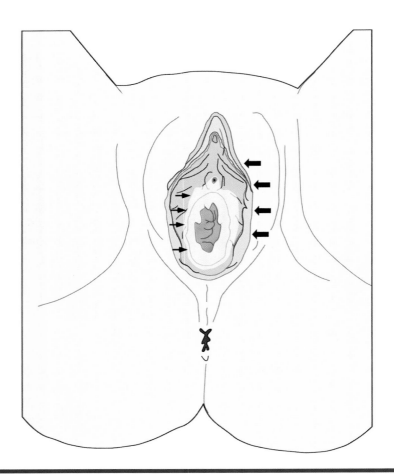

FIGURE 2.32 Normal vulva. The large arrows delineate the pilosebaceous line. The smaller arrows delineate Hart's line.

women. They diverge anteriorly and blend into the mons. The labia minora are small folds located medially to the labia majora. The labia minora have numerous sebaceous glands that are visible clinically as small, white, slightly elevated, smooth areas known as *Fordyce spots*. The labia minora fuse anteriorly to form the frenulum of the clitoris. The portion of the clitoris that is visible is a small cylindrical nodule about 0.5 cm in diameter. It contains erectile tissue and enlarges during sexual arousal, but it rarely exceeds 1 cm in diameter. Beneath the clitoris is the urethral opening or urinary meatus, a slit-like opening 0.5 cm in diameter.[33,34]

The hymeneal ring represents the remnant of the urogenital membrane. Prior to intercourse, the hymen is commonly a plate-like structure with small areas of perforation (Figure 2.33). After intercourse or vaginal delivery, small peripheral mucosal tags known as *myrtiform caruncles* represent the remnants of the hymeneal plate. Rare cases of imperforate hymen, in which the hymeneal plate remains intact,

lead to accumulation of both menstrual efflux and vaginal material known as hematocolpos.[34]

The vestibule contains numerous gland openings. The two Skene's ducts are located just inferior and lateral to the urethra. The two Bartholin's ducts are located lateral to the posterior fourchette. The Skene's and Bartholin's ducts are small (less than 0.5 mm in diameter), and are not recognizable clinically unless obstructed and secondarily infected. The minor vestibular glands are located in a semicircular area that approximates Hart's line. The number of minor vestibular glands varies from one to 100, but usually averages between 2 and 10 in examined vestibulectomy specimens. These glands are also not recognizable clinically unless inflamed, when they appear as reddened spots. Near the introitus are variable numbers of raised micropapillae, known as micropapillomatosis labialis. Although similar in appearance to a small vulvar condyloma, these structures do not consistently contain human papillomavirus DNA.

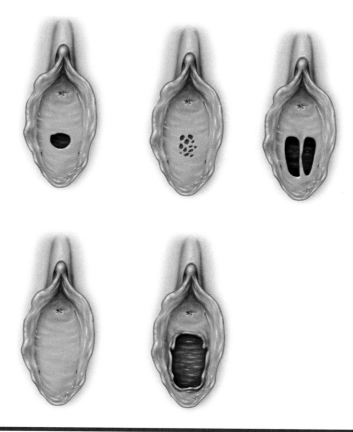

FIGURE 2.33 Types of hymeneal perforations. The size and shape are indicative of the amount of degeneration in the urogenital membrane. A lack of degeneration will result in a solid hymeneal plate, which can lead to a hematocolpos (collection of menstrual efflux in the vagina). Large perforations are usually the result of tampon insertion, intercourse or vaginal deliveries, but can occur spontaneously.

Hair growth begins at puberty and reaches adult amounts by late adolescence. Hair distribution over the vulva, or the escutcheon, is shaped like an inverted triangle, with the base located at the upper mons pubis. The hair shafts arise from the mons and the lateral labia majora. The medial labia majora and the labia minora do not contain pilosebaceous units. The amount of pubic hair decreases after menopause.

The arterial supply of the vulva is mainly through branches of the pudendal and hemorrhoidal arteries. In general, the venous drainage parallels the arterial vessels. The exception is the convoluted venous plexes of the vestibular bulb. The apex of this teardrop shaped bulb is the clitoral vein; the base is in the vicinity of Bartholin's gland. These plexes drain laterally into the labial and pudendal veins. The lymphatic drainage of the vulva is initially into the inguinal nodes, then subsequently into the femoral and pelvic nodes. Although not common, direct drainage into the femoral nodes has been reported. In addition, central structures such as the introitus and clitoris can rarely drain directly into the pelvic nodes using accessory channels over the symphysis pubis. Innervation of the vulva is through superficial branches of the pudendal and hemorrhoidal nerves from sacral roots 2, 3 and 4. The anterior portion of the vulva (mons) is supplied by branches of the ilioinguinal and genitofemoral nerves. (Figure 2.34).[8,33]

2.4.3 Histology

The majority of the vulva consists of keratinized skin. Because of its location and the fact that it is subject to various dermatological diseases, it is an area of interest to many diverse groups including gynecologists, family practitioners, dermatologists, general surgical pathologists, dermatopathologists, gynecological pathologists and other providers of women's health care.

The surface of the nonvestibular hair-bearing vulva is covered by keratinized stratified squamous epithelial cells or keratinocytes. Small projections of

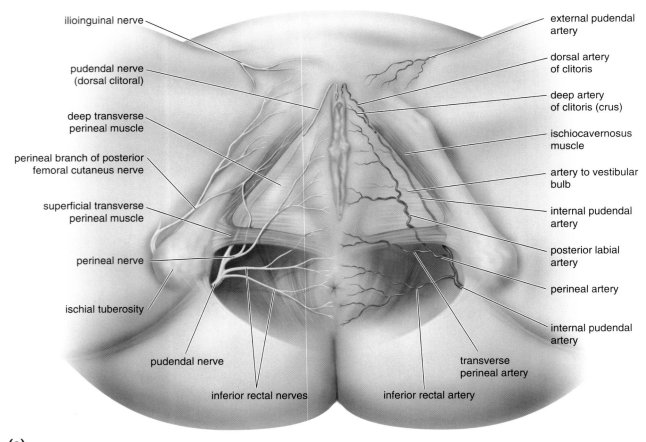

(a)

FIGURES 2.34a,b   (a) Arterial supply and innervation of the vulva and superficial perineum.

epidermal cells known as rete pegs extend into the superficial stroma or dermis.[35] Melanocytes are neuroepithelial cells responsible for producing protective pigmentation. They are distributed along the basal cell layer in a ratio ranging from 1:10 to 1:50 melanocytes to keratinocytes(Figure 2.35). Langerhans cells, associated with skin immunity, are located suprabasally in a distribution ratio of approximately 1 Langerhans cell to 5 keratinocytes (Figure 2.36). Merkel cells, which are neuroendocrine-type cells, can also be identified within the vulvar epithelium; their function is unknown.[34]

The dermis consists of collagen, capillaries, and myofibroblastic type cells. It is divided into two regions. The papillary dermis is that portion found between the rete pegs. The reticular dermis is the solid confluent area beneath the rete pegs. Within the reticular dermis are hair-bearing follicles with associated sebaceous glands, apocrine and eccrine glands. The apocrine glands are sensitive to hormonal stimulation and release material by cytoplasmic secretion. The eccrine glands produce a watery sweat. They secrete by release of material through myoepithelial

cell contraction into sweat ducts. These glands are not modulated by hormonal activity. Once the transition to non-hair bearing skin occurs, the dermis of the labia minora contains only sebaceous glands and rare eccrine glands (Figure 2.37).[34]

The epithelium overlying the vestibule and the portion of the labia minora within Hart's line also consists of stratified squamous cells. This epithelium, however, has no surface keratin and the mature squamous epithelial cells become glycogen rich (Figure 2.38). This is particularly true of the hymeneal squamous epithelium; mild nuclear enlargement and the impression of cytoplasmic clearing can lead to a false diagnosis of human papillomavirus cytopathic effect. The dermis is highly vascular and rich in elastic fibers and erectile tissue. Here, adnexal structures are essentially absent.

The periurethral or Skene's glands are typically no more than 1.5 cm in length. Like the urethra, the ducts are lined with transitional-type epithelium that merges with the stratified squamous epithelium of the vestibular surface. The glands themselves are lined by mucin-producing columnar epithelium.

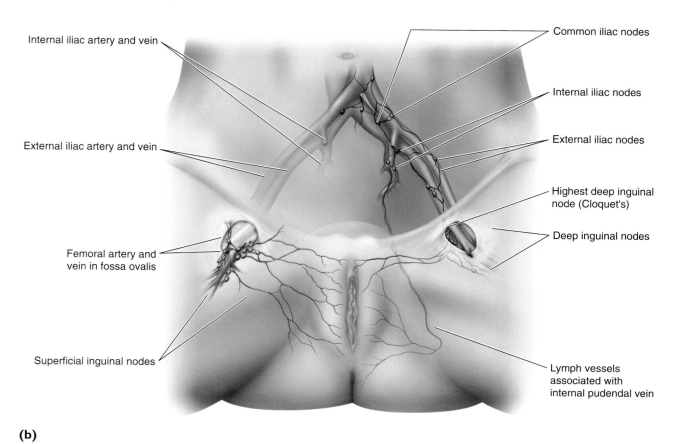

(b)

FIGURES 2.34a,b Continued. (b) Lymphatic drainage of the vulva and superficial perineum.

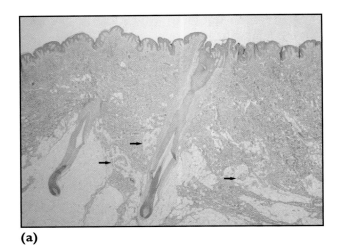

(a)

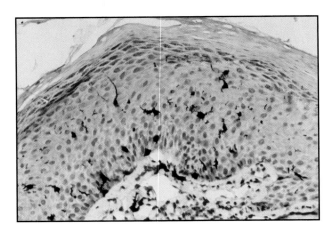

FIGURE 2.36 Langerhans cells. Individual dendritic type cells are scattered among the surface epithelial cells (immunperoxidase stain using antibodies against S100 protein, hematoxylin counter stain, high power magnification).

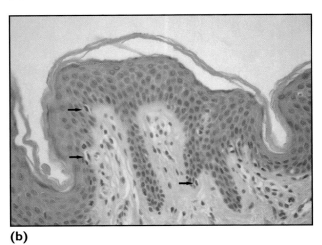

(b)

FIGURES 2.35a,b Vulvar surface covering the labia majora. **(a)** Low power. Note the epidermal evaginations or rete pegs that interdigitate between the papillary dermis. Two hair shafts are found in the more eosinophilic reticular dermis. Eccrine glands (arrows) are also present. Subcutaneous fat is present below the dermis (hematoxylin and eosin, low power magnification). **(b)** High power. Note the scattered melanocytes (arrows) in the epidermal basal layer (hematoxylin and eosin, high power magnification). ▬

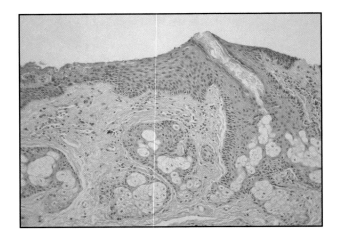

FIGURE 2.37 Vulvar surface covering the vestibule. Numerous sebaceous glands are present beneath the epidermis. There are, however, no accompanying hair shafts (hematoxylin and eosin, medium power magnification). ▬

The major vestibular or Bartholin's gland area consists of acini lined by columnar epithelium and of ducts lined by columnar and transitional cell type epithelium. As these ducts approach the surface, they are lined by stratified squamous epithelium. It is notable that the Bartholin's gland usually has multiple acini and ducts (Figure 2.39). Because of this, Bartholin's abscesses are usually multiloculated.[34]

The ducts of the minor vestibular glands exit directly into the mucosal surface around Hart's line. The tubular glands are shallow and have a maximum depth of 3 mm to 4 mm. They are lined by columnar-type mucin-producing epithelium (Figure 2.40). As they approach the surface, the epithelia transform into the stratified squamous cells of the vulvar epidermis. It is common for these glands to undergo squamous metaplasia. In some cases, the metaplasia may cause complete transformation of the vestibular gland into squamous epithelium, producing a cleft-like structure. The transitional type cells commonly seen in the major vestibular and periurethral glands are not present. Further information on the anatomy and histology of the vulva can be found in Chapter 15.

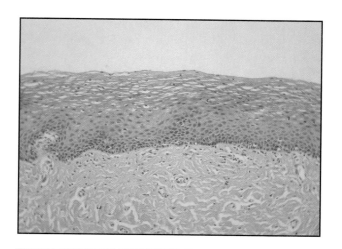

FIGURE 2.38 Vulva surface near the introitus. The epithelial surface is similar in appearance to the squamous mucosa of the vulva and vagina. Note the absence of rete pegs (hematoxylin and eosin, medium power magnification).

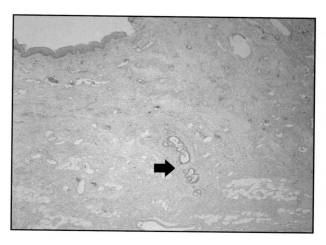

FIGURE 2.40 Minor vestibular glands. The small gland cluster (arrow) is found approximately 2 mm to 3 mm beneath the surface (hematoxylin and eosin, low power magnification).

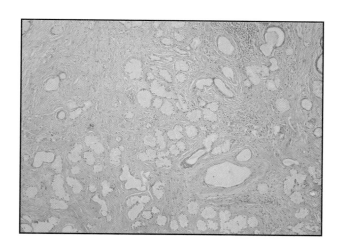

FIGURE 2.39 Major vestibular (Bartholin's) glands. Numerous acini lined by mucinous type epithelial cells are present. Scattered larger ductal structures are lined by urothelial-type cells (hematoxylin and eosin, medium power magnification).

2.5 Biopsy Specimen Collection, Processing and Interpretation

Various instruments have been designed to obtain cervical biopsies. All have scissors-like tips that can excise a 3-mm to 5-mm tissue fragment. The lower blade is slightly extended and can be placed into the cervical canal to stabilize the instrument. Little or no discomfort is felt if the forceps blades are sharp; dull blades cause tissue pulling, crushing, and subsequent cramping. Instruments designed to obtain endocervical material have the appearance of small baskets or rakes. The tissue is scraped off the canal surface, resulting in tiny tissue fragments in blood and mucus. Specimens obtained using loop excisional devices are similar in shape to large-shave biopsies. Biopsies of the vagina and vulva can be somewhat difficult to obtain because of their relatively flat surface. Cervical biopsy instruments can be used for raised lesions at these sites. For vaginal lesions that are flat, the mucosal surface can be tented using small hooks. Macular vulvar lesions can be removed using a Keyes punch, which is a trephine-cutter type instrument that removes a cylinder of surface epithelium and underlying dermis. Tissue from the proximal vagina adjacent to the cervix can be removed without anesthesia. Biopsies from the distal vagina and vulva usually require local anesthetic injection.

After removal, the tissue pieces are placed in formalin-filled containers labeled with the patient's name and the type of specimen submitted ("cervix biopsy," "labial biopsy," "ECC"). At the same time, a requisition form should be completed. This should include the patient's name, age, and pertinent history. Helpful additional information includes pregnancy status, hormone usage, the colposcopic impression, cytology result, and any prior lower genital tract abnormalities and treatment.

If biopsy location is important to the colposcopist, individual tissue fragments can be submitted in separate labeled containers. To assist in specimen orientation, the biopsy pieces can be placed on pieces of paper or Gelfoam®. Larger loop excision fragments can be oriented by dotting the surface with ink or by placing a small suture and noting the location on the requisition. If margin involvement is important, the colposcopist should indicate the order in which multiple fragments are removed so that the pathologist can determine which fragments represent the true ecto- and endocervical margins.

Once received in the laboratory, the specimen is logged and assigned an accession number, which usually represents the number of specimens received up to that point for a particular year. The specimen is then examined and described by a pathologist or an assistant, who notes the size, number, color, and consistency of the tissue pieces for a particular container.

Larger tissue pieces, such as those removed during loop excisional procedures, are cut into smaller serial cross sections, a process known as "bread-loafing" (Figure 2.41). The fragments are then placed in small rectangular plastic cassettes. The process of describing and transferring the tissue into cassettes is known as prosection, "grossing" or "cutting-in" the material.

After grossing is completed, a histotechnologist places the individual cassettes in a tissue processor that dehydrates the tissue and replaces any water with a medium that allows for optimal tissue cutting. This procedure is time dependent and takes approximately 4 to 9 hours. The tissue is then embedded into a modified paraffin material and sectioned by a microtome into small 5-μm ribbons. Before embedding, the histotechnologist must orient the biopsy specimen by hand; the larger the fragment, the easier it is to obtain sections that include surface epithelium and underlying stroma. The wax strips are then transferred to glass slides, stained using hematoxylin and eosin dyes, and coverslipped (Figure 2.42). Preparing biopsy material for microscopic examination takes about 6 to 10 hours. The pathologist then examines the glass slide after consulting the matching pathology requisition form for any pertinent clinical information and reports the result as a microscopic or final diagnosis. This process is known as "signing out" the specimens. The total process from specimen receipt and accession by the laboratory to provision of a diagnostic report to the colposcopist takes on average 24 hours (Figure 2.43).[36]

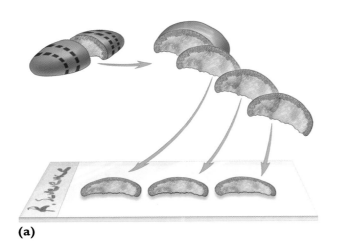

(a)

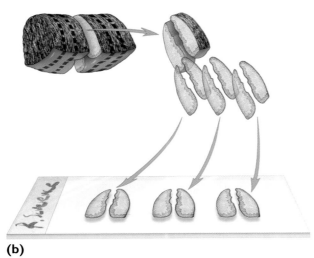

(b)

FIGURES 2.41a,b Specimen preparation. **(a)** Sectioning small biopsy specimens for microscopic examination. **(b)** Sectioning larger specimens obtained by means of cone and loop excision for microscopic examination.

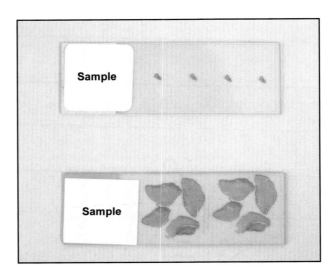

FIGURE 2.42 Glass slides stained with hematoxylin and eosin. The slide with the smaller pieces represents a cervical biopsy. The slide with the larger sections represents a loop excision.

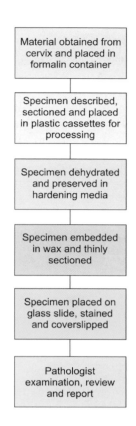

```
┌─────────────────────┐
│ Material obtained from│
│ cervix and placed in │
│ formalin container   │
└─────────────────────┘
          │
┌─────────────────────┐
│ Specimen described,  │
│ sectioned and placed │
│ in plastic cassettes for│
│ processing           │
└─────────────────────┘
          │
┌─────────────────────┐
│ Specimen dehydrated  │
│ and preserved in     │
│ hardening media      │
└─────────────────────┘
          │
┌─────────────────────┐
│ Specimen embedded    │
│ in wax and thinly    │
│ sectioned            │
└─────────────────────┘
          │
┌─────────────────────┐
│ Specimen placed on   │
│ glass slide, stained │
│ and coverslipped     │
└─────────────────────┘
          │
┌─────────────────────┐
│ Pathologist          │
│ examination, review  │
│ and report           │
└─────────────────────┘
```

FIGURE 2.43   Processing of histology material by a pathology laboratory.

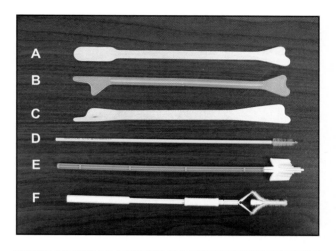

FIGURES 2.44a–f   Different cervical cytologic sampling devices. **(a–c):** Spatulas; **(d)** Cytobrush®; **(e)** Cervex-Brush® or Papette®; **(f)** Accellon Combi® device.

Since a single random 5-μm thin section may miss a dysplasia that partially covers a 3-mm to 4-mm biopsy fragment, most surgical pathology laboratories will cut two to three strips through different layers of the fragment, called "levels" or "step sections." Occasionally, a pathologist will request additional levels if diagnostic questions are raised during the initial microscopic interpretation or the specimen is maloriented. In addition, special stains may be ordered if the presence of bacterial or fungal organisms is suspected, or to better clarify a specific abnormality. When this occurs, the pathologist will often generate a preliminary diagnosis, with a comment noting that a final diagnosis will be forthcoming after further evaluation of additional material.

2.6 Cytology Specimen Collection, Processing, and Interpretation

At present, two types of cytologic specimens can be obtained. The conventional Pap smear involves direct application of the cellular material collected from the cervix or vagina onto a glass slide. The slide is then sprayed or immersed in an alcohol fixative. Newer liquid processing systems permit the transference of the collected cellular specimen into a solution for transport to the laboratory, where the material is then mechanically dispersed and a representative thin layer of cells is transferred to a glass slide (see Chapter 3, section 3.4.2.1). The majority of providers use three types of sampling devices for specimen collection: the Ayre spatula (Surgipath Medical Industries Inc., P.O. Box 528, Richmond IL 60071), the Cytobrush® (Cooper Surgical, Inc., 95 Corporate Drive, Trumbull, CT 06611), and the Cervex-brush® (Unimar, Inc. 475 Danbury Rd., Wilton, CT 06897) or Papette® (Wallach Surgical Devices, Inc. 235 Edison Rd., Orange, CT 06477) (Figure 2.44).

The spatula is widely available, inexpensive, causes minimal discomfort and only rarely causes cervical trauma. It cannot, however, sample a SCJ located in the endocervical canal. Therefore, the original Ayre tip has been lengthened in some devices, and plastic spatulas have been introduced to improve cell capture and transfer. Use of the spatula is straightforward. It is placed against the cervix, rotated 360° at least once, and the collected material spread across a glass slide. In some cases, however, the long end of the spatula is not always placed into the os. For women with a large ectropion, the spatula should be placed laterally in order to sample the red-to-pink interface representing the SCJ. Transfer of the material to the slide must be quick and deliberate to minimize cell distortion by air-drying. If a liquid processing system is used, the material is obtained by a plastic spatula and then vigorously stirred in the solution for at least 10 seconds.

The Cytobrush® has perpendicular pliable plastic bristles at the end of a thin wire applicator. For maximal sampling of the entire cervix, it should be used in conjunction with the spatula. The narrow tip of the cytobrush can be inserted into a narrowed cervical os to sample the endocervical canal. To minimize bleeding, the brush should be rotated only one fourth (90°) to one half (180°) of a complete turn. Optimal cell transfer is accomplished by rolling the brush across a slide. If a liquid preparation system is used, the brush is stirred in the preservative for 10 seconds and then rolled around the wall of the collection jar at least 10 times. Some providers will also scrape the bristles with a spatula to improve cell transfer. Recent studies have shown that the Cytobrush® is safe for use during pregnancy, but this is not approved by the manufacturer.[37] The Cytobrush® has replaced the cotton swab or cotton-tipped applicator, as the cotton fibers of the latter cause cell trapping and may result in insufficient cell transfer (Figure 2.45).[38]

The Cervex-brush® or Papette® has bristles that are softer, thicker, and longer centrally than those of the Cytobrush®. The device resembles a paintbrush, except that the central bristles are longer than the shorter lateral bristles. The longer bristles are inserted into the canal, while the shorter strands spread over the portio and lateral ectocervix. Because of its shape, many clinicians refer to this device simply as "the broom." The technique for using this device is the most meticulous of the four. The cervix must first be wiped with a large cotton swab in order to remove any mucus adherent to the external cervical os. The Cervex-brush® is applied to the cervix with the central bristles inserted into the canal and rotated five times in a clockwise fashion. It is then smeared longitudinally across the glass slide in a single motion, turned to the opposite side, and again swept across the slide. If a liquid preparation system is used, the broom is stirred in the solution for at least 10 seconds, pressed against the bottom and then stirred again for 10 seconds. Some systems require that the broom tip be removed and sent in the liquid container.

Many comparative studies have evaluated the efficacy of different collection devices. Most have concluded that the combination of a Cytobrush® and spatula is the best technique for sampling the cervix, followed by the broom.[39,40] A recent evidenced-based review evaluated different sampling devices to determine the best technique to detect the presence of cervical dysplasia.[41] Although not universally accepted, this review concluded that dysplasia was much more likely to be detected when individual

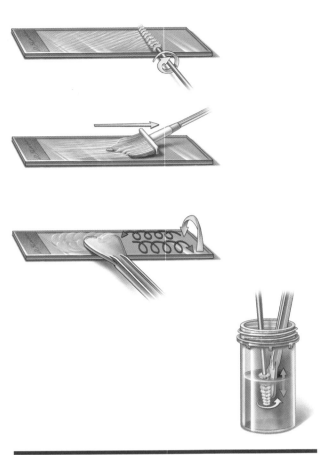

FIGURES 2.45a,b   (a) Transfer of cervical material to glass slides for preparation of conventional smears. **(b)** Transfer of cervical material to liquid medium for preparation of monolayer smears.

smears contained endocervical cells, and the proportion of smears with endocervical cells increased progressively with the severity of dysplasia. While the extended tip spatula, Cervex-brush®, and the Cytobrush® were better than the classic Ayre spatula for sampling the canal, the best technique for identification of cervical dysplasia was a combination of the spatula and Cytobrush®.[41]

In general, women should not douche, use vaginal creams, or have intercourse within 24 hours of specimen collection. The cytologic specimen should be obtained before other cervical and uterine specimens and before the bimanual examination. Water or a thin film of water-soluble gel can be used as a speculum lubricant. Once the smear is obtained, the slide should be quickly fixed using an alcohol-based solution, labeled with the patient's name, and submitted to a laboratory with a requisition sheet that also includes the patient's name and any pertinent history. Important information for optimal smear interpretation includes the specimen source, the patient's age, her last menstrual period, any hormonal usage or, if pregnant, gestational age. Any history of prior abnormal cytologic specimens or treatment of cervical or vaginal abnormalities.

Once received by the laboratory, conventional and liquid processed slides are stained by the Pap method, which uses variable combinations of hematoxylin, eosin and orange G dyes, and coverslipped.[42] They are then screened by a cytotechnologist, an individual specifically trained to examine cytologic specimens. The cytotechnologist either reports the smear as normal, after which a report is generated, or identifies possible abnormalities that require final interpretation by the pathologist. In addition, laboratories are required by the U.S. Federal Clinical Laboratory Improvements Amendments (CLIA) of 1988 to randomly review 10 percent of all slides initially reported as normal. This is commonly done by a second senior cytotechnologist. As the screening of slides is tedious and labor intensive, laboratories are limited by law to the number of slides that can be screened by individual cytotechnologists over a 24-hour period. Most laboratories set a limit of 50 to 80 slides per day for each technologist. Because of this, the time from receipt of the cytologic specimen by the laboratory to the rendering of a final diagnostic report to the colposcopist can extend over several days, depending on the volume of slides reviewed by the laboratory and the number of cytotechnologists (Figure 2.46).

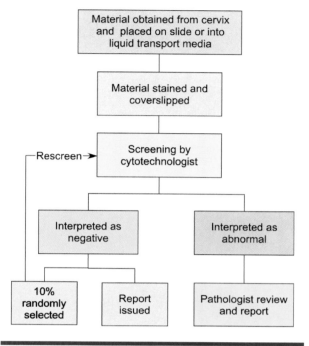

FIGURE 2.46   Processing of cytology material by a pathology laboratory.

References

1. Robboy S J, Bernhardt P F, Parmley T. Embryology of the female genital tract and disorders of abnormal sexual development. In: Kurman R J, ed. *Blaustein's Pathology of the Female Genital Tract* (4th ed). New York: Springer-Verlag, 1994:8–10.
2. Larsen W J. *Human Embryology*. New York: Churchill Livingstone, 1993:253–258.
3. Hendrickson M R, Kempson R L. Uterus and fallopian tubes. In: Sternberg S S, ed. *Histology for Pathologists*. New York: Raven Press, 1992:801–8.
4. Linhartova A. Extent of columnar epithelium on the ectocervix between the ages of 1 and 13 years. *Obstet Gynecol* 1978;52:451–6.
5. Robboy S J, Bentley R C. Vagina. In: Sternberg S S, ed. *Histology for Pathologists* (2nd ed.). Philadelphia-New York: Lippincott-Raven Publishers, 1997:867–79.
6. Wright T, Ferenczy A. Anatomy and histology of the cervix. In Kurman R J, ed. *Blaustein's Pathology of the Female Genital Tract*. (5th ed.) New York: Springer-Verlag, 2002:207–224.
7. Singer A. Anatomy of the cervix and physiological changes in cervical epithelium. In: Fox H, Well M. eds. *Haines and Taylor Obstetrical and Gynaecological Pathology*. New York: Churchill Livingstone, 1995:225–48.
8. Hellman L M, Pritchard J A. *Williams Obstetrics* (14th ed), New York: Appleton-Century-Crofts, 1970:19–30.
9. Kurman R J. Norris H J, Wilkinson E. Tumors of the Cervix, Vagina and Vulva. Atlas of Tumor Pathology (Series 3, Volume 4). Bethesda: Armed Forces Institute of Pathology (monograph), 1992:1–12.
10. Vooijs G P. Benign proliferative reactions, intraepithelial neoplasia and invasive cancer of the uterine cervix. In: Bibbo M, ed. *Diagnostic Cytopathology* (2nd ed.). Philadelphia: W B Saunders Co., 1997:161–8.
11. Feldman D, Romney S L, Edgcomb J, Valentine T. Ultrastructure of normal, metaplastic, and abnormal human uterine cervix: Use of montages to study the topographical relationship of epithelial cells. *Am J Obstet Gynecol* 1984;150:573–688.

12. Kupryjanczyk J. Epidermal growth factor receptor expression in the normal and inflamed cervix uteri: a comparison with estrogen receptor expression. *Int J Gynecol Pathol*. 1990;9:263–71.

13. Gigi-Leiter O, Geiger B, Levy R, Czernobilsky B. Cytokeratin expression in squamous metaplasia of the human uterine cervix. *Differentiation* 1986:31:191–205.

14. Maddox P, Szarewski A, Dyson J, Cuzick J. Cytokeratin expression and acetowhite change in cervical epithelium *J Clin Pathol* 1994;47:15–7.

15. Smedts F, Ramaekers F, Leube R E, Keijser K, Link M, Vooijs P. Expression of keratins 1,6,15,16 and 20 in normal cervical epithelium, squamous metaplasia, cervical intraepithelial neoplasia and cervical carcinoma. *Am J Pathol* 1993;142:403–12.

16. Cullen T S. *Cancer of the Uterus*, New York: D. Appleton and Co. 1900:180–7.

17. Fluhmann C F. *The Cervix Uteri and Its Diseases*. Philadelphia: W B Saunders, 1961:56–78.

18. Lawrence W D, Shingleton H M. Early physiologic squamous metaplasia of the cervix: light and electron microscopic observation. *Am J Obstet Gynecol* 1980;137:661–71.

19. Burke L, Antonioli D A, Ducatman B S. *Colposcopy, Text and Atlas*. Norwalk, CT: Appleton and Lange, 1991:29–59.

20. Smedts F, Ramaekers F, Troyanovsky S, et al. Basal-cell keratins in cervical reserve cells and a comparison to their expression in cervical intraepithelial neoplasia. *Am J Pathol* 1992;140:601–12.

21. Szamborski J, Liebhart M. The ultrastructure of squamous metaplasia in endocervix. *Path Europ* 1973;1:13–20.

22. Vooijs G P. Benign proliferative reactions, intraepithelial neoplasia and invasive cancer of the uterine cervix. In: Bibbo M, ed. *Diagnostic Cytopathology* (2nd ed.) Philadelphia: W B Saunders Co., 1997:169–74.

23. Autier P, Coibion M, Huet F Grivegnee A R. Transformation zone location and intraepithelial neoplasia of the cervix uteri. *Br J Ca* 1996;74:488–90.

24. Moscicki A-B, Burt V G, Kanowitz S, et al. The significance of squamous metaplasia in the development of low grade squamous intraepithelial lesions in young women. *Cancer* 1999;85:1139–44.

25. Gould P R, Barter R A, Papadimitriou J M. An ultrastructural, cytochemical and autoradiographic study of the mucous membrane of the human cervical canal with reference to subcolumnar basal cells. *Am J Pathol* 1979;95:1–16.

26. Tsutsumi K, Sun Q, Yasumoto S, et al. In vitro and in vivo analysis of cellular origin of cervical squamous metaplasia. *Am J Pathol* 1993;143:1150–8.

27. Hare M J, Toone E, Taylor-Robinson D, et al. Follicular cervicitis—colposcopic appearances and association with *Chlamydia trachomatis*. *Br J Obstet Gynaecol* 1981;88:174–80.

28. Papanicolaou G N, Traut H F, Marchetti A A. *The Epithelia of Woman's Reproductive Organs*. New York: The Commonwealth Fund, 1948:30–6.

29. Prins R P, Morrow C P, Townsend D E, Disaia P J. Vaginal embryogenesis, estrogens, and adenosis. *Obstet Gynecol* 1976;48:246–250.

30. Patton D L, Thwin S S, Meier A, Houston TM et al. Epithelial cell layer thickness and immune cell populations in the normal human vagina at different stages of the menstrual cycle. *Am J Obstet Gynecol* 1976;183:967–73.

31. Schaller G, Lengyel E, Pantel K, et al. Keratin expression reveals mosaic differentiation in vaginal epithelium. *Am J Obstet Gynecol* 1993;169:1603–7.

32. Speroff L, Glass R H, Kase N G. *Clinical Gynecologic Embryology and Infertility* (5th ed.) Baltimore: Williams and Wilkins, 1994:326–9.

33. Wilkinson E J. Benign diseases of the vulva. In: Kurman R J, ed. *Blaustein's Pathology of the Female Genital Tract* (4th ed.). New York: Springer-Verlag, 1994:31–87.

34. Wilkinson E J, Hart N S. Vulva. In: Sternberg S S, ed. *Histology for Pathologists*. New York: Raven Press, 1992:865–81.

35. Lever W F, Lever-Schaumburg G. *Histopathology of the Skin* (6th ed.) Philadelphia: J B Lippincott, 1983:90–3.

36. Prophet E B, Mills B, Arrington J B, Sobin L H, eds. *Laboratory Methods in Histotechnology*. Armed Forces Institute of Pathology, American Registry of Pathology, Washington, DC., 1992:25–45.

37. Lieberman R W, Henry M R, Laskin W B, et al. Colposcopy in pregnancy: directed brush cytology compared with cervical biopsy. *Obstet Gynecol* 1999; 94:198–203.

38. Rubio C A. The false negative smear II. The trapping effect of collecting instruments. *Obstet Gynecol* 1976;49:576–9.

39. Boon M E, de Graff Guilloud J C, Rietveld W J. Analysis of five sampling methods for the preparation of cervical smears. *Acta Cytol* 1988;33:843–8.

40. Germain M, Heaton R, Erickson D, et al. A comparison of the three most common Papanicolaou smear collection techniques. *Obstet Gynecol* 1994;84:168–73.

41. Martin-Hirsch P, Jarvis G, Ketchener H, Lilford R. Collection devices for obtaining cervical cytology samples. The Cochrane Library, 1999;2:1–25.

42. Mikel U V, ed. Advanced Laboratory Methods in Histology and Pathology (monograph). Armed Forces Institute of Pathology, American Registry of Pathology, Washington, DC, 1994:221–4.

The Cytology and Histology of Cervicovaginal Abnormalities

Table of Contents

3.1 Introduction

Cervicovaginal neoplasia has generated considerable attention throughout the past century. Much of this interest has resulted from easy access to clinical inspection, the discovery of a premalignant condition, and the slow progression from a normal healthy mucosa to invasive carcinoma (see Chapter 1). This chapter details the specific benign, premalignant and malignant alterations that can occur in the cervix and vagina.

3.2 Histology of Squamous Abnormalities

The diagnostic specimens usually submitted by colposcopists for histologic examination are directed biopsies, loop excision or conizations specimens, and endocervix curettings. Although small, these samples can supply a great deal of valuable information.

Colposcopically directed biopsies of the cervix are examined for the presence of the transformation zone (TZ). By convention, this is defined as the

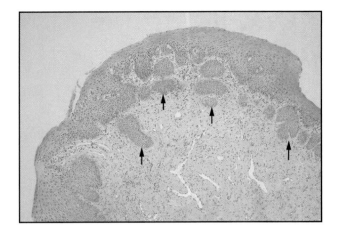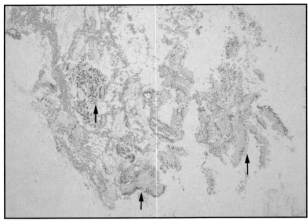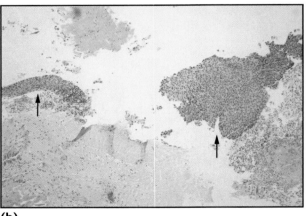

FIGURE 3.1   Cervical biopsy with squamous metaplasia. Although no endocervical cells are seen, the presence of immature squamous cell nests in the superficial stroma (arrows) is consistent with squamous metaplasia (hematoxylin and eosin, medium-power magnification).

(a)

(b)

FIGURES 3.2a,b   Endocervical curettings. **(a)** Scattered fragments of normal endocervical gland epithelia (arrows) are seen in a background of mucus and red blood cells (hematoxylin and eosin, medium power magnification). **(b)** Fragments of detached dysplasia (arrows) are present. As there is no surface or basement membrane, an accurate grade cannot be given. Nevertheless, the proliferation of squamous cells with enlarged atypical nuclei and scant cell cytoplasm suggests a high-grade dysplasia (hematoxylin and eosin, medium-power magnification).

presence of endocervical gland elements adjacent to or beneath squamous epithelium. In some cases, non-glycogenated immature squamous cells replacing superficial glands can also represent squamous metaplasia (Figure 3.1). Orientation of the fragment is important; ideally, an intact basement membrane and surface should be identifiable. This is necessary for the purpose of grading any surface dysplasia, as the severity of dysplasia is determined by assessing the amount of basaloid dysplastic cells extending from the basement membrane toward the surface. Because curettage specimens contain small unoriented fragments, the pathologist usually can indicate only that dysplasia is either present or absent (Figure 3.2).

Unless stated to be an excisional biopsy, a pathologist will consider small biopsy specimens to be diagnostic only and will not comment on the presence or absence of abnormalities at the resection margins. On the other hand, by convention, all loop and conization specimens are considered excisional unless stated otherwise. Because multi-pass loop excisional specimens often cut through dysplasia, it can be difficult to determine the true resection margins unless specifically marked on the specimen by the clinician or illustrated on the requisition form. The presence of thermal artifact (char) along the edge of a loop excision specimen is useful to identify the line of excision (Figure 3.3). Traditional conization

specimens are marked with colored ink along the nonmucosal cut edge before the specimen is sectioned for processing. When seen under the microscope, the presence of ink along a tissue edge differentiates a true resection margin from one created by tissue processing.

A pathologist should provide the following information on a diagnostic biopsy: degree of dysplasia if

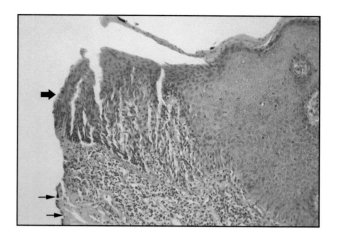

FIGURE 3.3   Loop excisional procedure. There is high-grade dysplasia that extends to the specimen edge. The presence of black ink on the surface (small arrows) and thermal damage (cell distortion—large arrow) marks this edge as a resection margin (hematoxylin and eosin, medium-power magnification).

the specimen is oriented; histologic type and grade; and presence or absence of lymphatic and vascular space invasion by tumor cells, if invasive carcinoma is identified. For excisional biopsies, such as a loop excision or conization specimen oriented by the colposcopist, the pathologist should report the degree of dysplasia, its extent (usually reported as numbers on a clock face), and completeness of excision. If invasive squamous cell carcinoma is identified, the histologic type, grade, depth of invasion, horizontal extent, apparent completeness of excision, and presence of lymphatic and vascular space invasion should be reported.

While it is generally assumed that pathologists can accurately differentiate benign from dysplastic and malignant abnormalities, it must be remembered that the result rendered on a histologic report represents only a best impression based on the history provided, the quality of submitted material, and the experience and expertise of the pathologist. While reproducibility of diagnoses among pathologists is best for high-grade dysplasias and invasive carcinomas, it can be only fair to poor for low-grade dysplasias.[1,2] In the future, it is possible that biomarkers such as Ki-67 (MIB-1) and p16(INK4a), which represent antigens often selectively expressed in intraepithelial neoplasias, may become useful in separating true dysplasias from markedly reactive epithelial changes.[3]

3.2.1 Reactive and reparative changes

It is common for areas of metaplasia to demonstrate evidence of acute or, more frequently, chronic inflammation. The changes are generally nonspecific but can be related to specific infectious organisms. In some instances, lymphoid follicles can be identified in the superficial stroma, a condition known as chronic follicular cervicitis.[4] Depending on the degree of inflammation, the surface epithelium can slough (erosive cervicitis). Immature metaplastic squamous cells quickly replace the lost squamous or glandular epithelia through a process known as repair. Typically, these cells have larger nuclei than the usual metaplastic cell. Nuclear chromatin is more granular and nucleoli are prominent. These reactive squamous changes can be distinguished from squamous dysplasia by the presence of smooth nuclear borders, general uniformity of nuclear size, presence of distinct cell borders, and lack of nuclear overlap. Mitoses are uncommon and, if present, are usually found along the basal cell layer. No abnormal mitotic forms are identified (Figure 3.4).[4,5]

3.2.2 Intraepithelial lesions

Squamous intraepithelial abnormalities, also referred to as squamous dysplasias, are associated with the presence of human papillomavirus (HPV). The degree of surface abnormality reflects the type of viral interaction with the immature squamous cell. In mild degrees of dysplasia, HPV produces proteins that direct the host cell to undergo maturation and cell death. The end result is a cell that exfoliates, disintegrates, and releases large numbers of intact viral particles. Higher degrees of dysplasia reflect actual disruption of the HPV DNA and integration into the host cell genome. Unregulated production of oncogenic viral proteins result in transformation and proliferation of the immature basal or parabasal cells that contain the viral DNA (see Chapter 5 for a more detailed explanation of this process). Squamous dysplastic cells commonly contain cytokeratins 10, 11, 13, and 16, which reflect the squamous origin of these cells. As dysplasia worsens, however, the cytokeratin distribution becomes more consistent with those found in immature metaplastic cells.[4]

The hallmark of surface dysplasia is the presence of variable abnormal cytologic features in the squamous epithelial cells. These dysplastic cells may extend into and fill superficial endocervical glands (Figure 3.5). The basement membrane, nevertheless,

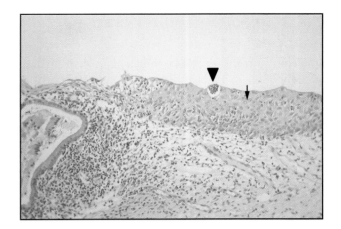

FIGURE 3.4   Reactive cervicitis. The immature metaplastic cells (small arrow) have enlarged nuclei and prominent nucleoli. Considerable cytoplasm is present and cell borders are recognizable. Acute inflammatory cells are present in the epithelium, and there is a small microabscess (arrowhead) (hematoxylin and eosin, medium-power magnification).

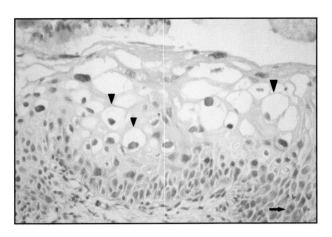

FIGURE 3.6   Mild dysplasia (cervical intraepithelial neoplasia or CIN 1). Basal cell proliferation extends through one third of the squamous surface. Note the mitosis (small arrow). The remaining two thirds contain koilocytotic cells (arrowheads) (hematoxylin and eosin, high-power magnification).

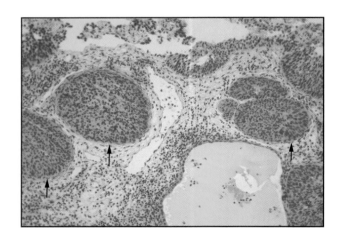

FIGURE 3.5   Squamous dysplasia present in superficial endocervical glands. Although highly cellular, the basement membrane (arrows) is intact. Dysplasia is also present on the surface (hematoxylin and eosin, medium-power magnification).

3.2.2.1 Cervical/vaginal intraepithelial neoplasia grade 1

The hallmark cell of CIN/VAIN 1 or mild dysplasia is the *koilocyte* (Figure 3.6). This cell reflects marked degeneration of a mature squamous cell with a nucleus filled with particles of HPV. Koilocytes are located in the upper two thirds of the squamous surface and are characterized by superficial or intermediate type cells with nuclei that are enlarged at least three times the size of a normal intermediate cell nucleus. The nuclei are dark and contain coarse chromatin that fills the nucleus or aggregates in the periphery (vesicular change). Nucleoli usually are not seen. The nuclear membrane is markedly wrinkled, giving the enlarged nucleus a raisin-like appearance. Often a single cell will contain multiple nuclei. The area adjacent to the nucleus appears transparent because the cytoplasm aggregates in the periphery, giving the appearance of a perinuclear halo.[11,12] The remaining peripheral cytoplasm is condensed into a border at the edge of the halo. Electron microscopic imaging of koilocytes indicates that the nuclei are filled with numerous encapsulated papillomavirus virions. The cytoplasm alterations represent aggregation of cytoskeleton filaments and organelles into the periphery. Koilocytosis signifies an intermediate step toward cell death. Therefore, the diagnosis of koilocytosis can be made only when the nuclei demonstrate unmistakable abnormal cytologic features.[12]

remains intact along the affected surface and around the involved glands. The World Health Organization (WHO) recognizes two general classification systems: cervical or vaginal dysplasia. graded as mild, moderate, and severe, and carcinoma in situ (CIS), or cervical or vaginal intraepithelial neoplasia (CIN/VAIN) graded as 1, 2, and 3.[5-10]

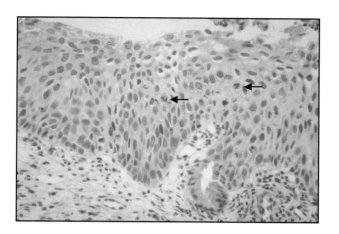

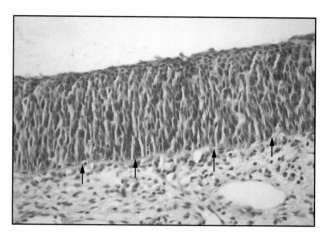

FIGURE 3.7 Moderate dysplasia (cervical intraepithelial neoplasia or CIN 2). The basal proliferation of dysplastic cells extends through approximately one half of the surface epithelium. Mitoses are also present at the epithelial surface midpoint (arrows). Koilocytic cells are still present near the surface (hematoxylin and eosin, high-power magnification).

FIGURE 3.8 Severe dysplasia/carcinoma in situ (cervical intraepithelial neoplasia or CIN 3). There is proliferation of immature dysplastic cells throughout the squamous epithelium from the base to the surface. The basement membrane (arrows), however, remains intact (hematoxylin and eosin, high-power magnification).

At the base, there is proliferation of the immature basal and parabasal cells; however, the degree of proliferation is limited to the lower third of the epithelial surface. Mitoses can be seen, but the mitotic figures are limited to the layer of proliferation. Abnormal forms are absent.[12]

3.2.2.2 Cervical/vaginal intraepithelial neoplasia grade 2

In CIN/VAIN 2 or moderate dysplasia, the degree of proliferation among the basal and parabasal cells increases to the point where the layer of abnormal cells reaches up to two thirds of the epithelial surface.[8,9,13] Very commonly, the proliferation occupies half of the surface epithelium. Cytologically, the nuclei within these immature cells are enlarged and irregular in shape. The nuclear size varies among the cells and nuclear overlapping is common. The nuclear membrane is irregular and nuclear chromatin is dark and granular. Nucleoli are small or absent. Mitotic figures now extend to one half of the epithelial surface, and abnormal forms (tripolar or ring shapes) are now present. Koilocytes can be found in the upper portion of the epithelial surface (Figure 3.7).

3.2.2.3 Cervical/vaginal intraepithelial neoplasia grade 3

In CIN 3, VAIN 3 or severe dysplasia/CIS, the proliferation of immature cells almost completely fills the epithelial surface (Figure 3.8). The cytologic appearance of these cells is similar to those seen in CIN 2. Mitoses, including abnormal forms, are now found at or near the top of the epithelial surface. In the past, the differentiation between severe dysplasia and CIS was felt to be significant. However, it is related to the presence of one or two residual layers of mature cells at the upper surface. The ability to differentiate a persistent layer of mature cells from degenerated superficial dysplastic cells is not consistent among pathologists, and the prognostic significance of a few residual "mature" cells is unclear. Consequently, most pathologists prefer the designation CIN 3 or VAIN 3 to include all proliferations of abnormal immature cells that occupy more than two thirds of the epithelial surface.[8,9,13]

3.2.3 Invasive carcinoma

Invasion is characterized by disruption of the basement membrane between the epithelial surface cells and the underlying stroma. Invasion initially occurs as finger-like extensions of malignant cells from adjacent epithelium into the stroma or as irregularly shaped nests of malignant cells throughout the stroma. A rim of fibrosis and inflammation known as desmoplasia is commonly seen around these malignant nests. The malignant cells are often larger than the adjacent dysplastic cells. The nuclei are also large with dense peripheral chromatin and prominent

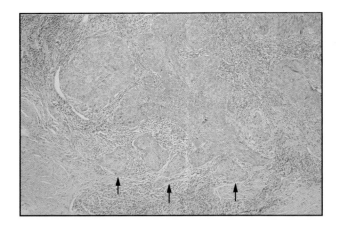

FIGURE 3.9 Early invasive squamous cell carcinoma. In contrast to the small cells in the surface squamous dysplasia, the invasive squamous cells have larger nuclei and abundant eosinophilic cytoplasm. The borders are irregular as small malignant nests (arrows) extend into the surrounding stroma. If the depth of invasion and horizontal spread was less than 5 mm and 7 mm, respectively, and the lesion was completely excised, the focus would qualify as a microinvasive squamous cell carcinoma (hematoxylin and eosin, medium-power magnification).

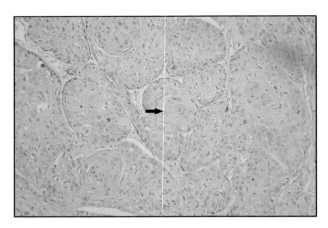

FIGURE 3.10 Keratinizing squamous cell carcinoma. Keratininzing pearls (arrow) are present in the malignant nests (hematoxylin and eosin, medium-power magnification).

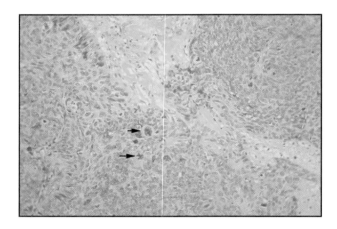

FIGURE 3.11 Poorly differentiated non-keratinizing squamous cell carcinoma. Note the absence of keratin pearls in the nests of malignant cells. Numerous mitotic figures, including abnormal forms (arrows), are easily seen. The surrounding stroma demonstrates a fibrotic (desmoplastic) response (hematoxylin and eosin, medium-power magnification).

nucleoli. The cytoplasm is eosinophilic and contains keratins 5, 8, 10, 13, 18 and 19, signifying squamous differentiation. The overall appearance suggests a process of "cellular maturation in the wrong direction," as the larger malignant cells are directed away from the surface (Figure 3.9).[5]

Squamous cell carcinomas are separated into keratinizing and nonkeratinizing types. Keratinizing tumors are characterized by the presence of squamous pearls in tumor nests (Figure 3.10). Carcinoma grading is based on the ability of the malignant cells to resemble normal squamous epithelium, as well as cell size, morphology, and the interface between the invasive neoplasm and the adjacent stroma. Well-differentiated carcinomas are usually keratinizing types that have large cohesive cells with a pushing interface. Poorly differentiated squamous carcinomas are usually nonkeratinizing and characterized by small cells that lack cohesion and infiltrate throughout the surrounding stroma (Figure 3.11).[14]

Because depth of invasion and horizontal spread have treatment and prognostic implications, small nests of invasive squamous cell carcinomas found in excisional biopsies should be measured with an ocular micrometer. The depth of invasion is measured from the nearest basement membrane of origin, which, in some cases, may be an endocervical gland that contains CIN. The measured tumor size, however, can be considered accurate only if any existing cancer and dysplasia are completely excised. The pathologist should report the presence of any lymphatic and vascular space invasion by tumor cells (Figure 3.12).[9,14,15]

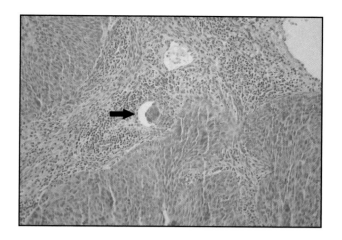

FIGURE 3.12 Lymphatic and vascular space invasion by tumor cells. The centrally located capillary-like space contains a cluster of malignant cells (arrow) (hematoxylin and eosin, medium-power magnification).

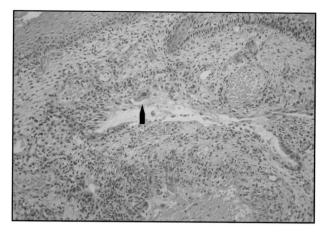

FIGURE 3.13 Reactive endocervical cells. The reactive cells (arrow) have slightly enlarged, irregularly shaped hyperchromatic nuclei. Features of adenocarcinoma in situ (mitoses, stratification), however, are absent (hematoxylin and eosin, medium-power magnification).

3.3 Histology of Glandular Abnormalities

Although glandular lesions can arise anywhere along the endocervical canal, the majority are found in the area of the TZ. Nonetheless, glandular lesions can occur outside the TZ and can be multifocal. If adenocarcinoma in situ (AIS) is noted in an excisional specimen, the two-dimensional extent of the abnormality should be measured, its location in relation to the TZ should be reported, and the presence of abnormal glands at a resection margin should be noted. If invasive adenocarcinoma is found, the pathologist should report the cell type, tumor grade, lesion size, margin status, and presence of lymphatic and vascular space invasion. The following represents brief morphologic descriptions of the more common glandular abnormalities. Additional information regarding glandular abnormalities can be found in Chapter 11.

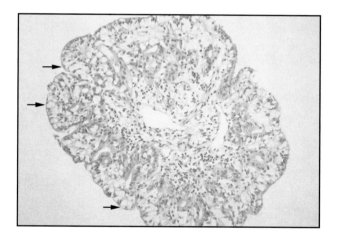

FIGURE 3.14 Endocervical polyp. The rounded polyp contains endocervical cells forming multiple small glands (microglandular hyperplasia-arrows) (hematoxylin and eosin, medium-power magnification).

3.3.1 Reactive changes

These changes are similar to those identified in squamous metaplastic cells. The nuclei of the affected glandular cells are enlarged and multinucleation can occur. The nuclear membranes, however, are smooth and the nuclear shapes are generally round to oval. Micronuclei are present. Mitotic activity generally is not found (Figure 3.13).[4,5]

Microglandular hyperplasia is a condition commonly seen in women who are pregnant or who use oral contraceptives. Commonly seen in endocervi-

cal polyps and areas of immature metaplasia, the glandular cells proliferate and coalesce to form small lumens. Individual cells also demonstrate small intracellular gland-like spaces. Although the pattern appears architecturally neoplastic, the nuclei are small and uniform, and mitoses are rare.[16] In some cases, microglandular hyperplasia will form polypoid masses (Figure 3.14). These endocervical polyps contain central fibrovascular cores with surface glandular proliferation and immature metaplasia.[17]

3.3.2. Intraepithelial lesions

Endocervical AIS is characterized by endocervical glands that, in general, are architecturally normal in size and location but contain cells that are cytologically abnormal (Figure 3.15). The cells contain less cytoplasm than do normal glandular cells. The nuclei are enlarged, nonuniform in size and shape, and dark, with dense granular chromatin. Nucleoli are difficult to identify. The cells stratify and mitoses are common. In some cases, the proliferating cells form bridges, resulting in a cribriform pattern (multiple small round glands within a larger single gland). The basement membrane, however, is always intact.[14,18]

Although the majority of AIS is confined to the TZ, approximately 20% of these lesions can be multifocal. For excisional specimens, the pathologist should report the extent of the AIS and whether the margins are free of glandular abnormalities, but the colposcopist must remember that this information does not necessarily imply completeness of excision.[14,18]

3.3.3 Invasive adenocarcinoma

As with invasive squamous cell carcinoma, invasive adenocarcinoma implies disruption of the basement membrane and infiltration of abnormal glandular cells into the surrounding stroma. As with AIS, invasive endocervical adenocarcinoma can be multifocal and can originate anywhere along the endocervical canal.

In invasive adenocarcinoma, the malignant cells contain enlarged, irregular shaped nonuniform nuclei with dense chromatin, commonly aggregated along the nuclear periphery (vesicular change) (Figure 3.16). Prominent nucleoli are present, and mitoses, including abnormal forms, are common. A desmoplastic stromal response is present and helps to identify these glands as malignant. Because the malignant cells have the potential to recapitulate the lining cells of various crypts and tubules of the genitourinary and gastrointestinal tracts, the different malignant cell types can include mucinous (colonic), endometrioid (endometrium), clear cell (renal tubule), and serous (fallopian tube).[14,18]

Endocervical adenocarcinomas are graded according to architectural appearance and the ability of the malignant cells to form recognizable glands. Well-differentiated adenocarcinomas contain numerous regular glands with minimal stratification and infrequent mitotic figures. Poorly differentiated adenocarcinomas, on the other hand, have solid sheets of malignant cells with few recognizable glands. Bizarre nuclei are common and mitoses are frequent. Special types of well-differentiated endocervical adenocarcinoma include the minimum-deviation adenocarcinoma (or adenoma malignum) and the villoglandular types. Minimum-deviation adenocarcinomas consist of deeply infiltrating glands with bland, almost normal-appearing cells. They can be diagnosed only in cervices removed by conization or hysterectomy and are often associated with polyposis syndromes and sex cord-stromal ovarian neoplasms. Villoglandular adenocarcinomas are superficial

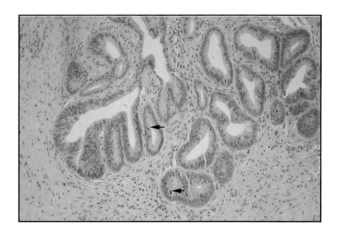

FIGURE 3.15 Endocervical adenocarcinoma in situ. There is stratification of the dysplastic glandular cells and numerous mitotic figures (arrows). The gland architecture, however, is normal and the basement membrane is intact (hematoxylin and eosin, medium-power magnification).

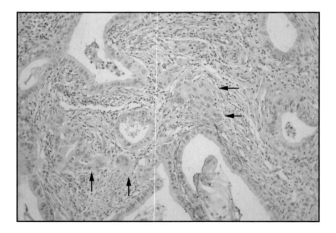

FIGURE 3.16 Invasive endocervical adenocarcinoma. Nests of malignant glandular cells (arrows) are present in the reactive endocervical stroma (hematoxylin and eosin, medium-power magnification).

neoplasms characterized by thin villous outgrowths (Figure 3.17).[14]

It is unclear whether superficially invasive endocervical adenocarcinomas have the same prognostic significance as microinvasive squamous cell carcinomas. Regardless, the pathologist can provide useful information in excisional specimens by estimating the size of the invasive carcinoma (reporting tumor depth measured from the surface and width using an ocular micrometer), its location in relation to the TZ, and whether AIS or invasive adenocarcinoma involves a resection margin. This information should always be qualified by the fact that these lesions can be multifocal. Lymphatic and vascular space involvement by adenocarcinoma should also be reported.

Although most adenocarcinomas of the cervix arise from the endocervical glands, extension to the cervix from endometrial adenocarcinomas, or metastases to the cervix from extrauterine sites, such as the fallopian tubes or ovaries, can occur. These can also be identified by cervical biopsy or endocervical curettage.

In addition to squamous cell carcinomas and adenocarcinomas, there are other less common malignancies that can occur in the cervix. These include adenosquamous carcinomas, small cell carcinomas, sarcomas and lymphomas.

3.4 Cytology of Cervicovaginal Abnormalities

The ability to identify atypical cells that represent squamous cell carcinoma in patients with abnormal vaginal bleeding was first reported separately by Babes and Papanicolaou in 1928.[19,20] The concept was revisited in a monograph by Papanicolaou and Traut in 1942.[21] The introduction of a sampling device by Ayre led to the possibility of sampling asymptomatic women in the hopes of identifying small cancers or preinvasive lesions. Regional population-based trials such as those conducted in central Kentucky confirmed the value of examining cervicovaginal cells as a screening test.[22] Eventually the Papanicolaou (Pap) smear or Pap test became widely accepted in this country as the prototypical technique for the early detection of cervical dysplasia and cancer.

The Pap test is based on a relatively simple principle. Cells from squamous epithelium exfoliate over time. Thus, the cells removed for cytologic examination represent epithelial cells, normal or abnormal, found at the surface. Large numbers of cells with abundant cytoplasm and small nuclei would be compatible with superficial cells found in an area of glycogenated mature squamous epithelium. Smaller cells with slightly enlarged nuclei would suggest sampling over an area of squamous metaplasia, or removal of exfoliated cells from an estrogen-deprived cervix where the epithelial surface consists of parabasal cells. In the case of CIN 1, the exfoliated cells mostly consist of koilocytic cells. Increasing degrees of intraepithelial neoplasia result in exfoliation of rising numbers of immature dysplastic cells. When squamous cell carcinoma occurs, rapid tumor growth results in exfoliation of abnormally shaped malignant cells (Figure 3.18). Endocervical cells tend to be more cohesive and are usually removed in clumps from the endocervical canal.

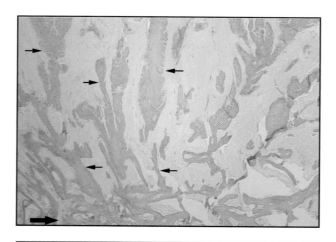

FIGURE 3.17 Villoglandular adenocarcinoma. Eosinophilic mucin separates thin villous-like extensions (small arrows) that arise from the superficial endocervix (large arrow) (hematoxylin and eosin, low-power magnification).

3.4.1 The Bethesda System

Since the initial detailed descriptions of methods to examine exfoliated cervicovaginal cells, attempts have been made to simplify the reporting of various cellular abnormalities. Papanicolaou introduced the earliest classification system by condensing different cell descriptors into five categories or classes. Class I represented nonatypical or normal cells; Class 2 included atypical cells that were not suspicious for malignancy; Class 3 included atypical cells that were suspicious for malignancy (dyskaryosis); Class 4 contained cells that suggested malignancy (CIS); and Class 5 represented cells that were diagnostic for malignancy. Over time, the Papanicolaou Class 3 evolved into the concept of dysplasia, or abnormal cell proliferation. Cervical dysplasia eventually included a spectrum of changes that began as mild cytologic changes in the early stages and subsequently evolved into the cells seen in the Papanicolaou Class 4, or

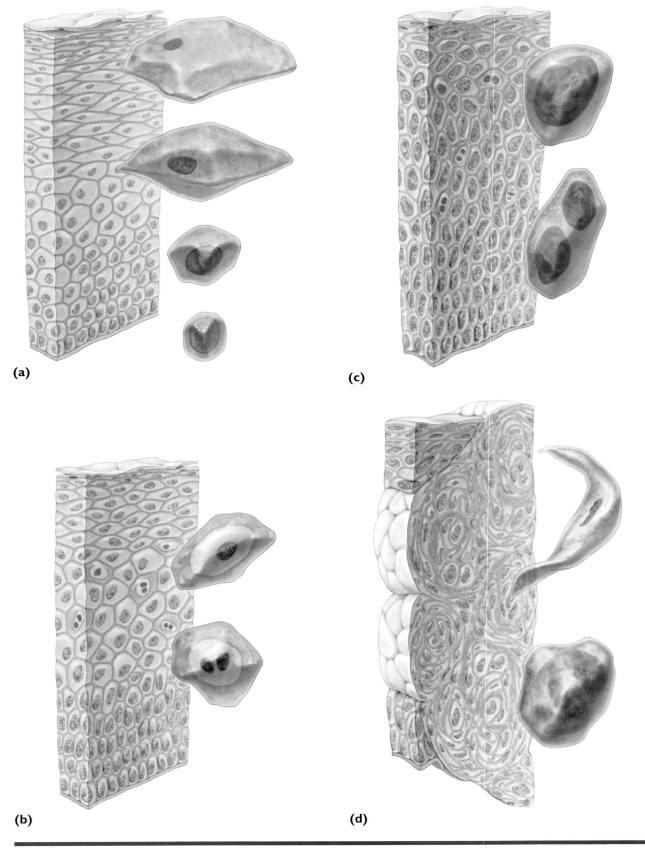

FIGURES 3.18a–d The cytology of individual normal and abnormal squamous cells and their histologic counterparts. **(a)** Normal squamous epithelium and corresponding superficial, intermediate, parabasal, and basal cells. **(b)** Low-grade squamous dysplasia and corresponding low-grade squamous intraepithelial cells. **(c)** High-grade squamous dysplasia and corresponding high-grade squamous intraepithelial cells. **(d)** Squamous cell carcinoma and corresponding malignant squamous cells.

CIS.[8] Over time, the Papanicolaou Class 3 was divided into mild, moderate and severe dysplasia. Later, the CIN classification system grouped the four separate categories of dysplasia and CIS into three grades.[8]

The discovery that HPV was associated with lower genital lesions directed investigators to reevaluate many lesions originally considered early dysplasias and reclassify them as pure viral infections, or koilocytotic or condylomatous atypias.[11] Table 3.1 compares the different classification systems used from 1950 until 1988 (for further information on the evolution of cervical cytology terminology, see Chapter 1).

The subsequent association of HPV with high-grade CIN and cervix cancers created confusion about how HPV related to various cervicovaginal abnormalities and how they should be classified.[23,24] As a result, individual laboratories used their own unique classification systems, which were not reproducible. As the problem of multiple diagnostic terms in cervicovaginal cytology became pervasive, a workshop was convened in 1988 on the campus of the National Institutes of Health in Bethesda, Maryland, to standardize the reporting system for Pap tests. The result of this meeting and subsequent ones in 1991 and 2001 became known as the Bethesda System for reporting cervicovaginal cytologic abnormalities.[25,27] In its present form, a Pap test is interpreted as either negative for intraepithelial lesions or malignancy or as demonstrating an epithelial cell abnormality. This latter category is subdivided into atypical squamous and glandular cells, low- and high-grade squamous intraepithelial lesions (SIL), endocervical AIS, and squamous and glandular malignancies. Additionally, the Bethesda System requires comments on the specimen quality, using terms such as *satisfactory*, and *unsatisfactory* to indicate the interpretability of a submitted slide. Table 3.2 summarizes the Bethesda System currently in use.[28]

3.4.1.1 Quality of the specimen

Specimen quality can affect the sensitivity of a cytologic specimen to identify cervicovaginal abnormalities.[29] The Bethesda System originally introduced three descriptors for the quality of the Pap test: *Satisfactory for Examination*, *Less than Optimal*, and *Unsatisfactory for Examination*.[25] Over time, *Satisfactory for Examination but Limited* replaced the term *Less than Optimal*.[26] Although the latter term was considered more clinically useful than *Less than Optimal*, confusion persisted among providers that a satisfactory Pap test would still be limited in some way and, therefore, not be completely acceptable. This confusion led to the most recent revision of the Bethesda System terminology: elimination of this intermediate category altogether. Even if the specimen is satisfactory for examination, however, the reviewer should note whether a cellular component representing the transformation zone (at least 10 metaplastic or 10 endocervical cells) is present. In addition, partially obscuring blood or inflammation, poor preservation of the cellular material, or lack of relevant clinical information can be noted as *Quality Indicators*.[28]

Reasons to label a specimen *Unsatisfactory for Examination* include the receipt of a broken slide, a slide with no patient identification (designated as *Rejected for Examination*), complete obscuration by blood or inflammation, or less than the minimally acceptable amount of cellular material on the slide. In the past, the amount of evaluable material on a slide was measured in percentages, with 10% being the minimum acceptable cellular amount, provided that

---

Table 3.1   Comparison of the Different Cytologic Classification Systems for Cervicovaginal Abnormalities Prior to 1988

Papanicolaou	Dysplasia	Cervical Intraepithelial Neoplasia	Papillomavirus
Class 1		Normal	
Class 2		Atypical	
Class 3	Mild dysplasia	CIN 1	Koilocytotic atypia
			CIN 1
	Moderate dysplasia	CIN 2	
	Severe dysplasia	CIN 3	
Class 4	Carcinoma in situ		
Class 5		Malignancy	

Table 3.2 The Bethesda System Classification for Cervicovaginal Abnormalities (2001)

Specimen Type

I. Conventional
II. Liquid-based thin-layer preparation
III. Other

Specimen Adequacy

I. Satisfactory for evaluation (describe presence or absence of endocervical/transformation zone component and any other quality limiting factors)
II. Unsatisfactory for evaluation (specify reason)
III. Specimen rejected (specify reason)
IV. Specimen processed and examined, but unsatisfactory for evaluation of epithelial abnormality (specify reason)

General Categorization (Optional)

I. Negative for intraepithelial lesion or malignancy
II. Other: see interpretation/diagnosis (e.g., endometrial cells in a woman 40 years of age or older)
III. Epithelial cell abnormality: see interpretation/diagnosis (specify "squamous" or "glandular," as appropriate)

Automated Review

If case is examined by automated device, specify device and result.

Ancillary Testing

Provide a brief description of the test methods and report the result so that the clinician easily understands it.

Descriptive Interpretations/Results

I. Negative for intraepithelial lesion or malignancy (when there is no cellular evidence of neoplasia, state this in the General Categorization above and/or in the Interpretation/Diagnosis section of the report, whether or not there are organisms or other non-neoplastic findings)
II. Organisms:
   A. *Trichomonas vaginalis*
   B. Fungal organisms morphologically consistent with *Candida spp*
   C. Shift in vaginal flora suggestive of bacterial vaginosis
   D. Bacteria morphologically consistent with *Actinomyces spp.*
   E. Cellular changes associated with herpes simplex virus
III. Other Non-Neoplastic Findings (optional to report; list not inclusive)
   A. Reactive cellular changes associated with
      1. Inflammation (including typical repair)
      2. Radiation
      3. Intrauterine contraceptive device (IUD)
   B. Benign-appearing glandular cells status post-hysterectomy
   C. Atrophy
IV. Other
   Endometrial cells (in a woman 40 years of age or older, specify if "negative for squamous intraepithelial lesion")

50% to 75% of cells were well preserved.[27] Since the introduction of specimens prepared using a liquid-based system, it has been recommended that an absolute number of cells be used as a minimally acceptable amount. For conventional specimens, the acceptable number is considered to be 10,000–12,000 well-preserved cells; for liquid-based monolayer specimens, the minimal number is 5000 cells.[28]

If abnormalities are identified on a specimen that would otherwise be considered unsatisfactory,

Table 3.2 Continued.

Descriptive Interpretations/Results

V. Epithelial Cell Abnormalities
    A. Squamous Cell
        1. Atypical squamous cells
            a. Of undetermined significance (ASC-US)
            b. Cannot exclude a high-grade squamous intraepithelial lesion (ASC-H)
        2. Low-grade squamous intraepithelial lesion (LSIL)
            Encompassing human papillomavirus cytopathic effect/mild dysplasia/cervical intraepithelial neoplasia (CIN) 1
        3. High-grade squamous intraepithelial lesion (HSIL)
            a. Encompassing: moderate and severe dysplasia, CIN 2, CIN 3 and carcinoma in situ (CIS)
            b. With features suspicious for invasion (if invasion is suspected)
        4. Squamous cell carcinoma
    B. Glandular Cell
        1. Atypical
            a. Endocervical cells (not otherwise specified)
            b. Endometrial cells (not otherwise specified)
            c. Glandular cells (not otherwise specified)
        2. Atypical
            a. Endocervical cells, favor neoplastic
            b. Glandular cells, favor neoplasitc
        3. Endocervical adenocarcinoma in situ (AIS)
        4. Adenocarcinoma
            a. Endocervical
            b. Endometrial
            c. Extrauterine
            d. Not otherwise specified
    C. Other Malignant Neoplasms (specify)

Educational Notes and Recommendations (Optional)

Suggestions should be concise and consistent with clinical follow-up guidelines published by professional organizations (references to relevant publications may be included).

---

the Bethesda System stipulates that they be reported rather than ignored even though the specimen is otherwise compromised.[26]

3.4.1.2 Negative for squamous intraepithelial lesions or malignancy

In the past, the descriptor *Benign Cellular Change* was used to describe epithelial cell alterations that reflect changes in the cervicovaginal environment from hormonal variations, shifts in pH, inflammation, overgrowth of vaginal flora, and exposure to external factors such as radiation and foreign material.[26] Although irritative in nature, these changes are not thought to be premalignant and, therefore, are considered *benign*. Nondysplastic epithelial cells that did not show these minimal variations were considered *Within Normal Limits*. *Benign Cellular Change* represented a compromise for pathologists who desired a category that encompassed cellular changes outside the realm of normal yet did not represent premalignant potential. However, clinicians have found the category confusing because the cells in question are qualified as not being normal. As a result, the most recent Bethesda System Workshop has recommended combining the general categories *Within Normal Limits* and *Benign Cell Change* into one general negative statement: *Negative for Intraepithelial Lesion or Malignancy*. This statement can then be qualified by descriptors indicating the presence of various organisms or nonspecific reactive or reparative changes. The category of reactive and reparative cellular changes is used to identify slides that require review and interpretation by a pathologist.[28,30]

3.4.1.3 Organisms

The cervicovaginal surface is polymicrobial and contains a large number of obligate and facultative organisms. Normally, the *Lactobacillus acidophilus* (Döderlein's bacillus) is present in large numbers and helps maintain an acidic pH (3.5 to 4.5). Organisms seen in fewer numbers include *Streptococcus viridans, Staphylococcus epidermatitis, Bacteroides faecalis, Gardnerella (Hemophilus) vaginalis,* and *Candida albicans.* These organisms vary depending on the hormonal milieu and pH of the vagina. Foreign material, such as tampons and intrauterine contraceptive device (IUD) strings, also can affect the number and type of organisms present. If there is an overgrowth of certain organisms normally found in the vagina, or if other pathogenic organisms are introduced by sexual activity, symptoms of a vaginal infection (discharge, odor, pruritis) may develop. In many cases, the causative organism or cellular changes indicative of a specific infection can be identified cytologically.[27,31]

Monilia or yeast infections are characterized by vaginal pruritis and a clumpy "cottage cheese" discharge. The etiologic agents are *Candida albicans* and, to a lesser extent, *Candida glabrata.* Other species can infect the vulvovaginal area, but they are seen less frequently. The presence of these organisms is usually confirmed by examination of potassium hydroxide-treated wet mounts of the discharge or by culture. In a Papanicolaou-stained specimen, *Candida albicans* appears as pseudohyphae with buds. Epithelial cells cluster around the yeast forms in a rouleau formation. *Candida glabrata* are usually present in budding forms only. The presence of yeast forms on Pap tests correlates highly with wet mount preparations in patients with symptomatic monilia infections (Figure 3.19).[31]

Bacterial vaginosis is characterized by a malodorous gray adherent discharge; vaginal itching is variable. An increase in the vaginal pH leads to an overgrowth of the initiating organism, which is usually *Gardnerella vaginalis* (a gram-negative coccobacillus), and associated anaerobic vaginal flora. On wet mounts and cytologic specimens, the characteristic feature is the *clue cell* or bacteria-covered squamous epithelial cell. For positive diagnosis, the bacteria must completely cover the cell and extend beyond the cell border, which gives the cell a moth-eaten appearance. In addition, the background is filmy or granular. If strict criteria are used to identify clue cells, bacterial vaginosis can be confirmed in 90% of patients with symptoms (Figure 3.20).[31,32]

Trichomonas vaginitis is characterized by vaginal itching and a greenish frothy discharge. Of the four Trichomonas species (*T. tenax, T homonis,* *T. fecalis, T. vaginalis*), *Trichomonas vaginalis* is most commonly associated with vaginal infections. The organism is sexually transmitted with an incubation time of 4 to 28 days. Factors that encourage proliferation of the trichomonads include endocervical mucus and associated vaginal flora. Clinical diagnosis consists of identifying the characteristic discharge and occasional ecchymoses (small hemorrhages) on the cervix surface ("strawberry cervix") along with motile organisms on wet-mount examination. On Pap tests, the organisms appear as pale

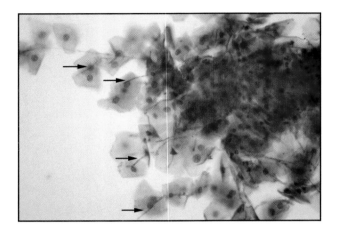

FIGURE 3.19 Candida. Branching hyphae (arrows) are seen in a cluster of superficial and intermediate cells (liquid preparation, Papanicolaou stain, high-power magnification).

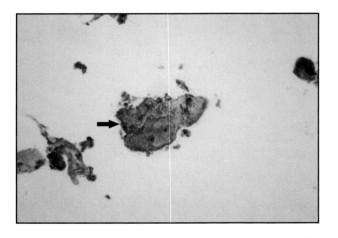

FIGURE 3.20 Bacterial vaginosis. A cluster of squamous cells (arrow) is covered by bacterial organisms (clue cells), giving the cytoplasm a "moth-eaten" appearance (liquid preparation, Papanicolaou stain, high-power magnification).

amphophilic oval unicellular structures 100 μm in size. The nucleus is elongated and acentric and the cytoplasm contains red granules in well-preserved specimens. The trichomonads tend to cluster around the edges of epithelial cells. Additionally, a cluster of leukocytes ("BB shot clusters") and a granular background are present. There is a high correlation among wet-mount preparations and vaginal cultures with trichomonads if strict criteria are used to identify Trichomonas vaginalis on cytologic specimens (Figure 3.21).[27,31,33]

Although often considered a fungus, the different actinomyces organisms (*A. israelii, A. bovis, and A. naeslundii*) actually represent higher-order bacteria that also include the *Mycobacteriaceae* and *Streptomycetaceae*. Actinomyces infections are usually associated with foreign objects. Ten percent of women with IUDs develop the infection, and the organism may persist for 12 months after its removal. Clinically, actinomyces infections are characterized by small yellow granules (sulfur granules). On cytologic specimens, small basophilic cotton ball clusters are identified on low-power examination; high-power inspection demonstrates acute angle branching of thin filamentous organisms (Figure 3.22).[31]

In the cervix, herpes virus infects the immature squamous, metaplastic, or columnar cells. Once infected, the epithelial cells enlarge and fuse as a result of alterations in the cell membranes. The nuclei also enlarge and the nuclear membranes are accentuated because of margination of the nuclear chromatin. The nuclei cluster and the nuclear membranes compress each other. The chromatin-

parachromatin interphase is lost and the chromatin material disperses. Pap tests from patients with herpetic infections will demonstrate multinucleated giant cells with nuclear molding, prominent nuclear membranes, and a homogenous "ground-glass" nucleoplasm (Figure 3.23).[27,31]

3.4.1.4 Reactive or reparative changes

In the past, nonspecific cellular alterations were classified as *cytologic atypias*. Atypia is a descriptive pathologic term that means "not in the range of normal."

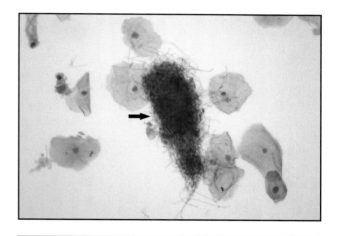

FIGURE 3.22   Actinomyces. A central mass of thin filamentous strands (arrow) is present (liquid preparation, Papanicolaou stain, high-power magnification). ▬▬

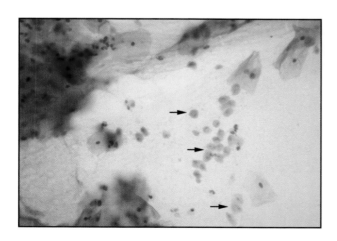

FIGURE 3.21   Trichomonas. The small protozoa (arrows) are characterized by a cyanophilic cytoplasm and eccentric round to oval nuclei (conventional preparation, Papanicolaou stain, high-power magnification). ▬▬

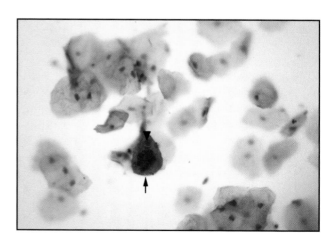

FIGURE 3.23   Herpes simplex virus. A single teardrop-shaped squamous cell (small arrow) contains multiple nuclei with prominent central (Cowdry A) bodies (arrowhead). Nuclear molding is also present (liquid preparation, Papanicolaou stain, high-power magnification). ▬▬

Cellular atypia could represent a number of conditions, including benign factors (inflammatory atypia, reactive atypia). However, clinicians in the past have equated atypia with premalignant changes. The confusion over different implications of the word atypia led to the introduction of the descriptive diagnosis *reactive or reparative change* as a substitute for atypical changes from benign processes.

Cytologically, reactive change caused by inflammation can occur in squamous or glandular cells and is usually represented by nuclear enlargement. In squamous cells, the enlargement is minimal—usually about 1.5 to 2 times the size of a normal intermediate cell nucleus. Glandular nuclei can show significant enlargement, along with multinucleation. The nuclei are hyperchromatic but lack coarseness. Mild cytoplasmic vacuolization is present, but there is no peripheral cytoplasmic accentuation (Figure 3.24). Hyperkeratosis and parakeratosis represent abnormal keratin production by mature and immature squamous epithelial cells. Cytologically, hyperkeratosis is characterized by the presence of mature orangophillic or polychromatic squamous cells that lack nuclei ("ghost cells"). Parakeratotic cells are small orangeophillic cells with dark pyknotic nuclei. Reparative changes represent a healing process seen after severe or erosive inflammation and correspond histologically to early metaplasia. The cells are arranged in sheets with recognizable cell borders. The nuclei are enlarged and hyperchromatic with slightly coarse chromatin. Nucleoli are recognizable (Figure 3.25).[31]

Postmenopausal women not using hormone therapy can demonstrate reactive changes related to atrophy, which is characterized by sheets of parabasal cells with mild nuclear enlargement in an inflammatory background. Because of drying artifact in a significant number of these specimens, the nuclei can be moderately enlarged and have smudged chromatin. Naked nuclei, which consist of basophilic amorphous material ("blue blobs"), represent degenerated parabasal cells. These changes can resolve with the application of a short course of topical estrogen.[34] Pap test results for patients who have undergone radiation treatment to the cervix and vagina

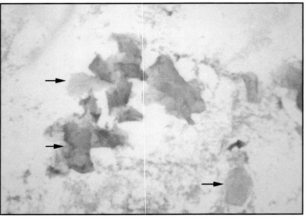

(a)

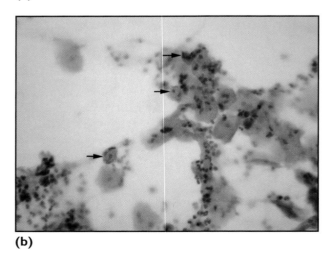

(b)

FIGURES 3.25a,b   **(a)** Hyperkeratosis. A group of orangeophilic squamous cells (arrows) that lack nuclear material is present (conventional preparation, Papanicolaou stain, high-power magnification). **(b)** Parakeratosis. Individual small orangeophilic cells (arrows) with pyknotic ("dot-like") nuclei are present (conventional preparation, Papanicolaou stain, high-power magnification). ∎

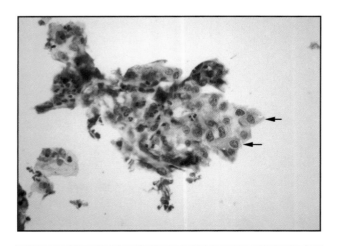

FIGURE 3.24   Reactive squamous cells. A cohesive sheet of metaplastic-type cells (arrows) demonstrates nuclei that are mildly enlarged with peripheral chromatin clumping and prominent nucleoli (liquid preparation, Papanicolaou stain, high-power magnification). ∎

will show increased cell size, multinucleation, and bizarre cell shapes. The cytoplasm is vacuolated and polychromatic. The nuclei demonstrate chromatin smudging and prominent single or multiple nucleoli (Figure 3.26).[27]

In addition to actinomycosis, specimens from women with IUDs will show metaplastic cell clusters with high nuclear-to-cytoplasmic ratios and prominent nucleoli. The cells will have large cytoplasmic vacuoles that displace the nucleus. Psammomatous-type calcifications are occasionally seen. IUDs can also generate small endometrial-like cells known as IUD cells.[31]

3.4.1.5 Cytologic evidence of vaginal glandular cells or normal endometrial cells

In the past, endocervical-type cells seen on vaginal specimen were considered a cytologic form of adenosis and were classified as a glandular cell abnormality. Since it is now known that women with normal endocervical cells on a vaginal specimen do not necessarily have underlying vaginal dysplasias or malignancies, this finding is no longer considered atypical. It is important for the provider, however, to record the precise source of the specimen so that glandular cells from the endocervix are not interpreted as vaginal cells.[5]

Normal endometrial cells are characterized cytologically as small cell clusters with diminutive round nuclei and minimally apparent nucleoli (Figure 3.27).[27] Traditionally, the presence of endometrial cells on a cytologic specimen was considered abnormal if these cells were present in the luteal phase of a reproductive age woman, or in a postmenopausal woman. It was thought that the presence of these cells indicated abnormal proliferation of the endometrium and could represent endometrial atypias or malignancies. However, the ability of the Cytobrush®, with its narrow tip, to easily remove endometrial cells from the lower uterine segment, along with the presence of endometrial cells in postmenopausal women using HRT, made the presence of these cells unreliable in predicting uterine abnormalities. While most women with normal endometrial cells found on a Pap test will have no underlying abnormalities,[35] a number of published studies have indicated that a small number of women age 40 or older with these cells may have underlying endometrial hyperplasias and carcinomas.[36–38] The present Bethesda System revision, therefore, has recommended the reporting of normal endometrial cells in a woman age 40 years or older, regardless of whether she is cycling normally or using hormonal therapy.[28]

3.4.1.6 Atypical squamous cells

Cytopathologists have long understood that there is a category of squamous epithelial cells that exhibit nuclear and cytoplasmic variations that, while not normal, do not clearly represent morphology consistent with either benign cell changes or dysplasia. In other words, the behavior of these groups of cells

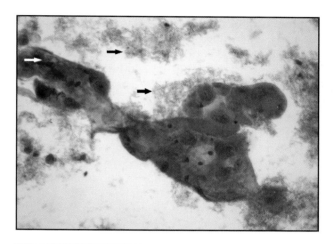

FIGURE 3.26 Radiation change. A central cluster of large cells with enlarged round nuclei containing prominent nucleoli is seen. Cytoplasmic vacuoles are present (white arrow). The background contains numerous lysed red blood cells (dark arrows) (liquid preparation, Papanicolaou stain, high-power magnification). ▬

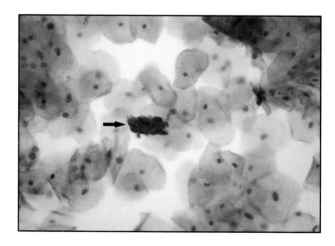

FIGURE 3.27 Endometrial cells. A small cluster of round cells (arrow) with sparse cytoplasm and round- to oval- basophilic nuclei is present (liquid preparation, Papanicolaou stain, high-power magnification). ▬

cannot be determined by the usual assessment of cytologic features. Because of this, category *Atypical Squamous Cells (ASC)* was created.[26] Categories of this type have existed in other areas of gynecologic pathology. Epithelial ovarian borderline tumors, vulvar aggressive angiomyxomas, and uterine smooth muscle tumors of uncertain malignant potential are neoplasms with similar atypical features. Although they are considered abnormal, their histologies are not sufficient to warrant a malignant diagnosis. The cervicovaginal cells in this group were originally named *Atypical Squamous Cells of Undetermined Significance;* qualifiers such as "favor reactive" and "favor neoplastic" were used to suggest potential behavior.[26,27,39] Presently, there are two categories of ASC: *Atypical Squamous Cells of Undetermined Significance (ASC-US)* and *Atypical Cells, Cannot Exclude a High-Grade Squamous Intraepithelial Lesion (ASC-H).*[28]

As defined by the Bethesda System, cells categorized as ASC-US have nuclear enlargement that is 2.5 to 3 times the normal intermediate cell nucleus. There is mild variation in nuclear size and shape and mild to moderate hyperchromasia of the nucleoplasm, but the chromatin is evenly distributed. The cytoplasm can show evidence of mild clearing, but the peripheral halo borders are poorly defined (Figure 3.28). In atrophy, the nuclei can show significant enlargement, irregular shapes, and hyperchromasia; however, these features usually resolve with topical estrogen treatment. ASC-US also encompasses atypical or pleomorphic parakeratosis, which consists of irregularly shaped orangophillic cells with enlarged darkly stained nuclei.[27] Unfortunately, in spite of established morphologic changes, the diagnosis of ASC-US is poorly reproducible, as different pathologists use uniquely personal criteria to signify this diagnosis.[2]

Recently, cytopathologists have recognized that ASC characterized by small immature metaplastic cells with dark irregular nuclei, often called *atypical immature metaplasia* or *atypical cells-suspicious for a high-grade squamous intraepithelial lesion,* may indicate a greater potential for finding significant underlying cervical and vaginal abnormalities.[40,41] Analysis of a completed National Cancer Institute-sponsored prospective trial has shown that women whose cytologic specimens contain these cells have a higher percentage of high-grade CIN on colposcopically directed biopsy and a higher prevalence of oncogenic HPV DNA than do women with cells consistent with ASC-US.[42] Consequently, the qualifier ASC-H was introduced in the present Bethesda System Classification (Figure 3.29).[28]

3.4.1.7 Low-grade squamous intraepithelial lesions

The finding of dysplastic cells on a Pap test indicates the presence of these cells on the surface of the cervix or vagina. For any degree of dysplasia, the hallmark

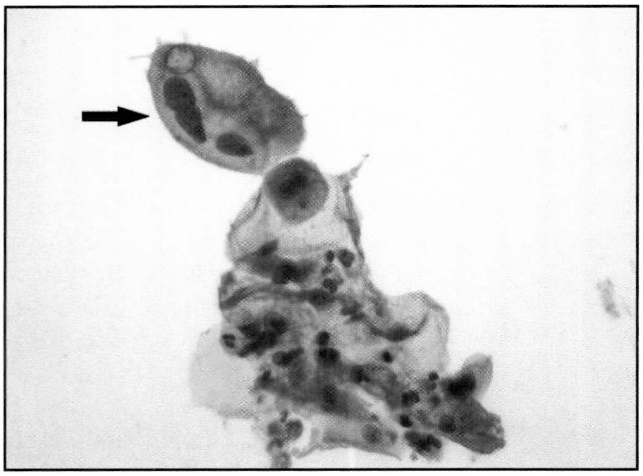

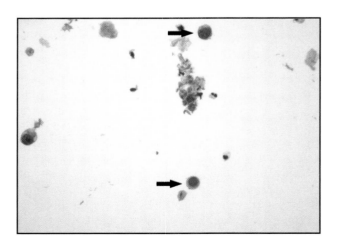

FIGURE 3.28 Atypical squamous cells of undetermined significance. A multinucleate cell (arrow) was found in this Pap specimen. The nuclei are mildly enlarged and irregularly shaped. However, the nuclear membranes are smooth and the chromatin is uniform (liquid preparation, Papanicolaou stain, high-power magnification). ■

FIGURE 3.29 Atypical squamous cells, cannot exclude a high-grade squamous intraepithelial lesion. Two immature squamous cells (arrows) with decreased cytoplasm and hyperchromatic nuclei with mild nuclear enlargement are present. The membranes are otherwise smooth to slightly irregular (liquid preparation, Papanicolaou stain, high-power magnification). ■

cytologic feature is abnormal nuclear transformation. The nucleus enlarges, there is wrinkling of the nuclear membrane, and the chromatin becomes more distinct (coarse). If mild air-drying is present, the nuclear chromatin will appear hyperchromatic and smudged. As with histologic evidence of dysplasia, the degree or grade of dysplasia is dependent cytologically on the size the dysplastic cell and, to a lesser extent, the number of dysplastic cells. The latter will be related to cell sampling, which reflects the skill of the examiner, the size of the abnormality, and type of processing. The interval between serial Pap tests may also affect cell yield. Low-grade dysplasias are characterized by the transformation of mature (superficial or intermediate) epithelial cells, whereas high-grade dysplasias are characterized by transformation of immature (metaplastic or parabasal/basal) cells.

The term *low-grade squamous intraepithelial lesions* (LSIL) encompasses the categories of mild dysplasia, CIN 1, and various descriptors indicating the presence of HPV, such as condylomatous dysplasia or koilocytotic atypia. The category LSIL reflects evidence that women whose Pap tests contain these diverse descriptors demonstrate the same decreased progression rates when compared to Pap tests with significant abnormalities (high-grade CIN or carcinoma), and that pathologists cannot easily differentiate mild dysplasias from supposedly pure HPV infections.

In LSIL, the nuclear size is at least three times that of a normal intermediate cell or polymorphonucleocyte nucleus. The nuclear appearance is "raisinoid," with irregular nuclear shapes and membrane wrinkling. The nucleoplasm demonstrates hyperchromasia and smudging. Multinucleation along with variation of nuclear size is also present. Nucleoli are absent. LSIL is confined to intermediate or superficial-type cells; although enlarged, the nucleus occupies only one third the total cell area. Many of these cells will have perinuclear clearing and aggregation of the cytoplasm into the cell periphery, consistent with koilocytosis. As with koilocytes seen in biopsy specimens, the border between the clear space and the cytoplasm is distinct (Figure 3.30).[5,27]

3.4.1.8 High-grade squamous intraepithelial lesions

The term *high-grade squamous intraepithelial lesions (HSIL)* encompasses the categories of moderate and severe dysplasia, CIN 2 and 3, and CIS. The primary reason given to combine these categories is the impression that, while the degree of dysplasia may

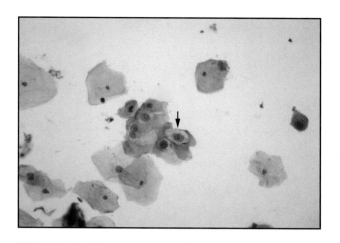

FIGURE 3.30 Low-grade squamous intraepithelial lesion. The nuclei in these dysplastic cells are moderately enlarged compared to the nuclei of the adjacent normal squamous cells. In addition, there is perinuclear clearing and accentuation of the peripheral cytoplasm (koilocytosis-arrow). The cell size is equivalent to a mature squamous cell (liquid preparation, Papanicolaou stain, high-power magnification).

appear slightly different histologically for each group, their behavior is similar.[43] Because this concept is not universally accepted, the histologic grading of high-grade dysplasia remains separated into three major tiers,[9] and, in the past, cytologists have been given the option to qualify a diagnosis of HSIL as a moderate dysplasia (CIN 2), severe dysplasia (CIN 3), or CIS.[25,27]

Cytologic specimens from patients with CIN 2 consist of cells with nuclear features similar to those in LSIL. The cell size, however, is the equivalent to that of an immature metaplastic cell. The nucleus can occupy up to half the total cell area. Because of this decrease in cytoplasmic amount, the nuclear-to-cytoplasmic ratio (N/C ratio) is increased. The cells are arranged singly, in sheets, or in syncytial-like aggregates (Figure 3.31). Specimens from patients having CIN 3 contain cells that are similar to parabasal or reserve cell in size. Although the nuclei have dysplastic features similar to those of LSIL, the nuclear size is smaller. Because of the smaller cell size and the relatively large nuclear area in relation to the amount of cell cytoplasm, the N/C ratio is markedly increased. The cells are either isolated or have a characteristic linear arrangement. Cells with negligible cytoplasm ("stripped nuclei") or large syncytial aggregates containing mostly nuclei ("microtissue fragments") are cytologically consistent with CIS (Figure 3.32).[5,27]

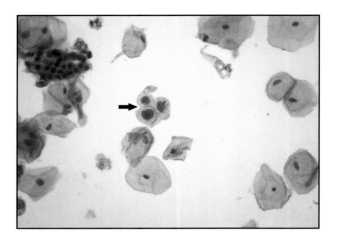

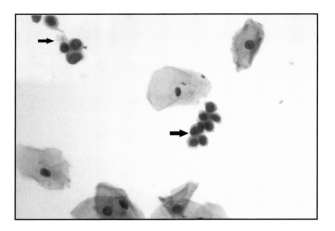

FIGURE 3.31 High-grade squamous intraepithelial lesion (moderate dysplasia). The centrally located dysplastic cells (arrow) have enlarged, abnormally shaped hyperchromatic nuclei with irregular nuclear borders. The cell size is equivalent to a metaplastic cell. A cluster of endocervical cells is in the upper left portion of the photomicrograph (liquid preparation, Papanicolaou stain, high-power magnification).

FIGURE 3.32 High-grade squamous intraepithelial lesion (severe dysplasia or carcinoma in situ). Two clusters of dysplastic cells from different areas are present (arrows). The small basaloid cells have minimal cytoplasm, and the irregularly shaped hyperchromatic nuclei are enlarged relative to the overall cell size. The nuclear to cytoplasmic ratio, therefore, is markedly increased (liquid preparation, Papanicolaou stain, high-power magnification).

3.4.1.9 Invasive squamous cell carcinoma

Invasive squamous cell carcinoma indicates disruption of the basement membrane and invasion into the underlying stroma. For this to occur, the squamous cells proliferate rapidly and may outgrow their blood supply. This may lead to necrosis or a tumor diathesis. The background of a specimen with invasive carcinoma is often described as "dirty." There is marked inflammation, hemorrhage, and fragments of degenerated cytoplasmic and nuclear material. The diathesis in a liquid-based specimen is subtler; and the degenerated elements are more condensed. Their appearance is described as having a "cotton candy" consistency (Figure 3.33). Squamous cell carcinomas that invade between 3 mm and 5 mm can also demonstrate cytologic evidence of a tumor diathesis.[44]

The individual malignant cells reflect the capability to invade adjacent stromal tissues or to metastasize. This is particularly true in microinvasive squamous cell carcinoma, which is often localized in a background of CIN. Specifically, the cells are arranged in syncytial aggregates similar to that in CIS. In contrast to CIS, however, nucleoli are present; macronucleoli can also be seen but are infrequent.[5]

In invasive squamous cell carcinoma, the cells have abnormal forms. The shape is dependent on the surface tension, the viscosity of the cytoplasm, and the rigidity of the cell membrane, and abnormal shapes are more common in the keratinizing squamous cell carcinomas. Non-keratinizing squamous cell carcinomas have cells that are arranged in syncytial masses with indistinct borders; nucleoli are usually present. The nuclear area is twice that of a normal cell. Keratinizing squamous cell carcinomas will have orangeophilic cytoplasm. The nuclei are dark and contain dense chromatin; nucleoli are not seen. Cytologic examination may not be helpful in the identification of very well differentiated squamous carcinomas, such as those with verrucous histology. Poorly differentiated squamous cell carcinomas will have small round cells that consist almost entirely of nuclei with dense coarse granular chromatin.[5]

3.4.1.10 Atypical glandular cells/ adenocarcinoma in situ

The category of atypical glandular cells (AGC) represents cytologic changes not recognized prior to the introduction of the Bethesda System. As with ASC, AGC represents glandular cells with morphologic variations that cannot easily be classified as benign, premalignant, or malignant.[25–28] Under

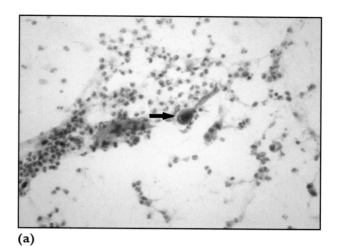

(a)

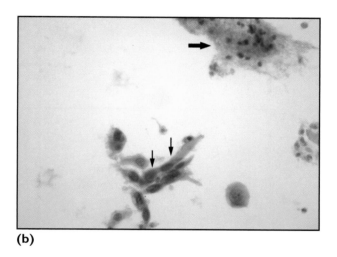

(b)

FIGURES 3.33a,b   Squamous cell carcinoma. **(a)** A tadpole-shaped (caudate) cell is present in the center of the field (arrow) (conventional preparation, Papanicolaou stain, high-power magnificaiton). **(b)** A cluster of elongated cells (small arrows) that have enlarged nuclei with distinct nucleoli are present. Focal orangeophilic staining indicates abnormal keratin production. There is also patchy ("cotton-candy") necrosis in the upper right of the photomicrograph (large arrow) (liquid preparation, Papanicolaou stain, high-power magnification).

the present Bethesda system revision, any atypical glandular cells should be categorized as either endocervical or endometrial in origin, if possible.[28] Also, it should be noted if a glandular dysplastic process is favored. As with ASC, the reproducibility of this diagnosis is also poor.[45] Sensitive and specific biomarkers may have future discriminatory use similar to that of squamous atypias and intraepithelial neoplasias.[46]

In conventional specimens, atypical endocervical cells tend to shed in sheets or clusters. However, the cell borders and consistent spacing normally seen between benign glandular cells are lost. The nuclei are enlarged and demonstrate mild variation in size and shape. The chromatin is increased in density, nucleoli are usually not seen, and mitoses may be noted. The overall nuclear-to-cytoplasmic ratio is increased because of nuclear enlargement; however, a reactive endocervical cell can also show a marked increase in nuclear size.[48] Other differential interpretations include degenerative changes in immature metaplastic cells caused by infections such as trichomoniasis, lower uterine segment endometrial cells that are commonly obtained post conization, cervical endometriosis, and reactive change due to vigorous rotation of the cytobrush®. In the past, the cytologic diagnosis of AIS had been included in the broad category of AGC. Recently, however, specific cytologic features (nuclear rosettes that "feather" or palisade peripherally) that are unique to AIS have been described. This interpretation can now be reported separately from AGC (Figure 3.34).[28]

AGC of endometrial origin are seen in small clusters usually containing five to ten cells. The nuclei are slightly enlarged and the nuclear-to-cytoplasmic ratios are increased. Nucleoli are usually present (Figure 3.35).[27]

3.4.1.11 Invasive adenocarcinoma

Invasive adenocarcinoma can be cytologically similar to AIS, but in the former, nucleoli are readily evident and the nuclear chromatin is irregular in consistency (Figure 3.36). There also may be considerable variation in nuclear size, and a tumor diathesis may be present. Specialized endocervical adenocarcinomas, such as clear cell and serous change, may appear as poorly differentiated carcinomas. Minimum deviation adenocarcinoma, or adenoma malignum, is a well-differentiated adenocarcinoma with malignant cells that have bland features. Because of this, cytologic changes useful to diagnose this entity have not been consistently described.[27,47]

In endometrial adenocarcinomas, the malignant cells are in small clusters (Figure 3.37). Although comparatively small, there is variation in nuclear size, and nucleoli are evident. Poorly differentiated carcinoma cells in a clean background characterize adenocarcinomas that are metastatic to the cervix.[47]

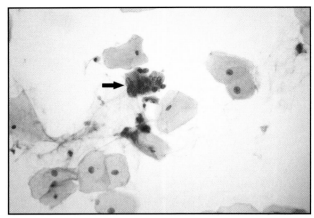

(a)

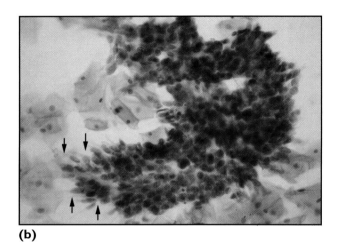

(b)

FIGURES 3.34a,b Atypical endocervical cells. **(a)** A small central cluster of atypical glandular cells is present (arrow). The nuclei are slightly enlarged and the chromatin is coarse (liquid preparation, Papanicolaou stain, high-power magnification). **(b)** A large group of atypical glandular cells. Note the peripheral palasading known as "feathering" (arrows). These features are indicative of an endocervical adenocarcinoma in situ (conventional preparation, Papanicolaou stain, high-power magnification). ▬▬▬

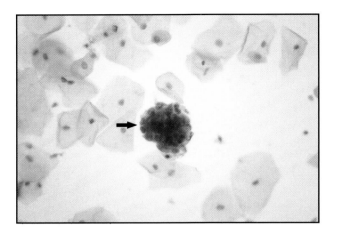

FIGURE 3.35 Atypical endometrial cells (arrow). In contrast to benign endometrial cells, the nuclei are enlarged and irregularly shaped. In addition, the chromatin is coarse and small but distinct nucleoli can be detected (liquid preparation, Papanicolaou stain, high-power magnification). ▬▬▬

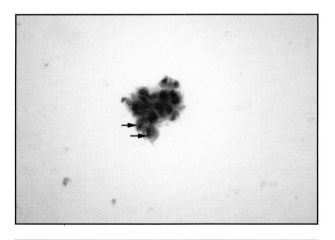

FIGURE 3.36 Endocervical adenocarcinoma. The malignant cells maintain a rounded glandular shape. Note the prominent nucleoli (arrows) (liquid preparation, Papanicolaou stain, high-power magnification). ▬▬▬

3.4.2 New technologies in cervicovaginal cytology

In the past decade, various ancillary technologies have been developed to augment the way cervical cytologic specimens are prepared and screened. Technologies in use today fall into two general categories: specimen preparation (liquid-based, thin-layer systems) and computerized systems. The latter have been divided into methods that target certain slide areas for manual interpretation (digital imaging systems) and those that identify slides requiring manual rescreening for potential abnormalities (computer-assisted screening).

3.4.2.1 Processing systems

Presently, there are two systems approved for Pap test preparation: ThinPrep™ (Cytyc Corporation, Boxborough, MA, Figure 3.38) and AutoCyte PREP™ or SUREPATH™ system (TriPath Corporation,

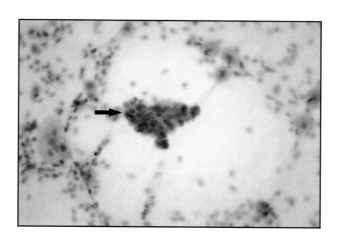

FIGURE 3.37 Endometrial adenocarcinoma (arrow). The cells are smaller than malignant endocervical cells, but they maintain their glandular shape. The nuclei are enlarged, irregularly shaped, have coarse chromatin, and have distinct but small nucleoli (liquid preparation, Papanicolaou stain, high-power magnification). ▬

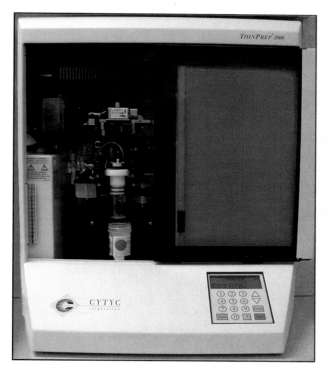

FIGURE 3.38 ThinPrep™ processing machine (T-2000). The device can only process one specimen at a time; staining is completed in the usual fashion. It takes about 1 to 2 minutes to transfer the material from the liquid container to a glass slide (Cytyc corporation, Boxborough, MA; used with permission). ▬

Burlington, NC, Figure 3.39). Collection devices approved for ThinPrep include the Cervex-Brush® or Papette®, or a combination of a Cytobrush® and plastic spatula. The Cervex-Brush® or Papette® is the only device approved to collect material for processing by the SUREPATH™ system. Both systems use a cell-preservative solution (Figure 3.40). For ThinPrep™, stirring the devices in the solution transfers the material. For SUREPATH™, the device tip is also sent in the solution to the laboratory. The transfer of cells from the solution to the slide differs for the two systems. With ThinPrep, the material is dispersed by spinning, suctioned onto a nuclepore filter to remove debris, and transferred onto a glass slide. For SUREPATH™, the cells are dispersed by withdrawing the material into a syringe containing a cell enrichment solution. The material is then centrifuged and vortexed to remove debris. Finally, the cells are transferred to a glass slide through gravitation. Regardless of the preparation method, the slides are screened in the conventional fashion (Figure 3.41). Presently, slides prepared by SUREPATH™ are approved for computer-assisted screening.

There are obvious advantages to liquid-based, thin-layered specimens. Air-dried and obscured slides can be eliminated. The material is well preserved and abnormal cells are easily recognizable. Numerous split-sample (preparing a conventional smear and a liquid-based monolayer slide from material obtained from the same cervix) and

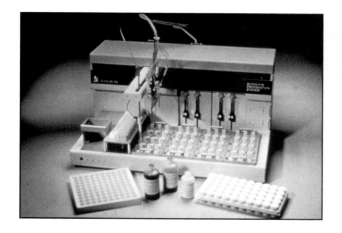

FIGURE 3.39 SUREPATH™ processing machine. The device can process and stain up to 48 specimens at one time, but the slides and liquid tubes have to be individually loaded by hand. (TRIPATH Corporation, Burlington, NC; used with permission). ▬

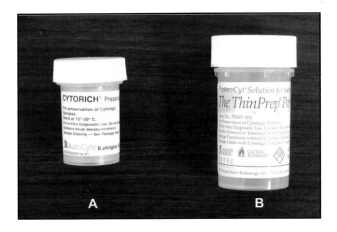

FIGURES 3.40a,b Liquid preservatives. **(a)** Cytorich™ solution (TRIPATH Corporation, Burlington, NC; used with permission). **(b)** Preservcyt™ solution (Cytyc corporation, Boxborough, MA; used with permission).

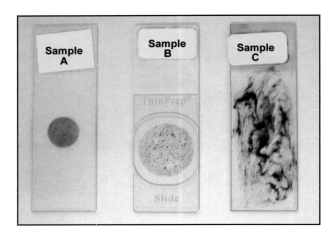

FIGURES 3.41a–c Liquid-based slides. **(a)** SUREPATH™ slide. The button is approximately 13 mm in diameter (TRIPATH Corporation, Burlington, NC; used with permission). **(b)** ThinPrep™ slide. The button is approximately 22 mm in diameter (Cytyc corporation, Boxborough, MA; used with permission). **(c)** Conventional slide. Note the uneven thickness and staining.

direct-to-vial (all material placed in the liquid medium) studies have shown a decrease in the number of specimens that were limited by obscuring blood, inflammation, or drying artifact.[48–50] Some investigators have also reported a decrease in the number of specimens interpreted as ASC and a corresponding increase in SIL in these cases, corresponding to an increase in CIN on colposcopically directed biopsy.[51,52] Additionally, the suspension can be used

to create multiple slides if outside consultation is necessary or if additional studies, such as HPV DNA typing or screening for chlamydia and gonococcal organisms, are requested.

There are, however, disadvantages to both systems. Cytotechnologists and pathologists need additional training to screen and interpret these slides. Screening must be deliberate, as fewer normal and abnormal cells are available for review. These systems are expensive for laboratories to institute, and the continuous use of disposables (filters, vials with preservatives, collection devices, slides) leads to additional costs. These expenses may be offset by the decrease in the number of patient visits necessary for reevaluation of Pap tests with unclear results.[53]

3.4.2.2 Digital imaging systems

These systems use an optical scanner to examine a specimen and identify areas of the slide with cells that require further evaluation. These areas are then captured as a digital image and presented on a computer monitor for examination. If needed, the glass slide can also be examined and correlated with the computer images. Numerous studies using an early model system consistently demonstrated the accuracy and effectiveness of digital image analysis.[54–56] The advantage of such a system is the ability of cytotechnologists to direct their attention only to those areas identified by the computer as potentially abnormal. Overall, screening time for a particular slide could be reduced. However, the equipment has been expensive to install and maintain, and cytotechnologists and pathologists need additional training to operate the equipment and interpret the slides.[57] None of these systems is presently commercially available, but numerous companies are developing new imaging products that will be less expensive and easier for individual laboratories to use.

3.4.2.3 Computer analysis and reporting systems

The only system approved for commercial use is AutoPap™ (TriPath Corporation, Burlington, NC, Figure 3.42). AutoPap™ uses a high-resolution digital scanner to image individual cells on a Pap test. The computer uses a Bayesian Belief Network Technology to classify cells as normal or abnormal. It then quantifies ("scores") the degree of abnormality to a threshold percentage programmed by the company or the laboratory (10%, 20%, 30%). This represents a percentage of slides that the scanner will identify for manual screening.[58] In a typical laboratory setting, the AutoPap™ can substitute as a primary screening

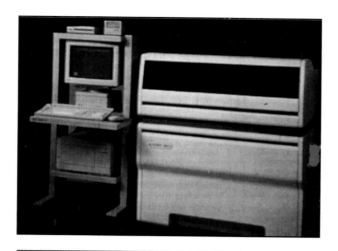

Figure 3.42 AutoPap™ computer assisted screener (TRI-PATH Corporation, Burlington, NC; used with permission).

four-fold improvement over manual rescreening of specimens originally interpreted as normal.[59,60] The AutoPap™ screening system, using a threshold percentage of 20%, has also been approved for primary screening of low-risk patients and can now screen liquid-based monolayer slides prepared using SUREPATH™ technology. Major disadvantages include the considerable purchase and maintenance expense for this device, which is unaffordable to all but the largest laboratories.

Much concern has been expressed recently over the cost of these various new technologies and whether they should be considered standard of care.[61–63] Various cost-efficiency models have been developed to compare liquid-based screening, digital imaging, and computer-assisted screening methods to each other and to various other screening and preventative systems. Most have demonstrated that the new technologies can be of value in reducing the ill-defined costs of patient visits for evaluation and management of poor-quality Pap tests and unclear diagnoses.[53,64–66] Whether these cost savings will translate into reduction in the overall incidence of cervical cancer is unclear. It must be remembered that the most reliable way to reduce deaths from this malignancy is to encourage women to participate in a periodic screening program.

system in low-risk patients at a setting of 20% manual screen threshold, and for a random rescreening system of 10% normal tests. In the latter, the AutoPap™ can rescreen all normal Pap tests. Using a threshold percentage point of 10%, it would identify slides requiring manual rescreening. Initial studies evaluating the AutoPap™ system demonstrated a three- to

References

1. Kato I, Santamaria M, De Ruiz P A, et al. Inter-observer variation in cytological and histological diagnoses of cervical neoplasia and its epidemiologic implication. *J Clin Epidemiol* 1995;48:1167–74.
2. Stoler M H, Schiffman M. Interobserver reproducibility of cervical cytologic and histologic interpretations: realistic estimates from the ASCUS-LSIL Triage Study. *JAMA* 2001;285:1500–5.
3. Keating J T, Cviko A, Riethdorf S, et al. Ki-67, cyclin E, and p16INK4 are complimentary surrogate biomarkers for human papilloma virus-related cervical neoplasia. *Am J Surg Pathol* 2001;25:884–91.
4. Wright T C, Ferenczy A. Benign Diseases of the Cervix. In: Kurman R J, ed.: *Blaustein's Pathology of the Female Genital Tract.* New York: Springer-Verlag, 1994:205–6.
5. Voorjis P G. Benign Proliferative Reactions, Intraepithelial Neoplasia and Invasive Cancer of the Cervix. In: Bibbo M. *Comprehensive Cytopathology* (2nd ed.) Philadelphia: WB Saunders Company, 1997:161–230.
6. Wright T C, Kurman R J, Ferenczy A. Precancerous Lesions of the Cervix. In: Kurman R J, ed.: *Blaustein's Pathology of the Female Genital Tract.* New York: Springer-Verlag, 1994:229–32.
7. Reagan J W, Seidemand I L, Saracusa Y. The cellular morphology of carcinoma in situ and dysplasia or atypical hyperplasia of the uterine cervix. *Cancer* 1953;6:224–35.
8. Richart R M. Cervical Intraepithelial Neoplasia: A Review. In: Sommers S C, ed.: *Pathology Annual.* New York: Appleton-Century-Crofts, 1973:301–28.
9. Scully R E, Bonfiglio T A, Silverberg S G. *Histologic Typing of Female Genital Tract Tumours.* World Health Organization International Histological Classification of Tumours (2nd ed.) New York: Springer-Verlag, 1994:39–46.
10. Zaino R J, Robboy S J, Bentley R, Kurman R J. Diseases of the Vagina. In: Kurman R J, ed. *Blaustein's Pathology of the Female Genital Tract.* New York: Springer-Verlag, 1994:156–70.
11. Meisels A, Fortin R. Condylomatous lesions of the cervix and vagina I: cytologic patterns. *Acta Cytol* 1976;20:505–9.
12. Wright T C, Kurman R J, Ferenczy A. Precancerous Lesions of the Cervix. In: Kurman R J, ed.: *Blaustein's Pathology of the Female Genital Tract.* New York: Springer-Verlag, 1994:245–9.
13. Wright T C, Kurman R J, Ferenczy A. Precancerous Lesions of the Cervix. In: Kurman R J, ed.: *Blaustein's Pathology of the Female Genital Tract.* New York: Springer-Verlag, 1994:249–53.

14. Kurman R J, Norris H J, Wilkinson E. Tumors of the cervix, vagina and vulva. In: *Atlas of Tumor Pathology* (Third Series: Fascicle 4). Washington D.C.: American Registry of Pathology, Armed Forces Institute of Pathology, 1992:37–157.

15. Wright T C, Ferenczy A, Kurman R J. Carcinoma and Other Tumors of the Cervix. In: Kurman R J, ed.: *Blaustein's Pathology of the Female Genital Tract.* New York: Springer-Verlag, 1994:280–97.

16. Wright T C, Ferenczy A. Benign Diseases of the Cervix. In: Kurman R J, ed.: *Blaustein's Pathology of the Female Genital Tract.* New York: Springer-Verlag, 1994:212–4.

17. Wright T C, Ferenczy A. Benign Diseases of the Cervix. In: Kurman R J, ed.: *Blaustein's Pathology of the Female Genital Tract.* New York: Springer-Verlag, 1994:218–9.

18. Wright T C, Ferenczy A, Kurman R J. Carcinoma and Other Tumors of the Cervix. In: Kurman R J, ed.: *Blaustein's Pathology of the Female Genital Tract.* New York: Springer-Verlag, 1994:300–9.

19. Tasca L, Östör A G, Babes V. History of Gynecologic Pathology XII: Aurel Babes. *Int J Gynecol Pathol* 2002;21:198–202.

20. Vilos G A. The history of the Papanicolaou smear and the odyssey of George and Andormache Papanicolaou. *Obstet Gynecol* 1998;91:479–83.

21. Papanicolaou G N, Traut H F. *Diagnosis of Uterine Cancer by the Vaginal Smear.* New York: The Commonwealth Fund, 1943:19–45.

22. Christopherson W M. Parker J E, Drye J C. Control of cervical cancer: preliminary report on community program. *JAMA* 1962;182:179–82.

23. Fujii T, Crum C, Winkler B, Fu Y S, Richart R M. Human papillomavirus infection and cervical intraepithelial neoplasia: histopathology and DNA content. *Obstet Gynecol* 1984;63:99–104.

24. Loning T, Ikenberg H, Becker J, Gissmann L, Hoepfer I, zur Hausen H. Analysis of oral papillomas, leukoplakias, and invasive carcinomas for human papillomavirus type related DNA. *J Invest Dermatol* 1985;84:417–20.

25. The 1988 Bethesda System for reporting cervical/vaginal cytologic diagnoses. Developed and approved at the National Cancer Institute Workshop, Bethesda, Maryland, U.S.A., December 12–13, 1988. *Acta Cytol* 1989;33:567–74.

26. The revised Bethesda System for reporting cervical/vaginal cytologic diagnoses: report of the 1991 Bethesda workshop. *Acta Cytol* 1992;36:273–6.

27. Kurman R J, Solomon D. *The Bethesda System for Reporting Cervical/Vaginal Cytologic Diagnoses.* New York: Springer-Verlag, 1994;99:1–81.

28. Solomon D, Davey D, Kurman R, et al. The Bethesda System 2001: terminology for reporting the results of cervical cytology. *JAMA* 2002; 287:2114–9.

29. Mintzer M, Curtis P, Resnick J C, Morrell D. The effect of quality of Papanicolaou smears on the detection of cytologic abnormalities. *Cancer Cytopathol* 1999;87:113–7.

30. Allen K A, Zaleski S, Cohen M B. Laboratory use of the diagnosis "reactive/reparative" in gynecologic smears: impact of CLIA 88. *Mod Pathol* 1995;8:266–9.

31. Gupta P K. Microbiology, Inflammation and Viral Infections. In: Bibbo M. *Comprehensive Cytopathology* (2nd ed.) Philadelphia: WB Saunders Co, 1997:125–41.

32. Davis J D, Connor E E, Clark P, Wilkinson E J, Duff P. Correlation between cervical cytologic results and Gram Stain as diagnostic tests for bacterial vaginosis. *Am J Obstet Gynecol* 1997;177:532–5.

33. Weinberger M W, Harger J H. Accuracy of the Papanicolaou smear in the diagnosis of asymptomatic infection with Trichomonas vaginalis. *Obstet Gynecol* 1993;82:425–9.

34. Keebler C M, Wied G L. The estrogen test: an aid in differential cytodiagnosis. *Acta Cytol* 1974;18:482–93.

35. Montz F J. Significance of "normal" endometrial cells in cervical cytology from asymptomatic postmenopausal women receiving hormone replacement therapy. *Gynecol Oncol* 2001;81:33–9.

36. Gomez-Fernandez C R, Ganjei-Azar P, Behshid K, Averette H E, Nadji M. Normal endometrial cells in Papanicolaou smears: Prevalence in women with and without endometrial disease. *Obstet Gynecol* 2000;96:874–8.

37. Cherkis R C, Patten S F, Andrews T J, et al. Significance of normal endometrial cells detected by cervical cytology. *Obstet Gynecol* 1998;71:242–4.

38. Gondos B, King E B. Significance of endometrial cells in cervicovaginal smears. *Ann Clin Lab Sci* 1977;7:486–90.

39. Sheils L A, Wilbur D C. Atypical squamous cells of undetermined significance. Stratification of the risk of association with, or progression to, squamous intraepithelial lesions based on morphologic subcategorization. *Acta Cytol* 1997;41:1065–72.

40. Geng L, Connolly D C, Isacson C, Ronnett B C, Cho K R. Atypical immature metaplasia (AIM) of the cervix: is it related to high-grade squamous intraepithelial lesion (HSIL)? *Human Pathol* 1999;30:345–51.

41. Sherman M E, Tabbara S O, Scott D R, et al. "ASCUS, rule out HSIL": cytologic features, histologic correlates, and human papillomavirus detection. *Mod Pathol* 1999;12:335–42.

42. Sherman M E, Solomon D, Schiffman M for the ALTS Group. Qualification of ASCUS: a comparison of equivocal LSIL and equivocal HSIL cervical cytology in the ASCUS LSIL Triage Study. *Am J Clin Pathol* 2001;116:386–94.

43. Kurman R J, Malkasian G D Jr, Sedlis A, Solomon D. From Papanicolaou to Bethesda: the rationale for a new cervical cytologic classification. *Obstet Gynecol* 1991;77:779–82.

44. Ng A B P, Reagan J W, Lindner E A. The cellular manifestations of microinvasive squamous cell carcinoma of the uterine cervix. *Acta Cytol* 1972;16:5–13.

45. Raab S S, Snider T E, Potts S A, McDaniel H L, Robinson R A, Nelson D L, et al. Atypical glandular

cells of undetermined significance: diagnostic accuracy and interobserver variability using select cytologic criteria. *Am J Clin Pathol* 1997;107:299–307.

46. Liao S Y, Stanbridge E J. Expression of MN/CA 9 protein in Papanicolaou smears containing atypical glandular cells of undetermined significance is a diagnostic biomarker of cervical dysplasia and neoplasia. *Cancer* 2000;88:1108–21.

47. Pacey N F, Ng A B P. Glandular Neoplasms of the Uterine Cervix. In Bibbo M. *Comprehensive Cytopathology* (2nd ed.) Philadelphia: WB Saunders Co., 1997:231–50.

48. Lee K R, Ashfaq R, Birdsong G G, et al. Comparison of conventional Papanicolaou smears and a fluid-based, thin-layer system for cervical cancer screening. *Obstet Gynecol* 1997;90:278–84.

49. Corkill M, Knapp D, Martin J, Hutchinson M L. Specimen adequacy of ThinPrep sample preparations in a direct-to-vial study. *Acta Cytol* 1997;41:39–44.

50. Vassilakos P, Saurel J, Rondez R. Direct-to-vial use of the AutoCyte PREP liquid based preparation for cervical-vaginal specimens in three European laboratories. *Acta Cytol* 1999;43:650–8.

51. Papillo J L, Zarka M A, St. John T L. Evaluation of the ThinPrep pap test in clinical practice: a seven month, 16,314-case experience in northern Vermont. *Acta Cytol* 1998;42:203–8.

52. Vassilakos P, Schwartz D, de Marval F, Yousfi L et al. Biopsy-based comparison of liquid based, thin-layer preparations to conventional Pap smear. *J Reprod Med* 2000;45:11–6.

53. Evaluation of cervical cytology. Evidence Report/Technology Assessment #5. Washington D.C.: Agency for Health Care Policy and Research. AHCPR Publication 99-E010, 1999.

54. Sherman M E, Mango L J, Kelly D, et al. PAPNET analysis of reportedly negative smears preceding the diagnosis of a high-grade squamous intraepithelial lesion or carcinoma, *Mod Pathol* 1994;7:578–81.

55. Ashfaq R, Salinger F, Solares B. Evaluation of the PAPNET system for prescreening triage of cervicovaginal smears. *Acta Cytol* 1997;41:1058–64.

56. Michelow P M, Hlongwane N F, Lieman G. Simulation of primary cervical cancer screening by the PAPNET system in an unscreened, high-risk community. *Acta Cytol* 1997;41:88–92.

57. O'Leary T J, Tellado M, Buckner S, Ali I S, Stevens A, Ollayos C W. PAPNET assisted rescreening of cervical smears: cost and accuracy with a 100% manual rescreening strategy. *JAMA* 1998;279:235–7.

58. Sedlacek T V. Automated cervical cytology. *The Colposcopist.* 1996;27:1–4.

59. Colgan T J, Patten S F, Lee J S J. A clinical trial of the AutoPap 300 QC system for quality control of cervicovaginal cytology in the clinical laboratory. *Acta Cytol* 1995;39:1191–8.

60. Wilbur D C, Bonfiglio T A, Rutkowski M A, et al. Sensitivity of the AutoPap 300 QC system for cervical cytologic screening. *Acta Cytol* 1996;40:127–32.

61. Brown A D, Garber A M. Cost effectiveness of three adjunctive methods to enhance the sensitivity of papanicolaou testing. *JAMA* 1999;281:347–53.

62. Statement on technical devices for innovation in cervical cytology screening (editorial). *Am J Clin Pathol* 1996;169:441.

63. Bartels P H, Bibbo M, Hutchinson M L, et al. Computerized screening devices and performance assessment: development of a policy towards automation (IAC Task Force summary). *Acta Cytol* 1998;42:59–68.

64. Hutchinson M L. Assessing the costs and benefits of alternative rescreening strategies. *Acta Cytol* 1996;40:4–7.

65. Radensky P W, Mango L J. Interactive neural network-assisted screening: an economic assessment. *Acta Cytol* 1998;42:246–52.

66. Schechter, C B. Cost-effectiveness of rescreening conventionally prepared cervical smears by PAPNET testing. *Acta Cytol* 1996;40:1272–82.

Cervical Cancer
Epidemiology and Etiology

Table of Contents

4.1 Introduction

During the last 3 decades, our understanding of the epidemiology and pathogenesis of invasive cervical cancer has changed dramatically. This change has occurred as a result of the integration of new virological approaches to studying the disease with classic epidemiology and pathology. For many years, it has been recognized that women who had multiple sexual partners, who began sexual activity at an early age, and who were of lower socioeconomic class were at greatest risk for cervical cancer. At the other end of the spectrum, virgins and women with limited sexual exposure were recognized to be at low risk. These observations strongly suggested that a sexually transmitted agent was responsible for invasive cervical cancer. However, the identity of that agent proved elusive until modern molecular biologic methods were used to study the pathogenesis of cervical cancer. Based on the results of both molecular and epidemiologic studies it is now known that infection with specific types of human papillomavirus (HPV) is necessary in the development of invasive cervical cancer.

4.2 Descriptive Epidemiology

4.2.1 Prevalence of invasive cervical cancer worldwide

Worldwide, cervical cancer is the second most common cancer among women. It is estimated that the number of new cases per year is approximately 437,600 and that cervical cancer comprises 12% of all cancers diagnosed in women.[1] Other squamous cell malignancies of the lower genital tract account for another 150,000 cases. Cervical cancer results in approximately 200,000 deaths worldwide each year.[2] It occurs in relatively young women, accounting for an average of 17 potential years of life lost for every death from invasive cervical cancer occurring before the age of 70. Therefore, approximately 3.4 million women-years of life before age 70 are lost yearly from cervical cancer throughout the world.

The impact of cervical cancer is greatest in developing counties[3,4] (Table 4.1). Cervical cancer is the most common cancer of women in many developing areas of Africa, Central and South America, and Asia, where it constitutes 20% to 30% of all cancers

Table 4.1 Percentage of Population that Is HPV DNA Positive, Percent with Condyloma and Incidence of Invasive Cervical Cancer for All Regions in the World

	HPV DNA	Genital Warts Women >15	Age Specific Incidence of Cervical Cancer (ASIR)			
			15–44	45–54	55–64	>65
World	15.8%	1.4%	9.5	44.9	51.8	41.9
More developed	10.0%	1.0%	11.9	22.4	23.8	26.3
Less developed	15.0%	1.5%	9.0	53.6	65.0	53.8

From: Table 2 (Modified): Bosch FX, De Sanjose S. Chapter 1: human papillomavirus and cervical cancer-burden and assessment of causality. *J Natl Cancer Inst Monogr.* 2003;31:3–13. With permission, Oxford University Press.

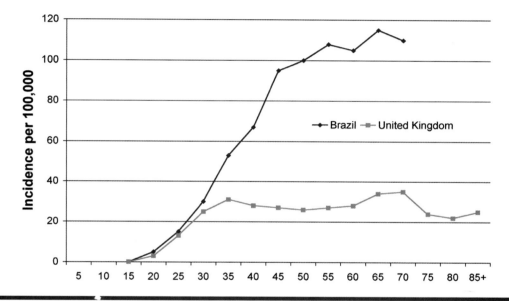

FIGURE 4.1 Age-specific incidence rates of cervical cancer in Brazil and in the UK demonstrate the excess burden of invasive cervical cancer in developing countries. Compiled by IARC for the years 1985, 1990 and 2000. Modified from Fig. 2 : Bosch FX, De Sanjose S. Chapter 1: human papillomavirus and cervical cancer-burden and assessment of causality. *J Natl Cancer Inst Monogr* 2003;(31):3–13. With permission, Oxford University Press.

among women. The absolute greatest number of cervical cancer cases comes from Asia (nearly 250,000 new cases annually) followed by countries in Central and South America.[5,6] Africa and Europe each account for 65,000 to 70,000 new cases annually. The Caribbean, and Central and South American countries have the highest incidence of invasive cancer, along with countries in Eastern and Southern Africa.[5,6] The lowest rates registered are in the southeastern and western regions in Asia, Australia, New Zealand and the northern countries in North America, where cervical cancer accounts for only 4% to 6% of cancers in women. Compared with other cancers, the prevalence of cervical cancer in Eastern European

women is intermediately placed. Age standardized incidence rates (ASIR) for all regions in the world show an increasing trend with age to reach a plateau after ages 45–50 in most countries. Screening has very little effect on cervical cancer incidence before the age of 30 as demonstrated here by the nearly identical curve for women of young age in a well-screened population (UK) and one with minimal screening (Brazil) (Figure 4.1). Identical rates before age 30 also indicate similar levels of exposure to HPV and in some developed countries cervical cancer incidence is higher for young women aged 15–44 than for age-matched women in less developed countries. However, for women age >45 in less developed countries cervical cancer incidence is more than double that found in more developed countries,[5] for after age 30 the shape of the curve is highly dependent on the screening efforts. This divergence in the incidence of cervical cancer in a well developed and screened country (UK) is dramatically evident in the comparison to that documented in Brazil with no organized screening activity.

Invasive cervical cancer is predominately a disease of women older than age 30 years. In the United States, the Surveillance, Epidemiology and End Results (SEER) Program of the National Cancer Institute (NCI) has monitored the incidence, mortality, and age distribution of invasive cervical cancer since 1973.[7] From 1991 to 1995, the age-specific incidence rates of invasive cervical cancer were 2.6 cases per 100,000 for women 20 to 24 years old, 7.8 cases per 100,000 women 25 to 29 years old, 8 to 14 cases per 100,000 women 30 to 39 years old, and 15 to 17 cases per 100,000 women in the age groups of 40 years and over (Figure 4.2). In the United States, approximately 25% of cases of cervical cancer occur in women older than age 65, approximately 12,800 new cases of cervical cancer are diagnosed every year, and approximately 4,500 women succumb to this disease annually.

4.2.2 Time trends and impact of cytologic screening

During the last four decades, there have been dramatic reductions in the incidence of invasive cervical cancer in North America and Western Europe. Much of the reduction in incidence and mortality rates for cervical cancer reflects the availability of cytologic screening. The incidence of cervical cancer in the US has decreased 75% and mortality has decreased 74% since the implementation of Papanicolaou (Pap)

smear screening in 1949.[7] Between 1973 and 1996, the age-adjusted incidence rates for squamous cell carcinoma declined by 41.9% (9.45 to 5.49 per 100,000 women) although an upward trend in squamous cell carcinoma rates was temporarily noted in the late 1980s in the UK.[8] In contrast, the age-adjusted incidence rates for adenocarcinoma increased 29.1% during the same period, from 1.34 to 1.73 per 100,000 women.[9] Similar increases have been reported in other countries with well developed screening activities.[4,5,10–12] Several theories have been proposed to explain the increasing rate of adenocarcinoma. Because abnormal cells from early glandular lesions are less easily detected by cytology,[5] some have deduced that the increased rate of adenocarcinoma is only relative compared to the more easily detected screened-out preinvasive squamous lesions. However, the increased rate appears to be absolute and may reflect new environmental influences on the columnar epithelium, such as oral contraceptive use, and the possibility that the prevalence of HPV 18 may be increasing.[5]

The impact of nationwide screening programs is also clearly demonstrated by the Scandinavian experience.[13–15] In Finland, a national screening program to prevent cervical cancer, begun in the 1950s, dramatically lowered rates of cervical cancer to 5.5 cases per 100,000 women and the experience in Sweden was similar. In contrast, Norway, which only recently developed a nationwide screening program, has a much smaller reduction in cervical cancer rates and continues to have a rate of cervical cancer that is three times higher (15.6 per 100,000) than that of Finland (Figure 4.3). In contrast to the experience in Nordic countries, cervical screening in countries without organized programs for screening call and recall have had mixed results. Cervical screening with cytology

FIGURE 4.2 HPV age-specific rates of cervical HPV infection and associated disease in the U.S. Modified from: Lowy D R, Howley P M. Papillomaviruses and their replication. In: *Fields' Virology.* Knipe D M, Howley P M, eds. Philadelphia: Lippincott Williams & Wilkins, 2001:2231–64. With permission.

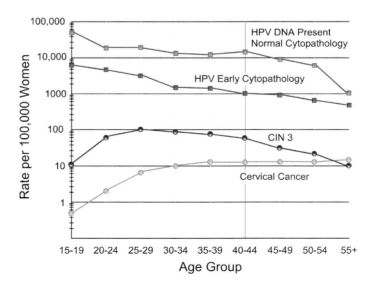

started in England in 1964 but failed to achieve sufficient coverage or follow-up of women with positive results until the establishment of a national call and recall system in 1988.[16,17] Following the establishment of organized screening, coverage for all women aged 25 to 64 rose from 45% in 1988 to 85% in 1994 and has remained steady since. The dramatic change in incidence and mortality since 1990 has been attributed to this increase in coverage.[16] From 1971 to the mid-1980s, incidence remained steady at 14 to 16 per 100,000, then fell steadily to 10 per 100,000 by the mid-1990s. Total mortality fell at a steady rate of approximately 1.5% per year prior to the onset of adequate coverage of the population, but following the implementation of widespread screening, mortality declined at a threefold rate, reaching 3.7 per 100,000 by 1997.[17] The high age-specific incidence rates (ASIRs) for cervical cancer in countries late to enter organized screening, such as the UK and Denmark, when compared to countries beginning such screening decades earlier, are demonstrated in Figure 4.4. Comparison of estimated incidence rates

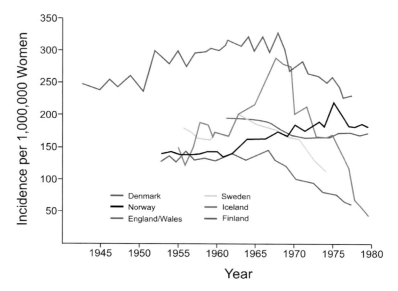

FIGURE 4.3   Decreasing incidence of invasive cervical cancer in those Scandinavian countries that introduced national call and recall screening programs (Finland, Sweden and Iceland) demonstrates a much steeper fall-off in cervical cancer rates than in those countries where organized screening was introduced recently or not at all (Denmark, Norway, England and Wales). From: Campion M J, Ferris D G, di Paola F M, Reid R I. *Modern Colposcopy: A Practical Approach.* ASCCP, Hagerstown, MD. 1991;pp. 4–2.

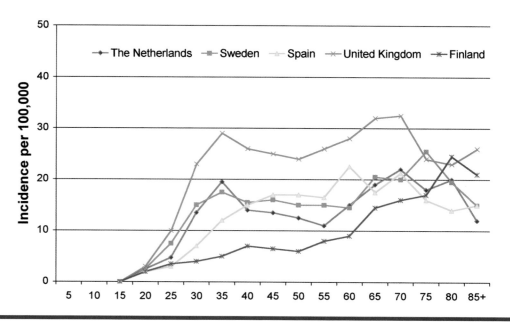

FIGURE 4.4   Age-specific incidence rates of cervical cancer in six European countries reflect primarily differences in screening policy noted over time. From Fig. 2C Bosch F X, De Sanjose S. Chapter 1: human papillomavirus and cervical cancer-burden and assessment of causality. *J Natl Cancer Inst Monogr* 2003;31:3–13.. With permission, Oxford University Press.

from 1985 and 2000 demonstrates a slight reduction in the total number of cases in developed countries and an increase in developing regions, particularly in Africa, the Caribbean and Central and South America.[5] Substantial reduction in the mortality from cervical cancer has been reported in China.[18]

Variability of cervical cancer incidence within populations in a given geographic area is also partly dependent on differences in the use of cytologic screening. Between 1960 and 1974, the incidence of cervical cancer in white women in the United States decreased by 43% from 21 to 12 cases per 100,000 women-years. However, during the same time period, the incidence among African-American women decreased by only 16%, from 37 to 31 per 100,000 women-years. This dichotomy was attributed to a difference in the penetrance of cytologic screening among the two populations. During the last two decades, cytologic screening has become more common among African-American women in the United States, and the difference in the incidence of cervical cancer between the groups has narrowed but still remains significant (Figure 4.5). Additionally, white women continue to be more likely to have cervical carcinoma diagnosed at an earlier stage [1A-1] than are age-matched African-Americans or Hispanics.[19]

Women who fail to have regular Pap smears are particularly vulnerable to cervical cancer. The lifetime risk that a woman in the US who has never been screened will develop cervical cancer is estimated to be 3.7%, or 3,748 cases per 100,000 women.[20] With annual cytologic screening, the lifetime risk drops to 0.3%, or 305 cases per 100,000 women. Based on these results, the Pap test has clearly been the most successful cancer preventive test to date.

4.2.3 Other factors affecting geographic variations

In addition to the availability of cytologic screening, other factors relating to sexual behavior and socioeconomic status influence geographic variations in the rate of invasive cervical cancer. Low rates of cervical cancer are typically found in countries characterized by conservative sexual behavior, regardless of the widely varying levels of economic development.[21] The age-adjusted incidence rates of invasive cervical cancer in Spain, Italy, Ireland, Israel, China, and Kuwait are all under 10 cases per 100,000 women-years.[1] Because all of these countries are well known for their conservative sexual mores, this low rate suggests that sexual behaviors play an important role. Further support for

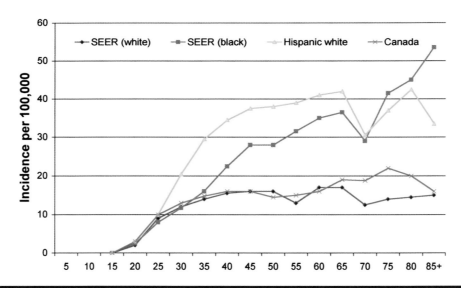

FIGURE 4.5 Data on white populations from the SEER and Canadian registries show that cervical cancer incidence rises steeply between ages 20 and 35 and stays stable in the middle age groups, with some slight increase after 55–60. In contrast, for Blacks, Hispanic and Chinese, the incidence increases steadily throughout lifetime, reaching 2 to 3 times the incidence among whites in the most advanced age groups. These statistics reflect the impact of socioeconomic and racial differences in cervical cancer rates primarily as a function of access to screening. Data compiled by IARC for the year 1985, 1990 and 2000 for Canada and SEER statistics for the same years. From: Bosch F X, De Sanjose S. Chapter 1: Human papillomavirus and cervical cancer-burden and assessment of causality. *J Natl Cancer Inst Monogr* 2003;31:3–13. With permission, Oxford University Press.

the role of sexual behavior comes from the finding that an increase in cervical cancer incidence rates occurs among women who were in their early reproductive years during periods of social upheaval. This cohort effect has been best documented for women who were in their early reproductive years during either World War I or World War II.[22] These women had a higher risk for cervical cancer throughout their lives than did the cohorts of women who experienced their early reproductive years during the periods immediately before or after the wars. The increased risk of developing cervical cancer in these age cohorts may be attributable to a relaxation of sexual mores during the two wars. Similarly, the increase in cervical cancer mortality in young women observed in the United States and Europe starting in the 1980s is often attributed to changes in sexual behavior that began in the 1960s.[5]

Epidemiological studies by Bosch and colleagues[3] have clearly demonstrated that part of the geographic variation in cervical cancer incidence is attributable to differences in the sexual behaviors of men. These investigators conducted a series of epidemiological analyses using population-based surveys to evaluate socioeconomic, medical, and sexual factors.[23-25] The studies found that, although there are marked variations in the average number of lifetime sexual partners of women in different areas, these variations were insufficient to explain the geographic variations in cervical cancer. Moreover, there was no statistically significant correlation between the age-adjusted incidence rate of invasive cervical cancer and the average number of lifetime sexual partners women had. In the majority of these countries, women traditionally had only one to very few partners. In contrast, there was a strong correlation between the incidence of cervical cancer and the estimated average number of lifetime sexual partners of men in the different geographic locations.[3]

The importance of socioeconomic factors is evidenced by the declining incidence of cervical cancer in many developed countries prior to the introduction of widespread cytologic screening (Figure 4.6). For example, in the late 1940s, the incidence of invasive cervical cancer in the United States was 33 cases per 100,000 for white women and 70.4 per 100,000 for African-American women. By 1969, the incidence had dropped to 16.5 and 35.7, respectively, for the two groups of women. Although some of this decline is undoubtedly secondary to the onset of cervical screening in the 1950s, the decrease in incidence is higher than would be expected prior to the period of widespread cytologic screening.[22] In wealthier countries, mortality rates from cervical cancer tend to be higher among women in lower socioeconomic groups. Although part of this difference is attributable to differences in access to cervical cancer screening, some of it may be related to differences in diet, cigarette smoking, or sexual exposures. For example, studies of women in Spain and Colombia have demonstrated a higher prevalence of genital HPV infections in women from lower, compared with higher, socioeconomic strata.[24,25] Similarly, African-American women in the United States have had up to a 2.7-fold risk for developing cervical cancer compared with that for white women. This difference is associated with an increase of a similar magnitude in the prevalence of risk factors for cervical cancer, including multiple sexual partners, low income level, and multiparity.[26] In the United States, high rates of invasive cervical cancer are also observed in Vietnamese, Hispanic, Alaskan Native American, and Korean women.[27]

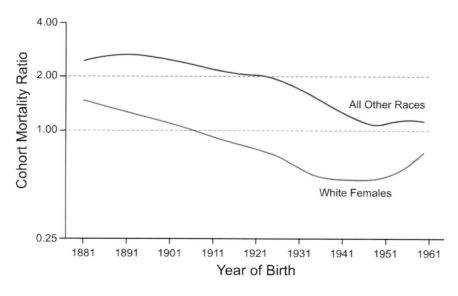

FIGURE 4.6 Incidence of invasive cervical cancer in the U.S. began to decline before the introduction of cervical screening with the Pap, indicating that socioeconomic forces also play a role in the cohort risk for this cancer. Decline was seen in all races but mortality was always lower with white females. From: Campion MJ, Ferris DG, di Paola FM, Reid RI. *Modern Colposcopy: A Practical Approach*, 1991. ASCCP, Hagerstown, MD.

4.3 Risk Factors for Invasive Cervical Cancer

There are numerous behavioral and environmental determinants of cervical cancer incidence (Table 4.2). These include demographic factors, such as a woman's age, where she lives, and her socioeconomic status. Sexual behaviors are significant risk factors. These include both a woman's sexual behavior as well as the behavior of her partner(s), her history of sexually transmitted diseases, and her age at first sexual intercourse. Behavioral and medical factors, including cigarette smoking, access to medical care for screening, oral contraceptive use, parity, and history of immunosuppression, are also important. Finally, a woman's nutritional status and genetic background may influence her risk for developing cervical cancer. However, the most important risk factor is anogenital infection with specific types of human papillomavirus (HPV).

Table 4.2 Environmental and Behavioral Determinants of Cervical Cancer Incidence at the Population Level

	HIGH RISK FACTORS	LOW RISK FACTORS
HPV PREVALENCE	HPV prevalence in the 35+ age groups at or above 10 %	HPV prevalence in the 35 + age groups at or below 5%
FEMALE SEXUAL BEHAVIOR	• Early age at sexual initiation • Multiple sexual partners	• Delayed age at sexual initiation • Monogamy
PROSTITUTION AND GROUPS PRACTICING HIGH RISK SEXUAL BEHAVIOR	Frequent	Limited
MALE SEXUAL BEHAVIOR	• Favor multiple partners • Use of prostitution services common • Condom use not reinforced	• Favor monogamy • Use of prostitution services rare • Condom use reinforced
PREVALENCE OF CO-FACTORS (Smoking, Hormonal Contraception, HIV, Other STDs)	High and sustained over a long time	Rare, recent introduction
PARITY	High	Low
SCREENING PRACTICES	• Low or non-organized • Quality control of screening activity irregular or non-existent • Screening events related to social class • Follow up of cervical lesions irregular	• Centrally organized, quality-controlled screening programs • Universal coverage sustained • Screening events unrelated to social class or migration • Follow-up of cervical lesions ensured at high standard
GENETIC SUSCEPTIBILITY OF THE POPULATION	Unknown	Unknown

From: Bosch FX, De Sanjose S. Chapter 1: human papillomavirus and cervical cancer-burden and assessment of causality. *J Natl Cancer Inst Monog.* 2003;31:3–13. With permission, Oxford University Press.

4.3.1 Sexual behavior

4.3.1.1 Female sexual behaviors

Cervical cancer has many of the epidemiologic characteristics of a sexually transmitted disease (STD). There is a strong association between the temporal, occupational, social, and geographic distributions of STDs at a national level and the mortality from invasive cervical cancer.[21] Women with a history of having acquired an STD, such as genital warts, herpes genitalis, gonorrhea, Trichomonas, chlamydia, or pediculosis pubis (crab lice), are at increased risk for developing cervical cancer.[28–34]

Early age at first sexual intercourse has been identified as a significant risk factor for invasive cervical cancer in most case-control studies. Women who have their first sexual intercourse before the age of 16 years have approximately twice the risk of developing cervical cancer when compared to women who begin sexual activity after the age of 20 years.[29–31,35,36] The finding that sexual exposure at an early age increases a woman's risk of subsequently developing invasive cervical cancer has been interpreted as indicating that the cervix is more susceptible to carcinogenic influences when the transformation zone is evolving.

A woman's risk of developing cervical cancer is also influenced by her marital status and her lifetime number of sexual partners. In general, the incidence of invasive cervical cancer is less in never-married women than in those who are divorced or widowed.[37] Women with invasive cancer are more likely to report multiple male sexual partners than control women.[29,30,37,38] Similarly, the risk of developing a high-grade squamous intraepithelial lesion (HSIL) has been shown to increase in a stepwise fashion with increases in number of sexual partners. For example, the risk for carcinoma in situ in one study increased to 4.5 for women with two to three partners compared with women who had only one partner. For women with seven or more partners, the risk increased to 8.1.[39]

4.3.1.2 Male sexual behaviors

The concept of a male role in the development of cervical cancer has been extensively investigated.[23,37,40–43] In 1935, Handley[40] recognized that the lower rates of cervical cancer in Moslems compared with Hindus living in the Fiji Islands might be attributable to a protective effect of circumcision. Handley also suggested that circumcision of male partners might explain the low rates of invasive cervical cancer among Jewish, compared with non-Jewish women. Several decades later, a study by Kessler[37]

clearly demonstrated the importance of the "high-risk" male in the development of cervical cancer. The study compared two groups of women; one group married to men whose previous wives had developed cervical cancer and another demographically similar control group married to men without such a history. The cohort of women who were married to high-risk males had almost a three-fold risk for cervical cancer compared with the control cohort. Recently, a case-control study of the male partners of women with either invasive cervical cancer or CIN 3 has been reported from Spain and Colombia.[23,36,43] In Spain, the husbands' number of extramarital partners, exposure to prostitutes, presence of serum antibodies to Chlamydia trachomatis and detection of penile HPV were all associated with cervical neoplasia in the wife. However, baseline sexual activity of males in Colombia was so high that associations between male sexual behavior and cervical neoplasia could not be made, for there were too few males with low-baseline sexual activity for comparison.

Similar findings in earlier studies were widely interpreted to indicate that certain high-risk men harbored a sexually transmitted agent involved in the development of cervical cancer. The epidemiologic and molecular evidence that this STD was likely to be HPV began to accumulate in the early 1980s. The concept of the high-risk male is important because it helps explain why selected female populations exhibit high rates of cervical cancer, despite rather conservative female sexual behavior.[42,43] Evidence that lack of circumcision definitively increased risk was demonstrated by the International Agency for Research on Cancer (IARC) pooled data from seven case-control studies of cervical carcinoma in situ and cervical cancer in five countries.[43] Male circumcision was shown to be associated with a reduced risk of penile HPV infection and, in the case of men with a history of multiple sexual partners, a reduced risk of cervical cancer in their current female partners.

4.3.2 Human papillomavirus

Once it was recognized that cervical cancer had the epidemiological characteristics of a STD, a search began for the sexually transmitted agent. Rotkin stated in 1962 that "further studies now isolate ages 15–20 as the susceptible period. Speculation suggests a male contribution that becomes established in adolescent girls, who are most susceptible. The agent may be a substance, organism, or particle not related to the ejaculate, perhaps borne on the unsanitary male organ or contraceptive, and remaining dormant for a mean latent period of 30 years before developing into carcinoma."[44] A number of potentially

Relative Risk for HPV and Cervical Cancer in Comparison With the Relative Risk for Smoking and Lung Cancer

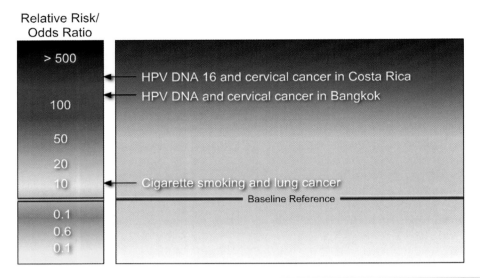

FIGURE 4.7   The relative risk of high-risk HPV infection for cervical cancer is many times greater than the association of smoking with lung cancer. For example, the risk of HPV 16 infection and cervical cancer in the NCI study in Costa Rica was greater than 25 times that noted for smoking and lung cancer. Modified from: Bosch F X, Lorincz A, Munoz N, Meijer C J, Shah K V. The causal relation between human papillomavirus and cervical cancer. *J Clin Pathol* 2002;55:244–65. With permission, Oxford University Press.

mutagenic sexually transmitted agents have been considered and subsequently rejected as being the cause of cervical cancer, although some may contribute to the promotion of cellular abnormality by the STD (HPV), now known to cause cervical cancer. These agents include smegma, sperm, various bacteria, protozoa, and viruses including herpes simplex virus type 2 (HSV 2).

Specific types of HPV have now been classified as human carcinogens. Over 99% of invasive cervical cancers are associated with these specific "high-risk" types of HPV, indicating that HPV is a necessary cause of cervical cancer.[45–49] Based on an IARC finding of sufficient evidence of carcinogenicity in humans for HPV-16 and HPV-18 and limited evidence of carcinogenicity in humans for other HPVs types, such as HPV-31 and 33, high-risk human papillomaviruses (HPV) have been nominated for listing in the Report on Carcinogens by the National Institute of Environmental Health Sciences (NIEHS).[50] In fact, high-risk HPV types, particularly HPVs 16 and 18, demonstrate a relative risk for cervical cancer that is many times that noted for the association of lung cancer and smoking (Figure 4.7). In 1000 cervical cancers collected worldwide by IARC the most prevalent HPV types detected were HPV 16 (53%), HPV 18 (15%),

HPV 45 (9%), HPV 31 (6%), and HPV 33 (3%) (Figure 4.8).[45] HPV 16 was the most common type in all geographical regions, followed by HPV 18, which was particularly common in South-East Asia. In addition, high-risk types of HPV are found in association with a high proportion of other invasive anogenital cancers, including those of the penis, vulva, vagina, and perianal region. The wealth of molecular data supporting the hypothesis that specific types of HPV are causal in the etiology of cervical neoplasia is discussed in Chapter 5. It is this association between cervical cancer and infection with specific types of HPV that results in invasive cervical cancer having the epidemiological characteristics of a STD.

There is very little definitive information on the incidence of genital HPV infection in the United States, but the most comprehensive population study demonstrated an increase in the incidence of genital warts from 13 per 100,000 in the early 1950s to 106 per 100,000 in the late 1970s.[50] Genital warts represent only a fraction of the HPV infections transmitted (Figure 4.9). Several prospective studies of women have reported 18–36 month acquisition rates for new HPV infection of 38% to 44%[50–53] and the lifetime likelihood of infection with HPV is estimated to be up to 80%. Multiple HPV types often coexist. Populations at high-risk of cervical cancer and populations with high rates of HIV tend to show higher proportions of multiple types, but risk for cervical cancer does not appear to be increased for women testing positive for multiple types.[54] In the IARC multicenter study, 8.2 % of the HPV positive cancers and 13.9 % of the HPV positive controls were positive for multiple types.[5,45]

The strength of the causality of the association of HPV with cervical cancer is based upon an understanding of the molecular biology of HPV as well as upon its epidemiology. Proof of causality requires that the association does not conflict with what is known of the natural history and biology of the disease (Table 4.3).[5] The evidence for the causal role of HPV in the induction of cervical cancer may be briefly summarized as:[5] 1) The regular presence of HPV-DNA in cervical cancer specimens; 2) Demonstration of viral oncogene expression E6 and E7 in

cervical cancer cells but not in cells from the adjacent stroma; 3) Transforming properties of these genes; 4) Requirement for E6 and E7 expression for maintaining the malignant phenotype of cervical carcinoma cell lines; 5) Interaction of viral oncoproteins with growth-regulating host-cell proteins and 6) Epidemiological studies pointing at these HPV infections as the major risk factors for cervical cancer development.[55] The mechanism is now so well described that it serves as the model for understanding viral-mediated oncogenesis. The HPV viral and host interactions leading to cell transformation and malignancy are described in several reviews,[46,48] and in more detail in Chapter 5.

Until the mid-1990s only 60 to 70% of invasive cervical cancer cases were reported to have detectable HPV DNA, and many theorized that the disease could also be secondary to non-HPV mechanisms. However, improved HPV testing has now documented HPV

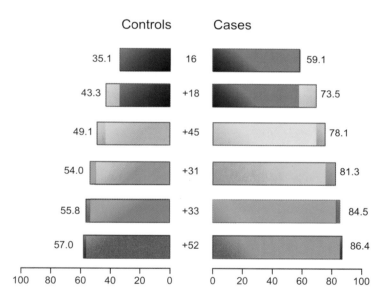

FIGURE 4.8   Cumulative prevalence of HPV types in cervical cancer (cases) and in HPV positive women with normal cervical cytology (controls) included in the International Agency for Research on Cancer (IARC) multicenter study. From Fig 1: Bosch F X, De Sanjose S. Chapter 1: human papillomavirus and cervical cancer-burden and assessment of causality. *J Natl Cancer Inst Monogr* 2003;31:3–13. With permission, Oxford University Press. ▬

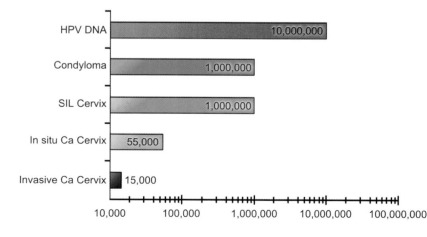

FIGURE 4.9   HPV prevalence estimates of genital tract HPV infections and of HPV-associated diseases in U.S. women. Modified from: Howley P M, Lowy D R. Papillomaviruses and their replication. In: *Fields' Virology.* Knipe D M, Howley P M, eds. Philadelphia: Lippincott Williams & Wilkins, 2001:2197–229. With permission.

Table 4.3 Criteria for Proof of Causality Are All Fulfilled in Terms of the Relationship of High-risk HPV with Cervical Cancer

CRITERIA	CONCEPT
Time Sequence	Exposure must precede disease
Experimental (Prevention)	Reduction of disease following reductions in exposure
Strength and Consistency	Highly associated with the disease in different settings
Biological Plausibility and Coherence	Mechanisms consistent with previous knowledge
Dose - response	Risk of disease is related to level of exposure

From: Table 4: Bosch FX, De Sanjose S. Chapter 1: human papillomavirus and cervical cancer-burden and assessment of causality. *J Natl Cancer Inst Monogr* 2003;31:3–13. With permission, Oxford University Press.

viral markers in 95 to 100 % of cervical cancers.[47,49] Based upon the strength of evidence of multiple studies it has been proposed that HPV DNA is a necessary cause of cervical cancer and that HPV DNA is also an environmental sufficient cause.[5] Initially it was not considered possible that HPV could be a sufficient cause, i.e. that HPV alone could induce cervical cancer, because most HPV infections are transient and do not result in significant disease. The implication was that cofactors must modulate the evolution of HPV infections that result in neoplastic lesions. However, the finding that HPV is the only environmental factor identified in approximately 25% of cases challenges the necessity for cofactors other than permissive host immunity.[5]

4.3.3 Cofactors to HPV-induced oncogenesis

Co-factors to HPV in cervical carcinogenesis may act in at least three ways: (1) by influencing the acquisition of HPV infection; (2) by increasing the risk of HPV persistence; and (3) by increasing the risk of progression from HPV infection to CIN 2,3 and cancer.[56] Nested case-control studies carried out in Denmark[57] and the UK[58] suggest that risk factors for HPV infection/CIN 1 are not necessarily the same as those for CIN3 and cancer.

4.3.3.1 Other STDs

4.3.3.1.1 Chlamydia trachomatis and cervical inflammation A number of cervical factors, such as infection by sexually transmitted pathogens other than HPV, have been proposed as cofactors that may influence the natural history of HPV infection along the pathways of persistence and progression or of resolution.[59,60] In theory, any factor that increases cervical cell turnover and repair might promote viral persistence and transformation by altering the balance between an HPV infection and host immunity. Geni-

tal tract infections with Chlamydia trachomatis and herpes simplex virus type 2 [HSV-2] both may cause intense cervical inflammation and are the most suspect cofactor STDs. After adjusting for race, marital status, parity, number of sexual partners, and history of other STDs, exposure to Chlamydia trachomatis, as assessed by serological assays, has been found to be a significant and independent risk factor (2.0 to 2.5-fold increased risk) for cervical neoplasia in some studies.[34,61–64].

Except for HSV and Chlamydia, the potential roles of other STDs as cofactors in HPV oncogenesis have not been well-evaluated. These include gonorrhea, bacterial vaginosis, cytomegalovirus and Epstein-Barr virus (EBV).[59,38] Any effects these agents may have on the development of cervical cancer, is most likely secondary to the effects of decreased mucosal immunity or reparative metaplasia induced by the acute and chronic cervicitis that frequently occurs in women with these disorders. Co-infection with HPV and C. trachomatis in cervical tissue may result in a more profound inflammatory state, as manifested by increased expression of proinflammatory cytokines over levels present during either infection alone.[65] In fact, HPV infections alone do not induce an inflammatory state.

Chronic inflammation promotes oncogenesis in cervical, vulvar and other anogenital tumors.[66] High rates of cervical cancer are found in populations with endemic and epidemic cervicitis,[59] and CIN 2/3 is more common among high-risk HPV-infected women with cervicitis.[66] Demonstration of increased cycloxygenase-2 (COX-2) expression in human cervical cancer,[67] also suggests that inflammation is linked to cervical carcinogenesis, as this is a prostaglandin G/H synthetase that is specifically upregulated in inflammatory processes.[68,69] By upregulation of COX-2, Chlamydia also may promote HPV persistence through functional down-regulation of dendritic cells, the predominant antigen-presenting cells of cell-mediated immunity.[59,70]

4.3.3.1.2 Herpes simplex virus type 2 (HSV 2)

In the 1970s, HSV 2 received considerable attention as a possible etiologic agent for invasive cervical cancer and its precursor lesions. HSV 2-associated antigens were identified by immunofluoresence in exfoliated cervical cancer cells, and the virus was identified using electron microscopy in cultured cervical carcinoma cells.[71] It was shown that HSV 2 could transform cells in culture, and HSV RNA was identified in biopsies of CIN by in situ hybridization.[72] When carefully examined, patients with cervical cancers and high-grade precursors have been found to be more likely to have antibodies against HSV 2 than do controls,[73,74] as confirmed by a large recent multi-center case-control study.[75] However, it is now accepted that HSV 2 is not the etiologic agent for cervical cancer.[76] This is because HSV 2 DNA sequences are detected using modern molecular techniques in only a small percentage (10 to 30%) of invasive cervical cancers, and prospective serologic studies have found no significant association between exposure to HSV 2 and the subsequent development of cervical disease.[76–78]

These data suggest that HSV 2 might be a cofactor for the development of cervical cancer in high-risk HPV-infected women, although the data continue to be sparse. If HSV has any role as a cofactor, the most likely mechanism involves cervical inflammation and repair leading to genetic damage and chromosomal alterations of HPV-infected cells without maintaining HSV 2 DNA within the modified host cell genome.[79]

4.3.3.2 Cofactors and variables other than STDs

High parity, smoking, and long-term OCP use are cofactors that may modulate the risk of progression from HPV infection to CIN 2/3 and to cervical cancer. The strength of the evidence ranges from strong and consistent (smoking), to moderate (parity) and less consistent (OCP use).[56] Risk factors for CIN 3 and cervical cancer are similar.[80] The strength of these associations may eventually influence screening and management recommendations, promoting closer surveillance and less expectant management for women who are multiparous, are smokers, and/or are long-term users of OCPs.[56]

4.3.3.2.1 Multiparity Multiparity has been found in most case-control studies to be associated with both cervical cancer and CIN3, with risk rising with increasing number of pregnancies. The effect of multiparity is independent of sexual behavior and socioeconomic variables.[56,81–84] For example, women from Panama, Costa Rica, Mexico, and Colombia were found to have a 5.1–fold risk of invasive cervical cancer associated with having had 14 or more births compared with zero to one birth.[83] In this study, an increase in risk with increasing parity was observed in all four countries. Similarly, a 4.4-fold relative risk for invasive cervical cancer was demonstrated among women with five or more live births compared with nulliparous women[83], a finding similar to the International Agency for Research on Cancer (IARC) pooled analysis that demonstrated an OR of 4.0 for women with 7 or more full-term pregnancies compared to that in nulliparous women.[84]

Pregnancy-induced alterations in nutritional status, the effects of hormones on the cervix or on HPV expression, an increased susceptibility to potential mutagens, or the effect of trauma at delivery could all play a role in the increased risk for cervical cancer associated with multiparity.[56] A new dynamic phase of immature metaplasia occurs with pregnancy-induced eversion of columnar epithelium. Multiparity maintains this enhancement of the transformation zone on the exocervix for many years,[85] facilitating the direct exposure to HPV and possibly other cofactors.[56] Increased permissiveness of cell-mediated immunity to HPV during pregnancy also may play a role, resulting in increased shedding of HPV.[84,86] Nutritional changes that occur during pregnancy may be important. Pregnancy is known to deplete maternal folate stores, which may be involved in immune suppression.[87] However, the similar increased risks of multiparity with OCP use suggest that hormonal influences may be of primary importance in the promotion and persistence of HPV.[56,88] Increased progesterone during pregnancy may promote integration of HPV DNA into the host cell's genome and so promote progression to malignancy.[89]

4.3.3.2.2 Cigarette smoking Among environmental cofactors, cigarette smoking is a significant and independent risk factor for the development of CIN 3 and squamous cell carcinoma of the cervix, increasing relative risk from 2 to 5-fold.[90,91] Furthermore, risk increases with increased intensity and duration of smoking (pack-years) and is more significantly associated with CIN 3 than CIN 1, suggesting that tobacco containing carcinogens promote neoplastic progression in HPV-infected cells.[56,92,93] The risk associated with cigarette smoking was originally thought to merely reflect confounding by other risk factors, particularly sexual behavior variables. However, even though cigarette smokers are more likely to begin intercourse earlier and to have more sexual partners, cigarette smoking remains as a significant risk factor for squamous cell carcinoma of the cervix after adjusting for sexual variables.[90,91] Even three hours of passive smoking (second-hand smoke) per day may confer an increased risk of cervical abnormalities.[94]

Two mechanisms have been postulated for the increased risk imposed by cigarette smoking. The first is secretion of chemical carcinogens, such as cotinine, nicotine, phenols, and hydrocarbons, at highly concentrated levels into the cervical mucus of women who smoke.[95-97] Cigarette smoke condensate has been proven to induce malignant transformation of HPV 16-immortalized human endocervical cells,[56,98] suggesting that a direct mitogenic effect causing DNA damage is likely to be responsible for malignant transformation of cervical cells by tobacco carcinogens, just as it is for bronchial, bladder, oral and other areas with high exposure to these carcinogens.

The second proposed mechanism is a reduction in the density and functionality of antigen-presenting Langerhan's cells in the cervices of women who smoke. Reduced Langerhan's cells decreases the host's ability to mount an effective local immune response against HPV,[99-101] thereby allowing HPV infections to become persistent. Smokers maintain cervical HPV infections significantly longer and have a lower probability of clearing oncogenic infections than women who never smoked.[56,102] One interventional study has correlated reduction in the size of minor grade lesions with cessation of smoking.[103] Although both mechanisms may contribute to the increased risk of cervical cancer, the secretion of carcinogens into cervical mucus is probably unimportant in the absence of HPV infection, since celibate women who smoke are not at increased risk.[90]

4.3.3.2.3 Oral contraceptive pills (OCPs) An increased incidence of squamous cell carcinoma of the cervix has been observed in women taking oral contraceptives (OCPs) in some, but not all, studies.[104-107] The strongest evidence comes from an IARC multicenter case control study demonstrating only a moderate association with cancer risk (OR=1.4).[107] However, there was a strong dose-response relationship with duration of use.[56] When compared with patients who have never used OCPs, those who had used them for less than 5 years did not have increased risk of cervical cancer (odds ratio [OR] 0.73), but longer-term use of oral contraceptives in HPV-positive women increased the OR to 2.82 for 5 to 9 years and to 4.03 for 10 or more years. These risks did not vary by time since first or last use. These data controlled for possible confounding factors, including higher frequency of cytologic screening among pill users, which might decrease the risk of cervical cancer by early detection and treatment of precursor lesions; lower use of barrier contraceptives, which might increase exposure to HPV; and potentially greater

numbers of sexual partners among pill users.[56] Therefore, it is now generally accepted that use of OCPs conveys a measurable increase in risk for squamous cell carcinoma, and perhaps an even greater risk of developing invasive adenocarcinoma of the cervix.[108] It is less clear whether a similar association of OCPs with CIN exists. Although several studies have failed to find an increased risk for CIN in women with long-term OCP usage, others observed an increased incidence of all grades of CIN.[109-113] The only prospective study of OCP use in women with CIN3 and cervical cancer did not find an association.[92]

OCPs have several physiologic effects on cervical epithelium that might explain their association with cervical neoplasia. OCPs produce an eversion of the columnar epithelium, thus activating HPV-vulnerable immature squamous metaplasia. OCPs also appear to exert a weak immunomodulatory effect and to cause megaloblastic changes in cervical epithelial cells by decreasing blood folate levels.[114] Both of these effects have been associated with an increased incidence of CIN and invasive cervical cancer.[89] Hormone-related mechanisms also may promote progression from CIN to invasion by promoting integration of HPV DNA into the host genome.[56] Integration results in deregulation of E6 and E7 expression,[46] and estradiol may stimulate the transcription of these open reading frames, thereby promoting malignant transformation.[115] OCPs also may promote the expression of HPV oncoproteins.[88] Steroid hormone response elements are present in the HPV genome, and both glucocorticoids and progesterone act as transcriptional promoters for several genital HPV types.[116,117]

Progesterone has also been shown to increase the efficiency of transformation of rodent cells by HPV 16 in vitro.[118] Taken together, these effects suggest that the weak association observed in epidemiological studies between OCP use and cervical cancer and its precursor lesions has biologic plausibility. However, the small increased risk associated with OCPs is not felt to warrant their abandonment since the morbidity associated with the increased risk of pregnancy in women who discontinue hormonal contraceptives greatly outweighs the risk of developing cervical cancer. In contrast, women on hormonal contraceptives in countries without cervical cancer screening programs may be at greater risk, intensifying the urgency to implement screening for all women.[107]

4.3.3.2.4 Barrier methods of contraception Use of barrier methods of contraception, including diaphragms and male condoms, has been associated with a reduced risk of cervical cancer.[119-121] However, the magnitude of the effect of barrier contraceptives has been small. Since condoms are only partially effective in reducing the sexual transmission of HPV, they may only partially reduce invasive cervical cancer risk. One recent meta-analysis of 20 studies did not demonstrate consistent evidence that condom use reduces a woman's risk of becoming HPV DNA-positive.[120] However, risks for genital warts, CIN 2 or 3, and invasive cervical cancer were somewhat reduced. The protective effects of diaphragm usage may be attributable to the concurrent use of spermicides, which can reduce the risk of sexual transmission of a number of infectious agents, including some viruses.[121]

4.3.3.2.5 Nutritional factors Changes in nutritional factors, particularly reduction in serum levels of vitamin C, vitamin A, folate, and carotinoids have been suggested to increase risk of invasive cervical cancer. However, the majority of studies examining the relationship of diet and nutrient status with cervical neoplasia did not control for HPV or for factors such as smoking and oral contraceptive use that are related to cervical cancer.[59] Only six studies have controlled for HPV. These have demonstrated an inverse association between serum beta-carotene and risk for CIN[122-124] and invasive cervical cancer.[59,125-127] Carotenoids other than beta-carotene have also been inversely associated with invasive cervical cancer.[125-129] Vitamin E concentrations also have been shown to be inversely associated with risk for CIN[127,128,130,131] and invasive cervical cancer,[129] but other studies have not found this relationship.[122,132]

Despite the apparent increased risk for cervical neoplasia with decreased dietary and serum levels of carotinoids and vitamin E, interventional chemoprevention trials have failed to demonstrate benefit.[133] Only one topical retinoic acid trial resulted in increased resolution or improvement of CIN.[134] Two folic acid and five beta-carotene Phase 3 trials have failed to show a treatment effect.[59] However, several problems inherent to all interventional trials may have adversely affected the results. Possible issues include not administering the nutrient at the critical point in oncogenesis, treating for too short a period of time with single nutrients, and using pharmacological rather than dietary concentrations of the nutrient.[59] If anti-oxidant nutrients reduce the risk of cervical neoplasia, the mechanism may be through reduction in the risk of persistence of HPV. Among young U.S. women, dietary lutein (a carotinoid), vitamin E, and circulating concentrations of lycopene have been shown to be inversely associated with decreased high-risk HPV persistence.[133] Additionally, lower serum beta-carotene, beta-cryptoxanthin, and lutein concentrations were associated with HPV persistence[134] as was vitamin C.[135] The majority of the data suggest that some dietary carotinoids may influence the natural history of HPV infection, however, not all studies have consistently found this association.[136]

The possibility that anti-oxidants reduce HPV persistence is biologically plausible.[59] Tipping the oxidant: anti-oxidant balance in favor of reactive oxidants, as occurs with smoking and inflammation, may directly promote HPV transcriptional activity. In addition to directly damaging cellular proteins and DNA, reactive oxygen species appear to have a central role in cell signaling by activating transcription factors, cell proliferation, and by suppressing apoptosis.[137] These activities could promote HPV viral replication (viral load), transcriptional activity (expression of HPV 16 E6 and E7 proteins), cell proliferation and accumulation of mutations by inhibiting apoptosis, all pivotal events in cervical carcinogenesis.[59]

4.3.3.2.6 Immunosuppression and HIV A strong association between HIV, HPV and cervical neoplasia has been documented in a meta-analysis of the literature,[138] and other studies have confirmed similarly increased risk for HPV and cervical neoplasia with both primary immunodeficiency and iatrogenic immunosuppression.[8,139,140] The most likely mechanism for this association is the inability of immuno-compromised women to clear HPV, increasing susceptibility to HPV and oncogenicity. Additionally, a direct molecular interaction between HPV and HIV may be contributory.[50] However, HIV and HPV viruses do not co-infect cervical epithelial cells or co-localize in cervical tissues. Therefore, any direct interaction between the two viruses is likely to be mediated by extracellular factors.[141]

Female renal transplant recipients have a 16-fold increased incidence of CIN, genital warts and other lower genital tract and anal neoplasia.[142,143] Moreover, anal warts and other anal HPV-induced disease are more common and persistent in men who are HIV-infected than in men who do not have HIV, with the rate of anal disease varying inversely with the CD4 level.[144] In HIV-infected women, the prevalence of cervical HPV infection has ranged from two to four times greater than that observed in HIV-uninfected control women.[141,145-148] These increases in prevalence are observed for all types of HPV.[146] Additionally, HPV infections are significantly more likely to be persistent in HIV-infected women and the prevalence and severity of HPV-associated lesions, including CIN, is higher.[149,150] The risk for developing CIN increases as levels of immunosuppression increase. In HIV-infected women, intraepithelial disease is typically multifocal, demonstrating high rates of persistence after standard therapy.[148-150] Although invasive cervical cancer has been designated an AIDS-defining illness, associations between HIV-infection and invasive cervical cancer are less strong than are associations with CIN,[151,152] but women infected with HIV-1 do have a two- to three-fold risk for invasive cervical cancer compared with women in the general population.[153,154] Increased rates of invasive squamous cell carcinomas of the anus have also been reported in HIV-infected homosexual males, as have vulvar cancers in HIV-infected women.[145,155]

Subtle alterations in immune responses also may be an important risk factor for cervical neoplasia. Some women have chronic, recalcitrant HPV-associated lesions without having clinical immuno-suppression or other manifestations of a malfunction of their immune system.[156] Although these women have normal immune responses in all other respects, a significant reduction of the suppressor-cytotoxic/helper T-cell ratio has been observed in some, suggesting that these women have an idiopathic syndrome associated with a reduced immuno-competence to HPV. The finding of familiar clustering of these women suggests the possibility that the syndrome has a genetic component.

4.3.3.2.7 Genetic factors

Some of the differences in rates of cervical cancer observed between whites, African-Americans, and Native Americans may be attributable to genetic differences. The critical role of the human leukocyte antigen (HLA) system in presenting peptides to antigen-specific T-cell receptors may explain why only some HPV-infected women progress to cervical cancer.[157] An association between specific HLA haplotypes and cervical cancer has been demonstrated in a number of studies.[157-164] Some class I HLA antigens are down-regulated in both preinvasive and invasive lesions associated with HPV.[50] For example, increased risks of cervical squamous cell carcinoma have been shown to be associated with DRB1*1001, DRB1*1101, and DQB1*0301, and decreased risks have been associated with DRB1*0301 and DRB1*13.[157] These results add to the evidence that certain HLA class II allele combinations, or genes linked to them, make some women more susceptible to squamous cell carcinoma. Three large studies from the United States and Costa Rica noted an increased risk for cervical neoplasia among women with HLA-CW*0202.[158] These findings support the hypothesis that a single allele may be sufficient to confer protection against cervical neoplasia. Because natural killer cells (NK) have been shown to be influenced by HLA-C and its receptors, the role played by HLA-haplotypes in cervical neoplasia may reflect a direct effect on the efficiency of the immune response to HPV.[158]

4.4 Summary: Epidemiologic Evidence for the Etiology of Cervical Cancer

The evidence implicating specific HPV types in the etiology of cervical cancer is now strong enough to establish a causative role for HPV.[46-48] Other risk factors for cervical cancer, such as a history of other STDs, most likely represent surrogate markers for increased sexual exposure and risk of exposure to HPV. Immature squamous metaplasia within the cervical transformation zone appears to be the epithelium at greatest risk for cellular transformation by HPV. Metaplasia appears to be a maladaptive response to chronic irritation in many organs, but in the cervix, metaplasia is a ubiquitous finding among sexually active women.[165,166] Risk for incident LSIL has been shown to be related to the rate of active metaplasia rather than to the size of the transformation zone.[167] This suggests that dynamic changes in the transformation zone over time may facilitate the cellular manifestations of HPV infection.[165] One mechanism proposed for the association between higher parity and cancer risk is the repeated eversion of endocervical cells onto the portio increasing exposure of the transformation zone to carcinogenic influences. Exposure of this epithelium to HPV establishes its potential for subsequently developing into a cervical cancer precursor. The most active phases of metaplasia occur during fetal life, in the adolescent years immediately following puberty, and during pregnancy,[166] which explains why both early age at first intercourse and multiparity are risk factors for cervical neoplasia.

Cervical neoplasia originates as a complex interplay between HPV and the immature squamous metaplastic epithelium of the cervical transformation zone. Exposure to HPV is an extremely common event, especially in sexually active young women.[51,167] However, despite the fact that HPV infections are common in young women who are at greatest risk for having immature squamous metaplasia, invasive cervical cancer occurs relatively uncommonly, even in unscreened women, suggesting that additional events or cofactors are required for the development of cervical cancer.

The role of cofactors in the development of cervical neoplasia is just beginning to be understood. As described in Chapter 5, the natural history of most HPV infections is exposure, followed by a variable period of non-expression, then the development of a productive viral infection for many that is not always associated with a lesion (i.e., a genital wart or CIN), followed by the induction of host-cell immunity against HPV, resolution of the lesion, and development of long term HPV-specific immune suppression or clearance. The eventual inability of even the most sensitive tests to detect HPV in most women indicates that clearance of the HPV infection may be a possibility. In contrast, the latter events do not occur in women who develop invasive cervical cancer. Instead, HPV infections become persistent, and other, probably random events occur that help promote malignancy.[168,169] Cofactors such as cigarette smoking, nutritional factors, and infection with HIV appear to act by impairing the ability of mucosal cellular immunity to permanently suppress or eliminate HPV. Impaired immune surveillance may permit the long-term persistence of infection required for the development of invasive cancer. Other cofactors, such as oral contraceptives, may directly alter the natural history of HPV infections. The commonness of this virus and the relative rarity of these cancers highlight the complexity of the natural history of HPV. The comprehensive understanding of HPV so recently established enables us to tell the story of the natural history of HPV, but as in the dialogue between the King and the white rabbit in Lewis Carroll's wonderful "Alice in Wonderland," we might ask: "Where shall I begin, please, your majesties?" Like the King we will say, "Begin at the beginning and go until you come to the end. Then stop!"

References

1. Ferlay J, Bray F, Pisani P, Parkin D M, editors. Globocan 2000: Cancer incidence, *Mortality and Prevalence Worldwide,* Version 1.0. IARC CancerBase No. 5. IARC Press; 2001.

2. Pisani P, Parkin D M, Ferlay J. Estimates of the worldwide mortality from eighteen major cancers in 1985. Implications for prevention and projections of future burden. *Int J Cancer* 1993;55:891–903.

3. Bosch F X, de Sanjose S, Castellsague X, Munoz N. Geographical and social patterns of cervical cancer incidence. In: Franco E, Monsonego J, eds. *New Developments in Cervical Cancer Screening and Prevention.* London: Blackwell Science Ltd, 1997:23–33.

4. Cancer Incidence in Five Continents, vol. VII. Lyon: International Agency for Research on Cancer; 1997.

5. Bosch F X, De Sanjose S. Chapter 1: human papillomavirus and cervical cancer-burden and assessment of causality. *J Natl Cancer Inst Monogr.* 2003;31:3–13.

6. Parkin D M, Pisani P, Ferlay J. Estimates of the worldwide incidence of eighteen major cancers in 1985. *Int J Cancer* 1993;54:594–606.

7. SEER Program - National Cancer Institute, USA. http://www-seerimsncinihgov/ScientificSystems/ 1999.

8. Farmery E, Gray J A M. Report of the first five years of the NHS cervical screening program. Oxford: National Coordinating Network, 1994.

9. Smith H O, Tiffany M F, Qualls C R, Key C R. The rising incidence of adenocarcinoma relative to squamous cell carcinoma of the uterine cervix in the United States-a 24-year population-based study. *Gynecol Oncol* 2000 78:97–105.

10. Vizcaino A P, Moreno V, Bosch F X, Muñoz, N, Barros-Dios X M, Parkin D M. International trends in the incidence of cervical cancer: I. Adenocarcinoma and adenosquamous cell carcinomas. *Int J Cancer* 1998;75:536–45.

11. Vizcaino A P, Moreno V, Bosch F X, Muñoz N, Barros-Dios X M, Borras J, et al. International trends in incidence of cervical cancer: II. Squamous-cell carcinoma. *Int J Cancer* 2000;86:429–35.

12. Sasieni P, Adams J. Changing rates of adenocarcinoma and adenosquamous carcinoma of the cervix in England. *Lancet* 2001;357:1490–3.

13. Hakama M. Screening for cervical cancer: experience in Nordic countries. In: Franco E and Monsonego J, eds. New Developments in Cervical Cancer Screening and Prevention. Blackwell Science, London. 1997;190–9.

14. Hakama M, Magnus K, Petterson F et al. Effect of organized screening on the risk of cervical cancer in Nordic countries. In: Miller A, Chamberlain J, Day Day N, Hakama M, Prorok P, eds. *Cancer Screening.* Cambridge; Cambridge University Press 1991:153–62.

15. Hristova L, Hakama M. Effect of screening for cancer in the Nordic countries on death, costs and quality of life up to the year 2017. *Acta Oncologica* 1997;36(suppl. 9):1–60.

16. Department of Health. Cervical screening program in England. 1994–95 to 1996–97. London DoH. 1996–97 (Statistical Bulletin 1996/3, 1996/26, 1997/27).

17. Quinn M, Babb P, Jones J, Allen E, UK Association of Cancer Registries. Effect of screening on incidence and mortality from cancer of the cervix in England: evaluation based on routinely collected statistics. *BMJ* 1999;318:904–8.

18. Li H, Jin S, Xu H, Thomas D B. The decline in the mortality rates of cervical cancer and a plausible explanation in Shandong, China. *Int J Epidemiol* 2000;29:398–404.

19. del Carmen M G, Montz F J, Bristow R E, Bovicelli A, Cornelison T, Trimble E. Ethnic differences in patterns of care of stage 1A(1) and stage 1A(2) cervical cancer: a SEER database study. *Gynecol Oncol* 1999;75:113–7.

20. Cox J T. Management of cervical intraepithelial neoplasia. *Lancet.* 1999 Mar 13;353:857–9.

21. Beral V. Cancer of the cervix: a sexually-transmitted disease? *Lancet* 1974;i:1037–40.

22. Kessler II. Cervical cancer epidemiology in historical perspective. *J Reprod Med* 1974;12:173–85.

23. Bosch FX, Castellsague X, Munoz N, et al. Male sexual behavior and human papillomavirus DNA: key risk factors for cervical cancer in Spain. *J Natl Cancer Inst* 1996;88:1060–7.

24. de Sanjose S, Bosch FX, Munoz N, et al. Socioeconomic differences in cervical cancer: two case-control studies in Colombia and Spain. *Am J Public Health* 1996;86:1532–8.

25. Cuello C, Correa P, Haenszel W. Socio-economic class differences in cancer incidence in Cali, Colombia. *Int J Cancer* 1982;29:637–43.

26. Schairer C, Brinton LA, Devesa SS, Ziegler RG, Fraumeni JF, Jr. Racial differences in the risk of invasive squamous-cell cervical cancer. *Cancer Causes Control* 1991;2:283–90.

27. Monograph S. Racial/ethnic patterns of cancer in the United States, 1988–1992. Bethesda, MD: National Cancer Institute, 1995.

28. Lynge E, Jensen OM. Cohort trends in incidence of cervical cancer in Denmark in relation to gonorrheal infection. *Acta Obstet Gynecol Scand* 1985;64.

29. Herrero R, Grinoton LA, Reeves WC, et al. Sexual behavior, venereal diseases, hygiene practices, and invasive cervical cancer in high risk population. *Cancer* 1990; 65:380–6.

30. Brinton LA, Tashima KT, Lehman HF, et al. Epidemiology of cervical cancer by cell type. *Cancer Res* 1987;47:1706–11.

31. La Vecchia C, Franceschi S, DeCarli A, et al. Sexual factors, venereal diseases, and the risk of intraepithelial and invasive cervical neoplasia. *Cancer* 1986;58:935–41.

32. Slattery ML, Overall JC, Abbott TM, French TK, Robison LM, Gardner J. Sexual activity, contraception, genital infections, and cervical cancer: support for a sexually transmitted disease hypothesis. *Am J Epidemiol* 1989;130:248–58.

33. Chichareon S, Herrero R, Munoz N, et al. Risk factors for cervical cancer in Thailand: a case-control study. *J Natl Cancer Inst* 1998;90:50–7.

34. Wallin KL, Wiklund F, Luostarinen T, Angstrom T, Anttila T, Bergman F, et al. A population-based prospective study of Chlamydia trachomatis infection and cervical carcinoma. *Int J Cancer* 2002;101:371–4.

35. Peters RK, Chao A, Mack TM, Thomas D, Bernstein L, Henderson BE. Increased frequency of adenocarcinoma of the uterine cervix in young women in Los Angeles County. *J Natl Cancer Inst* 1986;76:423–8.

36. Munoz N, Bosch FX, de Sanjose S, et al. Risk factors for cervical intraepithelial neoplasia grade III/carcinoma in situ in Spain and Colombia. *Cancer Epidemiol Biomarkers Prev* 1993;2:423–31.

37. Kessler H. Etiological concepts in cervical carcinogenesis. *Gynecol Oncol* 1981;12:S7–24.

38. Brinton LA. Epidemiology of cervical cancer—an overview. In: Munoz N, Bosch FX, Shah K, Meheus A, eds. *The epidemiology of cervical cancer and human papillomavirus*. Vol. 119. Lyon: IARC Scientific Publications, 1992:3–23.

39. Brock KE, Berry G, Brinton LA, et al. Sexual, reproductive and contraceptive risk factors for carcinoma-in-situ of the uterine cervix in Sydney. *Med J Aust* 1989;150:125–30.

40. Handley WS. The prevention of cancer. *Lancet* 1936;i:987–91.

41. Skegg DCG, Corwin PA, Paul C, Doll R. Importance of the male factor in cancer of the cervix. *Lancet* 1982;ii:581–3.

42. de Sanjosé S, Bosch FX, Muñoz N, Shah K. Social differences in sexual behavior and cervical cancer. In: Kogevinas M, Pearce N, Susser M, Boffetta P, editors. *Social Inequalities and cancer.* Lyon: IARC; 1997. p. 309–18.

43. Castellsague X, Bosch FX, Munoz N, Meijer CJ, Shah KV, de Sanjose S, et al. The International Agency for Research on Cancer Multicenter Cervical Cancer Study Group. Male circumcision, penile human papillomavirus infection, and cervical cancer in female partners. *N Engl J Med* 2002;346:1105–12.

44. Rotkin ID. Relation of adolescent coitus to cervical cancer risk. *JAMA* 1962;179:486–91.

45. Bosch FX, Manos MM, Munoz N, et al. Prevalence of human papillomavirus in cervical cancer: a worldwide perspective. International biological study on cervical cancer (IBSCC) Study Group. *J Natl Cancer Inst* 1995;87:779–80.

46. IARC. Human Papillomaviruses. IARC monographs on the evaluation of carcinogenic risks to humans. Vol. 64. Lyon: IARC, 1995:407.

47. Munoz N. Human papillomavirus and cancer: the epidemiological evidence. *J Clin Virol* 2000;19:1–5.

48. Bosch FX, Lorincz A, Munoz N, Meijer CJ, Shah KV. The causal relation between human papillomavirus and cervical cancer. *J Clin Pathol* 2002;55:244–65.

49. Walboomers JMM, Jacobs MV, Manos MM, Bosch FX, Kummer JA, Shah KV, et al. Human papillomavirus is a necessary cause of invasive cervical cancer worldwide. *J Pathol* 1999;189:1–3.

50. ROC Background Document for HPV: Genital mucosal types. ntp-server.niehs.nih.gov/newhomeroc/roc11/HPV_RG2_Public.pdf

51. Ho GYF, Bierman R, Beardsley L, Chang CJ, Burk RD. Natural history of cervicovaginal papillomavirus infection in young women. *New Eng J Med* 1998;338:423–8.

52. Woodman CB, Collins S, Winter H, Bailey A, Ellis J, Prior P, et al. Natural history of cervical human papillomavirus infection in young women: a longitudinal cohort study. *Lancet* 2001;357:1831–36.

53. Franco, EL, Villa LL, Sobrinho JP, Prado JM, Rousseau MC, Desy M, et al. 1999. Epidemiology of acquisition and clearance of cervical human papillomavirus infection in women from a high-risk area for cervical cancer. *J Infect Dis* 180:1415–23.

54. Minkoff H, Feldman J, DeHovitz J, Landesman S, Burk R. A longitudinal study of human papillomavirus carriage in human immunodeficiency virus-infected and human immunodeficiency virus-uninfected women. *Am J Obstet Gynecol* 1998;178:982–6.

55. Sellors J W, Mahony J B, Kaczorowski J, Lytwyn A, Bangura H, Chong S, et al. Prevalence and predictors of human papillomavirus infection in women in Ontario, Canada. *CMAJ* 2000;163(5):503–8.

56. Castellsague X, Munoz N. Chapter 3: cofactors in human papillomavirus carcinogenesis-role of parity, oral contraceptives, and tobacco smoking. *J Natl Cancer Inst Monogr.* 2003;2003(31):20–8.

57. Kruger-Kjaer S, van den Brule A J, Svare E I, Engholm G, Sherman M E, Poll P A, et al. Different risk factor patterns for high-grade and low-grade intraepithelial lesions on the cervix among HPV-positive and HPV-negative young women. *Int J Cancer* 1998;76:613–9.

58. Deacon J M, Evans C D, Yule R, Desai M, Binns W, Taylor C, et al. Sexual behaviour and smoking as determinants of cervical HPV infection and of CIN3 among those infected: a case-control study nested within the Manchester cohort. *Br J Cancer* 2000;83:1565–72.

59. Castle P E, Giuliano A R. Chapter 4: genital tract infections, cervical inflammation, and antioxidant nutrients—assessing their roles as human papillomavirus cofactors. *J Natl Cancer Inst Monogr.* 2003;:29–34.

60. Schmauz R, Okong P, de Villiers E M, Dennin R, Brade L, Lwanga S K, Owor R. Multiple infections in cases of cervical cancer from a high-incidence area in tropical Africa. *Int J Cancer* 1989;43:805–9.

61. Schachter J, Hill E C, King E B. Chlamydia trachomatis and cervical neoplasia. *JAMA* 1982;248:2134.

62. Koskela P, Anttila T, Bjorge T, Brunsvig A, Dillner J, Hakama M, et al. Chlamydia trachomatis infection as a risk factor for invasive cervical cancer. *Int J Cancer* 2000;85:35–9.

63. Smith J S, Munoz N, Herrero R, Eluf-Neto J, Ngelangel C, Franceschi S, et al. Evidence for Chlamydia trachomatis as a human papillomavirus cofactor in the etiology of invasive cervical cancer in Brazil and the Philippines. *J Infect Dis* 2002;185:324–31.

64. Anttila T, Saikku P, Koskela P, Bloigu A, Dillner J, Ikaheimo I, et al. Serotypes of Chlamydia trachomatis and risk for development of cervical squamous cell carcinoma. *JAMA* 2001;285:47–51.

65. Rasmussen S J, Eckmann L, Quayle A J, Shen L, Zhang Y X, Anderson D J, et al. Secretion of proinflammatory cytokines by epithelial cells in response to Chlamydia infection suggests a central role for epithelial cells in chlamydial pathogenesis. *J Clin Invest* 1997;99:77–87.

66. Castle P E, Hillier S L, Rabe L K, Hildesheim A, Herrero R, Bratti M C, et al. An association of cervical inflammation with high-grade cervical neoplasia in women infected with oncogenic human papillomavirus (HPV). *Cancer Epidemiol Biomarkers Prev* 2001;10:1021–7.

67. Kulkarni S, Rader J S, Zhang F, Liapis H, Koki A T, Masferrer J L, et al. Cyclooxygenase-2 is overexpressed in human cervical cancer. *Clin Cancer Res* 2001;7:429–34.

68. Chan T A. Nonsteroidal anti-inflammatory drugs, apoptosis, and colon-cancer chemoprevention. *Lancet Oncol* 2002;3:166–74.

69. Thun M J, Henley S J, Patrono C. Nonsteroidal anti-inflammatory drugs as anticancer agents: mechanistic, pharmacologic, and clinical issues. *J Natl Cancer Inst* 2002;94:252–66.

70. Harizi H, Juzan M, Pitard V, Moreau J F, Gualde N. Cyclooxygenase-2-issued prostaglandin e(2) enhances the production of endogenous IL-10, which down-regulates dendritic cell functions. *J Immunol* 2002;168:2255–63.

71. Royston I, Aurelian L. Immunofluorescent detection of herpesvirus antigens in exfoliated cells from human cervical carcinoma. *Proc Natl Acad Sci, USA* 1970;67:204.

72. Galloway D A, McDougall J K. The oncogenic potential of herpes simplex viruses: evidence for a "hit and run" mechanism. *Nature* 1983;302:21–3.

73. Dale G E, Coleman R M, Best J M, et al. Class-specific herpes simplex virus antibodies in sera and cervical secretions from patients with cervical neoplasia: a multi-group comparison. *Epidem Inf* 1988;100:455–65.

74. Hildesheim A, Mann V, Brinton L A, Szklo M, Reeves W C, Rawls W E. Herpes simplex virus type 2: a possible interaction with human papillomavirus types 16/18 in the development of invasive cervical cancer. *Int J Cancer* 1991;49:335–40.

75. Smith J S, Herrero R, Bosetti C, Munoz N, Bosch F X, Eluf-Neto J, Castellsague X, Meijer C J, Van den Brule A J, Franceschi S, Ashley R; International Agency for Research on Cancer (IARC) Multicentric Cervical Cancer Study Group. Herpes simplex virus-2 as a human papillomavirus cofactor in the etiology of invasive cervical cancer. *J Natl Cancer Inst.* 2002;94:1604–13.

76. Lehtinen M, Koskela P, Jellum E, Bloigu A, Anttila T, Hallmans G, et al. Herpes simplex virus and risk of cervical cancer: a longitudinal, nested case-control study in the Nordic countries. *Am J Epidemiol* 2002;156:687–92.

77. Vonka V, Kanka J, Roth Z. Herpes simplex type 2 virus and cervical neoplasia. *Adv Cancer Res* 1987;49:149–91.

78. Di Luca D, Costa S, Monini P, et al. Search for human papillomavirus, herpes simplex virus and c-myc oncogene in human genital tumors. *Int J Cancer* 1989;43:507–7.

79. DiPaolo J A, Jones C. The role of Herpes Simplex 2 in the development of HPV-positive cervical carcinoma. *Papillomavirus Reports* 1999;10:1–8.

80. Moreno V, Munoz N, Bosch F X, de Sanjose S, Gonzalez LC, Tafur L, et al. Risk factors for progression of cervical intraepithelial neoplasm grade III to invasive cervical cancer. *Cancer Epidemiol Biomarkers Prev* 1995;4:459–67.

81. Brinton L A, Reeves W C, Brenes M M, et al. Parity as a risk factor for cervical cancer. *Am J Epidemiol* 1989;130:486–96.

82. Ngelangel C, Munoz N, Bosch F X, et al. Causes of cervical cancer in the Philippines: a case-control study. *J Natl Cancer Inst* 1998;90:43–9.

83. Parazzini F, La Vecchia C, Negri E, Cecchetti G, Fedele L. Reproductive factors and the risk of invasive and intraepithelial cervical neoplasia. *Br J Cancer* 1989;59:805–9.

84. Munoz N, Franceschi S, Bosetti C, Moreno V, Herrero R, Smith J S, et al. Role of parity and human papillomavirus in cervical cancer: the IARC multicentric case-control study. *Lancet* 2002;359:1093–101.

85. Autier P, Coibion M, Huet F, Grivegnee A R. Transformation zone location and intraepithelial neoplasia of the cervix uteri. *Br J Cancer* 1996;74:488–90.

86. Schneider A, Hotz M, Gissman L. Prevalence of genital HPV infections in pregnant women. *Int J Cancer* 1987;40:198.

87. Butterworth C E J, Hatch K D, Macaluso M, et al. Folate deficiency and cervical dysplasia. *JAMA* 1992;267:528–33.

88. Moreno V, Bosch F X, Munoz N, Meijer C J, Shah K V, Walboomers J M, et al. Effect of oral contraceptives on risk of cervical cancer in women with human papillomavirus infection: the IARC multicentric case-control study. *Lancet* 2002;359:1085–92.

89. Mittal R, Tsutsumi K, Pater A, Pater M M. Human papillomavirus type 16 expression in cervical keratinocytes: role of progesterone and glucocarticoid hormones. *Obstet Gynecol* 1993;81:5–12.

90. Castellsague X, Bosch F X, Munoz N. Environmental co-factors in HPV carcinogenesis. *Virus Res* 2002;89:191–9.

91. Szarewski A, Cuzick J. Smoking and cervical neoplasia: a review of the evidence. *J Epidemiol Biostat* 1998;3:229–56.

92. Castle P E, Wacholder S, Lorincz A T, Scott D R, Sherman M E, Glass A G, et al. A prospective study of high-grade cervical neoplasia risk among human papillomavirus-infected women. *J Natl Cancer Inst* 2002;94:1406–14.

93. Ho G Y, Kadish A S, Burk R D, Basu J, Palan P R, Mikhail M, et al. HPV 16 and cigarette smoking as risk factors for high-grade cervical intra-epithelial neoplasia. *Int J Cancer* 1998;78:281–5.

94. Slattery M L, Robison L M, Schuman K L, et al. Cigarette smoking and exposure to passive smoke are risk factors for cervical cancer. *JAMA* 1989;261:1593–8.

95. Schiffman M, Brinton L, Holly E, et al. Regarding mutagenic mucus in cervix of smokers. *J Natl Cancer Inst* 1987;78:590–1.

96. Schiffman M H, Haley N J, Felton J S, et al. Biochemical epidemiology of cervical neoplasia: measuring cigarette smoke constituents in the cervix. *Cancer Res* 1987;47:3886–8.

97. Prokopczyk B, Cox J E, Hoffmann D, Waggoner S E. Identification of tobacco-specific carcinogen in the cervical mucus of smokers and nonsmokers. *J Natl Cancer Inst* 1997;89:868–73.

98. Yang X, Jin G, Nakao Y, Rahimtula M, Pater M M, Pater A. Malignant transformation of HPV 16-immortalized human endocervical cells by cigarette smoke condensate and characterization of multistage carcinogenesis. *Int J Cancer* 1996;65:338–44.

99. Barton S E, Hollingworth A, Maddox P H, et al. Possible cofactors in the etiology of cervical intraepithelial neoplasia: an immunopathologic study. *J Reprod Med* 1989;34:613–6.

100. Barton S E, Maddox P H, Jenkins D, Edwards R, Cuzick J, Singer A. Effect of cigarette smoking on cervical epithelial immunity: a mechanism for neoplastic change? *Lancet* 1988:652–4.

101. Poppe W A, Ide P S, Drijkoningen M P, Lauweryns J M, Van Assche F A. Tobacco smoking impairs the local immunosurveillance in the uterine cervix. An immunohistochemical study. *Gynecol Obstet Invest* 1995;39:34–8.

102. Giulian A R, Sedjo R L, Roe D J, Harri R, Baldwi S, Papenfuss M R, Abrahamsen M, Inserra P. Clearance of oncogenic human papillomavirus (HPV) infection: effect of smoking (United States). *Cancer Causes Control* 2002;13:839–46.

103. Szarewski A, Jarvis M J, Sasieni P, Anderson M, Edwards R, Steele S J, et al. Effect of smoking cessation on cervical lesion size. *Lancet* 1996;347:941–3.

104. Beral V, Hermon C, Munoz N, Devesa S S. Cervical cancer. *Cancer Surv* 1994;19/20:265–85.

105. Irwin K L, Rosero-Bixby L, Oberle M W, et al. Oral contraceptives and cervical cancer risk in Costa Rica. Detection bias or causal association? *JAMA* 1988;259:59–64.

106. Brinton L A. Oral contraceptives and cervical neoplasia. *Contraception* 1991;43:581–95.

107. Moreno V, Bosch F X, Munoz N, Meijer C J, Shah K V, Walboomers J M, et al. International Agency for Research on Cancer. Multicentric Cervical Cancer Study Group. Effect of oral contraceptives on risk of cervical cancer in women with human papillomavirus infection: the IARC multicentric case-control study. *Lancet* 2002;359:1085–92.

108. Chilvers C, Mant D, Pike M C. Cervical adenocarcinoma and oral contraceptives. *BMJ* 1987;295:1446–7.

109. Parazzini F, LaVecchia C, Negri E, Fedele L, Franceschi S, Gallotta L. Risk factors for cervical intraepithelial neoplasia. *Cancer* 1992;69:2276–82.

110. Cuzick J, Singer A, De Stavola B L, Chomet J. Case-control study of risk factors for cervical intraepithelial neoplasia in young women. *Eur J Cancer* 1990;26:684–90.

111. Jones C J, Brinton L A, Hamman R F, et al. Risk factors for in situ cervical cancer: results from a case-control study. *Cancer Res* 1990;50:3657–62.

112. Negrini B P, Schiffman M H, Kurman R J, et al. Oral contraceptive use, human papillomavirus infection, and risk of early cytological abnormalities of the cervix. *Cancer Res* 1990;50:4670–5.

113. Lacey J V Jr, Brinton L A, Abbas F M, Barnes W A, Gravitt P E, Greenberg M D, et al. Oral contraceptives as risk factors for cervical adenocarcinomas and squamous cell carcinomas. *Cancer Epidemiol Biomarkers Prev* 1999;8:1079–85.

114. Whitehead N, Reyner F, Lindenbaum J. Megaloblastic changes in the cervical epithelium. Association of oral contraceptive therapy and reversal with folic acid. *JAMA* 1973;266:1421.

115. Mitrani-Rosenbaum S, Tsvieli R, Tur-Kaspa R. Oestrogen stimulates differential transcription of human papillomavirus type 16 in SiHa cervical carcinoma cells. *J Gen Virol* 1989;70:2227–32.

116. Pater M M, Mittal R, Pater A. Role of steroid hormones in potentiating transformation of cervical cells by human papillomaviruses. *Trends Microbiol* 1994;2:229–34.

117. Pater A, Belaguli N S, Pater M M. Glucocorticoid requirement for growth of human papillomavirus 16-transformed primary rat kidney epithelial cells: correlation of development of hormone resistance with viral RNA expression and processing. *Cancer Res* 1993;53:4432–6.

118. Pater M M, Pater A. Human papillomavirus types 16 and 18 sequences in carcinoma cell lines of the cervix. *Virol* 1985;145:313–8.

119. Thomas D B, Ray R M, Pardthiasong T, Chutivongse S, Koetsawang S, Silpisornkosol S, Virutamasen P, Christopherson W M, Melnick J L, Meirik O, Farley T M, Riotton G. Prostitution, condom use, and invasive squamous cell cervical cancer in Thailand. *Am J Epidemiol.* 1996;15;143:779–86.

120. Manhart L E, Koutsky L A. Do condoms prevent genital HPV infection, external genital warts, or cervical neoplasia? A meta-analysis. *Sex Transm Dis.* 2002 Nov;29(11):725–35.

121. Hatcher R A, Warner D L. New condoms for men and women, diaphragms, cervical caps, and spermicides: overcoming barriers to barriers and spermicides. *Curr Opin Obstet Gynecol* 1992;4:513–21.

122. Goodman M T, Kiviat N, McDuffie K, Hankin J H, Hernandez B, Wilkens L R, et al. The association of plasma micronutrients with the risk of cervical dysplasia in Hawaii. *Cancer Epidemiol Biomarkers Prev* 1998;7:537–44.

123. Brock K, Berry G, Mock P, MacLennan R, Truswell A, Brinton L. Nutrients in diet and plasma and risk of in situ cervical cancer. *J Natl Cancer Inst* 1988; 80:580–5.

124. Van Eenwyk J, Davis F, Bowen P. Dietary and serum carotenoids and cervical intraepithelial neoplasia. *Int J Cancer* 1991;48:34–8.

125. Potischman N, Herrero R, Brinton L A, Reeves W C, Stacewicz-Sapuntzakis M, Jones C J, et al. A case-control study of nutrient status and invasive cervical cancer. *Am J Epidemiol* 1991;134:1347–55.

126. Batecha A M, Armenian H K, Morris J S, Spate V E, Comstock G W. Serum micronutrients and the subsequent risk of cervical cancer in a population based nested case-control study. *Cancer Epidemiol Biomark Prev* 1993;2:335–9.

127. Palan P, Mikhail M, Goldberg G, Basu J, Runowicz C, Romney S. Plasma levels of beta-carotene, lycopene, canthaxanthin, retinol, and alpha-tocopherol in cervical intraepithelial neoplasia and cancer. *Clin Cancer Res* 1996;2:181–5.

128. Palan P, Mikhail M, Basu J, Romney S. Plasma levels of anti-oxidant b-carotene and a-tocopherol in uterine cervix dysplasia and cancer. *Nutr Cancer* 1991;15:13–20.

129. Nagata C, Shimizu H, Yoshikawa H, Noda K, Nozawa S, Yajima A, et al. Serum carotenoids and vitamins and risk of cervical dysplasia from a case-control study in Japan. *Br J Cancer* 1999;81:1234–37.

130. Cuzick J, de Stvola B, Russel M, Thomas B. Vitamin A, vitamin E, and the risk of cervical intraepithelial neoplasia. *Br J Cancer* 1990;62:651–2.

131. Kwasniewska A, Tukendorf A, Semczuk M. Content of tocopehrol in blood serum of human papillomavirus-infected women with cervical dysplasias. *Nutr Cancer* 1997;28:248–51.

132. Knekt P. Serum vitamin E level and risk of female cancers. *Int J Epidemiol* 1988;17:281–8.

133. Sedjo R L, Roe D J Abrahamsen M, Harris R, Craft N, Baldwin S, Giuliano A R. Vitamin A, carotenoids and risk of persistent oncogenic human papillomavirus infection. *Cancer Epi Biomark Prev* 2002;11:876–84.

134. Giuliano A R, Papenfuss M, Nour M, Canfield L M, Schneider A, Hatch K. Anti-oxidant nutrients: associations with persistent human papillomavirus infection. *Cancer Epidemiol Biomarkers Prev* 1997;6:917–23.

135. Giuliano A R, Siegel E M, Roe D, Ferreira S, Baggio M L, Galan L, et al. Dietary carotenoids, vitamins C and E, and risk of persistent type-specific HPV infection in Brazilian women: Results form the Ludwig-McGill HPV Natural History Cohort. *J Infect Dis.* 2003;188:1508–16.

136. Palan P R, Chang C J, Mikhail M S, Ho G Y, Basu J, Romney S L. Plasma concentrations of micronutrients during a nine-month clinical trial of beta-carotene in women with precursor cervical cancer lesions. *Nutr Cancer* 1998;30:46–52.

137. Palmer H J, Paulson K E. Reactive oxygen species and anti-oxidants in signal transduction and gene expression. *Nut Rev* 1997;55:353–61.

138. Mandelblatt, J S, Kanetsky P, Eggert L, Gold K. Is HIV infection a cofactor for cervical squamous cell neoplasia? *Cancer Epidemiol Biomarkers Prev* 1999;8:97–106.

139. Levi J E, Kleter B, Quint W G, Fink M C, Canto C L, Matsubara R, et al. High prevalence of human papillomavirus (HPV) infections and high frequency of multiple HPV genotypes in human immunodeficiency virus-infected women in Brazil. *J Clin Microbiol* 2002;40:3341–5.

140. Penn I. Tumors of the immunocompromised patient. *Ann Int Med* 1988;39:63–73.

141. Wright T C, Sun X-W. Anogenital papillomavirus infection and neoplasia in immunodeficient women. *Obstet Gynecol Clin North Am* 1996;23:861–94.

142. Penn I. Cancers of the anogenital region in renal transplant recipients. *Cancer* 1986;58:611–6.

143. Harwood, C A, Surentheran T, McGregor J M, Spink P J, Leigh I M, Breuer J, et al. Human papillomavirus infection and non-melanoma skin cancer in immunosuppressed and immunocompetent individuals. *J Med Virol* 2000;61:289–97.

144. Palefsky, J M Barrasso R. HPV infection and disease in men. *Obstet Gynecol Clin North Am* 1996;23:895–916.

145. Palefsky J M. Human papillomavirus infection and anogenital neoplasia in human immunodeficiency virus-positive men and women. *J Natl Cancer Inst* 1998;23:15–20.

146. Sun X-W, Ellerbrock R V, Lungu O, Chiasson M A, Bush R J, Wright T C. Human papillomavirus infection in human immunodeficiency virus-seropositive women. *Obstet Gynecol* 1995;85:680–6.

147. Sun X W, Kuhn L, Ellerbrock T V, Chiasson M A, Wright T C. Human papillomavirus infection in HIV-seropositive women; natural history and variability of detection. *New Eng J Med* 1997;337:1343–9.

148. Wright T C, Ellerbrock T V, Chiasson M A, Sun X W, Van Devanter N, Study NYCD. Cervical intraepithelial neoplasia in women infected with human immunodeficiency virus: prevalence, risk factors, and validity of Papanicolaou smears. *Obstet Gynecol* 1994;84:591–7.

149. Fruchter R G, Maiman M, Sedlis A, Bartley L, Camilien L, Arrastia C D. Multiple recurrences of cervical intraepithelial neoplasia in women with the human immunodeficiency virus. *Obstet Gynecol* 1996;87:338–44.

150. Wright T C, Koulos J, Schnoll F, et al. Cervical intraepithelial neoplasia in women infected with the human immunodeficiency virus: outcome after loop electrosurgical excision. *Gynecol Oncol* 1994;55:253–8.

151. Kuhn L, Sun X-W, Wright T C. Human immunodeficiency virus infection and female lower genital tract malignancy. *Current Opinion in Obstet Gynecol* 1999;11:35–9.

152. CDC. 1993 Revised classification system for HIV infection and expanded surveillance case definition for AIDS among adolescents and adults. *MMWR* 1993;41:1–20.

153. Chin K M, Sidhu J S, Janssen R S, Weber J T. Invasive cervical cancer in human immunodeficiency virus-infected and uninfected hospital patients. *Obstet Gynecol* 1998;92:83–7.

154. Chiasson M A, Wright T C. The gynecologic manifestations of HIV. In: Mandell GL and Mildvan D, eds. Atlas of Infectious Diseases. Vol. 1, 2nd Ed. Edinburgh: Churchill Livingstone, 1997:12.1–12.15.

155. Wright T C, Koulos J P, Liu P, Sun X-W. Invasive vulvar carcinoma in two women infected with human immunodeficiency virus. *Gynecol Oncol* 1995;60:500–3.

156. Okagaki T. Female genital tumors associated with HPV infection and the concept of genital neoplasia-papilloma syndrome (GEMP), *Pathol Ann* 1984;19:31–62.

157. Madeleine M M, Brumback B, Cushing-Haugen K L, Schwartz S M, Daling J R, Smith A G, et al. Human leukocyte antigen class II and cervical cancer risk: a population-based study. *J Infect Dis* 2002;186:1565-74.

158. Wang S S, Hildesheim A, Gao X, Schiffman M, Herrero R, Bratti M C, et al. Comprehensive analysis of human leukocyte antigen class I alleles and cervical neoplasia in 3 epidemiologic studies. *J Infect Dis* 2002 1;186:598–605.

159. Hildesheim A, Wang S S. Host and viral genetics and risk of cervical cancer: a review. *Virus Res* 2002;89:229–40.

160. Apple R J, Erlich H A, Klitz W, Manos M M, Becker T M, Wheeler C M. HLA DR-DQ associations with cervical carcinoma show papillomavirus-type specificity. *Nature Genetics* 1994;6:157–62.

161. Glew S S, Stern P L, Davidson J A, Dyer P A. HLA antigens and cervical carcinoma. *Nature* 1992;356:22–3.

162. Wank R, Thomssen C. High risk of squamous cell carcinoma of the cervix for women with HLA-DQw3. *Nature* 1991;352:723–5.

163. Gregoire L, Lawrence W D, Kukuruga D, Eisenbrey A B, Lancaster W D. Association between HLA-DQB1 alleles and risk for cervical cancer in African-American women. *Int J Cancer* 1994;57:504–7.

164. Gostout B S, Podratz K C, McGovern R M, Persing D H. Cervical cancer in older women: a molecular analysis of human papillomavirus types, HLA types, and p53 mutations. *Am J Obstet Gynecol* 1998;179:56–61.

165. Sherman M E. Chapter 11: future directions in cervical pathology. *J Natl Cancer Inst Monogr.* 2003;31:72–9.

166. Pixley E. Basic morphology of the prepuberal and youthful cervix: topographic and histologic features. *J Reprod Med* 1976;16:221–30.

167. Moscicki A, Burt V G, Kanowitz S, Darragh T, Shiboski S. The significance of squamous metaplasia in the development of low grade squamous intraepithelial lesions in young women. *Cancer* 1999;85:1139–44.

168. Schlecht N F, Kulaga S, Robitaille J, Ferreira S, Santos M, Miyamura R A, et al. Persistent human papillomavirus infection as a predictor of cervical intraepithelial neoplasia. *JAMA* 2001;286:3106–14.

169. Remmink A J J, Walboomers J M M, Helmerhorst T J M, Voorhorst F J, Rozendaal L, Risse E K J, et al. The presence of persistent high-risk HPV genotypes in dysplastic cervical lesions is associated with progressive disease: natural history up to 36 months. *Int J Cancer* 1995;61:306–11.

The Biology and Significance of Human Papillomavirus Infection

Table of Contents

5.1 Introduction

The relationship between human papillomavirus (HPV) and cervical cancer is now certain. HPV infection causes virtually all cases of CIN 3 and cervical cancer and a less-defined, smaller fraction of vaginal, vulvar, penile, and anal cancers.[1-6] By the mid-1990s, case control studies had demonstrated that the great majority of women with cervical neoplasia have detectable levels of HPV DNA.[2,7-9] Furthermore, the presence of high-risk HPV predicts an increased risk of high-grade intraepithelial neoplasia, whereas HPV infection in normal women is less likely to be with a high-risk type.[10-16] On a given day, approximately 5% to 27% of normal women will test positive for high-risk HPV DNA,[15,17-20] in contrast to 90% to 100% of women with a high-grade lesion.[20-24]

The study of the natural history and epidemiology of HPV infection has been severely hampered by the inability to culture the virus and the relative insensitivity of currently available serologic tests to determine exposure. The first molecular probes for the detection of HPVs were developed in 1983,[25,26] and the number of high-risk genital HPV types

detected have now grown to approximately 15, with three more listed as probable high-risk. In this short time, the DNA sequences have been mapped, RNA transcription and protein translations have been partially elucidated, and efficient, cost-effective tests have been developed. A clear understanding of the biology, morphologic expression, and natural history of cervical HPV infection is essential to the rational management of cervical neoplasia. This chapter outlines the present state of knowledge regarding the role of HPV in the development of neoplasia throughout the lower genital tract.

5.2 Description and Nature of Human Papillomavirus (HPV)

Papillomaviruses are small, double-stranded DNA viruses that infect epithelial cells and can induce a variety of benign and malignant tumors in humans and other species.[27] The viral genome is encased in a nonenveloped 72-sided icosahedral protein capsid (Figure 5.1) that usually exists in an episomal (circular) configuration with only one strand transcriptionally

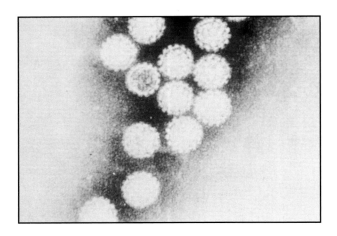

FIGURE 5.1　A highly magnified electronmicrograph demonstrates the icosahedral structure of the human papillomavirus virion. [From: Campion M J, Ferris D G, di Paola F M, Reid R I. Modern Colposcopy: A Practical Approach. ASCCP Hagerstown, MD. 1991;pp. 4–2]

active. The entire HPV genome comprises only about 8,000 base pairs with relatively few viral-specific functions. Each function is responsible for the production of a specific protein.[27] The HPV genome is divided into three regions: the long control region (LCR), the early region (E), and the late region (L) (Figure 5.2). The LCR is a noncoding region of the HPV genome that is responsible for regulation of viral replication and transcription of downstream sequences in the early region.[28] Functional papillomavirus units are found only on the early (E) and late (L) regions and are referred to as open reading frames (ORFs). Each ORF is read as a specific unit by RNA polymerase.[27] The early region encodes predominantly for proteins that are important in viral replication, which occurs "early" in the viral life cycle. The late region encodes for viral structural proteins necessary for capsid production, which occurs "late" in the viral life cycle.

The early region is responsible for maintaining high viral copy number through promotion of viral replication.[28,29] In HPV types that are associated with invasive cancer, this region also encodes for proteins that promote cellular transformation. Eight different ORFs that can encode for proteins have been identified in the early region of HPV; these are designated E1, E2, E3, E4, E5, E6, E7, E8 (Table 5.1).[30] The E1 ORF produces a protein that is responsible for genomic replication. The E2 ORF encodes for two DNA binding proteins that regulate transcription by exerting control over the expression of other early region ORFs.[31,32] These proteins bind-specific DNA sequences in the LCR. The larger of the two E2 transcription regulators encodes a protein that can stimulate transcription of the early region (transactiva-

tion), whereas the smaller E2 regulator encodes a protein that inhibits transcription of the early region (transrepressor). The function of the E3 protein is not known. The E4 ORF protein function is not well understood; however, the protein products from E4 are detected in large amounts in productive infections and may be important in altering the normal cytokeratin matrix of infected cells, allowing the release of viral particles from the cells.[27,33,34] The E5 protein has been shown to activate growth receptors, such as epidermal growth factor receptor and platelet-derived growth factor receptor.[27] The E6 and E7 ORFs are crucial in the process of oncogenesis, as they produce the proteins necessary for cellular proliferation and immortalization. The function of the E8 protein is not known.[27]

The two late regions, L1 and L2, encode for proteins involved in construction of the capsid of the infective HPV genome (Figure 5.3). The L1 capsid protein, which is the major capsid protein, is structurally but not antigenically constant in all the HPV types, whereas the minor capsid protein, produced by L2, is much more variable among HPV types.[35,36] However, because the antigenic response to L2 is more cross-reactive, the key epitopes do not follow the general level of conservation. Naked DNA is not infective.

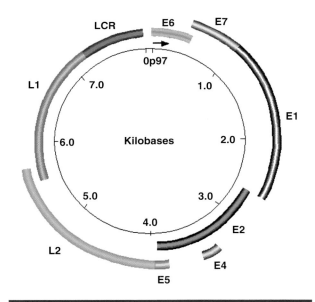

FIGURE 5.2　The nucleoside sequence of the human papillomavirus genome. The DNA exists in a double-stranded circular helix that can be divided into three regions: the long control region (LCR), the early region (E), and the late region (L). From: Shah KH, Howley PM. Papillomaviruses. In: Field's Virology. Fields BN, Knipe DM, Howley PM, eds. Philadelphia: Lippincott Raven, 1996; 2:2028. With permission.

Table 5.1　Functions of HPV Genes

Gene designation	Function
E1	initiation of viral DNA replication
E2	regulation of viral transcription with an auxillary role in DNA replication
E3	no known function
E4	disrupts cytokeratins
E5	transformation (animals only)
E6	transformation, targets degradation of p53 tumor supressor protein
E7	transformation, binds to the retinoblastoma protein
E8	no known function
L1	major capsid protein
L2	major capsid protein

From: Lowy DR, Howley PM. Papillomaviruses. In: Knipe DM, Howley PM, eds. *Fields Virology* (4th Edition). Philadelphia: Lippincott, Williams, & Wilkins; 2001:2231-64. With permission.

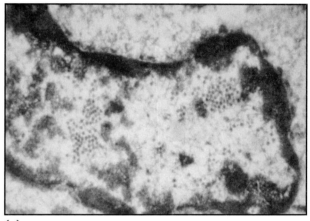

(a)

FIGURES 5.3　Electron microscopy of cells productively infected with human papillomavirus: an entire nucleus of a koilocyte in the upper epithelial layers of a low-grade lesion show clusters of HPV genomes. From: Campion M J, Ferris D G, di Paola F M, Reid R I. Modern Colposcopy: A Practical Approach. ASCCP, Hagerstown, MD. 1991;pp. 4–7

Hence, capsid production in terminal cells in the upper epithelial layers is critical if HPV is to pass from host to host. Transcription of L1 and L2 capsid proteins appears to be initiated by transcriptional regulators found only in differentiated host cells in the intermediate and superficial layers of the epithelium.[37] Large amounts of L1 and L2 encoded proteins can be detected in condyloma acuminata but only low amounts are present in CIN 3 and cancer.[37,38]

Although papillomaviruses are found in many animal species, human papillomaviruses do not infect any animal hosts. The species specificity of papillomaviruses enables their classification by their natural host species (e.g., human, bovine). The mechanism of species specificity has not been determined but is probably attributable to host regulatory proteins rather than to virus absorption and penetration.[27] Subclassification into types is done according to nucleotide sequence. The most common HPV types are listed in Table 5.2. Each papillomavirus type is highly tropic for a specific epithelium and has its own degree of oncogenicity. Although viral tropism is poorly understood, it is presumed to be secondary to differences in nucleotide structure and reflects interactions between viral- and host- encoded proteins at specific anatomic sites.[27]

HPV types are numbered in order of discovery. The original definition of a new HPV type required that the new HPV genome cross-hybridize with less than 50% of the genome of previously described types, but the more recent definition of a new HPV type is having less than 90% sequence homology with other HPV types in the E6, E7, and L1 ORFs.[27] More than 100 types of HPV have now been described, more than 40 of which have a predilection for the anogenital tract. Of these, approximately 15 have been found in cervical cancers and have therefore been termed "high-risk" (HPVs 16, 18, 31, 33, 35, 39, 45, 51, 52, 56, 58, 59, 68, 73, and 82).[6,39,40] Three additional HPV types have been classified as "probable high-risk" (HPVs 26, 53, and 66), and 12 have been classified as low-risk types (HPVs 6, 11, 40, 42, 43, 44, 54, 61, 70, 72, 81, and CP6108.[40] All of the genital HPVs are found in the Supergroup A (See Section 5.2.4) with most of the high-risk types in two clusters, one containing HPV-16 and one containing HPV-18.[27,41] Although genital HPV is a common term for this group, they may also infect several nongenital sites, including the upper airways, oral

Table 5.2   Major Clinical Association of Genital Tract and Other Mucosal HPVs

Clinical association	HPV Type
Genital tract	
Subclinical infection	all genital HPVs
Exophytic condyloma	6, 11
Flat condyloma	6, 11, 16, 18, 31, others
Bowenoid papulosis	16
Giant condyloma (Bushke-Lowenstein tumor)	6, 11
Cervical cancer	
Strong or moderate association	16, 18, 31, 33, 35, 39, 45, 51, 52, 56, 58, 59, 68
Weak or no association	6, 11, 26, 42, 43, 44, 53, 54, 55, 62, 66
Vulvar cancer	16
Penile cancer	16
Respiratory papillomas	6, 11
Conjunctival papillomas	6, 11
Oral cavity	
Infection with genital tract HPVs	6, 11, 16

From: Lowy DR, PM Howley. Papillomaviruses. In: Knipe DM, Howley PM, eds. *Fields' Virology* (4th Edition). Philadelphia: Lippincott, Williams, & Wilkins; 2001:2231-64. With permission.

mucosa, conjunctiva, and periungual tissues.[42] The principle reservoirs of infection, however, are the moist mucosa and adjacent cutaneous epithelia of male and female genitalia.

5.2.1 Low-risk viral types

HPV 6 and 11 are responsible for approximately 90% of the exophytic condylomata of the external genitalia, vagina, and cervix (Figure 5.4), for most recurrent respiratory papillomatosis and for less than 15% of low-grade lesions of the cervical transformation zone (Figure 5.5).[43] Mixed infections with both low-risk and high-risk viruses occur in 2% to 25% of women with CIN.[12,44] HPVs 42, 43, and 44 are related to HPVs 6 and 11 on both the nucleotide level and in their common lack of association with cervical cancer. These types have been found in only a small proportion of low-grade lesions of the vulva, cervix, and penis. Of 1000 cervical cancers evaluated worldwide, only a single cervical cancer tested positive for a low-risk viral type.[3] Other low-risk types, such as HPVs 53, 61, 70, and 71, are primarily associated with low-grade squamous intraepithelial lesions throughout the lower genital tract.[28,45]

5.2.2 High-risk viral types

The oncogenic risk of high-risk HPV types has been delineated by their close association with human tumors and by their ability to immortalize normal cells.[27] The relative risk for many of these genital

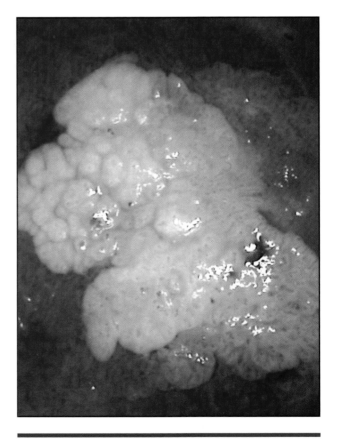

FIGURE 5.4   A clinically obvious condyloma acuminatum within the cervical transformation zone. Cervical condylomata are usually secondary to HPV 6 or 11, and are a relatively uncommon (3%) manifestation of cervical HPV. ■

HPVs for CIN 3 and cervical cancer has been well delineated.[39,40,43] Some 15 HPV types are involved in over 95% of cervical cancer cases. HPV 16 and 18, which are the most common types identified, respectively represent 40% to 70% and 10% to 40% of the viral types involved in invasive cancer (Figure 5.6).[39] Data pooled from 11 case-control studies from nine

countries documented that the most common HPV types in patients with squamous cell cervical cancer in descending order of frequency were types 16, 18, 45, 31, 33, 52, 58, and 35 (Table 5.3).[40] The most common types among women in the control group not having cancer were types 16, 18, 45, 31, 6, 58, 35, and 33. Therefore, the four most common types in the population are also the four most common types in women with cervical cancer.

The most common viral type detected in both high-grade CIN and invasive cancers is HPV 16, which is found in over 50% of squamous intraepithelial lesions and carcinomas of the cervix[3] and in approximately one third of adenocarcinomas (Figure 5.7).[46] HPV 16 is also detected in at least 85% of HPV-related intraepithelial neoplasias of the vulva (VIN), vagina (VAIN), penis (PIN), and anus (PAIN) (Figure 5.8).[46] Although HPV 16 is considered a high-risk viral type, it is detected in at least 40% of minor low-grade lesions of the vulva and penis, 30% of minor-grade cervical lesions, 10% of external condylomata acuminata, and in up to 7% of cytologically normal young women.

This wide clinical variability associated with HPV 16 indicates that women infected with this virus, although at greater risk for HPV-associated malignancies, most commonly remain normal or develop lesions that do not progress to invasive cancer. It is still not understood why some HPV 16-associated CIN may progress to invasion, whereas others do not. One possibility is that there may be individual

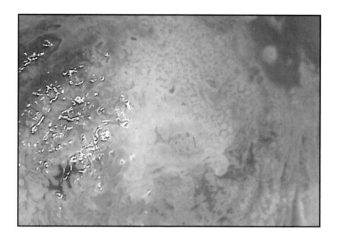

FIGURE 5.5   A low-grade HPV associated lesion of the cervix that tested positive for HPV 6. Although exophytic condylomas are virtually always secondary to low-risk HPV types, these same types also may present as flat lesions characterized by an irregular margin, indistinct acetowhitening and a trivial vascular pattern. The differential for minor HPV changes, as demonstrated here, is with normal immature metaplasia.

Distribution of Human Papillomavirus Types Worldwide

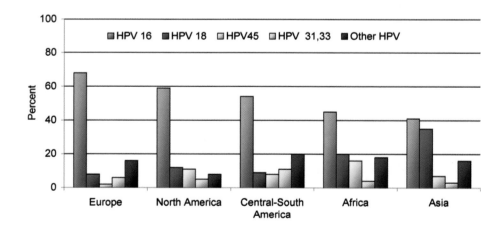

FIGURE 5.6   HPV 16 is responsible for approximately 50% of invasive cervical cancers worldwide. Geographic variations do occur, with just over 40% of cervical cancers in Asia testing positive for HPV 16 and almost 70% HPV 16 positive in Europe. From: Bosch F X, Manos M M, Munoz N, et al. Prevalence of human papillomavirus in cervical cancer: a worldwide perspective. *J Natl Cancer Inst* 1995;87:796–802. With permission, Oxford University Press.

Table 5.3 Distribution of HPV Types in 1918 Women with Histologically Confirmed Squamous-cell Cervical Cancer and 1928 Control Women. Data Pooled from 11 Case-control Studies in Nine Countries

HPV type	Cases		Controls		OR (95% CI)*	
	No.	%	No.	%		
negative	46	3.39	1091	84.44	1.00	
HPV 16	685	50.52	42	3.25	434.34	(278.30–677.87)
HPV 18	177	13.05	17	1.32	248.56	(138.37–446.48)
HPV 31	36	2.65	8	0.62	122.16	(52.87–282.26)
HPV 33	14	1.03	1	0.08	368.34	(46.15–2939.53)
HPV 35	15	1.11	6	0.46	74.99	(26.82–209.72)
HPV 39	8	0.59	0	0	–	
HPV 45	74	5.46	9	0.7	197.46	(91.69–425.26)
HPV 51	13	0.96	4	0.31	65.65	(19.76–218.12)
HPV 52	37	2.73	4	0.31	198.99	(67.49–586.72)
HPV 56	9	0.66	5	0.39	45.24	(14.05–145.63)
HPV 58	31	2.29	6	0.46	115.64	(45.40–294.57)
HPV 59	17	1.25	1	0.08	418.60	(54.15–3236.17)
HPV 73	5	0.37	1	0.08	107.28	(11.52–999.43)

*OR adjusted for age and center

Adapted from: Munoz N, Bosch FX, de Sanjose S, Herrero R, Castellsague X, Shah KV, Snijders PJ, Meijer CJ. International Agency for Research on Cancer Multicenter Cervical Cancer Study Group. Epidemiologic classification of human papillomavirus types associated with cervical cancer. *N Engl J Med.* 2003;348:518–27. From: Bosch FX, De Sanjose S. Chapter 1: Human papillomavirus and cervical cancer burden and assessment of causality. J. Natl Cancer Inst (monograph) 2003: 31:3–13. With permission.

differences in the genetic capability of the host immune response to suppress HPV expression.[47] Another is the existence of unique variants of specific HPV types that may have significant clinical implications. An association between HPV 16 variants and the development of cervical cancer has been well documented. Excess risk is secondary to non-European variants.[48] Variants of other types are less well studied, but limited data available on types HPV 18 and 58 suggest that non-European variants of these types are also associated with increased risk of cervical cancer.[49–52] For example, some intratype gene variations of HPV 16 may be more prone to developing persistent infection.[53] These variants have deletions in transcriptional silencer elements, explaining their greater success in persisting. Cervical cancer derived from HPV 16 harbors almost exclusively E6 variants (94%), whereas CIN 3 demonstrates a more uniform distribution of variants (56%) and prototype (44%) (Figure 5.9). Variations that have been identi-

FIGURE 5.7 HPV 18 is more commonly associated with adeno- and adenosquamous carcinomas, in which it represents approximately 68% of the cancers. However, it is also found in approximately 25% of squamous cell cervical carcinomas.[3]

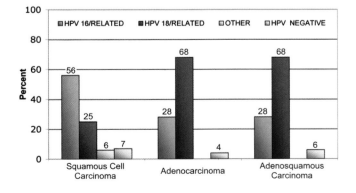

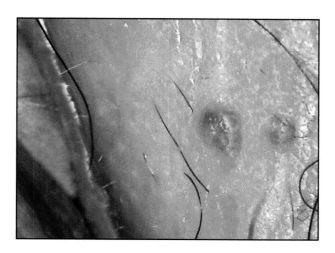

FIGURE 5.8 Two pigmented lesions on the left labium majus typed positive for HPV 16 and histologically interpreted as VIN 3. These lesions are relatively common in young women. Despite their association with a known oncogenic viral type and the high-grade morphologic appearance, these may occasionally be transient lesions with resolution occurring before treatment can be scheduled. ▬▬

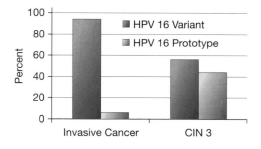

Distribution of Human Papillomavirus Type 16 and Variants in Cervical Intraepithelial Neoplasia and Invasive Carcinoma

FIGURE 5.9 HPV 16 variants have deletions in transcriptional silencer elements that may be responsible for the ability of some HPV 16 to persist. In contrast to the more uniform distribution of variants and prototype in CIN 3, demonstration of a virtual preponderance of HPV 16 variants in cervical cancer supports this significance. Modified from: Zehbe I, Wilander E, Delius H, Tommassino M. Human papillomavirus 16 E6 variants are more prevalent than the prototype. *Cancer Res* 1998;58:829–33. With permission. ▬▬

fied to date have been in areas likely to be important for protein-protein interaction with p53 or in areas of other immunologic significance. In contrast, E7 variations are rare. Such variation within HPV 16 may be partially responsible for the variability in risk noted for individuals infected with this viral type.[53,54]

HPV 18 is less frequently detected in any grade of CIN than would be expected, considering its place as the second most common (25%) viral type in invasive cervical cancers. This suggests that these cancers may arise *de novo* without traversing the intraepithelial spectrum or that they transit too rapidly to be detected by routine screening.[55] Adenocarcinomas in young women have been particularly suspect to fit this model as they are most commonly associated with HPV 18 and often fail to be detected in a timely manner by cytologic screening. Cancers associated with HPV 18 occur 2.6 times more frequently within one year of a negative smear than do cancers positive for HPV 16.[55] Additionally, detection of HPV 18 is possibly an adverse prognostic factor. The average age of women with HPV 18 cancers is 8 to 12 years younger than those with HPV 16 containing tumors, and recurrence rates are higher (45% versus 16%).[56] Finally, endocervical cells may be more susceptible to HPV 18.[57]

5.2.3 Infections with multiple HPV types

A large population study in the Netherlands documented multiple HPV types in 11.8% of HPV positive specimens with normal/ASCUS cytology, 34.5% of HPV-positive samples with CIN 1 and 2 and in 4.4% of the HPV-positive cancer specimens.[58] The increasing number of types found in women with CIN compared with women who have normal cytologic specimens likely reflects tolerance of HPV infection in individuals developing CIN, whereas dominance of single type in cancers reflects the known monoclonal development of HPV-induced cancer.[59,60] Permissive immunity would allow accumulation of HPV infections upon exposure to different types because of an inability to clear each infection as it occurs. Therefore, the accumulation of multiple HPV types could serve as a surrogate marker for increased risk for cervical neoplasia that reflects decreased immunocompetence and subsequent viral persistence.[61] In the rare cases in which multiple infections are found in carcinomas, additional other-type CIN lesions within the specimen may be the source.[58,61] An increased risk for persistence of HPV was demonstrated over a short period of 6 months (odds ratio [OR] 4.1) in young women with multiple HPV types.[17] However, persistence of HPV infection was independent of coinfection with other HPV types in another study that also observed that 82% of all coinfections consisted of only two HPV types. As in other studies, acquisition of multiple types was more likely in women with HPV 16.[62,63]

5.2.4 Functional differences between low-risk and high-risk types

Human and animal papillomaviruses can be grouped in a phylogenetic tree into Supergroups to demonstrate relatedness based on comparison of nucleotide sequences coding for the L1 capsid protein. HPVs and animal papillomaviruses in their own Supergroup are more closely related than they are to other HPVs and animal papillomaviruses in a different Supergroup.[28] (Figure 5.10) Mutations in these viruses are rare, and once present, they spread subsequently as markers in the phylogenetic tree.[64] For example, low-risk types appear to have developed within a single branch of the phylogenetic tree.[65] This viral stability and lack of significant genomic variation have important implications for vaccine development.

All papillomaviruses share the need to induce DNA synthesis in quiescent host cells in order to replicate viral DNA. This is commonly achieved by the interaction of the E7 protein with members of the retinoblastoma gene (pRb) family of the host, which would normally lead to the induction of growth arrest or apoptosis in the infected cell (Figure 5.11).[66] Although both low-risk and high-risk HPV types have the capability of prohibiting apoptosis in the proliferating cells of low-grade cervical intraepithelial lesions (CIN 1) and condylomata, only the E5, E6 and E7 proteins of high-risk HPV types neutralize cell cycle regulators responsible for inhibiting malignant proliferation.[45,67] E5 may have several possible transforming functions, including a role in EGF-related signal transduction and a role in the disruption of cell-to-cell communication, which is often observed in transformed cells.[27] HPV E6 and E7 proteins each have several individual effects on

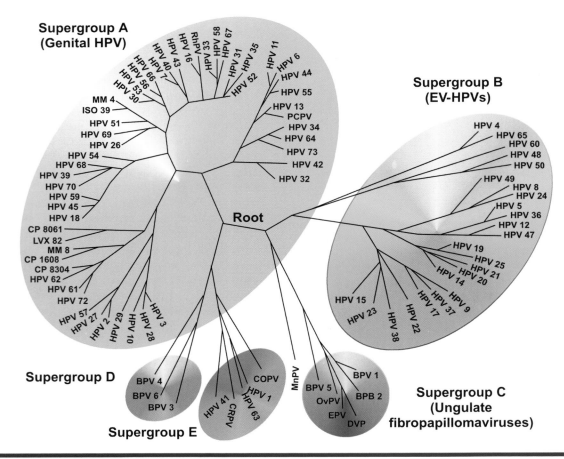

FIGURE 5.10 Phylogenetic tree for 92 human (HPVs) and animal papillomaviruses demonstrates that HPVs are more closely related to animal papillomaviruses in their Supergroup than to HPVs in a different Supergroup. Modified from: Chan S-Y, Delius H, Halpern AL, Bernard HU. Analysis of Genomic Sequences of 95 Papillomavirus Types: Uniting Typing, Phylogeny, and Taxonomy. *J. Virol*, 1995, 69:3074–83. Used with permission.

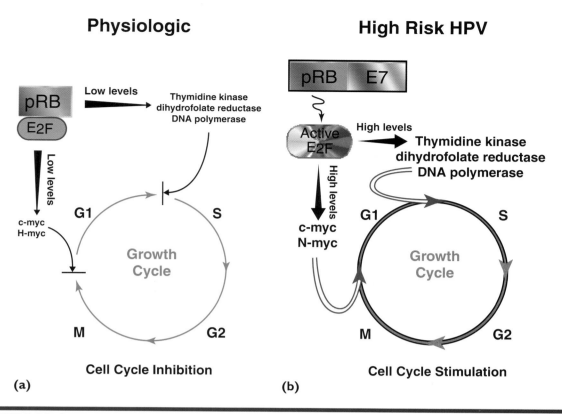

FIGURES 5.11a,b Both low- and high-risk viral types need to replicate by inhibiting apoptosis (cell death) in proliferating cells that would normally follow any abnormal cell growth. One mechanism by which HPVs accomplish this is by interaction of the E7 protein with protein produced by the pRb family of host genes responsible for ordering cell destruction. Demonstrated here are the interactions between HPV-16 E7, pRb and E2F-1: **(a) Physiologic:** G-1 phase growth arrested cell under physiologic conditions; **(b) High Risk HPV:** proliferating cell infected with high oncogenic-risk HPV type. From Park TW, Fujiwara H, Wright T C. Molecular biology of cervical cancer and its precursors. *Cancer* 1995;76:1902-13. Used with permission.

cell proliferation and genetic abnormalities, but both are necessary to initiate neoplastic transformation.[27] HPV E6 binds to and targets the degradation of p53 (Figure 5.12) while E7 binds and functionally inactivates cellular proteins produced by the retinoblastoma (Rb) gene, cyclin A, and p107. E6 proteins from low-risk HPV types cannot induce degradation of p53. Hence, low-risk HPV types do not have the capability to promote cellular immortalization, transformation, and oncogenesis.[27] While the primary function of E6 proteins of high-risk HPV types has long been considered to be primarily the inactivation of p53 tumor suppressor proteins, E6 proteins may also contribute to malignant transformation by their effect on telomerase, which promotes cell immortalization and on other proteins involved in regulating apoptosis, cytoskeletal structure, cell polarity, signal transduction, and differentiation.[27,68] The activity of the E6 oncoprotein is necessary for oncogenesis to occur because degradation of p53 and

subsequent blockage of the normal apoptotic response to inappropriate DNA replication depends entirely on the action of this protein.[69] Cell immortalization may also be promoted by continued addition of telomeric sequences secondary to the increased expression of telomerase.[27,70] Increased telomerase expression has been found in tissues infected with HPV 16 or 18 expressing HPV E6. Telomerase expression is significantly higher in cervical cancers (85%) and CIN 2 and 3 (61%) than in CIN 1 (10%) or normal histology (7%).[27]

HPV E7 from high-risk, but not from low-risk, types also interacts with cellular growth regulatory proteins that may contribute to cell transformation.[71,72] The protein product of E7 binds the tumor suppressor protein of pRb, as well as the pRb-related pocket proteins p107 and p130.[27] The retinoblastoma tumor suppressor protein is a critical regulator of the DNA synthesis (S) phase of cell division.[27] Normal epithelial cells have terminally withdrawn

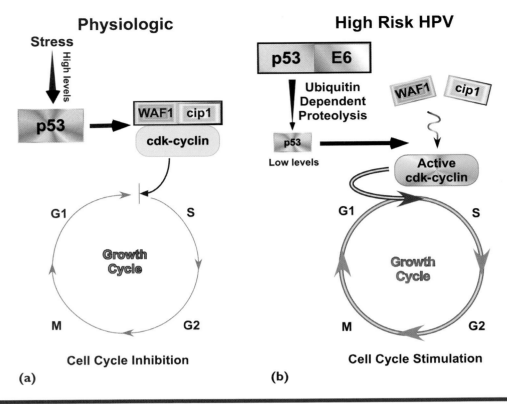

FIGURES 5.12a,b Interactions between HPV 16 E6 p53 and CDK-cyclin: **(a) Physiologic:** G1-phase growth-arrested cell that has been exposed to some form of cellular stress; **(b) High Risk HPV:** proliferating cell-infected high-oncogenic risk HPV type. From Park T W, Fujiwara H, Wright T C. Molecular biology of cervical cancer and its precursors. *Cancer* 1995;76:1902-13. Used with permission.

from cellular replication as only basal cells can replicate. Therefore, induction of epithelial proliferation by HPV requires that the pRb protein be suppressed.[73] High-risk HPV E7 proteins have a higher affinity for pRb proteins compared to the low-risk HPVs due to a single amino acid difference in the E7 protein of low-risk types.[74] This difference ensures that high-risk HPV E7 will increase cell proliferation, and thereby cellular transformation, by promoting transition from the G1 to the S phase.[75-77] Additionally, HPV E7 proteins can inactivate the cyclin-dependent kinase inhibitors p21[78,79] and p27[80], which are important in inducing growth arrest in cells.[73]

Therefore, the function of E7 in the oncogenic process may be to (1) override cell cycle checkpoint controls, (2) modulate the expression of cellular proteins, (3) deregulate cellular carbohydrate metabolism, and (4) modulate apoptosis.[27] Several interactions may be important. For instance, high-risk HPV-encoded E7 genes have been shown to interact with high-risk HPV E6 genes in cell immortalization, which is initially not tumorigenic but eventually becomes so following the chance occurrence of

mutations over time.[81] High-risk HPV E6 and E7 proteins are also individually able to induce genomic instability in normal human cells with E6 inducing gene amplifications and deletions and E7 inducing aneuploidy.[82-84] E6 and E7 proteins also can cooperate to induce centrosome-associated defects of mitotic spindle formation that may result in aneuploidy and chromosomal instability.[85] Low-risk HPV E6 and E7 proteins do not induce genomic instability.[86] Thus E7 may act as a mitotic mutator, resulting in the abnormal mitoses and genomic instability demonstrated in the malignant progression of HPV-associated lesions.[87,88] The absence of molecular plausibility for low-risk HPV types in the oncogenic process explains the segregation of HPV types into those found in malignancies and those that are not. The process involved in the development of rare malignancies associated with low-risk HPV types, such as HPV 6-associated Buschke-Lowenstein verrucous carcinomas, remains speculative.[89]

One function common to both low- and high-risk HPV types is their ability to evade host-immune recognition, which may be enhanced by HPV E7 suppression of the interferon signal. HPV 16 and HPV 11 E7 proteins mediate the suppression of IRF 1, a component of the anti-proliferative effect of interferons, perhaps facilitating immune evasion.[90] Therefore, expression of HPV E6 and E7 proteins may promote viral persistence and interruption of cellular growth pathways that normally would lead to growth arrest and cell death.[91] Apoptosis of DNA-damaged human keratinocytes is markedly reduced in cells expressing either HPV 16 E6 or E7 protein.[92] Such inhibition may render the cells susceptible to the accumulation of mutations necessary for carcinogenesis. HPV oncogenesis may require long-term persistence of the virus in order for the process to have the time to be exposed to random events that eventually lead to the accumulation of these mutations.

Viral integration appears to occur when poorly understood viral, host and cofactor interactions result in loss of host-cellular control and persistence of high-risk HPV.[93,94] Integration of HPV DNA into the host genome is a rare irreversible genetic alteration that is likely to initiate a chain of events involving the impairment of tumor suppressor genes (e.g., p53 and Rb) and subsequent genomic instability and cell immortalization.[95,96]

When HPV integrates, viral DNA most frequently breaks in the HPV E1/E2 gene region.[97] Disruption of the E2 ORF results in loss of the function of E2,[97] which normally produces an important regulatory protein of the major E6 and E7 oncogenes (Fig-

ure 5.13). Since the E2 protein is essential for control over both transcription and replication,[98] loss of E2 function can produce increased transcription of E6 and E7 oncogenes.[97] Keratinocytes containing integrated HPV 16 have been shown to have a growth advantage compared with those containing episomal HPV 16 because of the increased levels of HPV 16 E6 and E7 protein.[99] Expression of E6 and E7 is retained in cervical cancers, but E5 expression is commonly lost following viral integration.[27]

The frequency of HPV integration increases with increasing disease severity and therefore is likely to be an important and perhaps critical step in progression to invasion.[95,100] The discrepancy between the high rate of HPV infection and the low incidence of cervical cancer may be secondary to the relative infrequency of these interactions all occurring in an individual.

5.3 Natural History of Genital HPV Infection

5.3.1 Transmission

Cancers caused by genital tract HPVs have risk factors related to sexual practices, which are in large part surrogate measures for HPV exposure.[101] It is likely that the transmission of viral infection to nongenital sites occurs as a consequence of certain sexual behaviors, such as oral-genital contact, or by auto-inoculation

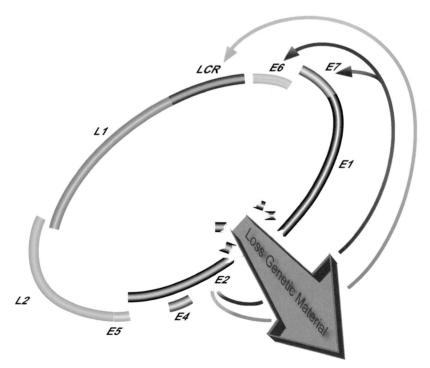

FIGURE 5.13 Loss of normal cell regulatory control occurs with integration of HPV DNA into the host chromosome. In the episomal state E2 has regulatory control over E6 and E7 (Blue arrow) and also regulates the long control arm (LCR) (Green arrow). Breakage of the chromosome between E1 and E2 prior to integration interrupts this control. ■

from a genital infection, and therefore will be captured by use of standard sexual behavior measures. Sexual behaviors known to be associated with HPV exposure include high number of lifetime sexual partners, young age at first intercourse, and a history of sexually transmitted disease(s). While other mechanisms of transmission are possible (intrapartum transmission, transmission through nonsexual or non-coital sexual contact such as deep kissing) they are likely to be less common sources of infection. Interactions between sexual behaviors and other known risk factors for cancers at a particular site must also be considered. For instance, in the case of oropharyngeal cancers, alcohol and tobacco use may confound analysis of sexual behavior.

5.3.1.1 Sexual transmission

Evaluations of large cohorts of initially virginal women have strongly confirmed the sexually transmitted nature of a HPV infection, which is essentially absent until the onset of sexual exposure.[102-104] Cervical cancer is the long-term sequelae of a sexually transmitted persistent HPV infection. Sexual activity is the most important risk factor for penile HPV lesions and for cervical carcinogenesis, and the sexual history of either partner is equally important in risk analysis. However, the contribution of "the male factor" has always been difficult to evaluate accurately.[105,106] An eight-fold difference in cervical cancer rates between Colombia (48/100,000 women) and Spain (6/100,000 women) is associated with dramatic differences in the sexual behavioral characteristics of males in each country.[107] The male population in Colombia, when compared to the male population in Spain, reported a 3.3-fold mean lifetime number of sexual partners and a 1.6-fold mean lifetime number of prostitutes, accounting for a 5-fold prevalence of penile HPV DNA in Colombia.

Genital tract papillomaviruses are readily transmitted by genital-to-genital contact. The length of the average incubation period from exposure to HPV to lesion expression varies greatly and may range from a few weeks to occasionally many years or decades.[108,109] About 24%[110] to 66%[108,109,111,112] of sexual partners of persons with genital condylomata acuminata develop similar lesions. Presumably, the 40% not proven to have lesions either do not become infected, never express disease, or develop lesions so transiently that they remain undetected. Altered epithelial immunity with increasing age may be a factor when the period between exposure and the development of an identifiable lesion is long.[113] The potential for a protracted period between exposure and the identification of a specific lesion eliminates for most individuals the possibility of determining when and where HPV exposure

occurred; however the strongest predictor of HPV detection and of new disease expression is a history of recent partner change.[101,104,114]

Transmission studies of clinically apparent condyloma acuminata have shown that lesions of recent origin are more likely to be infective than lesions present for longer duration.[108] Although the frequency with which HPV types induce clinically apparent condyloma acuminata has been documented, the proportion of partners who develop only subclinical disease is not known. The infectivity of subclinical HPV-induced disease also is poorly defined. Studies of the male consorts of women with subclinical HPV-associated cervical disease have shown that 64% to 70% will have histologically proven genital HPV infection.[111] Approximately one third of these will have clinically apparent lesions, and about two thirds will have only subclinical disease. Because histologic analysis is compromised by considerable subjectivity, complete and accurate diagnosis of subclinical HPV infection often requires HPV testing for confirmation.

Although condyloma acuminata are most often associated with HPV 6 and 11 infection, concurrent CIN is most frequently secondary to high-risk HPV types, particularly HPV 16. Therefore, multiple-type HPV infections are not uncommon. The treatment outcome of genital condyloma acuminata in women appears to be independent of adequate treatment of similar lesions in the sexual consort.[115] This is because clearance of virally induced lesions depends on an effective host-immune response and not on absence of reexposure to the same viral type. It is believed that successful treatment of genital HPV lesions reflects control until immune suppression eliminates expression of new disease. Evidence for this supposition is at least partially based upon differences in recurrence of HPV lesions posttreatment in individuals with normal immunity and those whose immunity is compromised. For example, recurrence in immunocompromised individuals is most commonly of the same HPV type, reflecting the inability of the host to suppress remaining HPV or to suppress reexposure to the same HPV type. In contrast, spontaneous or treatment-aided regression in the immunocompetent host is unlikely to be followed by reoccurrence secondary to the same HPV type.[115]

5.3.1.2 Extragenital and fomite transmission

Genital-oral transmission of specific HPV types is suggested by detection of HPV 6, 11, and 16 in oral specimens,[116] and transmission of HPV 6 or 11 has long been known to cause benign respiratory papillomas.[117] However, evaluation of a large cohort of young women only rarely found HPV in the oral cavity, and when it was detected, it was not associated with oral-penile contact.[114] Early studies of HPV involvement of cancers of the oral cavity, pharynx, and larynx gave widely varying results, both with respect to HPV prevalence and HPV type distribution.[117,118] However, recent studies have consistently identified high-risk HPV in approximately 25% of oropharyngeal cancers, particularly those found in the tonsils and at the base of the tongue.[117] HPV-associated oral cancers differ from similar cancers not found to have HPV by less frequent p53 mutations, more basaloid cell type and better prognosis.[119,120] The most common types identified in head and neck cancers are HPV-16, 31, and 33. The viral genome is specifically localized to the tumor cells and is transcriptionally active.[121,122] As further proof of the role of HPV in these cancers, the total number of lifetime sexual partners, young age at first intercourse, and a history of genital warts have all been documented to be risk factors for oral cancer, after adjustment for alcohol and tobacco exposure.[117,120]

In addition to the possible genital-oral transmission of HPV, HPV-induced extragenital skin lesions may occasionally serve as viral reservoirs. The potential for extragenital skin lesions to serve as viral reservoirs is illustrated by the detection of HPV 16 in periungual warts and squamous cell carcinomas[42] and of HPV 35-induced Bowenoid papulosis in association with a HPV 35 peri-ungual verrucae.[123] Nonsexual transmission of HPV types 6 and 11 to the conjunctiva and nose has also been reported.[124,125] Additionally, HPV 16 and HPV 18 E6 gene expression has been demonstrated in conjunctival cancers.[126] HPV infection of the conjunctiva most likely occurs by autoinocculation, although it has been speculated that intrapartum exposure of the fetus as it passes through an infected birth canal might be another possible route of exposure.[127] Additionally, fomite transmission may be responsible for some cases of nonsexual exposure. Transmission of non-genital HPV types to the genital area has been described from tanning beds and other fomites.[128,129] However, transmission from medical examination tables and instruments has yet to be documented, although viral DNA can be detected in the medical office setting.[130]

5.3.1.3 Vertical transmission

The contribution of vertical or peripartal transmission of HPV remains unclear, for there have not been any new important epidemiological studies on vertical transmission.[101] HPV seropositivity in children[131] and occasional cervical HPV DNA detection in some,[132] but not all,[104] studies of virgins raise the possibility of vertical transmission of genital HPV types. However, the virtual requirement of sexual intercourse as a prerequisite for cervical cancer indicates either that genital colonization at the time of birth with oncogenic HPVs does not occur, or if colonization does occur, cofactors transmitted sexually must be necessary for viral promotion. Most likely, the unfavorable hormonal milieu present in the neonate after clearance of maternal estrogen and progesterone is at least partly responsible for the absence of expressed HPV infection in the post-partal period. Alternatively, rapid transit through an infected birth canal may limit exposure. If vertical transmission of HPV were to result in even transient infection, such exposure could potentially influence later immune response at the time of sexual exposure.[101,133]

The only clinically expressed HPV disease known to be acquired at birth is respiratory papillomatosis. HPV types 6 and 11 may be transmitted vertically from mother to infant at the time of birth with an attendant risk of neonatal laryngeal papillomatosis.[134,135] Although HPV colonization may be quite common, expression of such disease is relatively uncommon, with estimates varying between 1/400 to 1/2000 infants born to women with condyloma present at the time of birth. It should be noted, however, that considerably higher risks have been estimated when genital warts develop late in pregnancy in a woman without a prior history. Most likely, HPV 6 and 11 are transmitted to the larynx of the neonate by amniotic fluid containing virion-laden squames from the maternal genital tract and inhaled at the time of birth.

HPV 16, as well as other viral types, may also be transmitted in this manner, but exposure may not equate with infection. HPV DNA has been detected in 33% of nasopharyngeal aspirates from neonates and has been found in amniotic fluid of women who were positive for cervical HPV.[136] Forty percent of male infants born to 10 HPV-positive mothers also tested positive for HPV DNA in either foreskin specimens or oral scrapings. Certainly, it is logical that HPV could be transmitted at birth, but susceptibility to the establishment of HPV infection remains unclear.

The presence of genital condylomata in children often initiates concern that HPV may have been transmitted by sexual molestation. However, some children with such lesions have not been sexually molested.[137,138] Further, genital condyloma acuminata may occur in virginal girls and perianal condyloma acuminata may occur in persons who deny heterosexual or homosexual contact. Although most genital HPV infection is sexually transmitted, the presumption of sexual transmission should never be absolute.

5.4 Life Cycle of HPV

A myriad of possibilities follows the transmission of HPV. Since a large percentage of the population is exposed cumulatively over time to HPV, yet the majority never develop detectable HPV-induced lesions, it would appear that clinically expressed disease is more often the exception than the rule.[139] Evaluation of newly diagnosed HPV in women with negative cytologic results suggests that only about 15% will have a subsequent abnormal Papanicolaou (Pap) test within 5 years.[140] Most of these infections appear to result in only transient expression, as a complex interplay of host, viral, and environmental factors most commonly result in immune dominance over the viral intruder.[5] For a relative minority of individuals, however, this complex interplay has far different results, as persistent expression may escape immune control and result in a variety of morphologic possibilities. The first step begins with viral entry.

5.4.1 Viral entry

HPV is transmitted in desquamated genital epithelial cells (Figure 5.14) that degenerate, leaving HPV capsids free to bind to a receptor on the basal keratinocytes that are most likely exposed in sites of microtrauma (Figure 5.15).[108,141,142] Therefore, areas most affected by trauma, such as the posterior fourchette and inner aspect of the labia minora in

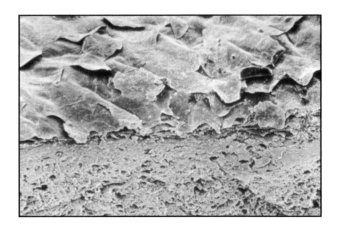

FIGURE 5.14 Hand-colored scanning electromicrograph of squamous epithelium, revealing squamous cells about to be shed from the surface epithelium. These shed squames contain the formed and infectious human papillomavirus particles. From: Campion M J, Ferris D G, di Paola F M, Reid R I. Modern Colposcopy: A Practical Approach. ASCCP, Hagerstown, MD. 1991; Color Plate 8. ▬▬▬

females and on the prepuce and frenulum in males, are the areas most commonly found to have genital warts. Once within the host cells, the viral genome is transported to the cell nucleus, where it establishes an episomal infection; i.e., HPV DNA exists as a self-replicating plasmid that is not integrated into the human chromosome. In order to ensure a persistent infection of the basal stem cells the genome is replicated once per cell cycle during S phase.[27] It is likely that HPV DNA may remain present but quiescent within cells either before or after active expression.[143,144] However, it is not clear whether this state of "quiescence" can be permanent or whether genomes involved in switching on viral replication typically do so soon after infection, with some resulting in expressed HPV disease and others suppressed by the host immune response too quickly to be detected. The traditional term for this state of quiescence is viral "latency," but it must be understood that this term indicates only that HPV cannot be detected by any conventional means, including molecular, cytologic, or visual methods.

5.4.2 Productive viral infection

A productive infection begins when HPV replicates independent of host chromosomal DNA synthesis (Figure 5.16). Since most HPV-induced cellular abnormalities are transient, it is still not known what proportion of infected individuals express HPV. Viral replication induces the host cells to proliferate abnormally, resulting in acanthosis, koilocytosis, nuclear atypia, and multinucleation. Lesional morphology may range from flat to papillary.[145] Although the exact factors that determine HPV expression are unknown, a complex interplay between host, viral, and environmental factors are most likely important.[145] Many individuals will never have detectable HPV-induced cellular changes, while others may manifest a wide range of disease expression, from transient minimally abnormal cytologic and colposcopic changes (Figure 5.17) to invasive cancer.

HPV DNA is present in low copy number in the basal cells of lesional tissue, but once DNA replication begins, approximately 50–100 HPV genomes are generated per cell (Figure 5.18).[27] HPV replication involves E1 and E2 proteins.[28] E4 also plays a role in productive infection by contributing to vegetative DNA replication or by facilitating viral release through its role in the disruption of the cytokeratin network.[27] Various growth factors and their receptors are also produced during HPV replication. These include the epidermal growth factor receptors [EGFr][146] and proliferating cell nuclear antigen [PCNA].[147] Once a productive lesion develops, viral

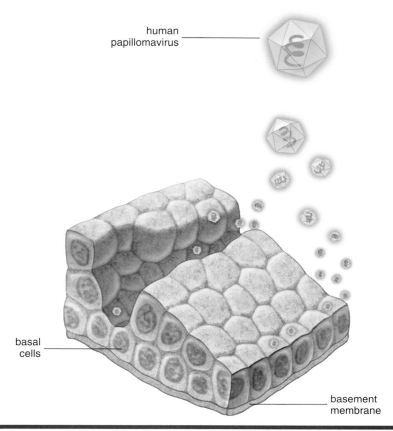

FIGURE 5.15   HPV DNA is released from the surrounding protein capsid and infects the basal epithelium in areas of microtrauma.

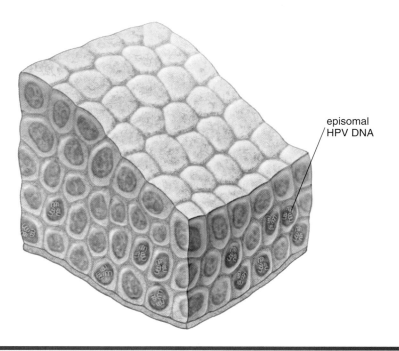

FIGURE 5.16   HPV begins to replicate in immature metaplasia.

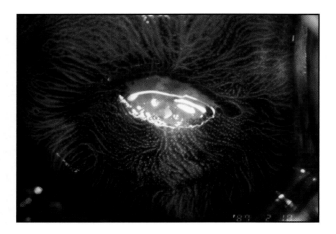

FIGURE 5.17   Minimal HPV expression may occasionally present as pinpoint acetowhite spots on the cervix and vagina often called minimally expressed papillomavirus infection (MEPI). Here these spots (reverse punctation) are demonstrated after the application of aqueous iodine solution. The findings are nonspecific, as they may be found in other inflammatory conditions. Campion M J, Ferris D G, di Paola F M, Reid R I. Modern Colposcopy: A Practical Approach. ASCCP, Hagerstown, MD. 1991; color plate 9. ▬

replication produces increasing numbers of viral genomes in cells that are closest to the surface (Figure 5.19). Hence, infected cells most likely to be desquamated contain the highest viral load. In the upper epithelial layers, HPV L1 and L2 capsid proteins are expressed in increased amounts.[142] The accumulation of these proteins and of complete HPV virions in the upper layers of lesions (Figure 5.20) produces the cytopathic effects of HPV, which include a hyperchromatic irregular "raisinoid" shaped nucleus and vacuolated cytoplasm (Figure 5.21). These cytopathic effects are termed koilocytosis.

Wound healing in abrasions may stimulate basal cell division and vascular proliferation that may accelerate viral replication.[141] Clinically, the reoccurrence of genital warts along the healing margins of ablated epithelial areas (the Koebner reaction) is a demonstration of the effects of such viral promotion during cell replication.[148] Whatever initiates viral

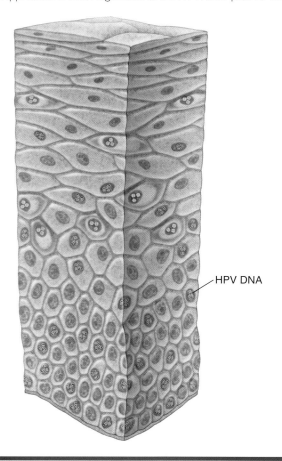

HPV DNA

FIGURE 5.18   Once vegetative DNA replication begins, approximately 50–100 HPV genomes are generated per cell with only the bottom layer of cells demonstrating cytopathic effects initially. Histology is CIN 1. ▬

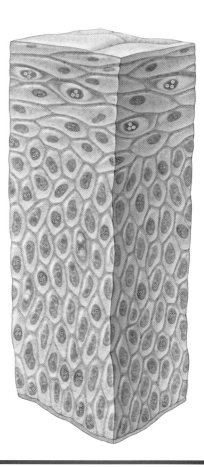

FIGURE 5.19   Viral replication works up through the epithelium as cells mature producing increasing numbers of viral genomes in cells that are closest to the surface. Here increasing numbers of abnormal cells with increased nuclear:cytoplasmic ratio extend two-thirds through the epithelium to produce a CIN 2. ▬

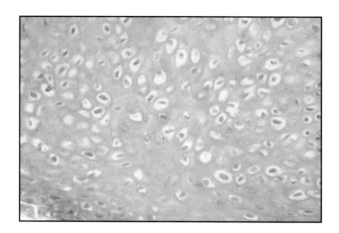

FIGURE 5.20   Histology of a low-grade lesion demonstrates koilocytes almost entirely in the upper layer of the epithelium where HPV replication occurs: histological features of a productive low-grade infection are demonstrated here. These include acanthosis, cytoplasmic vacuolization, nuclear atypia, and multinucleation. From: Campion MJ, Ferris DG, di Paola FM, Reid RI. Modern Colposcopy: A Practical Approach. ASCCP, Hagerstown, MD. 1991; Fig. 4.8. ▬

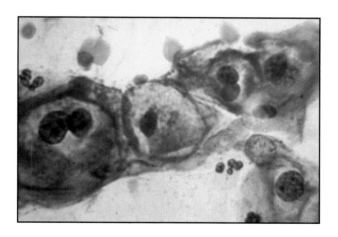

FIGURE 5.21   The cytopathic effects of HPV includes a hyperchromatic irregular "raisinoid" shaped nucleus and vacuolated cytoplasm, producing the classic koilocyte. Reprinted with permission from Wright VC. Color Atlas of Colposcopy— Cervix, Vagina and Vulva. Houston: Biomedical Communications, 2000. ▬

replication and a productive infection, once initiated the rapid epithelial and capillary proliferation that ensues is initially uninhibited by immunity. Epithelial proliferation results in acanthosis, hyperchromasia, and increased mitotic activity. Extensive vascular overgrowth, most commonly induced by HPV 6 or 11, results in the stromal projections of exophytic papillomas (Figure 5.22). In contrast, high-risk viral types are more likely to produce flat or slightly raised

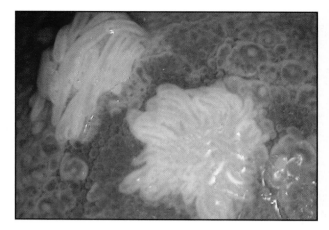

FIGURE 5.22   Exuberant stromal projections of exophytic papillomas dot this cervical ectopy in islands of metaplasia. ▬

lesions with capillary and stromal proliferation insufficient to produce the classic "cauliflower" shaped wart (Figure 5.23). When HPV-induced epithelial alterations do occur, there is enormous variability in the sites involved, disease extent, lesion morphology, clinical course, therapeutic response, and risk of neoplastic transformation. The complexity of possible disease presentations complicates management decisions.

5.4.3 Host containment

Whether disease persists or regresses, the extent and severity of the lesions, and the success of therapy ultimately depend primarily on the success of the host

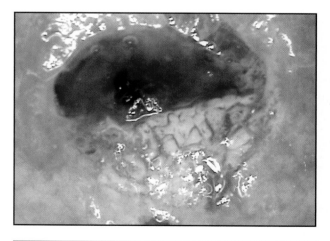

FIGURE 5.23   Subclinical, flat, high-grade lesion secondary to a high-risk HPV type. High-risk types generally do not produce stromal proliferation as is seen with low-risk types and, therefore, rarely have a papillary appearance. Vascular proliferation has resulted in both mosaic and punctation.

immune response. Emergence of a host immune response depends initially on recognition of the presence of HPV. Because HPV does not kill the epithelial cell that it infects and epithelial cells are not good antigen-presenting cells, the presence of HPV may not be recognized for a length of time that varies greatly from one individual to another but may be considerable. Once detected, the primary immunological response to HPV-infected epithelial cells is a cellular one. Antibodies are produced as part of the immune response but do not appear to be important in effecting regression of established HPV infections and related lesions.[95,149] Mononuclear cells predominate in the inflammatory response observed in regressing condylomas,[150] whereas individuals with impaired T-lymphocyte function do not manifest this containment stage, suggesting that cellular immunity plays the major role in host defense against HPV infection. Langerhan's cells are decreased in both CIN and in condylomas,[151] with the threshold for suppression varying by HPV type.[152] The activity of natural killer cells also appears to be related to HPV type, as HPV 6 and HPV 11-induced condylomas and verrucous carcinomas are associated with a decreased activity of natural killer cells and an increased production of interferon gamma and interleukin 2,[153] events that are not seen in HPV 16-induced lesions.[142]

Clinical condylomas will undergo spontaneous regression in as many as 20% of infected individuals during the first 3 months following recognized clinical expression, marking the end of any clinically apparent episodes.[154] In another 60% of patients, localized destruction of obvious vulvar condylomas leads to a lasting clinical remission. In the remaining 10% to 20%, HPV-induced lesions linger, proving refractory to standard office treatments (Figure 5.24). Control of these lesions typically may require a more comprehensive treatment approach that may include expensive outpatient procedures, such carbon dioxide laser, occasionally followed by immune-boosting regimens such as interferon or imiquimod.

Whether by spontaneous or treatment-aided remission, absence of recurrence is de facto evidence of type-specific immune memory. HPV antibody detection is a marker of current and/or past exposure to HPV.[95,155–157] Antibodies are likely to be protective against reinfection with the same type, particularly those antibodies that target the L1 and L2 proteins that comprise the virion capsid. T-cell responses to HPV, however, have not been demonstrated to be type-specific.[158,159] Therefore, T-cell responses generated post-infection may provide some protection from progression of HPV infection by new types into early lesions.[95] In a true state of sustained clinical remission, all disease expression ceases and the patient is no longer contagious, since viral capsid replication in the outer epithelial layers ends even though HPV genomes may remain in basal cells in a quiescent stage.[143] Evidence for the likely persistence of HPV in a quiescent state in some individuals after lesion regression comes from data on the expression of new HPV disease in a significant percentage of immunosuppressed transplant patients. If HPV returns to an undetectable, quiescent "latent" state, it may once again be found only in the basal cells, where only a limited number of viral genes are transcribed. The strong cell-mediated immunity that engenders regression of HPV infected lesions prevents recurrence of HPV expression from the basal cells in the majority of immunocompetent individuals.[143] Since the late genes (L1 and L2) required for forming infectious viral particles are not actively transcribed, such HPV persistence is not likely to be contagious unless rare release from immune suppression results in new HPV expression. In contrast, patients with subclinical disease may continue to shed virus and may remain contagious to other sex partners despite the absence of visible lesions.

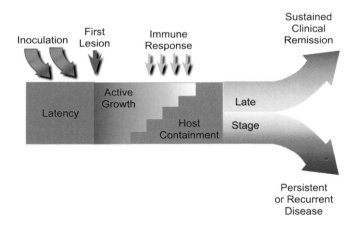

FIGURE 5.24 An overview of a typical expressed HPV infection: Following Inoculation a period of non-expression occurs, often termed "latency". Some individuals suppress or clear their HPV infection without ever having detectable HPV lesions, while others have HPV-induced cell proliferation that results in lesional development. "Host containment" follows immune recognition of the presence of HPV, resulting in sustained clinical remission for the majority. However, 10–20% will have lesions that do not clear due to the absence of an adequate immune response. Modified from: Campion MJ, Ferris DG, di Paola FM, Reid RI. Modern Colposcopy: A Practical Approach. ASCCP, Hagerstown, MD. 1991; Fig. 4-9. ◼

The 10% to 20% of patients who either persist in active disease expression or who "recur" after a lesion-free interval comprise the subset that is at risk for neoplastic progression. Presumably, most people in this subset have a reduced immunocompetence to HPV of unknown etiology, although some "persistence" or "recurrence" will represent exposure to new HPV types. For example, it has been demonstrated that individuals who recur within 6 months posttreatment usually harbor the same HPV type as their original lesion and probably represent an incomplete immune response, whereas those who recur after 6 months most often harbor a different HPV type.[160] Patients with ineffective responses to lesions caused by one HPV type may respond effectively to other HPVs. The rare hereditary skin disorder, epidermodysplasia verruciformis, provides an important insight into the nature and extent of HPV infection and the importance of immunity. Almost one half of the presently known HPV types have been isolated from the nongenital skin of these individuals, who have a disorder in local cellular immunity. The inability of immunity to clear these viruses permits the long-term persistence required for the malignant conversion of flat warts, which occurs in approximately 25% of patients and often at a young age.[95] The prevalence of numerous novel HPV types in individuals with this disorder indicates how ubiquitous HPV must be, since it is highly unlikely that these uncommon cutaneotropic viruses would persist in nature if they infected only immunocompromised hosts. That some individuals may be genetically more susceptible to HPV is also demonstrated by evidence that having a sister or mother with cervical cancer increases the risk for cervical cancer two-fold.[161] Thus, heritability might explain some of the variation in cervical cancer risk (See Chapter 4).[95,162]

5.5 Natural History of Cervical Intraepithelial Neoplasia

5.5.1 Development of low-grade disease

Although exposure to HPV is very common in the teens and twenties soon after initiation of intercourse, easily detectable clinically expressed HPV disease is relatively uncommon. For instance, 46% of women at a university health center tested positive for HPV DNA by PCR, yet at any one time, only about 4% to 6% of women at this young age had cytologic changes secondary to HPV.[163] However, very frequent screening would likely result in much higher rates. A 3-year follow up of young women by PCR and cytologic evaluation documented a 60% cumulative rate of infection with HPV, but most incident HPV infection was transient (Figure 5.25).[17,164] The median duration of detection of HPV infection was only 8 months. However, the median duration in a recent study was shown to be longer and type-dependent.[165] Low-risk HPV types persisted for a mean duration of only 13.4 months and high-risk HPV for 16.3 months. HPV 16 remained detectable for the longest period (mean duration, 18.3 months from first detection), followed by HPV 31 and HPV 53 (14.6 and 14.9 months, respectively). The transient nature of most HPV infections is also confirmed by

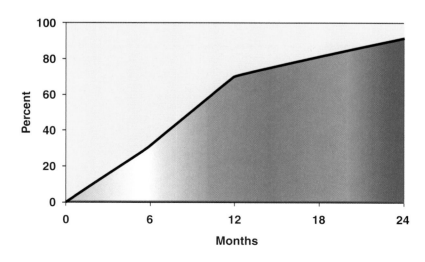

The Probability of Losing a Newly Acquired Human Papillomavirus Infection Over Time

FIGURE 5.25 In one study, the probability of losing a newly acquired HPV infection was very high (70%) in the first 12 months after detection of HPV, then dropped off so that only another 11% not already cleared at 12 months became HPV negative within 18 months. Only 9% remained HPV positive at 24 months.[17]

data documenting that the lifetime number of sexual partners is not as strongly related to HPV positivity as is the number of partners in the last 5 years.[166]

Therefore, it appears that one of three clinical pathways may subsequently occur (Figure 5.26). Most infections either remain permanently quiescent and undetectable by molecular, cytologic, and colposcopic means or only transiently produce cytologic changes missed by infrequent screening. Whether such undetectable HPV infections persist indefinitely or are permanently cleared is not known, but as dis-

cussed previously, the high rate of HPV expression in individuals immunosuppressed post-transplantation or by other immunosuppression argues that many immunocompetent individuals remain persistently infected with the virus held "in check" by the immune response.[167] Other women will develop HPV-associated cervical or vaginal disease, detectable by cytologic changes diagnostic of HPV infection, including koilocytotic atypia.[168] It is not known whether this group represents the majority of HPV infections and is just under-represented by the tran-

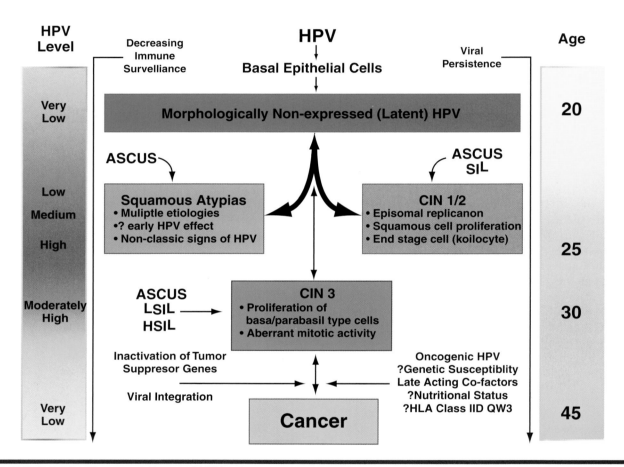

FIGURE 5.26   The natural history of HPV and cervical neoplasia. After HPV infects basal epithelial cells, morphologic changes may occur after varying lengths of latency. Cytologic findings may clearly indicate HPV expression (LSIL, koilocytotic atypia) or may be more difficult to interpret (ASC-US). Histology may demonstrate morphologic changes ranging from atypia suggestive, but not definitive for HPV, to CIN 1. Given time, most of these minor manifestations will actually regress spontaneously following immune recognition of the presence of HPV. A minority will develop a high-grade lesion, probably from monoclonal cellular changes that develop either within, or outside of, previous low-grade lesion development. High-grade lesional development does not preclude an immune response, but it does significantly decrease the probability of spontaneous resolution. The factors that promote transit from high-grade CIN to invasion are not completely understood, but a combination of a high-risk HPV type, perhaps some genetic susceptibility, late acting cofactors and possibly nutritional factors may all be important. Genomic instability results in inactivation of tumor suppressor genes and in viral integration into the host DNA. Modified from Cox JT. Epidemiology of CIN: what is the role of HPV? In: Jones HW, ed. *Cervical Intraepithelial Neoplasia.* Best Practice and Research Clinical Obstetrics and Gynecology (formerly Baillieres Clinical Obstetrics Gynecology) 1995 Elsevier Ltd. London:1–37.

sient nature of expression and infrequent opportunity for detection. Some will shed cells that demonstrate some but not all of the features of a HPV infection (e.g., atypical squamous cells of undetermined significance [ASCUS].[169] Most women with only minor atypia or low-grade intraepithelial neoplasia have lesions that will either regress spontaneously or persist unchanged. Those who develop high-grade CIN during follow-up remain persistently high-risk HPV DNA positive,[15,170] usually at high quantitative levels.[171] Intermittently HPV-positive women do not appear to be at risk for progression of disease, at least during short-term (24-month) follow up.[172]

The most comprehensive review of the literature on progression, regression, and persistence rates for cervical disease comes from a compilation of all studies on the natural history of CIN from 1952–1992 (Table 5.4).[173] Rates were shown to vary greatly depending on study size, length of follow up, and whether the diagnosis was established by histologic or only cytologic and colposcopic means. For low-grade lesions, the average rate of regression in all studies combined was approximately 60% and the average persistence rate approximately 30%. Progression to CIN 3 occurred in 11% and progression to invasion in 1%. Data from the ASCUS/LSIL Triage Study (ALTS) confirmed progression to CIN 2 or 3 over 2-year follow-up in 13.0% of women with CIN 1 detected after referral for the evaluation of a LSIL or a HPV-positive ASCUS Pap.[174] The findings were almost identical to the progression rate for women in the same study found to have either a completely normal cervix at colposcopy or an atypical transformation zone but normal findings on biopsy (11.2% and 11.6% subsequent detection of CIN 2 or 3 over 2-year follow-up, respectively).[174] These findings indicate that it is the presence of high-risk HPV and not the presence or absence of CIN 1 that determines risk for subsequent detection of CIN 2 or 3.

Because CIN was historically viewed as a progressive biological continuum leading to cervical

cancer,[175,176] older management protocols advocated aggressive treatment of all CIN lesions, including low-grade lesions. Recently, however, many have come to view CIN 1 as simply the acute manifestation of a usually transient HPV infection. In contrast, high-grade CIN 2 or 3 is generally considered to be a true precancer, with biologic potential for progression. Some studies have questioned whether CIN 1 lesions ever progress or are simply self-limited productive infections that may only persist or subsequently regress. The theory that CIN 1 progresses to CIN 2, which then progresses to CIN 3, has been replaced by data showing that patients who appear to progress actually have two adjacent concurrently established lesions with separate natural histories and different likelihoods of detection at given points in time.[176,177] These data could explain why developing high-grade lesions are almost always at the advancing new squamocolumnar junction (SCJ) and proximal to low-grade lesions. Additionally, Burghardt and Ostor[178] have shown that the abrupt transition between lesions of differing morphology and the occasional finding of normal tissue separating such lesions support the theory of adjacent development of distinct lesions of different clonal origins.

5.5.2 Progression to high-grade CIN

While the well-differentiated cytopathic effects of low-grade CIN are those classic for a replicative viral infection, high-grade lesions are characterized by undifferentiated cells classic for the neoplastic process. Characteristic findings of high-grade lesions include nuclear crowding, substantial pleomorphism, loss of tissue organization and cellular polarity, and abnormal mitotic figures.[27] Additionally, abnormal cells extend past the lower third of the epithelium in CIN 2 and 3. Most high-grade CIN results from persistent high-risk HPV infection. One longitudinal study of the natural history of HPV infection did not detect a single CIN 2 or 3 among women whose

Table 5.4 Ostor Evaluated All Natural History Studies Published Since 1950, Compiling These Statistics on Regression, Persistence and Progression of CIN.

	REGRESS	PERSIST	PROGRESS TO CIN3	TO CANCER
CIN 1	60%	30%	10%	1%
CIN 2	40%	40%	20%	5%
CIN 3	33%	<56%	—	>12%

From: Ostor AG. Natural history of CIN: A critical review. Int J Gynecol Pathol 1993;12:186–92.

infection had cleared by the third visit,[27,179] but some high-grade lesions were detected in another study without prolonged HPV exposure.[180]

Detection of CIN 3 increases with age up to 30 to 40 years.[181,182] Prevalence then decreases between the age of 40 and 65, with a second peak in prevalence of high-grade lesions in women over 65 years of age.[181] Although a majority of low-grade lesions are associated with high-risk HPV types, only a small number will develop CIN 3 or invasive cancer. Risk of progression to CIN 2 or 3 is clearly type-dependent. In a prospective cohort study of initially cytologically normal HPV 16- and 18-positive women, 39% developed CIN 2 or 3 within 2 years, in contrast to only 3% who were negative for all HPV types.[177] Women positive for HPV 31, 33, or 35 had an intermediate progression rate of 22%. In Ostor's comprehensive review of natural history studies,[173] CIN 3 was found to regress in 32% and to progress to invasion in more than 12%. The rates for progression or regression of CIN 2 were squarely between those for CIN 1 and CIN 3.

As discussed previously, the finding that there are different variants of HPV 16 and perhaps of other HPV types that may have different biologic potential may also play an important role in determining whether a lesion will regress or progress. For instance, the demonstration that some specific variants of HPV 16 may be more prone to developing persistent infection may partially explain why these variants are more prone to produce high-grade lesions.[53] Another variable that may separate lesions

likely to progress from those that are likely to regress may be the identification of inactivated tumor-suppressor genes in one or more of four chromosomal regions [3p, 4p, 4q, and 11q] (Figure 5.27).[183–185] Functional inactivation of these tumor-suppressor genes is assumed by detection of loss of hererozygosity (LOH) of the chromosomal region where they reside. LOH in tumor-suppressor loci has been documented in 0% of CIN 1 lesions, 22% of CIN 2 lesions, 41% of CIN 3 lesions, and 88% of invasive cancers.[183] Additionally, LOH studies of different regions of large or multifocal high-grade lesions in individual patients indicates loss of the same allele at each locus without exception. This finding strongly suggests that high-grade cervical intraepithelial lesions arise from a single precursor and that loss of specific tumor-suppressor genes is an early event in the development of high-grade lesions. Other cellular events that appear to be associated with progression are aneuploidy and HPV integration (See Chapter 4). A higher DNA index and aneuploidy are noted in CIN 3 as compared with CIN 1 and CIN 2 lesions.[186] HPV integration increases with increasing grade of CIN, and genomic instability and, consequently, aneuploidy are likely mediated through disruption of p53 gene activity. The dramatic increase in the frequency of LOH seen in the transition from CIN 2 to CIN 3 may reflect a similarly dramatic increase in HPV integration, ultimately leading to inactivation of p53.[183] Inactivation of p53 facilitates the subsequent accumulation of genetic damage, as evidenced by aneuploidy and

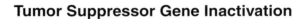

FIGURE 5.27 Functional inactivation of host tumor suppressor genes at 3p, 11q, 4q, and 4p gene loci are found with increasing frequency with increasing grade of CIN and invasive cancer. Occurrence of these genetic alterations may be important steps in the molecular basis of progression, at least for some lesions. Modified from: Larson A A, Liao S-Y, Stanbridge E J, et al. Genetic alterations accumulate during cervical tumorigenesis and indicate a common origin for multifocal lesions. *Cancer Res* 1997;57:4171–6.

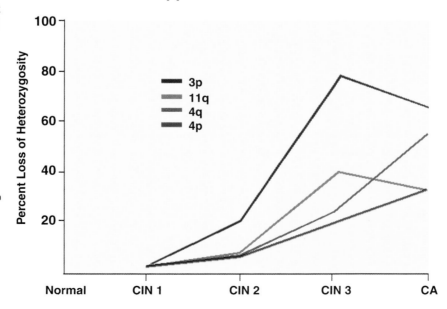

Tumor Suppressor Gene Inactivation

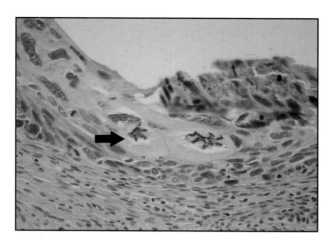

FIGURE 5.28 The only morphologic change reflecting the accumulation of genetic damage is aneuploidy, as demonstrated at the arrow.

LOH analyses (Figure 5.28). The long period of time required for progression to invasion most likely reflects the time necessary for these random genotoxic events to occur.

5.5.3 Progression to invasion

Many believe that, given a long enough period of observation, most CIN 3 will eventually progress to invasion.[187] Regression of CIN lesions is at least partly age-dependent, as CIN has been shown to regress in about 80% of women under 34 years and in about 40% of older women.[188] Whereas regression of CIN 3 may be an uncommon event, regression of CIN 2 is likely to be common, as demonstrated by a deficit in cumulative detection of CIN 2 in the ALTS trial in comparison with CIN 3.[189] Microinvasive squamous-cell cancer usually arises from high-grade CIN and is characterized by a single or multiple irregular tongues of highly atypical squamous epithelium penetrating no more than 3mm through the plane of the basal lamina and into the cervical stroma.[27] Invasive cervical cancer has the same histologic appearance but differs in that the depth of penetration into the stroma is >3 mm (Figure 5.29).

Cancer results from the loss of normal control over cell growth. Normal tissue maintenance is an orderly process of cell aging, cell death, and cell replacement. When this process goes awry because of mutations in the cell DNA or other genotoxic stress, the normal cell response is either growth arrest or the induction of programmed cell death (apoptosis). Apoptosis is a strategy used by organisms to counter malignant progression or tumorigenesis. Two tumor-suppressor proteins (p53 and the retinoblastoma susceptibility gene product, pRb) are produced when

a cell experiences DNA damage, when growth factors are limiting, or when oncogenes force the cell into a replicative state.[190] In response to DNA damage, an increase in p53 protein levels is observed.[191] This increase leads to either arrest in cell-cycle progression[191] or apoptosis, as described earlier in this chapter.[192] While these events are well described, many molecular events required for progression to cervical cancer are yet to be determined. For instance, although the inactivation of p53 and Rb gene products by E6 and E7 proteins are well known, the role of additional genes targeted by high-risk HPVs, such as C-MYC, RAS, and telomerase/hTERT, still need to be clarified.[95] Additionally, silencing of tumor suppressor genes via promoter hypermethylation in HPV-infected host cells has been demonstrated to be a frequent human epigenetic event.[95,193,194] In this process, a methyl group is attached to the promoter region of a gene, resulting in the suppression of gene expression. This process is common in human

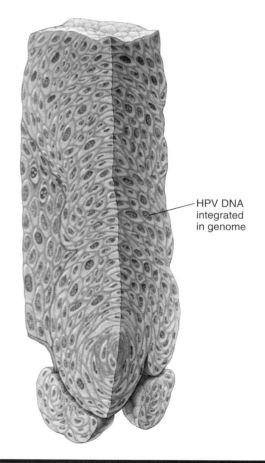

HPV DNA integrated in genome

FIGURE 5.29 Invasive cervical cancer has the same histologic appearance as microinvasive cancers in that single or multiple areas of invasion may occur, but differs in that the depth of penetration into the stroma is >3mm.

Cervical Cancer Incidence by Age

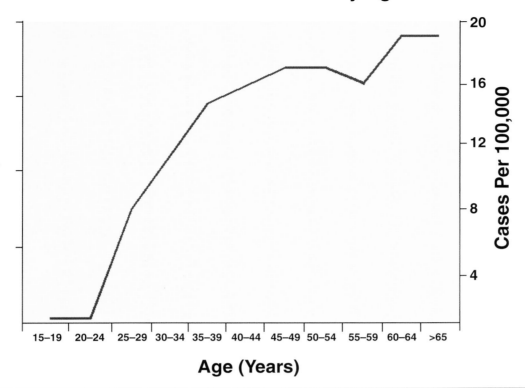

Age (Years)

cancers and suggests another potential role for HPV in the oncogenic pathway.

The incidence of invasive cervical cancer reaches a plateau in Caucasian U.S. women between the ages of 40 and 45 (Figure 5.30).[195] In most immunocompetent individuals, the complex steps involved in viral integration and cellular transformation must require this extended period of time from the earliest exposure to HPV to the development of invasive potential. Increasing time also permits the chance occurrence of secondary events that may be necessary for transformation (Figure 5.31). Such progression is most commonly monoclonal, usually involving integration of HPV DNA into the host genome.[196]

FIGURE 5.31 Schematic of a mutation arising in an otherwise normally functioning cell. Such mutations would normally result in increased p53 protein levels, which would lead to either cell death or arrest of cell division and replication.

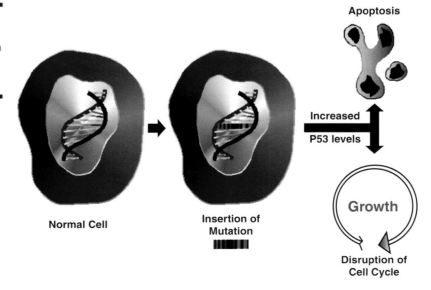

However, HPV 16 DNA may not always be integrated in carcinomas, as it has been detected in episomal or as a combination of episomal and integrated forms. Integration is rare in preinvasive disease and has never been reported in women not having dysplasia.[197]

Until the late 1990s, a definite percentage of cervical cancers had HPV-negative test results. Data suggested that these HPV-negative tumors were a distinct group that exhibited more aggressive behavior and worse prognosis.[198–200] and the detection of somatic mutations of p53 and pRb in some cervical cancers suggested that some might not be HPV-related.[201] However, newer HPV-testing technology has documented HPV in 99.7% of 1000 cervical cancers in the IARC study, strongly questioning the existence of non-HPV related squamous or adenocarcimonas of the cervix.[4,5] The presence of high-risk HPV appears to be necessary for genetic alterations brought about by dysfunction of p53 and pRb to accumulate and result in the molecular changes necessary for the multistep progression from CIN to cancer.[201]

5.6 New Biologic Markers

The high cost of cervical cytologic screening programs, interobserver variability in the interpretation of cytologic, colposcopic, and histologic images, and the trend toward expectant management of CIN 1 have increased the need for markers that more specifically separate women at risk for progression from those who are not at risk. Such risk stratification will be even more important if HPV testing is increasingly utilized in primary cervical screening. Since only a small proportion of women with high-risk HPV infection are at risk for development of cervical cancer, more specific markers for risk of progression must be identified if cervical cancer screening is to become significantly more cost effective. Although CIN 2, 3 and cervical cancer have been shown in some cross-sectional studies to have a consistently higher viral load,[202–204] difficulties with sampling variability, controlling testing for cell count, and the existence of high viral load in some low-grade lesions detract from the potential utility of measuring viral load as a risk marker.[95,204,205] Even if viral load can be determined using new PCR methods, such as kinetic PCR,[206] interpretation of the significance of high viral load will be hampered by inability to predict whether the result represents long-term persistent HPV infection or recent infection. Significance of the former is likely to be much higher than high viral load associated with recent infection.

Viral persistence is one marker that is established as a predictor of risk for progression and is the only

marker other than high-risk HPV types presently utilized in clinical guidelines.[15,207] Unfortunately, testing for persistence to stratify risk necessarily delays determination of risk, which may prolong anxiety for some women and occasionally may delay diagnosis of a significant lesion. Clearly, other markers need to be identified.

Markers presently under study include identification of HPV integration into the host genome, expression of p16, telomerase, and 3q amplification, measurement of HPV transcripts and their ratios, proliferation (Ki67), aneuploidy, and HPV variants (Figure 5.32).[208] Studies on gene and protein expression using microarray technology and laser-capture microdissection are one area of basic research that may lead to the identification of clinically useful markers. These studies may identify gene families that are upregulated or downregulated at varying stages of cervical carcinogenesis.[95,209,210] Microarray technology allows the examination of thousands of genes at a time, facilitating the comparison of genetic events at different stages of the pathogenic process, thereby not only increasing the understanding of the oncogenic process but also potentially identifying markers for progression. Areas to be evaluated for comparison of genetic events include cancer versus CIN 3 and CIN 3 versus HPV infection, comparison of adenocarcinomas and squamous cell carcinomas, and comparison of different HPV types and variants.[95]

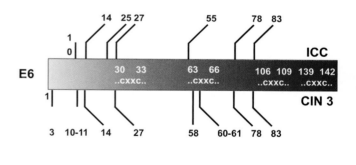

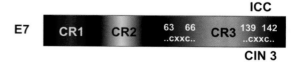

FIGURE 5.32 The location of gene loci variations between prototype HPV 16 and variant HPV 16. Such variations may be useful as molecular markers for risk for progression. Modified from: Zehbe I, Wilander E, Delius H, Tommassino M. Human papillomavirus 16 E6 variants are more prevalent than the prototype. *Cancer Res* 1998;58:829–33. With permission. ■

A marker's clinical utility will likely vary by whether the marker is to be used for screening, diagnosis, or prognosis, and whether the population is already screened heavily, rarely, or not at all. For instance, a marker will need to be highly specific in well-screened populations in order to prevent overtreatment of HPV-infected women, most of whose lesions will regress,[95] whereas screening in developing countries will require increased sensitivity even at the expense of specificity and will need to be inexpensive. p16[INK4a] is a marker of oncogenic HPV expression that has shown some promise for the identification of high-grade CIN,[95,211] but further study will be required to evaluate its utility in predicting risk for subsequent development of CIN 3.

Markers evaluating the prognosis of cervical cancers are also being evaluated. Among the major prognostic factors are stage, depth of invasion and grade of tumor, histologic type, lymphatic spread, and vascular invasion.[212] At this time, no clinically useful markers have been identified beyond those classically used in staging.

5.7 Prospects for HPV Vaccines
5.7.1 Prophylactic vaccines

If introduced worldwide, vaccination against HPV 16 alone could prevent a large proportion of the nearly one-quarter million deaths that occur annually from cervical cancer. A quadravalent vaccine including types 6, 11, 16, and 18 could theoretically prevent 90% of genital warts and 75% of cervical cancers. The potential is not only in reduction of morbidity from genital warts and cervical cancer and mortality from the latter but in the possibility that physical, psychological, and financial costs associated with screening, follow-up, and treatment might be significantly decreased.[213] Two different categories of vaccines are presently under development or testing: prophylactic and therapeutic. Prophylactic vaccines are directed toward preventing attachment of the viral capsid to the host upon exposure. Therapeutic vaccines are designed to either eliminate HPV infections in patients already infected or to kill high-grade CIN and invasive cancer cells.

Although the potential benefits of vaccination for HPV have long been understood, the inability to propagate HPV in culture and the oncogenic risk of introducing an attenuated or inactivated virus containing oncogenes delayed efforts until it was possible to develop a subunit vaccine not containing the viral DNA. However, successful vaccines developed for animal papillomaviruses provided the prospect that similar success could be achieved with human papillomavirus vaccines. For example, calves vaccinated with bovine papillomavirus wart extract develop protective neutralizing antibodies.[214] These animals are then protected against papillomavirus infection when challenged with live virions.

In the mid-1990s, it was recognized that recombinant technology could be used to develop genetically engineered, immunologically active virus-like particles (VLPs).[215,216] These particles are made by cloning the L1 and L2 ORFs (regions encoding for capsid proteins) of specific types of HPV into insect vectors, yeast, or a bacculovirus system. These vectors then produce L1 and L2 proteins that are capable of folding correctly and forming empty, DNA-free capsids (VLPs) that have three-dimensional and antigenic properties identical to native HPV virions.[213] This led to the development of vaccines based on these VLPs. L1 VLPs have been shown to induce high levels of neutralizing antibodies in both animals and in humans.[213] For example, a strong HPV 11 L1 IgG antibody response has been elicited in green monkeys after vaccination with HPV 11 L1 VLPs.[217] The antibodies were detected in both serum and at the mucosa, suggesting that vaccination with L1 VLPs may protect against HPV infection by preventing virus from adhering to basal cells. The most compelling data reported to date on VLP vaccination in humans demonstrated that women who received HPV-16 VLP and were followed for a median of 17.4 months after completing the vaccination regimen did not test positive for HPV 16 or develop HPV-16 CIN.[218] In contrast, the incidence of persistent HPV 16 infection was 3.8 per 100 woman-years among recipients of the placebo, and all nine cases of HPV-16 CIN in this study occurred in the placebo group, yielding 100 percent efficacy. If this result can be duplicated in the quadravalent vaccine studies, it may then be technically feasible to produce a polyvalent HPV vaccine with all genital HPV types. Doing so would require proof that the presence of additional HPV types neither alters the safety profile of the vaccine nor interferes with the immunologic response to the more prevalent HPV types present in the original vaccine.[213]

VLP vaccines presently under study will be relatively expensive to produce and will require three injections, similar to vaccination for Hepatitis B, in order to achieve peak immune response.[213] Additionally, because papillomavirus-neutralizing antibodies against L1 are type-specific, it is expected that vaccination will be protective for only those types included in the vaccine. Several randomized HPV VLP vaccine trials are presently underway with recommendation by the FDA that, to prove efficacy, reduction in CIN 2 and 3 and in HPV type-specific persistence must be documented. Persistence is defined as at least two consecutive positive HPV DNA tests separated by at least 6 to 12 months.[213] The trials must also determine whether the vaccine is safe through administration to large numbers of individuals, whether protection is type-specific, whether protection is against incident infection, and whether protection is equal against variants of the HPV types in the vaccine. As with the release of other new vaccines, long-term protection beyond the short 3 to 5 years expected for vaccine study will not be guaranteed until long after vaccine release, when population administration facilitates longer analysis.[213]

HPV vaccines containing the minor capsid protein L2 might have the potential to confer protection against multiple HPV types since L2 has been shown to have cross-reacting epitope(s) with other types.[213] However, the L2 epitope is not as immunogenic as the L1 neutralization epitopes and, therefore, may not achieve levels of neutralizing antibodies that are high enough to be protective.

Prophylactic HPV vaccines will need to be administered before infection in order to elicit neutralizing antibodies that would inhibit either attachment or entry. Because HPV is easily and frequently transmitted soon after sexual debut, the target population for prophylactic HPV vaccination will necessarily be children who have not attained the age of sexual maturity.

5.7.2 Therapeutic vaccines

Cell-mediated immune responses appear to be crucial for the regression of HPV-induced lesions. T lymphocytes identify and eliminate virally infected cells by recognizing viral peptides displayed at the cell surface in association with major histocompatability complex (MHC) class I molecules. Therefore, a vaccine designed to stimulate cell-mediated immunity would need to prime for CD8+ cytotoxic T lymphocytes (CTL) responses, in the context of MHC class.[219] Because both E6 and E7 appear to be required for transformation and for the continued proliferation of HPV-infected cells, the development of CTLs specific for these proteins might prove to be immune effectors in recognizing and destroying HPV-infected cells. For this reason, HPV 16 E6 and E7 proteins are prime targets for immunotherapy against cervical cancer.[220]

Recombinant live vectors have been shown to induce CTL responses, but their safety is still uncertain.[221] Recently, successful CTL priming by exogenous E7 protein antigen has been shown to stimulate

tumor-specific cell-mediated protective immunity to HPV-16 induced cancers.[220] Additionally, hybrid VLPs have been developed that induce both CTL responses and antibody production. Immunization with these hybrid VLPs has been shown to be capable of inducing complete protection against viral challenge.

A vaccine that could both prevent new infections and successfully treat established infections would be ideal. Hence, combining a prophylactic and a therapeutic HPV vaccine would most quickly reduce morbidity and mortality from cervical cancer and its precursors.[213] Unfortunately, the prospects for such a combined vaccine are presently not high because of the known difficulty in developing successful therapeutic vaccines. To date, all approved non-HPV vaccines in widespread use are prophylactic. One approach that has promise is the use of chimeric VLPs. Chimerics contain L1 VLPs plus polypeptides from one or more nonstructural viral proteins.[213] These are either incorporated into L1 or fused to L2. Because this is a VLP-based approach, it might successfully combine the prophylactic properties of L1 VLPs with the therapeutic potential of immunity directed against nonstructural viral determinants.[213] Although the prospects for the development of therapeutic vaccines are less promising than for prophylactic vaccines, use of chimerics or other novel approaches may eventually overcome these barriers.

5.8 Summary

There can no longer be any doubt regarding the role of specific HPV types in the etiology of essentially all cervical cancers and of many neoplasias of the vulva, vagina, anus, and penis. Specific high-risk types of HPV are found in association with nearly 100% of invasive cervical cancers. The interaction of high-risk papillomavirus and immature metaplastic epithelium initiates the process that leads to the development of cervical neoplasia in some women. Mature squamous epithelium is at lower risk for development of cancer or its precursors. However, exposure to HPV is an extremely common event, whereas the development of cervical cancer is uncommon.

This indicates that other factors must be important to disease progression. The increase in high-grade CIN and cervical cancer observed in immunosuppressed patients suggests that immune surveillance plays a critical role in preventing persistent infections and the subsequent development of high-grade and invasive lesions. Other possible factors may include a genetic propensity, infection by other microbial agents, the use of tobacco products, specific dietary deficiencies, and the effect of hormonal contraceptives and pregnancy. The long period between exposure and the development of cancer supports the concept that cervical cancer develops by a multistage model of carcinogenesis. Events that are probably important include alterations with LOH at tumor-suppressor gene loci, integration of HPV into the genome, hypermethylation products of HPV, and possibly specific mutations. Therefore, malignant progression, when it does occur, commonly takes many years or decades. Women presenting initially with only low-grade HPV-induced atypia are at low risk of progression to invasive cancer, yet such progression is reported. The term "progression" may be a misnomer, however, as "apparent" progression may really represent adjacent "de-novo" development of higher-grade CIN within an area of lower-grade disease.

Squamous epithelial cancers of the vulva, vagina, penis, anus, and oropharynx are often induced by HPV as well. However, only the anal area has a transformation zone that is nearly equivalent to that of the cervix. The increased vulnerability of the transformation zones in these two areas accounts for the significantly greater risk of HPV-induced cancers in the cervix and anus and for the similar virtually exclusive etiology. In contrast, malignancies of the vagina, vulva, and penis are among the rarest of cancers and are often not caused by HPV.

Because phylogenetic studies have provided evidence of minimal HPV genomic drift over the millennia, it may be assumed that HPV is a stable virus. The instigation of many vaccine trials offers hope that a successful vaccination program may profoundly reduce cervical cancer worldwide during the 21st century.

References

1. Franco E L. Cancer causes revisited: human papillomavirus and cervical neoplasia. *J Natl Cancer Inst* 1995;87:779–89.

2. Munoz N, Bosch F X, Sanjose S, et al. The causal link between HPV and invasive cervical cancer: a population based case-control study in Colombia and Spain. *Int J Cancer* 1992;52;743–9.

3. Bosch F X, Manos M M, Munoz N et al. Prevalence of human papillomavirus in cervical cancer: a worldwide perspective. *J Natl Cancer Inst* 1995;87:796–802.

4. Walboomers J M, Jacobs M V, Manos M M, Bosch F X, Kummer J A, Shah K V, Snijders P J, Peto J, Meijer C J, Munoz N. Human papillomavirus is a necessary cause of invasive cervical cancer worldwide. *J Pathol* 1999;189:1–3.

5. Bosch F X, Lorincz A, Munoz N, Meijer C J L M, Shah K V. The causal relation between human papillomavirus and cervical cancer. *J Clin Pathol* 2002;55:244–65.

6. Schiffman M, Kjaer S K. Chapter 2: natural history of anogenital human papillomavirus infection and neoplasia. *J Natl Cancer Inst* (monograph) 2003;31:14–9.

7. Morrison E A, Ho G F, Vermund S H, et al. Human papillomavirus infection and other risk factors for cervical neoplasia: a case-control study. *Int J Cancer* 1991;49:6–13.

8. Munoz N, Bosch F X, Shah V, et al, eds. *The Epidemiology of Cervical Cancer and Human Papillomavirus.* Lyon, France: International Agency for Research on Cancer (WHO);l992. IARC Scientific Publications No. 119.

9. Peng H Q, Liu S L, Mann V, et al. HPV types 16 and 33, Herpes Simplex Type 2, and other risk factors in cervical cancer in Sichuan Province, China. *Int J Cancer* 1991;47:711–6.

10. Jones C J, Brinton L A, Hamman R F, et al. Risk factors for in situ cervical cancer: results from a case-control study. *Cancer Res* 1990;50:3657–62.

11. Cuzick J, Terry G, Ho L, et al. Type specific HPV DNA as a predictor of high-grade cervical intraepithelial neoplasia. *Br J Cancer* 1994;69:167–71.

12. Terry G, Ho L, Jenkins D, et al. Definition of human papillomavirus type 16 DNA levels in low and high grade cervical lesions by simple PCR technique. *Arch Virol* 1993;128:123–33.

13. Konno R, Sato S, Yajima A. Progression of squamous cell carcinoma of the uterine cervix from cervical intraepithelial neoplasia infected with human papillomavirus: a retrospective follow-up study by in situ hybridization and polymerase chain reaction. *Int J Gynecol Pathol* 1992; 11:105–12.

14. Koutsky L A, Holmes K K, Critchlow C W, et al. Cohort study of risk of cervical intraepithelial neoplasia grade 2 or 3 associated with cervical papillomavirus infection. *NEJM* 1992;327:127–78.

15. Nobbenhuis M, Walboomers, J M, Helmerhorst T I. Rozendaal, L. Relation of human papillomavirus status to cervical lesions and consequences for cervical-cancer screening: a prospective study. *Lancet* 1999;354:20.

16. Jacobs M V, Zielinski D, Meijer C J, Pol R P, Voorhorst F J, de Schipper F A, Runsink A P, Snijders P J, Walboomers J M. I. A simplified and reliable HPV testing or archival Papanicolaou-stained cervical smears: application to cervical smears from cancer. *Br J Cancer* 2000;82:1421–6.

17. Ho G Y F, Bierman R, Beardsley L, Chang C J, Burk R D. Natural history of cervicovaginal papillomavirus infection in young women. *NEJM* 1998;338:423–8.

18. Van den Brule A J C, Walboomers J M M, Maine M D, et al. Difference in the prevalence of human papillomavirus in cytomorphologically normal cervical

smears is associated with a history of cervical intraepithelial neoplasia. *Int J Cancer* 1991;48:404–8.

19. Peyton C L, Gravitt P E, Hunt W C, Hundley R S, Zhao M, Apple R J, Wheeler C M. Determinants of genital human papillomavirus detection in a US population. *J Infect Dis* 2001;183:1554–64.

20. Clavel C, Masure M, Bory J P, et al. Human papillomavirus testing in primary screening for the detection of high-grade cervical lesions: a study of 7932 women. *Brit J Cancer* 2001; 89:1616–23.

21. Cox J T, Lorincz A T, Schiffman M H, et al. HPV testing by hybrid capture appears to be useful in triaging women with a cytologic diagnosis of ASCUS. *Am J Obstet Gynecol* 1995;172:946–54.

22. Manos M M, Kinney W K, Hurley L B, et al. Identifying women with cervical neoplasia: using human papillomavirus DNA testing for equivocal Papanicolaou results. *JAMA* 1999;281:1605–10.

23. Solomon D, Schiffman M H, Tarone R. Comparison of three management strategies for patients with atypical squamous cells of undetermined significance: baseline results from a randomized trial. *J Natl Cancer Inst* 2001;93:293–9.

24. The Atypical Squamous cells of Undetermined Significance/Low-Grade Squamous Intraepithelial Lesions Triage Study (ALTS) Group. Human papillomavirus testing for triage of women with cytologic evidence of low-grade squamous intraepithelial lesions: baseline data from a randomized trial. *J Natl Cancer Inst* 2000;92:1014–8.

25. Durst M, Gissmann L, Ikenberg H, zur Hausen H. A papillomavirus DNA from a cervical carcinoma and its prevalence in cancer biopsy samples from different geographic regions. *Proc Natl Acad Sci USA* 1983;80:3812–5.

26. Gissman L, Wolnik L, Ikenberg H, et al. Human papillomavirus types 6 and II DNA sequences in genital and laryngeal papillomas and in some cervical cancers. *Proc Natl Acad Sci USA* l983;80:560.

27. ROC Background Document for HPV: Genital mucosal types. ntp-server.niehs.nih.gov/newhomeroc/roc11/HPV_RG2_Public.pdf

28. Howley P M, Lowy D R. Papillomaviruses and their replication. In: *Fields' Virology.* Knipe D M, Howley P M, eds. Philadelphia: Lippincott Williams & Wilkins, 2001:2197–229.

29. Botchan M, Lusky M. Characterization of the bovine papillomavirus plasmid maintenance sequences. *Cell* 1984;36:391–401.

30. Broker T R. Structure and genetic expression of papillomaviruses. *Obstet Gynecol North Am* 1987;14:329–48.

31. Ward P, Coleman D V, Malcolm D B. Regulatory mechanisms of the papillomaviruses. *Trends Genet* 1989;5:97–8.

32. Bernard B A, Bailly C, Lenoir M C, et al. The human papillomavirus type 18 (HPV 18) E2 gene product is a repressor of the HPV 18 regulatory region in human keratinocytes. *J Virol* 1989;63:4317–24.

33. Doobar J. An emerging function for E4. *Papillomavirus Reports* 1991;2:145–7.

34. Palefsky J M, Winkler B, Rabanus J-P, et al. Characterization of in-vivo expression of the human papillomavirus type 16 E4 protein in cervical biopsy tissues. *J Clin Invest* 1991;87:2132–41.

35. Pilacinski W P, Glassman D L, Kazysek R A. Cloning and expression in E. coli of the bovine papillomavirus type L1 and L2 open reading frames. *Biotechnology* 1984;2:356.

36. Komly C A, Breitburd F, Croissant O, et al. The L2 open reading frame of human papillomavirus 1a encodes a minor structural protein carrying type-specific antigens. *J Virol* 1986;60:813–6.

37. Firzlaff J M, Kiviat N B, Beckmann A M, et al. Detection of human papillomavirus capsid antigens in various squamous epithelial lesions using antibodies directed against the L1 and L2 open reading frames. *Virology* 1988;164:467–77.

38. Kurman R J, Jenson A B, Sinclair C F, et al. Detection of human papillomaviruses by immunocytochemistry. In: *Advances in immunocytochemistry.* Chicago: Yearbook Medical Publishers,1984;45:201–21.

39. Bosch F X, De Sanjose S. Chapter 1: human papillomavirus and cervical cancer-burden and assessment of causality. *J Natl Cancer Inst* (monograph) 2003;31:3–13.

40. Munoz N, Bosch F X, de Sanjose S, et al. International Agency for Research on Cancer Multicenter Cervical Cancer Study Group. Epidemiologic classification of human papillomavirus types associated with cervical cancer. *NEJM* 2003;348:518–27.

41. Van Ranst M, Tachezy R, Burk R D. Human papillomaviruses: a never-ending story? In: Lacy C, ed.: *Papillomavirus Reviews: Current Research on Papillomaviruses.* Leeds, UK: Leeds University Press,1996:1–19.

42. Moy R L, Eliezri Y D, Nuovo G J, et al. Human papillomavirus type 16 DNA in periungual squamous cell carcinomas. *JAMA* 1989;261:2669–73.

43. Lorincz A T, Reid R, Jenson A B, et al. Human papillomavirus infection of the cervix: relative risk associations of 15 common anogenital types. *Obstet Gynecol* 1992;79:328–37.

44. Nuovo G J, Darfler M M, Impraim C C, Bromley S E. Occurrence of multiple types of HPV in genital tract lesions: analysis by in situ hybridization and PCR. *Am J Pathol* 1991;138:53–8.

45. Lowy D R, Howley P M. Papillomaviruses. In: *Fields' Virology.* Knipe D M, Howley P M, eds. Philadelphia: Lippincott Williams & Wilkins, 2001: 2231–64.

46. Schiffman M H, Burk R D. Human papillomaviruses. In: Evans A S, Kaslow R, eds. *Viral Infections of Humans.* 4th ed. New York: Plenum Press, 1995:345–92.

47. Ogagaki T. Female genital tumors associated with HPV infection and the concept of genital-neoplasia syndrome (GEMP). *Pathol Ann* 1984;19:31–62.

48. Hildesheim A, Wang S S. Host and viral genetics and risk of cervical cancer: a review. *Virus Res* 2002;89:229–40.

49. Villa L L, Sichero L, Rahal P, Caballero O, Ferenczy A, Rohan T, et al. Molecular variants of human papillomavirus types 16 and 18 preferentially

associated with cervical neoplasia. *J Gen Virol* 2000;81:2959–68.

50. Hecht J L, Kadish A S, Jiang G, Burk R D. Genetic characterization of the human papillomavirus (HPV) 18 E2 gene in clinical specimens suggests the presence of a subtype with decreased oncogenic potential. *Int J Cancer* 1995;60:369–76.

51. Lizano M, Berumen J, Guido M C, Casas L, Garcia-Carranca A. Association between human papillomavirus type 18 variants and histopathology of cervical cancer. *J Natl Cancer Inst* 1997;89:1227–31.

52. Chan P K, Lam C W, Cheung T H, et al. Association of human papillomavirus type 58 variant with the risk of cervical cancer. *J Natl Cancer Inst* 2002;94:1249–53.

53. Zehbe I, Wilander E, Delius H, Tommassino M. Human papillomavirus 16 E6 variants are more prevalent than the prototype. *Cancer Res* 1998;58:829–33.

54. Xi L F, Koutsky L A, Galloway D A, et al. Genomic variation of human papillomavirus 16 and risk for high-grade cervical intraepithelial neoplasia. *J Natl Cancer Inst* 1997;89:796–802.

55. Kurman R J, Schiffman M H, Lancaster W D, et al. Analysis of individual human papillomavirus types in cervical neoplasia: a possible role for type 18 in rapid progression. *Am J Obstet Gynecol* 1988;159:293–6.

56. Winkelstein W, Selvin S. Cervical cancer in young Americans. *Lancet* 1989;1:1385.

57. Yokoyama M, Tsutsumi K, Pater A, Pater M. Human papillomavirus 18 immortalized endocervical cells with in-vitro cytokeratin expression characteristics of adenocarcinoma. *Obstet Gynecol* 1994;83:197–204.

58. Kleter B, van Doorn L J, Schrauwen L, et al. Development and clinical evaluation of a highly sensitive PCR-reverse hybridization line probe assay for detection and identification of anogenital human papillomavirus. *J Clin Microbiol* 1999;37:2508–17.

59. Iftner T, Villa L L. Chapter 12: Human papillomavirus technologies. *J Natl Cancer Inst* (monograph) 2003;31:80–8.

60. Ponten J, Guo Z. Precancer of the human cervix. *Cancer Surv* 1998;32:201–29.

61. Wallin K L, Wiklund F, Angstrom T, et al. Type-specific persistence of human papillomavirus DNA before the development of invasive cervical cancer. *NEJM* 1999;341:1633–8.

62. Rousseau M C, Pereira J S, Prado J C M, Villa L L, Rohan T E, Franco E L. Cervical co-infection with human papillomavirus (HPV) types as a predictor of acquisition and persistence of HPV infection. *J Infect Dis* 2001;184:1508–17.

63. Liaw K L, Hildesheim A, Burk R D, et al. A prospective study of human papillomavirus (HPV) type 16 DNA detection by polymerase chain reaction and its association with acquisition and persistence of other HPV types. *J Infec Dis* 2001;183:8–15.

64. Ho L, Chan S Y, Chow V, et al. Sequence variants of HPV type 16 in clinical samples permit verification and extension of epidemiological studies and construction of a phylogenic tree. *J Clin Microbiol* 1991;29:1765–72.

65. Chan S-Y, Chew S-H, Kiyafumi E, et al. Phylogenetic analysis of the human papillomavirus type 2 (HPV-2), HPV-27, and HPV-57 group, which is associated with common warts. *Virology* 1997;239:296–302.

66. Elbel M, Carl S, Spaderna S, Iftner T. A comparative analysis of the interactions of the E6 proteins from cutaneous and genital papillomaviruses with p53 and E6AP in correlation to their transforming potential. *Virology* 1997;239:132–49.

67. Armstrong D L, Roman A. The relative ability of human papillomavirus type 6 and human papillomavirus type 16 E7 proteins to transactivate E2F-responsive elements is promoter- and cell-dependent. *Virology* 1997;239:238–46.

68. Thomas, M, Pim D, Banks L. The role of the E6-p53 interaction in the molecular pathogenesis of HPV. *Oncogene* 1999;18:7690–700.

69. Hengstermann A, Linares L K, Ciechanover A, Whitaker N J, Scheffner M. Complete switch from Mdm2 to human papillomavirus E6-mediated degradation of p53 in cervical cancer cells. *Proc Natl Acad Sci USA* 2001;98:1218–23.

70. Rapp L, Chen J J. The papillomavirus E6 proteins. *Biochem Biophys Acta* 1998;1378:F1–19.

71. Jones D L, Munger K. Analysis of the p53-mediated G1 growth arrest pathway in cells expressing the human papillomavirus 16 E7oncoprotein. *J Virol* 1997;71:2905–12.

72. Zwerschke W, Jansen-Dürr P. Cell transformation by the E7 oncoprotein of human papillomavirus type 16: interactions with nuclear and cytoplasmic target proteins. *Adv Cancer Res* 2000;78:1–29.

73. Alani R M, Münger K. Human papillomaviruses and associated malignancies. *J Clin Oncol* 1998;16:330–7.

74. Heck D V, Yee C L, Howley P M, Munger K. Efficiency of binding the retinoblastoma protein correlates with the transforming capacity of the E7 oncoproteins of the human papillomaviruses. *Proc Natl Acad Sci USA* 1992;89:4442–6.

75. Dyson N, Howley P M, Munger K, et al. The human papillomavirus 16 E7 oncoprotein is able to bind the retinoblastoma gene product. *Science* 1989;243:934–7.

76. Munger K, Werness B A, Dyson N, et al. Complex formation of papillomavirus E7 proteins with the retinoblastoma tumor suppressor gene product. *EMBO Journal* 1989;8:4099–105.

77. Gonzalez S L, Stremlau M, He X, Basile J R, Munger K. Degradation of the retinoblastoma tumor suppressor by the human papillomavirus type 16 E7 oncoprotein is important for functional inactivation and is separable from proteasomal degradation of E7. *J Virol* 2001;75:7583–91.

78. Funk J O, Waga S, Harry J B, Espling E, Stillman B, Galloway D A. Inhibition of CDK activity and PCNA-dependent DNA replication by p21 is blocked by interaction with the HPV-16 E7 oncoprotein. *Genes Dev* 1997;11:2090–100.

79. Jones D L, Alani R M, Münger K. The human papillomavirus E7 oncoprotein can uncouple cellular differentiation and proliferation in human

keratinocytes by abrogating p21Cip1-mediated inhibition of cdk2. *Genes Dev* 1997;11:2101–11.

80. Zerfass-Thome K, Zwerschke W, Mannhardt B, Tindle R, Botz JW, Jansen-Dürr P. Inactivation of the cdk inhibitor p27KIP1 by the human papillomavirus type 16 E7 oncoprotein. *Oncogene* 1996;13:2323–30.

81. Jones DL, Münger K. Interactions of the human papillomavirus E7 protein with cell cycle regulators. *Semin Cancer Biol* 1996;7:327–37.

82. Livingstone LR, White A, Sprouse J, Livanos E, Jacks T, Tlsty TD. Altered cell cycle arrest and gene amplification potential accompany loss of wild-type p53. *Cell* 1992;70:923–35.

83. Tlsty TD. Normal diploid human and rodent cells lack a detectable frequency of gene amplification. *Proc Natl Acad Sci USA* 1990;87:3132–6.

84. Duensing S, Munger K. Centrosome abnormalities, genomic instability and carcinogenic progression. *Biochem Biophys Acta* 2001;1471:M81–8.

85. Duensing S, Lee LY, Duensing A, et al.. The human papillomavirus type 16 E6 and E7 oncoproteins cooperate to induce mitotic defects and genomic instability by uncoupling centrosome duplication from the cell division cycle. *Proc Natl Acad Sci USA* 2000 97:10002–7.

86. Southern SA, Evans MF, Herrington CS. Basal cell tetrasomy in low-grade squamous intraepithelial lesions infected with high-risk human papillomaviruses. *Cancer Res* 1997;57:4210–3.

87. Duensing S, Duensing A, Crum CP, Munger K. Human papillomavirus type 16 E7 oncoprotein-induced abnormal centrosome synthesis is an early event in the evolving malignant phenotype. *Cancer Res* 2001;61:2356–60.

88. Skyldberg B, Fujioka K, Hellström AC, Sylvén L, Moberger B, Auer G. Human papillomavirus infection, centrosome aberration, and genetic stability in cervical lesions. *Mod Pathol* 2001;14:279–84.

89. Boshart M, zur Hausen H. Human papillomaviruses in Buschke-Lowenstein tumors: physical state of the DNA and identification of a tandem duplication in the noncoding region of a human papillomavirus 6 subtype. *J Virol* 1986;58:963–6.

90. Park JS, Kim EJ, Kwon HJ, Hwang ES, Namkoong SE, Um SJ. Inactivation of interferon regulatory factor-1 tumor suppressor protein by HPV E7 oncoprotein. Implication for the E7-mediated immune evasion mechanism in cervical carcinogenesis. *J Biol Chem* 2000; 275:6764–9.

91. White AE, Livanos EM, Tlsty T. Differential disruption of genomic integrity and cell cycle regulation in normal human fibroblasts by HPV oncoproteins. *Gene Develop* 1994;8:866–77.

92. Magal SS, Jackman A, Pei XF, et al. Induction of apoptosis in human keratinocytes containing mutated p53 alleles and its inhibition by both the E6 an E7 oncoproteins. *Int J Cancer* 1998;75:96–104.

93. zur Hausen H. Intracellular surveillance of persisting viral infections: human genital cancer resulting from a failing cellular control of papillomavirus gene expression. *Lancet* 1986;2:489–91.

94. zur Hausen H. Human papillomaviruses in the pathogenesis of anogenital cancer. *Virology* 1991;184:9–13.

95. Wang SS, Hildesheim A. Chapter 5: Viral and host factors in human papillomavirus persistence and progression. *J Natl Cancer Inst* (monograph) 2003;31:35–40.

96. Ferenczy A, Franco E. Persistent human papillomavirus infection and cervical neoplasia. *Lancet Oncol* 2002; 3:11–6.

97. Sang BC, Barbosa MS. Increased E6/E7 in HPV–18 immortalized human keratinocytes results from inactivation of E2 and additional cellular events. *Virology* 1992;189:448–55.

98. Turek LP. The structure, function and regulation of papillomaviral genes in infection and cervical cancer. *Adv Virus Res* 1994;44:305–56.

99. Jeon S, Allen-Hoffman BL, Lambert PF. Integration of human papillomavirus type 16 into the human genome correlates with a selective growth advantage of cells. *J Virol* 1995;69:2989–97.

100. Klaes R, Woerner SM, Ridder R, et al. Detection of high-risk cervical intraepithelial neoplasia and cervical cancer by amplification of transcripts derived from integrated papillomavirus oncogenes. *Cancer Res* 1999;59:6132–6.

101. Schiffman M, Kjaer SK. Chapter 2: Natural history of anogenital human papillomavirus infection and neoplasia. *J Natl Cancer Inst* (monograph) 2003;31:14–9.

102. Burk RD, Kelly P, Feldman J, et al. Declining prevalence of cervicovaginal human papillomavirus infection with age is independent of other risk factors. *Sex Transm Dis* 1996; 23:333–41.

103. Rylander E, Ruusuvaara L, Almstromer MW, Evander M, Wadell G. The absence of vaginal human papillomavirus 16 DNA in women who have not experienced sexual intercourse. *Obstet Gynecol* 1994;83 *(5 pt 1)*: 735–7.

104. Kjaer SK, Chackerian B, van den Brule AJ, et al. High-risk human papillomavirus is sexually transmitted: evidence from a follow-up study of virgins starting sexual activity (intercourse). *Cancer Epidemiol Biomark Prev* 2001;10:101–6.

105. Bosch FX, Castellsague X, Munoz N, et al. Male sexual behavior and human papillomavirus DNA: key risk factors for cervical cancer in Spain. *J Natl Cancer Inst* 1996;88:1060–7.

106. Munoz N, Castellsague X, Bosch FX, et al. Difficulty in elucidating the male role in cervical cancer in Colombia, a high risk area for the disease. *J Natl Cancer Inst* 1996;88:1068–75.

107. Castellsague X, Ghaffari A, Daniel RW, et al. Prevalence of penile human papillomavirus DNA in husbands of women with and without cervical neoplasia: a study in Spain and Colombia. *J Infect Dis* 1997;176:353–61.

108. Oriel JD. Natural history of genital warts. *Br J Vener Dis* 1971;47:1–13.

109. Barrett TJ, Silbar JD, McGinley JP. Genital warts—a venereal disease. *JAMA* l954;154:333–4.

110. Maymon R, Bekerman A, Werchow M, et al. Clinical and subclinical condyloma: rates among male sexual partners of women with genital human papillomavirus infection. *J Reprod Med* 1995;40:31–6.

111. Barasso R, de Brux, Croissant O, Orth G. High prevalence of papillomavirus-associated penile intraepithelial neoplasia in sexual partners of women with cervical intraepithelial neoplasia. *NEJM* 1987;317:916–23.

112. Schneider A, Sawada E, Gissmann L, Shah K. Human papillomaviruses in women with a history of abnormal Papanicolaou smears and in their male partners. *Obstet Gynecol* 1987;69:554–62.

113. Meanwell C A, Cox M F, Blackledge G, et al. HPV l6 DNA in normal and malignant cervical epithelium: implications for the aetiology and behavior of cervical neoplasia. *Lancet* l987;1:703–07.

114. Winer R L, Lee S K, Hughes J P, Adam D E, Kiviat N B, Koutsky L A. Genital human papillomavirus infection: incidence and risk factors in a cohort of female university students. *Am J Epidemiol* 2003;157:218–26.

115. Nuovo G J, Banbury R, Calayag P T. Human papillomavirus types and recurrent cervical warts in immunocompromised women. *Mod Pathol* 1991;4:632–5.

116. Jenison S A, Yu X P, Valentine J M, et al. Evidence of prevalent human papillomavirus types in adults and children. *J Infect Dis* 1990;162:60–9.

117. Gillison M L, Shah K V. Chapter 9: Role of mucosal human papillomavirus in nongenital cancers. *J Natl Cancer Inst* (monograph) 2003;31:57–65.

118. Steinberg B, DeLorenzo T. A possible role for human papillomaviruses in head and neck cancer. *Cancer Metastasis Rev* 1996;15:91–112.

119. Gillison M, Koch W, Capone R, et al. Evidence for a causal association between human papillomavirus and a subset of head and neck cancers. *J Natl Cancer Inst* 2000;92:709–20.

120. Schwartz S, Yueh B, McDougall J, Daling J, Schwartz S. Human papillomavirus infection and survival in oral squamous cell cancer: a population-based study. *Otolaryngol Head Neck Surg* 2001;125:1–9.

121. Klussmann J, Weissenborn S, Wieland U, et al. Prevalence, distribution, and viral load of human papillomavirus 16 DNA in tonsillar carcinomas. *Cancer* 2001;92:2875–84.

122. Wiest T, Schwarz E, Enders C, Flechtenmacher C, Bosch F. Involvement of intact HPV16 E6/E7 gene expression in head and neck cancers with unaltered p53 status and perturbed pRb cell cycle control. *Oncogene* 2002;21:1510–7.

123. Rudlinger R, Grob R, Yr Y X, Schnyder U W. Human papillomavirus 35-positive verruca with Bowenoid dysplasia of the periungual area. *Arch Dermatol* 1989;125:655–9.

124. Brandsma J, Abramson A, Sciubba J, et al. Papillomavirus infection of the nose. In: Steinberg B M, Brandsma J L, Taichman L B, eds. *Papillomaviruses:*

125. *Cancer Cells.* Vol 5. Cold Spring Harbor, NY: Cold Spring Harbor Laboratory, 1987;1115–9.

125. McDonnell P J, McDonnell J M, Kessis T, et al. Detection of human papillomavirus type 6/11 DNA in conjunctival papillomas by in situ hybridization with radioactive probes. *Hum Pathol* 1987; 18:115–9.

126. Scott I, Karp C, Nuovo G. Human papillomavirus 16 and 18 expression in conjunctival intraepithelial neoplasia. *Ophthalmology* 2002;109:542–7.

127. McDonnell J, Wagner D, Ng S, Bernstein G, Sun Y. Human papillomavirus type 16 DNA in ocular and cervical swabs of women with genital tract condylomata. *Am J Ophthalmol* 1991;112:61–6.

128. Perniciaro C, Kicker C H. Tanning bed warts. *J Am Acad Dermatol* 1988;18:586–7.

129. Rowson K E K, Mahy B W J. Human papova (wart) virus. *Bacteriol Rev* 1967;31:110–31.

130. Ferenczy A, Bergnon C, Richart R. HPV DNA in fomites on objects used for the management of patients with genital HPV infections. *Obstet Gynecol* 1989;74:950–4.

131. Galloway D. Serological assays for the detection of human papillomavirus antibodies. In: Munoz N, Bosch F X, Shah K V, Meheus A, eds. *The Epidemiology of Human Papillomavirus and Cervical Cancer.* New York: Oxford University Press; 1992:147–61.

132. Wheeler C M, Parmenter C A, Hunt C, et al. Determinants of genital papillomavirus infection among cytologically normal women attending the University of New Mexico student health center. *Sex Trans Dis* 1993;20:286–9.

133. Mant C, Cason J, Rice P, Best J M. Non-sexual transmission of cervical cancer-associated papillomaviruses: an update. *Papillomavirus Rep* 2000;11:1–5.

134. Cook T A, Brunschwig J P, Butel J S, et al. Laryngeal papilloma: etiologic and therapeutic considerations. *Ann Otol Rhinol Laryngol* 1973;82:649–55.

135. Quick C A, Watts S L, Krzyzek R A, et al. Relationship between condylomata and laryngeal papillomata. *Ann Otol Rhonol Laryngol* 1980;89:467–71.

136. Sedlacek T V, Lindheim S, Eder C, et al. Mechanism for human papillomavirus transmission at birth. *Am J Obstet Gynecol* 1989;161:55–9.

137. Vallejos H, Del Mistro A, Kleinhaus S, et al. Characterization of human papilloma virus types in condylomata acuminata in children by in situ hybridization. *Lab Invest* 1987;56:611–5.

138. Tang C, Shermeta D W, Wood C. Congenital condylomata acuminata. *Am J Obstet Gynecol* 1978;131:912–3.

139. Moscicki A B, Hills N, Shiboski S, et al. Risks for incident human papillomavirus infection and low-grade squamous intraepithelial lesion development in young females. *JAMA* 2001;285:2995–3002.

140. Castle P E, Wacholder S, Sherman M E, et al. Absolute risk of a subsequent abnormal Pap among oncogenic human papillomavirus DNA-positive, cytologically negative women. *Cancer* 2002;95:2145–51.

141. Taichman L B, La Porta R F. The expression of papillomaviruses in epithelial cells. In: Salzman N P, Howley P M, eds. *The Papovaviridae*. Vol 2. New York: Plenum Press, 1987:109–39.

142. Schneider A, Koutsky L A. Natural history and epidemiological features with genital HPV infection in the epidemiology of cervical cancer and human papillomavirus. In: Munoz N, Bosch F X, Shah K V, & Meheus A, eds. *The Epidemiology of Human Papillomavirus and Cervical Cancer*. New York: Oxford University Press; 1992:25–52.

143. Stanley M. Chapter 17: Genital human papillomavirus infections—current and prospective therapies. *J Natl Cancer Inst* (monograph) 2003;31:117–24.

144. Maran A, Amella C A, Di Lorenzo T P, Auborn K J, Taichman L B, Steinberg B M. Human papillomavirus type 11 transcripts are present at low abundance in latently infected respiratory tissues. *Virology* 1995;212:285–94.

145. Park T J, Fujihara H, Wright T C. Molecular biology of cervical cancer and its precursors. *Cancer* 1995;76:1890–1907.

146. Chapman W B, Lorincz A T, Willett G D, et al. Epidermal growth factor receptor expression and presence of human papillomavirus in cervical squamous intraepithelial lesions. *Int J Gynecol Pathol* 1982;11:221–6.

147. Dollard S C, Wilson J L, Demeter L M, et al. Production of human papillomavirus and modulation of the infections program in epithelial raft cultures. *Genes Develop* 1992;6:1131–42.

148. Papay F, Wood B, Coulson M. Squamous cell papilloma at the tracheo-esophageal puncture stoma. *Arch Otolaryngol Head Neck Surg* 1988;114:564–8.

149. Sun Y, Eluf-Neto J, Bosch F X, Munoz N, Walboomers J M, Meijer C J, et al. Serum antibodies to HPV16 proteins in women from Brazil with invasive cervical carcinoma. *Cancer Epidemiol Biomark Prev* 1999;8:935–40.

150. Rogozinski T T, Jablonska S, Jarzabek-Chorzelska M. Role of cell-mediated immunity in spontaneous regression of plane warts. *Int J Dermatol* 1988;27:322–6.

151. Tay S K, Jenkins D, Maddox P, et al. Lymphocyte phenotypes in cervical intraepithelial neoplasia and human papillomavirus infection. *Br J Obstet Gynaecol* 1987;94:16–21.

152. Hawthorn R J, Murdoch J B, MacLean A B, MacKie R M. Langerhans' cells and subtypes of human papillomavirus in cervical intraepithelial neoplasia. *BMJ* 1988;297:643–6.

153. Cauda R, Tyring S K, Grossi C E, et al. Patients with condyloma acuminatum exhibit decreased interleukin-2 and interferon gamma production and depresses natural killer activity. *J Clin Immunol* 1987;7:304–11.

154. Eron L J, Judson F, Tucker S, et al. Interferon therapy for condyloma acuminata. *NEJM* 1986;315:1059–64.

155. Schiller J T, Hildesheim A. Developing HPV virus-like particle vaccines to prevent cervical cancer: a progress report. *J Clin Virol* 2000;19:67–74.

156. Lehtinen M, Dillner J, Knekt P, Luostarinen T, Aromaa A, Kirnbauer R, et al. Serologically diagnosed infection with human papillomavirus type 16 and risk of subsequent development of cervical carcinoma: nested case-control study. *BMJ* 1996; 312:537–9.

157. De Sanjose S, Hamsikova E, Munoz N, et al. Serological response to HPV16 in CIN-III and cervical cancer patients. Case-control studies in Spain and Colombia. *Int J Cancer* 1996;66:70–74.

158. Tsukui T, Hildesheim A, Schiffman M H, et al. IL-2 production by peripheral lymphocytes in response to human papillomavirus-derived peptides: correlation with cervical pathology. *Cancer Res* 1996;56:3967–74.

159. Kadish A S, Timmins P, Wang Y, et al. Regression of CIN and loss of HPV infection is associated with cell-mediated immune responses to a HPV type 16 E7 peptide. *Cancer Epidemiol Biomark Prev* 2002;11:483–8.

160. Mitchell M F, Tortolero-Luna G, Cook E. A randomized clinical trial of cryotherapy, loop electrosurgical excision for treatment of squamous intraepithelial lesions of the cervix. *Obstet Gyneol* 1998;92:737–44.

161. Hemminki K, Li X, Mutanen P. Familial risks in invasive and in situ cervical cancer by histological type. *Eur J Cancer Prev* 2001;10:83–9.

162. Magnusson P K, Lichtenstein P, Gyllensten U B. Heritability of cervical tumours. *Int J Cancer* 2000;88:698–701.

163. Bauer H M, Ting Y, Greer C E, et al. Genital human papillomavirus infection in female university students as determined by PCR-based method. *JAMA* 1991;265:472–7.

164. Einstein M H, Burk R D. Persistent human papillomavirus infection: definitions and clinical implications. *Papillomavirus Report* 2001;12:119–23.

165. Richardson H, Kelsall G, Tellier P, Voyer H, Abrahamowicz M, Ferenczy A, Coutlee F, Franco E L. The natural history of type-specific human papillomavirus infections in female university students. *Cancer Epidemiol Biomarkers Prev.* 2003;12:485–90.

166. Svare E I, Kjaer S K, Worm A M, et al. Risk factors for HPV infection in women from sexually transmitted disease clinics: comparison between two areas with different cervical cancer incidence. *Int J Cancer* 1998;75:1–8.

167. Palefsky J M, Minkoff H, Kalish L A, et al. Cervicovaginal human papillomavirus infection in human immunodeficiency virus-1 (HIV)-positive and high-risk HIV-negative women. *J Natl Cancer Inst* 1999;91:226–36.

168. Meisels A. The story of a cell. *Acta Cytologica* 1983;27:584–96.

169. Schneider A. Sensitivity of the cytological diagnosis of cervical condylomata in comparison with HPV DNA hybridization studies. *Diag Cytopathol* 1987;3:250–5.

170. Meijer C J L M, van den Brule A J C, Snijders P J F, et al. Detection of human papillomavirus in cervical scrapes by the polymerase chain reaction in relation to cytology: possible implications for cervical cancer screening. In: Munoz N, Bosch F X, Shah K V, Meheus A I, eds. *The Epidemiology of Human Papillomavirus and Cervical Cancer.* Lyon: IARC Scientific Publications, 1992:271–81.

171. Ylitalo N, Sorensen P, Josefsson A M, et al. Consistent high viral load of human papillomavirus 16 and risk of cervical carcinoma in situ: a nested case-control study. *Lancet* 2000; 355:2194–8.

172. Moscicki A B, Palefsky J, Smith G, et al. Variability of human papillomavirus DNA testing in a longitudinal cohort of young women. *Obstet Gynecol* 1993;82:578–85.

173. Ostor A G. Natural history of CIN: a critical review. *Int J Gynecol Pathol* 1993;12:186–92.

174. Cox J T, Schiffman M, Solomon D; ASCUS-LSIL Triage Study (ALTS) Group. Prospective follow-up suggests similar risk of subsequent cervical intraepithelial neoplasia grade 2 or 3 among women with cervical intraepithelial neoplasia grade 1 or negative colposcopy and directed biopsy. *Am J Obstet Gynecol* 2003;188:1406–12.

175. Richart R M. Natural history of cervical intraepithelial neoplasia. *Clin Obstet Gynecol* 1968;10:748–84.

176. Kiviat N B, Koutsky L A. Do our current cervical cancer control strategies still make sense? *J Natl Cancer Inst* 1996;88:317–8.

177. Koutsky L A, Holmes K K, Critchlow C W, et al. Cohort study of risk of cervical intraepithelial neoplasia grade 2 or 3 associated with cervical papillomavirus infection. *NEJM* 1992;327:1272–8.

178. Burghardt E, Ostor A G. Site and origin of squamous cervical cancer: a histomorphologic study. *Obstet Gynecol* 1983;62:117–26.

179. Schlecht N F, Kulaga S, Robitaille J, et al. Persistent human papillomavirus infection as a predictor of cervical intraepithelial neoplasia. *JAMA* 2001;286:3106–14.

180. Woodman C B, Collins S, Winter H, et al. Natural history of cervical human papillomavirus infection in young women: a longitudinal cohort study. *Lancet* 2001;357:1831–6.

181. Herrero R, Hildesheim A, Bratti C, et al. Population-based study of human papillomavirus infection and cervical neoplasia in rural Costa Rica. *J Natl Cancer Inst* 2000;92:464–74.

182. Adam E, Berkova Z, Daxnerova Z, Icenogle J, Reeves W C, Kaufman R H. Papillomavirus detection: demographic and behavioral characteristics influencing the identification of cervical disease. *Am J Obstet Gynecol* 2000;182:257–64.

183. Larson A A, Liao S-Y, Stanbridge E J, et al. Genetic alterations accumulate during cervical tumorigenesis and indicate a common origin for multifocal lesions. *Cancer Res* 1997;57:4171–6.

184. Lazo P A. The molecular genetics of cervical carcinoma. *Br J Cancer* 1999; 80:2008–18.

185. Southern S A, Herrington C S. Molecular events in uterine cervical cancer. *Sex Transm Infect* 1998; 74:101–109.

186. Watanabe T. Flow cytometric evaluation of DNA ploidy pattern and cell heterogeneity in cervical dysplasia and carcinoma in situ. *Nippon Sanka Fujinka Gakkai Zasshi* 1993;45:1381–8.

187. Garnett G P, Waddell H C. Public health paradoxes and the epidemiological impact of a HPV vaccine. *J Clin Virol* 2000;19:101–11.

188. Herrero R, Muñoz N. Human papillomavirus and cancer. *Cancer Surv* 1999;33:75–98.

189. ASCUS-LSIL Triage Study (ALTS) Group. Results of a randomized trial on the management of cytology interpretations of atypical squamous cells of undetermined significance. *Am J Obstet Gynecol* 2003;188:1383–92.

190. Levine A J. P53, cellular gatekeeper for growth and division. *Cell* 1997;88:323–31.

191. Kuerbitz S J, Plunkett B S, Walsh W V, et al. Wild type p53 is a cell cycle checkpoint determinant following radiation. *Proc Natl Acad Sci* 1992;89:7491–5.

192. Lowe S W, Ruley H E, Jacks T, Houseman D E. P-53 dependent apoptosis modulate the cytotoxicity of anti-cancer drugs. *Cell* 1993;74:957–67.

193. Dong S M, Kim H S, Rha S H, Sidransky D. Promoter hypermethylation of multiple genes in carcinoma of the uterine cervix. *Clin Cancer Res* 2001;7:1982–6.

194. Virmani A K, Muller C, Rathi A, et al. Aberrant methylation during cervical carcinogenesis. *Clin Cancer Res* 2001;7:584–9.

195. Schiffman M H. Commentary. Recent progress in defining the epidemiology of HPV infection and cervical neoplasia. *J Natl Cancer Inst* 1992;84:394–8.

196. Cullen A P, Reid R, Campion M J, Lorincz A T. An analysis of the physical state of different human papillomavirus DNAs in preinvasive and invasive cervical neoplasia. *J Virol* 1991;65:606–12.

197. Shah K V. HPV and other biological markers in cervical cancer. In: Munoz N, Bosch F X, Shah K V, Meheus A, eds. *The Epidemiology of Human Papillomavirus and Cervical Cancer.* New York: Oxford University Press; 1992:209–18.

198. Riou G, Favre M, Jeannel D, et al. Association between poor prognosis in early-state invasive cervical cancer and non-detection of human papillomavirus DNA. *Lancet* 1990;335:1171–4.

199. Higgins G, Davy N, Roder D, et al. Increased age and mortality associated with cervical carcinomas negative for human papillomavirus DNA. *Lancet* 1991;338:910–3.

200. De Britton R C, Hildesheim A, De Lao S, et al. Human papillomavirus and other influences on survival from cervical cancer in Panama. *Obstet Gynecol* 1993;81:19–24.

201. Scheffner M, Munger K, Byrne J, et al. The state of the p53 and retinoblastoma genes in human cervical carcinoma cell lines. *Proc Natl Acad Sci USA* 1991;88:5523–7.

202. Schiffman M, Herrero R, Hildesheim A, et al. HPV DNA testing in cervical cancer screening: results from women in a high-risk province of Costa Rica. *JAMA* 2000; 283:87–93.

203. Healey S M, Aronson K J, Mao Y, et al. Oncogenic HPV infection and cervical lesions in aboriginal women of Nunavut, Canada. *Sex Trans Dis* 2001; 28:694–700.

204. Sherman M E, Schiffman M, Cox J T. Effects of age and HPV viral load on colposcopy triage: data from the randomized atypical squamous cells of undetermined significance/low-grade squamous intraepithelial lesion triage study (ALTS). *J Natl Cancer Inst* 2002; 94:102–7.

205. Gravitt P E, Burk R D, Lorincz A, et al. A comparison between real-time polymerase chain reaction and hybrid capture 2 for human papillomavirus DNA quantitation. *Cancer Epidemiol Biomark Prev* 2003;12:477–84.

206. Gravitt P E, Peyton C, Wheeler C, Apple R, Higuchi R, Shah K V. Reproducibility of HPV 16 and HPV 18 viral load quantitation using TaqMan real-time PCR assays. *J Virol Methods*. 2003;112:23–33.

207. Wright T C, Schiffman M H, Solomon D, et al. Interim guidance on the use of HPV DNA testing as an adjunct to cervical cytology. *Obstet Gynecol* 2004; 103:304–9.

208. Sherman M E. Chapter 11: Future directions in cervical pathology. *J Natl Cancer Inst* (monograph) 2003;31:72–9.

209. Liotta L, Petricoin E. Molecular profiling of human cancer. *Nat Rev Genet* 2000; 1:48–56.

210. Alizadeh A, Eisen M, Davis R E, et al. The lymphochip: a specialized cDNA microarray for the genomic-scale analysis of gene expression in normal and malignant lymphocytes. *Cold Spring Harb Symp Quant Biol* 1999;64:71–78.

211. Klaes R, Friedrich T, Spitkovsky D, et al. Overexpression of p16(INK4A) as a specific marker for dysplastic and neoplastic epithelial cells of the cervix uteri. *Int J Cancer* 2001;92:276–84.

212. Burghardt E. Prognostic factors. In: Burghardt E, ed. *Surgical Gynecologic Oncology*. 1st ed. Stuttgart: Thieme Medical Publishers, 1993:315–33.

213. Lowy D R, Frazer I H. Chapter 16: Prophylactic human papillomavirus vaccines. *J Natl Cancer Inst* (monograph) 2003;31:111–6.

214. Peh W L, Middleton K, Christensen N, et al. Life cycle heterogeneity in animal models of human papillomavirus-associated disease. *J Virol* 2002;76:10401–16.

215. Christiansen N D, Reed C A, Cladel N M, et al. Immunization with virus-like particles induces long-term protection of rabbits against challenge with cotton-tail rabbit papillomavirus. *J Virol* 1996;70:960–5.

216. Peng S, Frazer I, Fernando G J, Zhou J. Papilloma virus-like particles can deliver defined CTL epitopes to the MHC class I pathway. *Virology* 1998;240:147–57.

217. Lowe R S, Brown D R, Bryan J T, et al. Human papillomavirus type 11 (HPV-11) neutralizing antibodies in the serum and genital mucosal secretions of African green monkeys immunized with HPV-11 virus-like particles expressed in yeast. *J Infect Dis* 1997;176:1141–5.

218. *Koutsky L A, Ault K A, Wheeler C M, et al, and the Proof of Principle Study Investigators*. A controlled trial of a human papillomavirus type 16 vaccine. *NEJM* 2002;21;347:1645–51.

219. Tindle R W, Frazier I H. Immune response to human papillomaviruses and the prospects for human papillomavirus-specific immunization. *Curr Top Microbiol Immunol* 1994;186:217–53.

220. De Bruijn M L H, Schuurhuis D H, Vierboom M P M, et al. Immunization with human papillomavirus type 16 (HPV 16) oncoprotein-loaded dendritic cells as well as protein in adjuvant induces MHC Class I-restricted protection to HPV 16-induced tumor cells. *Cancer Res* 1998;58:724–31.

221. Londono L P, Chatfield S, Tindle R W, et al. Immunization of mice using Salmonella typhimurium expressing human papillomavirus type 16 E7 epitopes inserted into hepatitis B virus core antigen. *Vaccine* 1996;14:545–52.

CHAPTER 6

Colposcopic Equipment, Chemical Agents and Colposcopy Supplies; Colposcopy Image and Data Management

Table of Contents

6.1 Introduction

Colposcopy requires properly maintained equipment and the supplies needed to facilitate patient care. Colposcopists must ensure that the examination room is fully stocked with all necessary instruments, supplies, and properly functioning equipment prior to each scheduled colposcopic visit. Appropriate care and routine maintenance of colposcopic equipment and instruments are critical for optimum performance. This chapter includes a discussion of basic colposcopic equipment, instruments, chemical agents, and colposcopy supplies needed for routine colposcopy. Additionally, an overview of supplemental equipment, such as cameras, video equipment, digital imaging systems, and colposcopic image and data management systems that might be useful to clinicians with academic or busy colposcopic practices is provided.

6.2 Colposcopes

6.2.1 Overview

A colposcope is an optical instrument that permits illuminated and magnified examination of the lower genital tract. The intense light transilluminates the epithelium, and magnification allows for close examination of the surface epithelium and subepithelial blood vessels. There are two types of colposcopes: the traditional optical colposcope[1] and the newer video colposcope (Figures 6.1 and 6.2).[2] The video colposcope with monitor, which completely replaces the standard binocular optics of the traditional colposcope, enables colposcopists to view the cervix on a video monitor rather than directly through eyepieces. There are several factors to consider when using or purchasing a colposcope.

6.2.2 Objective lenses and focal length

Colposcopes have either a single or a double objective lens positioned in the front of the instrument. While colposcopes made with a single objective lens are adequate, colposcopes designed with double objective lenses provide true stereoscopic images since each eyepiece is linked visually to a separate complex of lenses. Objective lenses have a fixed focal length derived from the curvature of the lens. Focal length determines the distance between the objective lens and the cervix, or from a practical perspective, the *working distance* between the colposcope and the vaginal speculum when the cervix is in focus (Figure 6.3). Focal length corresponds to the space available between the colposcope and speculum for

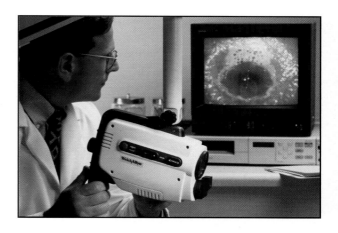

FIGURE 6.2 A video colposcope and high-resolution video monitor. The colposcopist views the examination indirectly on the monitor. ∎

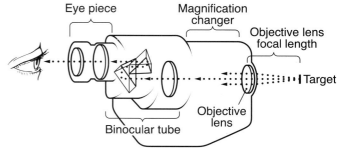

FIGURE 6.3 Diagram of the focal length of an objective lens. The eyepieces, binocular tubes and magnification complex are the other components of the optical colposcope (From: Ferris DG, Willner WA, Ho JJ. Colposcopes: a critical review. *J Fam Pract* 1991(33): 506–51. Reprinted with permission, Dowden Health Media.) ∎

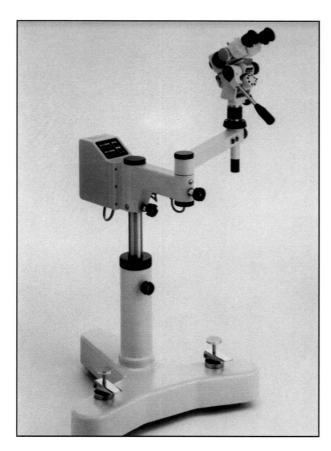

FIGURE 6.1 A traditional or optical colposcope. The colposcopist views the examination directly through the oculars. ∎

introducing and working with biopsy and treatment instruments; i.e., the shorter the focal length, the smaller the available working space. Most colposcopes have lenses with a 300-mm focal length. This focal length provides the greatest versatility and operator comfort when using biopsy instruments without compromising colposcopic detail. A 240-mm objective lens, although excellent for colpophotography, does not allow sufficient room between the colposcope and speculum to accommodate most biopsy instruments and hinders colposcopically directed laser surgery and electrosurgical loop excision procedures. One colposcope has an adjustable focal length of 200 mm to 350 mm. This allows focusing using a knob instead of moving the colposcope (Figure 6.4).

6.2.3 Illumination and filters

A colposcope should have a powerful light source capable of incremental adjustments to provide the desired amount of illumination. Some newer colposcopes automatically adjust the level of illumination.

There are many types of light sources, including incandescent bulbs, arc lamps, tungsten and halogen lamps. Tungsten, halogen and arc lamps provide brighter lighting and are superior for colpophotography, videocolposcopy, and computer-based digitized image capture (Figure 6.5). Different types of lamps provide different color hues. Incandescent bulbs provide a warm, reddish color, halogen bulbs and arc lamps emit a very white color, whereas other types of bulbs produce a cool, bluish hue.

A colposcope should provide illumination of the entire field of view at low magnification. In general, the amount of illumination decreases as the level of magnification increases; however, very intense light sources on newer colposcopes provide ample illumination at high magnification levels.[2] The position of the light source is also relevant because the bulb may generate considerable heat. If the light source is in the head of the colposcope, the heat can be uncomfortable for both the colposcopist and the patient. Several colposcopes have a small fan to direct heat away from the colposcope and patient. On other colposcopes, the bulb is placed away from the head of the scope and fiberoptic cable is used to deliver light to the colposcope head. The fiber optic cable should be enclosed within a protective sheath of flexible plastic or metal to protect it from potential damage (Figure 6.6). Otherwise, if twisted or bent, the small glass fibers within the cable may break, resulting in nonilluminated dark "spots" and overall reduced illumination. Spare light bulbs and fuses should be available and readily accessible during procedures.

A green or blue filter is a desirable feature because it increases contrast in the colposcopic image while

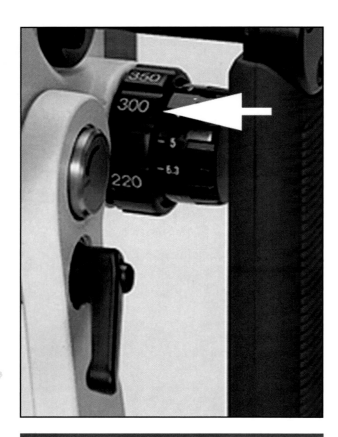

FIGURE 6.4 One colposcope has an adjustable focal length of 200 mm to 350 mm. This knob is used to focus instead of moving the colposcope.

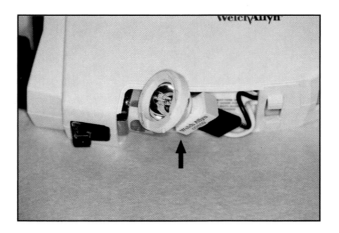

FIGURE 6.5 This arc lamp provides intense white illumination. The bulb (arrow) can be easily replaced.

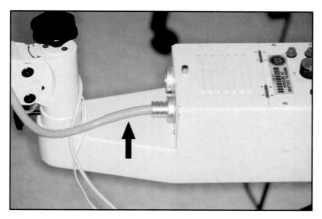

FIGURE 6.6   The fiber optic cable on this colposcope (arrow) can be plugged into one of two separate lamp receptacles. Such engineering allows a quick change to a new bulb if the other fails during a colposcopic examination.

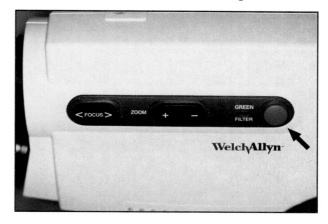

FIGURE 6.8   The video colposcope's electronic green filter is activated by depressing the small button at the rear of the operations panel.

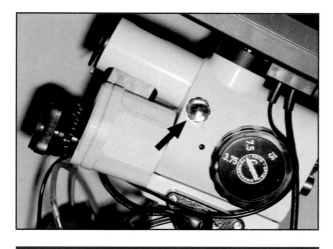

FIGURE 6.7   The green filter is selected by a small knob (arrow) centrally positioned on this colposcope.

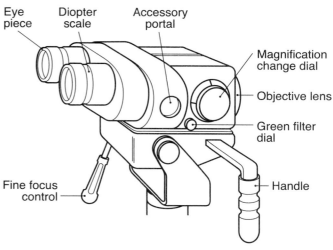

FIGURE 6.9   Components of an optical colposcope (From: Ferris DG, Willner WA, Ho JJ. Colposcopes: a critical review. *J Fam Pract* 1991(33): 506–51. Reprinted with permission, Dowden Health Media.)

only slightly reducing the overall illumination. Green filters block red light transmission, making blood vessels appear black. They also may modify contrast between acetowhite and nonacetowhite epithelium. It is easy to interpose filters between the light source or optics and the area viewed on both optical and video colposcopes. On optical colposcopes, a knob, lever, or sliding mechanism activates the green filter (Figure 6.7). On video colposcopes, a small touch button on the sides of the scope electronically activates the filter (Figure 6.8). Green filters, which are standard on most modern colposcopes, ideally should be encased within the colposcope to prevent dust accumulation.

6.2.4 Magnification

Colposcopic magnification is determined not only by the magnification lens but also by the objective lens and the oculars (Figure 6.9).[3] For example, if a single objective lens and magnification lens coupled with 10X oculars (eyepieces) produce a final magnification of 7.5X, the same objective and magnification lenses coupled with a 20X ocular would produce a final magnification of 15X. Colposcopes with a magnification range of approximately 2X to 15X are ideal for assessing the lower genital tract. A greater level of magnification is not necessary for routine colposcopy. A broad magnification range permits

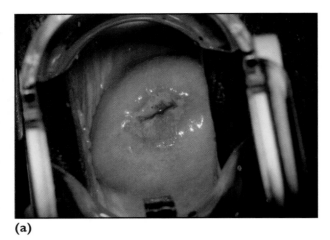

(a)

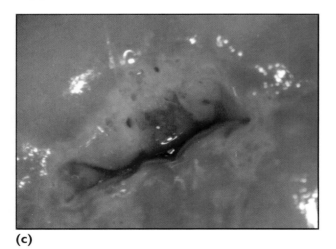

(b)

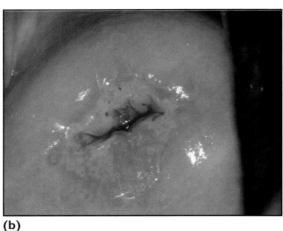

(c)

FIGURES 6.10a–c The cervix at **(a)** 3.5X, **(b)** 7.5X, and **(c)** 15X magnification.

low-power scanning of the external genitalia and allows for colposcopic visualization during biopsies and electrosurgical loop excisions. The entire cervix and vagina can be observed at 3.5X magnification (Figure 6.10a). At approximately 7.5X magnification, the average cervix will completely occupy the colpo-

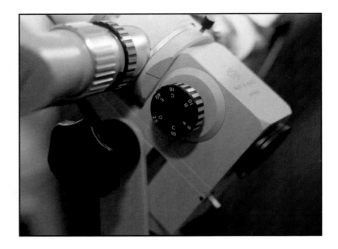

FIGURE 6.11 Colposcope with multiple fixed magnification changer.

scopic field of view (Figure 6.10b). Greater magnification (15X) permits partial but more detailed viewing of a smaller portion of the cervix (Figure 6.10c). Hence, as magnification is increased, the field of view (what is seen using the colposcope) decreases. Colposcopic examination of the cervix generally requires 7.5X to 15X magnification. Higher magnification, such as 20X to 30X, is less useful clinically but allows closer inspection of fine vascular detail (Figure 6.10c).

Colposcopes with only a single level of magnification (high or low) are not ideal because they severely restrict detailed examinations and are cumbersome to use. Colposcopes with either multiple fixed magnification or zoom magnification are preferable. Adjusting a knob achieves the desired level of magnification on colposcopes with multiple fixed magnification (Figure 6.11). Zoom magnification provides a continuous range of magnification from lowest to highest levels. Although the optical quality of the image obtained from zoom magnification colposcopes may be somewhat lower than that of fixed magnification colposcopes, the difference in image quality is neither perceptible by the human eye nor sufficient to impair clinical accuracy. Electronic or motorized zoom magnification operated by a foot pedal or button is a standard feature of the video colposcope and is available as an option on some zoom magnification optical colposcopes.

6.2.5 Oculars and monocular observation tubes

Interchangeable or fixed oculars (eyepieces) of various magnification permit adjustments in magnification and individual eyepiece focusing. The binocular tubes containing the oculars can be adjusted to accommodate

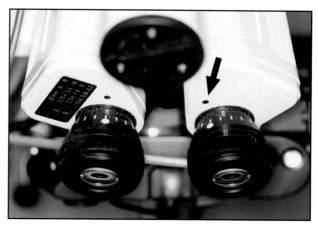

FIGURE 6.12 The diopter scales on each eyepiece are set to the 0 position when the dots on the eyepieces and colposcope (arrow) are aligned.

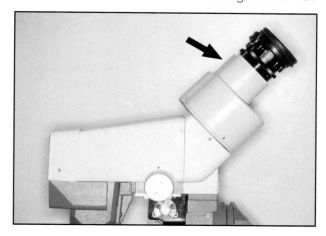

FIGURE 6.14 Inclined eyepieces (arrow) are preferred by some colposcopists.

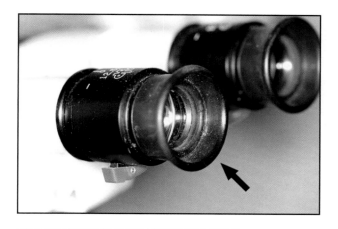

FIGURE 6.13 These ocular hoods (arrow) are extended and help prevent obscuring ambient light.

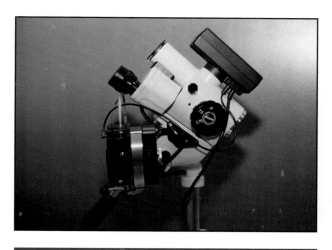

FIGURE 6.15 Colposcope with straight in-line oculars.

the colposcopist's interpupillary distance and vision. Diopter settings, which are present on some oculars, indicate the unique focus setting of each ocular (Figure 6.12). The midpoint, or "0" setting, is the default for colposcopists with normal or normal-corrected vision. For colposcopists who wear eyeglasses but choose not to use them during colposcopy, twisting the eyepieces toward the negative or positive diopter settings allows proper focus for colposcopists with myopia or hyperopia, respectively. Ocular hoods or eyepiece cups may be extended for colposcopists who wear contact lenses or have normal uncorrected vision (Figure 6.13). These may be inverted (flattened or removed) if the colposcopist prefers to wear glasses during the examination (Figure 6.12). One advantage to the use of eyepiece cups is that they reduce ambient light, which may be distracting.

The angle of the oculars or binocular tubes in relation to the direct line of sight from the eye to the cervix varies from inclined (45°) (Figure 6.14) to straight in-line tubes (180°) (Figure 6.15). Straight in-line oculars permit viewing directly toward the target. Thereby, a casual glance away from the oculars allows a nonmagnified observation of the same target. Clinicians who have difficulty focusing with binoculars may prefer a videocolposcope, which has no oculars.

A monocular observation tube attached to a colposcope portal permits viewing by a second person (Figure 6.16). In the teaching setting, the capacity for simultaneous observation by an inexperienced colposcopist has instructional value. However, in the non-teaching clinical setting, where this capacity is rarely needed, the monocular observation tube has limited usefulness. Since the monocular observation tube is awkward to use, offers no depth perception, and can be expensive, a video colposcopy system

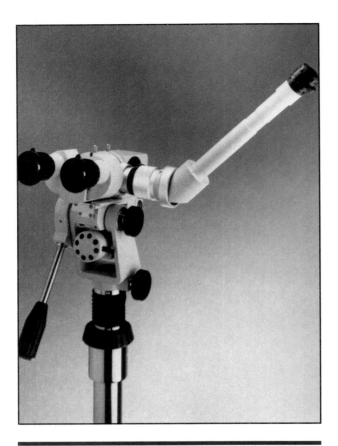

FIGURE 6.16   A monocular co-observation tube permits simultaneous observation of colposcopy by a single learner.

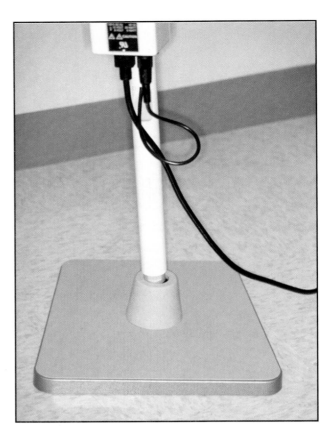

FIGURE 6.17   Colposcopists must place their feet on the foot platform for stability when using this colposcope.

with a monitor might be a better investment in settings where the capacity for joint observation by students, nursing assistants and patients is useful.

6.2.6 Mounting

Colposcopes can be affixed to an examination table, mounted on a stand, or fitted to a swivel arm attached to the wall or ceiling. Mobile colposcopes are usually the most practical since they permit easy transfer from room to room or within a room. Some colposcopes are mounted by a universal joint to a small, flat platform on a wheelless base that is stabilized by the colposcopist's feet (Figure 6.17). A weighted or wide colposcope base prevents inadvertent tipping of the scope and potential injury to the delicate optics. Since colposcopes mounted on wheels often depend on mobility for coarse focusing, wheel locks designed to prevent accidental rolling are rarely activated (Figure 6.18).

Types of supports available for the colposcope head include center-post, flexible articulating arm, or overhead boom-type (Figures 6.19 a-c). Of these three, center-post and flexible articulating arm scopes provide better stationary viewing. Overhead boom scopes often have unintended play, even though the

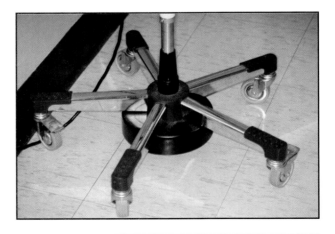

FIGURE 6.18   A wide, weighted base helps prevent accidental tipping of the colposcope.

tension at each joint is adjustable. When selecting a type of colposcope support, it is important to consider individual preference, available examination room space, frequency of colposcope transportation, and cost. Colposcopic head and platform stability are particularly important for laser-adapted colposcopes.

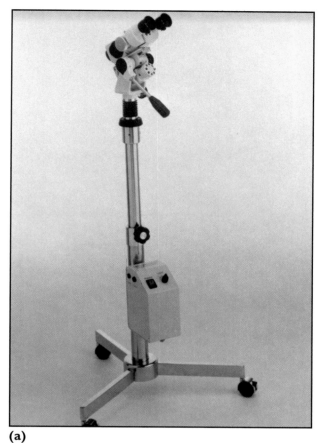

(a)

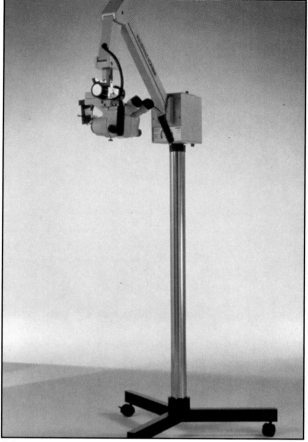

(c)

FIGURES 6.19a–c Colposcopes mounted on a **(a)** center post, **(b)** flexible articulating arm, and **(c)** overhead boom.

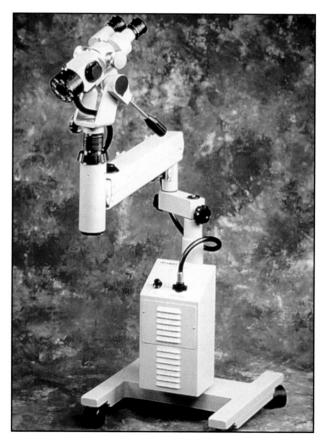

(b)

6.2.7 Focus controls

Colposcopes can be focused by both coarse and fine movement methods. When using an optical or video colposcope, adjusting the colposcope head in relation to the patient accomplishes coarse focus. If the colposcope is mounted on a center-post and wheels, coarse focus requires the entire unit to move. If the colposcope head is mounted on a flexible articulating arm or an overhead boom, the base remains stationary and only the head moves.

At low magnification, simply moving the head of the colposcope toward or away from the target or anatomical organ being examined achieves rapid focus. Manipulating a fine focus handle, knob or lever on the colposcope moves only the colposcope head in relation to the remainder of the colposcope (Figure 6.20). This minor adjustment allows for fine focus at both low and high magnification levels.

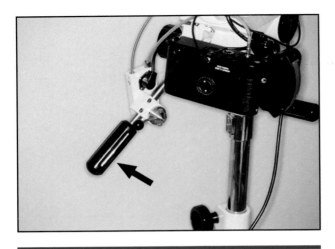

FIGURE 6.20   Fine focusing is accomplished by turning the fine focus handle (arrow).

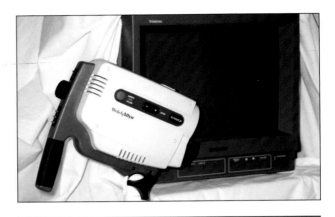

FIGURE 6.21   Components of the video colposcope include an electronic green filter, motorized zoom magnification changer, motorized fine focus control, light source, and handle mounted image management buttons.

Additionally, gentle manipulation of the vaginal speculum is useful for focusing at high magnification since most colposcopes have a narrow depth of field. Depth of field refers to the area in focus at a particular level of magnification. At low-level magnification, the depth of field is quite broad. At a high level of magnification, the depth of field is limited, and therefore, only several millimeters of movement brings an object into or out of focus. The video colposcope provides a bi-directional, button-activated, motorized fine focus similar to the same feature found on video camcorders. This fine-focus mechanism allows the external video colposcope to remain stable, with focus achieved solely by the movement of the internally positioned optics.

6.2.8 Cost

The cost of a colposcope varies from $4,000 to more than $20,000 depending on optical quality, sophistication of design, components, mounting system, and photographic and video capabilities. A higher purchase cost usually reflects better quality in colposcopes. A good rule of thumb is to buy the best colposcope the equipment budget can bear. Although most colposcopes are well constructed, it is important to have access to good, prompt service for problems with lighting, optics, or photographic reproduction quality. Accessible customer support is particularly important until the colposcope user becomes familiar with this relatively costly piece of equipment.

6.2.9 Colposcope care

Colposcopes require meticulous care and maintenance. When moving the scope a considerable distance, be careful not to bump or jar the optics out of alignment to avoid seriously compromising the colposcopic image. Cover the colposcope at the end of each day to prevent dust from accumulating on oculars and lenses. When the oculars or lens(es) become dusty, clean with lens paper. Adjust the tension of the support mechanism as needed. Protect fiberoptic light cables from trauma, twisting, or bending to avoid breaking the encased glass strands. Replace light bulbs and fuses as necessary. To remove potentially infectious bodily secretions and blood, routinely use a disinfectant to wipe portions of the colposcope that come in regular contact with clinicians. Be sure to choose a disinfectant that is safe for use on the surface materials of the instrument.

6.3 Video Colposcope

Video colposcopy is a relatively new method for examining the lower genital tract.[2] The video colposcope system includes a video colposcope (a video camcorder-type device) mounted on either a center pole stand or an overhead boom and a high-resolution video monitor (Figure 6.21). Because the video colposcope has no eyepieces, the technique differs from traditional optical colposcopy in that the colposcopist views only the target area shown on the video monitor. The video colposcope has an excellent light source, electronic green filter, and motorized, touch-activated controls for fine focus and zoom magnification. Touch-activated buttons on the handle electronically capture colposcopic images that are digitally saved in a computer or printed using a color video printer.

A modified colposcopy technique enhances depth perception. Observed shadows and light reflections

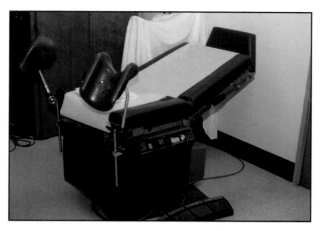

FIGURE 6.22 A mechanical or hydraulic patient examination table with leg supports facilitates the colposcopy examination.

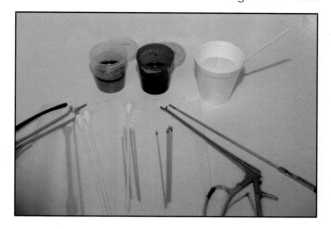

FIGURE 6.23 Setup for colposcopic instruments, chemicals, and supplies.

create an apparent three-dimensional image on the two-dimensional video monitor. "Point and see" is the best way to describe this visualization process. The colposcopist uses the handle to move the scope to the correct focal length and parallel with the axis of the vagina. The fine focus button allows the operator to further sharpen the video image, if necessary. The colposcopist accomplishes assessment and sampling by observing the image displayed on the video monitor. The video colposcope costs about the same as a good optical colposcope that does not include a beam splitter, adaptor, charged coupled device (CCD), camera, and video monitor.

6.4 Examination Table and Instrument Stand

Although a standard nonhydraulic gynecologic table is suitable for colposcopic examinations, the foot of the table may be too low for some examiners. Raising it slightly often provides a better view of the cervix. Raising the head of the table slightly may be more comfortable for the patient while allowing the colposcopist to optimize communication. Either padded heel supports or behind-the-knee leg supports are adequate for the colposcopic examination table, but more expensive leg supports can reduce patient fatigue during prolonged examinations or procedures. Some women, however, may prefer the sense of control foot stirrups provide. A mechanical or hydraulic table offers distinct advantages (Figure 6.22). Adjustment of the examination table height and the angle of the patient's pelvis in relation to the colposcope light source allows for better visualization of the cervix and vagina.

The colposcopist should have convenient access to a stable instrument stand, cart, or counter space for the instruments, supplies, and solutions required for a colposcopic examination. Figure 6.23 shows a standard setup of instruments, solutions, and supplies used by many colposcopists.

6.5 Colposcopic Instruments

6.5.1 Vaginal specula

Different-sized vaginal specula should be available: a small speculum for young girls and virginal women, a medium Pederson speculum for women with a narrow vagina, and medium and large Graves specula for most women. A short Cusco or Collins' speculum is ideal for examining the vaginal vault in posthysterectomy patients. A large metal Graves speculum is required for patients with vaginal wall laxity or prolapse, obese women, and most pregnant women. Use of the widest speculum tolerated by the patient usually provides the best cervical visualization. An extended or long Graves or Pederson speculum is the best choice for an extremely long vagina.

Metal and disposable plastic specula are both appropriate for colposcopy. When using plastic specula with independent light sources, an additional speculum light source is not necessary. Blackened specula are designed specifically for CO_2 laser surgery but are also ideal for colpophotography because they reduce reflection. Specula with an electrically resistant coating that are designed to hold smoke evacuation tubing are the best choice for electrosurgical loop excision procedures.

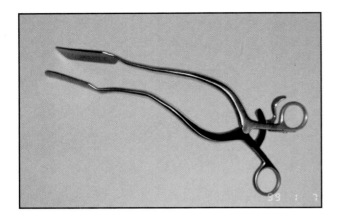

FIGURE 6.24 A lateral vaginal sidewall retractor. The instrument retracts prolapsing vaginal sidewalls that hinder colposcopic visualization.

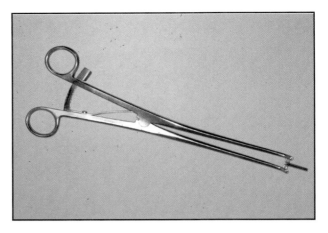

FIGURE 6.25 An endocervical speculum permits visualization of components of the transformation zone or cervical lesions positioned within the canal.

6.5.2 Lateral sidewall retractors

Lateral vaginal sidewall retractors may be helpful when examining patients who have lax vaginal walls that block the view of the cervix through the vaginal speculum (Figure 6.24). Vaginal sidewall retractors have long, narrow, rounded blades designed to be placed between the blades of a vaginal speculum. Use of these instruments requires caution to avoid pinching the wall of the vagina between the blades of the lateral sidewall retractor and the blades of the speculum. A large Graves speculum or a specially designed speculum with a wide introital opening is preferable because it allows the vaginal sidewall retractor to open fully. Another approach to retract the vaginal sidewalls is to cut off the distal end of either a condom or the middle finger of a rubber glove and place it over the vaginal speculum blades.

6.5.3 Endocervical specula

In some women, use of an endocervical speculum improves visualization of the squamocolumnar junction or cervical lesion extending deep within the endocervical canal (Figure 6.25). The endocervical speculum has narrow opposing blades that extend into the endocervical canal and open to gently retract the tissue for better visualization (Figure 6.26). Although the blades of most endocervical specula are 1.5 cm long, it is difficult to see to this depth within the canal. Endocervical specula generally allow good visualization of the first 5 mm to 10 mm of the endocervical canal. Many colposcopists have several different sizes of endocervical specula on hand to accommodate varying diameters of the os. Specula with wide blades are best for a patulous or average-sized cervical os, and specula with narrow blades are preferable for a stenotic os (Figures 6.27 a, b). Modified de

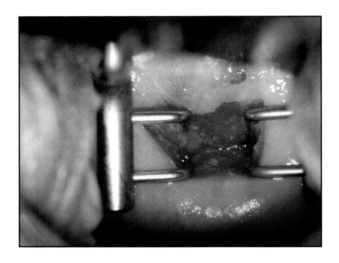

FIGURE 6.26 Endocervical speculum used in an examination of the squamocolumnar junction or proximal extent of neoplasia within the endocervical canal.

Jardin's gallbladder forceps, Campion endocervical forceps, long pickups, Kelly clamps, or even ring forceps also can be used to examine the distal part of the endocervical canal. These types of forceps are used to lift the anterior and posterior lips of the portio, permitting easy, relatively atraumatic access to the canal.

6.5.4 Biopsy forceps

Cervical biopsy forceps are designed specifically to permit relatively small (approximately 2 mm to 5 mm) tissue specimens to be obtained from the cervix (Figure 6.28). The many types of biopsy forceps all have their proponents. A few of the most commonly used types include the Tischler, baby Tischler, Eppendorfer, Burke, Kevorkian, Townsend, and the

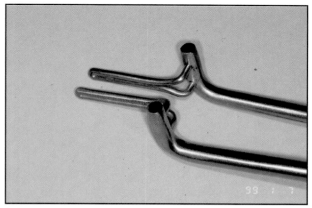

(a)

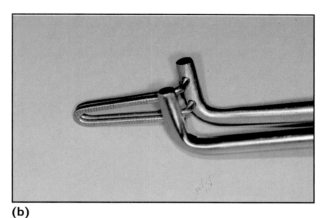

(b)

FIGURES 6.27a,b   Endocervical specula of two different sizes, **(a)** a narrow blade for a stenotic os and **(b)** a wider blade for a parous os.

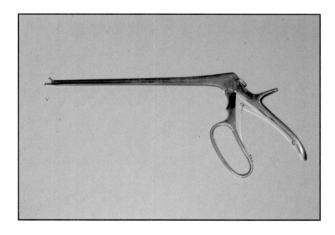

FIGURE 6.28   A mini-Townsend cervical biopsy forceps.

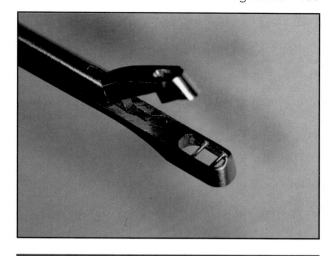

FIGURE 6.29   A Tischler-Morgan biopsy forceps with a single tooth and oval cutting interface.

mini-Townsend biopsy forceps. Because the different types of biopsy forceps remove varying amounts of cervical tissue, they have a range of clinical uses.

The standard Tischler-Morgan biopsy forceps has an oval cutting "cup" on the upper edge and a single tooth at the front to fix the cervix during the biopsy (Figure 6.29). The oval configuration and cutting cup make these forceps excellent for taking large biopsies: up to 5 mm in diameter and up to 4 mm in depth. Although the diagnosis of intraepithelial lesions seldom requires such large biopsies, they are useful when cancer is clinically suspected. Because the cutting surface is completely oval, small biopsies obtained with biopsy forceps of the Tischler-Morgan type are somewhat difficult to orient in the pathology laboratory. Specimen orientation is important so that the histologic sections can be cut perpendicular to the epithelial surface.

Biopsy forceps with square jaws or half-oval, half-square "bites" are designed to produce a biopsy specimen that is easy to orient correctly. There are numerous types of square-jawed biopsy forceps, including the Kevorkian, Tischler-Kevorkian, and Coppleson styles. Specimens obtained using these forceps have straight edges, allowing for easier orientation. Kevorkian forceps also have a distal row of teeth on the lower jaw designed to fix the cervix and facilitate tissue excision (Figure 6.30). One drawback of this design is that the four teeth make it difficult to obtain a deep biopsy.

Burke, baby Tischler, and mini-Townsend biopsy forceps have smaller heads and remove less tissue than do the Tischler-Morgan or standard Kevorkian biopsy forceps (Figure 6.31). Since 1-mm to 2-mm biopsy depth is usually adequate, these smaller biopsy forceps are commonly used in routine practice. Smaller biopsies are generally preferable to larger biopsies, except

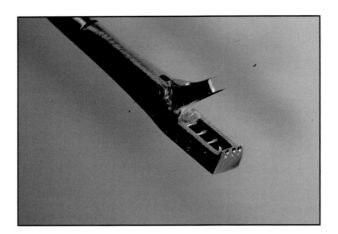

FIGURE 6.30 Kevorkian biopsy forceps with four teeth along the lower jaw. These teeth may impede biopsy collection.

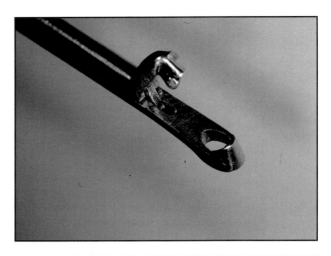

FIGURE 6.32 The Burke biopsy forceps with jaws that open widely.

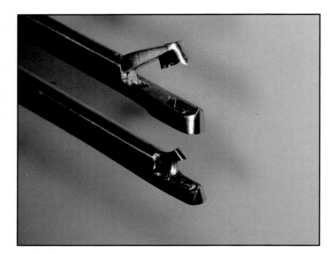

FIGURE 6.31 Comparison of cervical biopsy bite sizes, a large Tischler-Morgan bite (above), and the smaller mini-Townsend bite.

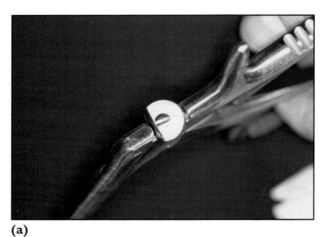

(a)

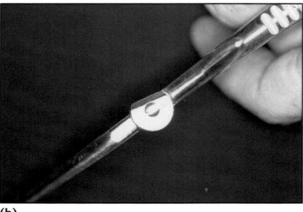

(b)

FIGURES 6.33a,b A thumb-activated locking mechanism on biopsy forceps seen in the **(a)** open and **(b)** locked position.

when cancer is suspected, because they produce less bleeding and pain. Smaller biopsy forceps are also easier to use for biopsies of lesions within the distal endocervical canal. The jaws of the Burke forceps open widely to facilitate biopsies of lesions in difficult-to-access regions (Figure 6.32). For difficult endocervical biopsies, consider the Eppendorfer forceps (without teeth). It optimizes biopsy of the flat portion of the cervix, and also may be used on the vulva and vagina.

Many biopsy forceps have a thumb-activated locking mechanism above the handle to close the forceps jaws securely once a biopsy has been taken (Figures 6.33 a,b). This device locks the jaws in a closed position to prevent the specimens from being lost as the biopsy forceps is withdrawn from the vagina. The locking mechanism also helps protect

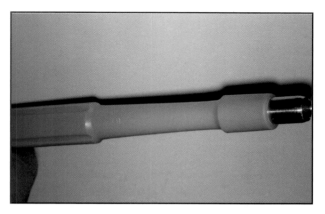

FIGURE 6.34   Keyes dermal biopsy punch to sample vulvar lesions.

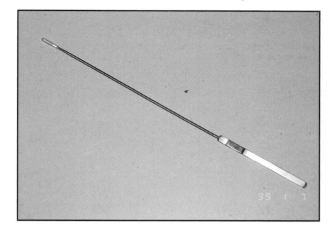

FIGURE 6.35   An endocervical curette used to obtain a histological sample from the endocervical canal. The distal cutting edge is aligned with the depression located in the handle.

the sharp cutting surfaces during sterilization. Since no single instrument is ideal for all situations, experienced colposcopists usually have several different types of biopsy forceps available. Additionally, many clinicians use small, round dermal (Keyes) biopsy punches to sample vulvar lesions (Figures 6.34).

Biopsy instruments eventually become blunt with use, particularly if autoclaved in metal trays and not wrapped individually before sterilization. Because dull instruments increase crush artifact in the specimen and cause more pain,[4] instruments should always be sharp and well maintained. A good test of instrument sharpness is to biopsy a piece of heavy typing paper or a thin plastic sheet. A sharp instrument cuts cleanly through the paper or plastic without fraying edges. Some instruments come with a lifetime resharpening service. If not, sharpening services for surgical instruments are available in most areas.

6.5.5 Endocervical curette

Endocervical curettes are used to obtain tissue samples from the endocervical canal. A cutting edge at the end of the long handle is scraped over the endocervix to remove tissue (Figure 6.35). A small depression in the handle denotes instrument alignment with the distal cutting edge. There are numerous different styles of endocervical curettes, the most common of which is the rectangular-shaped Kevorkian curette. Kevorkian curettes are available either with or without a specimen-retention grid, or "basket" (Figures 6.36a,b). The basket consists of metal wires or a perforated cage that traps mucus and tissue. Some clinicians prefer instruments with a basket because it increases the amount of material retained in the curette, while others prefer those without baskets since trapped material may be difficult to remove. As with cervical biopsy forceps, a sharp instrument yields more tissue and causes less discomfort than a dull curette.

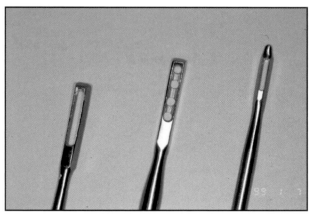

(a)

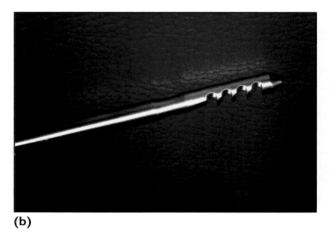

(b)

FIGURES 6.36a,b   An endocervical curette without a specimen retention grid (basket, left), with a specimen retention grid (center), and with a rounded end (right). A London curette with four cutting surfaces is seen in (b).

Additional styles of endocervical curettes include rounded rather than square cutting heads and small-diameter instruments that are useful for women with partially stenotic ora. A Cytobrush®, central long bristles of a CervexBrush®, or as a last resort, a saline-moistened, small, calcium alginate swab rotated in the endocervical canal may provide a suitable specimen for evaluation in women with cervical stenosis. Some clinicians routinely use cytobrushes instead of a metal curette to sample the endocervical canal. Chapter 7 includes a discussion of different approaches to sampling the endocervical canal.

6.5.6 Other instruments

Ring forceps, long-nosed forceps, and long pick-up forceps are useful for applying soaked cotton balls to the mucosal surfaces, removing tissue, mucus, and endocervical polyps. A skin hook is a small, curved hook with one or more sharp projections at the end of a long handle that can be used to stabilize or lift tissue. Several different types of skin hooks are available. Although seldom needed for routine cervical colposcopy, skin hooks are useful in special circumstances, such as everting the lateral corners of the proximal vaginal cuff in women who have had a prior hysterectomy or retrieving tissue that has slipped away from a biopsy instrument.

Long-handle scissors, needle drivers, medium-caliber absorbable suture on a cutting needle, and pick-ups are rarely needed, except when persistent bleeding at biopsy or surgical sites requires suturing (Figure 6.37). A thin sound or narrow round probe with a bulbous head is occasionally useful for identifying or gaining access to the endocervical canal. A set of small cervical dilators is also quite useful for dilating the endocervical canal in women with steno-sis. Some clinicians use a spray bottle to apply 5% acetic acid. A tenaculum is not required to perform colposcopy.

6.6 Chemical Agents and Supplies

6.6.1 Saline

Normal saline (Figure 6.38) is a commonly used moistening and cleansing solution. It does not modify the appearance of the cervical epithelium and is useful for cleaning the cervix when evaluating abnormal blood vessels and leukoplakia prior to the application of 5% acetic acid solution. Saline solution poured from a large stock bottle into smaller disposable cups or containers can be used for individual procedures.

6.6.2 Acetic acid solution

Application of acetic acid solution (Figure 6.38) enhances the detection of anogenital neoplasia during colposcopy. Acetic acid in a 3% to 5% solution is available either as white vinegar, purchased from a grocery store, or as a prepared solution from the pharmacy. It is important to know the acid content of the vinegar purchased from a consumer outlet, such as a grocery store, is usually 5%. Brands with less than 3% acidity are not suitable for colposcopy. Most colposcopists prefer 5% acetic acid solutions to 3% because the higher concentration produces a more rapid and longer-lasting tissue response. On the other hand, a 3% solution of acetic acid is less irritating and may be a better option when there is a possibility of vulvovaginitis and for examining the vulva of women with fair skin. When using acetic acid provided by a pharmacy, it is important to ensure it is a 3% to

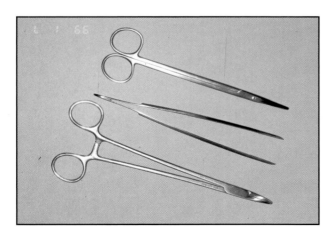

FIGURE 6.37   Long scissors, needle driver, and pickups are rarely required to achieve hemostasis.

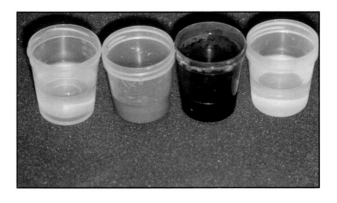

FIGURE 6.38   Chemical solutions used as epithelial contrast agents and hemostatics during colposcopy: normal saline, Monsel's paste, Lugol's iodine solution, and 5% acetic acid (from left to right).

5% solution, as 0.5% solutions are sometimes used in wound dressings and 85% trichloroacetic acid used to treat genital condylomas. Approximately 10 mL to 20 mL of 5% acetic acid solution poured into a separate small container or cup from a larger stock bottle is typically used for each patient and disposed of at the end of the procedure.

6.6.3 Lugol's solution

Aqueous Lugol's solution (Figure 6.39) is an iodine-based contrast solution (iodine and potassium iodide). It is essential for properly evaluating the vagina and is frequently used for cervical evaluation. The iodine in Lugol's solution transiently stains the glycogen in squamous cells, imparting a dark, mahogany brown color to normal glycogenated epithelium. In contrast, most neoplastic tissues do not contain glycogen and, thus, do not stain. Lugol's iodine is commonly diluted with tap water to a half-strength solution. The diluted solution is easier to apply, provides a better staining reaction, and causes minimal mucosal irritation. Full strength Lugol's solution is particularly useful when examining post-menopausal women who are not taking estrogen replacement therapy. Patients should *always* be asked if they have an iodine allergy before Lugol's solution is applied. Since patients may not know if they are allergic to iodine, it is important to ask about shellfish allergies. When using Lugol's solution, be careful to avoid staining the patient's clothing or your own, as iodine is difficult to remove. Topical benzocaine gel works effectively to "erase" or quickly remove iodine from unintentionally stained epithelium.

6.6.4 Monsel's solution

Monsel's (ferric subsulfate) solution (Figure 6.40) is a hemostatic agent that can be used after biopsy or surgical excisions. When mixed according to USP formulary, Monsel's solution is a thin, brown-colored liquid that performs best when allowed to dehydrate or dry to a thick, mustard-color, paste-like consistency. This consistency is achieved by placing the solution in a small open container where it is exposed to the air. After several days, a precipitate forms on the bottom of the container with an overlying thin, dark brown fluid. The dark-brown solution should be poured off the top and discarded. Once prepared, the paste should be stored in a closed container. Left alone, the Monsel's paste texture will slowly harden over time, but adding small amounts of Monsel's solution whenever the paste becomes excessively thick will maintain a proper paste-like consistency.

Because Monsel's paste is highly acidic (pH = 1), avoid excessive or inadvertent application to tissues not requiring hemostasis. Monsel's solution causes severe tissue artifacts that can preclude histologic evaluation; therefore, it is important to keep the solution away from tissues to be biopsied. This is particularly an issue for endocervical curettage since adverse histologic effects of Monsel's solution can persist for several weeks.

6.6.5 Silver nitrate sticks

Silver nitrate sticks provide hemostasis by chemical cautery. To stop bleeding, the head of the stick is applied to the biopsy site (Figure 6.41). Some women will experience a mild burning or cramping sensation when the stick is applied to the cervix.

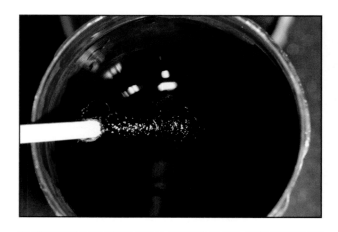

FIGURE 6.39 Lugol's solution used for colposcopic examination of the cervix and vagina.

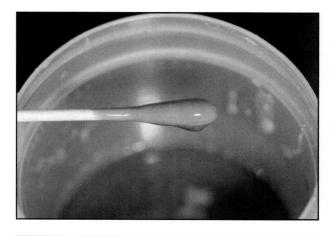

FIGURE 6.40 Monsel's paste used for hemostasis.

Because silver nitrate cauterizes tissue and produces an opaque white color, it should not come in contact with the surrounding epithelium. Excessive application may obscure adjacent acetowhite lesions. Subsequent histologic assessment of tissue obtained through an area of silver nitrate cautery will demonstrate a black precipitation of silver near the basement membrane, but this discoloration will not adversely affect the pathologic interpretation.

6.6.6 Bactericidal solutions for instrument care

Commercial bactericidal solutions containing glutaraldehyde may be used to sterilize instruments. These solutions should be used only in well-ventilated areas. A 70% alcohol solution or a 10% solution of bleach may be used to clean surfaces not amenable to sterilization techniques, keeping in mind that bleach solutions are quite damaging to biopsy forceps and other instruments, including colposcopes. Instruments may also be sterilized using a gas or steam autoclave.

6.6.7 Topical and local anesthetics

Cervical biopsy and endocervical curettage causes pain in some women. Although some colposcopists use topical anesthetics prior to cervical biopsy and endocervical curettage to minimize patient discomfort,[5] placebo-controlled trials have demonstrated that topical applications of xylocaine and benzocaine are ineffective in reducing pain in women undergoing colposcopy or endocervical curettage.[4,6,7] Therefore, the routine use of topical anesthetics during colposcopy is not recommended.

Injectable local anesthetics, such as 1% or 2% xylocaine or lidocaine with or without epinephrine, are an effective pain-relief measure for electrosurgical loop excisions and biopsies of the vagina, vulva, and penis. Many colposcopists use dental syringes to inject local anesthetics because the prefilled cartridges are convenient. A Campion syringe is also useful for injecting anesthetics into the cervix or proximal vagina (Figure 6.42). A topical mixed 5% lidocaine/prilocaine anesthetic cream (EMLA® or ELA-Max-eutectic mixture of local anesthetics) reduces the discomfort associated with injecting xylocaine or lidocaine into the vulva or penis, but in order to be effective to the depth of 2 mm, the application must remain under a nonbreathable barrier for at least 20 to 60 minutes.[8,9] While useful to minimize discomfort on the external genitalia, it is not used on the cervix.

6.6.8 Disposable supplies

Large and small cotton swabs and cotton balls are useful to apply solutions, to tamponade a bleeding site, to remove debris, solutions, or blood from the cervix or vagina, and to maneuver the cervix to obtain proper visualization. One-inch squares of brown paper or filter paper are useful to put biopsies on before submersion in fixative. Disposable protector pads placed beneath the patient's buttocks absorb dripping acetic acid and blood. Gauze pads (4″ × 4″) are useful for applying acetic acid solution to the introitus, vulvar, and perirectal areas, but because they are abrasive, they are not appropriate for the cervix. Sanitary napkins and tampons should be available, along with vaginal packs of tightly rolled gauze pads to tamponade bleeding sites.

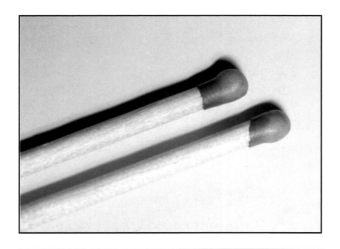

FIGURE 6.41 Silver nitrate sticks used for hemostasis.

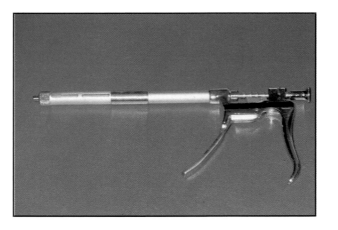

FIGURE 6.42 A Campion syringe used to inject anesthetics into the cervix or proximal vagina.

6.7 Video and Photographic Systems for Optical Colposcopes

6.7.1 Video systems

Video systems for optical colposcopes allow the patient and others to simultaneously view the procedure while the colposcopist looks through the colposcope. This capacity is particularly useful when training residents and students in colposcopy. Even in the nonteaching setting, video capacity helps patients better understand their cervical findings and aids in communicating with them about cervical disease. Additionally, video systems permit colposcopists to document their examination using videotapes, color video prints, CDs or DVDs.

Not all colposcopes adapt easily for image acquisition. Optical colposcopes that have a beam splitter (image diverter) and accessory portals permitting the attachment of different types of cameras provide the best video images and photographs (Figure 6.43).[10] The beam splitter ensures that the image viewed by the colposcopist is identical to the one appearing on the monitor. For colposcopes without beam splitters, attaching a small CCD video camera to the side of the colposcope allows image acquisition. Since this type of system operates independently of the colposcope, however, it requires separate magnification and focus-control adjustments.

Most video systems consist of a small CCD video camera attached to the colposcope's beam splitter by means of an adapter. Images captured by the CCD video camera are transmitted to a high-resolution video monitor. Video images can be printed easily by dedicated color video printers, or the image can be captured by the computer's frame-grabber card and then printed using a standard color computer printer. Because of their ease of use, these methods of capturing video images have largely replaced 35-mm colpophotography, even though resolution of images on video monitors or video color print images is not as detailed as those obtained using colpophotography. However, video technology is changing rapidly and cameras are constantly improving. If the budget for purchase of a colposcope does not permit a video camera and monitor, which can cost $5000 or more, it may be wise to purchase a colposcope capable of accommodating a beam splitter so that video can be added later.

6.7.2 Colpophotography

Some colposcopists like to document their examinations using colpophotography.[10] The availability of cervical images as either photographs or color video prints allows the clinician to reconcile clinical findings with the biopsy report, provides an excellent

form of self-education and quality control, documents pertinent findings and possible adverse events during clinical trials, and aids during the prospective follow-up of patients with an untreated low-grade squamous intraepithelial lesion (SIL) (CIN 1). For colpophotography, digital, Polaroid, or 35-mm cameras are attached to the colposcope's beam splitter (Figure 6.44). When in focus and correctly illuminated, colpophotographs obtained with digital and 35-mm cameras provide greater resolution than do images obtained with Polaroid cameras. Good colpophotography can be extremely challenging,

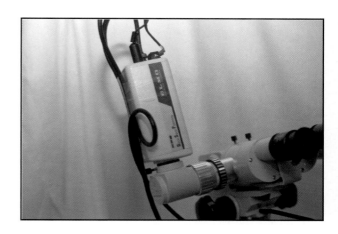

FIGURE 6.43 Optical colposcope with a beam splitter, adapter, and CCD video camera.

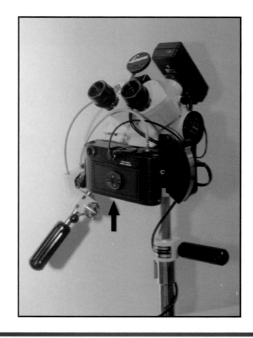

FIGURE 6.44 A 35-mm camera (arrow) system for colposcopic photography.

and many colposcopists question whether the extra expense for photographic capabilities, which is usually more than $2000 for camera and adapter, is justified outside referral centers or academic units.

6.8 Image, Data Management, and Patient Tracking Systems

Current computer-based systems are designed specifically to capture and store digitized colposcopic images, archive pertinent patient information, print visit information and color images for hard-copy documentation, provide patient tracking and recall services, and produce template or customized consultation letters (Figures 6.45 a–c). A colposcope and computer are combined as a single unit in one model (Figure 6.46). Immediate or delayed colposcopic consultation features are available. Linked colposcopy computer systems provide interactive distant telemedicine consultation by modem for less experienced clinicians and those who are geographically isolated.[11,12] These computer systems also enable procedure documentation and

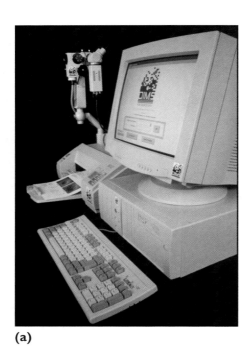

(a)

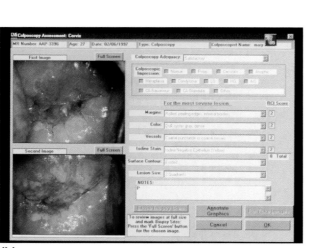

(b)

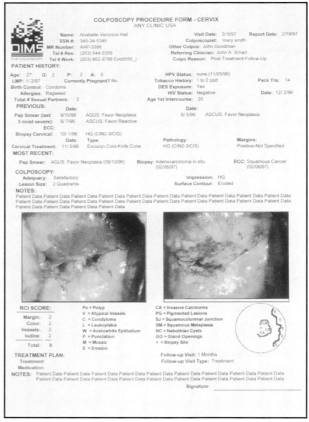

(c)

FIGURES 6.45a–c **(a)** An image management system for storing digitized colposcopic images and pertinent colposcopy data. The system includes a computer, monitor, keyboard, color printer, camera and custom software. **(b)** The colposcopic assessment screen of a computerized image management system with capacity for selective image enlargement. Colposcopic adequacy, colposcopic impressions, and lesion characteristics are accessible as drop-down options. **(c)** Colposcopy evaluation form with annotated cervical images produced by a digital imaging system and color printer. All data are recorded on the form. ▬

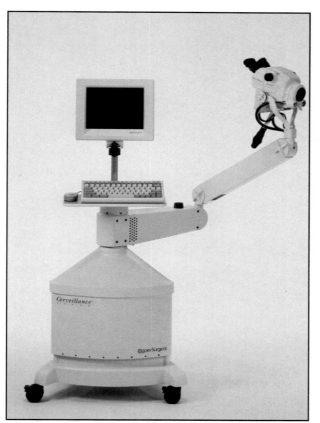

FIGURE 6.46 A colposcope and image management system combined as a single unit.

rapid retrieval of images obtained during colposcopic examinations. The ability to annotate images directly on the captured video image obviates the need for hand-drawn cervical findings (Figure 6.45c). Computerized image management systems also permit documentation of changes in lesion location, size, and volume. They provide objective outcomes in response to treatment or nontreatment, as well as monitor remote colposcopy practice for quality control purposes in clinical trials.

6.9 Summary

The quality of colposcopic equipment and supplies strongly influences the ease, efficiency, and safety of colposcopic examinations. The correct equipment, tools, and supplies should always be available. Inappropriate, outmoded equipment and improperly maintained instruments significantly increase patient discomfort, place an undue burden on the colposcopist, and compromise the safety of the procedure.

References

1. Ferris D G, Willner W A, Ho J J. Colposcopes: a critical review. *J Fam Pract* 1991;33:506–15.
2. Ferris D G. Video colposcopy. *J Lower Genital Tract Disease* 1997;1:15–8.
3. Wright V C. Understanding the colposcope optics, light path, magnification and field of view. In: Wright V C, ed. *Obstetrics and Gynecology Clinics of North America, Contemporary Colposcopy*. Philadelphia: Saunders, 1993.
4. Ferris D G, Harper D M, Callahan B, et al. The efficacy of topical benzocaine gel in providing anesthesia prior to cervical biopsy and endocervical curettage. *J Lower Genital Tract Disease* 1997;1:221–7.
5. Rabin J M, Spitzer M, Dwyer A T, Kaiser I H. Topical anesthesia for gynecologic procedures. *Obstet Gynecol* 1989;73:1040–4.
6. Prefontaine M, Fung-Kee-Fung M, Moher D. Comparison of topical xylocaine with placebo as a local anesthetic in colposcopic biopsies. *Can J Surg* 1991;34:163–5.
7. Clifton P A, Shaughnessy A F, Andrews S. Ineffectiveness of topical benzocaine spray during colposcopy. *J Fam Pract* 1998;6:242–6.
8. Wahlgren C F, Quiding H. Depth of cutaneous analgesia after application of a eutectic mixture of local anasthetics lidocaine and prilocaine (EMLA cream). *J Am Acad Dermatol* 2000; 42: 584–8.
9. Friedman P M, Fogelman J P, Nouri K, Levine V J, Ashinoff R. Comparative study of the efficacy of four topical anesthetics. *Dermatol Surg* 1999; 25:950–4.
10. Ferris D G, Willner W A, Ho J J. Colpophotography systems: a review. *J Fam Pract* 1991;33:633–9.
11. Ferris D G, Macfee M S, Miller J A, Litaker M S, Crawley D, Watson D. The efficacy of telecolposcopy compared with traditional colposcopy. *Obstet Gynecol* 2002;99:248–54.
12. Ferris D G, Litaker M S, Miller J A, Macfee M S, Crawley D, Watson D. Qualitative assessment of telemedicine network and computer-based telecolposcopy. *J Lower Genital Tract Dis* 2002;6:145–9.

The Colposcopic Examination

Table of Contents

7.1 Overview and Preparation for Colposcopy

7.1.1 Purpose of colposcopy

In most countries, colposcopy is used predominately to evaluate women with abnormal Papanicolaou (Pap) smears. The purposes of the colposcopic examination are to locate the source of abnormal cells identified in the Pap smear; diagnose, in conjunction with a colposcopically directed biopsy, the type and grade of lesions present; and delineate the extent of cervical lesions to determine the appropriate approach to treatment. Colposcopic examination involves use of a magnifying instrument to examine the epithelium and vasculature of the uterine cervix, lower genital tract and anogenital area for the purpose of detecting neoplasia, identifying abnormal tissue for biopsy, or affirming normality. Utilization of chemical solutions that aid in discriminating between normal tissue and abnormal lesions further enhances the procedure. Colposcopic examination and directed biopsies of the most abnormal appearing areas ensure histologic scrutiny of the most significant lesions. The results from the cytologic smear, the histologic evaluation of biopsied epithelium and the colposcopic impression of cervical abnormalities collectively derive the final diagnosis to determine appropriate patient management. Although individual colposcopic techniques vary somewhat, a systematic approach ensures inclusion of all critical steps. To become a competent colposcopist, a clinician needs to understand how to conduct a colposcopic examination, be knowledgeable about the visual features of cervical disease, and master the necessary psychomotor skills. This chapter includes background that will allow clinicians to perform a comprehensive colposcopic examination of female patients. Chapter 16 includes a discussion about examining the male patient.

7.1.2 Objectives of the colposcopic examination

Specific objectives of colposcopy ensure a proper colposcopic examination (Table 7.1). During each colposcopic examination, the colposcopist must: (1) visualize the cervix, vagina and vulva; (2) identify the squamocolumnar junction (SCJ) along its entire circumference (ie., 360°) and the encompassing transformation zone; (3) determine whether the colposcopic examination is satisfactory or unsatisfactory; (4) identify and assess suspected neoplastic lesions with respect to size, extent and severity of disease; (5) sample the endocervical canal by curettage or brush, when appropriate; (6) identify the most severe lesions and obtain biopsies; and (7) correlate the results of the Pap smear, cervical biopsies, and the colposcopic impression to determine appropriate patient management. Once the colposcopist has achieved these objectives, it will be evident whether cervical cancer, a cancer precursor or only normal findings are present. Communicating the clinical findings and their significance to the patient is also an integral part of every colposcopic examination.

7.1.3 Indications and contraindications

There are numerous indications for colposcopy (Table 7.2). The most common indication for colposcopy is an abnormal Pap smear. Colposcopy is indicated for women with Pap smear diagnoses of high-grade squamous intraepithelial lesions (HSIL), cancer, and for women with Pap smears suspicious for glandular neoplasia, or atypical glandular cells (AGC).[1] Colposcopy is also indicated for women with low-grade squamous intraepithelial lesions (LSIL), atypical squamous cells, favor high-grade (ASC-H), and is acceptable for women with atypical squamous cells of undetermined significance (ASC-US)[1]. Colposcopy is also indicated, along with cytology, for the followup of women with cervical intraep-

---

Table 7.1   Objectives of Colposcopy

- Visualize the cervix, vagina, vulva and perianal area
- Identify the squamocolumnar junction and transformation zone
- Determine whether the exam is satisfactory or unsatisfactory
- Identify and assess size, shape, contour, location and extent of neoplastic lesions
- Sample the endocervical canal (unless patient is pregnant)
- Identify and biopsy most severe lesions
- Correlate the Pap smear, biopsy and colposcopic impression
- Plan appropriate therapy
- Communicate findings to patient

Table 7.2   Indications for Colposcopy

Cytologic abnormality * (ASC-US, ASC-H, LSIL, HSIL, AGC, AIS, Cancer)

Gross or palpable cervical ulcer, mass, or growth

Positive screening tests including carcinogenic HPV, Cervigram™, speculoscopy (Pap Sure), visual or spectroscopic examination

Unexplained lower genital tract bleeding

History of in-utero diethylstilbestrol exposure

Partner with lower genital tract neoplasia

Multiple sexual partners

Post-treatment follow-up examination

Vulvar or vaginal HPV-associated lesion

See Chapter 18.

ASC-US denotes atypical squamous cells of undetermined significance; ASC-H, atypical squamous cells, cannot exclude HSIL; LSIL, low-grade squamous intraepithelial lesion; HSIL, high-grade squamous intraepithelial lesion; AGC, atypical glandular cells; AIS, Adenocarcinoma in-situ; and HPV, human papillomavirus.

---

ithelial neoplasia 1 (CIN 1) and a satisfactory colposcopic examination.[2] Chapter 18 includes an in-depth description of the guidelines for managing patients with an abnormal Pap smear result.

All women with grossly visible cervical lesions, ulcers, masses, or growths should be examined with the colposcope. Other possible indications for colposcopy include positive findings on a Cervigram™, a speculoscopy examination, a visual naked eye examination following acetic acid wash, or on a spectroscopic (optical biopsy) examination. Colposcopy is also recommended for women with high risk or carcinogenic human papillomavirus (HPV) detected using a DNA (hybrid capture or PCR) test. Women with recurrent "unsatisfactory" or "satisfactory with severe inflammation" Pap smear results may be candidates for colposcopy, particularly if they have increased risk factors for cervical neoplasia. Women with a history of in-utero diethylstilbestrol (DES) exposure, women whose sexual partners have genital condylomas, women who have been treated previously for cervical neoplasia, and patients with vulvar or vaginal HPV/neoplasia are also candidates for colposcopy. A history of unexplained abnormal vaginal bleeding or chronic postcoital bleeding should prompt a careful colposcopic examination. Finally, in some regions of the world (but not in the United States), women receive a colposcopy examination as part of routine cervical cancer screening.

There are no absolute contraindications for colposcopy. Although colposcopic examination is safe for women who take anticoagulant medication, it may be preferable to discontinue anticoagulants several days prior to the procedure and confirm a normal clotting profile before obtaining a cervical biopsy or performing endocervical curettage. Endocervical curettage, but not colposcopy, is contraindicated in pregnant women. In most cases, women with acute cervicitis or severe vaginitis should be evaluated and treated for specific infections prior to colposcopy since tissue fragility associated with infection, bleeding, and inflammatory changes can compromise the accuracy of the colposcopic evaluation. It is preferable not to perform colposcopy on women who are actively menstruating, but a successful examination is possible in women with minimal flow. Whenever future patient noncompliance is anticipated, colposcopy should be performed even under these visually obscuring conditions (Figures 7.1 a,b).

7.1.4 Patient preparation for colposcopy

Women are usually told that they should undergo colposcopy when they are notified of an abnormal Pap smear result. At that time, it is important to briefly describe colposcopy in order to prepare the patient and allay her anxiety. Explain that the examination takes approximately 15–20 minutes and may determine whether the results of the Pap smear are correct and, if so, may also identify the origin of the abnormal cells. A colposcopy education pamphlet may help clarify the procedure and serve as a resource for later reference. Although premedication

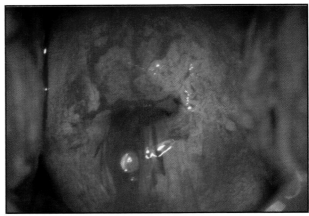

(a)

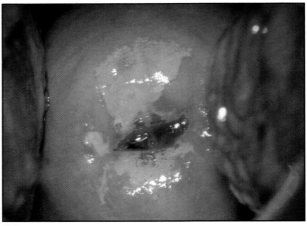

(b)

FIGURES 7.1a,b The cervix of a noncompliant woman who is menstruating and has a history of an high-grade squamous intraepithelial lesion on Papanicolaou smear **(a)**. Colposcopy was conducted regardless of her menses and high-grade acetowhite lesions of the anterior and posterior cervix can now be seen easily **(b)**.

is usually not required, selected women may benefit from a non-steroidal anti-inflammatory drug (NSAID) or, more rarely, an anxiolytic agent prior to the procedure. However, ibuprofen has been shown equivalent to placebo for pain prevention during colposcopy.[3]

Colposcopy can be performed at any point during the menstrual cycle, excepting days of maximum menstrual blood flow, but the best time to perform this procedure is during days 8 to 12 of the menstrual cycle, when the cervical mucus is clear and less viscous. Since such precise scheduling is not always possible, colposcopic examinations are often done randomly throughout the menstrual cycle. Postmenopausal women not receiving estrogen replacement therapy, and other women with atrophic epithelial changes (Fig. 7.2), may benefit from a two-to-three week course of estrogen (oral or topical) prior to their examination. A prior history of estrogen receptor-positive breast cancer is not an absolute contraindication for a short course of estrogen; however, if the patient's breast cancer diagnosis is recent, it may be advisable for the clinician to consult with a patient's oncologist prior to prescribing estrogen.

Instructions to patients should include avoiding intravaginal products, medications, douching, or sexual intercourse for 24 hours prior to colposcopy. Patients should have the option to have a friend or relative with them during the examination. This may be particularly helpful for consenting adolescents, excessively anxious women, and handicapped patients. Ideally, the colposcopist should explain the procedure in depth to the patient prior to performing the examination. Explain that a speculum will be inserted in the same manner as is done for her Pap smear following which a microscope like device or colposcope, positioned outside her body, will be used to look closely at the surface of the cervix. Vinegar, and often iodine, will then be applied to the cervix using soft cotton applicators. Application of the 5% acetic acid or vinegar (a weak acid) may cause a mild external burning sensation, particularly when vulvovaginal inflammation is present. Any abnormal lesions that may be present will temporarily appear white. The colposcope magnification and chemical solutions help identify the source of the abnormal cells found on the Pap smear. If a potentially abnormal area is identified, a biopsy or small tissue sample will be obtained. Reassure the patient that many women (approximately 50%) feel no sensation, but others may note a mild, transient pinch-like discomfort during the biopsy. Severe pain is quite unusual.[3] The examination might also necessitate another procedure known as endocervical curettage. Endocervical curettage usually causes a brief menstrual-like cramping pain. An examination of the vagina and vulva may also be necessary, but biopsies from these areas are seldom required. Be sure that the patient understands that simply taking a biopsy does not imply that she has cervical cancer, or even a precancerous lesion.

It may be advisable to obtain informed consent prior to colposcopy, cervical biopsy and endocervical curettage. As with informed consent for any medical procedure, informed consent for colposcopy should be in writing, following a thorough explanation by the clinician and an opportunity for the patient to ask questions. The consent form should include the nature of the disease, the procedure to be performed, reasonable risks involved, the prognosis with and

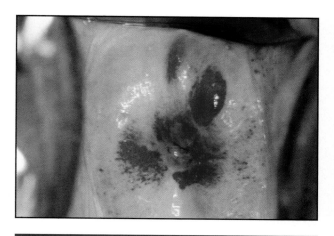

FIGURE 7.2 Atrophic changes of the cervix may complicate the colposcopic examination.

without evaluation or treatment, possible alternative procedures, permission to submit pathologic specimens for evaluation, and acknowledgement of the opportunity to ask questions about the procedure. The patient, a witness, and clinician should all sign and date the informed consent form.

7.1.5 Initial clinic work-up

Prior to performing a colposcopic examination, it is important to obtain a gynecologic history focusing on several key areas, including a history of in-utero DES exposure; immunosuppression, whether from steroid medication, post transplantation medication, diabetes mellitus or acquired immunodeficiency syndrome (AIDS); a hemorrhagic diathesis or use of anticoagulants, which might increase the risk of excessive bleeding; tobacco use; date of most recent menstrual period, and if pregnant, estimated gestational age; method of contraception; history of pelvic inflammatory disease (PID) and current symptoms of vaginitis or acute cervicitis. The clinician should inquire about a prior history of sexually transmitted disease, particularly HPV infection, and premalignant or malignant cervical disease and treatment. It is also important to specifically elicit any history of abnormal vaginal bleeding or postcoital bleeding, since these entities indicate the possibility of occult invasive disease.

7.2 Colposcopic Technique

A systematic approach to colposcopy is essential. The colposcopic examination consists of four distinct and orderly tasks: visualization, assessment, sampling and correlation. Colposcopists initially obtain proper visualization of the cervix and lower genital tract, assess the normal landmarks and any abnormal epithelium, and selectively sample areas of possible neoplasia, as indicated. Finally, colposcopists must correlate their colposcopic impression with the initial Papanicolaou smear and the results of their histologic sampling to determine appropriate management.

7.2.1 Visualization

7.2.1.1 Visualizing the cervix

Adequate visualization of the cervix is essential during colposcopy. Novice colposcopists sometimes fail to adequately visualize the cervix, resulting in frustrating examinations and inadvertent errors. The widest speculum that does not cause patient discomfort should be used to maximize visualization. On initial insertion of the speculum, the ectocervical portion of the cervix is the main area visible (Figure 7.3). As the blades of the speculum are opened, the anterior and posterior lips of the cervix separate, and the external os and part of the endocervical canal become visible (Figure 7.4). Therefore, it is important to open the speculum blades as widely as possible without producing discomfort. Increasing the speculum aperature at the yoke enlarges the introitus, allowing a greater amount of colposcopic illumination of the cervix and maximum visualization.

Prolapsing vaginal walls, common in obese, pregnant or elderly women, may hinder proper visualization of the cervix. A latex glove finger "tube", condom, or lateral sidewall retractor may be helpful in such patients to keep the vaginal sidewalls from obscuring visualization of the cervix (Figures 7.5 a,b). Visualization is greatly facilitated by the combination of a hydraulic or mechanical examination table and an adjustable stool (See Chapter 6, Figure 6.22). The hydraulic table and adjustable stool allow colposcopists to adjust the height of the patient and their position relative to the cervix. Proper patient/colposcopist positioning minimizes posturally induced back strain for the colposcopist.

The position of the cervix relative to the examiner can be changed by placing a large moistened cotton swab in the proximal fornix (alongside the cervix) and then applying gentle cephalad pressure (Figures 7.6 a,b). This action moves the cervix toward the swab, permitting better visualization of both an eccentrically oriented cervix and the vaginal fornix. This approach reduces the risk of the cotton swab causing abrasion-induced bleeding of the surface of the transformation zone. Another method of atraumatically maneuvering the cervix in the anterior and posterior directions is to gently move the speculum blades up or down. A moistened swab placed gently

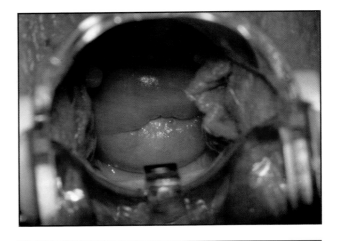

FIGURE 7.3 Only the ectocervix is visible on initial insertion of the speculum. Notice the slightly prolapsing vaginal sidewalls and the lack of complete illumination of the cervix. ■

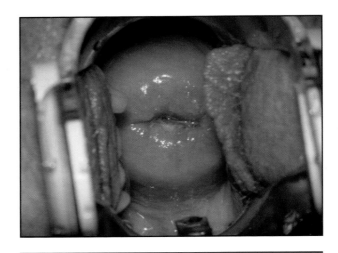

FIGURE 7.4 Once the speculum blades are opened with tolerance, the external os and distal endocervical canal are visible. The ectocervix is also well illuminated. ■

on the ectocervix outside the transformation zone can also be used to reposition the cervix (Figure 7.7).

7.2.1.2 Focusing the colposcope

The colposcopic examination begins by initially viewing the entire cervix through the colposcope at low power (2× to 4×) magnification (Figure 7.8). At low magnification, coarse focus can be achieved by simply moving the colposcope closer or farther away from the cervix. The distance between the colposcope objective lens and the cervix in focus equates to the focal length of the objective lens. A 300-mm objective lens, available on most modern colposcopes,

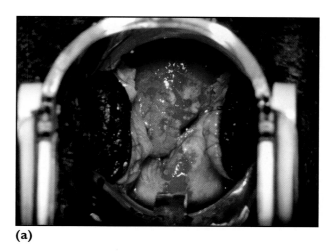

(a)

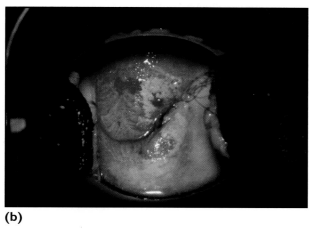

(b)

FIGURES 7.5a,b Use of a latex glove finger "tube" placed over the vaginal speculum blades limits vaginal side-wall prolapse. **(a)** Colposcopic view without use of "tube" and **(b)** with use of tube. ▬

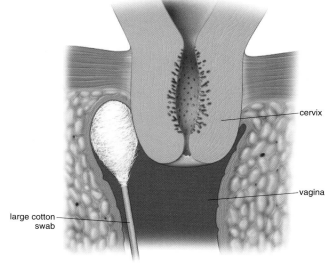

(a)

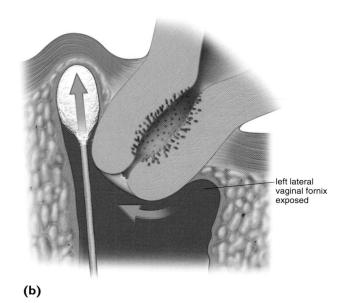

(b)

FIGURES 7.6a,b To move a cervix deviated toward the left fornix to the patient's right side or center vaginal position, place the moistened cotton swab in the right proximal vaginal fornix (at 9 o'clock position), and push forward gently toward the patient's head **(a)**. The cervix will move toward the swab (patient's right side) without actually touching the cervix, permitting visualization of the left side of the cervix and left proximal vaginal fornix **(b)**. ▬

enables sufficient space between the patient and colposcope for instrument manipulation. Once coarse focus is achieved, minor adjustments can be made by manipulating a fine focus handle or lever that moves only the optical colposcope head. In the case of a video colposcope, a bi-directional button accomplishes fine focus while the colposcope remains stationary. The entire cervix is visible at approximately 7× to 8× magnification. More detailed examination of small colposcopic features requires incremental increases to a higher power magnification (~10× to ~15×) (Figure 7.9). Magnification greater than 15× is generally not required for colposcopy, but it may further accentuate delicate vascular changes.

Novice colposcopists occasionally have difficulty focusing. The problem may be attributable to the eyepieces of an optical colposcope being set at diopter settings that do not conform to focus for both eyes. Alternatively, one interchangeable eyepiece may not be seated fully within the eyepiece-housing receptacle (binocular tubes), hence, contributing to a blurred image. Reliance solely on the fine focus handle or button when the target is either too close or too far away from an optical or video colposcope may cause focusing problems. Setting both

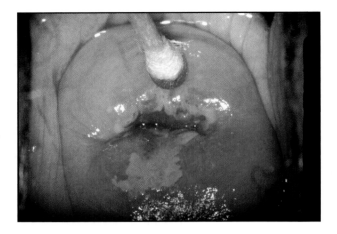

FIGURE 7.7   A small swab placed on the ectocervix to assist with positioning. An acetowhite CIN 2 is noted on the ectocervix. The examination is satisfactory because the entire SCJ and lesion are clearly seen.

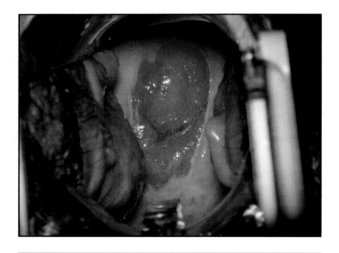

FIGURE 7.8   Low-power magnification of the cervix and proximal vagina. A normal ectropion is present, viewed as the central reddish portion of the cervix.

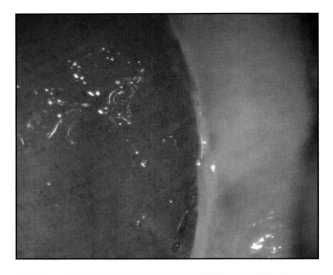

FIGURE 7.9   A high-power magnification of the cervix from Figure 7.8 demonstrating a highly magnified view of the squamous and columnar epithelium and the squamocolumnar junction.

eyepiece diopter settings at "0" or a central mark (dot) may correct diopter problems for a colposcopist having 20/20 vision. If not, another method is to first focus the colposcope using only one eye and eyepiece. Then look through only the opposite eyepiece with the other eye open and focus by turning the diopter ring for only the other eyepiece. Make sure that both eyepieces are completely seated within their respective eyepiece receptacles.

Focusing is best accomplished by first looking at the lateral field of view to see what is in focus. If the speculum or vaginal wall is clearly visible, use a coarse-focus positioning to move the colposcope forward, closer to the cervix. If the image is completely blurred, the colposcope is too close to the target, and it should be pulled back. If withdrawing the colposcope does not correct the problem, be sure that the oculars are set at your interpupillary distance to avoid seeing a double image. When both hands are occupied, colposcopes on a wheelbase can be focused easily by placing the feet atop the base and using them to adjust the position of the entire scope. Fine focus at a high-power magnification level can be achieved by gently pulling or pushing the vaginal speculum to obtain a clear view of the cervix.

7.2.1.3 Papanicolaou and microbiologic test collection

Repeating the Pap smear at the time of colposcopy provides little additional clinical information and can occasionally strip away the epithelium from the stroma and precipitate bleeding. If the patient's most recent Pap smear was collected within three months, is available to the pathologist, and does not indicate AGC, it may be preferable not to collect a repeat smear prior to colposcopy. If it is necessary to perform a Pap smear, it should be obtained before applying normal saline or 5% acetic acid to the cervix.

Specimens for viral and bacterial testing should be obtained at this point in the examination, prior to application of saline or 5% acetic acid. Excessive vaginal or endocervical canal discharge should be noted, and appropriate specimens obtained for culture, Gram stain, saline and potassium hydroxide (KOH) wet mount preparation, whiff test, pH determination and other relevant microbiologic tests (i.e. *Neisseria gonorrhoeae, Chlamydia trachomatis*). Colposcopy should be rescheduled following treatment if a severe cervical or vaginal infection is present, since these infections can significantly complicate the examination.

7.2.1.4 Removing obscuring blood and mucus

Blood and mucus may obscure the cervix, particularly when located within the endocervical canal. A small, cotton-tipped applicator soaked in 5% acetic acid and placed within the endocervical canal will frequently stop bleeding from this area. A larger, acetic acid-soaked swab placed on the ectocervix also works well to control bleeding on the portio. Hemostatic agents should not be used prior to colposcopic assessment since they distort the appearance of the epithelium. Dry cotton swabs should be avoided except for absorbing and removing obscuring blood, pooling

contrast solutions, or applying Monsel's paste because they can be abrasive when rubbed across or rotated on columnar epithelium. Mucus protruding from the os and obscuring a portion of the ectocervix, can often be moved from side to side with a small, moistened swab, allowing the underlying epithelium to be viewed. In other cases, mucus can be removed using a small forceps or a Cytobrush. Otherwise, it may be simply pushed into the endocervical canal with a small, moistened cotton swab or a moistened calcium alginate swab at the end of a thin wire shaft.

7.2.1.5 Application of normal saline

Once the cervix is positioned, normal saline is used to moisten the epithelium and remove obscuring mucus and cellular debris. The examination should focus on two important findings at this point: leukoplakia and abnormal blood vessels. Leukoplakia (Figures 7.10a,b,c,d) is a white, thickened area of

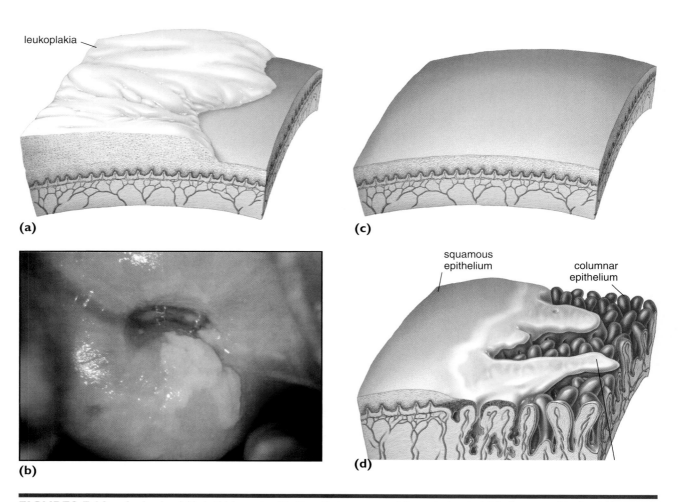

FIGURES 7.10a–d Leukoplakia is thickened epithelium that appears white and elevated **(a)**. An area of leukoplakia noted on the cervix following the application of normal saline, but prior to use of acetic acid **(b)**. The thickened epithelium appears white during initial inspection. Leukoplakia can be contrasted with normal squamous epithelium that has a pink color and is macular in topography **(c)**, and immature metaplasia **(d)** that is very thin and translucent. ■

epithelium that is visible before the application of acetic acid (Chapter 8). Leukoplakia sometimes disappears after the application of acetic acid, or thin sheets of loosely adhering superficial epithelium may be dislodged from the underlying thickened white patch when acetic acid is applied. Leukoplakia should always be biopsied, but not until after the colposcopic assessment is completed.

Small abnormal vessels are best visualized after the application of normal saline and prior to acetic acid application. Acetic acid causes tissue edema that exerts a mild, transient, vasoconstrictive effect on fine caliber blood vessels, which can frequently cause tiny abnormal vessels to become inapparent. A green filter (Figures 7.11 a,b) which enhances angioarchitec-

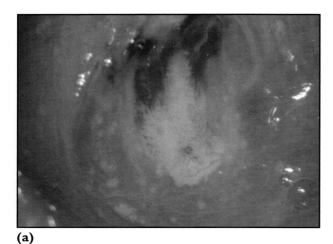

(a)

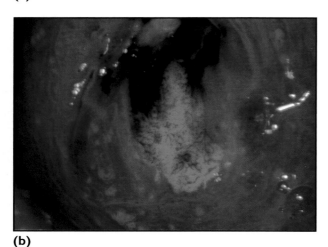

(b)

FIGURES 7.11a,b A green-filter examination of the cervix enhances recognition of the cervical vasculature. The green filter absorbs red light causing the blood vessels to appear black. A cervical lesion of the posterior cervical lip after 5% acetic acid application **(a)** and as seen with the green filter **(b)**.

ture, is often used during the saline examination of the cervix. The green filter absorbs red light, causing blood vessels to appear black, making them easier to discern against a green background. Many colposcopists omit the normal saline assessment of the cervix. Skipping this step may be unwise, particularly for the beginner, because atypical vascular patterns, which are visible after saline application, can be obscured transiently after the application of 5% acetic acid. When saline is not used, approximately 5 minutes is required following acetic acid application to fully appreciate the unmodified vasculature.

7.2.1.6 Application of 3% to 5% acetic acid

Two chemical solutions are then applied separately to the cervix to help discriminate normal from abnormal epithelium. The first is 3% to 5% acetic acid. This weak acid is applied liberally and frequently to the cervix using cotton balls and ring forceps, large cotton swabs, or using a spray technique (Figures 7.12 a,b). Gauze pads (4″ × 4″) should not be used to apply solutions to the cervix because of their abrasive properties. Some clinicians find that the use of a spray bottle to apply acetic acid onto the cervix limits epithelial abrasion, particularly during pregnancy. Irrespective of how the acetic acid is applied, the amount must be sufficient to elicit an optimal acetowhite reaction. Less experienced colposcopists commonly make the mistake of applying too little acetic acid or not waiting long enough for the full effect to take place. These errors can cause significant lesions to escape detection. Saturated cotton balls held with sponge-holding ring forceps apply a large volume of acetic acid to the cervix and help insure a good acetic acid effect. If cotton-tipped applicators are used, they must be large and fully soaked with acetic acid. Twirling a large cotton-tipped applicator in the container of acetic acid will cause partial unraveling of the cotton, producing a mop-like applicator similar to that of a well-soaked cotton ball. A second application of acetic acid ensures that sufficient time has elapsed (a total of 1 to 2 minutes) for the acetic acid reaction to occur. Since the effects of acetic acid are transitory, frequent repeated applications are necessary to retain an acetowhite effect. A red color in columnar epithelium indicates the need for additional acetic acid application (Figures 7.13 a,b). Normally, columnar epithelium blanches slightly white following acetic acid application, but this effect is quite brief. Once the blanched white color reverts to red, acetic acid should be reapplied. When applying acetic acid, avoid rotating or scouring motions to prevent bleeding. Steady direct application or gentle dabbing of acetic acid on the transformation zone is more effective.

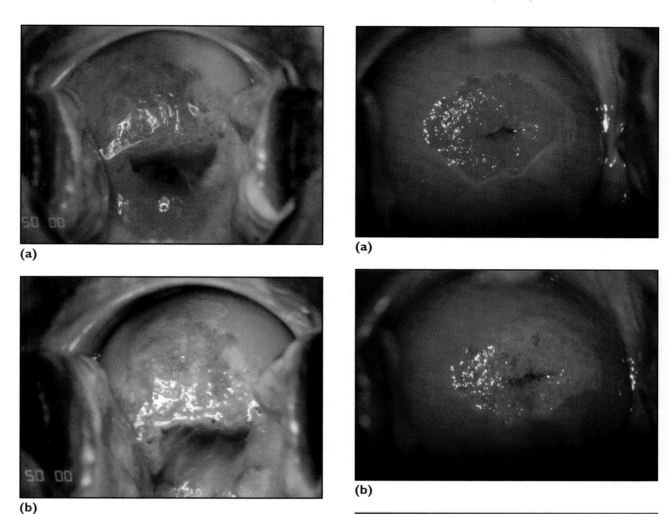

(a)

(b)

(a)

(b)

FIGURES 7.12a,b   The cervix before **(a)** and after **(b)** application of 5% acetic acid demonstrating an easily observed acetowhite CIN 3 lesion on the anterior cervix noted only following acetic acid application. ▬▬▬▬▬▬

FIGURES 7.13a,b   Columnar epithelium is red prior to 5% acetic acid application **(a)** and blanches faintly white after 5% acetic acid application **(b)**. ▬▬▬▬▬▬

Acetic acid interacts with both normal and neoplastic epithelium causing them to swell and change color. Following acetic acid application, both normal and abnormal tissues composed of cells with an increased nuclear-to-cytoplasmic ratio appear transiently white (acetowhite). Surrounding normal squamous epithelium retains its usual pink color. The rate of appearance and disappearance of the acetic acid effect varies with different types of lesions. Therefore, it is important to view the cervix through the colposcope while applying acetic acid. An adequate acetic acid response is indicated by faint acetowhite blanching of the normally red columnar epithelium (when visible). Fine vascular patterns initially become less distinct after the application of acetic acid. However, as the acetic acid reaction begins to subside, the capillary patterns become

more distinct against a white background (Figures 7.14 a,b,c). At this time, the vascular patterns of cervical neoplasia are most vivid. In general, the acetowhite color develops faster and persists longer in more severe grades of neoplasia.

Following application of acetic acid, the cervix and vaginal fornices should be systematically examined at low-power magnification (2× to 5×) to allow any acetowhite lesions to be identified. When areas of acetowhite epithelium are identified, the colposcopist should be careful to complete the systematic low-magnification inspection of the entire cervix, and vaginal fornices before proceeding to higher-power magnification (Figure 7.15) to ensure that additional lesions are not overlooked. After this low-magnification examination, all abnormal areas should be examined at high power (10× to 15×). The site and extent of all abnormal epithelia must be noted carefully.

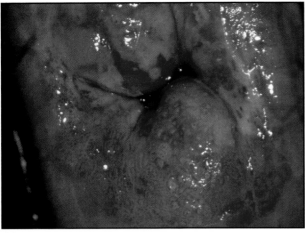

(a)

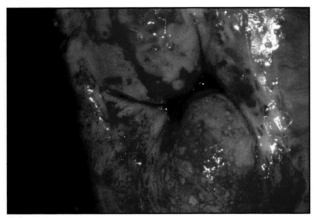

(b)

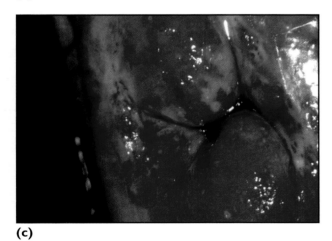

(c)

FIGURES 7.14a–c Time-lapsed colpophotography of a cervical lesion (CIN 3) immediately following **(a)**, three minutes after **(b)**, and more than five minutes after 5% acetic acid application **(c)**. Dense acetowhite epithelium and coarse punctation are visible. The vessels become more prominent as the acetic acid effect fades **(b)**.

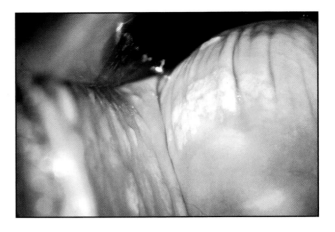

FIGURE 7.15 Vaginal neoplasia located in the proximal vaginal fornix in a woman with an abnormal Papanicolaou smear result.

7.2.1.7 Application of diluted Lugol's iodine solution

Half-strength Lugol's iodine is another contrast solution often used during colposcopy. Provided the patient is not allergic to iodine, Lugol's solution is applied in the same fashion as 5% acetic acid. Lugol's iodine stains intracellular glycogen dark brown (see Chapter 6). Original squamous epithelium of postpubertal women and areas of mature metaplasia are heavily glycogenated and will appear mahogany brown following the application of Lugol's solution. In estrogen-deficient women, there is less glycogenization of the squamous epithelium and the epithelium stains a tan or light-brown color. Schiller's iodine solution is 15 times more dilute than Lugol's solution, and therefore, it is rarely used during colposcopy.

Neoplastic epithelium, normal columnar epithelium, immature squamous metaplastic epithelium, and leukoplakia contain little or no glycogen and do not stain with Lugol's solution (Figures 7.16 a,b). Columnar or immature metaplastic epithelium appears reddish pink or light yellow. Neoplastic epithelium can have a range of staining patterns. Usually, HSIL or cervical intraepithelial neoplasia 2,3 (CIN 2,3) will appear as either a white-yellow or a mustard-yellow color and low-grade squamous intraepithelial lesion (LSIL or CIN 1) will appear a brighter orange-yellow color. This color difference may assist in differentiating low-grade from high-grade lesions. Some squamous intraepithelial lesions have small, randomly dispersed areas of glycogen within larger areas of neoplastic epithelium lacking glycogen, which produces a variegated yellow-brown ("tortoise-shell") staining pattern. Inflammatory lesions, including acute ectocervical and vaginal infections such as trichomoniasis, pro-

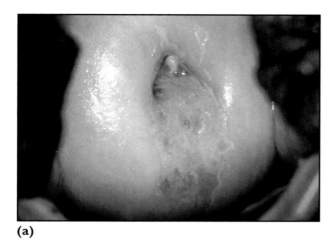

(a)

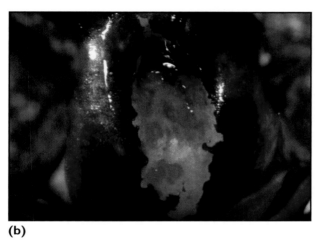

(b)

FIGURES 7.16a,b The cervix before **(a)** and after Lugol's iodine application **(b)**. The acetowhite lesion on the posterior lip of the cervix is not readily apparent **(a)**. However, a yellow-appearing cervical lesion is easily contrasted against a normal mahogany brown background of squamous epithelium **(b)**.

duce small, diffuse patches of glycogen-free epithelium that also do not stain after application of aqueous iodine. When inflammation is severe and the epithelium is denuded, the underlying stroma appear pink. Otherwise, inflammation produces patchy mustard-yellow areas.

Iodine staining is an optional colposcopy procedure for examining the cervix. It is not used by all colposcopists and even those who use it do not do so for all patients. However, iodine staining is critical for assessing the severity of cervical disease using some colposcopic scoring systems (See Chapter 9).[4,5] It is also quite helpful for detecting small HSIL (CIN 2,3) that can otherwise be missed. For example, inexperienced colposcopists commonly overlook HSIL (CIN 2,3) within a larger low grade lesion. In these cases, iodine staining may make the high-grade disease

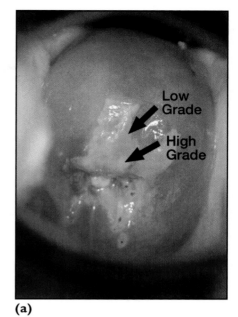

(a)

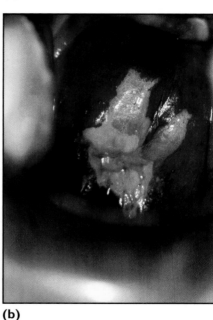

(b)

FIGURES 7.17 a,b An acetowhite lesion is seen on the anterior lip of the cervix **(a)**. A high-grade yellow lesion (arrow) positioned within a larger variegated low-grade lesion is better-appreciated following Lugol's iodine application **(b)**. The lesions are seen at the 12 o'clock position. The iodine provides a more distinct contrast between the centrally positioned high-grade lesion and the low-grade lesion in the periphery.

more visible. Iodine staining highlights the internal margin between the mustard-yellow, significant lesion and the variegated, partially stained low-grade lesion (Figures 7.17a,b). Sometimes a faint acetowhite lesion on the ectocervix or vagina is not obvious until

Lugol's solution is applied, producing a more vivid yellow/brown contrast. Therefore, the iodine examination may be beneficial when the source of a woman's abnormal cytology cannot be ascertained following the acetic acid examination. In the colposcopic examination of the vagina, iodine staining of the mucosa is invaluable, and probably mandatory, because vaginal lesions are more difficult to see following the use of acetic acid. Vaginal intraepithelial neoplasia (VAIN) assumes a mustard-yellow color against a surrounding brown color of normal vaginal epithelium when estrogenized (Figures 7.18 a,b).

There are numerous issues to consider with the routine use of iodine staining. It must be stressed that both normal immature epithelium and high-grade precursor lesions reject iodine and stain mustard-yellow. Thus, iodine-staining patterns are relatively nonspecific. Iodine application prevents assessment of the underlying vasculature and other colposcopic signs. Therefore, colposcopic examination with 3% to 5% acetic acid must be done before applying iodine. Additionally, areas selected for biopsy prior to the application of iodine may be difficult to relocate after staining because iodine staining hides vascular changes and subtle acetowhite differences necessary for accurate biopsy placement. Therefore, colposcopists need to maintain a mental image of how the cervix appeared after the application of acetic acid in order to biopsy the correct areas. When Lugol's iodine staining complicates the remainder of the examination and histologic sampling process, topical benzocaine gel works well to quickly "erase" unwanted iodine staining.

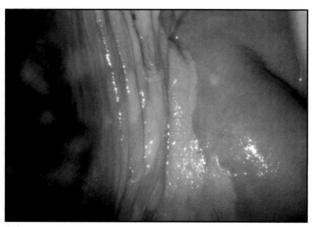

(a)

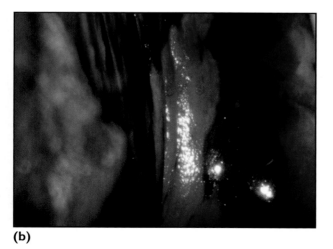

(b)

FIGURES 7.18a,b An acetowhite vaginal intraepithelial neoplasia 3 (VAIN 3) lesion of the proximal fornix **(a)**, and the same VAIN 3 noted following Lugol's iodine solution application **(b)**. Note the mustard-yellow lesion surrounded by mahogany brown normal squamous epithelium.

7.2.2 Assessment

Following colposcopic visualization of the cervix, colposcopists must assess their visual findings. Assessment includes identification of squamous and columnar epithelium, the squamocolumnar junction (SCJ) and transformation zone, recognition of neoplastic lesions, and estimation of the linear extent, size and degree of severity of neoplastic lesions, if present.

7.2.2.1 Concept of the "satisfactory" colposcopic examination

Prior to the introduction of colposcopy, women with abnormal Pap smears had cold-knife conizations to rule out invasive cancer. Colposcopy provided a less traumatic and more cost-efficient method of ruling out invasive cancer based on the colposcopic appearance and a small selective biopsy, but it has limitations. Invasion can only be ruled out if the entire transformation zone and all lesions, are colposcopically visible in their entirety. Therefore, early colposcopists developed the concept of the "satisfactory" colposcopic examination to identify patients who were candidates for outpatient conservative management.

When an examination is classified as "satisfactory", the entire transformation zone has been visualized with the colposcope. In practice, this means that 360 of columnar epithelium, 360° of squamous epithelium, and consequently, 360° of the current SCJ can be seen. Additionally, if a cervical lesion is present, the entire lesion, including both the distal and proximal margins, must be colposcopically visible in order for the examination to be classified as "satisfactory" (Figure 7.7). When 360° of columnar epithelium and the squamocolumnar junction, or lesion cannot be visualized in their entirety, the examination is classified as "unsatisfactory" and an excisional conization may be necessary (Figures 7.19 a,b).

7.2.2.2 Identification of the transformation zone

The first step during colposcopic assessment is to try to identify the limits of the transformation zone. This requires identification of both the original and the current SCJ. The approximate area of the original

squamocolumnar junction can sometimes be identified in younger women in whom gland openings and Nabothian cysts often remain visible in areas of squamous metaplasia. However, the original junction can be difficult, if not impossible, to identify in older women. Although it is helpful to identify the original SCJ, it is important to remember that the region immediately adjacent to the new or current SCJ is the region most likely to contain cervical neoplasia (Figure 7.20). Because complete visualization of the SCJ and columnar epithelium denotes a satisfactory colposcopic examination, colposcopists should always determine and indicate in the clinical record whether the entire SCJ and transformation zone were observed. This clinical notation will document whether the examination was satisfactory or unsatisfactory.

In many young women, including those who currently are or have recently been pregnant, the current or new SCJ is positioned in full colposcopic view on the ectocervix (Figure 7.21a). The thin SCJ appears transiently white following acetic acid application. In postmenopausal women and in those who have previously received cervical ablative or excisional therapy, the junction and columnar epithelium are more commonly located at the external os, or deep within the endocervical canal (Figure 7.21b). Colposcopic assessment of postmenopausal women was unsatisfactory for 57% in one study.[6] If the SCJ is not easily visualized when positioned in the endocervical canal, the colposcopist should attempt to visualize the entire junction without inducing bleeding. This can be accomplished in any one of several ways. To evert a patulous cervix, open the vaginal speculum blades widely within tolerance; push large, moistened cotton applicators cephalad in the anterior and

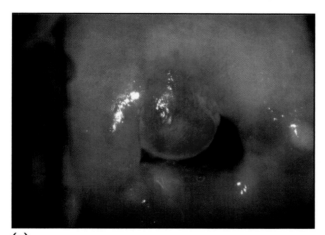

(a)

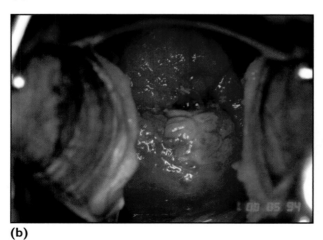

(b)

FIGURES 7.19a,b An unsatisfactory examination because the squamocolumnar junction cannot be seen **(a)**. A large nabothian cyst is seen on the right anterior cervical lip. Its presence obscures viewing the entire squamocolumnar junction. A cervical lesion extends up the endocervical canal beyond full view **(b)**. The examination is unsatisfactory because the proximal extent of the lesion cannot be identified. ■

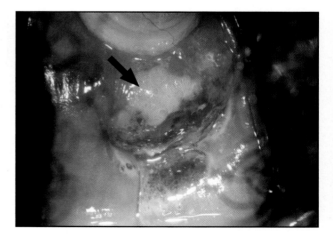

FIGURE 7.20 An acetowhite low-grade cervical lesion (arrow) adjoining the squamocolumnar junction. ■

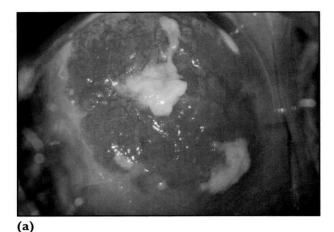

(a)

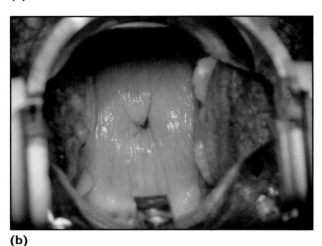

(b)

FIGURES 7.21a,b A low-grade cervical lesion seen in a young woman with a cervical ectropion **(a)**. The entire squamocolumnar junction is visible. The squamocolumnar junction is not seen following electrosurgical loop excision of the cervix **(b)**.

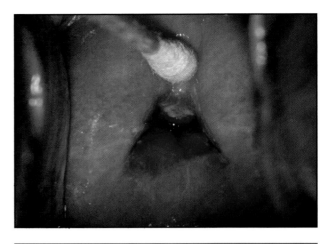

FIGURE 7.22 A high-grade cervical lesion with the squamocolumnar junction visible at the external os. The proximal limit of the lesion is seen clearly using a cotton tip applicator to evert the endocervix. The examination is satisfactory.

41 women whose entire SCJ could not be seen initially, had satisfactory colposcopy examinations 4 hours after Lamicel was placed in the endocervical canal.[7]

7.2.2.3 Identification of epithelial abnormalities

The second step during colposcopic assessment is to identify the source of the abnormal cells present on the Pap smear. In most instances, a lesion that accounts for the Pap smear findings will be readily apparent. When a cervical lesion is not seen, or if the lesion that is identified does not explain the cytologic abnormality, a systematic colposcopic assessment will usually identify the source of the abnormal smear result. Following application of acetic acid or Lugol's iodine solution, neoplastic lesions exhibit typical features that allow them to be identified. These features are derived from alterations in (1) color, (2) vascular caliber and pattern, (3) margins and (4) surface contour. Chapters 8 and 9 include a detailed description of these alterations. The process of colposcopic assessment involves carefully visualizing the transformation zone to identify abnormal appearing areas and evaluating these areas for each of these four parameters. Following evaluation of these parameters, the colposcopist then formulates a colposcopic impression that equates to the expected histologic composition of a given area. Colposcopic assessment also involves looking for the warning signs of invasive cervical cancer. Chapter 10 includes a description of these signs.

Some colposcopists use a colposcopic index or grading system to predict the severity of squamous disease and to aid in formulating their colposcopic

posterior vaginal fornices; or lift or push the tissue near the cervical os with small moistened cotton tipped applicators (Figure 7.22). Another method is to gently open the external os and inspect the distal endocervical canal using an endocervical speculum (Figures 7.23 a,b). For estrogen-deficient women, a short course of estrogen therapy may result in a satisfactory examination at subsequent colposcopy. In other women, the endocervical margin of cervical neoplasia cannot be identified (Figure 7.23 a). Some colposcopists dilate the external os using laminaria, but this approach often strips the epithelium from the stroma, making the subsequent colposcopic assessment impossible. In one study, Lamicel (a compressed polyvinyl alcohol sponge impregnated with magnesium sulfate) was used in women with unsatisfactory colposcopic examinations. Twenty-nine, of

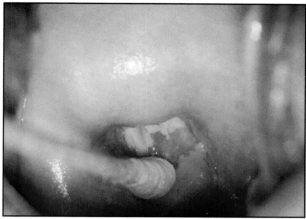

(a)

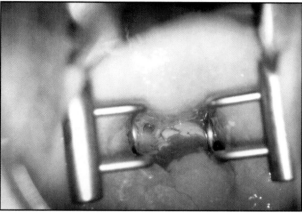

(b)

FIGURES 7.23a,b   A densely acetowhite cervical lesion that extends within the endocervical canal. The upper limit of the lesion could not be seen using a small cotton swab **(a)** or an endocervical speculum **(b)**. The examination is unsatisfactory.

impression.[4,5] These systems provide a structured, objective appraisal instead of a subjective approach, and are useful in assessing cervical lesions, especially for beginning colposcopists. Lesions can be colposcopically categorized as normal or non-neoplastic, low-grade disease (CIN 1, HPV), high-grade disease (CIN 2, CIN 3/CIS [carcinoma-in-situ]), or cancer (squamous or adenocarcinoma). Chapter 9 addresses colposcopic grading.

7.2.2.4 Determining the size, shape, contour, location and extent of cervical lesions

Once the colposcopic impression has been formulated, the next step in the assessment is to determine the size, shape, contour, location and extent of cervical lesions. Cervical lesions range from very small (only several millimeters in diameter) (Figure 7.22) to large (four quadrant) (Figure 7.14b). Generally speaking, the larger the size and linear length of the neoplasia, the greater the severity. However, four-quadrant condylomas or low grade lesions, frequently seen in immunocompromised women, do not conform to this adage. The shape or borders of a cervical lesion may indicate the severity of disease (Chapter 9). Lesions with irregular margins generally represent low-grade disease, while lesions with more regular or smooth edges are likely to be high grade. Similarly, lesion contour may reflect the level of neoplasia; for example, raised, exophytic lesions may be either condyloma or cancer. The source of the abnormal Pap smear may be located in the vagina and/or in variable positions on and within the cervix (Figures 7.24 a,b). Lesions may be focal (solitary) or multifocal (diffusely distributed). Size, shape, contour and location of cervical neoplasia influence the selection of the most appropriate treatment; therefore, colposcopists should appraise these lesion characteristics before selecting a type of treatment.

Determining the peripheral margin of a cervical lesion is usually easy, especially after staining the cervix with Lugol's iodine solution. Occasionally, transformation zones and lesions extend beyond the portio and into the vaginal fornices (especially in DES-exposed patients). Isolated vaginal lesions are sometimes of a higher grade than are the lesions on the cervix. Identifying a cervical lesion's proximal margin is one of the most important tasks for a colposcopist. Careful attention to the endocervical margin ensures that excisional procedures rather than ablative modalities are used to manage lesions extending beyond colposcopic view within the endocervical canal. In young women, the SCJ is located usually on the portio, distal or peripheral to the external os. In these patients, identifying the proximal or endocervical margins of cervical neoplasia is quite easy (Figure 7.25). In older patients (Figure 7.26), or in patients who have been treated previously for cervical neoplasia , the SCJ can be located at or proximal to the external os. In these women, identifying the proximal or endocervical margin of a lesion can be difficult. For estrogen-deficient women with atrophic changes, a short course of therapy with estrogen may alter the anatomy sufficiently to permit a satisfactory examination on a subsequent colposcopy. In some cases, use of a cotton-tip applicator or endocervical speculum allows the inner margin of a lesion to be identified (Figure 7.22). In other women, simple approaches are inadequate to identify the endocervical margin of cervical neoplasia (Figures 7.23 a,b).

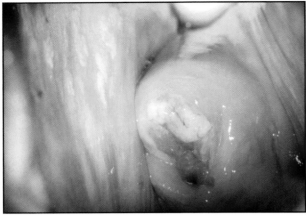

(a)

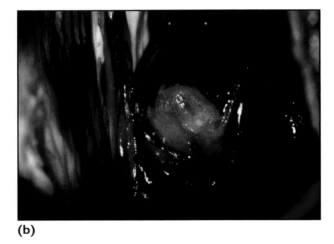

(b)

FIGURES 7.24a,b Lesions of both the cervix (CIN 1) and vagina (VAIN 1) in this woman following application of 5% acetic acid **(a)** and Lugol's iodine **(b)**.

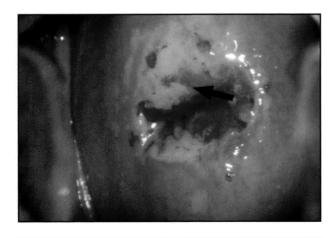

FIGURE 7.25 A CIN 2 on the ectocervix. The proximal lesion margin is seen easily (arrow). The colposcopic examination is satisfactory.

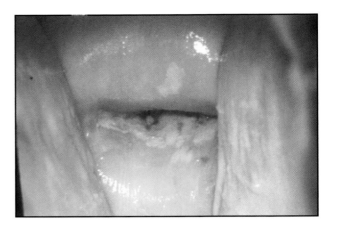

FIGURE 7.26 A low-grade lesion is seen on the posterior lip of the cervix in this older woman. The upper extent of the lesion and the squamocolumnar junction are not visualized. The examination is unsatisfactory.

7.2.3 Sampling

Colposcopists must collect an adequate and representative histologic sample of the most severe disease located on the ectocervix, within the endocervical canal, or elsewhere in the lower genital tract, when indicated. Histologic sampling of cervical lesions is useful in confirming the colposcopic assessment, determining the grade of neoplasia (if present), and ensuring that occult invasive cancer is not present. Histologic sampling consists of endocervical curettage and cervical biopsy.

7.2.3.1 Endocervical curettage (ECC)

Endocervical curettage (ECC) is performed to evaluate non-visualized areas of the endocervical canal, as indicated (Figure 7.27). In women with satisfactory colposcopic examinations, an ECC allows for detection of glandular neoplasia (sometimes multifocal) and rare "skip lesions" (isolated areas of squamous neoplasia, not contiguous with the SCJ found primarily in women who have had prior cervical surgery). In women with unsatisfactory colposcopic examinations and minor cytological abnormalities, an ECC can also help detect neoplastic lesions that are beyond colposcopic view within the endocervical canal.

7.2.3.1.1 Selective use of ECC in colposcopic practice Many colposcopists today are reconsidering the role of ECC. In the 1970's, ECC was considered an essential component of the colposcopic examination. The necessity for an ECC was based on an analysis by Townsend and Richart's of women who developed invasive cervical cancer after having

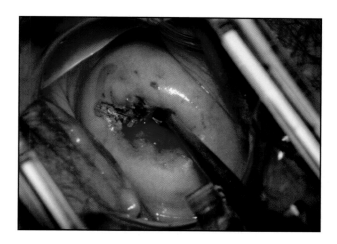

FIGURE 7.27 Endocervical curettage with a metal curette requires a representative sampling of the endocervical canal. ■

undergone colposcopic evaluation and cryosurgery.[8] An analysis revealed that the omission of ECC when otherwise indicated was the most common potential error in this series. This finding led to the following recommendation: before being considered eligible for ablative therapy, a woman should have not only a satisfactory colposcopic examination, but also a negative ECC.

The potential distribution of cervical lesions must be understood when considering collecting an ECC. Isolated areas of SIL within the endocervical canal (e.g.. "skip lesions") are extremely uncommon in women who have not been previously treated for cervical neoplasia. Therefore, a routine ECC in a woman with a satisfactory colposcopy examination is unlikely to detect an unsuspected lesion unless an occult glandular neoplasia is discovered. A routinely collected ECC may also inadvertently sample an ecto-cervical lesion when no neoplasia resides in the endo-cervical canal. Such an error would prompt an unnecessary conization. Since an ECC is usually uncomfortable and increases the cost of histologic evaluation, most colposcopists now feel that there is little reason to routinely perform it in women with satisfactory colposcopic examinations. However, other colposcopists continue to perform a routine ECC since they believe that it serves as a fail-safe measure, especially for colposcopists with limited experience. An ECC may detect glandular lesions that are difficult to recognize colposcopically. A negative ECC may also serve as a potential aid for medico-legal defense, should a cancer be subsequently diagnosed.

Despite the controversy about the routine use of ECC in women with satisfactory colposcopic examinations, there is little controversy that it is an essen-tial part of the colposcopic examination for some women. This group includes those being evaluated for an abnormal Pap smear who have a previous history of treatment for cervical neoplasia, women with glandular abnormalities on Pap smears, and women with significantly abnormal Pap smears and unsatisfactory colposcopic examinations.[9] Novice colposcopists should probably perform an ECC on all non-pregnant patients. Experienced colposcopists may be more selective in their use of ECC.

7.2.3.1.2 Obtaining an ECC Debate exists on whether or not to obtain the ECC prior to or after the cervical biopsy. Traditionally, an ECC was obtained prior to cervical biopsies. This sequence is followed hypothetically to reduce the risk of obtaining a false-positive ECC. Once a cervical biopsy is taken, CIN 2,3 at the edge of the biopsied area may peel away or fragment from the underlying stroma and possibly slide to the external os and mix with endocervical tissue fragments as they are collected from the external os. However, the vast majority of false-positive ECCs more likely result from accidentally nicking an ecto-cervical CIN adjacent to the external os. Another reason some colposcopists obtain the ECC first is that after a cervical biopsy, bleeding is sometimes significant enough to either obscure the colposcopist's view or make it difficult to collect the endocervical curet-tings. Following specimen collection, bleeding that obscures remaining procedures is rarely an important factor, if biopsy sites are cauterized immediately. It should be noted that many colposcopists advocate taking the cervical biopsy before the ECC because they believe the first priority is to sample the most severe lesion, which is usually visible on the ectocervix.

Just as there is controversy about when to perform an ECC, there is also controversy about whether to use an endocervical curette or a Cytobrush® to sample the endocervical canal. A conventional endocervical curette provides tissue for histological evaluation. The sheets or strips of epithelium have been shown to provide greater test specificity than does a Cytobrush® sample.[10,11] In contrast, a vigorous Cytobrush® sampling of the endocervical canal followed by cytologic assessment of the exfoliated calls is more sensitive for detecting CIN than is a conventional ECC (Figures 7.28 a,b). However, Cytobrush® cytologic samples have a high false-positive rate, which many colposcopists consider a weakness since it leads to unnecessary conization for some women. The high false-positive rate results from accidental sampling of ectocervical lesions when the endocervical canal is free of neoplasia.

Prior to performing the ECC, the examiner should inform the woman that the ECC will produce

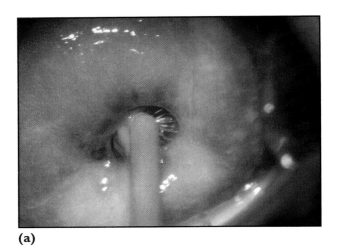

(a)

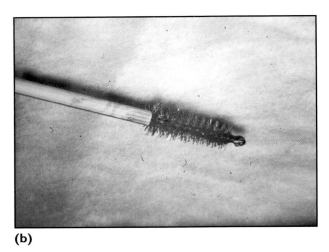

(b)

FIGURES 7.28a,b   A Cytobrush® used **(a)** to take an endocervical histologic specimen **(b)**.

brief uterine cramping pain. Topical anesthetics are ineffective in reducing the pain associated with endocervical curettage,[3,12,13] but use of sharp curettes may reduce the discomfort.[12] We prefer to obtain the ECC while looking through the colposcope at low magnification in order to carefully guide the curette into the endocervical canal. Holding the endocervical curette like a pencil, advance it at least 15 mm up the endocervical canal or just short of the internal os. While pressing the distal cutting tip firmly against the tissue,

move the curette using short "to and fro" strokes, rotating the tip of the curette simultaneously in a circular fashion so that the entire canal is sampled in a "corkscrew" fashion (Figure 7.29). An alternative sampling technique is to draw the curette repeatedly toward the external os along the canal while rotating the curette radially after each withdrawal until the entire canal circumference is sampled (Figure 7.30). Satisfactory sampling has been accomplished when mucus, tissue, and blood appear at the external os

FIGURE 7.29   Screw-type endocervical sampling performed with "to and fro" scraping motions while rotating the curette.

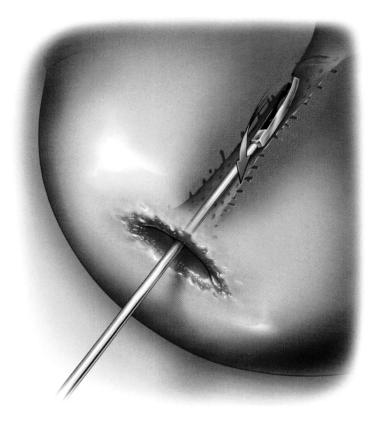

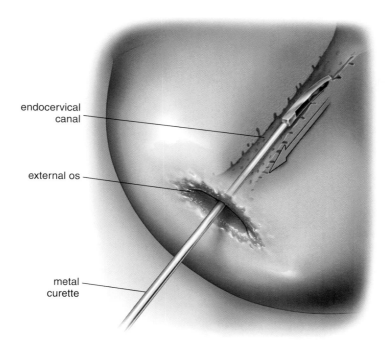

endocervical
canal

external os

metal
curette

FIGURE 7.30   Hoeing-type endocervical sampling by withdrawing the curette along the canal, then replacing the curette near the internal os, rotating slightly, and then withdrawing until all of the canal is sampled.

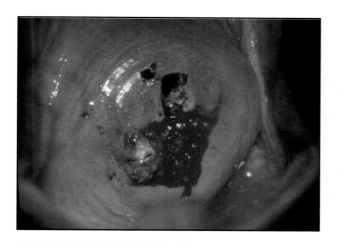

FIGURE 7.31   The endocervical specimen at the cervical os following curettage.

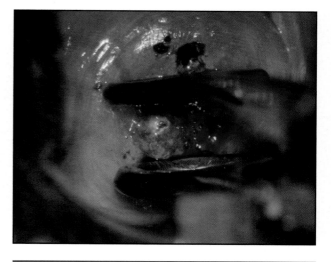

FIGURE 7.32   Retrieving the endocervical specimen using ring forceps.

(Figure 7.31). When removing the curette, it is important to avoid inadvertently sampling ectocervical lesions that extend close to the external os. Whenever possible, withdraw the curette so that the cutting edge faces an area of normal epithelium. Avoid sampling endometrial tissue located above the internal os, approximately 30 mm to 35 mm from the external os.

Prior to removing the open chamber curette, rotate it rapidly to trap cellular elements, mucus and blood within it. If the curette is removed straight from the canal, mucus and cellular material may be pulled out of each side of the curette, leaving the specimen within the canal and the curette chamber empty. Specimen retrieval is usually not a problem when a curette with a retention grid is used. Frequently, much of the endocervical tissue remains entrapped in blood at the external os. Forceps or a Cytobrush® can be used to retrieve this material from the os (Figure 7.32). A Cytobrush® evacuation of remaining tissue fragments from the canal following curette sampling actually increases cellular yield of the sample.[14] A Cytobrush® can also be used to retrieve material from the curette basket. The ECC specimen may be placed on a square of telfa, teabag or brown paper, and dropped into a separately

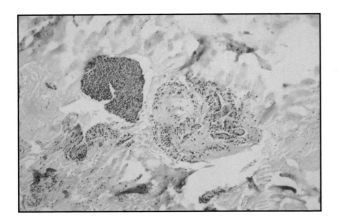

FIGURE 7.33 A positive endocervical curettage specimen demonstrating neoplasia. (Hematoxylin-eosin stain; medium power magnification)

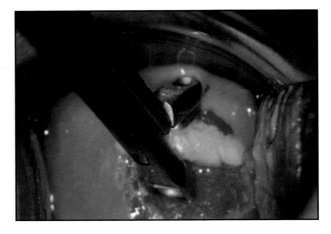

FIGURE 7.34 Obtaining a cervical biopsy from the ectocervix using sharp cervical biopsy forceps. The fixed jaw of the biopsy forceps is usually positioned closer to the cervical os.

labeled ("ECC") specimen container of fixative. Depending upon the pathologist's preference, the ECC specimen may also be placed directly into formalin and the sample centrifuged into a pellet or strained through filter paper in the laboratory.

As mentioned earlier, some clinicians prefer to use a Cytobrush® instead of a curette. When using this method, introduce the Cytobrush® into the canal and rotate vigorously. When withdrawn, cut off the end of the Cytobrush® and place it into a container of formalin for histologic interpretation (Figure 7.33). The cellular material and mucus can also be stripped from the bristles into formalin using an Ayre's spatula or filter paper. Alternatively, roll the Cytobrush® specimen across a glass slide and fix with a 95% ethanol solution, or place it in a liquid cytology medium, and then submit the specimen for histologic interpretation. If a cytology specimen is submitted, it is important to note on the requisition form that material represents a diagnostic, and not a screening specimen.

7.2.3.2 Cervical biopsy

In a majority of cases, cervical biopsy begins with the selection of the most abnormal-appearing areas for sampling regardless of cervical location. The exception is when multiple biopsies will be taken and hemostasis is not secured immediately following each biopsy. Under these circumstances, it may be preferable to obtain biopsies from the posterior cervical lip first to keep blood from an anterior lip biopsy from obscuring biopsy sites on the posterior lip. Since the most prominent areas of colposcopic change do not necessarily coincide with the areas of greatest histological abnormality, colposcopists are always at risk of not selecting the most abnormal sites for biopsy. Large peripheral acetowhite areas are readily recognized, but focal, more severe coexisting disease is often over-

looked. Therefore, representative biopsies should be taken from all areas with significant colposcopic findings. Usually, the area closest to the SCJ is biopsied since this is the region of maximum disease severity. The number of biopsies taken from an individual patient depends on the size, severity and number of lesions present, but generally, one to three biopsies are needed. Cervical biopsies are best obtained while looking through the colposcope at low-power magnification. After selecting the biopsy site, orient the opened biopsy forceps so that the fixed jaw end of the biopsy forceps is positioned closer to or within the os (Figure 7.34). The biopsy forceps should be positioned directly over the lesion to be biopsied. It is unnecessary to obtain normal adjoining epithelium with biopsy of a neoplasia. However, if an ulceration is being biopsied, it is important to include abnormal epithelium adjacent to the ulcer with the specimen. Necrotic, nondiagnostic material may occupy the center of an ulceration, hence, the necessity for supplying surrounding abnormal histology for review. When biopsying a lesion on the posterior lip, hold the biopsy instrument handles upside down. Lifting the biopsy handles upward prior to biopsying an anterior lip lesion places the lesion in the center of the jaws, reducing the risk of slippage. Pushing the cervix backward with the opened biopsy forceps until the cardinal ligaments prevent further cephalad uterine motion also helps keep the forceps from slipping off the biopsy site. A sharp biopsy forceps minimizes slippage. A specimen is obtained by quickly squeezing the forceps handles together, then locking the jaws (if so equipped) prior to passing the forceps to an assistant. In most instances, biopsies need to be only 2 mm deep. Deeper biopsies are only needed when invasion is suspected.

After taking a biopsy, it is best to confirm colposcopically that the intended area was adequately sampled. If an adequate or representative sample was not obtained, another biopsy should be attempted immediately. Hemostasis can then be accomplished by pressing a cotton swab against the biopsy site or applying silver nitrate or Monsel's paste (ferric subsulfate) (Figures 7.35 a,b). Monsel's paste or silver nitrate must directly contact the actual biopsy site in order to be effective. If applied to a bloody surface, these agents only coagulate extravasated blood and do not produce hemostasis. The entire base and sides of the biopsy site must be cauterized, including the epithelial wound edges, which tend to bleed a moderate amount. Monsel's paste or silver nitrate sticks must be applied precisely and only to the biopsy site(s). Imprecise application of silver nitrate can obscure other adjoining acetowhite areas that also require biopsy. Furthermore, improper use of these hemostatic agents can ruin the histology of subsequent biopsy specimens and ECC if collected within the next 3 weeks. Sutures are rarely required following biopsy, but in the event they are, the necessary supplies and instruments should be readily available. This same biopsy process is then repeated for other abnormal lesions, if present. Alternately, some colposcopists secure all cervical biopsies prior to applying hemostatic agents. However, in performing a biopsy on the cervix of a pregnant patient or one with invasive cancer, excessive bleeding can be prevented by placing a cotton-tipped applicator soaked in Monsel's paste against the site immediately following removal of the biopsy forceps. When hemostatic agents are not sufficient to stop bleeding, or when hemostatic agents are not available, a single strand of gauze packing may be inserted against the cervix after the procedure and removed by the patient several hours later. After all biopsies are obtained, blood, 5% acetic acid, and excess hemostatic agents should be removed from the distal vagina with care taken to not interfere with hemostasis at the biopsy sites.

The biopsy specimen should be oriented on paper and placed into a bottle containing fixative. Specimens mounted on paper prior to fixation are more likely to be optimally oriented, have a preserved SCJ, and have intact surface epithelium than are specimens placed directly into fixative.[15] Some pathologists, however, accept biopsy samples submitted directly in fixative. Ideally, clinicians who are learning colposcopy should place each cervical biopsy in a separate container, or in a single container in which each biopsy is secured and labeled separately. This procedure allows the colposcopist to compare each specific histologic result with their colposcopic impression at each biopsy site. Cervical biopsies should always be separated from the ECC specimen.

7.2.4 Complications during colposcopy

The most common minor complication of colposcopy is excessive bleeding following cervical biopsy. Brief, mild-to-moderate bleeding should always be anticipated following collection of a histologic specimen. Significant bleeding is likely when a biopsy is taken from pregnant patients and those with acute cervicitis or cervical cancer. Since pressure and rapid application of silver nitrate or Monsel's paste work effectively, hemostasis rarely requires sutures. Thin epithelium in women with atrophic changes due to estrogen deficiency is easily traumatized, resulting in ecchymosis, superficial lacerations, avulsions and pain. These complications and discomfort can be prevented easily by prescribing a short course of topical estrogen for several weeks prior to the colposcopic examination. Premedication with a

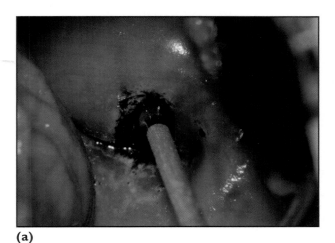

(a)

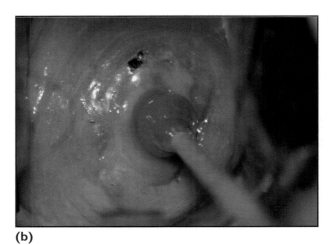

(b)

FIGURES 7.35a,b Hemostasis is achieved following cervical biopsy using silver nitrate sticks **(a)** or Monsel's paste **(b)**.

short-acting NSAID can minimize temporary uterine cramping discomfort invoked by cervical biopsy and ECC. Proven, specific medications for each woman's dysmenorrhea may work best for pain prophylaxis. Inadvertent burns or cauterization of surrounding normal epithelium (cervix, vaginal or vulva) may occur when hemostatic agents are applied imprecisely. Excessive generalized use of hemostatics is not necessary and may adversely affect pathologic interpretation of multiple submitted specimens. Common management errors result from inability or failure to visualize the entire SCJ or proximal extent of a lesion, failure to sample the endocervical canal or failure to formulate a colposcopic impression. Chapter 20 includes a discussion of common management errors.

7.3 Examining the Vagina and the Vulva

7.3.1 Vaginal examination

Because of the potential multicentric effects of HPV infection, the colposcopic examination should include the entire lower genital tract. All patients should have a brief colposcopic vaginal inspection. A more comprehensive vaginal examination is necessary when a woman presents with an abnormal Pap smear and no cervical lesion is found to explain the cytologic findings. A careful colposcopic examination of the vagina is also indicated for women with an abnormal Pap smear and a previous hysterectomy or a history of DES exposure. Prior to cervical conization or hysterectomy, it may be prudent to conduct a comprehensive vaginal examination to detect coexisting or even primary occult vaginal neoplasia.

With proper visualization, a comprehensive colposcopic examination of the vagina is fairly simple (see also Chapter 14). The colposcopic examination should also include inspection of the entire vagina, including the fornices and cul-de-sac, following application of 5% acetic acid. The vagina should be re-examined after applying half-strength Lugol's iodine solution (Figure 7.36). The lateral walls of the vagina may be difficult to visualize because of rugae and the parallel orientation to the light source. Opening the speculum widely tends to flatten rugae in young women. Small, moistened cotton-tipped applicators may also be used to manipulate these vaginal folds (Figure 7.37). Gentle lateral displacement of the speculum handle to the same side and slight repositioning of the colposcope to the opposite side will make it easier to view the sidewall. The examination should also include the anterior and posterior vaginal walls obscured by the blades of the speculum. This can be done by inspecting them as

the speculum is withdrawn slowly in the anterior/posterior plane. Alternatively, the vaginal speculum blades may be rotated to a lateral alignment to observe the anterior and posterior walls. In order to prevent unnecessary discomfort (urethral trauma and superficial lacerations), the speculum blades should be relaxed prior to rotation.

Vaginal biopsies should be obtained from all significant acetowhite or iodine negative colposcopic lesions, including vaginal ulcerations or grossly exophytic lesions. A vaginal biopsy is obtained in a manner similar to that of a cervical biopsy, except that a shallower specimen is collected and local anesthesia (i.e., subcutaneous lidocaine) is required if the lesion is located in the distal one-third of the vagina adjacent to the introitus. If the biopsy forceps are unable to grasp the stretched vaginal mucosa, relax the vaginal speculum blades to reduce sidewall tautness and facilitate

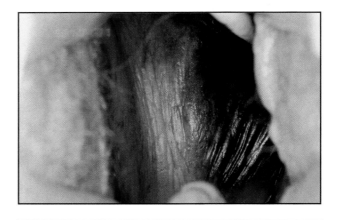

FIGURE 7.36   Vaginal lesion noted following Lugol's iodine solution application. The lesion is yellow and the surrounding brown epithelium is normal.

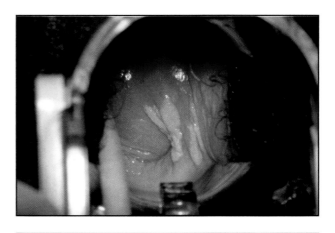

FIGURE 7.37   A moistened, large cotton swab is used to help examine an acetowhite lesion of the left lateral vaginal fornix.

biopsy. Skin hooks are usually not needed, but they can facilitate eversion of the lateral corners of the vaginal cuff in women who have undergone a hysterectomy. The biopsy forceps are aligned as closely as possible to perpendicular to the mucosa with the movable jaw more distally positioned. This orientation permits the colposcopist to observe where the biopsy will actually be taken. Vaginal biopsy rarely causes significant bleeding. Monsel's paste or silver nitrate may be used as necessary for hemostasis. Vaginal biopsies are submitted separately in a fashion similar to that for cervical histologic interpretation and labeled appropriately (e.g., proximal right lateral vagina).

7.3.2 Vulvar, perineal, perianal and bimanual examinations

A careful inspection of the vulva and perianal areas should be performed after the speculum is removed. The vulva, perineum and perianal areas may be examined using the naked eye, a hand-held low-power magnification device, or the colposcope (at 2× to 4×). Although colposcopy with acetic acid application is not required in all women, in some instances, use of this solution facilitates the identification of small lesions. If acetic acid is used, it should be applied to the external genitalia using cotton balls, 4" × 4" gauze pads, or a spray mist for 3 to 5 minutes. Because the epithelium external to Hart's line or the vulva is keratinized, it takes longer for acetowhitening to occur. Lesions around or beneath the clitoral hood, within the distal urethra, in the minor vestibular glands, beneath hymeneal remnants, and in the perianal region are frequently overlooked (Figures 7.38a,b,c,d). Colposcopically significant acetowhite, non-acetowhite, red, or pigmented lesions, as described in Chapter 15, are biopsied using a cervical biopsy forceps, a knife for superficial "shave" excision, or a Keyes punch following administration of an anesthetic. Specimens are then submitted for

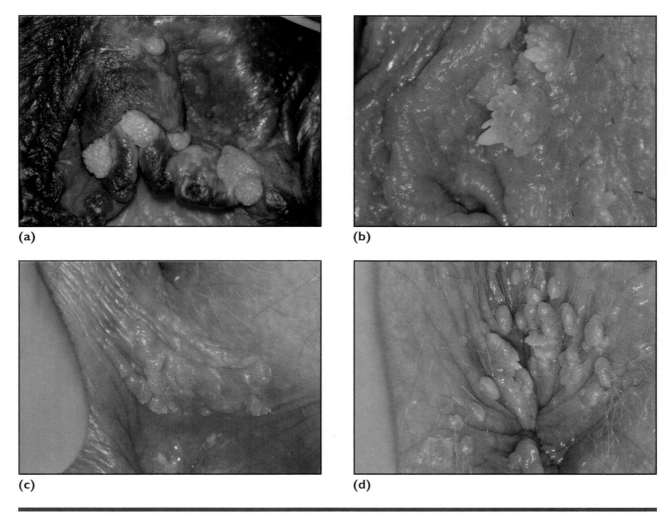

(a)

(b)

(c)

(d)

FIGURES 7.38a–d Examination of the vulva and perirectal areas revealing condylomas of the clitoral hood **(a)**, vulva **(b)**, posterior forchette **(c)**, and the perianal regions **(d)** induced by human papillomavirus.

pathologic interpretation in separately labeled bottles. Other indications for biopsy of vulvar lesions are listed in Chapter 15.

Because a majority of women will have had a recent pelvic examination performed when the Pap smear was obtained, the bimanual examination may not be necessary at the time of colposcopy, although some colposcopists perform a pelvic examination after each colposcopic examination. This is particularly true when the patient has been referred and not previously seen by that colposcopist. Occasionally, a patient will present with negative colposcopic findings but have a palpable cancer of the endocervix, vagina, or lower bowel. Colposcopic evidence of invasive cancer of either the cervix or vagina should mandate a careful bimanual examination. When a bimanual examination follows a cervical biopsy, the examination should be gentle enough not to precipitate bleeding.

7.4 Examining the Anorectal Region

Colposcopy is also used to examine the anorectal region or anorectal transformation zone for the presence of anal intraepithelial neoplasia (AIN) and squamous cell cancer (Figures 7.39a,b).[16] The proce-

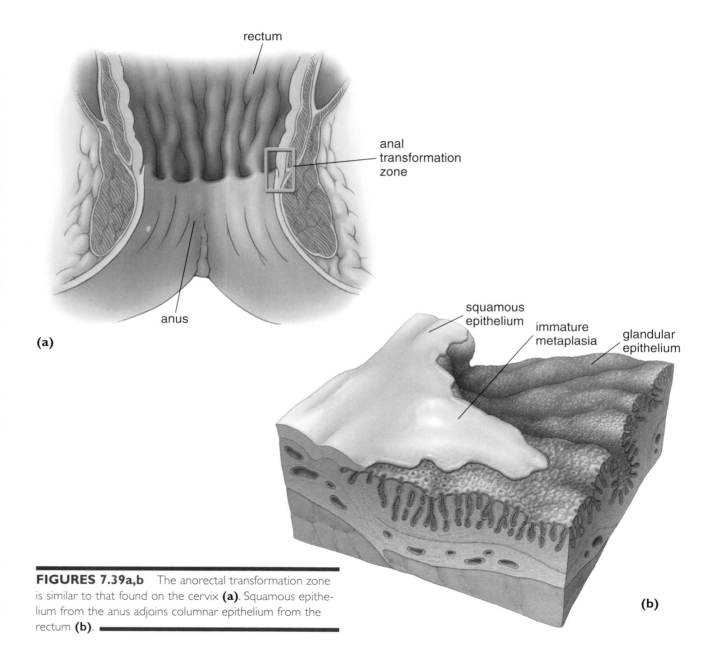

FIGURES 7.39a,b The anorectal transformation zone is similar to that found on the cervix **(a)**. Squamous epithelium from the anus adjoins columnar epithelium from the rectum **(b)**.

dure has been advocated particularly for HIV-positive patients, who have a higher prevalence of anorectal oncogenic HPV, AIN and cancer than do HIV-negative patients.[17] As with cervical neoplasia surveillance, an abnormal cytologic result prompts evaluation using colposcopy.

Patients considered at risk can be screened for anorectal neoplasia using an anorectal cytologic specimen. To collect a cytologic specimen, a moistened dacron swab is inserted deeply within the anal canal to sample the anal transformation zone, a squamous (anal)/columnar (rectal) cellular interface, analogous to the cervical transformation zone. The specimen is submitted, processed and examined like a Pap smear of the cervix. Patients with abnormal cellular changes consistent with a SIL or cancer are then examined by colposcopy.

7.4.1 Colposcopy of the anorectal region

Colposcopy of the anal transformation zone is quite similar to colposcopy of the lower genital tract, except for minor procedural differences. A 3% acetic acid-soaked gauze-wrapped dacron swab is inserted through an anoscope to the anal canal and the anoscope is withdrawn. After several minutes, the swab is removed and the anoscope is reinserted to begin the colposcopic examination. The anal transformation zone is first inspected. Anal low-and high-grade lesions resemble comparable lesions of the cervix except that fine mosaic and punctation are found uncommonly (Figures 7.40 a,b,c).[18] Lesions are typically flat, acetowhite and have coarsely dilated vessels. Papillary and exophytic condylomas may also be encountered. Shallow biopsies are collected and submitted in the usual fashion for histologic interpretation.

7.5 Documentation

7.5.1 Documenting colposcopic findings

The findings of the colposcopic examination should be fully documented. A standardized reporting form is an essential part of that documentation (Figures 7.41a,b). The form should include pertinent history, clinical findings, colposcopic impression, and management plans. A diagrammatic representation of the colposcopic findings that can be understood by other clinicians is an essential part of documentation. A large circle typically represents the cervix with

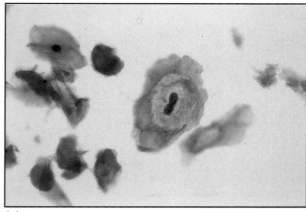

(a)

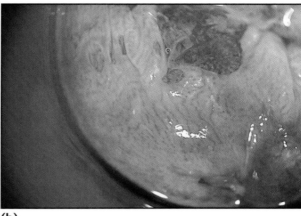

(b)

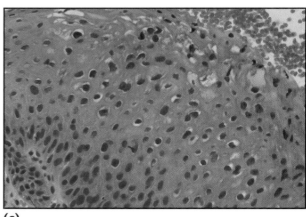

(c)

FIGURES 7.40a–c   Anal Pap smear that demonstrates LSIL **(a)** (Papanicolaou stain, high power magnification). The anal colposcopic exam reveals an acetowhite lesion along the SCJ. Diffuse punctation is observed **(b)**. Histology **(c)** from a biopsy of this lesion that demonstrates AIN 1 (Hematoxylin-eosin stain; medium power magnification). Photos courtesy of Drs. Teresa Darragh and Joel Palefsky.

the external os indicated in the center as a smaller circle. A stamp or preprinted form facilitates documentation. The current SCJ should be indicated as a solid line. The clinician should draw the colposcopic lesions to scale and describe key features such as color, margin, contour and vascular pattern. Symbols can be used to indicate specific features and biopsy sites (Figures 7.41b). The written documentation should also clearly state whether the colposcopic examination was satisfactory.

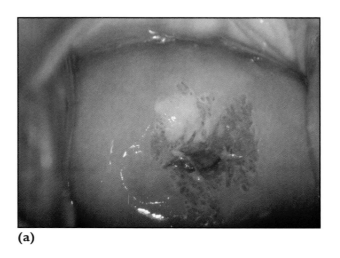

(a)

(b)

FIGURES 7.41a,b   An example of proper documentation of colposcopic examination findings **(a)**. The cervical findings are documented in **(b)**.

Photodocumentation (Polaroid, video print, 35 mm, videotape, and digital image) assists patient education, management, clinician education and follow-up monitoring. Colposcopic documentation may also be accomplished using a computer-based data/image management system (See Chapter 6, Figure 6.45a). A patient/laboratory/management-tracking log should be maintained to ensure appropriate care and follow-up. Computerized colposcopy tracking software programs facilitate appropriate recall, communication, and education. Photographic documentation of colposcopic findings may also provide valuable medicolegal documentation, if necessary.

7.5.2 Correlation of cytology, histology and colposcopy findings

Colposcopy, along with cervical cytology and histology, are collectively useful in diagnosing and determining the appropriate management of cervical neoplasia. The results of all three should agree within one degree of severity (Figures 7.42a,b,c). The first step in resolving discrepancies is a review of the cytology and histology by one pathologist, preferably an individual with an interest in lower genital tract abnormalities (Figures 7.43a,b,c). If the original diagnoses are deemed correct, reexamination of the patient with additional histological sampling may be necessary. In difficult cases, it may be prudent to refer the patient to an expert colposcopist. On reexamination of the patient, the endocervical canal and proximal vagina require particular attention. If the second examination does not resolve the discrepancy, other procedures, such as cervical conization, may be indicated when the unexplained cytologic finding is of significant concern.

7.6 Post-Procedure Instructions

After undergoing colposcopy and cervical biopsy (Figures 7.44a,b,c,d,e,f,g) women should receive specific patient instructions. Patients occasionally need to take NSAIDs for transient cramping or discomfort. Vaginal bleeding heavier than a normal menstrual period is rare following cervical biopsy and should be evaluated and treated. Reapplication of Monsel's paste or silver nitrate will usually restore hemostasis. Patients should be told to expect a slight serous, mildly blood-tinged, vaginal discharge with a brown or black (Monsel's paste, silver nitrate) color for sev-

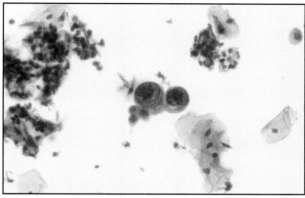

(a)

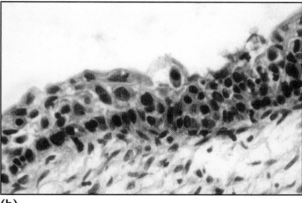

(b)

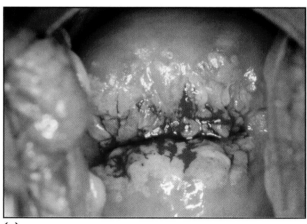

(c)

FIGURES 7.42a–c   Agreement of the cytology (HSIL) **(a)** (Papanicolaou stain, high power magnification), histology (CIN 3) (Hematoxylin-eosin stain; high power magnification) **(b)** and colposcopic impression (high-grade lesion/CIN 3) **(c)** permits conservative therapy. ▬▬▬

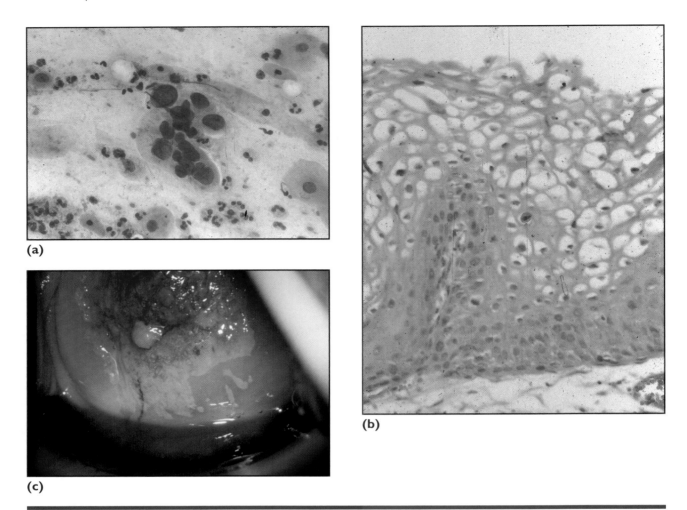

FIGURES 7.43a–c   Lack of agreement of the cytology (cancer) **(a)** (Papanicolaou stain, high power magnification), histology (Hematoxylin-eosin stain; medium power magnification) (CIN 1) **(b)** and colposcopic impression (low-grade lesion/CIN 1) **(c)** mandate review of the laboratory results, endocervical curettage, inspection of the proximal vagina, and further evaluation by conization, if otherwise unexplained.

eral days following cervical biopsy. It is generally best for women to refrain from sexual activity for a day or two after a biopsy to prevent bleeding from the biopsy site. Explain that the histology report may not return for several days, or weeks, and that you will notify the patient of the results as soon as they are available. Finally, tell your patient what you have found or expect to find based on the colposcopic examination. When appropriate, reassure the patient that she does not have evidence of a cervical cancer. This helps to relieve her anxiety while awaiting the pathology results.

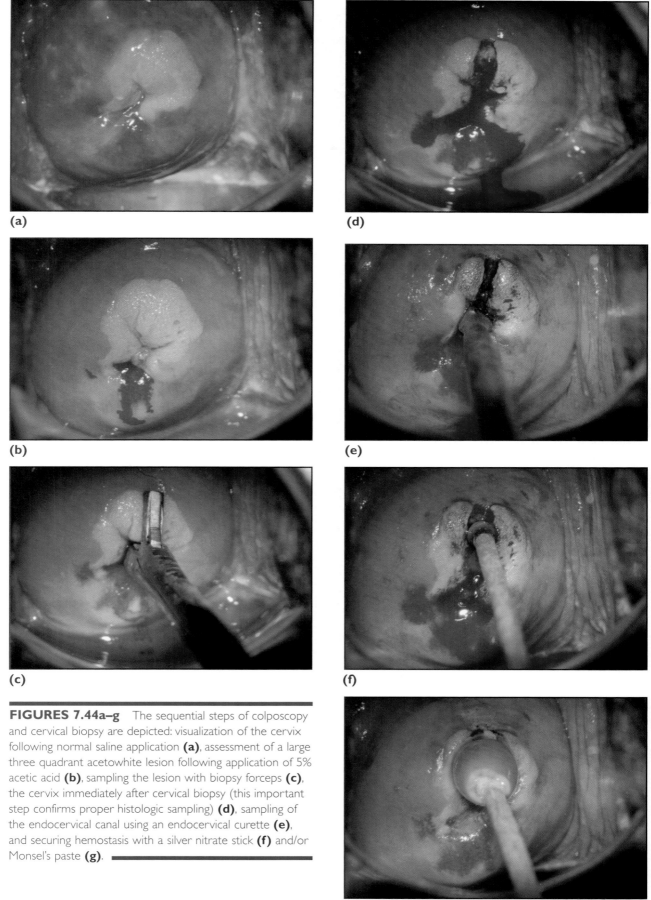

FIGURES 7.44a–g The sequential steps of colposcopy and cervical biopsy are depicted: visualization of the cervix following normal saline application **(a)**, assessment of a large three quadrant acetowhite lesion following application of 5% acetic acid **(b)**, sampling the lesion with biopsy forceps **(c)**, the cervix immediately after cervical biopsy (this important step confirms proper histologic sampling) **(d)**, sampling of the endocervical canal using an endocervical curette **(e)**, and securing hemostasis with a silver nitrate stick **(f)** and/or Monsel's paste **(g)**.

References

1. Wright T C, Cox J T, Massad L S, Twiggs L B, Wilkinson E J. 2001 Consensus guidelines for the management of women with cervical cytologic abnormalities. *JAMA* 2002;287:2120–9.

2. Wright T C, Cox J T, Massad L S, Carlson J, Twiggs L B, Wilkinson E J. 2001 Consensus guidelines for the management of women with cervical intraepithelial neoplasia. *J Lower Genital Tract Disease* 2003;7:154–67.

3. Church L, Oliver L, Dobie S, Madigan D, Ellsworth A. Analgesia for colposcopy: double-masked, randomized comparison of ibuprofen and benzocaine gel. *Obstet Gynecol* 2001; 97:5–10.

4. Ferris D G, Greenberg N M. Reid's Colposcopic Index. *J Fam Pract* 1994;39:65–70.

5. Reid R, Scalzi P. Genital warts and cervical cancer. VII. An improved colposcopic index for differentiating benign papillomaviral infections from high-grade cervical intraepithelial neoplasia. *Am J Obstet Gynecol* 1985; 153:611–8.

6. Toplis P J, Casemore V, Hallam N, Charnock M. Evaluation of colposcopy in the postmenopausal woman. *Br J Obstet Gynaecol* 1986;93:843–51.

7. Johnson N, Crompton A C, Wyatt J, Buchan P C, Jarvis G J. Using Lamicel to expose high grade cervical lesions during colposcopic examinations. *Br J Obstet Gynaecol* 1990;97:46–52.

8. Townsend D E, Richart R M, Marks E, Nielsen J. Invasive cancer following outpatient evaluation and therapy for cervical cancer. *Obstet Gynecol* 1981; 57:145–9.

9. Cox J T. ASCCP Practice Guidelines: Endocervical curettage. *J Lower Genital Tract Disease* 1997;1:251–6.

10. Anderson W, Frierson H, Barber S, Tabbarah S, Taylor P, Underwood P. Sensitivity and specificity of endocervical curettage and the endocervical brush for the evaluation of the endocervical canal. *Am J Obstet Gynecol* 1988; 159:702–7.

11. Hoffman M S, Sterghos S Jr, Gordy L W, Gunasekaran S, Cavanagh D. Evaluation of the cervical canal with endocervical brush. *Obstet Gynecol* 1993; 82:573–7.

12. Ferris D G, Harper D M, Callahan B, et al. The efficacy of topical benzocaine gel in providing anesthesia prior to cervical biopsy and endocervical curettage. *J Lower Genital Tract Disease* 1997;1:221–7.

13. Clifton P A, Shaughnessy A F, Andrew S. Ineffectiveness of topical benzocaine spray during colposcopy. *J Fam Pract* 1998; 46:242–6.

14. Tate K M, Strickland J L. A randomized controlled trial to evaluate the use of the endocervical brush after endocervical curettage. *Obstet Gynecol* 1997; 90:715–7.

15. Heatley M K. A comparison of three methods of orienting cervical punch biopsies. *J Clin Pathol* 1999;52:149–50.

16. Sonnex C, Scholefield J H, Kocjan G, Kelly G, Whatrup C, Mindel A, et al. Anal human papillomavirus infection: A comparative study of cytology, colposcopy and DNA hybridization as a method of detection. *Genitourin Med* 1991;67:21–5.

17. Sobhani I, Vuagnat A, Walker F, Vissuzaine C, Mirin B, Hervatin F, et al. Prevalence of high-grade dysplasia and cancer in the canal in human papillomavirus-infected individuals. *Gastroenterology* 2001;120:857–66.

18. Jay N, Berry M, Hogeboorn C J, Holly E A, Darragh T M, Palefsky J M. Colposcopic appearance of anal squamous intraepithelial lesions. *Dis Colon Rectum* 1997;40:919–28.

Normal and Abnormal Colposcopic Features

Table of Contents

8.1 Introduction

Once the cervix can be visualized clearly through the colposcope, the colposcopist's attention is directed at identifying the squamocolumnar junction (SCJ) and the surrounding transformation zone (Figure 8.1). When the examination follows the discovery of abnormal cytologic findings, the colposcopic mission becomes one of detecting the source of the abnormal screening test. Assuming a cervical etiology, the deviant cells most likely evolved from an alteration within the epithelium of the transformation zone. Thus, recognition of abnormalities within the transformation zone is the most critical objective of colposcopy. The real value of colposcopy lies in the ability of the experienced colposcopist to recognize a variety of quite different morphologic appearances, all of which are consistent with specific histologic diagnoses. Within the cervical epithelium, neoplasia can produce visibly striking changes, which can be assessed colposcopically according to severity, size, and location, thereby providing the basis for planning a therapeutic approach.

In addition to cytologic and histologic findings, proper patient management depends upon the colposcopic impression, which evolves directly from critical assessment of unique characteristics of the epithelium and vasculature. The discrimination of normal from abnormal colposcopic findings is not always simple. Although some solitary colposcopic signs can be interpreted as normal or abnormal, the combination of multiple signs or appearances may be confusing. Only ample training and sufficient experience permit colposcopists to discern subtle differences, such as those noted between normal variants and low-grade lesions, and between low-grade lesions and high-grade lesions. This chapter describes the colposcopic features that allow for discrimination of normal from abnormal and various levels of abnormality.

8.2 The Normal Transformation Zone

A detailed description of the development and histology of the normal transformation zone is given in Chapter 2. In order for the colposcopist to better discriminate normal from abnormal colposcopic findings, a brief review is given here. A detailed description of epithelial and vascular colposcopic findings of the normal transformation zone is presented later in the chapter.

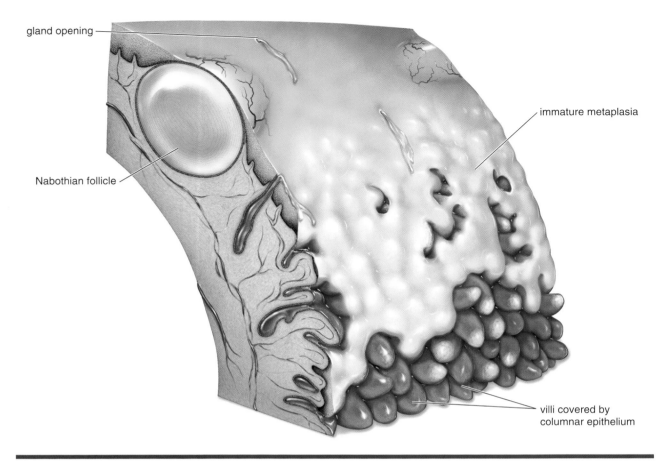

gland opening

Nabothian follicle

immature metaplasia

villi covered by columnar epithelium

FIGURE 8.1 The normal transformation zone includes immature and mature metaplastic epithelium, Nabothian follicles and gland openings.

The cervix is covered by three different types of epithelium: squamous, columnar, and immature and mature metaplasia (Figure 8.2). Squamous and columnar epithelium form the two boundaries of the transformation zone. Nonkeratinized stratified squamous epithelium extends from Hart's line, or the embryologic junction between the vagina and vulva (Figure 8.3), to the SCJ on the cervix at the woman's birth. Squamous epithelium contains four types of cells: basal, parabasal, intermediate, and superficial (Figures 8.4a,b). Basal cells differentiate and mature through the other three cellular stages as they ascend from the basement membrane to the surface. Columnar epithelium is a single cell layer of tall mucus-secreting cells (Figure 8.4). Cervical columnar epithelium courses proximally from the SCJ and within the endocervical canal to the internal os. Columnar epithelium covers villi, small polypoid

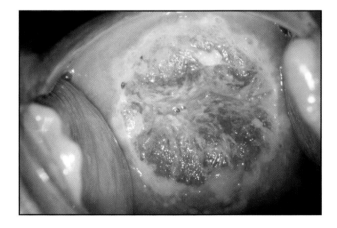

FIGURE 8.2 The normal cervix and transformation zone with pink squamous epithelium, white immature metaplasia, and red columnar epithelium.

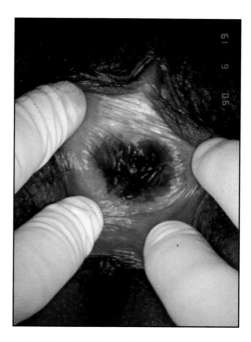

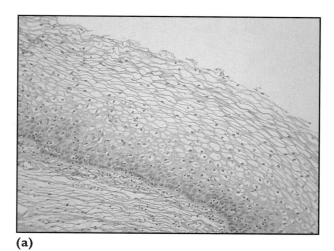

(a)

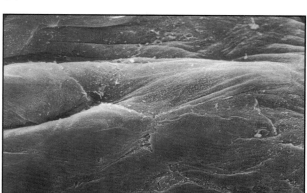

(b)

FIGURE 8.3 Hart's line or the junction between glycogenated vaginal epithelium and keratinized vulvar squamous epithelium. This interface represents the most distal portion of the vagina.

FIGURES 8.4a,b **(a)** Squamous epithelium contains basal, parabasal, intermediate and superficial cells that differentiate from the basement membrane in that order (Hematoxylin-eosin stain; medium power magnification). **(b)** A surface scanning electron micrograph of squamous epithelium. Notice the overlapping of cells creating an impenetrable surface.

projections that contain central loop capillaries (Figures 8.5a–e). Metaplastic epithelium lies between the squamous and columnar epithelium. Metaplastic epithelium is formed when metaplastic cells replace columnar cells. These cells eventually differentiate to become squamous epithelium. Metaplasia is a normal process that occurs naturally in all women.

The position of the squamocolumnar junction on the ectocervix at birth is known as the original SCJ. The squamocolumnar junction noted in young adults at the time of colposcopy is called the new SCJ or simply "SCJ" (Figures 8.6a–d). At this phase in life, it is variably positioned on the ectocervix, closer to the external os or slightly within the endocervical canal. Later in life, the SCJ may not be easily identified colposcopically since the cellular interface may be hidden deeply within the endocervical canal (Figure 8.7). Between the original SCJ and the advancing new SCJ lies an area of continuously changing epithelium. This area has been termed the transformation zone in recognition of the apparent transformation of columnar cells to squamous cells. The dynamic nature of this process results in a mix of immature and then mature metaplastic epithelium. These metaplastic cells comprise the transformation zone.

Although some transformation begins during fetal life as a consequence of exposure to maternal estrogen, the estrogen surge that begins at puberty and ends at menopause is responsible for the changes noted during a woman's reproductive life. This estrogen surge at puberty initiates glycogen storage in epithelial cells and subsequent colonization of *Lactobacillus acidophilus* within the vagina. In addition to producing H_2O_2 to limit opportunistic pathogens, the *Lactobacilli* produce lactic acid that reduces the vaginal pH to less than 4.5. This highly acidic environment may minimally damage

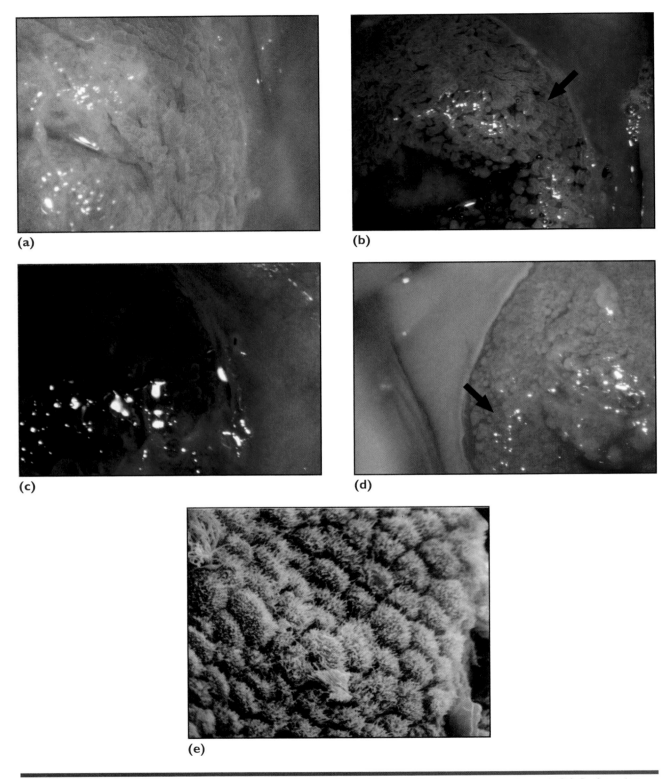

(a)

(b)

(c)

(d)

(e)

FIGURES 8.5a–d Villi covered with columnar epithelium. Central loop capillaries can be seen (arrow). **(e)** Surface electron micrograph of columnar epithelium. Notice the microvilli projecting from the cell's surfaces.

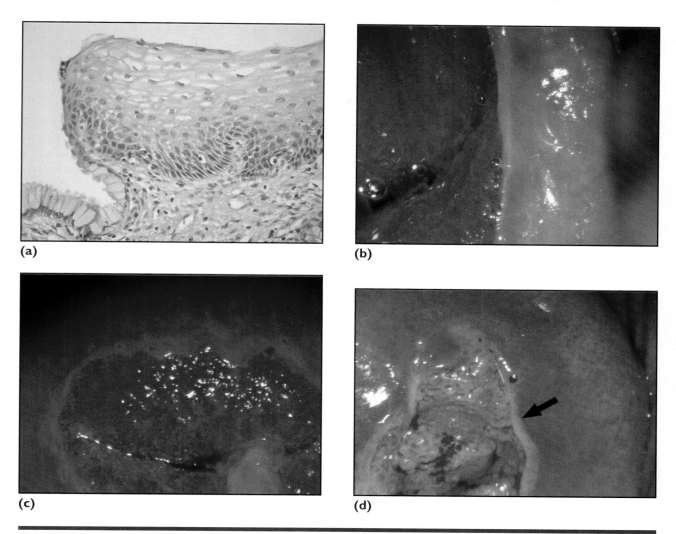

FIGURES 8.6a–d **(a)** Histologic section of the squamocolumnar junction (Hematoxylin-eosin stain; high power magnification). **(b–d)** The squamocolumnar junction (SCJ) separates pink squamous epithelium from red columnar epithelium. The SCJ (arrow) appears as a thin white line after 5% acetic acid application to the cervix.

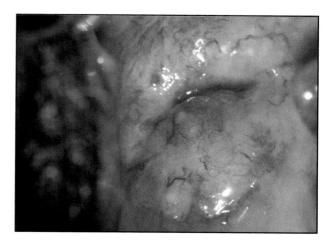

FIGURE 8.7   The squamocolumnar junction is located within the endocervical canal and cannot be seen in this postmenopausal patient. However, remnants of the transformation process and Nabothian follicles are apparent. The epithelium is thin and, therefore, prominent blood vessels can be easily seen. This epithelium is mature metaplasia.

superficial squamous cells, which are continuously replaced within the multilayered squamous epithelium. Mucus secretion by columnar epithelium serves both reproductive and vaginal hygienic purposes. However, the mucus is an inefficient protective shield from the acidic environment. Because the columnar epithelium is thin and fragile, it is easily traumatized by the acid. In contrast to squamous epithelium, columnar epithelium is without multiple underlying replacement cell layers. Consequently, the cellular injury from lactic acid may help stimulate a defensive transformation of the susceptible single-cell layer columnar epithelium to a more resilient multicell-layer metaplastic epithelium. However, it is not known whether the acidic environment actually causes metaplasia.

Transformation may occur by means of one of two mechanisms. With the first, the traumatized acid-burned columnar epithelium is replaced by small, round, nuclear, dense reserve cells positioned beneath the columnar epithelium. These cells eventually proliferate and differentiate to form a thin replacement layer of immature metaplastic epithelium, then a multicell-layer of mature metaplastic epithelium. Initially, this metaplastic cellular change appears on the exposed tips of columnar villi (Figures 8.8a–e). Next, the immature metaplastic epithelium fuses or bridges with immature metaplastic epithelium on adjoining villi. Finally, opalescent sheets of immature metaplasia are formed that extend as tongue-like projections toward the os. The second method of transformation (squamous epithelialization) involves an advancing immature metaplastic epithelium that undermines columnar epithelium. As the columnar epithelium is lifted from the underlying stroma, it is replaced by a thin metaplastic layer. The epithelial transformation process is episodic but progressive, starting in the periphery of the transformation zone and advancing concentrically toward the os and extending up the endocervical canal in later life. Noncontiguous islands of immature metaplasia may be seen proximal to the advancing SCJ. These eventually coalesce with broad sheets of immature metaplasia along the SCJ (Figures 8.9a–e). Maximal transformation zone activity is seen in late fetal life, at the onset of the estrogen surge, during the first pregnancy, and in women taking oral contraceptive drugs. Cellular alterations arise in this immature metaplasia, resulting in cervical squamous neoplasia. Consequently, colposcopists direct their examinations at this susceptible tissue.

Mature metaplasia lies between immature metaplasia and the original SCJ. Mature metaplastic epithelium is a multicell layer of fully differentiated squamous epithelium. This epithelium differs from immature metaplasia in that the latter contains only a few layers of mainly undifferentiated cells. However, mature metaplasia has two unique features (gland openings and Nabothian cysts) that are not found in original squamous epithelium but are often apparent by histologic and sometimes colposcopic examination. If advancing metaplastic epithelium surrounds the cleft on the surface but does not completely replace all the columnar epithelium and fill the space between columnar villi, a gland opening results (Figures 8.10a,b). Mucus produced by the deeply confined, remaining columnar cells protrudes to the surface through this opening. Should the cleft become occluded by metaplastic epithelium at the surface, the mucus produced by the retained columnar cells becomes trapped beneath, resulting in a Nabothian cyst or follicle (Figures 8.11a–f). The normal transformation zone is recognized colposcopically and histologically by the presence of mature and immature metaplastic epithelium, along with Nabothian follicles and gland openings, which are remnants of the transformation process.

8.2.1 Neoplastic alteration of the normal transformation zone

The normal transformation zone, a dynamic region of epithelium, consists of both mature and immature metaplastic epithelium. Immature metaplasia is more susceptible to cellular insult that may divert it from the normal maturation process. Infection of these immature cells by human papillomavirus (HPV) is the cellular insult that appears to be uniquely necessary in the process of neoplastic transformation. A complex series of cellular events (Chapter 5) may ensue, leading to various degrees of cellular abnormality. As lesions evolve, epithelial and vascular morphologic characteristics of the normal transformation zone assume a wide range of abnormal colposcopic features.[1-5] However, progressive cellular and vascular evolution is neither universal nor unidirectional, as certain low-grade neoplasias may persist unaltered or, more commonly, may regress to normal tissue. A complicated interaction involving immature metaplastic epithelium and local immunity, oncogenic HPV, and various cofactors determine whether the outcome will be normal or variably abnormal. Neoplastic growth requires all three components. The process for deviation to an abnormality occurs in very immature, unstable metaplastic epithelium of the normal transformation zone.

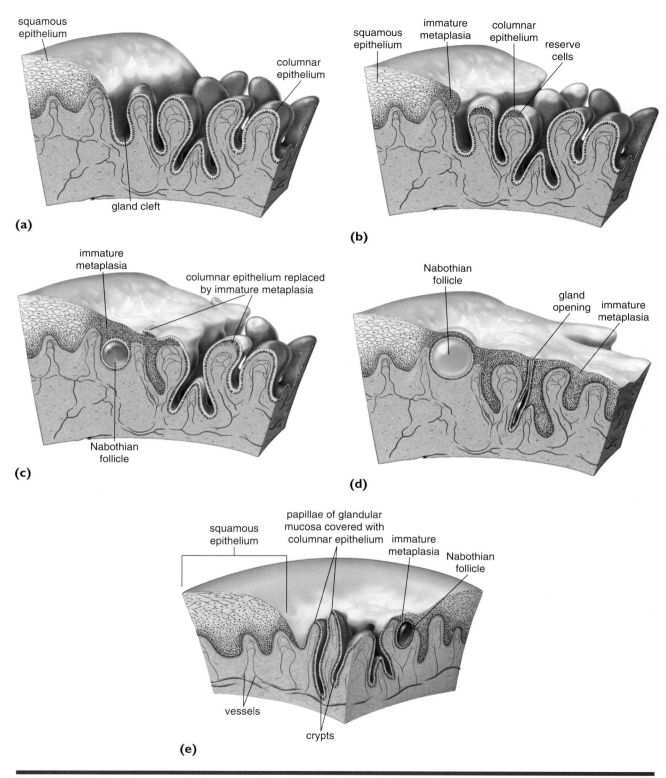

FIGURES 8.8a–e   The transformation process is depicted in these five figures. **(a)** Normal squamous and columnar epithelium are seen. **(b)** Reserve cells are now noted beneath some columnar cells on the tips of the villi. These villi tips blanch white following 5% acetic acid application. **(c)** A Nabothian follicle is seen to form. **(d)** Finally, the columnar epithelium has been replaced by metaplastic epithelium **(e)**.

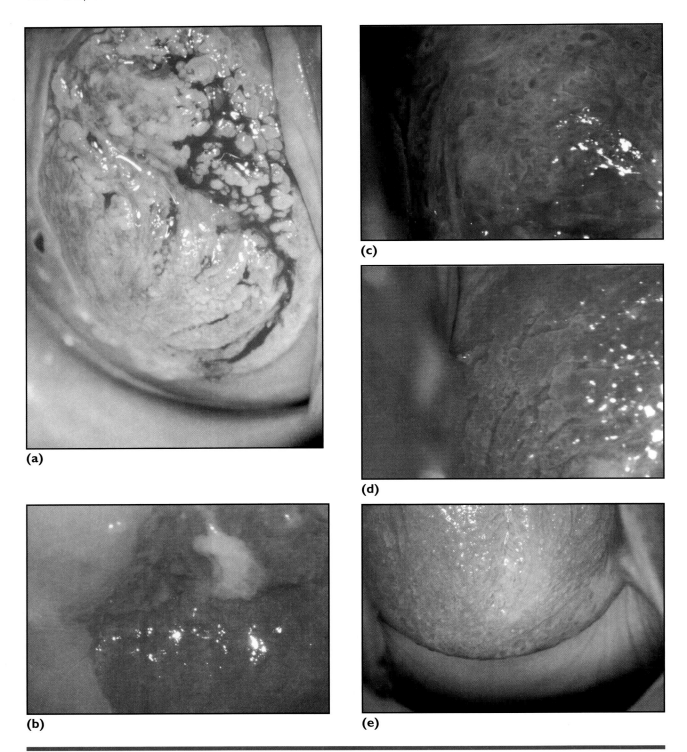

(a)

(b)

(c)

(d)

(e)

FIGURES 8.9a–e   Various stages of the metaplastic process are seen from blanching of the villi tips to bridging across villi and finally to opalescent sheets of metaplasia.

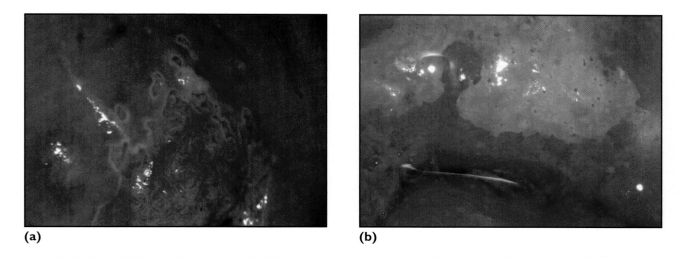

FIGURES 8.10a,b   Gland openings can be seen above the contiguous SCJ. Each gland opening has a thin white SCJ with a central reddish color indicating retained columnar epithelium **(a)**. Small gland openings are seen in this area of immature metaplasia **(b)**.

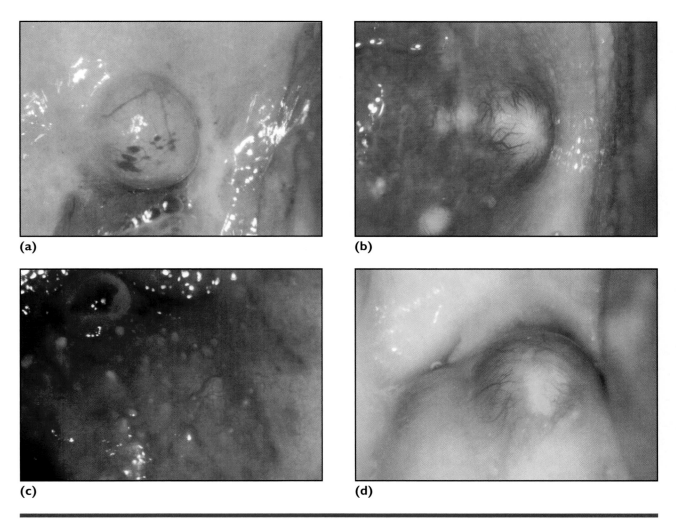

FIGURES 8.11a–f   Amber-yellow round Nabothian cysts with overlying dilated, but normal branching blood vessels.

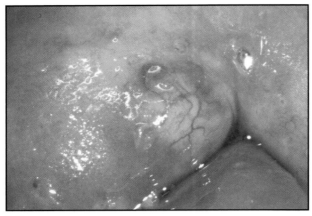

(e)

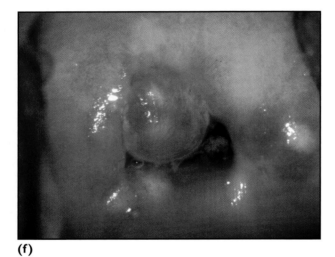

(f)

FIGURES 8.11a–f Nabothian cysts. **Continued**

8.3 The "Abnormal" Transformation Zone

The "abnormal" transformation zone, although not recognized officially as an international colposcopic term, represents an alteration of the normal transformation zone, usually initiated in immature metaplastic epithelium, whereby the normal regimented and progressive differentiation of squamous cells is modified to an epithelium lacking cell maturation and increasing cellular atypia or neoplasia. The cellular changes may be limited to various levels of the epithelium, or when a malignancy evolves, they may extend beneath the basement membrane and beyond. Diverse modifications of the normal supporting vasculature also emerge. These vascular changes result from interaction with the dynamic epithelium or from proliferation stimulated by angiogenic factors associated with viruses or malignancy.[6–12]

The most significant neoplastic lesions initiate near the new or current SCJ. Squamous neoplasias originate in metaplastic epithelium along the SCJ. They appear to extend distally from the SCJ. In contrast, glandular neoplasias arise in columnar epithelium near the SCJ and appear to extend proximally from the SCJ. Abnormal colposcopic features arise through epithelial and vascular alterations of normal colposcopic findings. Potentially abnormal epithelial features include leukoplakia, acetowhite epithelium, and iodine-negative epithelium. Epithelial absence, in the form of an ulceration or erosion, may be considered abnormal. Epithelial proliferation that causes a raised contour with respect to the normal adjoining surface also may represent an abnormality. Punctation, mosaic, and atypical blood vessels are all potentially abnormal vascular colposcopic signs. All of these epithelial and vascular colposcopic features associated with the abnormal transformation zone also may be seen in the normal transformation zone.

8.4 Colposcopic Findings
8.4.1 Critical colposcopic considerations

There is no single colposcopic sign or anatomical feature detected within the cervical transformation zone that differentiates disease from normality or provides definitive evidence of the presence of premalignant or early invasive neoplasia. Any condition that causes increased cellular division, decreased cellular maturation, increased or decreased thickness of epithelium, abnormal cellular metabolism, or increased vascularization can produce atypical colposcopic findings. Because no solitary colposcopic sign permits independent differentiation of the normal transformation zone from the spectrum of cervical neoplasia, colposcopic impressions should not be based on any single colposcopic sign.

Abnormal colposcopic features may occur in normal variants seen during the early estrogen surge, during pregnancy, with use of oral contraceptives, after in-utero exposure to Diethylstilbestrol (DES), and with estrogen withdrawal. Benign conditions such as squamous metaplasia, regeneration, repair, inflammation, and infection also may produce dramatic vascular and epithelial colposcopic changes. In order to minimize the risk of interpreting benign conditions as abnormal, the full complement of colposcopic signs must be considered collectively in deriving a reasonable colposcopic impression with a high degree of reliability and validity. For example, the same colposcopic features noted in areas of immature squamous metaplasia may also be seen in women with inflammation, repair, low-grade cervical neoplasia and cervical cancer.

8.4.2 Identification of colposcopic signs

Normal and abnormal colposcopic findings may involve all or part of the transformation zone. These findings can extend distal to the original SCJ to affect the peripheral cervix and vagina. Alternatively, the colposcopic findings may involve epithelium of the endocervical canal. Shifting of the transformation zone over time means that normal and abnormal colposcopic findings need be neither site specific nor location dependent.

The intense illumination and magnification of the colposcope permit assessment and differentiation of normal and abnormal colposcopic features. Except for leukoplakia, the more common abnormal colposcopic signs are not apparent on naked-eye observation. Certainly, grossly nodular malignancies or large exophytic condylomas of the cervix may be clearly visible and readily palpable. However, proper recognition of less apparent and less severe degrees of neoplasia is necessary to identify CIN. Tiny capillary anomalies can be more fully appreciated using the visual enhancements provided by a modern colposcope. Contemporary management of women with lower genital tract neoplasia requires expertise in the recognition of these subtle abnormal colposcopic features.

The chemical solutions used during colposcopy permit visualization, identification, and discrimination between certain normal and abnormal areas of the transformation zone. Saline should be used initially to moisten the cervix and to permit the nontraumatic removal of obscuring debris. Additionally, saline facilitates visualization of the vasculature prior to the application of acetic acid. Acetic acid (3% to 5%) permits a transient observation of immature portions of the normal transformation zone and detection of more persistent acetowhite changes noted with epithelial abnormalities. Lugol's iodine solution contrasts normal glycogenated epithelium from nonglycogenated immature normal or abnormal epithelium. The green filter, which blocks red light transmission, enhances the recognition of blood vessels, and is most important in the identification of abnormal vessels associated with severe neoplastic transformation. By filtering out the red color, vessels appear black against a light green epithelial background. The surface contour of the cervix varies vastly. Normal and abnormal topography may be smooth or flat, papillary, nodular, papular, uneven, raised, or ulcerated. The edges of normal epithelia or abnormal lesions can also assume a multitude of patterns. Margins may be extremely irregular, delicately feathered, nearly indistinct, almost straight, rounded, curved, complex, or visibly peeling.

8.5 Normal and Abnormal Colposcopic Signs

Leukoplakia, acetowhite epithelium, ulceration, punctation, mosaic, and atypical vessels are the colposcopic signs seen in both normal and abnormal epithelium of the lower genital tract. Colposcopic signs that collectively, in whole, in part, singly, or in combination, represent normal and abnormal epithelium are shown in Table 8.1, which also includes the theoretical reasons for the colposcopic signs.

The colposcopic features that are considered most important for differentiating normal from abnormal conditions and discriminating levels of abnormality may be grouped systematically as follows:

- Epithelial color: before and after the application of normal saline, 3% to 5% acetic acid, or Lugol's iodine solution
- Vasculature: type of vessel, vessel pattern, vessel caliber, and intercapillary distances
- Surface topography: flat, ulcerated or raised surfaces
- Margin characteristics: border shape of discrete epithelial lesions

8.5.1 Epithelial color
8.5.1.1 Before application of 3% to 5% acetic acid and Lugol's iodine solution

8.5.1.1.1 Normal cervix As described in Chapter 2, healthy mature squamous epithelium can be distinguished easily from columnar epithelium or immature squamous epithelium based on color tone. This is accomplished following normal saline application but before the application of 5% acetic acid or Lugol's iodine solution. Color is derived colposcopically by the interaction of transmitted colposcopic light with the epithelium and stroma (Figures 8.12a,b). Certain wavelengths of the colposcope's white light are either reflected back to the observer immediately or absorbed, then emitted as specific wavelengths of light that convey a unique color. The nuclear-to-cytoplasmic ratio of epithelial cells and epithelial thickness affect the intensity of reflected white light. As each increases, the amount of white light returned to the colposcopist increases and the amount of red color emitted from transilluminated blood vessels decreases.

Healthy mature nonkeratinized stratified squamous epithelium (whether original squamous epithelium or mature metaplastic epithelium) has a pink

Table 8.1   Normal and Abnormal Colposcopic Signs

TYPE OF TISSUE	COLPOSCOPIC SIGN	ETIOLOGY
Epithelial	Acetowhite epithelium	Increased cellular and nuclear density
		Intracellular protein agglutination
		Abnormal intracellular keratins
		Intracellular dehydration
	Leukoplakia	Traumatically induced, thickened superficial epithelium
		Abnormal keratin production from a viral or neoplastic process
	Ulceration	Absence of epithelium caused by trauma, infection, medications, or neoplasia
Vascular	Punctation and Mosaic	Alterations in epithelial capillaries due to:
		(a) proliferative effect of the normal immature metaplastic process
		(b) capillary proliferative effect of HPV
		(c) intraepithelial pressures exerted by expanding blocks of neoplastic epithelium
	Atypical blood vessels	Very immature metaplastic epithelium
		The proliferative effect of vascular endothelial growth factor and angiogenin, tumor angiogenesis factors noted in invasive cancer
		Catabolic oxygen demands of invasive cancer
		Random invading directions of cancer
		Postradiation angiogenesis
		Granulation tissue

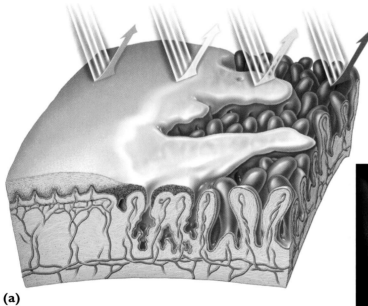

(a)

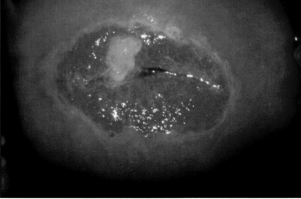

(b)

FIGURES 8.12a,b   **(a)** The color of the normal cervix is derived from the interaction of the colposcope light with the tissue; **(b)** squamous epithelium is pink and columnar epithelium red prior to the application of 5% acetic acid.

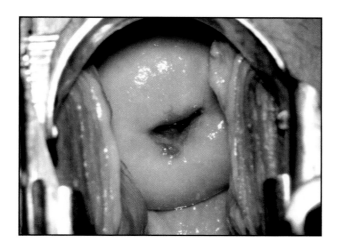

FIGURE 8.13 Stratified squamous epithelium of the cervix, demonstrating a pink color.

color (Figure 8.13). The epithelium appears pink because a network of capillaries underlies stratified squamous epithelium, which may be 10 to 15 cell layers thick. A majority of the white light from the colposcope, combined with a small amount of red color from deeply positioned capillaries, blends to emit a pink tone (Figure 8.14). A more pale pink color may be seen in postmenopausal women not receiving estrogen replacement therapy because of a thinner epithelium (Figure 8.15). When observed through the colposcope at high-power magnification, tiny, wispy, superficially located dark red blood vessels can be detected against the homogeneous pink background (Figures 8.16a,b). These loop capillaries in stromal papillae penetrate into the lower one third of the squamous epithelium to nourish the maturing cells. The reduced epithelial thickness over the loop capillaries allows greater transmission of a focal red color.

Both columnar epithelium and immature metaplastic epithelium appear red (Figures 8.17a,b) at initial inspection. Columnar epithelium may be "beefy" red or dull red, depending on the amount, turbidity, and viscosity of overlying mucus, and vascular prominence secondary to inflammation. The red color is derived from the interaction of the colposcope light with the thin tissue. The close proximity of the underlying loop capillaries, which are covered by only a single cell layer of columnar epithelium, emits a predominant red hue from the transilluminated light. The color of immature metaplastic epithelium varies depending on its stage of maturation. Very immature metaplasia is quite thin, composed of only a few cell layers; consequently, prior to acetic acid application, this epithelium appears a moderate red color (Figures 8.18a,b,c,d). The red color is not as intense as that seen with columnar epithelium because the capillaries lie slightly deeper beneath the thin maturing

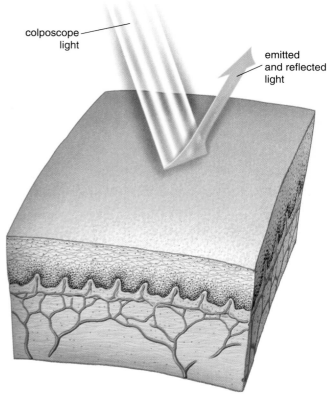

FIGURE 8.14 Squamous epithelium appears pink because the white light of the colposcope combined with a small amount of red color from the deeply residing capillaries blend to produce a light pink color.

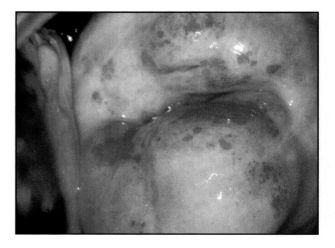

FIGURE 8.15 An atrophic cervix is pale pink. The epithelium is thin. Consequently, small subcutaneous hemorrhages induced by minor contact trauma are seen.

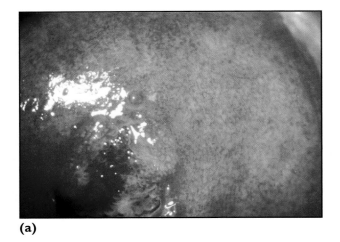

(a)

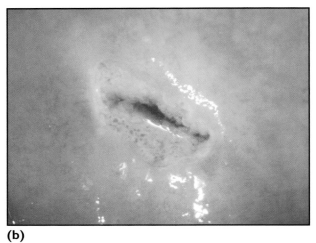

(b)

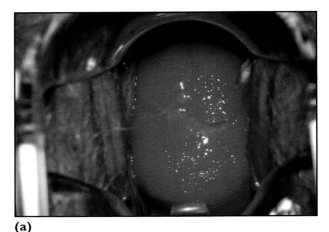

(a)

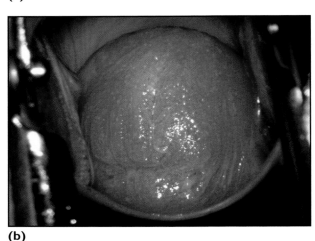

(b)

FIGURES 8.16a,b   Tiny, small network capillaries of normal squamous epithelium. Photograph **(a)** courtesy of Dr. Kenneth L. Noller.

FIGURES 8.17a,b   Columnar epithelium of an ectropion of the cervix, demonstrating a red color. The red color of columnar epithelium prior to the application of 5% acetic acid is derived from the interaction of the colposcope light with the tissue and underlying vessels.

epithelium. As the epithelium matures and thickens, less red color can be appreciated. With complete metaplastic differentiation, the epithelium assumes a characteristic pink color similar to that observed in original squamous epithelium.

Amber yellow, round Nabothian cysts may be observed in metaplastic epithelium (Figures 8.11a–f). Nabothian cysts evolve from the transformation process when advancing metaplastic epithelium seals a gland cleft opening, thereby trapping mucus secreted from columnar epithelium recessed deeply within the gland cleft. An abundance of retained mucus slowly stretches the overlying epithelium and stroma. The epithelium becomes compressed and thinned as the trapped mucus accumulates. The bulging, gently rounded amber protrusion conveys a translucent quality upon colposcopic illumination. Prominent, readily transilluminated blood vessels will usually be apparent in the epithelium overlying

the cysts. Although these vessels appear dilated, they exhibit normal arboreal branching. Because these large-caliber vessels are associated with a contour change, they may be mistaken for atypical blood vessels seen with invasive cancer. However, the smooth, yellow, translucent contour and the dichotomously branching vessels are characteristic of Nabothian cysts.

During pregnancy, the normal cervix assumes a bluish hue (Figure 8.19). This discoloration results from hormonally mediated vascular congestion. Cervical changes during pregnancy are discussed further in Chapter 12.

8.5.1.1.2 Abnormal cervix
8.5.1.1.2.1 Leukoplakia
Definition   The term *leukoplakia* means "white patch" and is defined as an epithelium that appears

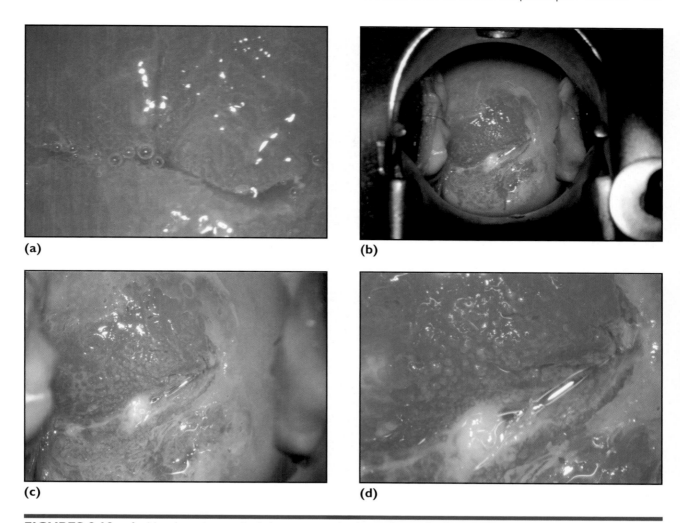

(a)

(b)

(c)

(d)

FIGURES 8.18a–d   Very immature metaplasia appears red prior to the application of 5% acetic acid. The color results from the interaction of the white light of the colposcope with the epithelium and underlying blood vessels.

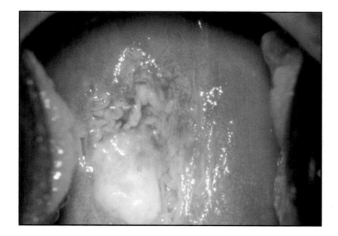

FIGURE 8.19   The cervix during pregnancy, demonstrating a bluish hue, thick mucus, and eversion of columnar epithelium.

white when viewed with the naked eye or with the colposcope prior to the application of 5% acetic acid (Figure 8.20). When considering leukoplakia, it is necessary to remember that a variety of histologic processes can appear as white areas on the cervix. Most commonly, regions of leukoplakia are associated with an increase in the amount of keratin at the surface of the epithelium. This histologic process is referred to as "hyperkeratosis" (Figure 8.21). When the hyperkeratotic material retains pyknotic cell nuclei, it is referred to as "parakeratosis" (Figure 8.22). Thus, the term *keratosis* has been used to refer to areas of leukoplakia. However, not all leukoplakias demonstrate benign hyperkeratosis or parakeratosis. Some represent neoplastic or acanthotic (thickening of the intermediate and superficial layers of the squamous epithelium) processes and appear white because of the increased nuclear density of underlying neoplastic cells and the thickened epithelium, which reflects a substantial amount of white

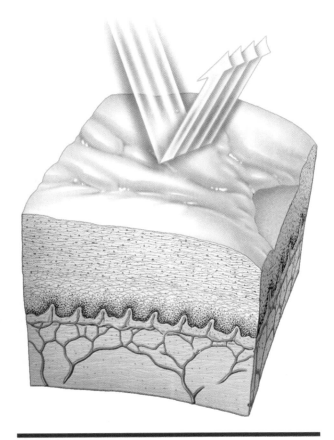

FIGURE 8.20 The white color of leukoplakia results from the reflection of the white colposcope light back to the colposcopist.

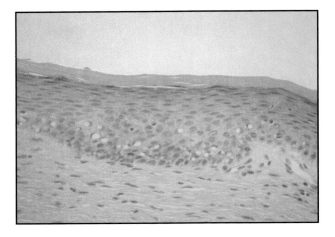

FIGURE 8.21 A histologic specimen demonstrating hyperkeratosis (Hematoxylin-eosin stain; Medium power magnification).

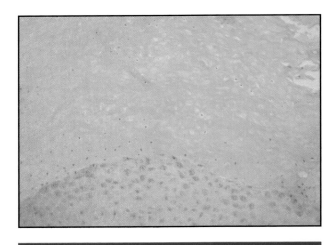

FIGURE 8.22 A histologic specimen demonstrating parakeratosis in which nuclei are retained in the superficial cells (Hematoxylin-eosin stain; High power magnification).

light back to the colposcopist (Figure 8.20). The current International Federation of Cervical Pathology and Colposcopy (I.F.C.P.C.) colposcopic terminology (Table 8.2) uses the term *keratosis* instead of *leukoplakia* even though not all white lesions of the cervix demonstrate hyperkeratosis or parakeratosis on histologic examination.

Etiology Leukoplakia results from a variety of noxious stimuli, including HPV infection, trauma (particularly chronic irritation), and neoplasia (both preinvasive and invasive). However, many cases are idiopathic, especially those occurring in young women. When associated with chronic trauma, leukoplakia may be thought of simply as an epithelial response to irritation, such as might occur with use of a diaphragm, retained tampon, or pessary. Normal epithelium must protect underlying structures from external injury, penetration, and hence, infection. By defensively thickening the epithelium, either through hyperkeratosis or acanthosis, leukoplakia provides a protective barrier that can better withstand insult and protect epithelial integrity. This form of leukoplakia is sometimes referred to as dystrophic leukoplakia, since it represents a dystrophic

process. It is usually associated with hyperkeratosis and mild or minimal acanthosis.

Colposcopic appearance Leukoplakia appears as a white, thickened, raised epithelium observed prior to the application of 3% to 5% acetic acid (Figures 8.23a,b). It may be seen with the naked eye but is better appreciated after saline application and using the colposcope. Leukoplakia occurs on the cervix, both within and outside the transformation zone. Leukoplakia may also be seen elsewhere in the lower genital tract. The location of leukoplakia is important since it may reflect the underlying etiology. When leukoplakia occurs in original squamous epithelium, it usually represents a benign condition (Figures 8.24a,b). When leukoplakia occurs within the

Table 8.2   International Federation of Cervical Pathology and Colposcopy (IFCPC)
Colposcopic Terminology

I. Normal Colposcopic Findings
    Original squamous epithelium
    Columnar epithelium
    Transformation zone
II. Abnormal Colposcopic Findings
    Flat acetowhite epithelium
    Dense acetowhite epithelium*
    Fine mosaic
    Coarse mosaic
    Fine punctation
    Coarse punctation*
    Iodine partial positivity
    Iodine negativity*
    Atypical vessels*
III. Colposcopic features suggestive of invasive carcinoma
IV. Unsatisfactory colposcopy
    Squamocolumnar junction not visible
    Severe inflammation, severe atrophy, trauma
    Cervix not visible
V. Miscellaneous findings
    Condylomata
    Keratosis
    Erosion
    Inflammation
    Atrophy
    Deciduosis
    Polyps

*Major changes.

Walker P, Dexeus S, DePalo G, Barrasso R, Campion M, Girardi F, et al. International terminology of colposcopy: An updated report from the International Federation for Cervical Pathology and Colposcopy. *Obstet Gynecol* 2003;101:175–7. Reprinted with permission.

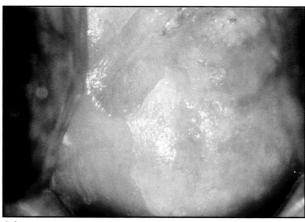

(a)

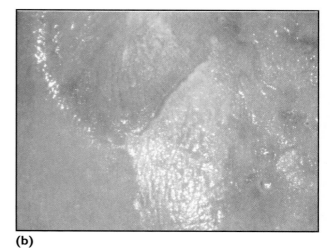

(b)

FIGURES 8.23a,b   Leukoplakia of the cervix, demonstrating white, thickened, raised epithelium prior to the application of 5% acetic acid.

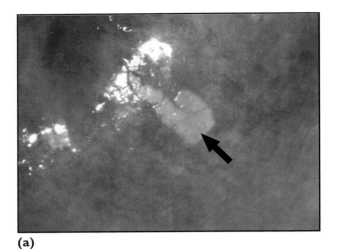

(a)

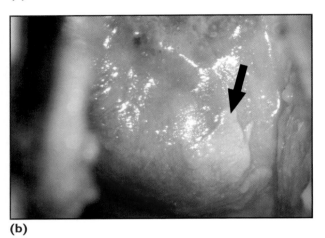

(b)

FIGURES 8.24a,b Leukoplakia noted outside the cervical transformation zone (arrow). Such lesions are not likely to be associated with a neoplastic process.

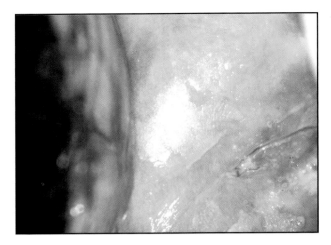

FIGURE 8.25 An irregularly shaped area of leukoplakia located at the 10 o'clock position.

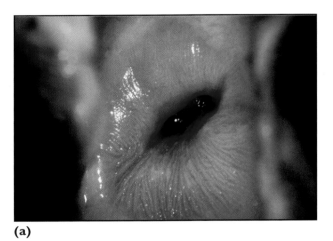

(a)

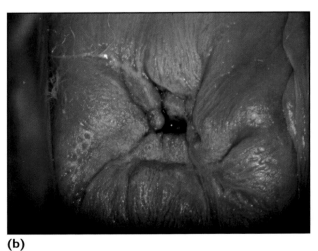

(b)

FIGURES 8.26a,b Parakeratosis noted after loop excision of the cervix. Pinpoint, white elevations of the epithelium are noted. The normally flat squamous epithelium assumes a "grainy," pebbled texture.

transformation zone, severe underlying neoplastic conditions, including cancer, should be considered.

Leukoplakia varies in color, size, distribution, and contour (Figure 8.25). Leukoplakia is snow-white to silver-white in color. Areas of leukoplakia are frequently well demarcated and can appear as multiple small areas, focal lesions, or as large confluent patches with smooth or irregular borders. Leukoplakia may be macular or raised, but it typically has an elevated smooth or mildly irregular contour. The surface may have a waxy or shiny texture. Consequently, saline and acetic acid solutions may be repelled from the surface much like water interacts on the surface of a newly waxed automobile. Tiny pinpoint white elevations are commonly noted in women who have had previous ablative or excisional procedures of the cervix (Figures 8.26a,b). These micropapular projections may assume an intermittent linear pattern, radiating from the os much like spokes of a bicycle wheel. Each small elevation represents focal benign parakeratosis overlying a loop capillary. Large elevated patches of keratosis that are referred to as "iceberg leukoplakia" are occasionally seen and may indicate chronic irritation, such as occurs in women using pessaries to prevent uterine prolapse through the vagina (Figures 8.27a–c).

Usually, no vascular pattern is observed on the surface of leukoplakia. It is important to stress that it is impossible to predict the nature of the epithelium underlying leukoplakia with any degree of certainty by colposcopic visualization. Highly abnormal vascular patterns can be hidden if located sufficiently deep beneath an overlying thickened keratin layer. Peeling away the keratotic tissue frequently produces bleeding that obscures the underlying tissue. In cases of leukoplakia associated with chronic irritation, peeling away the keratotic layer may reveal an underlying fine red punctation.

Colposcopic examination of the tissue surrounding an area of leukoplakia may indicate the source of the keratotic area. For instance, leukoplakia associated with neoplasia may partially cover or abut a large area of abnormal acetowhite epithelium (Figure 8.28). However, an adjoining premalignant epithelium is usually visible only following 5% acetic acid application. In many cases, it is possible to detect cancers with leukoplakia prior to 5% acetic acid application.

Clinical significance Leukoplakia is generally thought to be a benign epithelial process, but it is possible for areas of leukoplakia to completely cover and obscure underlying neoplastic lesions. Clinicians should consider all the probable causes of leukoplakia to derive a satisfactory explanation. Colposcopists may initially confuse leukoplakia with cervical candidiasis. However, gentle swabbing will not remove leukoplakia entirely—only perhaps the most superficial layers. Trauma, viral effects, neoplasia, or idiopathic processes must be entertained as possible etiologies for leukoplakia. Leukoplakia is a clinical diagnosis. While a cervical cytologic report of hyperkeratosis or parakeratosis might suggest the presence of lower genital tract leukoplakia, it is not considered an indication for colposcopy in the absence of other cellular abnormalities. However, leukoplakia, observed during clinical examination of the cervix or when obtaining a Pap smear, is an indication for a colposcopic examination. Although most cases of leukoplakia represent a benign process, even lesions presenting in the original squamous epithelium can occasionally indicate a serious neoplastic condition,

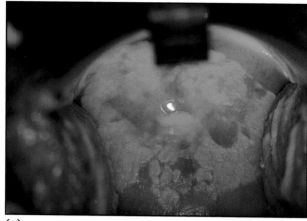

(a)

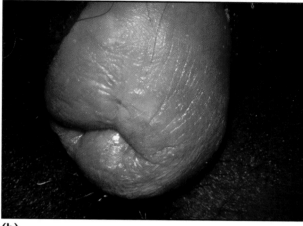

(b)

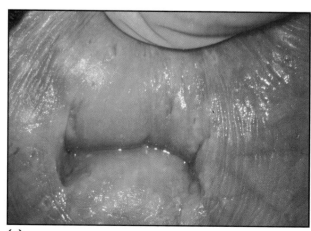

(c)

FIGURES 8.27a–c **(a)** Leukoplakia seen in a woman who wore a pessary to prevent uterine prolapse. **(b,c)** Hyperkeratosis of the cervix is seen in another woman with uterine prolapse. The tissue thickened in response to the chronic irritation caused by the continual trauma.

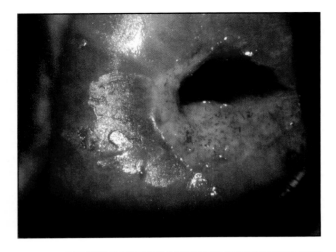

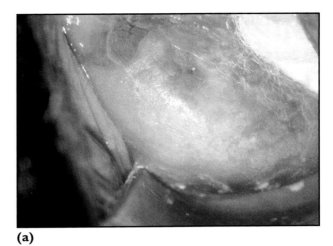

(a)

FIGURE 8.28   Leukoplakia associated with neoplasia abutting against an area of abnormal acetowhite epithelium.

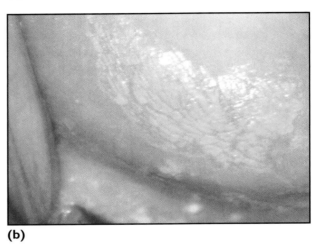

(b)

FIGURES 8.29a,b   This area of leukoplakia was associated with an abnormal Pap smear. Therefore, biopsy is mandatory to exclude an underlying occult neoplasia. ▬

such as a keratinizing invasive squamous cell carcinoma. Leukoplakia obscures meaningful colposcopic evaluation of other abnormal colposcopic signs. Therefore, regardless of the localization of the area of leukoplakia, a biopsy must be taken to exclude underlying neoplasia (Figures 8.29a,b).

8.5.1.1.2 Neoplasia   Unless accompanied by leukoplakia, most premalignant lesions of the cervix cannot be discriminated from normal epithelium based solely on color. Epithelial contrast solutions are generally required to provide sufficient recognition. In contrast, many invasive cancers are recognized by their color following saline application. Advanced cancers may be yellow or red with varying shades of either color. Cancers may also exhibit a "glassy" or gelatinous appearance. Areas of necrotic epithelium may appear brown or black. However, many early cervical cancers appear pink prior to the application of contrast solutions. Cancers may have coexisting areas of leukoplakia that will impart a white color before application of 5% acetic acid.

8.5.1.2 After application of 3% to 5% acetic acid

8.5.1.2.1 Background   The use of 3% to 5% acetic acid during colposcopy was introduced to remove the thin film of mucus that adheres to and may obscure the cervical epithelium. We now recognize its more important role as a contrast agent used to help identify neoplasias of the lower genital tract. To simplify terminology, 5% acetic acid will be used throughout the text to denote the use of 3% to 5% acetic acid.

8.5.1.2.2 Normal and abnormal cervix   The appearance of mature nonkeratinized squamous epithelium does not change after the application of 5% acetic acid. Healthy, mature stratified epithelium, whether it is original squamous epithelium or mature metaplastic epithelium, retains its pink-tan color after the application of 5% acetic acid (Figure 8.30a). In contrast, the dark red color of columnar epithelium becomes somewhat blanched, assuming a transient, translucent white color (Figure 8.30b). This transient white color persists for only several minutes, returning then to the original red color. Any persisting acetowhite color after this time represents immature metaplasia or neoplasia (Figure 8.30c). Furthermore, following 5% acetic acid application, each villus covered by columnar epithelium assumes a more distinct outline, appearing as grape-like or

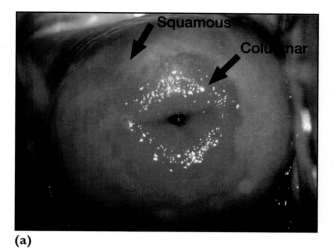

(a)

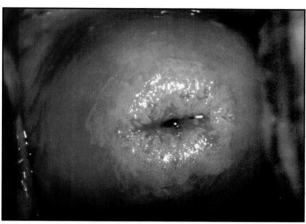

(b)

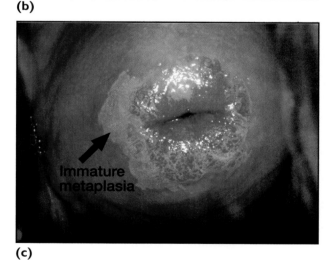

(c)

FIGURES 8.30a–c **(a)** Before acetic acid application, the squamous epithelium is pink (arrow), and columnar and immature metaplasia are red (arrow). **(b)** Immediately following acetic acid application, squamous epithelium remains pink, columnar epithelium blanches a faint white color, and immature metaplasia becomes translucent white. **(c)** The columnar epithelium returns quickly to a red color, while the area of immature metaplasia remains white (arrow).

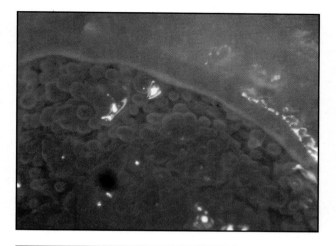

FIGURE 8.31 A high-magnification colpophotograph of columnar epithelium demonstrating grape-like villous structures covered by columnar epithelium. The acetic acid application makes the villi appear more distinct.

narrow polypoid structures (Figure 8.31). Normal fine caliber capillaries, spaced uniformly about 0.1 mm apart, may not be as readily apparent immediately following 5% acetic acid application. Slowly, the tiny vessels will become visible at high-power magnification of the colposcope once the acetic acid reaction begins to fade. Nabothian cysts do not change color after acetic acid application (Figures 8.11a–f). They retain their amber yellow color. Prominent branching vessels may be seen overlying the transilluminated thinned epithelium. Gland openings may be seen near the SCJ as round openings in immature metaplasia. The openings are surrounded by a thin rim of acetowhite epithelium (Figure 8.10). A red color is seen in the center of the gland openings because columnar epithelium remains in the deep gland clefts.

8.5.1.2.2.1 Acetowhite epithelium

Definition Acetowhite epithelium refers to epithelium that transiently changes color from pink or red to white after the application of 3% to 5% acetic acid. The temporary reaction is noted in immature metaplastic, reparative, and neoplastic epithelium. The changes may be seen on the cervix, vagina, vulva, or anorectal areas. Acetowhite epithelium is the most common colposcopic feature observed. Although acetowhite epithelium is seen in all cases of cervical intraepithelial neoplasia (CIN), it is also seen in 57% of normal cervices.[13] Prior to the application of acetic acid, immature metaplasia and many neoplastic lesions appear a reddish-pink or normal color. However, seconds to minutes after 5% acetic acid is applied, these epithelia assume a variably white color

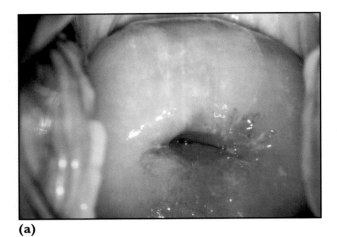

(a)

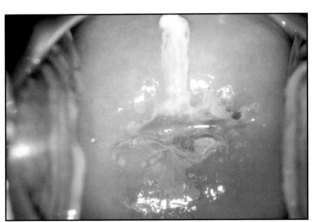

(b)

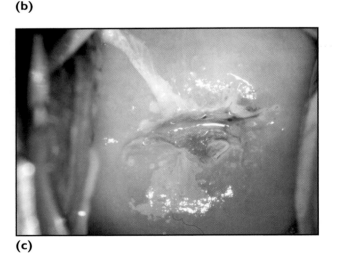

(c)

FIGURES 8.32a–c   The cervix **(a)** before and **(b,c)** after acetic acid application. An acetowhite low-grade lesion gradually appears on the posterior lip of the cervix. ▬▬▬

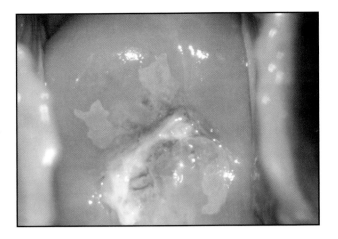

FIGURE 8.33   Areas of CIN 1, demonstrating a transparent acetowhite color. ▬▬▬

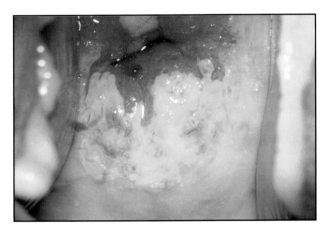

FIGURE 8.34   Acetowhite epithelium associated with CIN 3 that demonstrates an opaque acetowhite color. ▬▬

(Figures 8.32a–c). The acetowhite effect is transitory and disappears relatively rapidly (2 to 10 minutes) after discontinuing the application of acetic acid.

The acetowhite color can present with different shades of white. Furthermore, the opacity or translu-cency of the acetowhite response varies across the spectrum of CIN. Normal immature metaplasia and low-grade cervical lesions (CIN1) usually appear faintly acetowhite or slightly translucent (Figures 8.32b,c). The acetowhite response of high-grade lesions appears more opaque. The amount of white-ness has been shown to be proportional to severity of disease.[14] For example, immature metaplasia and low-grade lesions are frequently described as having a "snow-white" or faintly white appearance that is quite transparent after the application of acetic acid (Figure 8.33). In contrast, high-grade colposcopic lesions (CIN 2,3) may have a "dirty" white appear-ance that is quite opaque to transillumination of the colposcope light (Figure 8.34). These findings vary depending on patient age. Women older than 35 years old have CIN lesions that are thinner than women younger than 35 years old.[15] Consequently,

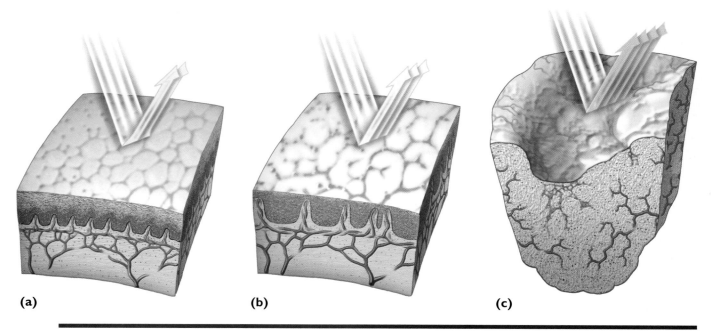

(a)   **(b)**   **(c)**

FIGURES 8.35a–c After 5% acetic acid has been applied to the cervix, the resulting acetowhite color is determined by the interaction of the colposcope light with the epithelium and blood vessels. The white color of CIN 1 is **(a)** more translucent white and not as opaque as that seen with **(b)** CIN 3, or **(c)** invasive cancer.

older women's lesions may not be as acetowhite as those in younger women. Evaluating the cervix for acetowhite color is a critical part of every colposcopic examination since it allows identification of the presence and distribution of cervical lesions.

Etiology Tissues that reflect the majority of the projected white light from the colposcope back to the colposcopist or temporarily absorb the white light but emit most of the white light back appear acetowhite (Figures 8.35a–c). The exact mechanism responsible for the transient acetic acid-induced color change is unknown and, therefore, continues to be debated. However, there are several potential mechanisms for the acetowhite color. Acetic acid may produce osmotic changes in the tissue that cause a diffusion of intracellular fluid to the extracellular space. The transient transfer of fluid from within the cells to the extracellular space causes tissues to temporarily assume a greater nuclear-to-cytoplasmic ratio. Consequently, the intracellular cytoplasm becomes concentrated, less free water is present, and the cells become more reflective to white light. Increasing nuclear density results in less absorption and more reflection of light. Another postulated explanation is that acetic acid may induce conformational changes in either intracellular proteins (especially intermediate filaments such as cytokeratin proteins) or the nuclear matrix that render selective tissues more reflective to white light.

Colposcopic appearance Acetowhite areas are visualized colposcopically as transient but colposcopically distinct regions of white epithelium within normal surrounding pink or red epithelium (Figure 8.36). Acetowhite epithelium may be unifocal or multifocal, positioned within or outside the cervical transformation zone. The shade of white can include translucent white, snow-white, off-white, gray, and yellow, with varying degrees of luster and opacity. Color depends on the cellular nuclear-to-cytoplasmic ratio; thickness and type of epithelium; underlying type, caliber, and spacing of the vasculature; and duration, concentration, and coverage of acetic acid.

The rates of development and persistence of acetowhite color vary depending on whether the tissue is normal or abnormal, and whether 3% or 5% acetic acid is used. The acetowhite effect observed in normal immature metaplastic epithelium develops most rapidly. Since more time is required for abnormal epithelium to turn acetowhite, colposcopists must always observe the cervix for several minutes to ensure that the maximum acetowhite effect is observed. A second acetic acid application aids and hastens the onset of the acetowhite color. On second application, one should usually allow 1 to 2 minutes for the full development of an acetowhite color to occur. High-grade lesions (especially regions of severe dysplasia and carcinoma in-situ) retain the acetowhite effect for a longer time (5 to 10 minutes) than do less-severe grades of neoplasia.[14] In order to

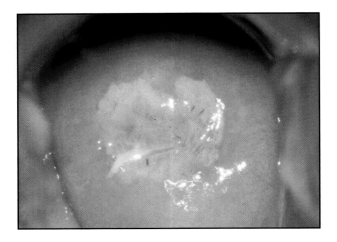

FIGURE 8.36 Acetowhite epithelium of the cervix. ▬

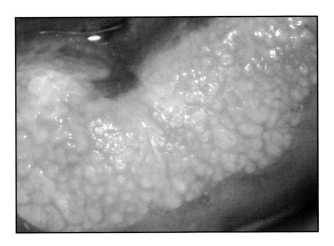

FIGURE 8.38 A snowy-white lesion within a field of normal pink surrounding squamous epithelium. The lesion is characteristic of cervical condyloma. ▬▬

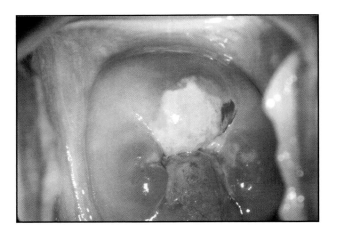

FIGURE 8.37 CIN 3 on the anterior cervical lip and an area of translucent acetowhite immature metaplasia is seen on the posterior lip. The more opaque acetowhite color indicates the area that should be biopsied. ▬▬

maintain the acetowhite effect, many clinicians reapply acetic acid continuously during the entire colposcopic examination. A quicker, perhaps more pronounced, acetowhite response is noted with 5% acetic acid compared with the less concentrated 3% acetic acid. The transient color change persists for a greater duration when using 5% acetic acid, but the more concentrated solution may cause a slightly greater burning sensation when applied to women with fair complexions or women suffering from a lower genital tract inflammatory process, such as vaginitis or vulvitis.

Evaluation of specific colposcopic features of acetowhite epithelium—degree and opacity of whiteness, lesion edges or margin, size, and surface contour—facilitates the differentiation of acetowhite epithelium associated with normal tissue from acetowhite epithelium associated with pathologic conditions (Figure 8.37). For example, most neoplastic lesions have a distinct margin with a greater degree of acetowhite color than does immature metaplasia. Moreover, the surface epithelium of neoplastic lesions may appear thicker, raised, and more opaque or "dense". Lesion size is useful in determining the nature of observed acetowhite changes. As lesion surface area increases, so does lesion severity.[16] The linear extent of CIN 3 generally does not exceed 15 mm.[17] Furthermore, the larger and more severe the lesion, the greater the extent of the lesion into gland clefts. Specific colors, degree of surface luster or shine, and duration of the acetic acid reaction all reflect the severity of the underlying disease process. Although it has been traditionally taught that degree of whiteness correlates with severity of underlying disease, many low-grade HPV-induced lesions will produce a prominent, vivid, snow-white acetic acid reaction (Figure 8.38).

The acetowhite color of normal immature metaplastic epithelium develops rapidly and fades rapidly. It may be difficult to reestablish the acetowhite effect by reapplying more acetic acid once the initial acetowhite color has faded. The white color appears translucent, especially in regions of very immature metaplasia (Figure 8.39). As these regions mature, the epithelium may retain the distinctive appearance and contour of the early phases of metaplasia until late in the process. Hence, a gently pebbled texture reflecting the underlying villous remnants may be observed. Frequently, the margins

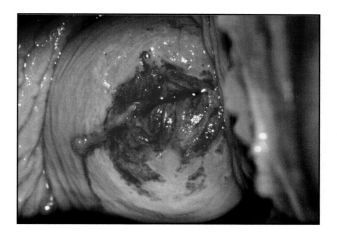

FIGURE 8.39 A translucent acetowhite color on the anterior and posterior cervix, depicting very immature metaplasia.

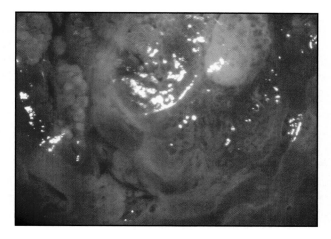

FIGURE 8.40 Colpophotograph of acetowhite areas from a woman with a low-grade squamous intraepithelial lesion and a similar acetowhite area demonstrating immature metaplasia. The low grade lesion is seen in the upper right corner of the photograph.

of immature metaplasia are indistinct, as the acetowhite epithelium tends to blend gradually with the adjacent squamous epithelium or mature metaplastic epithelium.

The acetowhite effect observed in regions of low-grade lesions is frequently similar or identical to that observed in regions of immature metaplasia (Figure 8.40). In other instances, the acetowhite effect observed in low-grade lesions appears more opaque white. Reliable discrimination between low-grade lesions and immature metaplasia based on acetowhite color alone is a difficult task for even an expert colposcopist (Figures 8.41a–c). Recognizing slight differences in the margins of the two may facilitate differentiation. The margins of low-grade lesions, compared with those of metaplasia, are usually more clearly demarcated from the adjacent normal or abnormal epithelium. An asymmetrical, focal acetowhite distribution along the SCJ is more likely indicative of low-grade lesions than of immature metaplasia (Figures 8.42a,b).

The acetowhite color observed in regions of high-grade lesions (Figure 8.43) and cancer (Figure 8.44) is usually more intense and more persistent than color seen in regions of low-grade lesions or metaplasia. With increasing disease severity, the acetowhite color tends to be more opaque than that seen in lower-grade lesions.[14] A dull appearance, sometimes referred to as "dirty" or "oyster" white, may be noted in the highest-grade lesions. The margins of high-grade acetowhite lesions are almost always well defined, often raised and "rolled," and distinct from surrounding normal and sometimes adjacent mildly abnormal tissue. Therefore, color contrast is easiest to detect in these lesions.

Clinical significance Acetowhite epithelium may represent a wide histologic spectrum from simply normal epithelium (i.e., immature squamous metaplasia, inflammation, repair) to invasive cancer. The clinical significance of acetowhite epithelium in a particular patient depends on various factors, including patient age, associated cytologic findings and, perhaps most importantly, other colposcopic features. An easily visualized active, normal, immature transformation zone in a young woman may be confused with a low-grade neoplastic process, particularly when the Pap smear that prompted the examination indicated low-grade lesion or atypical squamous cells. Since an active metaplastic process is rarely seen in postmenopausal women because the active transformation zone is not present on the ectocervix, acetowhite epithelium noted in older women may more commonly represent a neoplastic process. Similarly, regions of acetowhite color in women with high-grade lesion on Papanicolaou (Pap) smears should be viewed carefully. In general, large prominent acetowhite areas are more likely to represent significant lesions than are small, nonconfluent acetowhite regions.[16] However, large, symmetrical, circumferential acetowhite areas of the cervix in young women may represent simply a normal "congenital" transformation zone (Figures 8.45a,b) (see Chapter 2).[1]

It is important for all colposcopists to appreciate that acetowhite epithelium does not universally equate with neoplastic tissue. Although acetowhite epithelium quickly captures the attention of the

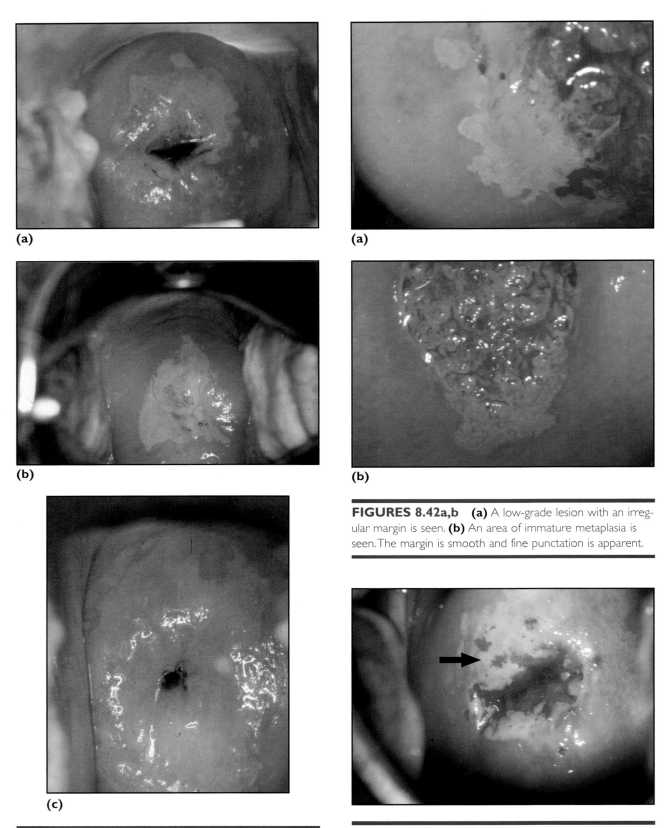

(a)

(b)

(c)

(a)

(b)

FIGURES 8.42a,b **(a)** A low-grade lesion with an irregular margin is seen. **(b)** An area of immature metaplasia is seen. The margin is smooth and fine punctation is apparent.

FIGURES 8.41a–c These areas of acetowhite immature metaplasia are difficult to discriminate from CIN 1.

FIGURE 8.43 A high-grade squamous intraepithelial lesion of the cervix following 5% acetic acid application. The area of CIN 2 (arrow) can be contrasted with the less opaque areas of immature metaplasia.

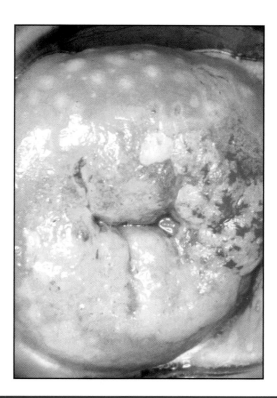

FIGURE 8.44 Acetowhite epithelium of cervical cancer. Photo courtesy of Dr. Vesna Kesic. ▬

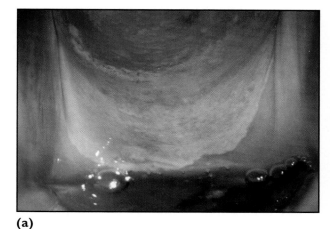

(a)

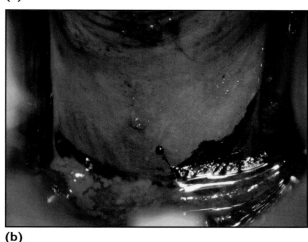

(b)

FIGURES 8.45a,b A congenital transformation zone extends into the posterior vaginal fornix. This area may mimic a low-grade squamous intraepithelial lesion or areas of immature metaplasia **(a)**. This area is also seen following the application of Lugol's iodine solution **(b)**. ▬

colposcopist during colposcopy, its presence alone remains a nondiagnostic entity. Determining indications for biopsy based solely on the presence of acetowhite epithelium promotes nonspecific sampling of many regions of entirely normal epithelium. This is particularly true for young women with cervical ectropions and active immature transformation zones clearly visualized on the ectocervix.[13]

8.5.1.3 After application of Lugol's iodine solution

8.5.1.3.1 Background Iodine solutions temporarily stain different epithelial types to assist colposcopic identification and discrimination. Lugol's iodine solution is a stain for glycogen.[2] For clinical use, Lugol's solution is generally diluted to one half to one quarter strength to avoid possible skin irritation.

8.5.1.3.2 Normal cervix
8.5.1.3.2.1 Lugol's iodine-negative and iodine-positive epithelium
Definition Iodine-negative or Lugol's-negative epithelium does not contain glycogen. Hence, nonglycogen-containing normal immature metaplasia appears yellow and normal columnar epithelium appears pink following Lugol's iodine application. In

contrast, iodine-positive epithelium contains glycogen and, therefore, normal original nonkeratinized squamous epithelium and mature metaplastic epithelium assume a transient mahogany-brown color following Lugol's iodine application. Although maximum glycogen deposition in squamous epithelium is seen in the late follicular phase, immediately prior to ovulation, the brown color response varies little in fully estrogenized women.[18] When positive, the iodine color changes persist for a longer duration than does the more abbreviated white color modification noted following application of 5% acetic acid to other epithelia.

Etiology The presence of intracellular glycogen determines iodine absorption within tissues. Iodine

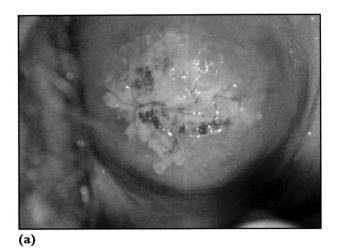

(a)

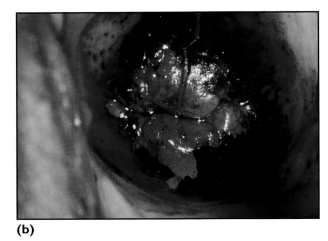

(b)

FIGURES 8.46a,b Mature metaplastic epithelium **(a)** appears pink following 5% acetic acid application. Since it contains glycogen it stains a rich mahogany brown color **(b)**. The iodine negative areas that are yellow represent immature metaplastic epithelium following Lugol's iodine solution application **(b)**.

has an affinity for glycogen. Normal, fully mature metaplastic cells and original squamous cells contain sufficient stores of glycogen and, hence, stain brown, indicating the benign nature of the tissues. Immature metaplastic cells, although benign, reject iodine uptake and consequently appear yellow. Since most neoplastic epithelia have no glycogen, they also stain yellow instead of brown. Just as acetowhite epithelium may denote either benign or neoplastic tissue, Lugol's iodine-negative epithelium may indicate benign or neoplastic tissue.

Colposcopic appearance During the reproductive years, the original squamous epithelium of the cervix and vagina, as well as areas of mature metaplastic epithelium, are well-glycogenated and stain dark brown after the application of Lugol's iodine solution. In contrast, endocervical columnar epithelium and immature metaplastic epithelium do not contain significant amounts of intracellular glycogen and, therefore, appear red or slightly yellow after Lugol's iodine solution is applied (Figures 8.46a,b).

Clinical significance Because Lugol's iodine solution evokes a transient, nonspecific, iodine-negative response, it is not possible to discriminate normal from neoplastic epithelium based only on absence of staining with Lugol's solution alone. Because a yellow color may indicate immature metaplasia, leukoplakia, or neoplasia, other colposcopic signs must be considered to formulate an accurate colposcopic impression. A mahogany-brown color response indicating iodine uptake, however, denotes an invariably benign epithelium, suggesting to the colposcopist

that areas previously expected to be suspicious for neoplasia are of little concern.

8.5.1.3.3 Abnormal cervix

8.5.1.3.3.1 Lugol's iodine-negative and iodine-positive epithelium

Colposcopic appearance Neoplastic epithelium always appears yellow (iodine negative) following application of Lugol's iodine solution. Some large low-grade lesions display a variegated yellow/brown patchy uptake, denoting areas of mild neoplasia intermingled with small areas of normal epithelium. Otherwise, low-grade lesions tend to appear uniformly more orange or darker yellow (Figures 8.47a,b). High-grade lesions can assume a blanched, whitish-yellow color in comparison (Figures 8.48a,b). This variation in yellow color may be appreciated when examining women with large, complex or mixed lesions. Some neoplasias also have a large amount of hyperkeratotic material at the epithelial surface, which turns a characteristic bright yellow color after Lugol's staining. However, attempting to differentiate low-grade CIN from high-grade CIN simply on the basis of variations in the color of iodine-negative epithelium is not productive, as normal immature metaplastic epithelium also appears yellow or iodine negative following Lugol's iodine application.

While iodine-positive epithelium (mahogany brown) is never considered abnormal, normal-appearing brown epithelium may infrequently obscure dysplastic epithelium residing deeply within gland clefts. Iodine-positive epithelium may also cover the entire ectocervix, falsely conveying a "normal" examination to the colposcopist, while iodine-

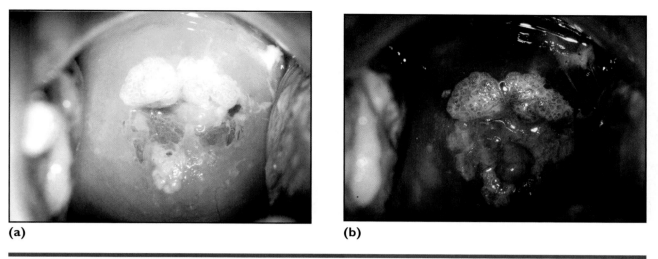

(a)   **(b)**

FIGURES 8.47a,b   An iodine-negative color corresponding to the acetowhite lesions is noted. CIN I **(a)** after 5% acetic acid application and **(b)** following Lugol's iodine application.

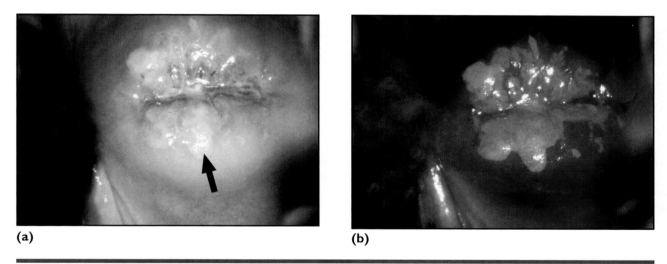

(a)   **(b)**

FIGURES 8.48a,b   A high-grade cervical lesion following **(a)** acetic acid (arrow) and **(b)** Lugol's iodine application. A bland whitish-yellow color indicates the absence of glycogen.

negative abnormal epithelium may be hidden within the endocervical canal or in the vagina.

Clinical significance   Iodine-negative epithelium should be considered along with other colposcopic findings, particularly following 5% acetic acid application, in order to derive a meaningful colposcopic impression. Even though the contrast agents are complementary, not all colposcopists use Lugol's iodine solution routinely. Postmenopausal women and some premenopausal women who use progestin-only contraceptives and are estrogen deficient have little glycogen in the thinner original squamous epithelium and mature metaplastic epithelium. Hence, the atrophic epithelial response to iodine staining will be a light

brown to tan color instead of a positive dark mahogany-brown. This limited uptake can initially be confused with an iodine-negative response. The sharp contrast between iodine-negative and iodine-positive epithelium, consequently, is diminished. A two- to three-week course of estrogen therapy to augment glycogen deposition in normal epithelium will allow for easier discrimination during a repeat colposcopic examination.

Iodine-negative epithelium seen during colposcopy, although not independently predictive of neoplasia, should be considered suspicious in women with abnormal cervical cytologic findings. This is particularly true for older women and women who have had prior therapy for cervical neoplasia and in whom the SCJ is located within the endocervical canal. Typically, neoplastic iodine-negative epithelium will correspond to areas of acetowhite epithelium (Figures 8.47, 8.48). Both 5% acetic acid and Lugol's iodine react well on the cervix of fully estrogenized women, but Lugol's iodine seems to deliver a more distinct contrast between normal and abnormal vaginal epithelia.

Use of Lugol's iodine solution may be useful when the findings of the colposcopic examination are discordant (i.e., the Pap smear indicates significant dysplasia, but the colposcopic examination using 5% acetic acid is unable to detect similar disease). For example, occasionally, a significant iodine-negative lesion is observed colposcopically on the cervix when no acetowhite lesion can be appreciated. In these rare cases, the source of cytologic abnormality is identified only by use of Lugol's iodine solution.

Since acetowhite effects are generally more difficult to appreciate, Lugol's iodine solution is also particularly helpful in evaluating the vagina (Figures 8.49a,b). A careful Lugol's iodine examination of the vagina may identify lesions that explain discordance between a positive cytologic finding and a negative cervical examination. Therefore, Lugol's iodine examinations of the vagina are critical prior to conization for discordant pathology/colposcopy findings. Lugol's iodine helps to demarcate pertinent tissues before therapy. For example, Lugol's iodine is typically used as an epithelial contrast agent prior to electrosurgical loop excision. All areas that appear yellow (indicating neoplasia and immature metaplasia) must be excised, including an encompassing ring of normal brown epithelium to provide normal margins (Figures 8.50a,b).

Although staining with Lugol's iodine solution is helpful in delineating the size and distribution of many lesions and invasive cancers, iodine staining has a number of drawbacks that limit its usefulness. One problem is that a number of non-neoplastic conditions produce nonstaining areas. These include areas of immature metaplasia, regions of hyperkeratosis, congenital transformation zones, and atrophy. Sometimes, the thinly stretched normal mature metaplastic epithelium overlying a Nabothian follicle will appear as an iodine-negative round area with indistinct margins. The same area will not appear white following 5% acetic acid application. The most significant problem is that iodine staining will mask most other colposcopic signs, including the vascular pattern and variations in acetowhite color. Vascular patterns are critical to the recognition of invasive cancers. Therefore, Lugol's iodine staining should be performed only after a careful colposcopic assessment has been performed using saline and 5% acetic acid.

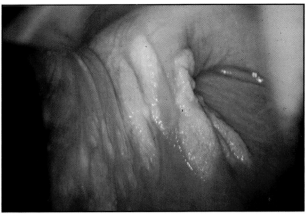

(a)

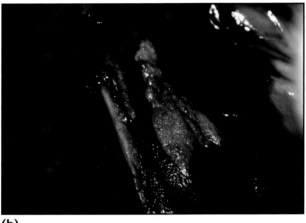

(b)

FIGURES 8.49a,b This woman's cervix appeared normal with colposcopic examination. However, her Pap smear was reported as LSIL. Examination of the vagina using **(a)** 5% acetic acid and **(b)** Lugol's solution detected the source of the abnormal cytologic findings.

If Lugol's solution is to be applied to the cervix prior to biopsy, colposcopists must visually remember the most abnormal area in order to direct biopsy placement. If necessary, topical benzocaine gel can be used to quickly remove iodine from glycogen-containing epithelium.

8.5.2 Vasculature

8.5.2.1 Background

Blood vessels of various types can be observed easily through high-power magnification (10× to 15×) of the colposcope (Figure 8.51). The specific vessel pattern, vessel caliber, and intercapillary distance between these vessels help differentiate normal from abnormal vessels.[19] Because of the vasoconstrictive

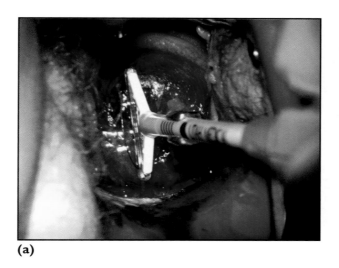
(a)

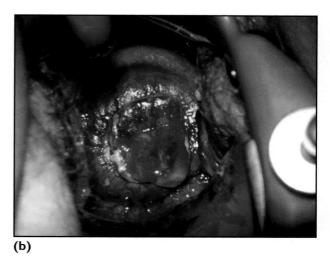
(b)

FIGURES 8.50a,b   All yellow iodine-negative areas of the cervix **(a)** are excised using the loop electrode. After removing the specimen **(b)**, no iodine-negative areas are seen indicating that all immature metaplasia and neoplasia have been removed from the ectocervix.

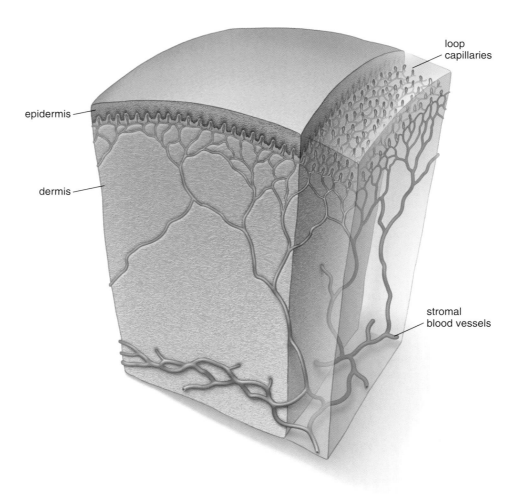

FIGURE 8.51   The vascular supply to the cervical epithelium. Small loop capillaries terminate in the lower one third of squamous epithelium.

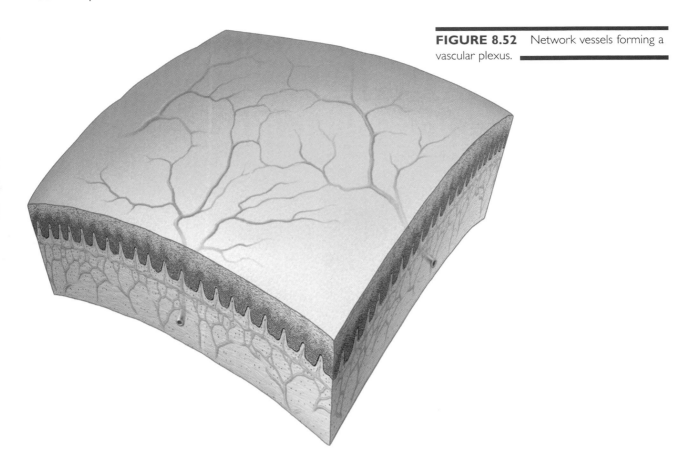

FIGURE 8.52 Network vessels forming a vascular plexus.

effects of 5% acetic acid, vessels are best studied after the application of normal saline and before 5% acetic is applied. Although a 5% acetic acid application may transiently diminish the vascular pattern, the ensuing vessel contrast against a white background often enhances colposcopic inspection of vessels. Vessel visualization may be accentuated by use of the colposcope's green filter, which causes the red vessels to appear black. The resulting contrast between the black vessels and the light green background highlights small delicate vessels that might otherwise blend into the pink background. At times, abnormal vessels resemble normal vessels. Normal vessels may also mimic abnormal vessels. In order to identify alterations in blood vessels and vascular patterns that are most indicative of disease, colposcopists must recognize vascular patterns that occur under normal conditions.

8.5.2.2 Vasculature of the normal cervix

As outlined in Chapter 2 (The Normal Cervix), the original squamous epithelium has two types of blood vessels, referred to as network and hairpin capillaries.[3,4] Network vessels form a vascular plexus that lies in the submucosal stroma beneath the basement membrane (Figure 8.52). When viewed

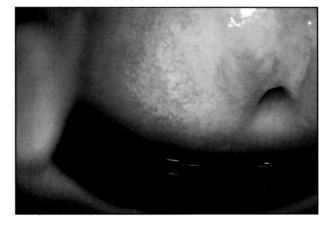

FIGURE 8.53 Network vessels of the normal cervix, demonstrating a fine reticular network of small terminal vessels that are haphazardly arranged. Photo courtesy of Dr. Kenneth L. Noller.

through the colposcope, the vascular plexus appears as a fine reticular network of small terminal vessels that are haphazardly arranged (Figure 8.53). The network vessels underlying the original squamous epithelium are most prominent when they become hyperemic and dilated during pregnancy or as a result of cervicovaginal infections. Additionally, these vessels are seen readily in patients who take oral contraceptives and when connective tissue papillae extending into the squamous epithelium decrease in height, as in postmenopausal women. Under these conditions, the vessels appear to form vascular pseudo-anastomoses, which can be seen under the squamous epithelium (Figure 8.54). The second type of vessels, hairpin terminal vessels, extend toward the epithelial surface in the connective tissue papillae. These vessels have both afferent (arterial) and efferent (venous) branches (Figure 8.55). When viewed along the vessel axis, they appear as fine red dots or punctation. When viewed obliquely, the afferent and efferent capillaries resemble hairpins or fine loops. Capillaries in normal epithelium are closely spaced and uniformly distributed. The intercapillary distance ranges from 50 μm to 250 μm with an average distance of 100 μm.[19].

The vessels underlying the metaplastic epithelium of the transformation zone vary depending on the degree of maturation of the transformation zone. In zones of immature metaplasia, prominent long parallel vessels or branched vessels that are oriented radially to the external os are often seen (Figures 8.56a,b,c,d). Parallel vessels are somewhat dilated and course horizontally for rather long distances near the surface of the epithelium. Branched vessels taper along their course and have a regular or orderly appearance. Branches from the long terminal vessels usually

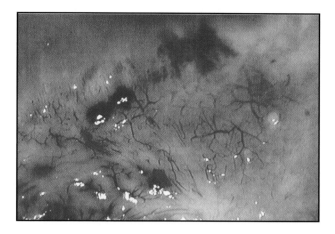

FIGURE 8.54 Network vessels demonstrating psuedoanastamoses beneath the squamous epithelium. ▬▬

FIGURE 8.55 Hairpin terminal vessels obliquely oriented toward the surface of the epithelium, demonstrating afferent and efferent capillary loops. ▬▬

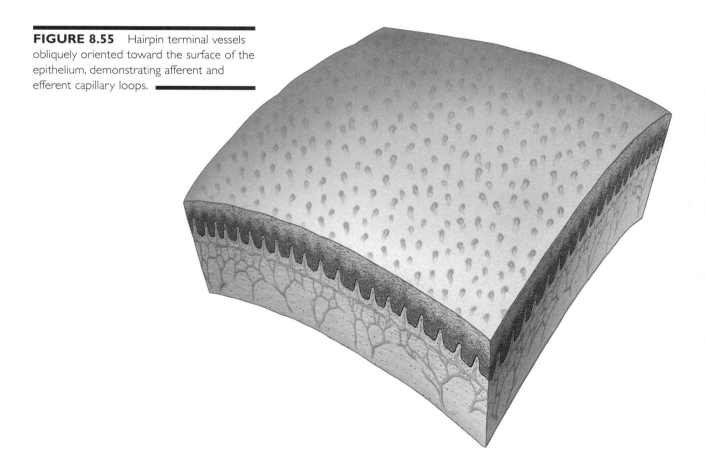

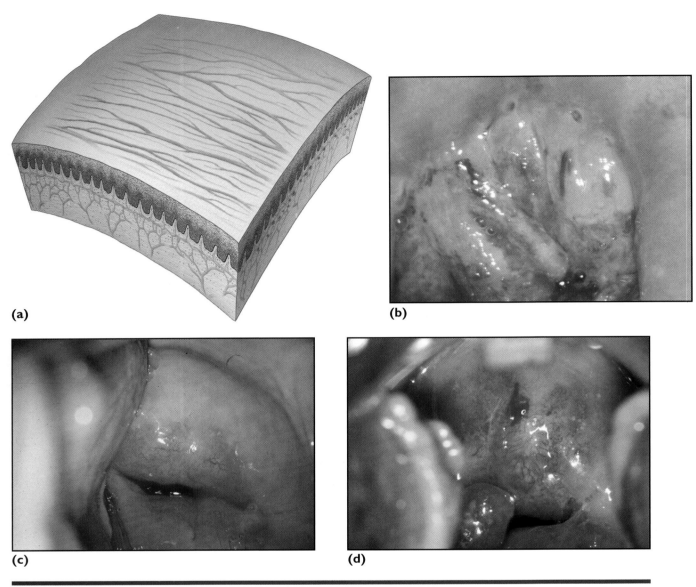

(a)

(b)

(c)

(d)

FIGURES 8.56a–d   **(a)** Long parallel blood vessels usually seen in **(b)** immature metaplasia. **(c,d)** Branched vessels are also more commonly seen in immature metaplasia.

emerge at an acute angle, much like branches projecting from a tree trunk. These branches have a smaller diameter than the parent vessel. Each succeeding branching vessel is of a smaller caliber (Figure 8.57). At the end of the long terminal vessels, a network of fine capillaries that have a normal intercapillary distance can be seen. These tree-like branched vessels can be observed, greatly dilated, overlying Nabothian cysts or cervical polyps (Figures 8.58a,b). In addition to long terminal vessels, the transformation zone also has network vessels under the surface epithelium, and hairpin capillaries that can project into stromal papillae of the maturing metaplastic epithelium in a manner similar to that seen in the original squamous epithelium.

The vessels of the endocervix consist of afferent and efferent loops of terminal vessels that extend toward the surface in the lamina propria of each of the columnar cell-covered endocervical villi. When viewed tangentially at high magnification, these vessels also appear as hairpin loops. Endocervical vessels are not easily discerned by casual colposcopic inspection, however, especially if viewed end-on.

8.5.2.3 Specific vasculature
8.5.2.3.1 Punctation
Definition   The term *punctation* is used to refer to the appearance of single-looped terminal capillaries

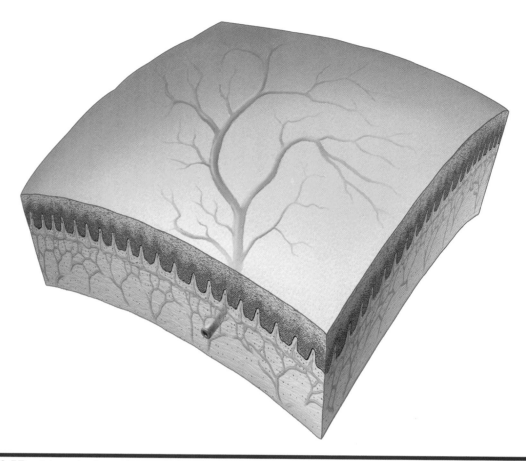

FIGURE 8.57   A branched vessel appears much like a tree with a trunk, branches and twigs. The caliber of the vessels gradually constrict towards the terminal vessels.

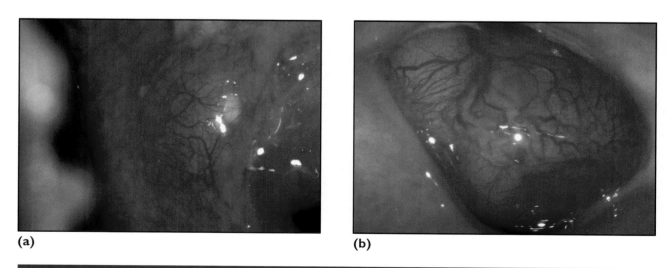

(a)   **(b)**

FIGURES 8.58a,b   Tree-like vessels greatly dilated overlying **(a)** a Nabothian cyst and **(b)** a cervical polyp.

within stromal papillae of either the original squamous epithelium or the transformation zone. These twisted vessels run perpendicularly or obliquely toward the epithelial surface. The vessels are a variation of hairpin capillaries. When viewed end-on (longitudinally) through the attenuated epithelium overlying them, these capillaries appear as reddish points or dots. The stippled appearance of punctation corresponds to the tops of simple or complex capillary loops. Punctation was formerly referred to as "grund der Leukoplaki" or "ground structure."[5] Most colposcopists currently classify punctation as being either fine punctation or coarse punctation, depending on the vessel caliber.

Etiology   Punctation is a nondiagnostic colposcopic finding, since it may represent either a normal vascular pattern or an abnormal modification of existing vascular architecture. All normal cervices have stromal papillae containing single-looped capillaries both within the original squamous epithelium and within the metaplastic epithelium of the transformation zone. Vessels within the stromal papillae extend within the lower third of the epithelium to perfuse differentiating cells. The stromal papillae observed in the original squamous epithelium are formed during embryogenesis and remain throughout life. When cervicitis is present, especially when it is associated with *Trichomonas vaginalis* infection, the hairpin capillaries become dilated and appear to extend higher into the connective tissue papillae, immediately underneath the surface. Marked inflammation, such as that induced by *Trichomonas vaginalis*, will often result in hairpin capillaries with two or more loops at the top. This particular manifestation of hairpin capillaries has been referred to as staghorn or double-capillaries (Figure 8.59). When present on the cervix, others have called the resulting appearance the "strawberry" cervix. Punctation secondary to inflammation is diffuse or clustered in distribution and usually not confined within sharply bordered areas (Figures 8.60a,b,c,d,e). However, it should be noted that

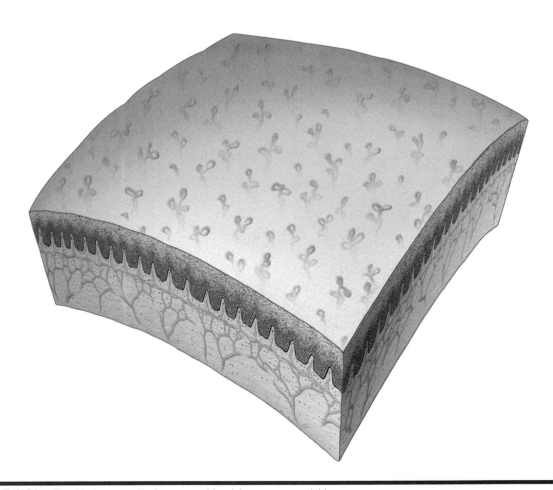

FIGURE 8.59   Double-loop capillaries seen with trichomonas cervicitis.

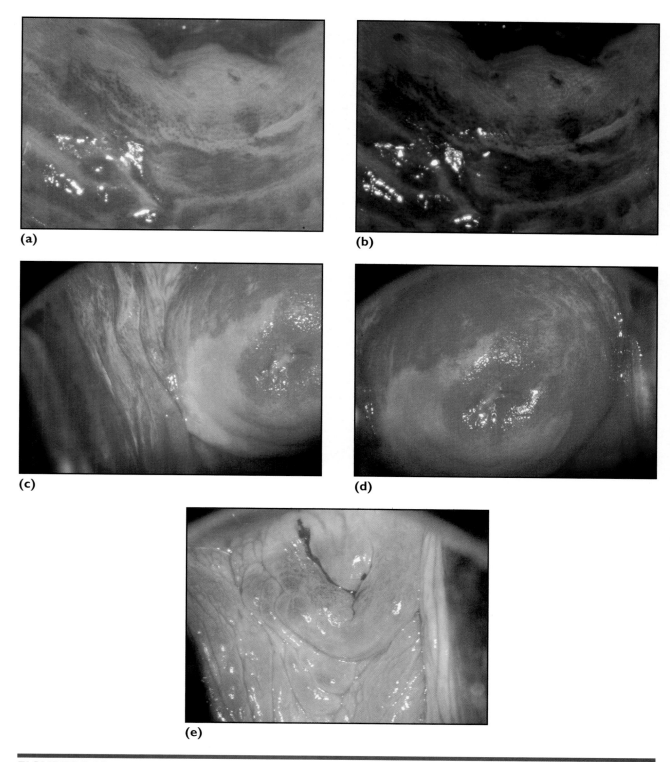

FIGURES 8.60a–e   Staghorn hairpin loop capillaries associated with *Trichomonas vaginalis* infection of the cervix. These diffuse punctate vessels are seen **(a)** without and **(b)** with use of the green filter. In another patient, diffuse punctuation is noted in the vagina **(c)** and on the cervix **(d)** caused by an inflammatory process. The last patient also has a diffuse vascular inflammatory response on the cervix and in the vagina **(e)**.

double capillaries can also be observed in regions of high-grade lesions (CIN 2,3).

Punctation occurring in the transformation zone is derived from hairpin capillaries in stromal papillae that invaginate perpendicular to the epithelial surface. In the transformation zone, these papillae arise during the development of squamous metaplasia. Prior to the development of squamous metaplasia, the region that will become the transformation zone is covered by columnar villi, each of which have a central afferent and efferent loop capillary. During the transformation process, the clefts or folds between the villi become filled by immature metaplastic epithelium (Figures 8.8c,d). Initially, the original afferent and efferent capillary loop remains central within each villus. As the clefts fill with metaplastic epithelium, the vessels and encompassing stroma develop into stromal papillae, similar to those of the original squamous epithelium. The vessels in the stromal papillae adjacent to the blocks of immature metaplastic squamous epithelium can appear as a fine vascular punctation pattern when viewed through the colposcope. When examined histologically, the epithelium usually demonstrates "epithelial pegs" with adjacent prominent stromal papillae that are elongated and extend almost to the epithelial surface. The "epithelial pegs" are of a variable width and often branch. The immature metaplastic epithelium usually forms a sharp histologic junction with mature metaplastic epithelium. This explains why regions of punctation, even when associated with normal epithelium, are usually sharply delineated colposcopically within contrasting acetowhite epithelium. As regions of metaplastic epithelium mature, the stromal papillae become less prominent, more flattened, and extend for a shorter distance toward the epithelial surface. These alterations eliminate the punctation vascular pattern seen in mature metaplastic epithelium.

The punctation that occurs in regions of neoplasia can be thought of as an accentuation of the process by which fine punctation arises in the transformation zone during the development of squamous metaplasia (Figure 8.61a). Proliferating blocks of neoplastic epithelium may cause compression of these vessels. Initially, laterally expanding epithelial compressive forces may impede venous return and cause a dilatation of the loop capillaries (Figure 8.61b). Further growth and epithelial expansion cause complete arterial occlusion of some of the capillaries, now surrounded by expanding cellular blocks of neoplasia, and lateral displacement of

remaining loop capillaries. The resulting obliteration and displacement of some of the central capillaries creates a greater intercapillary distance, or space, between adjoining vessels (Figure 8.61c). The surrounding vessels also dilate more and are referred to as coarse punctation. Histologically, the neoplastic epithelium forms epithelial pegs, that are wider and more irregular than those formed by immature metaplastic epithelium. Between these nests of neoplastic epithelium, tall stromal papillae containing the loop capillaries extend to just beneath the surface.

Punctation occurring in regions of neoplasia can evolve independently of the underlying villous angioarchitecture. For example, it has been suggested that changes of the stroma and blood vessels producing epithelial pegs almost invariably accompany the neoplastic process.[5] This suggestion is based on the fact that punctation is often observed in high-grade neoplastic lesions of the vulva, penis, and vagina, which lack a preexisting papillary endocervical configuration. Furthermore, HPV-induced condylomas at mucosal sites other than the cervix frequently contain punctation. Although controversial, recent evidence suggests that subepithelial angiogenesis may occur in premalignant as well as malignant lesions.[6]

Colposcopic appearance Punctation appears as tiny red dots of variable dimensions usually present within an area of acetowhite epithelium. The acetowhite effect that occurs after the application of acetic acid provides an excellent background against which red punctation is seen. However, when there is a strong acetowhite effect in the surface epithelium, the acetowhite epithelium can reflect so much light that the underlying vascular pattern is obscured. Additionally, 5% acetic acid causes temporary vasoconstriction. Hence, it is easier to initially overlook fine punctation than coarse punctation. In cases wherein the acetowhite effect obscures the vascular pattern, the underlying red vascular pattern will reappear as the acetowhite effects begin to fade, enabling visualization of coarse and particularly fine punctation (Figure 8.62).

In some instances, however, punctation is better seen prior to the application of acetic acid. Although punctation can also be observed after normal saline is applied to the cervix, novice colposcopists may have difficulty observing fine punctation prior to applying acetic acid because of the lack of contrast provided by an acetowhite background. Coarse

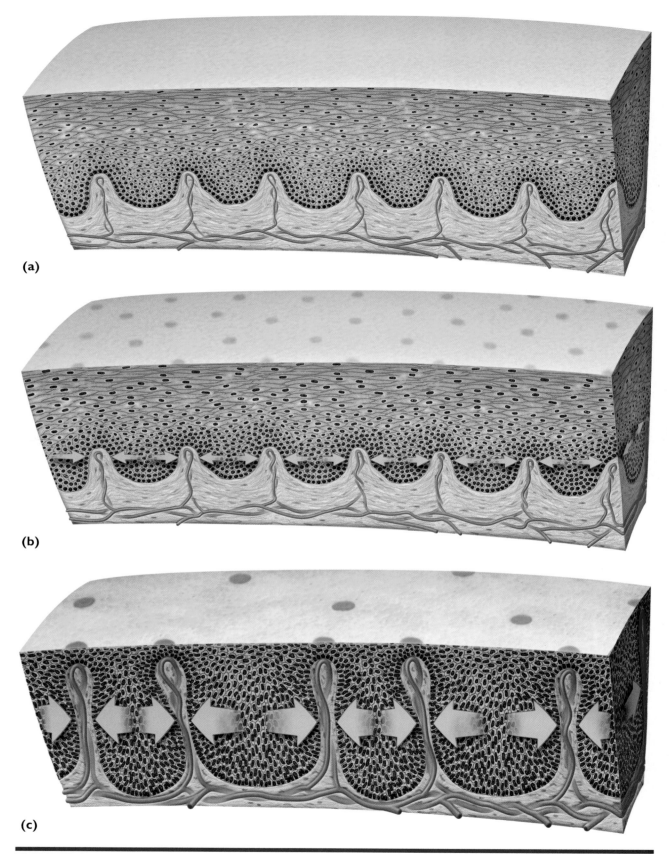

FIGURES 8.61a–c **(a)** Loop capillaries are of normal fine caliber, with uniform distribution and narrow intercapillary spacing prior to any neoplastic process. **(b)** Once neoplastic cells develop, they expand to perhaps exert pressure on these capillaries. Venous occlusion causes the vessels to dilate. With CIN 1, the intercapillary spacing and distribution remain similar to that seen in normal epithelium. However, with CIN 3, the vessels dilate further because of greater venous occlusion. **(c)** As the blocks of neoplastic tissue grow, the vessels are displaced outwards and some arterioles become occluded. Now the intercapillary distance is increased and randomly distributed.

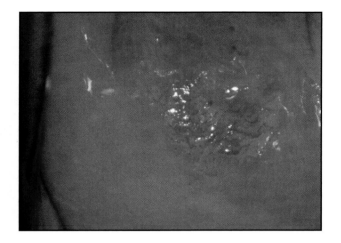

FIGURE 8.62   Fine punctation seen against faintly ace-towhite epithelium.

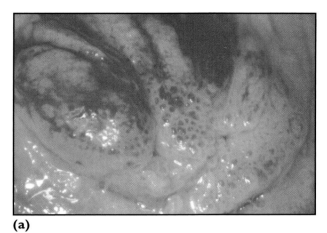

(a)

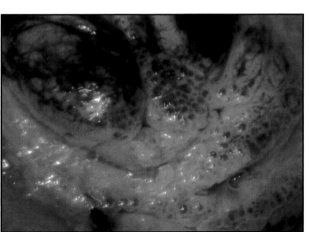

(b)

FIGURES 8.63a,b   **(a)** Coarse punctation of the cervix, demonstrating large-caliber vessels with wide inter-capillary distances. **(b)** These vessels are prominent when viewed using the green filter.

punctation is more readily apparent following saline application to the cervix. The green filter makes it easier to recognize the punctation, which appears as small black dots (Figures 8.63a,b).

Both the size or diameter of punctation (caliber of the loop vessels) and the distance between punctation (intercapillary distance) vary depending on the severity of underlying disease. Usually, as the caliber of the loop capillaries forming punctation increases, so does the intercapillary distance and the severity of the underlying disease.[19,20] Fine punctation is a regular pattern of looped capillaries of narrow diameter, usually closely and uniformly spaced (Figure 8.64). In fine punctation, the intercapillary distance more closely resembles the distances found between villi of the original columnar epithelium (Figures 8.65a,b). Since the distance between each capillary is minimal, fine punctation appears as a delicate stippling when present in a circumscribed acetowhite lesion (Figure 8.66). Fine punctation often occurs together with a fine mosaic vascular pattern (Figure 8.67).

In coarse punctation, the capillaries appear more pronounced because the loop capillaries are dilated and the intercapillary distance is greater. Furthermore, coarse punctation is more irregularly or chaotically spaced (Figure 8.68). The intercapillary distances in normal epithelium rarely (1.8%) measure more than 300 μm.[19] With progressive severity of neoplasia, the percentage of capillaries found to be separated by greater than 300 μm increases significantly. In CIN 3 lesions, 57% of vessels exhibit intercapillary distances of more than 300 μm.[19]

These coarse, dilated capillary loops are usually evident to experienced colposcopists prior to acetic acid application. After acetic acid application, very dilated capillaries (papillary punctation) may appear to project above the surface of the surrounding, densely acetowhite epithelium. The dilated capillaries are separated from each other by randomly wide intercapillary distances (Figure 8.69). Microinvasion should be considered when these large diameter vessels also visibly dilate above the surface of the epithelium, rendering a pin-cushion—like surface. These vessels individually reflect the tangential colposcope light to resemble a field of tiny white stars. Evaluation of this papillary punctation at higher colposcopic magnification may reveal tiny

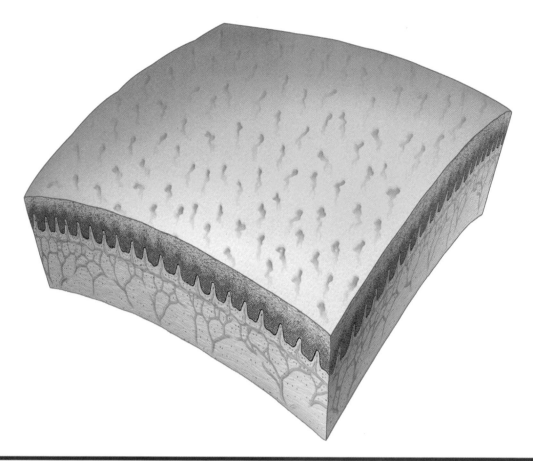

FIGURE 8.64   Fine caliber punctation demonstrating a uniformly spaced pattern in CIN 1. The intercapillary distance is considered narrow.

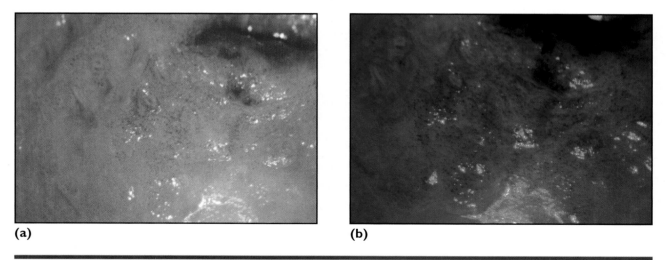

(a)

(b)

FIGURES 8.65a,b   **(a)** Fine punctation of the cervix seen following acetic acid application. Punctation enhanced by use of the green filter **(b)**.

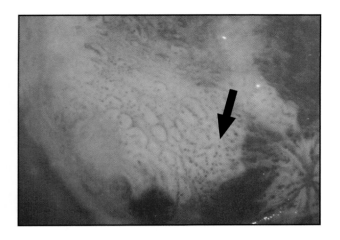

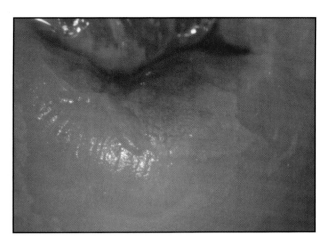

FIGURE 8.66 Fine punctation (arrow) of the cervix following acetic acid application. Acetowhite epithelium makes a good background to contrast the vessel changes. ━━

FIGURE 8.67 Fine punctation vascular pattern. ━━

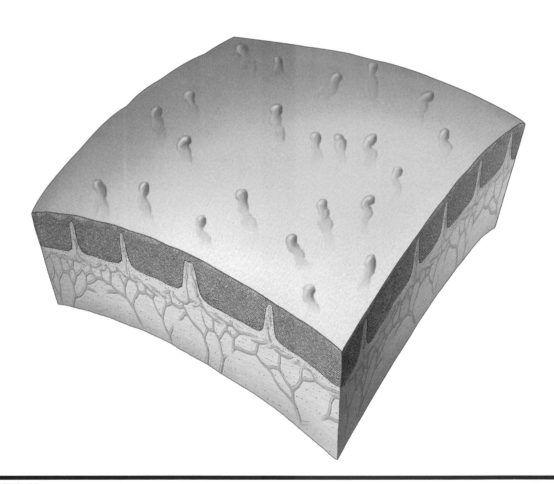

FIGURE 8.68 Coarse punctation with dilated loop capillaries, randomly distributed vessels and a wide intercapillary distance. ━━

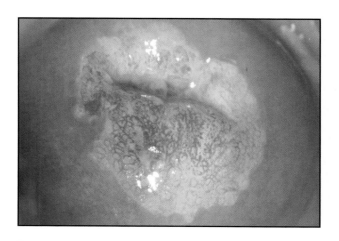

FIGURE 8.69   Coarse punctation demonstrating irregularly spaced vessels.

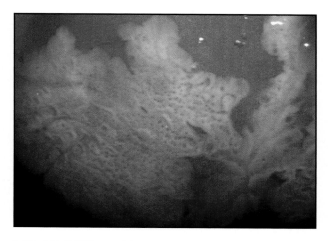

FIGURE 8.71   Fine punctation observed in an area of immature metaplasia that mimics a low-grade squamous intraepithelial lesion.

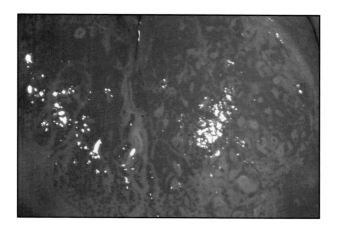

FIGURE 8.70   A coarse punctation and coarse mosaic vessel pattern in a patient with CIN 3.

corkscrew-shaped capillaries, not to be confused with atypical blood vessels. Coarse punctation often occurs together with a coarse mosaic vascular pattern (Figure 8.70).

Clinical significance Punctation was originally described when vascular changes were observed following removal of the keratin layer overlying invasive cancer. Therefore, early colposcopists equated punctation with the matrix of cancer. Punctation became a key criterion for defining the atypical transformation zone, which was erroneously considered to be a unique entity with malignant potential. Today, most colposcopists recognize that the vascular changes of punctation can occur in normal epithelium, inflammatory epithelium, and the full spectrum of squamous neoplasia. Therefore, it is not simply the presence or absence of punctation but

rather vessel caliber, uniformity of distribution, and intercapillary distance of punctation that predict disease severity.

Fine punctation can occur in a variety of conditions, including immature metaplasia, congenital transformation zones, infections, and low-grade lesions (CIN 1). When fine punctation is caused by inflammation, the punctation is diffuse without borders, and neither the application of 5% acetic acid nor that of Lugol's iodine will demonstrate a well-defined lesion (Figures 8.60a,b). Biopsy is usually required to exclude low-grade lesions, particularly if the patient has been referred for the evaluation of an abnormal Pap smear. When fine punctation is confined to an abnormal acetowhite lesion within a field of immature metaplasia, it is usually indicative of a low-grade lesion (CIN 1)(Figure 8.71). When fine punctation is confined to an abnormal acetowhite lesion on the original squamous epithelium, it may represent either a HPV-induced lesion or a variation of the normal metaplastic process.

A vascular pattern of coarse punctation usually indicates a high-grade lesion, or CIN 2,3 (Figure 8.72, Figures 8.73a,b), and possibly early invasion. Microinvasion should always be considered when the capillaries of coarse punctation visibly dilate at the surface of a high-grade CIN or sprout a small side vessel resembling a tadpole. However, most CIN 2,3 demonstrates neither coarse punctation nor coarse mosaic. Instead, most high-grade lesions have no colposcopically apparent vessels. In fact, the absence of vessels noted within a densely opaque acetowhite lesion generally denotes the presence of carcinoma in-situ (see Chapter 9). Frequently, a complex vessel pattern may be seen in CIN 3 lesions in which coarse

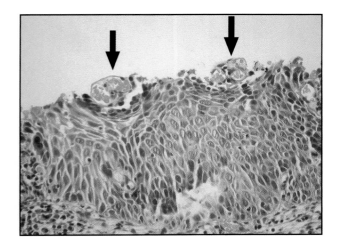

FIGURE 8.72 Histophotograph of punctation (arrow) within a cervical neoplasm (Hematoxylin-eosin stain; medium power magnification). These vessels appear very dilated. ▄▄

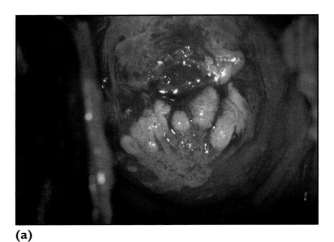

(a)

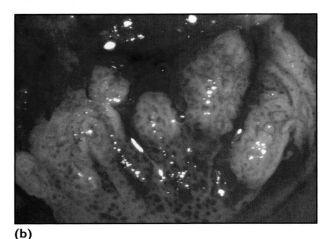

(b)

FIGURES 8.73a,b **(a)** Coarse punctation associated with a high-grade squamous intraepithelial lesion. **(b)** With closer inspection, these vessels are randomly distributed and have a wide intercapillary distance. ▄▄

punctation is intermingled with areas with a coarse mosaic pattern or without vessels.

8.5.2.3.2 Mosaic

Definition The term *mosaic* refers to a vascular pattern produced when capillaries in stromal papillae are arranged parallel to the epithelial surface and form a basket-like structure around blocks or pegs of epithelium. When viewed through the surface epithelium overlying the stromal papillae, the vessels form a chicken-wire or honeycomb pattern encompassing blocks of acetowhite epithelium, resulting in a mosaic tile or cobblestone-like appearance (Figures 8.74a–c). Mosaic (*felderung* in German) was initially considered to be a pathologic finding. However, it is now realized that although mosaic is an important attribute of neoplastic epithelium, it may also be seen in normal immature metaplastic epithelium. In current colposcopic terminology, mosaic is subdivided into fine mosaic and coarse mosaic, depending on vessel caliber and intercapillary spacing.

Etiology Like punctation, mosaic may occur in either a normal pattern or an abnormal modification of preexisting, normal vascular architecture. The etiology of punctation and mosaic are similar. Both develop from single-looped hairpin capillaries within stromal papillae adjacent to epithelial pegs of immature squamous metaplasia or neoplastic squamous epithelium in the transformation zone. As mosaic develops, the epithelial pegs remain discrete; it is the stromal papillae encompassing the loop capillaries that interconnect to form a peripheral vascular rim around the isolated pegs. When the epithelium is cut parallel to the surface of epithelium, the connected vessels can be observed histologically as separated from each other by plates of stroma.

The formation of mosaic has been studied extensively by Kolstad and Stafl,[4] who described three different patterns of mosaic, each of which represents a variation in the way stromal vessels encompass the adjacent avascular epithelial fields. One pattern arises when rows of hairpin capillaries coursing perpendicular to the epithelial surface form avascular epithelial fields (Figure 8.75). This pattern typically produces a fine mosaic and is most commonly associated with immature metaplasia or CIN 1. Another pattern is formed when relatively thin-caliber terminal vessels run parallel to the surface and surround endocervical gland openings in large areas of normal immature metaplasia. The third pattern, which is associated with neoplasia, is formed when terminal vessels in the stromal papillae produce a "basket-like" network around epithelial pegs. The terminal vessels tend to be dilated and irregular in caliber and the epithelial

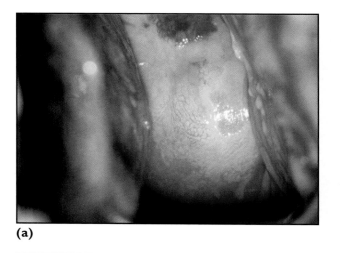

(a)

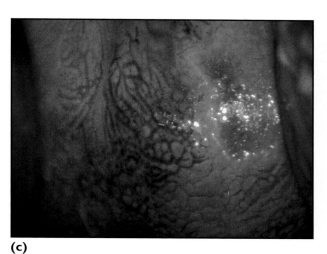

(b)

FIGURES 8.74a–c **(a)** Mosaic vessels of the cervix, demonstrating blocks of acetowhite epithelium surrounded by blood vessels in a honeycomb or chicken wire pattern. **(b,c)** This vascular pattern is readily seen by use of a green filter.

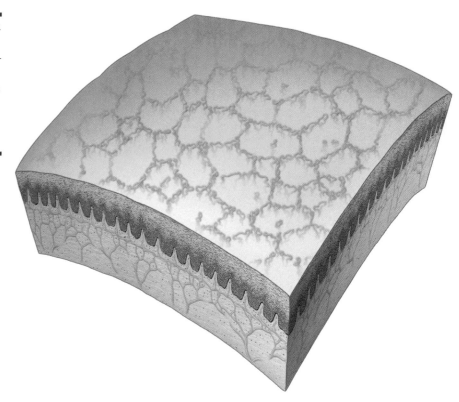

(c)

FIGURE 8.75 One example of a fine mosaic pattern wherein rows of hairpin capillaries coursing perpendicular to the epithelial surface produce a central avascular epithelial field. This pattern is seen in immature metaplasia and CIN 1. The intercapillary distance is narrow and the vascular distribution is uniform.

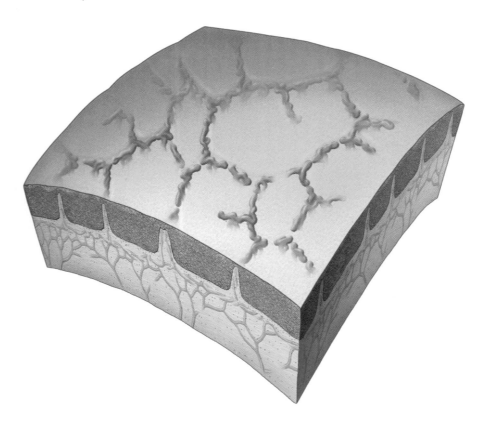

FIGURE 8.76　Mosaic vascular pattern seen in CIN 3. The vessels are dilated, the intercapillary distance is increased and the vascular distribution is quite random. ━━

pegs composed of neoplastic epithelium are typically large and irregular in shape. The process produces the coarse mosaic that is associated with high-grade lesions (CIN 2,3) and microinvasive carcinoma (Figure 8.76). It is possible that enlarging epithelial pegs exert compressive and occlusive forces on the surrounding vessels. Pronounced compressive forces from expanding blocks of dysplasia may obliterate some small arterioles and laterally displace others. Vessels may also dilate when low-level venous capillary compression occludes blood flow return. Therefore, vessels may dilate, occlude, or be displaced depending on how the venous or arterial capillaries are affected by varying levels of pressure and forces exerted by the expanding blocks of neoplastic epithelium.

Colposcopic appearance　Mosaic vasculature appears colposcopically as a red tile-like, polygonal grid viewed within an area of acetowhite epithelium (Figures 8.77a,b,c,d). The small blocks of epithelium, or epithelial pegs, encompassed by the mosaic vessels vary in size, shape, and uniformity. The intercapillary distances between mosaic vessels vary depending on the severity of neoplasia. In general, as vessel caliber and intercapillary distance increase, the severity of neoplasia also increases. More nonuniformly shaped epithelial blocks surrounded by mosaic vessels also appear as neoplasias become increasingly

more severe. Although definitive diagnosis requires biopsy, the type of mosaic pattern, when considered with other abnormal colposcopic signs, assists in clinically predicting the state of disease (Figures 8.78a,b). Mosaic vessels are present in both normal and abnormal epithelium. A mosaic vessel pattern may be detected in a normal congenital transformation zone, in normal immature metaplasia or in cervical lesions of any level of neoplasia. Mosaic vessels are categorized colposcopically as fine or coarse, based on their diameter. Because 5% acetic acid exerts a vasoconstrictive response soon after application, vessel caliber classification is made prior to its application or as the acetic acid effects wane (Figure 8.79).

A fine mosaic pattern is a closely interwoven, lacy, delicate network of capillaries of nearly normal caliber, dispersed perpendicularly in stromal ridges resembling red grouting between small white ceramic tiles. A uniformly consistent small intercapillary distance may be seen with immature metaplasia, a congenital transformation zone (Figures 8.45a,b), and CIN 1 lesions (Figures 8.80a,b). These narrow diameter vessels are usually not apparent by colposcopic examination prior to acetic acid application. The network of pale, narrow red lines confined within an area of acetowhite epithelium may not display a mosaic pattern throughout, and thus, the pattern

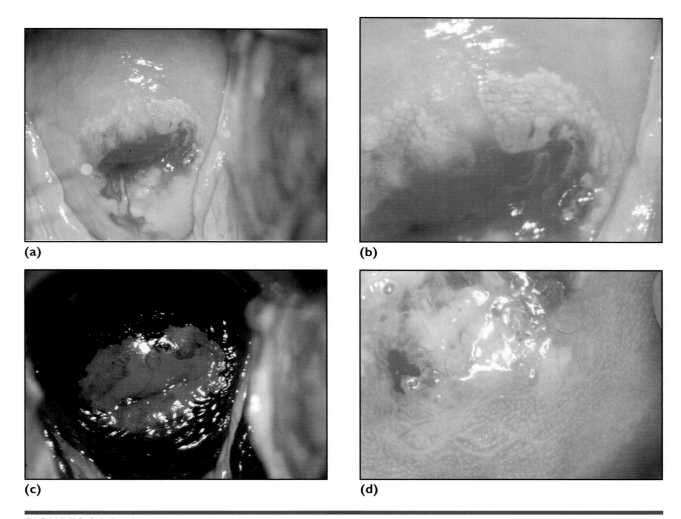

FIGURES 8.77a–d   A mosaic pattern is seen against acetowhite epithelium **(a,b)**. However, this vascular pattern is not seen following the application of Lugol's iodine solution **(c)**. The developmental stages of a mosaic pattern can be seen in **(d)**. A translucent acetowhite low-grade lesion with a fine mosaic pattern lies along the SCJ. In the periphery, a fine mosaic can be seen but no acetowhite epithelium. Beyond this area, small fine punctate vessels associated with a subclinical HPV infection are noted. Some of these vessels are arranged in a linear pattern that will start the development of a mosaic. The other vessels appear diffusely and randomly arranged.

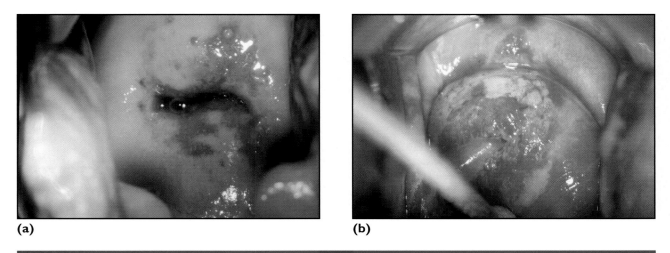

FIGURES 8.78a,b   **(a)** Several areas of mosaic on the posterior lip of the cervix are seen. **(b)** A very small but coarse mosaic vessel pattern is seen in the lesion at 1 to 2 o'clock.

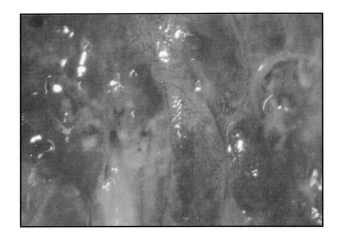

FIGURE 8.79 A very fine mosaic vascular pattern is noted following 5% acetic acid application. These vessels are nearly indistinct. ▬▬▬

may be interrupted and scattered. Coexisting areas of punctation may intermingle among the mosaic patterns. A solitary punctate capillary is sometimes seen surrounded by a mosaic vessel pattern. Colposcopists have used the term *umbilication* to describe this.

A coarse mosaic vascular pattern is characterized by dilated, varicose vessels that enclose larger diameter, irregularly shaped mosaic epithelial blocks (Figure 8.76). The abnormal coarse vascular pattern is also confined invariably to a well-demarcated, dense acetowhite lesion. This mosaic network of capillaries is more pronounced and is an intense red color; it may be seen readily during some colposcopic examinations using saline (Figures 8.81a,b). The epithelial pegs between the vessels are larger and more varied in shape, reflecting irregularity and an increase in

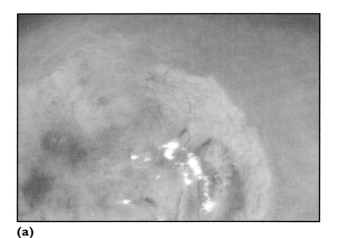

(a)

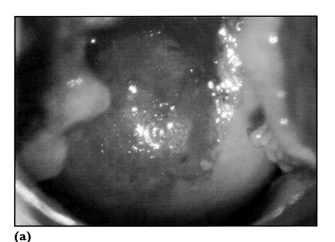

(a)

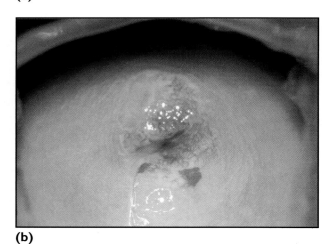

(b)

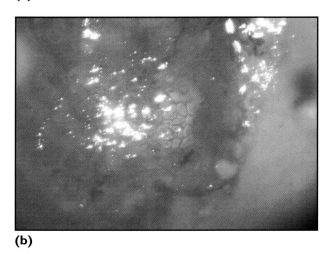

(b)

FIGURES 8.80a,b A fine mosaic pattern is seen against an acetowhite background in these two patients. ▬▬▬

FIGURES 8.81a,b A mosaic vascular pattern of the cervix seen at low and high magnification following saline application. The vessels are not as clearly recognized prior to the application of 5% acetic acid. ▬▬▬

intercapillary distance (Figures 8.82a,b). A wide, irregular, nonuniform intercapillary distance and coarse-caliber vessels would be typical of a mosaic pattern seen with CIN 3 (Figure 8.83). Mosaic vessels associated with CIN 3 are occasionally dilated above the surface plane of surrounding epithelium. When this occurs, a surface topography that appears "pock-marked" can be seen.

Mosaic vessels are generally not seen in frankly invasive cancer but may be in surrounding CIN. Yet, a focal area of microinvasive cancer may erupt within a field of coarse mosaic vessels associated with a high-grade lesion. Careful colposcopic inspection may reveal a microinvasive cancer where the usually regular and uniform mosaic is incomplete or interrupted.

Mosaic vessels are primarily restricted to the cervix and are not usually found in vaginal intraepithelial neoplasia (VAIN). However, a mosaic pattern may be observed in the vagina in women whose congenital transformation zone extends into the vaginal fornices. A mosaic may also be seen in vaginal adenosis undergoing metaplasia; and, a mosaic pattern observed in the vagina may indicate prior in-utero exposure to Diethylstilbesterol (DES).

Clinical significance Mosaic blood vessels are recognized quickly by colposcopists because of the unique capillary arrangement, but the pattern alone has no specific meaning. When appraised critically of capillary diameter, intercapillary distance, and uniformity of spacing, however, the analyzed mosaic provides insight into the nature of the epithelium being inspected. For example, the mean intercapillary distance between mosaic vessels in CIN 2 is significantly less than that seen in CIN 3 (0.06 mm vs. 0.12 mm).[21] Consideration of the distribution of a mosaic vessel pattern further helps to determine the type of epithelium observed. In a study of intercapillary distances measured by computer, the mean perimeter of a mosaic was 0.25 mm for CIN 2 and 0.44 mm for CIN 3.[21] The mosaic network also may be incomplete and patchy, as segments of the mosaic appear to be missing. Large fields of dense acetowhite epithelium may be interposed between sections of a rather loose mosaic arcade with severe neoplasia and early microinvasive cancer.

8.5.2.3.3 Atypical blood vessels

Definition Atypical blood vessels are superficial vessels that exhibit bizarre variation in diameter, course, spacing, and branching patterns when compared with normal blood vessels (Figure 8.84). These vessels are generally very dilated in comparison with other typical capillaries seen on the cervix. They traverse

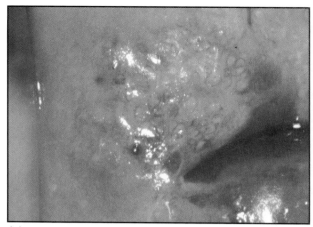

(a)

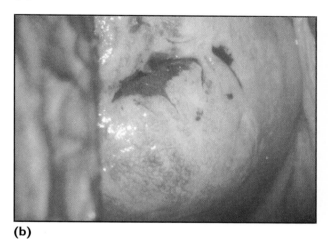

(b)

FIGURES 8.82a,b   A coarse mosaic pattern with a variably wide intercapillary distance and dilated vessels is seen. Both patients had CIN 3.

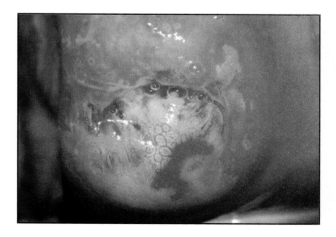

FIGURE 8.83   A coarse mosaic pattern on the posterior lip of the cervix in this woman with CIN 3.

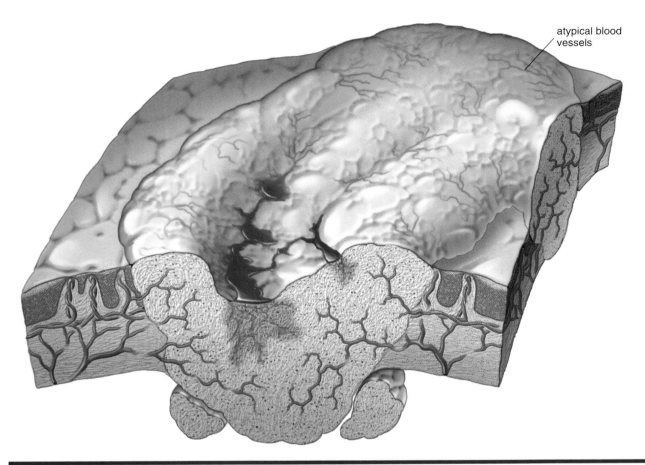

atypical blood vessels

FIGURE 8.84 Atypical blood vessels associated with a cervical cancer. The cancer depicted has contour changes, with both exophytic growth and ulceration due to tissue necrosis.

superficially within the epithelium, often oriented parallel to the surface. Although normal variants may be seen, atypical vessels are most commonly associated with invasive cancer and should be assumed so until proven otherwise by histologic sampling (Figures 8.85a–g).

Etiology Atypical vessels associated with malignancies develop in response to vascular endothelial growth factor and angiogenin, tumor angiogenesis factors (TAF), or substances secreted by cancers. These agents promote endothelial proliferation and capillary formation by stimulating the growth of new vessels necessary to support an enlarging tumor.[9] Elevated levels of vascular endothelial growth factor and angiogenin are seen in tissues only after premalignant lesions have been transformed into cancer.[11,12] Moreover, levels of vascular endothelial growth factor are significantly greater in tumors larger than 4 cm, and those with deep stromal invasion, lymphovascular emboli, parametrial invasion, and pelvic lymph node metastasis.[11] Rapid and uncontrolled growth of solid tumors requires neovascularization.[8] As evidence of neovascularization in the early stages of cancer, histologic specimens from microinvasive cancer contain more stromal microvessels than normal or dysplastic tissue.[9] Cancer spreads in chaotic, unpredictable and random directions, in contrast with normal epithelium. In abnormal epithelium, the supporting vessels must assume abnormally novel routes (Figure 8.86). The rapid cancer growth and accompanying vascular response supercede the usual orderly deposition of blood vessels in normal cervical tissue. Both the development of new vessels and enlargement of existing capillaries characterize the vascular modifications associated with cancer. When cancer growth exceeds the distribution of the existing normal vasculature, neovascularization follows. Consequently, new vessels may be seen within the nodular contour of an exophytic cancer. Deep atypical vessels within an endophytic tumor are not usually transilluminated. In addition, large bore vessels develop to deliver more blood to rapidly proliferating neoplastic tissue. The focal catabolic demand of cancer stimulates creation

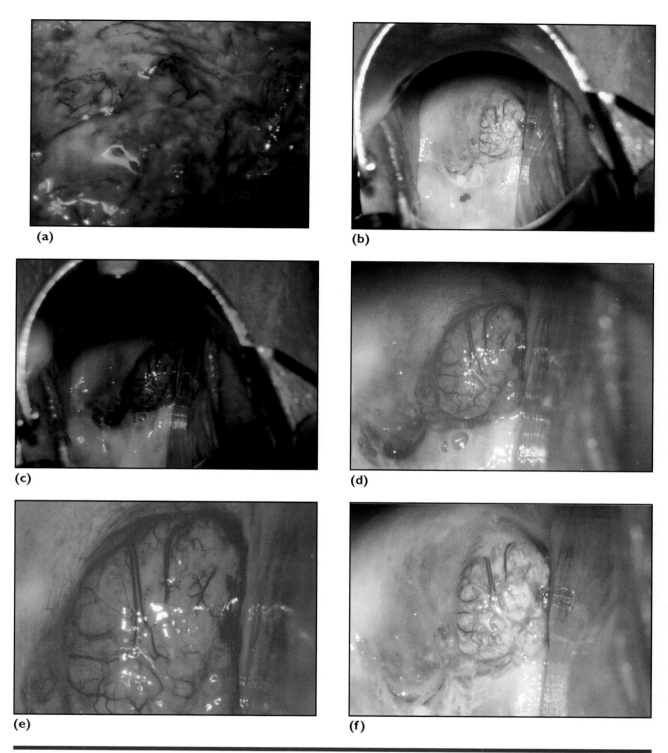

FIGURES 8.85a–g Atypical blood vessels in a squamous cell cancer **(a)**. The next patient has a very rare neuroendocrine cancer seen at 2 o'clock **(b–g)**. The tumor is easily seen at both low **(b,c)** and mid level magnification **(d)** following the application of normal saline. The very long, dilated atypical blood vessels are best appreciated at high magnification **(e)**. Following the application of 5% acetic acid, the epithelium appears opaque acetowhite **(f,g)**.

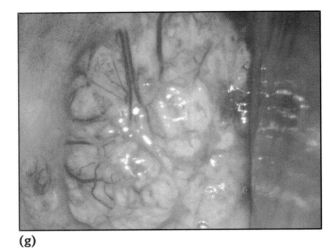

(g)

FIGURES 8.85g Continued.

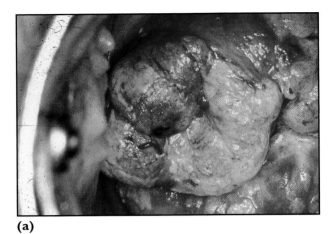

(a)

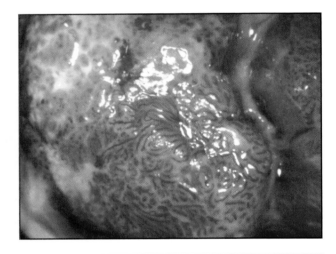

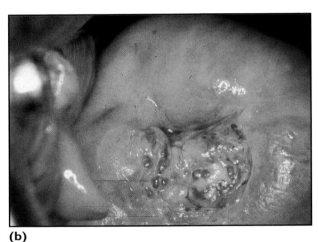

(b)

FIGURES 8.87a,b Very dilated atypical blood vessels located superficially on large exophytic cervical cancers. Photos courtesy of Dr. Vesna Kesic.

FIGURE 8.86 Atypical blood vessels are dilated and do not demonstrate normal branching patterns.

of pipeline-like vessels in an attempt to supply sufficient oxygen and energy to maintain the rapidly expanding tissue. Failure to deliver leads to anoxia and subsequent tissue necrosis. These extremely large-diameter vessels can make abrupt direction changes or traverse straight, prolonged distances.

Colposcopic appearance Blood vessels in benign epithelia branch in a dichotomous or tree-like fashion with wide trunks gradually giving rise to large, then smaller branches, followed by tiny twig-like branches. Terminal branches of atypical vessels often show no uniform taper or gradual decrease in diameter. While usually maintaining an overall varicosity, atypical vessels may display an abrupt change in diameter or irregularly varied caliber. These vessels

also exhibit a noticeably random course, changing direction suddenly. Moreover, atypical vessels are characteristically unique. In exophytic tumors, atypical vessels are superficially positioned and covered by very few cell layers of epithelium (Figures 8.87a,b). As such, these large blood vessels transilluminate readily and may be appreciated at low-power magnification. The vessels remain horizontal to the surface, are frequently elongated, and exhibit minimal branching. When present, the branching is irregularly spaced and varied in branching angle. Intercapillary distances are greater, leaving large avascular epithelial spaces between vessels. Early cancers may demonstrate normal to slightly increased vessel spacing (decreased overall vascularity),[4] whereas advanced cancers usually favor the latter pattern.[19,22] In fact, in invasive cancer, most capillaries (85.5%) are spaced more than 300 µm apart.[19] Furthermore, as the stage of invasive cancer increases, the percentage of cancers

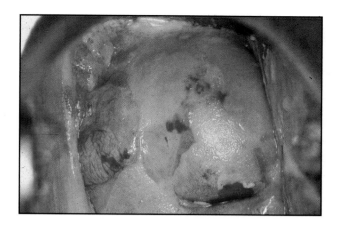

FIGURE 8.88 Elongated spaghetti-like atypical vessels are seen on the right side of the cervix. An opaque CIN 3 lesion without visible vessels covers the majority of the ectocervix. Photograph courtesy of Dr. Vesna Kesic. ▬

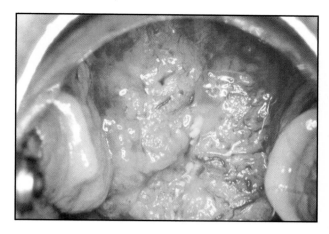

FIGURE 8.89 Very dilated atypical blood vessels are seen to abruptly terminate without tapering or branching in this woman with Adenocarcinoma. Photo courtesy of Dr. Vesna Kesic. ▬

with intercapillary distances greater than 450 μm increases proportionally (Stage I—23.1%, Stage II—36.4%, and Stages III/IV—54.5%).[1,23] In addition to very wide intercapillary spacing, atypical vessels are distributed randomly or nonuniformly.

The number of atypical blood vessels increases as the severity of cancer increases. In early-stage ectocervical cancers, only a few atypical vessels may be noted. Kolstad demonstrated that atypical blood vessels are rare (0.7%) in dysplasia, but more common in CIN 3 (16.7%), microinvasive carcinoma (76.9%), and invasive carcinoma (96.6%).[19] In another study, atypical blood vessels were detected in 2.8% of women with CIN 3, 50% of women with microinvasion, and 92% of women with invasive cancer.[24] Sugimori et al[25] detected atypical blood vessels in 9% of women with CIN 3. A meta-analysis by Hopman et al[13] found atypical blood vessels in 44% of women with microinvasion and 84% of women with invasive cancer. Sillman[24] determined that 82% of women with atypical vessels had invasion. No atypical vessels may be seen colposcopically with endophytic and strictly endocervical cancers.[24]

Atypical blood vessels associated with cancer have been categorized as resembling corkscrews, tadpoles, hairpins, spaghetti, and other unusual configurations (Figure 8.88). The atypical blood vessels of adenocarcinoma have been described (Chapter 11) as resembling tendrils, roots, willow branches, and waste threads.[3,26] Atypical blood vessels, particularly those associated with adenocarcinoma, may arise from alterations of central loop capillaries within columnar villi. Single corkscrew vessels with sharp, tortuous, irregular bends may be associated with

squamous cancers. Branching, network and hairpin atypical vessels, considered variants of normal, are also seen in squamous cancers. Branching vessels may exhibit a fairly prolonged, gently curved or straight course. However, abrupt vessel constriction can occur followed by immediate dilation. Extremely varicose atypical vessels may terminate suddenly without the gradual narrowing seen in normal vessels (Figures 8.89). These vessels may encircle large areas of otherwise avascular appearing epithelium. Network atypical vessels demonstrate variable caliber changes and abrupt side branching of much smaller-caliber vessels (Figures 8.90a–d). A coarse interlaced pattern with large intercapillary distances, various constrictions, and dilations may be seen. Hairpin atypical vessels are dilated, rounded hairpin capillaries. They are usually widely spaced. Depending on their orientation to the surface of the epithelium (vertical, horizontal or tangential), the entire loop may be seen or only portions thereof.

Atypical vessels are described by some as a variance of the normal network, hairpin, and branching blood vessels.[23] However, the pattern of atypical vessels is completely chaotic, with no regularity of the normal vasculature.[27] Succinctly stated, atypical vessels display an unlimited spectrum of expression. A lack of symmetry and uniformity in caliber, branching, and spacing best describe atypical vessels. Chapters 10 and 11 include further discussion of atypical vessels as one of the warning signs for invasive cancer.

Clinical significance Atypical vessels must be considered to be caused by cancer until proven otherwise by biopsy. This is particularly true for atypical vessels

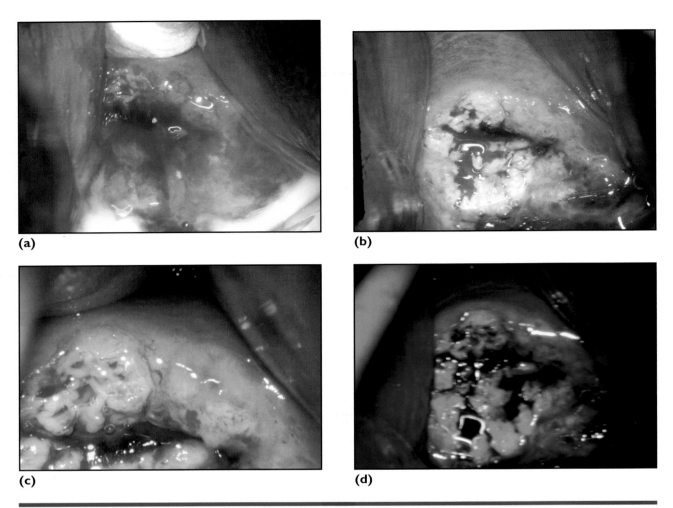

(a)   **(b)**

(c)   **(d)**

FIGURES 8.90a–d   Atypical blood vessels are seen in this patient following **(a)** saline, **(b,c)** 5% acetic acid application, and **(d)** using the green filter.

seen in women with abnormal cervical cytologic find-ings or a history of cervical neoplasia. The presence of other associated abnormal colposcopic signs, along with dense, dull, thickened acetowhite epithelium, ulceration, yellow friable necrotic epithelium and an exophytic mass, strongly implies the malignant nature of observed atypical blood vessels. Novice col-poscopists, fearful of uncontrollable bleeding, fre-quently question whether atypical vessels should be biopsied. Contrary to this concern, atypical vessels and the surrounding epithelium should be sampled without reservation and to a sufficient depth to allow an accurate histologic diagnosis.

There are several causes for benign atypical ves-sels not associated with a malignancy. Occasion-ally, normal atypical vessels may be observed in areas of very early immature metaplasia (Figures 8.91a–d). These vessels are covered by a thin layer of very translucent epithelium. The vessels exhibit

an increased caliber compared with other normal surrounding vessels and may extend parallel to the epithelial surface for rather long distances. Their course is usually fairly straight with minor varia-tion of direction. Tiny vessels may diverge from the main vessel, displaying normal branching of decreasing-caliber capillaries. Absence of other col-poscopic warning signs of cancer, along with a faint, translucent, extremely transient acetowhite background and young patient age, would suggest a benign mimic (Figures 8.92a–c). In addition, atyp-ical vessels are frequently encountered in women who have previously received local radiation ther-apy of the lower genital tract (Figures 8.93a,b). Because the epithelium is usually atrophic and thin, these rather bizarre vessels are readily appar-ent. Since these women also have a history of local cancer, it can be extremely challenging to discrimi-nate postradiation atypical vessels from recurrent

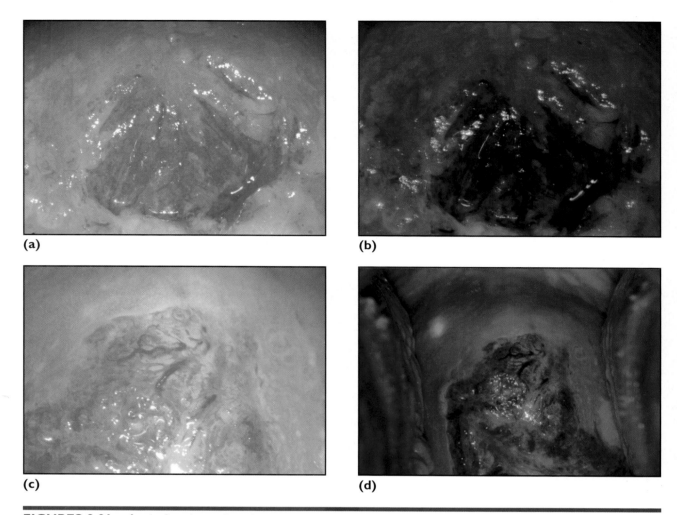

(a)

(b)

(c)

(d)

FIGURES 8.91a–d   At first glance, these large blood vessels in both patients appear to be atypical. However, with closer inspection, the vessels lie in immature metaplastic epithelium and do taper with some branching.

cancer-associated atypical vessels. Again, no evidence of other warning signs for invasive cancer suggests the benign nature of postradiation therapy atypical vessels. Histologic sampling must be done if there is any uncertainty of etiology. Atypical blood vessels may also be seen in decidual tissue associated with pregnancy (Chapter 12). Atypical blood vessels may be seen in tissue undergoing active reparative change, such as that seen during the healing phase following surgery of the cervix (Figures 8.94a,b,c). Finally, very bizarre vessels may be seen in granulation tissue. The reddish tissue color, tissue friability, and raised contour of granulation tissue may make discrimination from cancer difficult. Most granulation tissue is seen in the proximal vaginal cuff area in women following hysterectomy. Histologic confirmation may be particularly warranted in women who have had a hysterectomy for neoplastic indications.

8.5.3 Surface topography

8.5.3.1 Ulceration, erosion

Definition   An ulceration or erosion of the cervix is defined as a focal or multifocal absence of epithelium (Figure 8.84). A well-defined, circumscribed area void of cervical epithelium is noted, and only the underlying papillary or reticular stroma remains visible. Because the term *ulceration* is nearly synonymous with erosion, clinicians often use the terms interchangeably even though an ulceration is deeper than a more superficial erosion. The term *erosion* is also commonly confused with ectropion even though each denotes a distinctly different colposcopic finding, with the latter representing the normal eversion of columnar epithelium on the ectocervix. The two terms may be interchanged mistakenly because both appear colposcopically as red areas of the cervix displaying mildly irregular

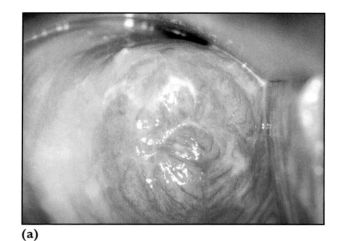

(a)

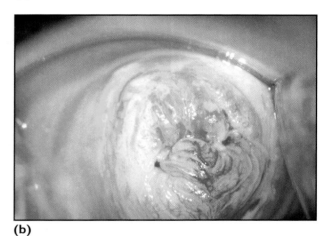

(b)

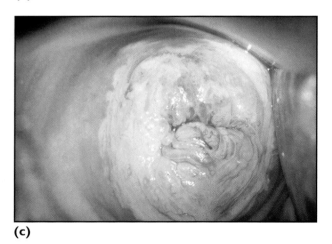

(c)

FIGURES 8.92a–c **(a)** Very dilated non-branching blood vessels are seen on the posterior lip of the cervix during the saline examination. These appear to be atypical vessels. **(b,c)** Following 5% acetic acid application, a large area of acetowhite epithelium is noted. The epithelium of the posterior cervix is translucent white especially in the area of the large vessels. This represents immature metaplasia. It is easy to overlook the opaque acetowhite epithelium at 9 o'clock with coarse punctation that represents CIN 3.

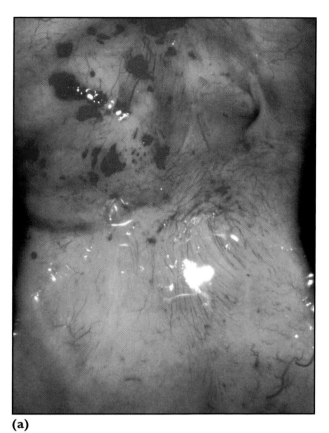

(a)

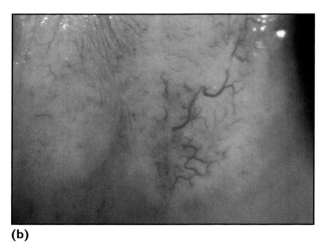

(b)

FIGURES 8.93a,b Atypical blood vessels seen in a woman following radiation therapy of the lower genital tract. The epithelium is atrophic and subcutaneous hemorrhages can be seen. There was no recurrence of cancer.

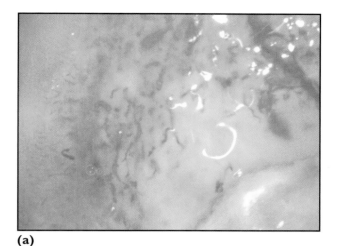

(a)

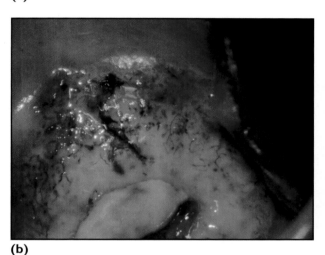

(b)

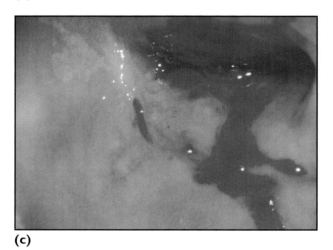

(c)

FIGURES 8.94a–c   These bizarre corkscrew-like blood vessels were seen in a patient approximately two weeks following a loop excision procedure **(a,b)**. The vessels lie in reparative tissue along the wound margin. The next patient **(c)**, has a straight dilated atypical appearing vessel at 8 o'clock. She also has an area of recurrent CIN 1 at 9 o'clock. ▬▬

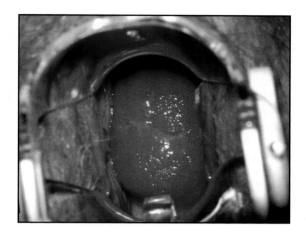

FIGURE 8.95   An ectropion of the cervix or eversion of columnar epithelium onto the ectocervix that is mistaken as an erosion. ▬▬

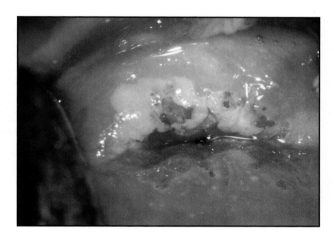

FIGURE 8.96   Ulceration of the cervix demonstrating a well-demarcated area without visible surface epithelium. The ulceration lies within a CIN 3 on the anterior lip of the cervix. ▬▬

contours (Figure 8.95). The red villous projections of an ectropion are rounded, uniform in distribution, and assume a faint acetowhite blush following 5% acetic acid application. The surface is pebbled and has a slightly depressed relationship to the elevated surrounding squamous and metaplastic epithelium. An erosion base may be friable, variably irregular in contour, and nonacetowhite following application of 5% acetic acid. The demarcation between a superficial erosion and surrounding epithelium may be gradual and somewhat imperceptible. In contrast, ulcerations exhibit a rather distinct, recessed, steep interface with the surrounding normal or neoplastic epithelium (Figure 8.96). Both erosions and ectropions may bleed easily following casual contact with moistened cotton applicators. This is especially true when an inflammatory process is present. While an ectropion is considered normal and is found mainly in young women, especially those taking oral contraceptive pills, an erosion is abnormal, just not necessarily neoplastic. In fact, if an erosion is observed in a woman who has a prior abnormal Pap smear, or a history or risk of cervical neoplasia, the erosion and surrounding epithelium should be considered to be associated with a potential severe neoplasia or malignancy until proven otherwise by colposcopic examination and histologic sampling (Figure 8.97).

Etiology   Ulcerations develop for a variety of reasons, including trauma, infection, and cancer. A direct sharp shearing force applied to healthy epithelium may cause an acute abrasion or erosion. Chronic pressure on the epithelium may produce an ulceration, a process similar to what occurs in the vagina when a tampon is retained for a prolonged time. Ulcerations may also result from other intravaginal devices or from an adverse response to intravaginal medications. The probability of inadvertent epithelial injury is greater when epithelium becomes thin, as in estrogen-deficient women with atrophy. Cervicitis promotes tissue fragility, increasing the likelihood of traumatic ulceration which is usually benign. However, an ulcer may be induced unintentionally in previously intact, severely neoplastic epithelium because of the propensity of hemidesmosomes (tiny papillary structures that bind the basal cells and cytoskeleton to the underlying stroma)[28] to lose their adhesive properties in the neoplastic process. Consequently, one should never assume that all epithelial trauma associated with the introduction of the vaginal speculum blades is benign.

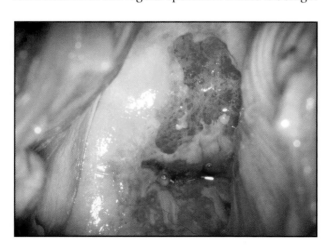

FIGURE 8.97   A large red recessed erosion is seen on the anterior lip of the cervix. The surrounding acetowhite epithelium was diagnosed histologically as CIN 2. It is important that the biopsy contain some abnormal epithelium if an ulceration adjoins the abnormal tissue. ▬▬

Focal cytopathic effects from viral or bacterial infections may cause ulcerations. Herpes simplex virus (HSV) produces multiple clusters of small, irregular ulcerations (Figures 8.98a,b). Syphilis and chancroid ulcerations are more likely to be larger, well circumscribed, and solitary. Abnormal vaginal discharge may accompany ulcerations caused by infectious organisms.

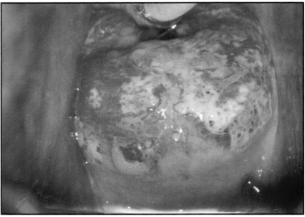

(a)

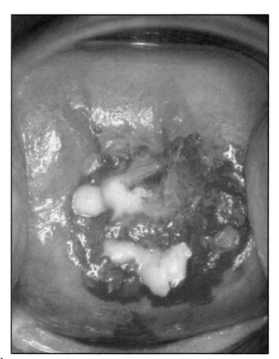

(b)

FIGURES 8.98a,b   (a) Herpes cervicitis can mimic invasive cancer **(b)**. Both are erythematous and friable. An associated exudate is also seen in each case. Photo **(b)** courtesy of Dr. Vesna Kesic. ▬▬

More importantly, ulcerations may evolve in epithelial areas invaded by rapidly proliferating cancers (Figures 8.99a,b). Under these circumstances, the rate of tumor growth may exceed oxygen delivery capacity by the enlarged but widely spaced blood vessels. Focal hypoxic ischemia and tissue necrosis ensue when intercapillary distance exceeds 350 μm.[23] As intercapillary distances of invasive cancer surpass 450 μm, superficial necrosis of the cervical epithelium occurs in 94.1% of women.[23] Intravascular pressure also determines tissue viability. For example, the oxygen tension of capillary blood in normal tissue measures 66 mm Hg, but it is reduced to a mean of 58.6 mm Hg in invasive cancer.[23]

Colposcopic appearance When viewed through the colposcope, ulcerations appear as well-demarcated, recessed, red, raw areas without visible surface

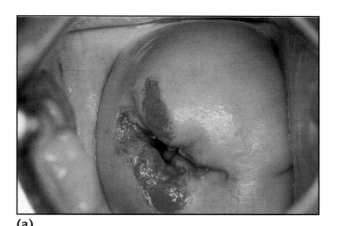

(a)

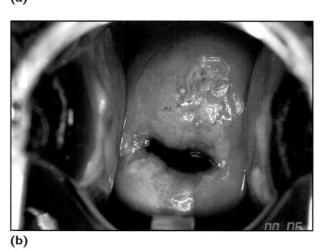

(b)

FIGURES 8.99a,b Ulcerations are also frequently seen in conjunction with invasive cervical cancers. Photo **(a)** courtesy of Dr. Vesna Kesic.

epithelium. They may be encompassed by normal or neoplastic epithelium (Figures 8.96–8.99). The type of surrounding epithelium indicates whether the ulceration is likely to be associated with a benign or neoplastic process. A dull, thickened, adjoining epithelium suggests neoplasia. Tissue friability is suspicious for infection or neoplasia. Associated hemorrhage, blood clots, and serous drainage may fill and obscure an underlying ulceration. If the ulceration is benign and due to trauma, ecchymosis may be observed in adjoining, otherwise normal epithelium, and a flap of freshly avulsed, normal-appearing epithelium may remain at the ulcer margin. When ulceration is associated with infection, tiny vesicles or pustules may be seen in the periphery.

The epithelial border of the ulceration may offer clues to the etiology of the ulcer. A raised margin, elevated above the surrounding epithelial surface, or an adjoining dense acetowhite epithelium may indicate a neoplasia. A well-defined, rolled ulcer margin or edge may be seen with infection caused by *Treponema pallidum* or in a patient with a retained vaginal tampon. An irregular border may indicate HSV infection or cancer. A tear of colposcopically normal appearing tissue may simply indicate benign trauma.

Ulcerations may occur as small or large solitary ulcers, or as multifocal ulcers of various sizes. The number of ulcerations and size are determined by the etiology. Diffuse ulcerations may be caused by viral agents or adverse reactions to intravaginal products or medications. Solitary ulcers may result from bacterial infection, neoplasia, or trauma. The size of ulcerations can vary for specific infections, trauma, and neoplasia.

Healing ulcerations may exhibit various stages of metaplasia and repair. An intense, flame-shaped erythematous band of inflammatory tissue may be noted in the epithelium that borders a healing ulcer. This red area surrounding an ulcer actually represents tiny closely spaced capillaries and sometimes extravasation of erythrocytes into the stroma.[27] Because of the abundant neovascularization in a healing ulcer, solitary capillaries may not be appreciable.

The shape and depth of ulcerations may offer etiological clues. Round ulcers may indicate infection, and irregularly shaped ulcers may suggest neoplasia. Trauma may produce frayed or sharply demarcated edges, depending on the health of the epithelium and source of injury. Deep, necrotic ulcerations may be more likely observed secondary to cancer, while shallow ulcers are more often a result of minor trauma or infection.

Clinical significance Definitive diagnosis of ulcerations is best made in conjunction with patient history and laboratory testing. Because the primary objective of colposcopy is to identify lower genital tract neoplasia, all ulcerations must be assessed. Previous abnormal cervical cytologic findings increase the probability of neoplasia. However, an intense inflammatory process may accompany a cancer to the extent that the cancer cells are obscured on the Pap smear. Therefore, a normal or inflammatory Pap smear result in a woman with a cervical ulceration does not exclude malignancy. Large, deep biopsies of the ulcer *and* adjoining epithelium are necessary to diagnose neoplasia.

Swab sampling of a fresh ulcer base or adjoining intact vesicles for culture or dark-field examination helps to confirm ulcers caused by HSV and syphilis, respectively. Herpes is usually seen early as a cluster of vesicles or pustules on erythematous bases (Figure 8.100). These vesicles ultimately rupture, producing small, superficial ulcerations, infrequently accompanied by abnormal serous vaginal discharge. Coexisting ulcers of the vulva and buttock regions may be seen in conjunction with cervical ulcerations (Figures 8.101a,b). In the case of externally located ulcerations, the woman may be aware that she has previously had a herpes infection. Unfortunately, some women experience only herpes cervicitis and remain virtually asymptomatic, increasing the likelihood that she will transmit the infection to sexual partners. Since detecting infection by means of dark-field examination is difficult from an access and interpretive perspective, serologic testing may be essential to confirm a diagnosis of syphilis.

Trauma may be the source of ulcerations. Ulcerations from use of intravaginal medication are suspected by history and distribution. While trauma is likely to occur in atrophic epithelium, cancers are also more prevalent in older women. Finally, trauma produced during insertion of a vaginal speculum may cause an acute ulceration with fresh bleeding. An iatrogenic ulcer usually involves normal, thin, or atrophic epithelium. Biopsy is not necessary if the colposcopist can be absolutely sure that the patient has no risk factor or clinical and laboratory evidence of neoplasia, but if any doubt exists as to the possibility of a neoplasia, a biopsy must always be taken. One must remember that iatrogenic ulcers are more likely to occur in friable epithelium (atrophic or neoplastic) that is susceptible to trauma. Although lower genital tract ulcerations may be associated with a broad spectrum of entities, cancer must always be ruled out, particularly if associated with abnormal cervical cytologic findings.

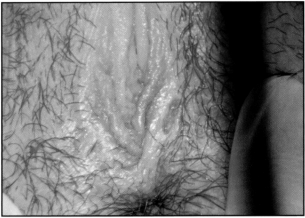

(a)

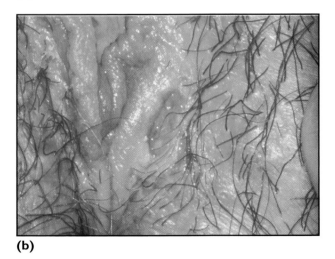

(b)

FIGURES 8.101a,b Primary herpetic ulcerations in the posterior forchette. These lesions were particularly painful and large. ■

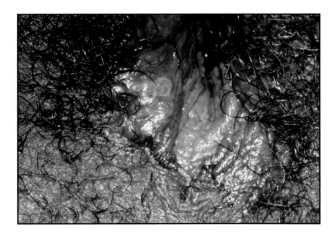

FIGURE 8.100 A cluster of herpetic vesicles on the vulva.

8.5.3.2 Epithelial elevations

Definition Variation of surface contour may be found in normal cervical epithelium of the ectocervix. While native squamous and mature metaplastic epithelia are generally flat or macular, columnar epithelium is distinctly villiform (Figure 8.5). Nabothian follicles may project above the epithelial surface as gently rounded, yellow mounds (Figure 8.11). These cysts may enlarge enough to be mistaken for tumors by clinicians unfamiliar with normal cervical anatomy. Immature metaplasia assumes a continuum of topography, initially adopting a villiform, then a pebbled, undulating, or papular, and finally a macular contour. The contour of the normal endocervical canal is irregular. When the SCJ is located near the external os, deep radial recesses from gland clefts may be seen to fold 5 mm beneath the surface. When the SCJ is positioned above the external os, the visible portion of the distal canal may appear smooth. A small percentage of women have papillary projections from tissue of the medial labia minora and introitus region known as micropapillomatosis labialis (MPL). The filiform surface can be confused with vulvar condyloma (Figure 8.102). A symmetrical distribution and absence of acetowhite color favor MPL. Similar, normal papillary projections (Figures 8.103a,b,c) can be found in the normal vagina (a) and cervix (b). Small, transient vesicular eruptions of the cervix or vagina caused by HSV, bullous or emphysematous vaginitis (Figure 8.104), or allergic reactions can occur but are infrequent.

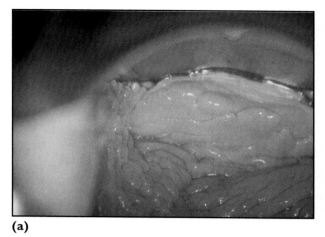

(a)

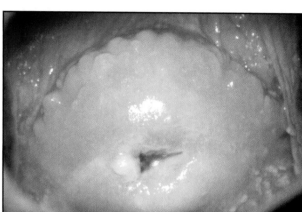

(b)

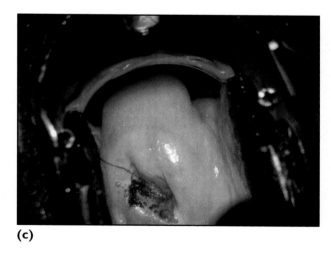

(c)

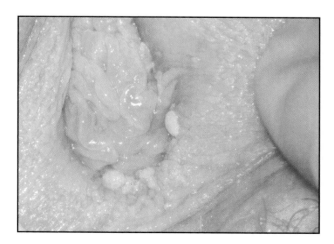

FIGURE 8.102 The normal papillary projections of micropapillomatosis labialis should not be confused with the condyloma seen at the posterior forchette.

FIGURES 8.103a–c Normal papillary projections are occasionally seen **(a)** in the vagina and **(b)** on the cervix. The projection from the anterior cervix **(c)** is called a cock's comb deformity. Although associated with exposure in-utero to DES, in this case the findings represent a variant of normal.

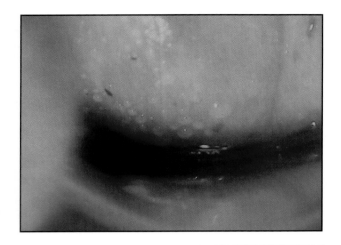

FIGURE 8.104 Bullous cervicitis seen in an elderly woman.

More profound epithelial contour changes may be observed in the abnormal cervix. Some of the greatest morphologic variation is seen with HPV lesions or CIN 1 of the cervix. Micropapillary, papillary, cerebriform, papular, plaque-like, and grossly exophytic lesions are all possible raised presentations of cervical HPV (Figures 8.105a–g). Some CIN 3 lesions are raised and plaque-like. Greater elevation may be seen if coexisting leukoplakia is present. The morphologic expression of cervical cancer varies depending on cell type, location, and whether the invasion is primarily endophytic or exophytic. Exophytic tumors are nodular, raised, or papular (Figures 8.106a–d). Advanced, large tumors may be readily seen without a colposcope and are easily palpated during bimanual examination. Because the ectocervix is predominately flat, particularly for most women older than 40 years of age, epithelial elevations of the ectocervix in these women should be suspect for neoplasia. Contour changes emanating from the endocervical canal may be benign or associated with a malignancy. Micro-glandular hyperplasia, papillary adenocarcinoma in situ, polyps, fibroids, deciduas, and adenocarcinoma can produce striking contour changes within columnar epithelium.

Etiology Elevations of the epithelium are caused by many factors, including trauma, infection, and benign and malignant tumors. Chronic, focal trauma to the cervix may produce circumscribed, plaque-like elevations of keratosis or leukoplakia (Figure 8.107). Tiny, diffuse, multiple pinpoint elevations may be seen after cervical surgery (Figures 8.108a,b,c).

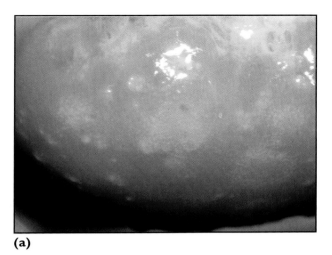

(a)

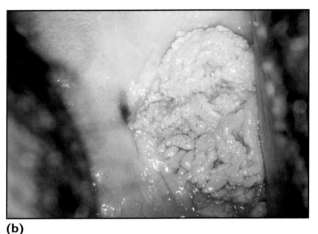

(b)

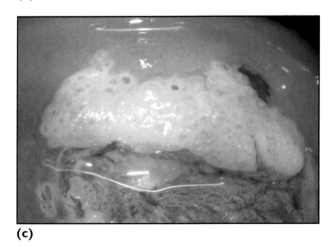

(c)

FIGURES 8.105a–g Different expressions of cervical human papillomavirus infection, which include **(a)** micropapillary, **(b)** papillary, **(c)** cerebriform (continued).

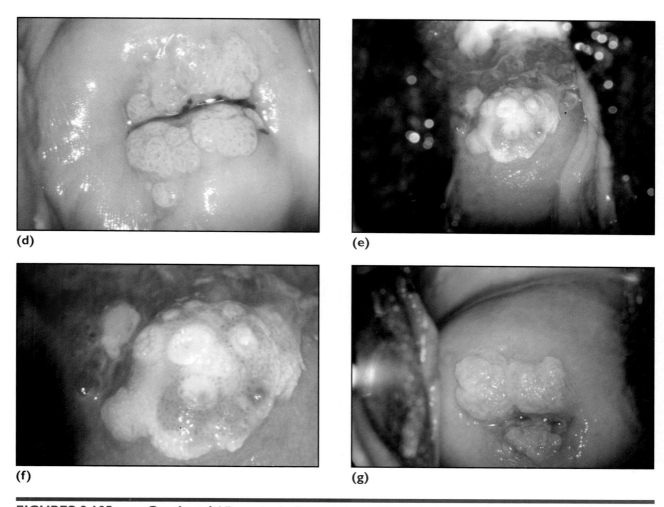

(d)

(e)

(f)

(g)

FIGURES 8.105a–g Continued (d) papular, **(e,f)** inverted, and **(g)** exophytic morphology.

HPV types 6 and 11 cause papillary or exophytic epithelial elevations (Figure 8.105). The virus may stimulate capillary proliferation and growth whereby the afferent and efferent loop capillaries, normally restricted within the lower one third of the squamous epithelium, expand within elongated rete pegs. Narrow, long, finger-like papillary projections may erupt (Figures 8.109a,b). Subclinical HPV infection may produce shorter epithelial projections, called asperities or micropapillae. When present, asperities impart a mildly irregular surface contour that can be appreciated only with high-power colposcopic magnification. Vesicular eruptions associated with infection or allergy result from the accumulation of a transudate beneath the superficial epithelium.

In addition to HPV-induced condylomas, nodular, papular, exophytic, or raised lesions may represent severe grades of cervical neoplasia. Raised plaque-like epithelial contour is suggestive of CIN 3 or cancer (Figures 8.110a–c). Once cells become malignant, their normal feedback mechanism to inhibit uncontrolled growth is lost. When one normal cell abuts against an adjoining cell, normal tactile intercellular feedback dictates recognition of the occupied space. Cancer cells do not retain this important feedback control and, thus, continue to divide and proliferate without regard to the adjoining cells. Such rampant growth causes nodular, exophytic lesions that extend above the surface of the epithelium and invade deeply within and below the epithelium as endophytic tumors. Vascular endothelial growth factor (VEGF) and angiogenin (AGN) that are present in cancer cause proliferation of new and large-caliber blood vessels that permit cellular expansion beyond the normal integrity of the epithelium. If the cancer exceeds its necessary vascular supply, ulcerations develop and the exophytic mass may assume an even more irregular contour.

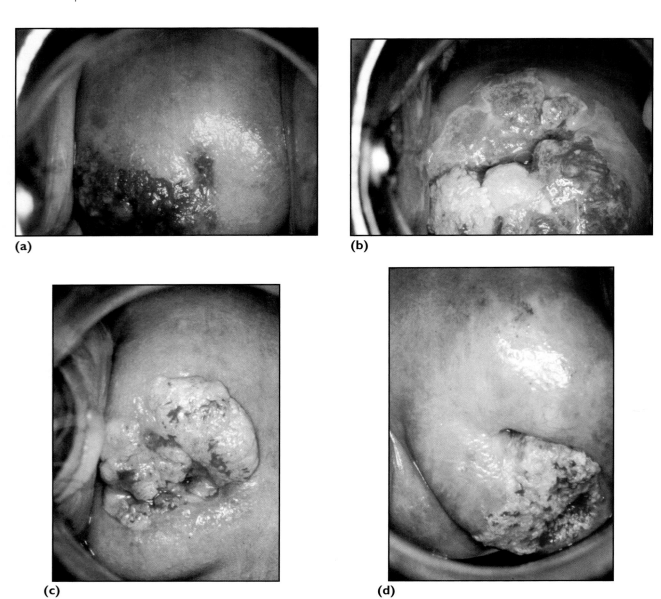

(a)

(b)

(c)

(d)

FIGURES 8.106a–d   Exophytic adenocarcinomas **(a,b)** and squamous cell carcinomas of the cervix **(c,d)**. Photos courtesy of Dr. Vesna Kesic.

FIGURE 8.107   Leukoplakia or a plaque-like white patch on the cervix prior to 5% acetic acid application.

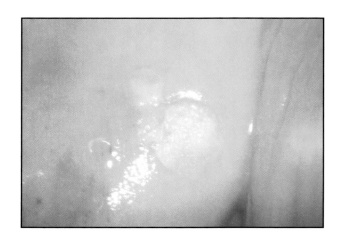

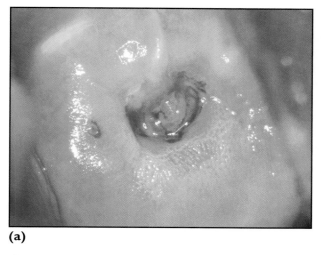

(a)

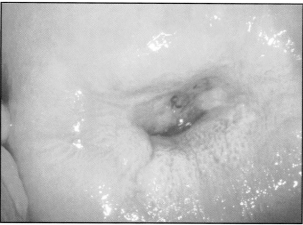

(b)

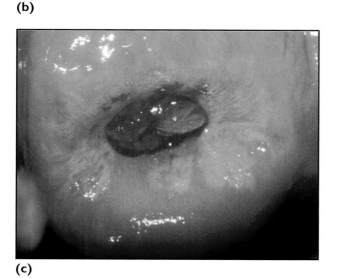

(c)

FIGURES 8.108a–c Parakeratosis seen on the posterior cervix following loop excision **(a)**. Tiny nonacetowhite elevations are noted. Parakeratosis is also seen in another patient **(b)** following cryotherapy. This should be contrasted with parakeratosis seen following loop excision **(c)** but with acetowhite lesions also. Biopsy indicated CIN 1.

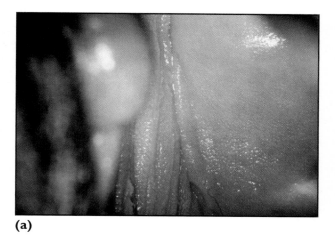

(a)

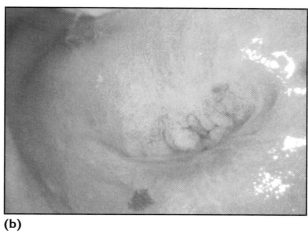

(b)

FIGURES 8.109a,b Micropapillae or asperities of the vagina produced by human papillomavirus infection **(a)**. Tiny raised capillaries associated with HPV infection are also seen in **(b)**.

Colposcopic appearance Elevations are best observed colposcopically when using a stereoscopic colposcope. Because many colposcopes do not permit stereoscopic viewing, associated shadows, contrasting tangential light reflections, and color hue and shades can be used to determine contour changes. Light reflection from surface irregularity is perhaps the best indication of contour elevation. Gentle manipulation of the cervix also helps the colposcopist discern subtle surface variations. Elevations of the cervix may be unifocal or multifocal, confined to the cervix, or present diffusely within the lower genital tract. Large, focal lesions or tiny, dispersed elevations may indicate HPV infection. The causative agent determines the contour, height, surface area, number, shape, and color of epithelial elevations.

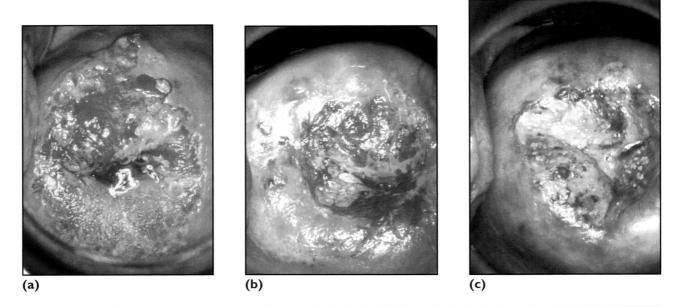

(a)   **(b)**   **(c)**

FIGURES 8.110a–c   Raised lesions of the cervix representing **(a)** adenocarcinoma and **(b,c)** squamous cell carcinoma. Photographs courtesy of Dr. Vesna Kesic.

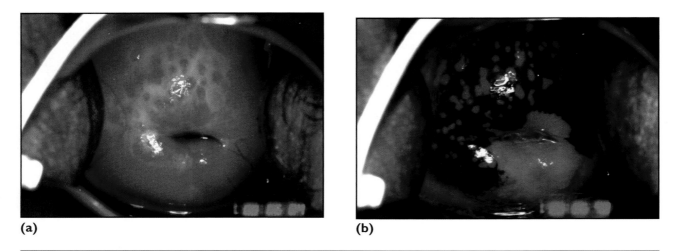

(a)   **(b)**

FIGURES 8.111a,b   Trichomonas cervicitis following **(a)** acetic acid application and **(b)** application of Lugol's iodine application. Notice the small red dots correspond with the yellow iodine negative dots.

Following 5% acetic acid application, micropapillae or asperities caused by HPV produce a pebbled, acetowhite epithelial appearance much like sand imbedded in paint (Figure 8.109). Small-loop capillaries may be seen in these tiny epithelial projections when viewed at high-level magnification. Application of Lugol's iodine greatly assists the identification of asperities, which appear as tiny yellow surface elevations (peaks) against a mahogany brown background. The colposcopic appearance resembles a "starry night" pattern unique to subclinical HPV infection.

Although similar tiny iodine negative dots, streaks, and patches may be seen with other inflammatory conditions, they are usually flat or macular. Trichomonas cervicitis or vaginitis is characterized grossly by small red patches that, with closer inspection, appear as randomly diffuse clusters of fine punctation (Figures 8.111a,b). These clusters may be mildly elevated as a gradually rounded tapered mound. Following application of Lugol's iodine, multiple well-circumscribed clusters of small yellow irregular patches or dots that conform to the previous diffuse red patches may be seen colposcopically.

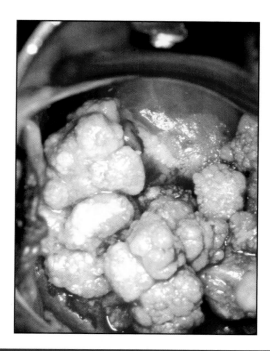

FIGURE 8.112 A large exophytic condyloma covers an occult cervical cancer hidden beneath it. A small opaque acetowhite high grade lesion is seen on the anterior cervix.

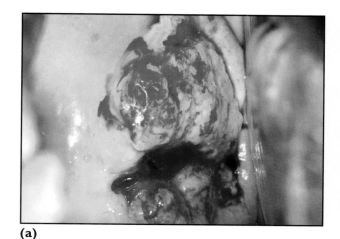

(a)

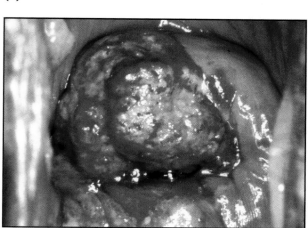

(b)

FIGURES 8.113a,b A large yellow cervical cancer can be seen eroding beneath the epithelium on the anterior cervix. **(a)** The normal epithelium is buckled forming a curved ridge secondary to the undermining. **(b)** A necrotic, friable exophytic cervical cancer is seen.

Papillary projections that appear as long, fili-form acetowhite clusters are caused primarily by HPV. Central afferent and efferent loop capillaries may be noted, especially as the acetic acid reaction fades. A brain-like surface contour may be seen, although it is rarely associated with HPV infection. This distinctive cerebriform contour change, how-ever, may also represent invasive cancer. Similarly, cauliflower-like growths may indicate either condy-lomas or cancer. Papular lesions can represent either extreme of the neoplastic spectrum, HPV infection or cancer, but the former etiology is favored. Although cervical dysplasia normally retains a macular con-tour, sometimes CIN 3 lesions may be elevated slightly or plaque-like. Leukoplakic plaques, which have sharply defined margins that rise abruptly from the surrounding epithelium, may be associated with a neoplastic process.

Because cervical cancer may appear papillary, it may be difficult to discriminate it colposcopically from a large condyloma (Figure 8.112). Cancer is typically more compact and focal than the long, finger-like papillae seen more commonly with HPV. Verrucous carcinoma can mimic a benign condy-loma. However, recognition of this similar morphol-ogy always demands histologic sampling to establish the correct diagnosis. Cancers more commonly pres-ent as nodular, papular, or raised exophytic growths

of the cervix. Coexisting atypical blood vessels, yel-low epithelium, ulcerations, bleeding, and friable, erythematous epithelium suggest cancer (Fig-ures 8.113a,b).

An elevated surface contour is never a normal colposcopic finding, provided the normal villiform pattern of columnar epithelium and Nabothian cysts are excluded. However, benign non-neoplastic eleva-tions may be seen. Mass-like protuberances from the external cervical os usually represent benign endo-cervical polyps (Figures 8.114a–j), occasionally pro-lapsing fibroids (Figure 8.115), and rarely neoplasia or products of conception. Polyps may be covered by columnar epithelium that imparts a pebbled, red surface. Otherwise, polyps are covered by varying degrees of smooth metaplasia. Surface irregularities

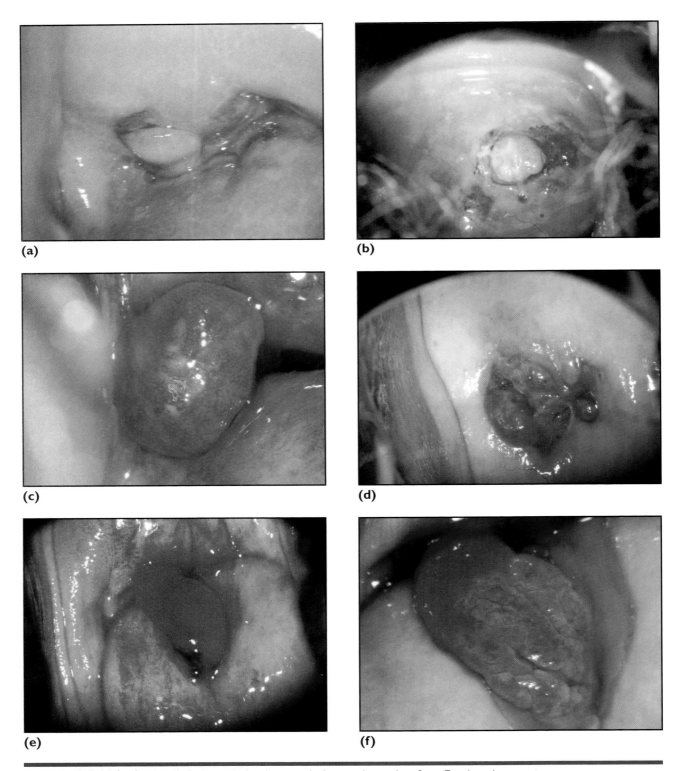

(a)

(b)

(c)

(d)

(e)

(f)

FIGURES 8.114a–j   (a–d) Endocervical polyps producing an elevated surface. Continued on next page.

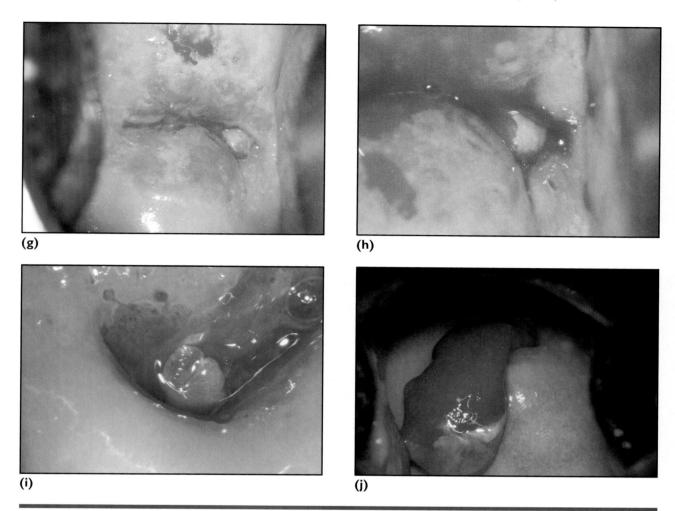

(g)

(h)

(i)

(j)

FIGURES 8.114a–j   Continued. A red polyp protruding from the os is seen **(e)** prior to and **(f)** following acetic acid application. The polyp seen at 3 o'clock in **(g)** is covered by opaque acetowhite epithelium. A coarse punctation can be seen at higher magnification **(h).** The histologic interpretation was CIN 2 and endocervical polyp. A small endocervical polyp **(i)** was noted during evaluation of a ASC-US Pap smear report. A large tongue-like endocervical polyp protrudes from the os in **(j).** This polyp in a 17-year-old woman was diagnosed as botryoid rhabdomyosarcoma, a malignant tumor. ▬

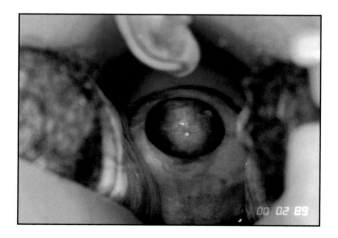

FIGURE 8.115   Fibroid prolapsing through the external os.

or projections may be seen as a cock's comb or cervical collar in women exposed to DES in utero. These changes are discussed in greater detail in Chapter 13. A red, fleshy protrusion covered by columnar epithelium surrounding the external os following excisional surgery of the cervix is known as a cervical button (Figures 8.116a,b,c). The protuberance results from an accelerated growth of columnar epithelium arising from the base of the surgical wound. This benign change may appear in conjunction with a fine radial punctation vessel pattern that extends centrally toward the os from the surgical excision margins. A slightly thickened, pebbled epithelial texture may be observed in the area of excision secondary to parakeratosis. The tiny surface projections usually correspond to and overlie the radial punctation vessels. A lack of surrounding acetowhite epithelium helps to

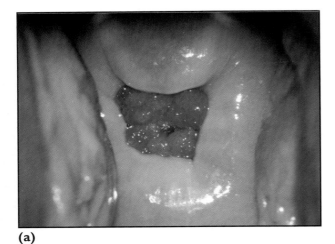

(a)

(b)

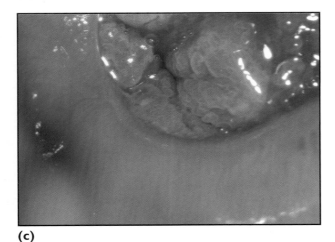

(c)

FIGURES 8.116a–c Cervical buttons resulting from healing following surgery of the cervix **(a,b)**. The button forms initially as columnar epithelium **(c)**.

distinguish this normal postoperative finding from neoplasia (Figures 8.117a–d). Small clusters of yellow vesicles or pustules, which are rarely observed, may represent a herpes simplex virus (HSV) infection. These can be differentiated from Nabothian follicles by the more fragile thin overlying epithelium and watery cyst fluid.

Clinical significance Contour elevations of the cervix may be normal, abnormal benign conditions or they may be caused by neoplasia. In the majority of cases, surface elevations should be considered abnormal. Neoplasia must be suspected, particularly when accompanied by abnormal cervical cytologic findings. A good colposcopist will also look for other abnormal colposcopic signs to assist the derivation of a clinically based colposcopic impression.

8.5.4 Margin characteristics of abnormal cervical epithelium

8.5.4.1 Abnormal cervix

8.5.4.1.1 Before application of 5% acetic acid and Lugol's iodine solution

Colposcopic appearance Sometimes, cervical lesions may be noted before epithelial contrast agents are applied to the cervix. In this circumstance, a raised margin or outline of the lesion will help determine the etiology. White areas of leukoplakia, pink condyloma, decidua, and exophytic cancers may be noted during the initial colposcopic inspection. Compared with the normal surrounding epithelium, leukoplakia is variably raised. The extent of elevation is determined by the amount of keratin accumulation. The raised interface or margin of leukoplakia may slope gradually or rise abruptly. A steep margin gives an impression that the area might be peeled off easily. The margins of leukoplakia are generally irregular or jagged, and rarely smooth or straight. Smaller surrounding satellite patches of leukoplakia may also be observed. Diffuse pinpoint areas of leukoplakia with steep margins can be best appreciated at high-power colposcopic magnification. These tiny areas may represent leukoplakia atop asperities or parakeratosis seen following surgery. Papillary or protuberant condyloma may be seen during cytologic sampling. These lesions with distinctive margins should be distinguished from decidual reaction of pregnancy, microglandular hyperplasia, and invasive cancer. Cervical cancers, especially when more advanced, can usually be seen without contrast solutions and colposcopy. A multitude of various abrupt or gradual margins can be encountered with cancer. The margins of all these abnormal

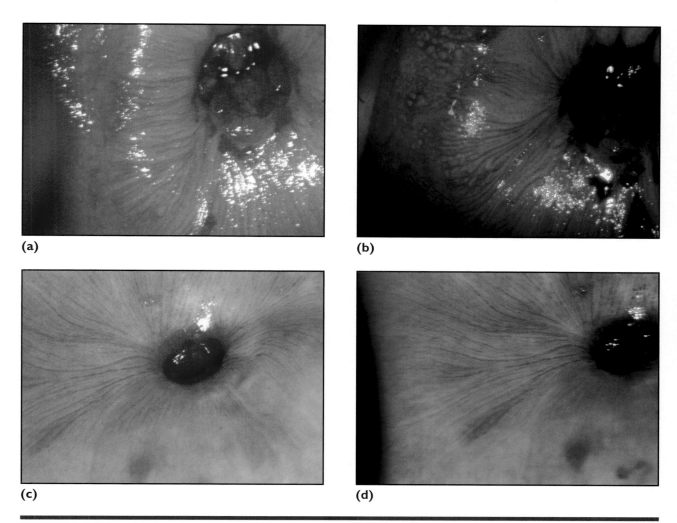

(a)

(b)

(c)

(d)

FIGURES 8.117a–d   Radial punctation blood vessels noted following surgery of the cervix in these two cases. There is no acetowhite epithelium present. This finding represents the normal healing vascular pattern of the cervix.

entities are also defined by their unusual elevated contour. It is the elevated contour, not necessarily margins, that most likely captures the attention of a colposcopist prior to the application of epithelial contrast solutions.

8.5.4.1.2 After application of 5% acetic acid or Lugol's iodine solution

Colposcopic appearance   The margins of most abnormal flat cervical lesions can be better appreciated following the application of both 5% acetic acid and Lugol's iodine (Figure 8.118). This demarcation allows appraisal of the margin characteristics. In most instances, acetowhite lesions of the cervix will exhibit the same margin as that seen following Lugol's iodine application (Figures 8.119a–c). In the case of macular, faintly acetowhite changes, Lugol's iodine will generally provide a more vivid and distinct contrast between different epithelial types. The observed

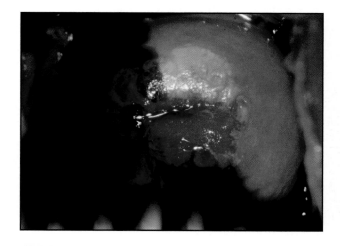

FIGURE 8.118   A large low-grade lesion is seen simultaneously after acetic acid and Lugol's iodine solution applications.

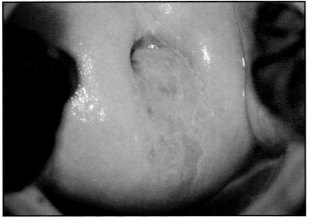

(a)

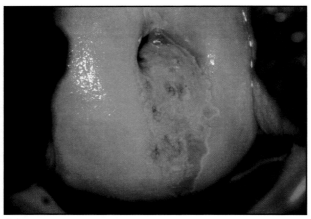

(b)

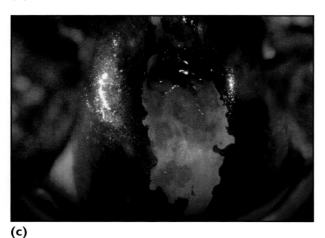

(c)

FIGURES 8.119a–c **(a)** An acetowhite lesion with an irregular margin is seen on the posterior cervix. **(b)** A fine mosaic vascular pattern is best seen using the green filter of the colposcope. **(c)** The iodine negative yellow epithelium corresponds to the acetowhite epithelium. The lesion also extends within the endocervical canal beyond colposcopic visualization. ■

margins between pink and white epithelium or between yellow and brown epithelium may vary tremendously. Occasionally, the margin interface may also exhibit a contour change, rendering them more easily detectable based on a color, margin, and topographic contrast.

Margins or staining interfaces may be noted between two different normal epithelia, between normal and abnormal epithelia, and between two different types of abnormal epithelium. Acetowhite or Lugol's iodine-negative immature metaplasia will generally form an irregular margin with mature metaplasia and columnar epithelium (Figure 8.120). An exception is the smooth margin between the epithelium of a congenital transformation zone and squamous epithelium. Normally, no visible margin between mature metaplasia and original squamous epithelium can be seen, even after application of contrast solutions. However, a faintly visible margin between normal epithelia may be appreciated in women following surgical excision procedures of the cervix. In this case, a slight variation in epithelial color, along with normal radial punctation and parakeratosis, may be noted. The excision line is not accentuated by contrast solutions, provided normal epithelium occupies each side of the line.

The margins between normal and abnormal epithelia assume a greater variation, from irregular to smooth, indistinct to sharp, and macular to elevated. Both immature metaplasia and CIN 1 lesions of the cervix exhibit similar margin types. Irregular, jagged, feathered, flocculated, or indistinct borders may be seen with either entity (Figure 8.121). The vague nature of these margins may be attributable to the

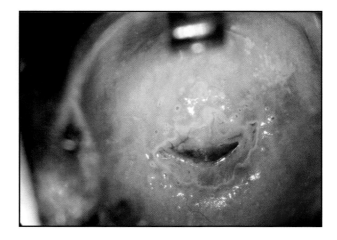

FIGURE 8.120 An irregular margin noted with immature metaplasia following acetic acid application. ■

effect of a poorly circumscribed viral infection in the case of CIN 1, or to the diffuse, varied reaction to acid-induced epithelial trauma noted with evolving immature metaplasia. Small satellite areas positioned in the periphery, away from large central lesions, also may be seen with immature metaplasia or CIN 1. These margin types are generally associated with macular epithelial areas and, therefore, no surface contour change can be appreciated. However, papillary condyloma, equivalent to CIN 1, should not be confused with immature metaplasia. Although very immature metaplasia may overlie a villus, which is normally covered by columnar epithelium, the villi and condyloma are not usually confused.

The margins associated with CIN 2 and CIN 3 are more uniform, typically straight or gently rounded (Figure 8.122). An abrupt histologic border between a severe dysplasia and normal epithelium conveys the sharp contrast seen colposcopically. These well-delineated high-grade lesion margins contrast readily with the sometimes diffuse, ill-defined margins of CIN 1 or immature metaplasia. The blocks of neoplastic epithelium are well circumscribed and segregated from dissimilar epithelium. With these grades of neoplasia, severely abnormal epithelium may appear slightly raised. The thickened epithelium may appear to be peeled from the stroma. An adenocarcinoma in situ may be less distinct with respect to colposcopic margins. These acetowhite lesions may be more apt to blend with the surrounding acetowhite blanched normal columnar epithelium or immature metaplasia.

However, some adenocarcinoma in situs are quite distinct (Figure 8.123).

The margins of advanced cancer are usually well delineated from the surrounding normal epithelium. The margins are perhaps less well defined from non-malignant areas of neoplasia if microinvasive cancer or an endophytic cancer coexists. However, this is not always the case (Figures 8.124a,b). Exophytic cancers have readily discerned margins that are very abrupt in relief. When palpated, the tumor may feel firm or hard when compared with the softer adjoining normal tissue. The margins demonstrate slight to moderate irregularity if the tumor is friable and necrotic. Otherwise, the margins of cancer are more discrete and smooth. Early adenocarcinoma margins may not

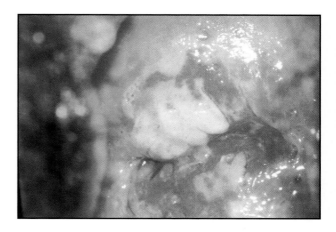

FIGURE 8.122 A fairly uniform straight lesion margin observed in a patient with CIN 3.

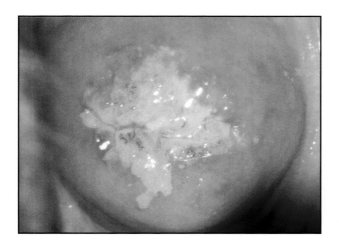

FIGURE 8.121 An irregular lesion margin noted in a CIN 1 lesion.

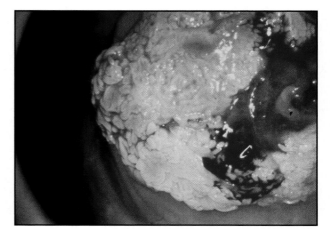

FIGURE 8.123 An obvious adenocarcinoma in situ with a distinct margin.

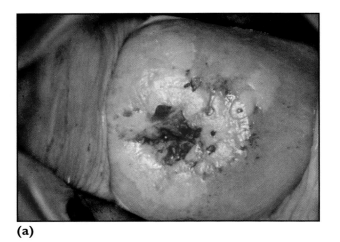

(a)

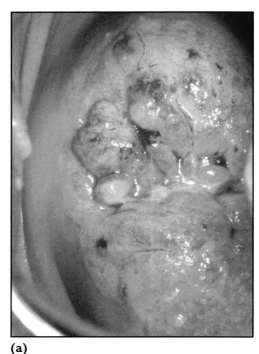

(a)

FIGURES 8.124a,b Two examples of microinvasive cervical cancer. These microinvasive lesions are associated with very large, high-grade lesions. Photos courtesy of Dr. Vesna Kesic.

be as readily recognized nor distinguished from normal columnar epithelium as squamous cancer is from adjoining squamous epithelium.

Unique margins between two different types of abnormal epithelium may be noted during the colposcopic examination. In this case, an acetowhite opaque, proximally positioned lesion may be distinguished from a more translucent peripherally located lesion. Sometimes a larger variegated lesion stained with Lugol's iodine will encompass a smaller, pale,

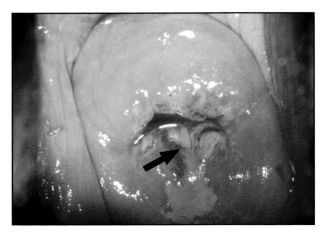

FIGURE 8.125 An internal margin or border located closer to the squamocolumnar junction (arrow), demarcating a high-grade cervical lesion near the os and a lower-grade lesion in the periphery.

iodine-negative lesion. Usually, the margin between these two areas is smooth or straight. Because both areas may be of similar color, the margin between abnormal epithelium may not be as well defined. Also, the more centrally positioned lesion may be quite small compared with the larger surrounding lesion. When a CIN 2 or CIN 3 is positioned within a larger CIN 1 lesion or area of immature metaplasia, an internal margin may be noted (Figure 8.125). This interface is an abnormal/abnormal margin. Moreover, an internal margin also may be noted between CIN 3 and an invasive cancer. At times, a surface contour change may help to further delineate the junction. If one area is raised (usually the central lesion) the demarcation should be more easily recognized. An associated surface ulceration also may be present. Coexisting squamous and glandular neoplasias may adjoin each other. Provided the glandular lesions are seen on the surface and are not confined to gland clefts, colposcopists may discern a colposcopically visible interface. However, because early glandular neoplasias can mimic immature metaplasia, the glandular lesion is likely to be less apparent.

Clinical significance Unique attributes of lesion margins should be noted during colposcopy. The margin characteristics of acetowhite or Lugol's iodine-negative epithelium help the colposcopist define normality and varying levels of abnormality. As such, lesion margin is considered a valuable colposcopic sign. Margin characteristics of neoplastic epithelium are discussed in greater detail in Chapter 9.

References

1. Coppelson M, Pixley E C, Reid B. *Colposcopy: A Scientific and Practical Approach to the Cervix, Vagina, and Vulva in Health and Disease,* 3rd ed. Springfield, IL: Charles C. Thomas, 1987.

2. Burke L, Antonioli D A, Ducatman B S. *Colposcopy Text and Atlas.* Norwalk, CT: Appleton and Lange, 1991.

3. Wright C V, Lickrish G M, Shier R M. *Basic and Advanced Colposcopy,* 2nd ed. Komoka, Ontario: Biomedical Communications, 1995.

4. Kolstad P, Stafl A. *Atlas of Colposcopy,* 3rd ed. Oslo: Scandinavian University Books, 1982.

5. Burghardt E, Ostor A G. *Colposcopy, cervical pathology. Textbook and Atlas.* New York: Thieme Stratton, 1984.

6. Maxwell G L, Sosson A P, Oster C, Miles P, Webb J, Carlson J. Subepithelial angiogenesis in cervical intraepithelial neoplasia. *J Lower Genital Tract Dis* 1998;2:191–4.

7. Folkman J, Merler E, Abernathy C, Williams G. Isolation of a tumor factor responsible for angiogenesis in tumor growth. *J Exp Med* 1971;133:275–88.

8. Folkman J. Anti-angiogenesis: new concept for therapy of solid tumors. *Ann Surg* 1972;175:409–16.

9. Abulafia O, Triest W E, Sherer D M. Angiogenesis in squamous cell carcinoma in situ and microinvasive carcinoma of the uterine cervix. *Obstet Gynecol* 1996;88:927–32.

10. Stafl A, Mattingly R F. Angiogenesis of cervical neoplasia. *Am J Obstet Gynecol* 1975;121:845–52.

11. Cheng W F, Chen C A, Lee C N, Chen T M, Hseik F J, Hseih C Y. Vascular endothelial growth factor in cervical carcinoma. *Obstet Gynecol* 1999; 93:761–5.

12. Bodnev-Adler B, Hefler L, Bodner K, Levdolter S, Frischmuth K, Kainz C, et al. Serum levels of angiogenin (ANG) in invasive cancer and in cervical intraepithelial neoplasia (CIN). *Anticancer Res* 2001; 21: 809–12.

13. Hopman E H, Kenemans P, Helmerhorst T J M. Positive predictive rate of colposcopic examination of the cervix uteri: an overview of the literature. *Obstet Gynecol Survey* 1998; 53: 97–106.

14. Sakuma T, Hasegawa T, Tsutsui F, Kurihara S. Quantitative analysis of the whiteness of the atypical cervical transformation zone. *J Reprod Med* 1985; 30: 773–6.

15. Zahm D M, Nidl I, Greinke C, Hoyer H, Schneider A. Colposcopic appearance of cervical intraepithelial neoplasia is age dependent. *Am J Obstet Gynecol* 1998;178:1298–304.

16. Tidbury P, Singer A, Jenkins D. CIN3: The role of lesion size in invasion. *Br J Obstet Gynecol* 1992; 99: 583–6.

17. Boonstra H, Aalders J G, Koudstaal J, et al. Minimum extension and appropriate topographic position of tissue destruction for treatment of cervical intraepithelial neoplasia. *Obstet Gynecol* 1990; 75:227–31.

18. Difiore M S H. *Atlas of Human Histology,* 4th ed. Philadelphia: Lea and Febiger, 1975.

19. Kolstad P. The colposcopic diagnosis of dysplasia, carcinoma in situ, and early invasive cancer of the cervix. *Acta Obstet Gynec Scand* 1964;43:105–8.

20. Follen M M, Lavine R U, Carillo E, Richart R M, Nuovo G, Crum C P. Colposcopic correlates of cervical papillomavirus infection. *Am J Obstet Gynecol* 1987;157: 809–14.

21. Mikhail M S, Romney S L. Computerized measurement of intercapillary distance using image analysis in women with cervical intraepithelial neoplasia: correlation with severity. *Obstet Gynecol* 2000; 95(suppl):S2–3.

22. Kolstad P. The development of the vascular bed in tumors as seen in squamous-cell carcinoma of the cervix uteri. *Br J Radiol* 1965;38:216–23.

23. Kolstad P. Intercapillary distance, oxygen tension and local recurrence in cervix cancer. *Scand J Clin Lab Invest* 1968; 106:145–57.

24. Sillman F, Boyce J, Fruchter R. The significance of atypical vessels and neovascularization in cervical neoplasia. *Am J Obstet Gynecol* 1981;139:154–9.

25. Sugimori H, Matsuyama T, Kashimura M, et al. Colposcopic findings in microinvasive carcinoma of the uterine cervix. *Obstet Gynecol Surv* 1979;34:804.

26. Wright V C. Colposcopy of adenocarcinoma in situ and adenocarcinoma of the uterine cervix: Differentiation from other cervical lesions. *J Lower Genital Tract Dis* 1999;3:83–97.

27. Johannison E, Kolstad P, Soderberg G. Cytologic, vascular, and histologic patterns of dysplasia, carcinoma in situ, and early invasive carcinoma of the cervix. *Acta Radiol* 1966;258(suppl):1–136.

28. Bloom W, Fawcett D W. *A Textbook of Histology,* 10th ed. Philadelphia: W. B. Saunders, 1975.

Colposcopy of Cervical Intraepithelial Neoplasia

Table of Contents

9.1 Introduction

The majority of colposcopy practice in the United States involves the evaluation of women with cervical cytologic changes that either ultimately are determined to be normal or confirmed to be cervical intraepithelial neoplasia (CIN). Since current triage thresholds indicate that women with solely minor cytologic changes, such as atypical squamous cells of undetermined significance (ASC-US) and low-grade squamous intraepithelial lesion (LSIL), need colposcopic examination, many women with entirely normal cervices are evaluated unnecessarily. Conversely, if screening thresholds were established at high grade squamous intraepithelial lesion (HSIL), fewer women would be referred unnecessarily but more disease would be missed. Yet, the value of cervical cytologic screening is indisputable. Where no cervical cytologic surveillance program exists, women present initially with advanced cervical cancer, obviating the need for colposcopy. On the other hand, in countries with a universal screening program, primary care clinicians infrequently encounter cervical cancer. Colposcopists who have gynecologic oncology, or mainly tertiary practices, care for the majority of women with cancer. Therefore, the majority of colposcopists will primarily diagnose and manage women with CIN.

Although microinvasive and occult invasive cervical cancer challenge the diagnostic skills of even very experienced colposcopists, most invasive cervical cancers are identified readily by colposcopy (Figure 9.1). However, accurate colposcopic diagnosis of distinct grades of CIN may be inherently more challenging. For example, differentiating CIN 2 from

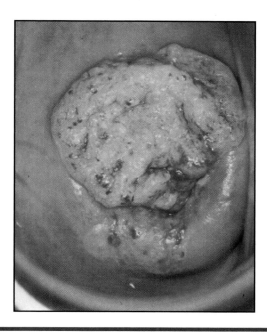

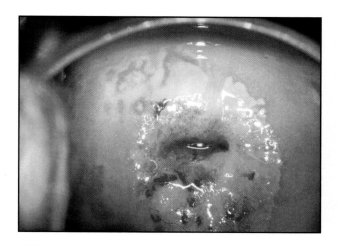

FIGURE 9.2   The acetowhite lesion may be called CIN 1 by one colposcopist and immature metaplasia by another. This is the most difficult discrimination for a colposcopist.

FIGURE 9.1   This microinvasive cancer could be easily confused with a large exophytic condyloma. Photo courtesy of Dr. Vesna Kesic.

a small area of CIN 3 by colposcopy can be nearly impossible. Detecting a small area of CIN 2 within a larger CIN 1 lesion summons considerable colposcopic expertise as well. Perhaps even more difficult is discriminating between CIN 1 and immature metaplasia of the normal cervix (Figure 9.2). This is confirmed by the fact that interobserver diagnostic reproducibility among colposcopists is better for CIN 2,3 than for CIN 1.[1] Primary care colposcopists who practice within a cervical neoplasia surveillance system, in which abnormalities are triaged at a low threshold, undoubtedly confront some of the most rigorous challenges of colposcopy, since divergent patient management options may be contingent upon a precise colposcopic diagnosis. In this chapter, we will discuss the analytic methods used to provide accurate colposcopic diagnoses and the colposcopic features of cervical intraepithelial neoplasia on which such a diagnosis is based.

9.2 Colposcopic Grading of Cervical Neoplasia

Colposcopy is the standard diagnostic procedure used to evaluate abnormal cervical cytologic changes in women. In order to manage cervical disease in patients properly, colposcopists must form a clinically based colposcopic impression. There are four basic colposcopic diagnoses: normal, low-grade lesion (CIN 1 and HPV), high-grade lesion (CIN 2,3) and invasive cancer. Even though these four colposcopic diagnoses are not internationally recognized terminology, they have become accepted clinical nomenclature by many colposcopists. This clinical terminology correlates directly with the Bethesda System of cervical cytology to facilitate interdisciplinary communication.[2] Some clinicians favor other more precise histologic CIN terminology (i.e., CIN 1,2,3). However, patient management is not modified by use of this more traditional, but less biologically appropriate, colposcopic terminology.

Before describing the colposcopic features of CIN, one must understand how colposcopists derive a clinical colposcopic diagnosis. Although a final diagnosis is ultimately based largely on the histologic interpretation of a tissue sample obtained from a colposcopically directed biopsy, the colposcopist's presumptive clinical diagnosis is an imperative part of proper evaluation and disease management. An accurate colposcopic impression helps to prevent adverse outcomes resulting from strict consideration of a potentially inaccurate histologic diagnosis. Considering both colposcopic and pathologic data enhances proper decision making about therapy.

Admittedly, much subjectivity remains in forming a colposcopic impression, just as some subjectivity exists in arriving at cytologic and histologic diagnoses. In a recent study, interobserver reproducibility for cervical cytologic diagnoses among pathologists was equivalent to the interobserver reproducibility for cervical histology (Kappa 0.46 and 0.46, respectively).[3]

This represents only a moderate level of interobserver agreement. Therefore, what is called CIN 2 by one pathologist may be diagnosed as CIN 1 or CIN 3 by another pathologist. In order to systematically categorize a multitude of colposcopic appearances that vary across the spectrum of disease states from normal to neoplasia, colposcopists have developed clinical indices or colposcopic grading systems to estimate disease severity. The goal of colposcopic grading is to provide an objective, reproducible, and meaningful clinical guide for gauging histologic severity.

9.2.1 Rationale for colposcopic grading

Pathologists evaluate certain cellular and epithelial criteria to make cytologic and histologic interpretations. For example, when forming a cytologic or histologic diagnosis, pathologists consider unique nuclear features, nuclear to cytoplasmic ratio, epithelial differentiation and maturation, and the extent of epithelial and stromal involvement by cellular atypia. By carefully considering these specific criteria and others, pathologists are able to derive diagnoses that are more accurate and reproducible. Similarly, colposcopists must form colposcopic impressions based on different macroscopic epithelial features within the same tissue. These colposcopic features include the color and opacity of the cervical lesion both before and following use of epithelial contrast solutions; the shape and character of lesion margins; the presence of blood vessels, their diameter, pattern, and branching characteristics; distances between adjoining capillaries; surface contour or topography; and duration of physiologic response to a 5% acetic acid solution.

Grading systems for colposcopy are systematic methods for predicting colposcopically the severity of cervical neoplasia by discriminatory analysis of unique colposcopic signs. Certain specific colposcopic signs or characteristics of abnormal epithelium within the transformation zone are considered sequentially by the colposcopist. Aggregate colposcopic signs are more accurately predictive of the

clinical severity of cervical disease than individual signs. For instance, the clinical consideration of only a single colposcopic sign, such as acetowhite epithelium, is fraught with potential for diagnostic error that can result in mismanagement. Normal immature metaplasia and areas of inflammation appear transiently acetowhite following the application of 5% acetic acid solution. In addition, all CIN lesions appear acetowhite. Therefore, if a colposcopist assumes incorrectly that all acetowhite areas indicate cervical neoplasia, then as many as 30% to 40% of women with normal cervices will receive an incorrect colposcopic diagnosis. This is particularly pertinent when performing colposcopy in young women, since the actively developing components of the transformation zone in these patients are readily apparent on the ectocervix. Furthermore, a biopsy taken from normal acetowhite immature metaplastic epithelium is frequently misdiagnosed histologically as CIN 2. These patients may undergo unnecessary treatment because of histologic overcall. Collectively considering other colposcopic signs increases the predictive accuracy of clinical colposcopic diagnosis.

To form a clinically based diagnosis, many colposcopists use a colposcopic index or grading system. Yet, other colposcopists fail to properly or consistently form a clinical colposcopic impression. Some form a colposcopic impression unconsciously, based on simple pattern recognition and many years of clinical experience. Others determine the severity of cervical disease merely by an ill-defined "gut reaction" or "wild guess". Of even greater concern, many colposcopists never form any kind of colposcopic impression and leave patient management decisions entirely in the hands of pathologists. As noted in Table 9.1, nonsystematic colposcopic impressions are inferior to systematic interpretations. Colposcopic scoring systems are consistently accurate, even for different population groups (e.g., HIV positive or pregnant patients) that may pose varied colposcopic challenges.[4] Furthermore, the attributes of colposcopic grading are confirmed biologically by the fact that colposcopic grading scores correlate better

Table 9.1   A Comparison of Systematic and Nonsystematic Colposcopic Interpretations

Criteria	Colposcopic Interpretations	
	Systematic	Nonsystematic
Critical Analysis	Structured	Arbitrary
Complexity Suitability	High	Low
Potential Accuracy	Maximal	Minimal
Reproducibility	Consistent	Erratic
Domain	Scientific	Artistic

among colposcopists when diagnosing lesions associated with high-risk types of human papillomavirus (HPV) compared with low-risk types.[5]

9.2.2 Importance of grading systems for colposcopy

Colposcopic grading systems are important because they provide a structured, systematic method to critically analyze cervical findings. Adherence to a structured evaluation method helps to prevent overlooking pertinent diagnostic features. A systematic approach, once learned and mastered, becomes routine and of extraordinary benefit to novice colposcopists. Colposcopic grading systems also allow colposcopists to form more accurate colposcopic impressions. After receiving histologic results, a colposcopic impression that was based on systematic criteria can be analyzed retrospectively to determine specific reasons for diagnostic discordance. This review may improve a colposcopist's ability to derive more accurate colposcopic impressions in the future. Well-designed colposcopic scoring systems enhance colposcopic reproducibility. Colposcopic grading systems are also helpful when attempting to select the most appropriate biopsy site, particularly when large, complex lesions of the cervix are encountered. In these cases, colposcopists can individually evaluate multiple lesions of the cervix to determine which area(s) contain(s) the most severe histologic change.

9.2.3 The colposcopic impression

By using a grading system, clinicians can form colposcopic impressions that can be compared with the cytologic and histologic diagnoses of pathologists. Only by forming a clinical colposcopic impression can the colposcopist determine whether discordance exists between the colposcopic findings and the laboratory diagnosis. Because cytologic and histologic interpretations are no more reproducible than colposcopic impressions,[3,6] a check and balance system to govern clinical and pathologic interpretation is essential. Significant disagreement between laboratory and clinical diagnoses indicates possible error by either party or both. Pathology/colposcopy discordance suggests a review of the cytology and histology by the same or a different expert gynecologic pathologist, a repeat colposcopy examination and/or histologic sampling by the same or a more expert colposcopist, or further diagnostic evaluation.

Routinely forming a colposcopic impression allows for quality control within the specialty. A unique quality control program in British Columbia monitors colposcopists by comparing their colposcopic impressions, which they indicate on their histology requisition forms, with the histologic diagnosis for each patient.[7] If a colposcopist's clinical impressions do not agree with the histologic interpretations at least 80% of the time, then the colposcopist receives remedial colposcopic training directed at improving clinical assessment of cervical lesions. More sophisticated quality control systems have been used for monitoring colposcopists in multi-site studies, such as the ASCUS/LSIL Triage Study (ALTS) funded by the National Cancer Institute.[8] In this study, the colposcopic impressions, biopsy intent, biopsy site selection, and cervical image adequacy of participating colposcopists were monitored by quality control colposcopy experts who remotely reviewed digitized cervical images from each patient, that were transferred by computer modem (Figure 9.3). A colposcopist who cannot adequately assess the severity of cervical lesions risks not obtaining the most abnormal tissue for pathologic interpretation.

The effective management of lower genital tract neoplasia depends on quality colposcopy. For example, an objective colposcopic impression is virtually indispensable when monitoring a woman with a previously diagnosed low-grade squamous intraepithelial lesion (LSIL) that was confirmed by biopsy but has not been treated. Although repeat cervical cytology is imperative when following these patients, a screening Papanicolaou (Pap) smear may be an insufficiently sensitive method for monitoring. Therefore, monitoring with colposcopy, in addition to cytology, may be essential for determining lesion progression. Good colposcopic skill minimizes the need for excessive or unnecessary biopsies that might increase the likelihood of poor patient compliance.

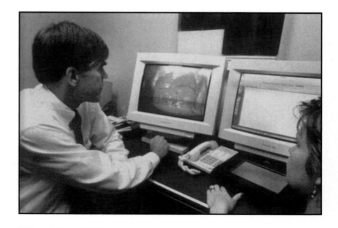

FIGURE 9.3   Remotely monitoring the quality of colposcopy practice using a computer image/data management system. ▬▬

Furthermore, critical analysis and selective sampling minimize diagnostic costs. Expert colposcopic evaluation of pregnant patients with minimally severe neoplasia minimizes the need for biopsy in the face of morphologic alterations of the cervix that occur during pregnancy.

9.2.4 Historical perspectives of colposcopic grading systems

9.2.4.1 Hinselmann colposcopic grading system

Although not commonly known, the importance of a colposcopic grading system was apparent to the inventor of the first colposcope, Dr. Hans Hinselmann. Just like any scientist who explores new frontiers, Dr. Hinselmann saw the need to scientifically categorize his new observations, the first colposcopic findings. He derived a novel, but rather crude, two-part colposcopic grading system which was subdivided into categories of "Simple Atypical Epithelium I and II," and "Highly Atypical Epithelium III and IV." Although now considered rudimentary, this early colposcopic grading system became the foundation that other renowned colposcopists modified based on their increased understanding of abnormalities within the transformation zone. No one colposcopic grading system is necessarily superior, but the historical evolution of grading systems has permitted further enhancements based on new knowledge in the field of cervical neoplasia.

9.2.4.2 Coppleson colposcopic grading system

Dr. Malcolm Coppleson, an Australian pioneer of colposcopy, devised another grading system in the 1960s.[9] The scheme underwent much revision, primarily as a result of the increasing recognition of low-grade SIL. The classification system is defined in Table 9.2.

In clinical practice, the majority of women with abnormal Pap smears have colposcopic grade I and II lesions. Few have grade III. The difficulty with the Coppleson grading system is that much attention became focused on color and density of acetowhitening, and the terms "grade I to III acetowhitening" became colposcopic jargon. However, CIN 1 may appear at times as a dense, shiny acetowhite lesion with a prominent vascular pattern. Thus, the severity of many low-grade lesions is overestimated using the system. The Coppleson system also failed to address the significance of findings involving the internal margins within an area of atypia, which usually indicate an area of more severe disease within a larger lesion. A coexisting, more severe lesion that was overlooked is a common explanation of a histologic diagnosis that is more severe than anticipated based on colposcopic findings. Most importantly, the Coppleson grading system remained somewhat subjective, and reproducibility was not assessed in a prospective study.

9.2.4.3 Stafl colposcopic grading system

In 1976, Dr. Adolph Stafl described a system for colposcopic grading based on four factors: surface pattern, color tone, intercapillary distance, and margin contour of the lesion with normal tissue.[10] His grading system was divided into normal, non-significant (inflammation), significant (CIN 1,2,3), and highly significant. Much emphasis was placed on the intercapillary distance within lesions, and a method was developed to objectively measure these very small distances. The original work of Kolstad had shown that increased intercapillary distance correlates with more significant histopathologic changes.[11] Problems with the Stafl grading system stemmed from four important weaknesses. First, the classic vascular changes within high-grade preinvasive neoplasia,

Table 9.2 The Coppleson Grading System

Grade I (insignificant, or suspicious)—Flat, acetowhite epithelium—borders not necessarily sharp; usually semitransparent with or without fine-caliber, regularly shaped vessels, often with ill-defined patterns; absence of atypical vessels; small intercapillary distance.

Grade II (significant, suspicious)—Flat, white epithelium of greater opacity with sharp borders; with or without dilated-caliber, regularly shaped vessels; defined patterns; absence of atypical vessels; usually increased intercapillary distance.

Grade III (highly significant, highly suspicious)—very white or gray opaque epithelium; sharply bordered; dilated-caliber, irregularly shaped, often coiled, often atypical vessels, increased but variable intercapillary distance; and sometimes irregular surface, microexophytic epithelium.

e.g., coarse punctation and a mosaic pattern, are relatively uncommon. Most CIN 3 lesions do not have prominent vascular patterns. Second, the epithelial and vascular proliferations associated with HPV infection can result in flat HPV lesions and CIN 1 lesions, both of which have prominent vascular patterns. It is not difficult for the experienced colposcopist to distinguish these patterns, but the emphasis on surface capillary patterns weakened the reproducibility of results using the Stafl grading system. Third, the Stafl system did not consider certain margin characteristics of lesions or the use of Lugol's iodine solution to visualize these characteristics. Finally, most colposcopists are unable to measure the very small intercapillary distances, which are one of the four criteria used in the Stafl grading system.

9.2.4.4 Burke colposcopic grading system

Dr. Louis Burke, a prominent Boston colposcopist, further refined the approach to grading cervical lesions by expanding the existing tri-part system.[12] The grading system, grades 1, 2 and 3, considered characteristics of lesion surface, margin, color, duration of acetowhite changes, and vessel characteristics (Table 9.3). Like Coppleson, but in contrast to Stafl, Burke realized the importance of surface contour. Furthermore, the Burke system superseded the Coppleson index by considering the duration of acetowhite

change that occurs in a lesion, which has now been proven to predict the severity of cervical disease. The Burke system also considers maximum intercapillary distance and the caliber of vessels when diagnosing CIN 3. As stated earlier, many of these lesions are characterized by a relative paucity of coarse vessels. Many practicing colposcopists were taught by Dr. Burke and, hence, still use this grading system.

9.2.4.5 Reid colposcopic index

In 1985, Dr. Richard Reid described the use of a new and less subjective colposcopic index to differentiate low-grade cervical disease from high-grade disease.[13,14] Consequently, the Reid Colposcopic Index (RCI) is not designed to discriminate premalignant from malignant cervical neoplasia. By defining specific aspects of certain colposcopic signs with which to accurately grade lesions, the index provides the most recent means of standardizing the evaluation of cervical neoplasia. Therefore, this index will be described in greater detail so that the RCI can be learned and used clinically.

9.2.4.5.1 RCI design The RCI is similar in design to the Apgar clinical scoring system used to assess the early health status of neonates. In contrast with the five categories of the Apgar scale, the RCI considers four colposcopic signs, which are margin or border

Table 9.3 Burke Colposcopic Grading System

Grade	Surface[1]	Margin	Color[2]	Time[3]	Vessels[4]	Pathology[5]
I	Flat	Indistinct	White	Slow/short	Fine, normal intercapillary distance	Insignificant infection, repair HPV
II	Flat	Distinct	Whiter	Average/average	Dilated punctation, mosaic, slight ↑ intercapillary distance	Significant HPV, CIN 1, CIN 2
III	Raised	Sharp	Whitest	Fast/long	Coarse, marked ↑ intercapillary distance, atypical vessels	Highly significant CIN 3, microinvasion or invasive cancer

Modified from Burke L, Antonioli D A, Ducatman B S, Colposcopy Text and Atlas. Norwalk, Connecticut. Appleton and Lange, 1991.
1. Contour of lesion
2. Color following application of 5% acetic acid
3. Onset of acetic acid effect/duration of acetic acid effect
4. Vessel caliber, intercapillary distance
5. Histology

Table 9.4   Reid Colposcopic Index

Colposcopic Sign	Zero Points	One Point	Two Points
Margin	Condylomatous or micropapillary contour Indistinct borders Flocculated or feathered margins Jagged, angular lesions Satellite lesions, acetowhite lesions outside the transformation zone	Regular lesions with smooth, straight outlines Sharp peripheral margins	Rolled, peeling edges Internal borders between lesions of different severity
Color	Shiny, snow white Transient, indistinct acetowhite, semi-transparent	Shiny, off-white Intermediate white	Dull, oyster grey Persistent, dense acetowhite
Vessels	Fine punctation or fine mosaic Uniform, fine caliber, nondilated capillary loops	Absence of surface vessels following acetic acid application	Coarse punctation or coarse mosaic Individual vessels dilated Wide intercapillary distance
Iodine Staining	Positive iodine uptake, producing a mahogany brown color Negative iodine uptake (mustard yellow) of a lesion recognized as low grade by above criteria ($\leq$ 2/6)	Partial iodine uptake Variegated, tortoise-shell appearance	Negative iodine uptake (mustard yellow) of a lesion considered high grade by above criteria ($\geq$ 3/6)
Total Reid Colposcopic Index Score:	0–2 = Normal or CIN 1	3–5 = CIN 1 or CIN 2	6–8 = CIN 2 or CIN 3

of lesion; color of lesion following application of 5% acetic acid solution; blood vessel characteristics within the lesion; and response of the lesion to the application of Lugol's iodine solution (Table 9.4). Each colposcopic sign is subdivided into three hierarchically distinct categories, each of which features unique characteristics that indicate specific stages of premalignant disease. Each category is assigned a numerical value from 0 to 2. Changes of human papillomavirus infection, CIN 1, and immature metaplasia are assigned a score of 0. A score of 1 represents the presence of CIN 1 to CIN 2, and a score of 2 reflects colposcopic findings predictive of CIN 3. Each of the four colposcopic signs is considered separately, and numerical scores are assigned respectively, depending on the severity of that characteristic within the detected cervical lesion. The scores for each of four colposcopic signs are added to establish a total RCI score (Table 9.5). The numeric value of the total score is then used to determine the estimated

severity of disease or clinical colposcopic impression (Table 9.6). The accuracy of the RCI is accomplished by deriving an aggregate diagnosis instead of considering only a solitary colposcopic sign.

9.2.4.5.2 The four RCI colposcopic signs The RCI considers unique morphologic and physiologic features of premalignant cervical lesions. The first three colposcopic signs are evaluated following proper application of an acetic acid solution (5%) to the cervix. The score for the final colposcopic sign is dependent on a preliminary subtotal score of the first three signs. The score for the fourth sign can only be determined after application of Lugol's iodine solution (one-half strength) to the cervix.

Margin The nature of a lesion margin, edge, or border varies depending on the severity of cervical neoplasia, making it an excellent indicator of the degree of cervical disease. Low-grade lesion

Table 9.5   Flow Sheet to Determine RCI Score

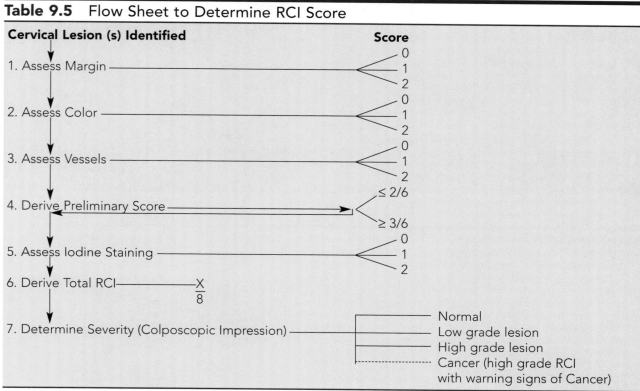

Cervical Lesion (s) Identified	Score

1. Assess Margin — 0 / 1 / 2

2. Assess Color — 0 / 1 / 2

3. Assess Vessels — 0 / 1 / 2

4. Derive Preliminary Score — $\leq 2/6$ / $\geq 3/6$

5. Assess Iodine Staining — 0 / 1 / 2

6. Derive Total RCI — $\dfrac{X}{8}$

7. Determine Severity (Colposcopic Impression) —
— Normal
— Low grade lesion
— High grade lesion
----- Cancer (high grade RCI with warning signs of Cancer)

Table 9.6   RCI Clinical Correlation

Total Colposcopic Sign Score	Colposcopic Impression
0–2	Normal or CIN 1 (Low Grade)
3–5	CIN 1 or CIN 2 (Intermediate Grade)[1]
6–8	CIN 2 or CIN 3 (High Grade)[2]

[1]Total colposcopic score of 3 likely represents a low grade lesion and a score of 5 predicts a high grade lesion.

[2]Maximum scores accompanied by colposcopic warning signs of cancer should invoke a colposcopic impression of cancer.

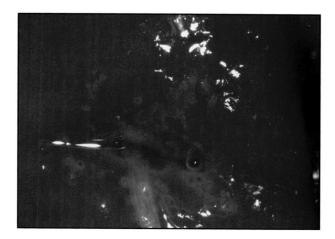

FIGURE 9.4   An irregular lesion margin at 2 o'clock noted in a woman with CIN 1. A score of 0 points is assigned for irregular margins.

(CIN 1 or HPV) margins may be irregular, flocculated, feathered (Figure 9.4), angular or "geographic" (Figures 9.5a,b), indistinct (Figures 9.6a,b) exophytic or micropapillary (condyloma-like) in contour (Figure 9.7), or surrounded by small "satellite" lesions (Figure 9.8). A score of 0 points is assigned to the lesion if these attributes are present. In contrast, smooth and fairly straight margins are characteristic of an intermediate lesion (CIN 1,2). A score of 1 point is assigned to the lesion when these margin characteristics are noted (Figure 9.9). High-grade lesions (CIN 3) may have raised, peeling epithelial edges (Figures 9.10a,b). Distinct lesions encompassed within a larger lower-grade lesion and located closer to the squamocolumnar junction may have an internal border that demarcates the area from the surrounding low-grade change (Figures 9.11a,b).

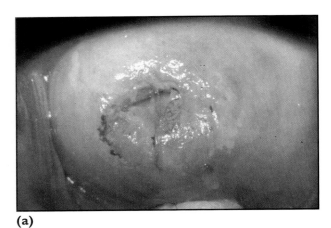

(a)

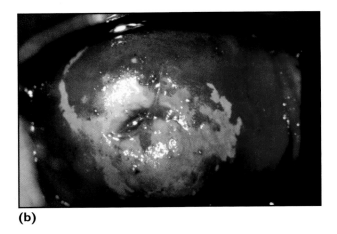

(b)

FIGURES 9.5a,b An angular or geographic lesion border that resembles the outline of an irregularly shaped country seen following application of acetic acid **(a)** and Lugol's iodine application **(b)**.

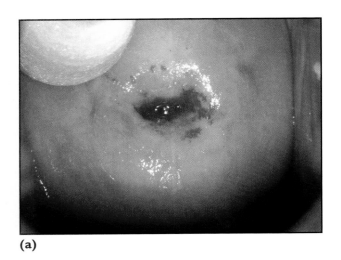

(a)

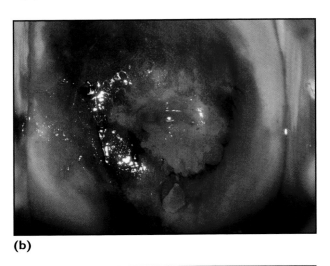

(b)

FIGURES 9.6a,b The margin of this acetowhite lesion **(a)** is fairly indistinct from the surrounding normal epithelium. The Lugol's solution stained cervix **(b)** more clearly displays the indistinct margin following application of acetic acid solution.

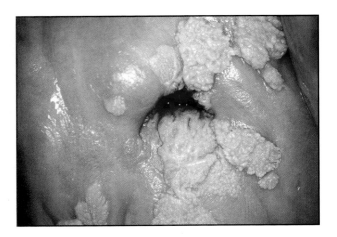

FIGURE 9.7 A papillary margin caused by human papillomavirus. This margin is given a score of 0 points.

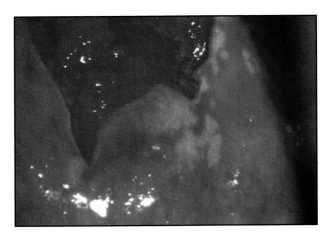

FIGURE 9.8 Small, diffuse and distant satellite lesions indicative of a low-grade CIN. Satellite lesions give a margin score of 0 points.

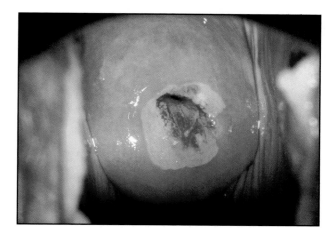

FIGURE 9.9 A distinct, smooth epithelial margin usually noted in CIN 2 or CIN 3. A straight margin is scored as 1 point.

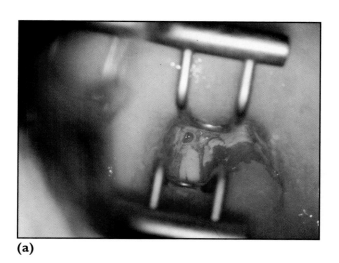

(a)

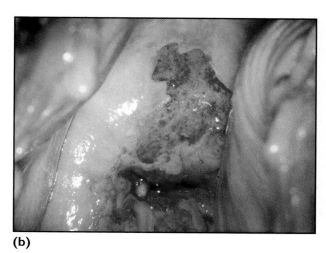

(b)

FIGURES 9.10a,b A raised, peeling lesion margin found in a woman with CIN 3 **(a)**. The acetowhite epithelium is very opaque and no vessels are apparent. The lesion extends into the endocervical canal beyond colposcopic view and thus the examination is unsatisfactory. Peeling epithelium and a large erosion are seen in **(b)**. The biopsy indicated CIN 2.

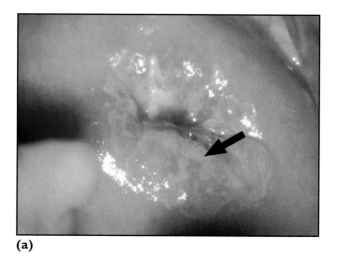

(a)

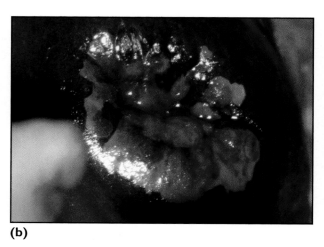

(b)

FIGURES 9.11a,b A large low-grade acetowhite lesion is readily observed on the cervix. However a high-grade lesion more proximally located near the external os on the posterior cervix is less apparent **(a)**. A demarcation line or internal border (arrow) separates the two lesions. This contrast is easily seen after application of Lugol's solution **(b)**. The yellow epithelium closest to the os represents CIN 3 and the brownish areas, CIN1.

Lesions with peeling edges or internal margins are likely to be CIN 3 and thus receive 2 points for their margin score. All cervical lesion margins are assigned a score prior to addressing the next colposcopic sign.

Color The color of the lesion following the application of 5% acetic acid solution determines the second colposcopic sign. Low-grade (CIN 1 or HPV) lesions are semitransparent, nearly translucent or a shiny snow-white in color (Figures 9.12a,b,c). These lesions are assigned 0 points for color. High-grade (CIN 3) lesions appear a dirty oyster-gray or very opaque in color after application of 5% acetic acid solution (Figures 9.13a,b). These lesions appear opaque white because the nuclear dense tissue of the lesion reflects much of the colposcope's light. They are assigned a score of 2 points for color. The opaque acetowhite color also persists for a longer period of time than does the translucent acetowhite color of CIN 1 lesions. An intermediate (CIN 1, 2) lesion is off-white, moderately opaque in color, and varies between the 2 extremes of the white color spectrum (Figures 9.14a,b). This is the most common category for color assignment and it is given a score of 1 point.

Vessels Blood vessel features are the third colposcopic sign considered in the Reid Colposcopic Index. Fine, narrow-caliber capillaries with small intercapillary distances characterize low-grade lesions. The small vessels may have either a punctation or a mosaic pattern. These vessels are not coarsely dilated and are configured in fairly loose, uniformly spaced arcades (Figures 9.15a–f). Zero points are assigned to lesions with these vessel characteristics. No superficial blood vessels are seen within acetowhite lesions of the intermediate category (Figures 9.16a,b,c,d). Thus, lesions with no visible vessels receive a score of 1 point. Coarsely dilated vessels present in areas of coarse punctation or coarse mosaic are present in high-grade (CIN 3)

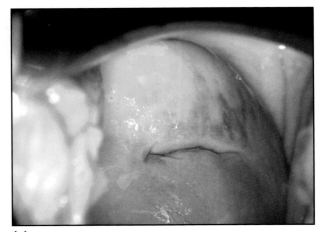

(a)

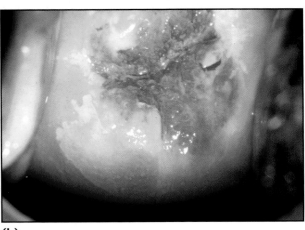

(b)

(c)

FIGURES 9.12a–c The color of the acetowhite lesions seen in **(a,b)** is very indistinct. A satellite lesion **(a)** is observed at 11 o'clock. Some low-grade lesions have a snow-white color **(c)**. Indistinct white and snow-white are scored as 0 points. ▬

lesions (Figures 9.17a–f). These vessels have a wide, irregular capillary pattern and are assigned a score of 2 points. The Reid Colposcopic Index pertains only to premalignant disease; thus, it does not include characteristics that may indicate more serious disease. Identifying coarsely dilated atypical blood vessels, a finding not listed in the RCI, during a colposcopic examination suggests the presence of invasive cancer.

Iodine The final colposcopic sign must be evaluated following staining of the cervix with Lugol's solution provided the patient has no known allergy to iodine. Normal original squamous epithelium and mature metaplastic epithelium contain glycogen, which has an affinity for iodine. Thus, these tissues transiently appear mahogany brown when stained with Lugol's iodine solution. Infrequently, low-grade (CIN 1 or HPV) lesions may absorb the iodine and appear a mahogany brown color or totally reject the iodine and appear a mustard-yellow color (Figures 9.18a–e). These lesions receive no points for iodine staining. A variegated yellow/brown or "tortoise-shell" appearance resulting from partial or inconsistent iodine uptake may occur in intermediate-grade CIN 1,2 lesions (Figures 9.19a–d). This

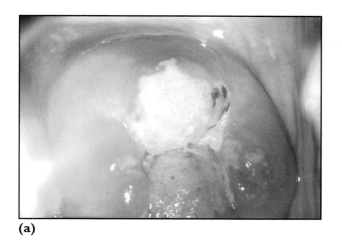

(a)

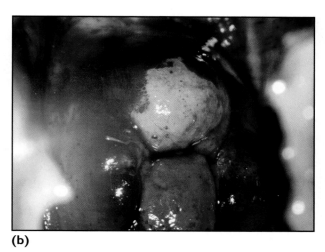

(b)

FIGURES 9.13a,b An opaque acetowhite lesion indicating CIN 3 on the anterior lip of the cervix **(a)**. Faint acetowhite epithelium representing immature metaplasia is noted on the posterior lip. The areas of CIN 3 and immature metaplasia are also noted following application of Lugol's iodine solution **(b)**. The CIN 3 lesion has a pale yellow color.

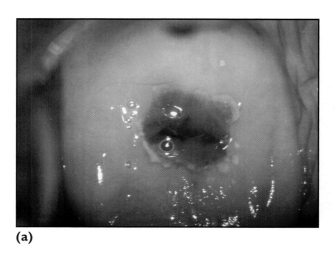

(a)

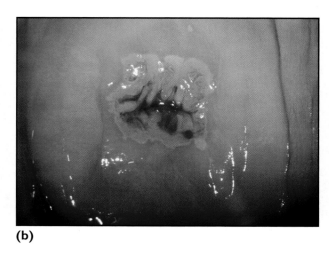

(b)

FIGURES 9.14a,b An intermediate acetowhite lesion of the cervix indicating CIN 2. The cervix is seen before acetic acid application **(a)** and after **(b)**. This color receives a score of one point.

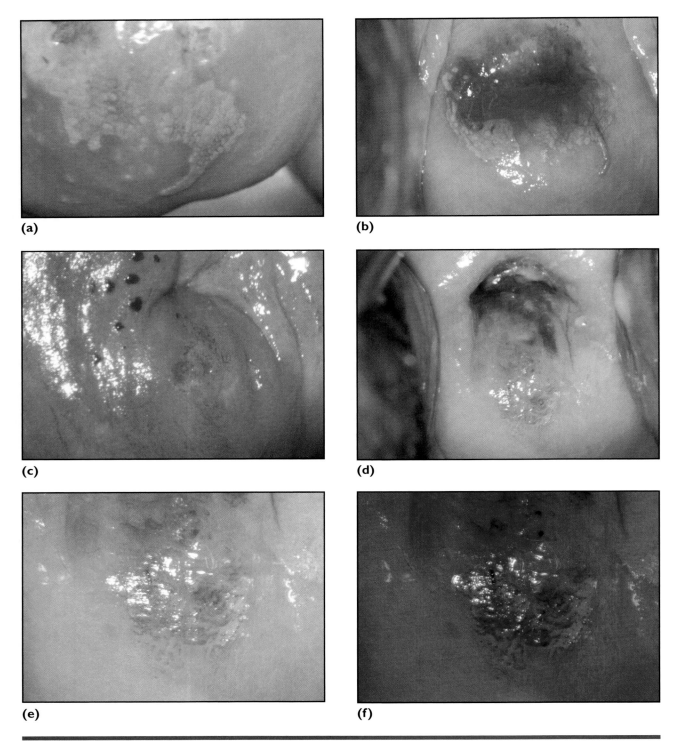

FIGURES 9.15a–f A fine-caliber mosaic vessel pattern is seen in **(a)** and **(b)**. The vessels are uniformly spaced with a narrow intercapillary distance. A fine punctation within a CIN 1 lesion on the posterior cervix is noted in **(c)**. There are acetowhite areas at 4 o'clock and 6 o'clock in **(d)**. With higher magnification of the lesion at 6 o'clock, fine punctation can be seen following acetic acid application **(e)** and with use of the green filter **(f)**. Fine vessels receive 0 points.

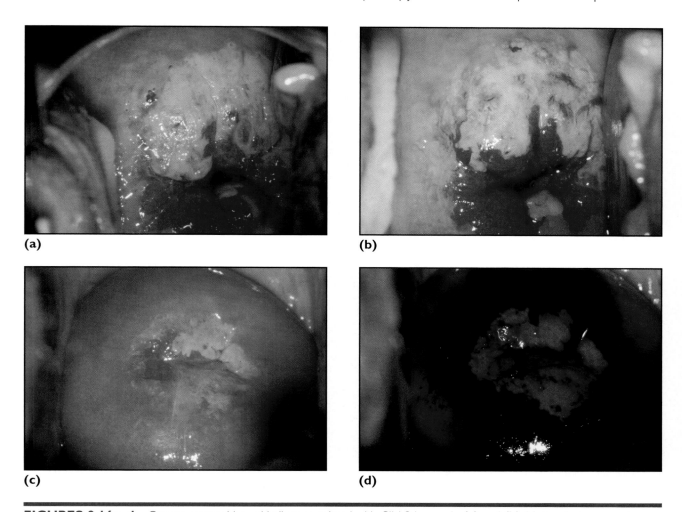

FIGURES 9.16a–d   Opaque acetowhite epithelium associated with CIN 3 is seen in **(a)** and **(b)**. Notice that no vessels are readily apparent. Another CIN 3 without visible vessels is seen in **(c)** and **(d)**. A score of 1 point is assigned if no vessels are apparent.

spotted response is assigned a score of 1 point. High-grade lesions (CIN 3) totally reject the iodine and briefly appear mustard-yellow against a mahogany background (Figures 9.20a–d). These severe lesions are assigned a score of 2 points. Some low-grade lesions, all high-grade lesions, and immature squamous metaplasia reject iodine uptake and appear mustard-yellow. Columnar cells reject iodine uptake and retain their reddish-pink color. Because all CIN appears yellow following Lugol's iodine application, and a score of 0 or 2 can be assigned for the same appearance, a subtotal of the points assigned to the lesion for the first three factors is used to determine the lesion's iodine score, as discussed in the next section.

9.2.4.5.3 Scoring the lesion   The total RCI score is reported as a ratio. The four scores derived from

evaluation of the four colposcopic signs are added to define the RCI numerator. The RCI denominator always remains constant at 8, but the numerator or total score fluctuates. The maximum possible total RCI score would be 8 and the minimum score would be 0.

Following application of 5% acetic acid solution to the cervix, the first three colposcopic signs are assessed and scored separately (Table 9.5). A preliminary subtotal score for these first three signs is summed before scoring the fourth sign. Lesions that reject iodine or turn mustard-yellow are assigned a score of 0 if the preliminary subtotal score of the first three colposcopic signs is 2 or less. Formerly acetowhite lesions that reject iodine and have a preliminary subtotal score of 3 or more receive 2 points. Lesions that turn a variegated color upon application of iodine receive a

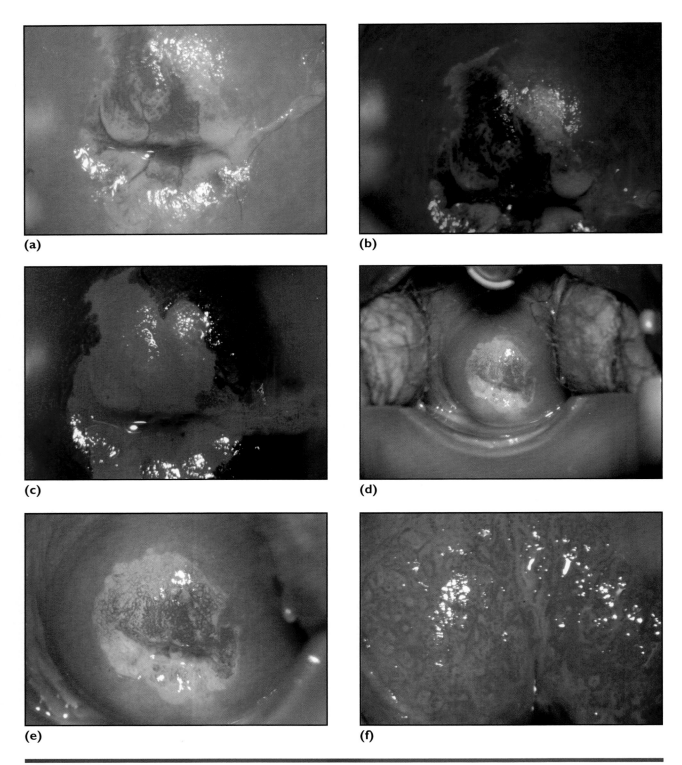

(a)

(b)

(c)

(d)

(e)

(f)

FIGURES 9.17a–f A coarse punctation is seen on the anterior cervix **(a)** following acetic acid application. A coarse vessel pattern is scored as 2 points. These coarse vessels are also seen using the green filter **(b)**. Usually application of Lugol's iodine solution obscures vessel patterns **(c)**. However, the coarse vessels can be seen at low magnification **(d)** and high magnification **(e)** in another woman with CIN 3. A very coarse mosaic and punctation vessel pattern is seen in **(f)**.

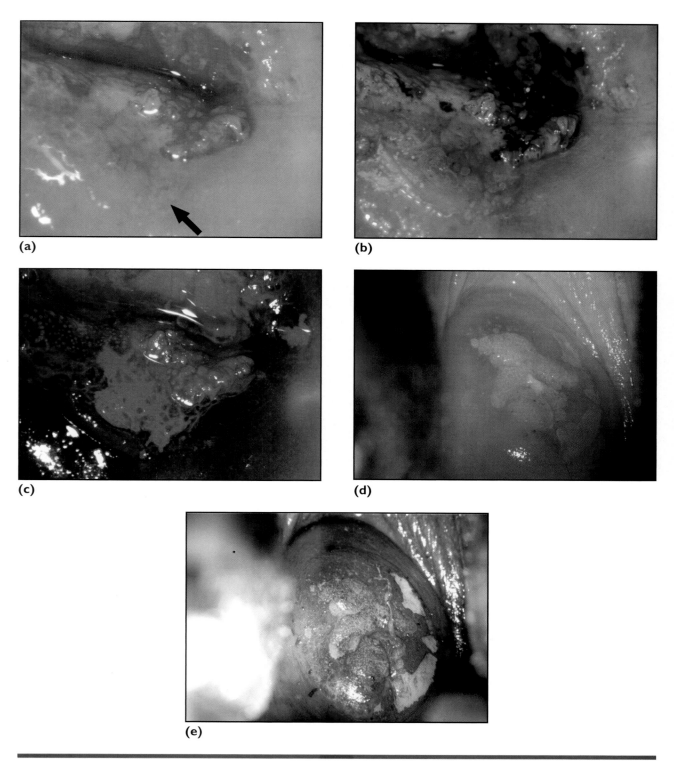

FIGURES 9.18a–e   The lesion on the posterior cervix **(a)** (arrow) has an irregular margin (0 points), a translucent ace-towhite color (0 points), and a fine-caliber mosaic seen in the green filter **(b)** (0 points). The preliminary score is 0/6. The same lesion totally rejects Lugol's iodine solution, and this is assigned 0 points for iodine **(c)**. This patient's cervical biopsy was diagnosed as CIN 1. The other lesion seen in **(d)** has an irregular margin with satellite lesions (0 points), an indistinct acetowhite color (0 points), and a fine mosaic pattern (0 points). The preliminary score is 0/6. The lesion picks up the iodine and appears brown (0 points) **(e)**. The total score of 0/8 suggests a low-grade lesion. The cervical biopsy was interpreted as CIN 1. ▬▬▬

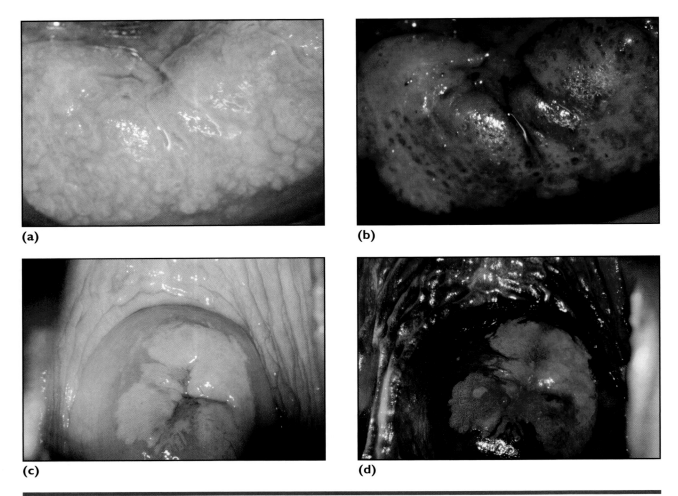

FIGURES 9.19a–d   The condyloma seen in **(a)** and **(b)** has a smooth margin (1 point), intermediate white color (1 point), and fine caliber mosaic vessels (0 points). There is variegated iodine uptake (1 point), resulting in a total score of 3/8. The biopsy indicated CIN 1. A large acetowhite lesion is seen in **(c)** and **(d)**. There is a low-grade lesion at 8 o'clock and a high-grade lesion at 2 o'clock. The former lesion has an irregular margin (0 points), a faint acetowhite color (1 point), and a fine mosaic (0 points). A variegated pattern of iodine uptake can be seen (1 point), earning the lesion a total score of 2/8 using the Reid Colposcopic Index. A biopsy was diagnosed as CIN 1. The lesion at 2 o'clock has a smooth margin (1 point), an opaque acetowhite color (2 points), and no visible vessels (1 point), resulting in a preliminary score of 4/6. Because it totally rejects the iodine, it is assigned 2 points for iodine staining. The total score of 6/8 indicates that it is a high-grade lesion. The cervical biopsy was interpreted as CIN 3.

score of 1 point. The total RCI score is then determined by adding the number of points scored for the fourth individual sign to the subtotal of the first three signs.

A degree of subjectivity exists in the scoring of each of the colposcopic signs. For example, one observer may examine a lesion and attribute it 0 points for color, while another observer may give the same lesion 1 point for color. This degree of subjectivity usually will not impact the overall colposcopic impression, since a highly subjective score for one sign will usually be counterbalanced by the scores for the other signs. The total score is based on 8 points, rather than 2 or 4 points. At first, scoring is a tedious exercise. However, with practice, the scoring of these four criteria will take no more than 15 to 30 seconds. Colposcopists who consistently use the RCI will notice marked improvement in their diagnostic accuracy.

9.2.4.5.4 The RCI clinical correlation   The RCI represents a weighted scoring system that helps colposcopists predict the severity of premalignant cervical lesions. As such, a low RCI score implies less serious cervical disease and a high RCI score indicates

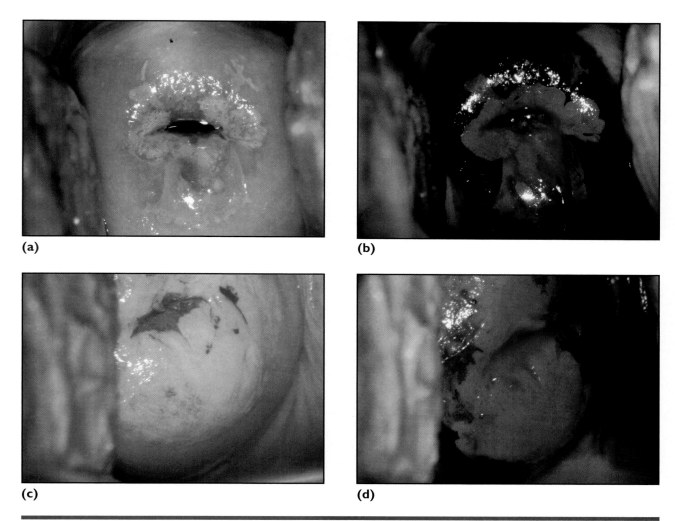

(a)

(b)

(c)

(d)

FIGURES 9.20a–d An opaque acetowhite, 3-quadrant lesion with a coarse punctation is seen in **(a)**. An internal margin separates this CIN 3 from a low-grade lesion at 6 o'clock. The low-grade lesion has an irregular margin, translucent white color, and fine mosaic vessel pattern. The high-grade lesion's preliminary score is (2,2,2) 6/6. It completely rejects iodine **(b)**, so its total score is 8/8. The low-grade lesion is scored as 0,0,0 for a preliminary score of 0/6. The pattern of iodine uptake is variegated; therefore, 1 point is assigned for iodine staining. The total score is 1/8 and this lesion is diagnosed as CIN 1. The large opaque acetowhite lesion **(c)**, with smooth margins and no visible blood vessels scores 1,2,1, for a preliminary score of 4/6. It completely rejects iodine and turns yellow **(d)**, so 2 points are assigned for iodine staining **(d)**. The total score is 6/8, indicating a high-grade lesion. The biopsy was interpreted as CIN 3.

more severe disease (Table 9.6). Numerator scores from 0 to 2 are predictive of CIN 1, human papillomavirus lesions, or normal immature metaplasia. Total RCI scores from 3 to 5 are suggestive of CIN 1 or CIN 2, with a score of 3 being more predictive of CIN 1 and a score of 5 more suggestive of CIN 2. An RCI score from 6 to 8 is predictive of CIN 2 to CIN 3. An RCI score of 8 for a cervical lesion demonstrating additional features considered to be warning signs for cervical cancer should be upgraded to a colposcopic impression of either microinvasive or invasive cancer.

The index does not result in scores that are 100% in agreement with histologic findings, but 100% correlation is not the aim. Colposcopic findings that are discordant with histologic findings will occur even when the most experienced colposcopist performs the examination. Nevertheless, use of the index results in more consistent agreement between colposcopic and histologic findings than would be achieved by a less systematic approach to colposcopic diagnosis.

9.2.4.5.5 Special considerations concerning the RCI

Some potential confusion with RCI may occur. Clinically obvious condylomas exhibiting a micropapillary or "cerebriform" (Figure 9.21) appearance of cervical HPV infection automatically score 0 points for peripheral margin, even though the margin is in fact raised above the surrounding epithelium. Although raised, these lesions do not appear as if they could easily be peeled away from the underlying stroma. Their margins are also still primarily irregular and not smooth in shape.

One of the most valuable aspects of the index is the concept of an internal margin within a larger lesion (Figures 9.22a–g). If in assessing a lesion colposcopically, the colposcopic disease pattern seen distally on the ectocervix is different than that seen proximally nearer the squamocolumnar junction, the internal lesion is almost invariably more severe. An internal margin usually indicates evolution of a new high-grade lesion within a larger, more stable, preexisting low-grade lesion. The high-grade lesion should adjoin the squamocolumnar junction. The internal margin between the two lesions is therefore a marker for centrally positioned high-grade disease and scores 2 points for margin. The one exception is when the internal lesion is a clinically obvious condyloma acuminata within a larger subclinical, HPV-induced lesion or larger area of immature metaplasia (Figure 9.23). Generally, this exception is also characterized by the position of the internal lesion near but not on the squamocolumnar junction. The larger, peripheral translucent acetowhite epithelium wraps around the internal lesion and contacts the squamocolumnar junction. In this scenario, the low-grade lesion or immature metaplastic epithelium actually adjoins the squamocolumnar junction.

A significant number of CIN lesions score 1 point for color. Indistinct or snow-white HPV-induced lesions do occur. A dull oyster-grey color predicts a high-grade lesion. These represent the two extremes and score 0 or 2 for color, respectively. They represent dichotomous translucent or opaque acetowhite colors. Most lesions exhibit a color in between, and score 1 point for color. This simple fact helps remove much of the subjectivity in scoring the

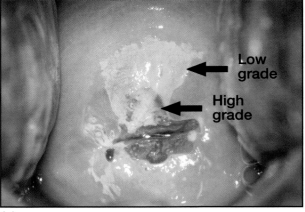

(a)

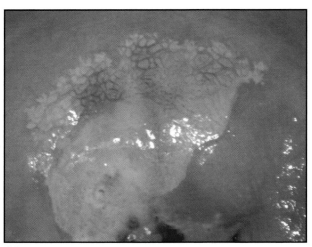

(b)

FIGURES 9.22a–g A large low-grade lesion (arrow) with a smaller high-grade lesion (arrow) positioned along the SCJ is seen in **(a)**. The high-grade lesion with coarse punctation is separated from the low-grade lesion by an internal margin. The low-grade lesion in the periphery **(b)** has a feathered margin, translucent white epithelium with a fine mosaic, and a punctation vessel pattern.

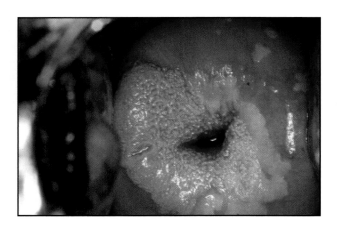

FIGURE 9.21 A HPV lesion that has a micropapilliferous appearance. The margin is scored 0.

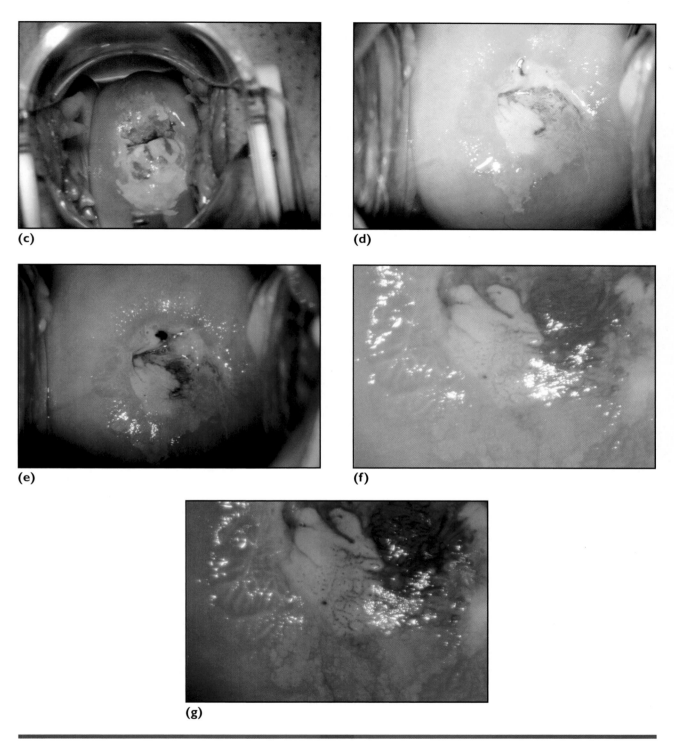

(c)

(d)

(e)

(f)

(g)

FIGURES 9.22a–g   Continued. There is a small high-grade lesion on the posterior cervix in **(c)**. It is separated by an internal margin from a larger low-grade lesion. A very opaque acetowhite lesion is separated from a large, translucent acetowhite lesion on the posterior cervix **(d–g)**. The larger low-grade lesion **(f,g)** has a geographic margin (0 points), a translucent color (0 points), and fine caliber vessels (0 points). The high-grade lesion has a coarse vessel pattern, opaque epithelium, and internal margin, which all score 2 points each.

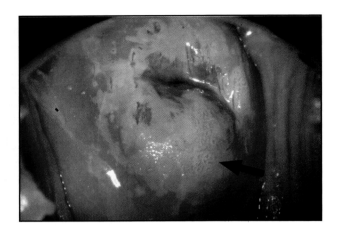

FIGURE 9.23 The exception to an internal margin whereby a condyloma (arrow) is positioned within a field of immature metaplasia but does not adjoin the squamo-columnar junction. ▬

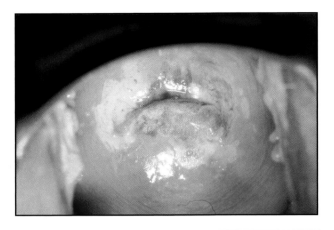

FIGURE 9.24 The lesion between 9 o'clock and 11 o'clock has no visible vessels and scores 1 point. The lesion at 6 o'clock has coarse vessels and scores 2 points for vessels. ▬

color of the lesion. In fact, indecision of greater than 15 seconds when assessing the color of cervical lesions should be quickly rectified by selecting a color score of 1 point.

Many lesions have no colposcopically apparent capillary pattern within the acetowhite lesion. A lesion with no visible blood vessels or absent vessels scores 1 point (Figure 9.24). If a vascular pattern is present, it is necessary to determine whether it represents a fine vascular pattern (score 0) or a coarse vascular pattern (score 2). The coarse vascular pattern is uncommon. Sometimes when vessels are moderately dilated, it is difficult to determine whether vessels should be considered fine or coarse caliber. For instance, pregnancy or cervicitis may cause normally small blood vessels of a low-grade lesion to dilate. Lesions in which the vessel pattern is difficult to score almost invariably occur within immature elements of the transformation zone. Lesions in the immature components of the transformation zone occasionally have an unexpected histologic diagnosis of CIN 2 when a low-grade morphology was expected based on colposcopic findings. For this reason, if there is difficulty ascribing a score for vessel pattern, some colposcopists choose to overestimate and assign the lesion a score of 2 points. If the lesion is in fact low-grade, it will receive lower scores for the other signs. Thus, the impression made based on the total RCI score will still be consistent with the histology results.

It is important to assess and score the first three characteristics of the lesion using a 5% acetic acid solution before assessing the last score using Lugol's

iodine solution. If the lesion scores 2 or fewer points for the first three signs, but rejects iodine staining and appears mustard-yellow, the lesion will be downgraded and scored 0 points for iodine staining (Figures 9.18a–e). The explanation for the negative iodine staining is that low-grade lesions occur within poorly or non-glycogenated, immature elements of the transformation zone. On the other hand, if the lesion has scored a total of 3 or more points on the previously assessed characteristics, and then stains mustard-yellow after application of Lugol's iodine solution, a score of 2 points is given for the iodine staining test (Figures 9.19c,d). In that lesion, the negative staining reflects a poorly differentiated high-grade lesion and a complete absence of glycogen in the superficial layers of epithelium.

Since the most prominent area of colposcopic change is not necessarily the area of greatest histologic abnormality, less experienced colposcopists may not select the most abnormal site for biopsy. Specifically, peripheral areas of prominent acetowhite epithelium are often overinterpreted, while the subtle acetowhite of a high-grade lesion or adenocarcinoma in situ are easily overlooked.

9.2.4.5.6 Reproducibility of the Reid Colposcopic Index In Reid's study, the overall diagnostic accuracy of colposcopy compared with histology was 97%, the high percentage of accuracy reflecting in part the skills of a most experienced colposcopist and a relatively small number of patients.[13] In another study of colposcopic accuracy using the RCI, a primary care colposcopist

achieved a 92% agreement rating between colposcopic impression and histologic diagnosis.[6] As these studies demonstrated, the use of such a system can greatly improve the accuracy of colposcopy. However, novice colposcopists should biopsy liberally since accuracy from these two referenced studies represents results from more experienced colposcopists.

9.3 Colposcopic Features of Cervical Intraepithelial Neoplasia (CIN)

The spectrum of variation in colposcopic signs is a nondistinct continuum that spans the three levels of CIN. Even at the ends of the CIN continuum, discrimination between normal immature metaplasia and CIN 1 or between CIN 3 and microinvasive cancer may still present a diagnostic challenge. Use of a colposcopic grading system enhances the colposcopist's ability to form colposcopic impressions. Only years of colposcopic experience, supplemented by feedback from histologic sampling, refines a colposcopist's skill in estimating the severity of cervical neoplasia.

The colposcopic appearance is determined by the architecture of the tissue being examined. Consequently, numerous combinations and various expressions of normal and abnormal tissue are possible within the transformation zone (leukoplakia, acetowhite epithelium, mosaic or punctation pattern, and atypical blood vessels) (Chapter 8). Because variation will occur, the colposcopic impression may differ with the cytologic and histologic interpretations within one degree of severity. In the next three sections, the colposcopic features of cervical intraepithelial neoplasia will be discussed.

9.3.1 Colposcopy of CIN 1

9.3.1.1 Location of CIN 1

The location of CIN 1 affects the colposcopist's ability to recognize and identify this level of disease. One of the greatest challenges in colposcopy is accurately diagnosing CIN in its first stage, particularly in young women in whom an abundance of immature portions of the cervical transformation zone are visible. The colposcopic prediction of ectocervical CIN 1 tends to be much easier in women with fully mature transformation zones, or in post-treatment and postmenopausal patients in whom areas of immature metaplasia are not seen. However, CIN 1 may be just as difficult to diagnose in the latter cases if the lesion is located entirely within the endocervical canal. A beginning colposcopist will initially have difficulty discriminating between immature metaplasia and some forms of CIN (Figures 9.25a–c). The problem may be further compounded by the fact that these viral or mildly neoplastic changes are usually adjacent to the squamocolumnar junction (SCJ) and engulfed in areas of immature metaplasia.

CIN 1 or satellite lesions outside the active transformation zone may be recognized against the normal, pink squamous epithelium (Figures 9.26a,b). CIN 1 may be found anywhere on the ectocervix, in the endocervical canal (Figure 9.27), or in both locations (Figure 9.28). Most neoplasia adjoins the squamocolumnar junction (Figures 9.29a,b). However, CIN 1 may be somewhat more inconsistent in this regard compared with CIN 2 or 3. Yet, most CIN 1 is found along the SCJ. As with other more severe CIN, it is mainly the position of the SCJ that determines the location of CIN 1.

9.3.1.2 Contour of CIN 1

In addition to location, the contour of CIN 1 lesions can vary tremendously. Many CIN 1 equivalents, represented by condylomas, have a wide but not unlimited range of morphologic expression, including micropapillary, papillary, papular, and raised contour. Although rare, a cerebriform or "brain-like" topography may be seen as well. Large exophytic condyloma occupying four quadrants of the cervix must be distinguished from invasive cancer by cervical biopsy (Figures 9.30a,b). These large HPV lesions normally have more distinct uniform papillary projections with centralized fine-caliber capillaries (Figure 9.31).

In contrast with elevated lesions, endophytic CIN 1 may be seen if the neoplastic epithelium extends within gland clefts. If this lesion is isolated to a gland cleft, a broad, slightly opaque acetowhite band of epithelium will be observed surrounding the gland opening (Figure 9.32). This periglandular cuffing is in contrast to the thin rim of acetowhite epithelium that surrounds normal, uninvolved gland openings. However, these sometimes occult endophytic lesions are usually associated with more apparent ectocervical lesions.

The majority of CIN 1 is macular in contour (Figure 9.33). In some cases, it may be maculopapular (Figure 9.34). Because of their lack of contrast with the surrounding normal, flat squamous epithelium, CIN 1 lesions are not generally apparent without the

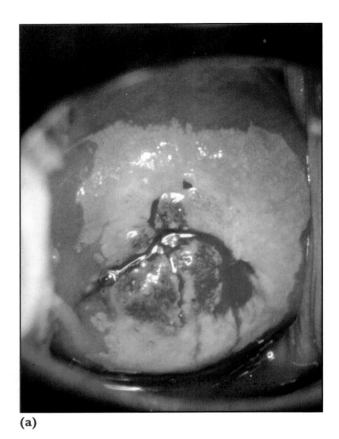

(a)

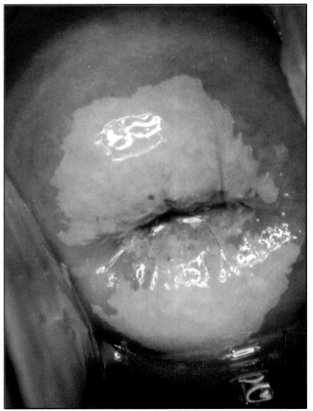

(b)

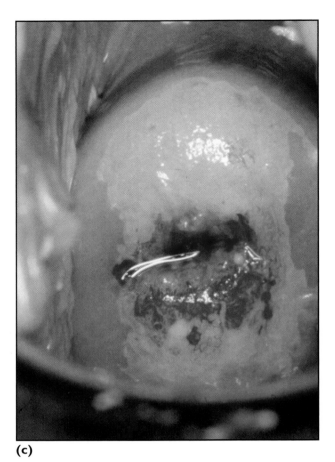

(c)

FIGURES 9.25a–c The large acetowhite areas on these three cervices were diagnosed as immature metaplasia by biopsy. Each one could be easily diagnosed clinically as CIN 1.

use of contrast solutions (Figures 9.35a,b). The one exception is when a slightly elevated area of leuko-plakia overlies a CIN 1 lesion. However, in this case, the keratinized epithelium is what is raised rather than the underlying CIN 1. A fine micropapillary surface contour may be seen with subclinical HPV infection of the cervix or vagina (Figures 9.36a,b,c,d,e). Tiny light reflections give the surface a slightly pebbled appearance. With close inspection, small capillaries may be observed inside the finger-like projections. This presentation is frequently seen in women with a LSIL Pap smear result and no discrete acetowhite lesion.

9.3.1.3 Margins of CIN 1

Because CIN 1 represents an acute epithelial HPV infection, these lesions tend to be diffuse and asymmetrical in shape (Figures 9.37a,b). The edges or

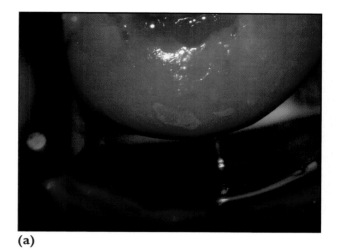

(a)

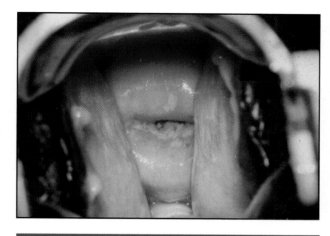

FIGURE 9.28   This CIN I is on the ectocervix, but it also extends within the endocervical canal.

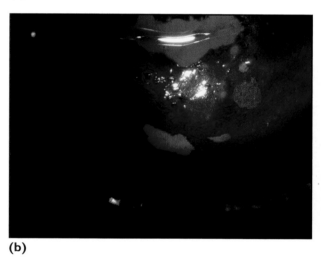

(b)

FIGURES 9.26a,b   A small CIN I located outside the transformation zone following application of 5% acetic acid solution **(a)** and Lugol's iodine **(b)**.

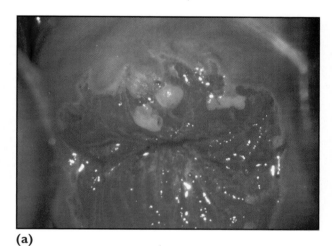

(a)

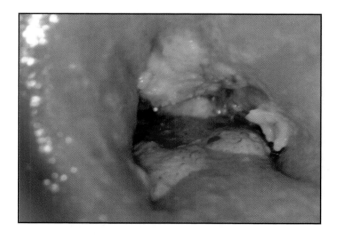

FIGURE 9.27   An exophytic condyloma within the endocervical canal. Fine vessels are seen on the posterior cervix.

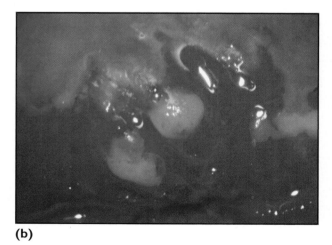

(b)

FIGURES 9.29a,b   These CIN I lesions are located on the squamocolumnar junction. These lesions would be considered at greater risk for progression than the lesion seen in Figure 9.26 **(a,b)**.

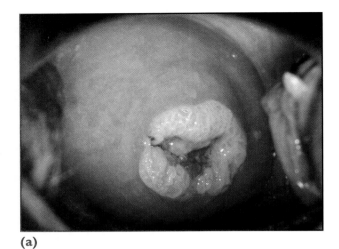

(a)

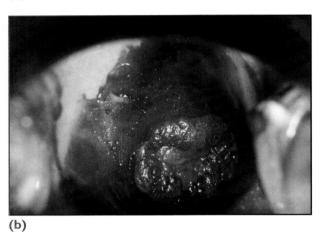

(b)

FIGURES 9.30a,b This large four quadrant acetowhite lesion of the cervix could be invasive cancer or an exophytic condyloma **(a)**. The lesion absorbs iodine and turns mahogany brown. Hence, the latter diagnosis is favored pending a histologic diagnosis **(b)**.

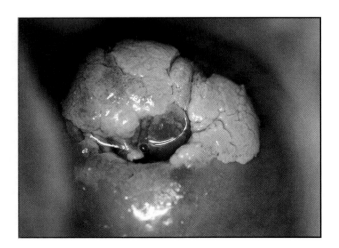

FIGURE 9.31 Fine vessels are noted in the papillary projections of this cervical condyloma.

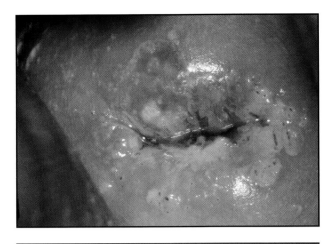

FIGURE 9.32 CIN 1 is seen within gland clefts at 5 o'clock. The normally thin translucent acetowhite rim around gland openings is broader and more opaque.

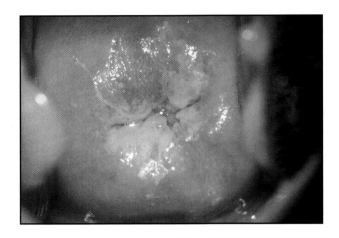

FIGURE 9.33 A macular CIN 1 on the anterior and posterior cervix.

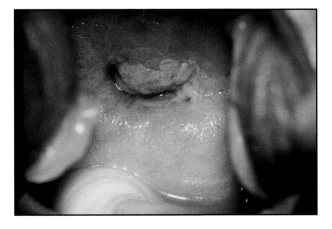

FIGURE 9.34 A maculopapular surface representing CIN 1.

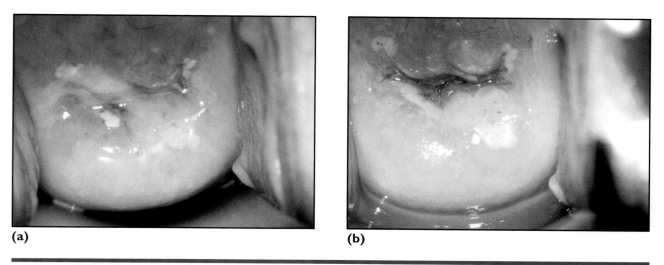

FIGURES 9.35a,b   Only a small area of leukoplakia is noted at 4 o'clock prior to the application of 5% acetic acid solution **(a)**. Following acetic acid application, a much larger acetowhite lesion is seen **(b)**.

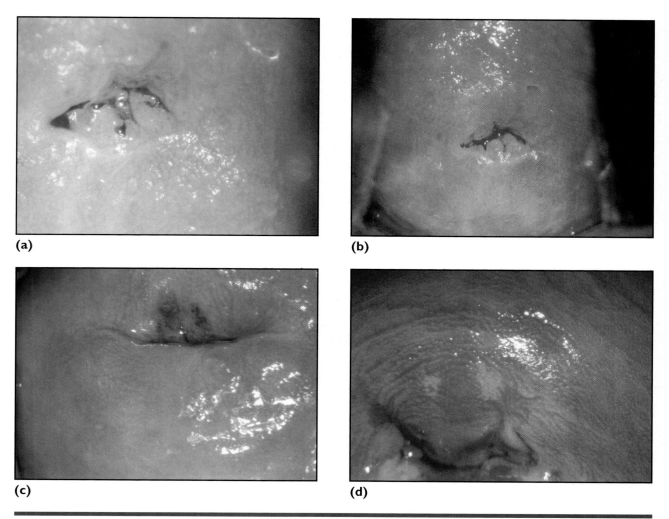

FIGURES 9.36a–e   Subclinical HPV infection can cause a fine micropapillary surface contour. Central loop capillaries may be observed within these tiny projections extending above the surface of the epithelium. (Continued)

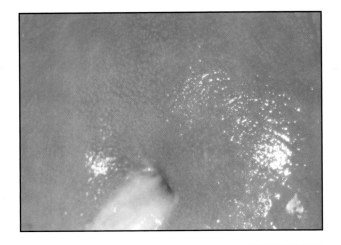

FIGURES 9.36a–e   Continued.

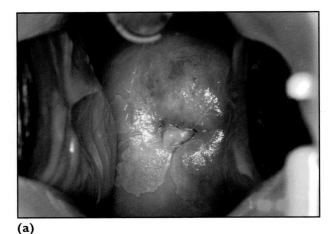

(a)

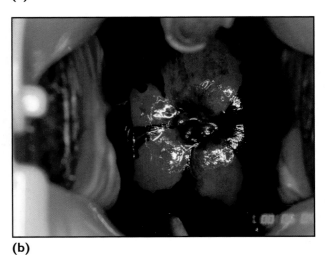

(b)

FIGURES 9.37a,b Diffuse, asymmetrical CIN 1 after application of 5% acetic acid solution **(a)** and Lugol's iodine solution **(b)**.

borders of CIN 1 are characteristically irregular (Figures 9.38a,b). These margins vary tremendously, assuming geographic, feathered, flocculated, or indistinct demarcations from the surrounding normal epithelium (Figures 9.39a,b). Multiple or solitary satellite lesions in the periphery of a central lesion support a diagnosis of CIN 1. Therefore, most CIN 1 margins are very uneven and crooked, reflecting the biologic nature of the lesion.

9.3.1.4 Color of CIN 1

Color is somewhat subjective, and therefore may be hard to classify. Variations of white can be even more difficult to describe. Glare also may influence the determination of color. The dilemma of color description is further affected by the varied illumination sources for colposcopes, which emit slightly different wavelengths or shades of white light. Regard-

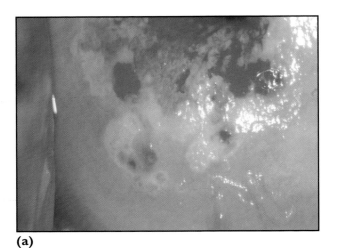

(a)

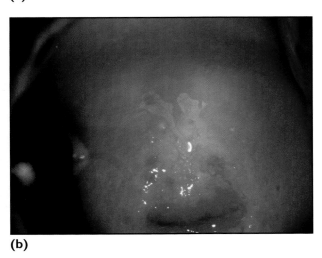

(b)

FIGURES 9.38a,b Irregular margins in 2 cases of CIN 1.

less, most CIN 1 lesions are transiently a light white following application of 5% acetic acid solution (Figures 9.40a-c). Prior to the application of an acetic acid solution, most CIN 1 lesions have a normal pink epithelial color. After the application of the 5% acetic acid, some lesions appear almost translucent white or faint white, but generally not as translucent as immature metaplasia or the transient white blush appearance of columnar villi (Figures 9.41a,b). Conversely, condylomas may be shiny white, conveying an opaque quality more typically seen in severe dysplasia. Virally induced leukoplakia reflects most of the colposcope's light, producing a more opaque white color than would be anticipated for the level of disease (Figures 9.42a,b). Because of the keratin, some condylomas also appear white prior to the application of 5% acetic acid solution.

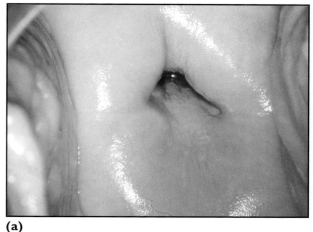

(a)

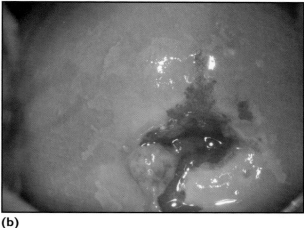

(b)

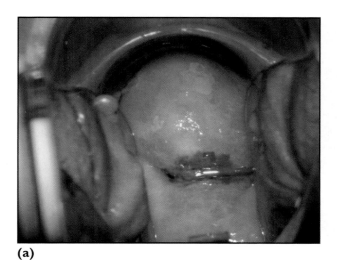

(a)

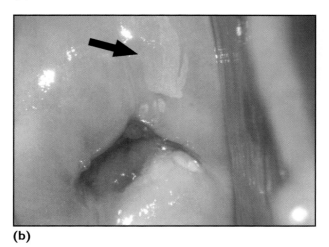

(b)

FIGURES 9.39a,b Geographic **(a)** and feathered **(b)** (arrow) margins indicate CIN 1.

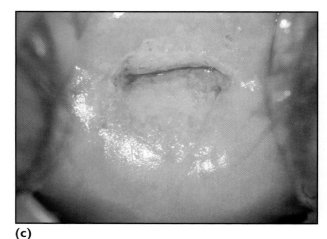

(c)

FIGURES 9.40a–c Translucent acetowhite lesions on the posterior **(a)** and anterior cervix **(b)**. The latter lesion has a geographic margin and fine caliber vessels. In the third patient **(c)**, translucent acetowhite lesions are present on the anterior and posterior cervix.

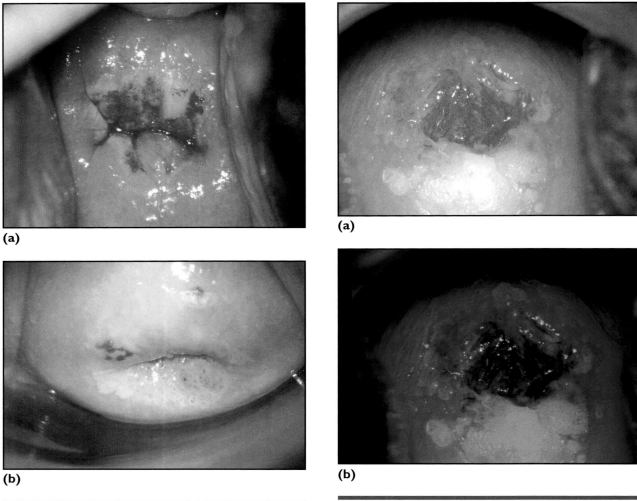

(a)

(b)

(a)

(b)

FIGURES 9.41a,b   These two CIN I lesions have a more opaque acetowhite color than those seen in Figures 9.40a,b.

FIGURES 9.42a,b   An area of leukoplakia within the central area of this CIN I **(a)**. The green filter does not enhance the colposcopic examination when vessels are not apparent **(b)**.

The degree of whiteness of cervical lesions and the duration of acetowhite effect of cervical neoplasia following the application of acetic acid has been quantitated previously.[15] Significant differences between the acetowhiteness of the 3 grades of CIN were detected, with CIN 1 having the lowest values and CIN 3 the greatest. Moreover, the resolution rates of acetowhite color 4 minutes after the application of acetic acid were 65% for CIN 1, 41% for CIN 2, and 29% for CIN 3. These progressively diminishing acetowhite effect rates document the tendency of CIN 1 to be very transiently acetowhite. Only the acetowhite color of squamous metaplasia resolved at a greater rate (78%) than CIN 1 within 4 minutes.[15]

9.3.1.5 Vessels of CIN 1

When blood vessels are noted colposcopically in CIN 1 lesions, they are invariably of a fine, narrow caliber

(Figures 9.43a-d). These vessels may be slightly more apparent than the small, wispy loop capillaries sometimes noted in native squamous epithelium (Figures 9.44a,b,c). A slightly increased intercapillary distance may be seen, but the vessel spacing is usually similar to that in normal tissue. The vessels of CIN 1 are arranged uniformly. Consequently, a mosaic vascular pattern associated with CIN 1 is homogeneous in distribution and appears delicate and lacy (Figures 9.45a,b, 9.46a,b, 9.47a,b). Punctation is observed as tiny red dots closely and uniformly distributed (Figures 9.48a,b). Fine caliber vessels may not be seen immediately following the application of 5% acetic acid solution. Although the tiny vessels contrast nicely against an acetowhite background, extremely narrow caliber vessels may not be visualized until the full acetowhite effect begins to diminish.

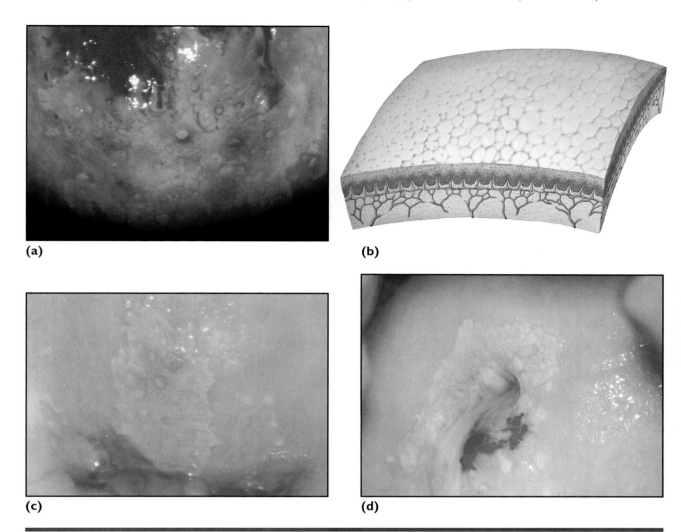

FIGURES 9.43a–d Fine punctation and mosaic in a CIN I **(a)**. An illustration of fine mosaic and fine punctation **(b)**. Another fine punctation is seen in a CIN I lesion **(c)**. A delicate, lacy, fine mosaic pattern is typical of CIN I **(d)**.

Atypical blood vessels are not seen in CIN 1. However, superficial, parallel atypical blood vessels not associated with cancer may be seen in areas of very immature metaplasia (Figures 8.91, 8.92), causing these areas to be easily confused with CIN 1 or cancer. These vessels are very coarse and horizontally positioned and have few branching vessels. In this case, the surrounding acetowhite change is minimal and extremely translucent.

9.3.1.6 Iodine staining of CIN 1

CIN 1 lesions are iodine negative with a mustard-yellow color after the application of dilute Lugol's iodine in areas that were formerly acetowhite (Figures 9.49a–h). Superficial keratin sometimes associated with CIN 1 also rejects iodine in areas that were white prior to application of 5% acetic acid solution (Figures 9.50a,b). Because CIN 1 is frequently positioned in a field of immature metaplasia, both areas will appear yellow following application of Lugol's iodine solution, and thus may blend together, making differentiation challenging.

Occasionally, there may be a variegated yellow and brown pattern noticed in focal epithelium that contains variable amounts of glycogen (Figures 9.51a,b; 9.52a,b). Because glycogen is usually found in intermediate and superficial layers of squamous epithelium and the atypical cellular changes of CIN 1 are found primarily in the basal and parabasal layers, it is not uncommon to see some degree of partial or even full iodine uptake in isolated areas of CIN 1.

9.3.1.7 Size and distribution of CIN 1

CIN 1 lesions tend to be relatively small (Figures 9.53a-c). The mean length of CIN 1 lesions is approximately 2.8 mm.[16] However, these lesions can reach a maximum length of 11.5 mm.[16] In comparison, CIN 2 and CIN 3 lesions are larger. The mean length of CIN 2 and CIN 3 are 5.8 mm and 7.6 mm, respectively. Their maximum lengths are 18.2 mm and 20.6 mm,

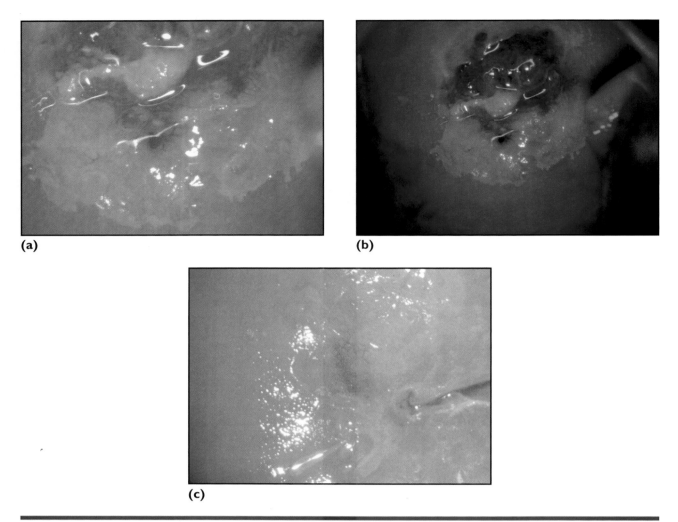

FIGURES 9.44a–c These fine vessels associated with CIN 1 are much larger than the small network capillaries of native squamous epithelium **(a,b)**. In the next case **(c)**, a translucent acetowhite lesion with geographic borders is noted near the os. There is a fine caliber mosaic vessel pattern. These colposcopic findings indicate a low-grade lesion.

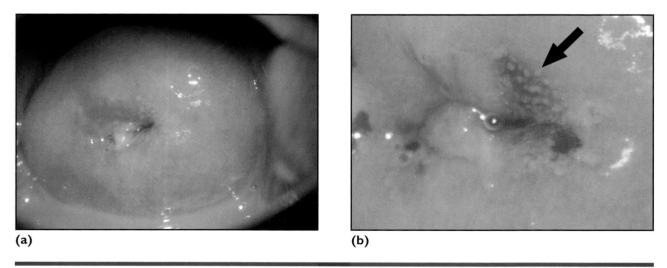

FIGURES 9.45a,b At low magnification an acetowhite lesion is seen at 2 o'clock **(a)**. The mosaic pattern (arrow) is better appreciated at higher magnification **(b)**.

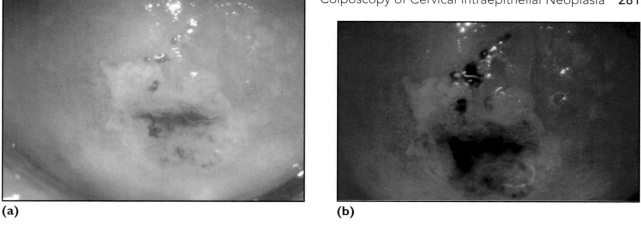

(a) **(b)**

FIGURES 9.46a,b   A delicate mosaic pattern is seen in the low-grade lesion at 10 o'clock **(a)**. The vessel pattern is accentuated by using the green filter **(b)**.

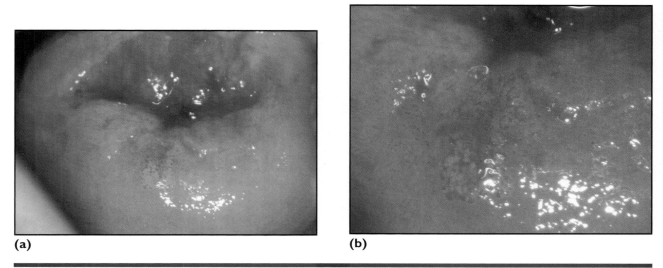

(a) **(b)**

FIGURES 9.47a,b   A small CIN 1 can be seen on the posterior cervix **(a)**. A fine mosaic pattern is noted in **(b)**. Also of interest, small HPV-induced papillary projections with central loop capillaries are observed surrounding the lesion.

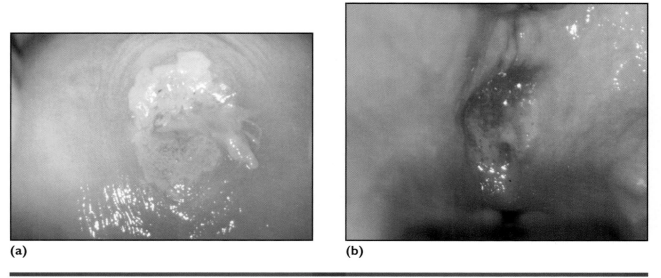

(a) **(b)**

FIGURES 9.48a,b   A fine punctation is seen in this CIN 1 **(a)**. Another fine punctation is noted in the CIN 1 following loop excision **(b)**.

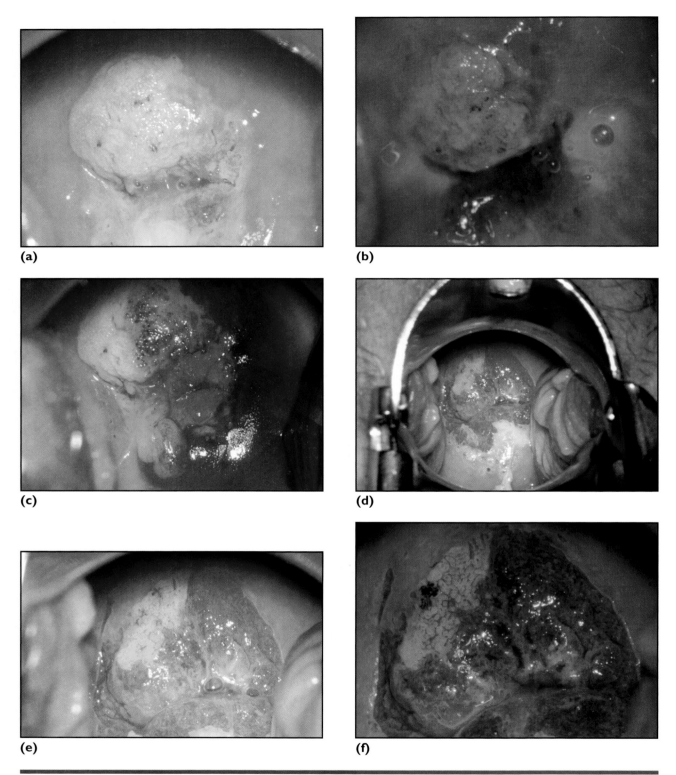

(a)

(b)

(c)

(d)

(e)

(f)

FIGURES 9.49a–h   A large condyloma occupies most of the anterior cervix **(a)**. Small punctate vessels are observed using the green filter **(b)**. Half of the lesion has been coated with application of Lugol's iodine solution **(c)**. The lesion rejects the iodine and appears yellow against the brown-staining, normal squamous epithelium. In another patient **(d-h)**, an acetowhite lesion can be seen at 10 o'clock along the SCJ **(d)**. This lesion has a fine mosaic pattern **(e,f,g)**. Lugol's iodine has been applied to a portion of the lesion **(h)** and the former acetowhite area now appears yellow.

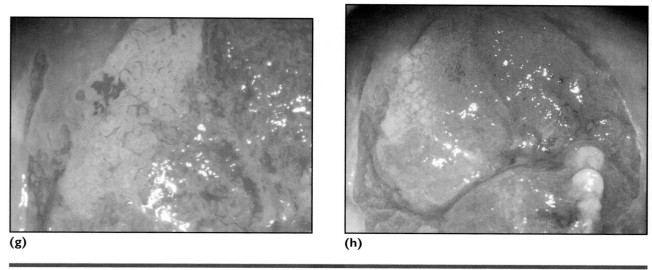

(g) **(h)**

FIGURES 9.49a–h Continued.

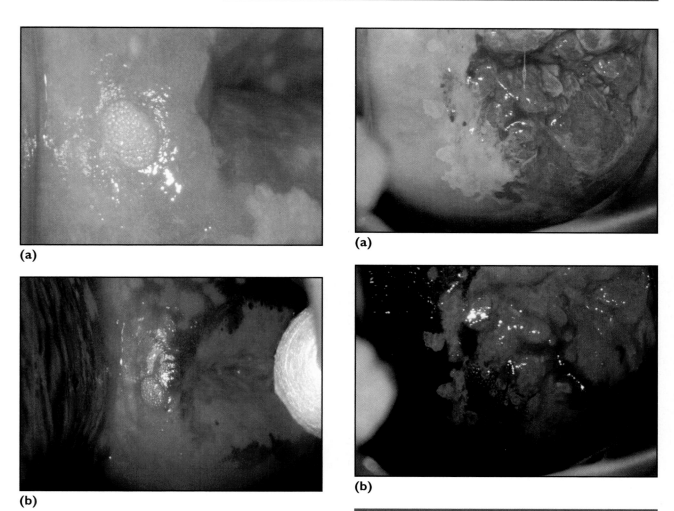

(a)

(b)

(a)

(b)

FIGURES 9.50a,b Leukoplakia covers this CIN 1 **(a)**. Consequently, the condylomatous lesion appears yellow following application of Lugol's iodine solution **(b)**.

FIGURES 9.51a,b The low-grade lesion with an irregular margin at 8 o'clock **(a)** has a variegated iodine-staining pattern. Some glycogen is present within the lesion.

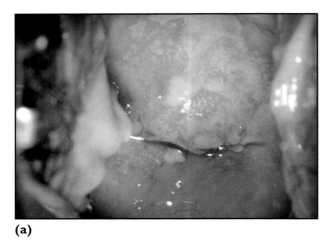

(a)

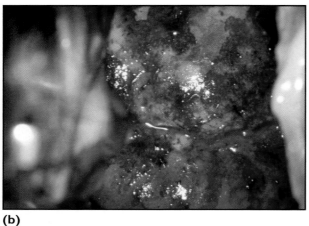

(b)

FIGURES 9.52a,b   This diffuse low-grade lesion also has a patchy variegated iodine uptake.

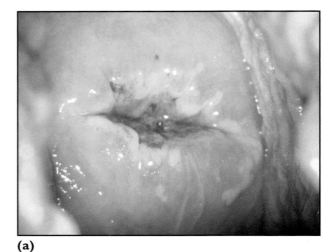

(a)

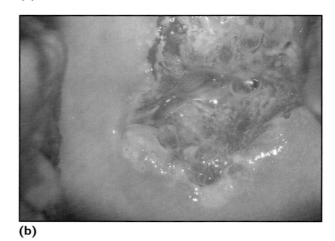

(b)

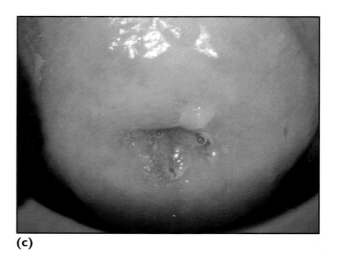

(c)

FIGURES 9.53a–c   Small CIN 1 **(a)**. Another small CIN1 located along the SCJ **(b)**. A small CIN 1 is seen at 6 o'clock **(c)**. Subclinical asperities caused by HPV can be seen in the periphery.

respectively.[6] Low-grade lesions may occupy only one quadrant of the cervix or a small percentage of the surface area of the ectocervix (Figures 9.54a,b,c,d). Occasionally, CIN 1 may involve multiple quadrants of the cervix particularly in immunocompromised women (Figures 9.55a,b). However, when what appears to be CIN 1 is present in all four quadrants of the cervix, it must be discriminated from a large congenital transformation zone, which may be similar in appearance. The latter normal acetowhite areas are usually more symmetrical than CIN 1 lesions, with less irregular margins.

The distribution of CIN 1 varies from unifocal to multifocal (Figures 9.56a–c). Multiple, distinct, small, randomly scattered lesions are characteristic of CIN 1. These may be located within or outside of the transformation zone (Figure 9.57). It is not uncommon to see coexisting HPV-related disease extending into the vagina in the form of

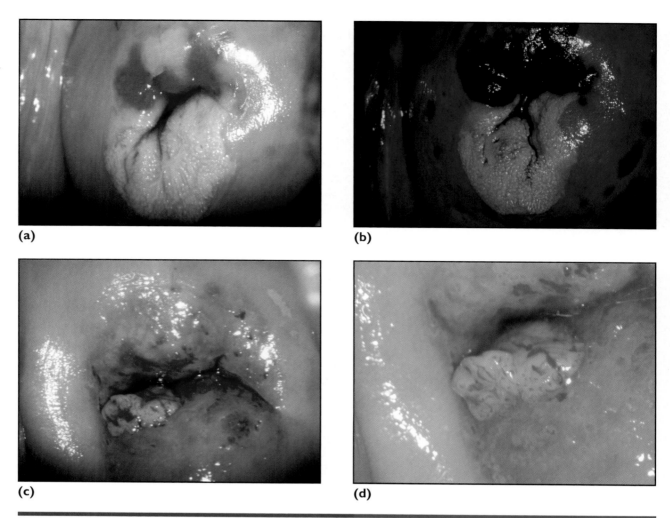

FIGURES 9.54a–d A large condyloma is seen occupying one quadrant of the posterior cervix **(a)**. This woman also has Trichomonas cervicitis **(b)**, as seen with the green filter. Otherwise, some lesions are quite small, as the one seen at 9 o'clock **(c,d)**. The fine capillaries of this condyloma are readily apparent **(d)**.

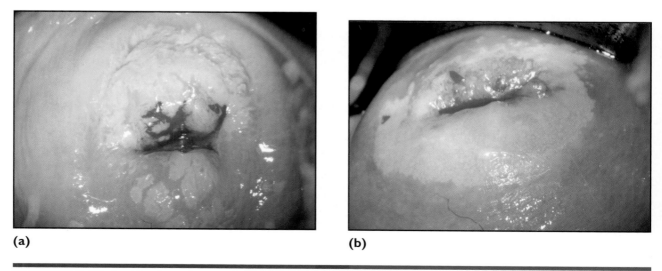

FIGURES 9.55a,b Two large, four-quadrant, low-grade lesions can be seen. The lesion in **(a)** occurred following electro-surgical loop excision.

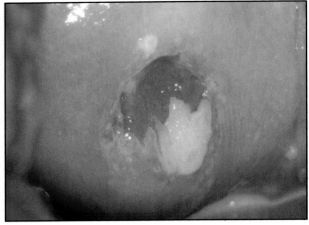

(a)

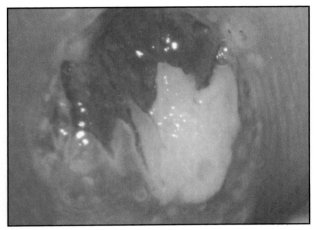

(b)

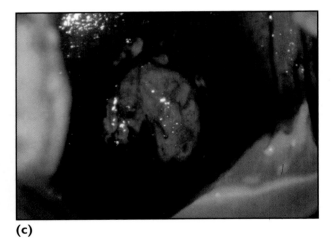

(c)

FIGURES 9.56a–c A unifocal CIN I is seen on the posterior cervix **(a,b)**. The lesion rejects Lugol's iodine solution and assumes a transient yellow color **(c)**. ▬

condyloma or vaginal intraepithelial neoplasia 1 (VAIN 1) (Figure 9.58). CIN 1 lesions tend to be relatively shallow. Rarely, does CIN 1 extend deeper than 2 mm into gland clefts.[16] The mean depth of CIN 1 gland cleft involvement is approximately 0.4 mm.[16]

9.3.2 Colposcopy of CIN 2

It can be extremely difficult to correctly diagnose CIN 2 (Figures 9.59a,b,c). For one reason, interobserver variability in the histologic diagnosis of CIN 2 is more than for CIN 1 or CIN 3. This relative lack of interobserver agreement between pathologists, and similarly poor intraobserver agreement, signifi-

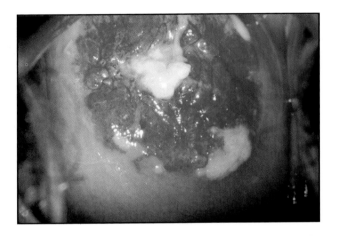

FIGURE 9.57 A CIN I along the SCJ and within the active transformation zone. This patient also has a large ectropion. ▬

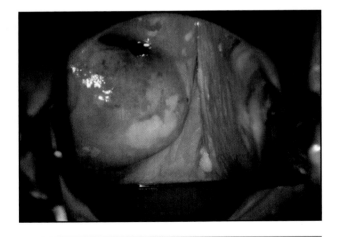

FIGURE 9.58 CIN I and VAIN I in this immunocompromised woman with both HIV and Hepatitis B. ▬

cantly influences agreement between the colposcopic impression and histologic diagnosis. Therefore, CIN 2 lesions may appear to have histologic and colposcopic characteristics more suggestive of CIN 1, but at times they may more closely mimic CIN 3, depending on histologic over- or under-interpretation. The colposcopic characteristics of CIN 2 should appear more like those of CIN 3 than CIN 1, but this is not always the case. A CIN 2 lesion may resemble a moderately severe CIN 1 lesion, or a CIN 1 lesion associated with an inflammatory response or pregnancy. A small CIN 2 lesion may also blend into a larger field of CIN 1 and remain unnoticed.

9.3.2.1 Location of CIN 2

Most CIN 2 lesions are located centrally on the cervix (Figure 9.60). Solitary CIN 2 lesions separated from the squamocolumnar junction are not typical. Almost always, CIN 2 will be found near or adjoining the squamocolumnar junction (Figures 9.61a,b), whether positioned on the ectocervix or within the endocervical canal (Figures 9.62a,b). The one exception is in the case of residual CIN 2 seen following ablative or excisional surgery of the cervix. In this case, the remaining CIN 2 will adjoin the healed surgical excision line, but may be separated from the new SCJ by immature and mature metaplastic epithelium.

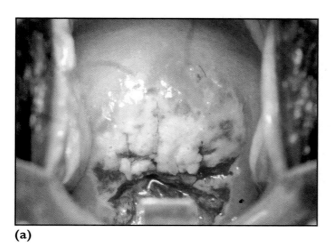

(a)

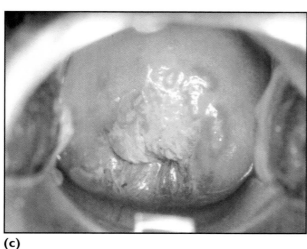

(c)

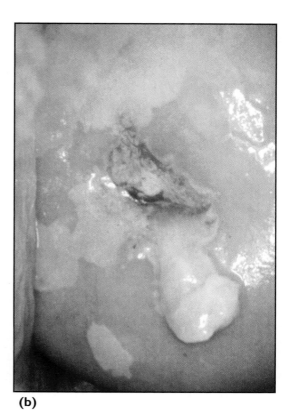

(b)

FIGURES 9.59a–c   Three CIN 2 lesions that demonstrate some features of CIN 1 and some features of CIN 3.

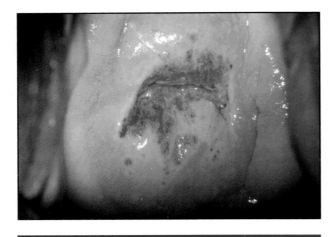

FIGURE 9.60 A centrally positioned CIN 2.

9.3.2.2 Contour of CIN 2

The unique contour of CIN lesions may assist colposcopists in deriving accurate colposcopic impressions. However, these lesions tend to be macular, although some are slightly thickened (Figure 9.63). As such, their contour may not help discriminate CIN 2 from CIN 1 or CIN 3. Irregular surface contour may be expected with HPV-related CIN 1 lesions that may be overrated histologically as CIN 2 lesions. Coexisting leukoplakia will also cause epithelial elevation, but this is generally an exception for CIN 2 (Figures 9.64a,b,c,d).

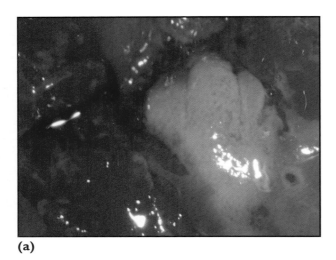

(a)

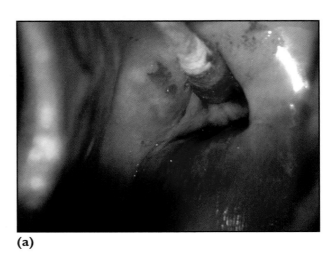

(a)

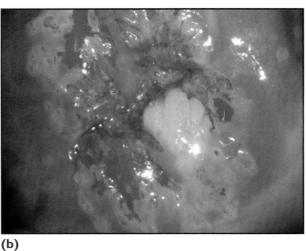

(b)

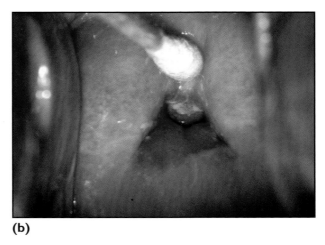

(b)

FIGURES 9.61a,b A CIN 2 located along the SCJ seen at high and low magnification.

FIGURES 9.62a,b A CIN 2 lesion located within the endocervical canal. The first examination was unsatisfactory **(a)**, but the upper extent of the lesion in **(b)** can be seen. Therefore, the colposcopic examination was satisfactory.

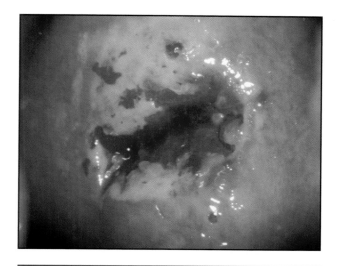

FIGURE 9.63   A macular CIN 2.

9.3.2.3 Margins of CIN 2

The margins of CIN 2 lesions tend to be less irregular or jagged in shape than those in CIN 1 lesions. Therefore, the margins are generally smooth, rounded, or straight with minor fine undulation (Figures 9.65a,b). The apparent external margin may resemble that of CIN 1 when a small focal area of CIN 2 is positioned within a larger CIN 1 lesion (Figures 9.66a,b). In this case, a distinct internal margin may not be seen clearly. CIN 2 may also form the peripheral rim around a more centrally positioned CIN 3. In this case, the margin is usually fairly straight with only minor variation.

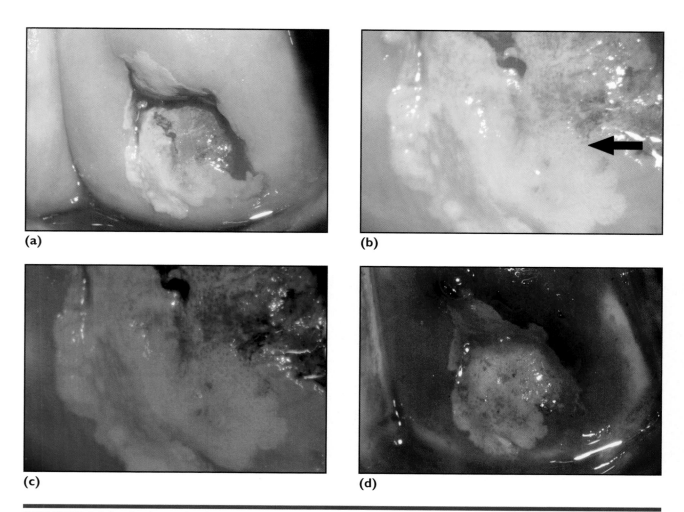

(a)

(b)

(c)

(d)

FIGURES 9.64a–d   A macular CIN 2 is seen between 6 o'clock and 8 o'clock **(a)**. However, an area of leukoplakia and acetowhite epithelium is also seen between 11 o'clock and 12 o'clock. An area of punctation (arrow) is noted alongside the area of leukoplakia **(b)**. The area of leukoplakia has an irregular contour. The punctation can be better seen using the green filter **(c)**. All areas of acetowhite epithelium and leukoplakia reject Lugol's iodine solution and appear yellow **(d)**.

9.3.2.4 Color of CIN 2

Basic white is the most common color seen in CIN 2 lesions following application of 5% acetic acid solution (Figure 9.67). This color can vary from off-white to medium white. CIN 2 lesions are not shiny or snow-white by nature. CIN 2 can be described as having an acetowhite color that is generally less translucent than that seen with CIN 1 lesions, but less opaque than with CIN 3 (Figure 9.68).[15] However, CIN 2 lesions tend to have an opaque white color derived from greater nuclear density in the epithelium. More CIN 2 lesions remain acetowhite for a longer time than the more transient acetowhite effect seen with CIN 1.[15] Accordingly, the acetowhite color noted in CIN 2 is more transient than that seen in CIN 3.[15]

9.3.2.5 Vessels of CIN 2

Fine to medium caliber vascular patterns of punctation and mosaic can usually be identified in CIN 2

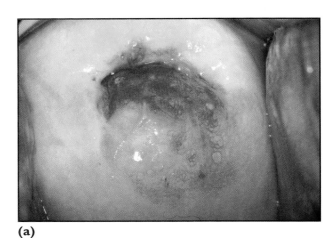

(a)

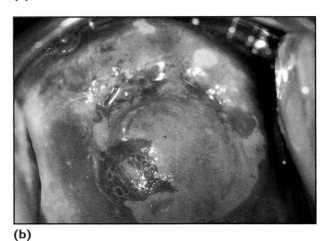

(b)

FIGURES 9.65a,b This CIN 2 lesion has an indistinct margin **(a)** and fine vessels. However, the margin is clearly smooth and not irregular as seen following application of Lugol's iodine solution **(b)**.

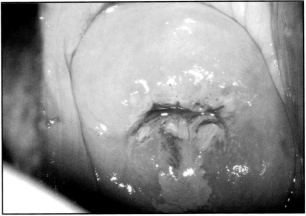

(a)

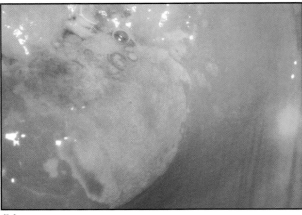

(b)

FIGURES 9.66a,b An internal margin is seen in the lesion on the posterior cervix **(a)**. A larger low-grade lesion is observed in the periphery. More opaque acetowhite epithelium of the CIN 2 demarcates the lesion from the less severe, more translucent CIN 1. In another patient **(b)**, fine vessels and translucent acetowhite epithelium indicate CIN 1 in the periphery. However, a more opaque acetowhite lesion with coarse vessels can be seen closer to the SCJ.

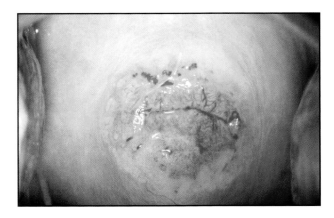

FIGURE 9.67 Intermediate acetowhite color of CIN 2.

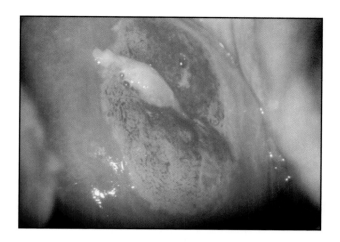

FIGURE 9.68 This acetowhite color of the CIN 2 is less translucent than CIN 2 and less opaque than CIN 3.

lesions (Figures 9.69a,b). The vessels tend to be of a smaller caliber, more similar to vessels seen in CIN 1 than those in CIN 3. Intercapillary distances may be similar or slightly greater than those in CIN 1, or they may infrequently approach the wider spacing noted with CIN 3. The vessels are also less uniformly spaced than in CIN 1 (Figures 9.70a,b). They assume a more random, heterogeneous distribution. Occasionally, blood vessels may not be apparent in CIN 2, particularly when observed immediately following application of 5% acetic acid solution (Figure 9.71a). However, these vessels will become apparent once the acetic acid effect begins to diminish (Figures 9.71b,c). Atypical blood vessels are not seen in CIN 2 lesions. Their presence indicates an invasive process that may coexist with the high-grade lesion.

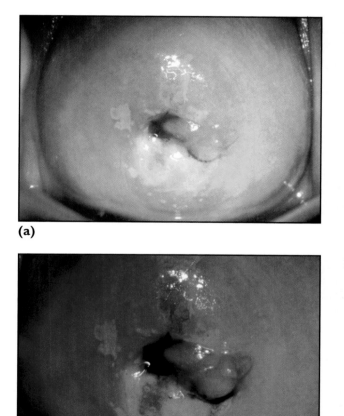

(a)

(b)

FIGURES 9.69a,b Medium caliber vessels seen in a CIN 2 lesion.

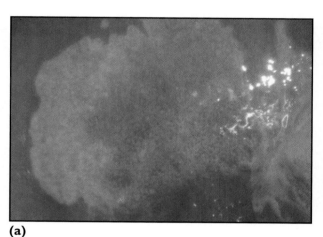

(a)

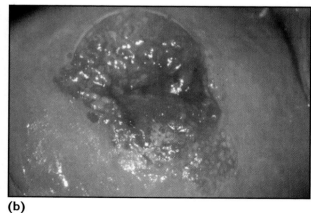

(b)

FIGURES 9.70a,b Medium caliber punctation **(a)** and mosaic **(b)** characteristic of CIN 2.

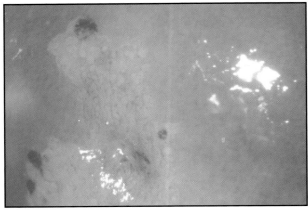

(a)

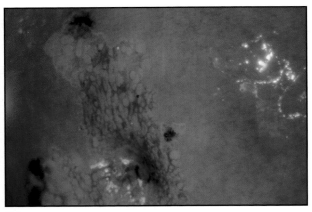

(b)

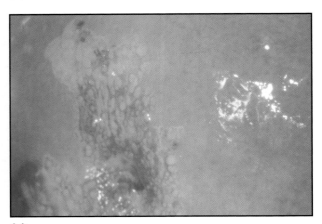

(c)

FIGURES 9.71a–c Immediately after acetic acid application, the mosaic pattern of this CIN 2 appears of narrow caliber **(a)**. This is better seen using the green filter **(b)**. After several minutes the vessels dilate slightly **(c)**.

9.3.2.6 Iodine staining of CIN 2

There is very little to no glycogen in the epithelium of CIN 2 lesions. Hence, a yellow iodine-negative color will invariably be present following application of Lugol's iodine solution (Figures 9.72a–e). Except for color, the outline of the iodine negative area should match the acetowhite area seen initially. A mahogany brown color never will be seen in a CIN 2 lesion. On rare occasions, a variegated yellow-brown iodine-stained pattern may be seen in CIN 2. Because both CIN 2 and CIN 3 have an iodine negative reaction, Lugol's iodine solution does little to help discriminate CIN 2 from CIN 3.

9.3.2.7 Size and distribution of CIN 2

In general, CIN 2 lesions are larger (mean 5.8 mm) than CIN 1 (mean 4.1 mm), but shorter than CIN 3 (mean 7.6 mm)(Figure 9.73).[16] CIN 2 lesions rarely exceed 18.2 mm in length. CIN 2 lesions can extend more deeply into gland clefts than CIN 1 (maximum depths 3 mm and 2 mm, respectively). CIN 2 is invariably seen within the transformation zone (Figure 9.74), in contrast to CIN 1, which may be found outside the transformation zone. CIN 2 may be multifocal (Figure 9.75), but a unifocal lesion is more common. Satellite lesions are not usually representative of CIN 2. Colposcopists will usually find CIN 2 along the SCJ, located either on the ectocervix or within the endocervical canal (Figure 9.76).

Colposcopists should not be discouraged when their colposcopic impression of a lesion was CIN 1, but the histologic diagnosis is CIN 2. This happens relatively frequently, even to more experienced colposcopists. Special attention to the lesion color (opacity) and vessel patterns may offer clues for rendering a more accurate clinical diagnosis. Knowledge of a screening Pap smear read as ASC-US or LSIL frequently biases colposcopic grading. Hence, there may be a tendency for the colposcopist to be swayed by minor cytologic results, and downgrade the colposcopic impression inappropriately. CIN 2 commonly resembles a CIN 1 lesion that looks slightly more severe than would be seen typically. However, as mentioned previously, CIN 2 may also be extremely difficult to discriminate from CIN 3 (Figures 9.77a,b).

9.3.3 Colposcopy of CIN 3

Once educated in the recognition of its classic colposcopic findings, colposcopists should be able to easily diagnose CIN 3 (Figures 9.78a–d). However, not all that appears to be CIN 3 is in fact CIN 3. Potentially serious errors can be made if rarely occurring

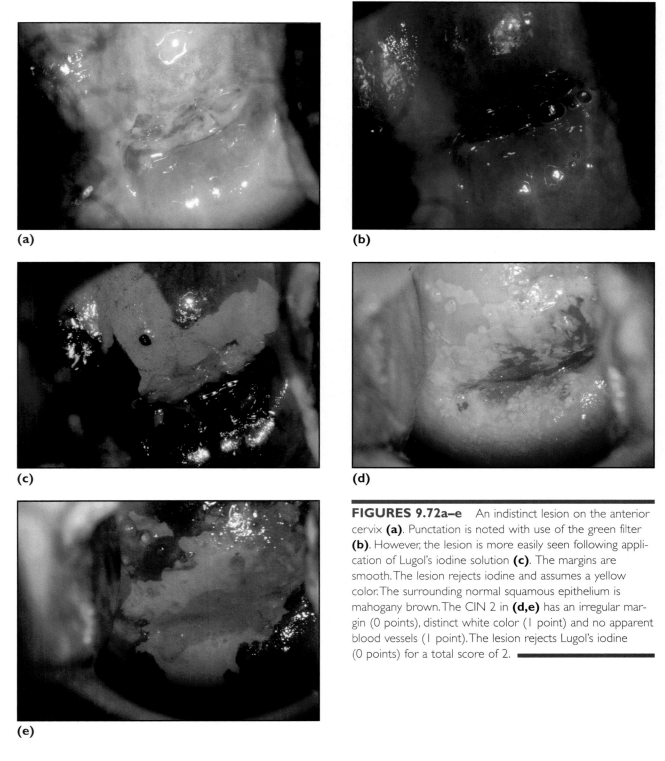

(a)

(b)

(c)

(d)

FIGURES 9.72a–e   An indistinct lesion on the anterior cervix **(a)**. Punctation is noted with use of the green filter **(b)**. However, the lesion is more easily seen following application of Lugol's iodine solution **(c)**. The margins are smooth. The lesion rejects iodine and assumes a yellow color. The surrounding normal squamous epithelium is mahogany brown. The CIN 2 in **(d,e)** has an irregular margin (0 points), distinct white color (1 point) and no apparent blood vessels (1 point). The lesion rejects Lugol's iodine (0 points) for a total score of 2.

(e)

small areas of occult, microinvasive cancer are mistaken for CIN 3. During a busy colposcopist's career such failures should be anticipated. It is extremely difficult to diagnose microinvasive cancer clinically, particularly when it is small and focal. Many times these lesions are hidden in large, especially severe, CIN 3 lesions. Yet, sometimes there is no way other than by careful histologic evaluation to tell that a small focal area has extended beneath the basement membrane less than 3 mm. This diagnostic error is particularly likely to occur when no coexisting warning signs of cancer (Chapter 10) are observed.

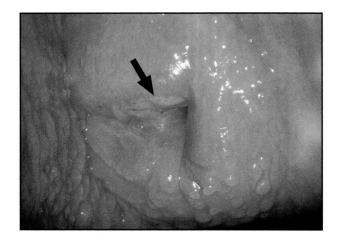

FIGURE 9.73 A small CIN 2 (arrow) on the anterior cervix. The papillary appearance of the cervix is a normal variant, which is rarely seen.

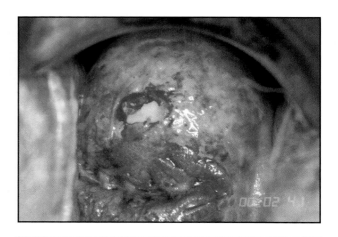

FIGURE 9.74 An opaque, small CIN 2 on the anterior cervix within the transformation zone.

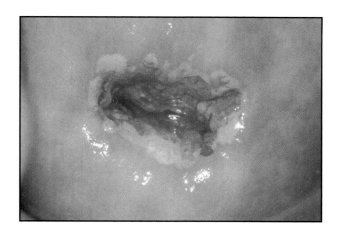

FIGURE 9.75 A multifocal CIN 2.

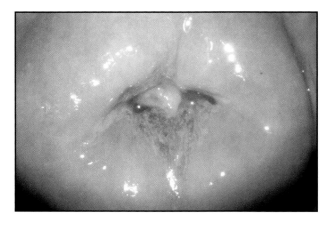

FIGURE 9.76 A CIN 2 along the SCJ and also extending within the endocervical canal.

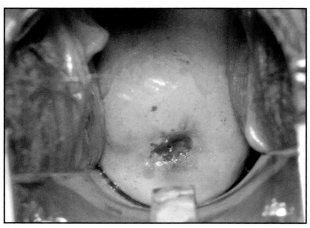

(a)

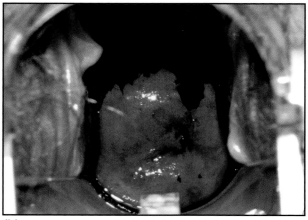

(b)

FIGURES 9.77a,b This large four-quadrant CIN 2 could be confused for a CIN 3 because of its size.

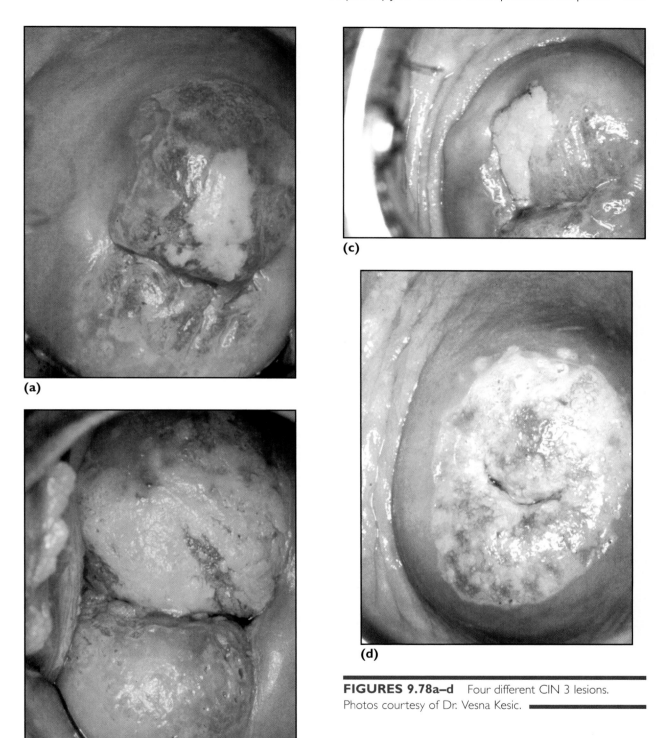

FIGURES 9.78a–d   Four different CIN 3 lesions. Photos courtesy of Dr. Vesna Kesic.

Consequently, excisional therapy may be preferred over ablative treatment of large or severe CIN 3 lesions. CIN 3 lesions should rarely, if ever, be misclassified as normal. Nevertheless, while learning colposcopy, and even occasionally after years of experience, some colposcopists will misidentify a CIN 3 lesion as a CIN 1 lesion.

9.3.3.1 Location of CIN 3

CIN 3 is invariably positioned along the SCJ, whether on the ectocervix or within the endocervical canal (Figures 9.79a,b; 9.80a,b, 9.81a-e). The one possible exception is in women who have residual CIN 3 lesions following surgery of the cervix (Fig-

ures 9.82a-e). These "skip" lesions may not adjoin the new squamocolumnar junction, but may instead lie proximally within the endocervical canal. When associated with a less severe neoplastic change, CIN 3 lesions are generally nearer to the squamocolumnar junction. Rarely, large CIN 3 lesions may also extend into the vaginal fornices.

9.3.3.2 Contour of CIN 3

The topography of CIN 3 lesions varies from macular (Figures 9.83a,b) to a generalized epithelial thickening that appears as if the intact abnormal epithelium could be peeled away from the underlying stroma (Figures 9.84a–d , 9.85a,b). Although, a

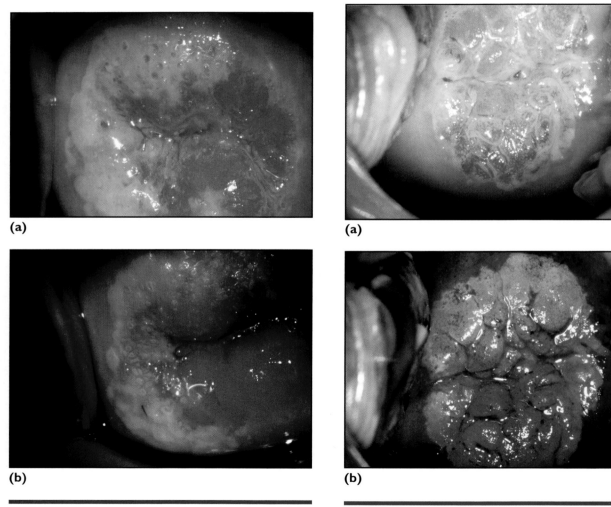

(a)

(b)

(a)

(b)

FIGURES 9.79a,b　A CIN 3 is seen along the SCJ **(a)**. With closer inspection at 9 o'clock **(b)**, the neoplasia extends deeply into the gland clefts causing periglandular cuffing.

FIGURES 9.80a,b　A large three quadrant CIN 3 extends from 12 o'clock to 9 o'clock **(a)**. A coarse mosaic vessel pattern is consistent with CIN 3. This area rejects Lugol's iodine solution and appears yellow **(b)**.

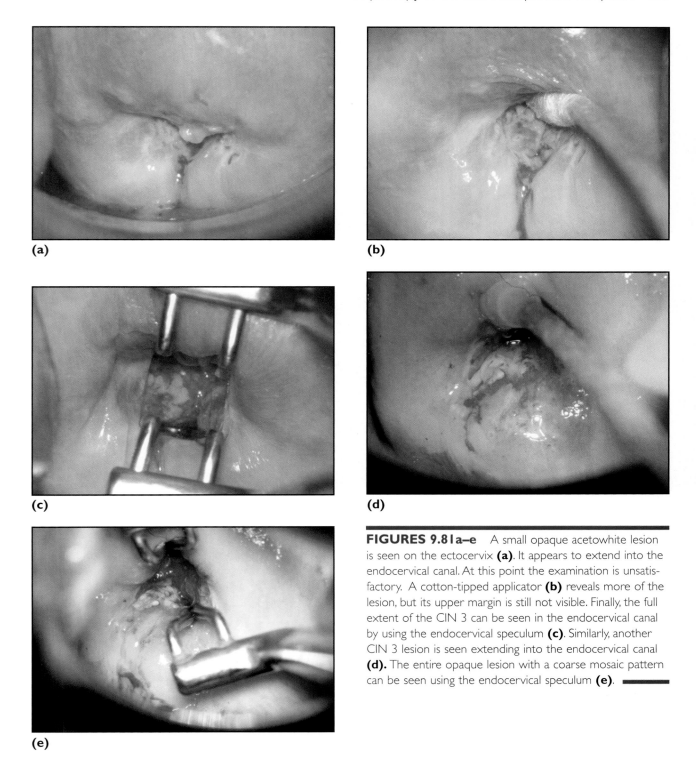

(a)

(b)

(c)

(d)

(e)

FIGURES 9.81a–e   A small opaque acetowhite lesion is seen on the ectocervix **(a)**. It appears to extend into the endocervical canal. At this point the examination is unsatisfactory. A cotton-tipped applicator **(b)** reveals more of the lesion, but its upper margin is still not visible. Finally, the full extent of the CIN 3 can be seen in the endocervical canal by using the endocervical speculum **(c)**. Similarly, another CIN 3 lesion is seen extending into the endocervical canal **(d).** The entire opaque lesion with a coarse mosaic pattern can be seen using the endocervical speculum **(e)**.

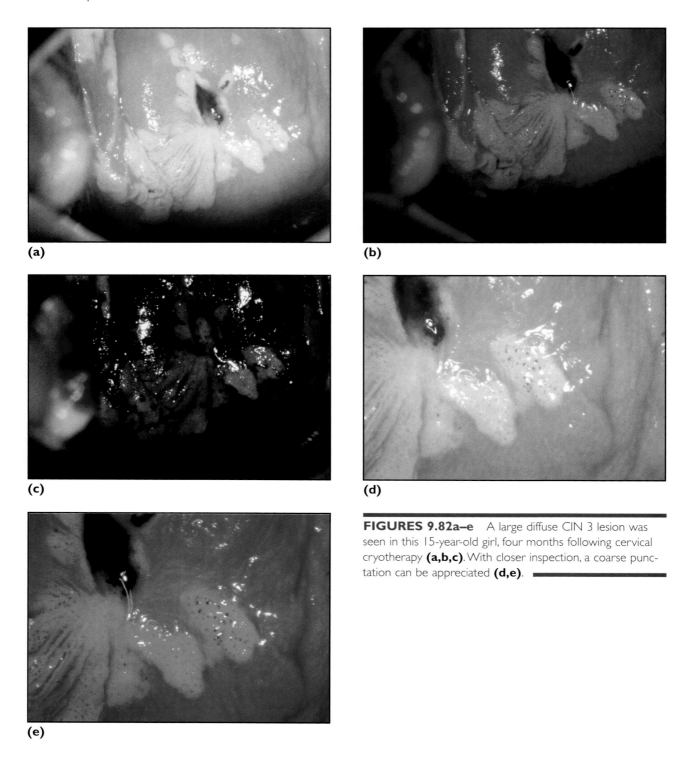

(a)

(b)

(c)

(d)

(e)

FIGURES 9.82a–e   A large diffuse CIN 3 lesion was seen in this 15-year-old girl, four months following cervical cryotherapy **(a,b,c)**. With closer inspection, a coarse punctation can be appreciated **(d,e)**.

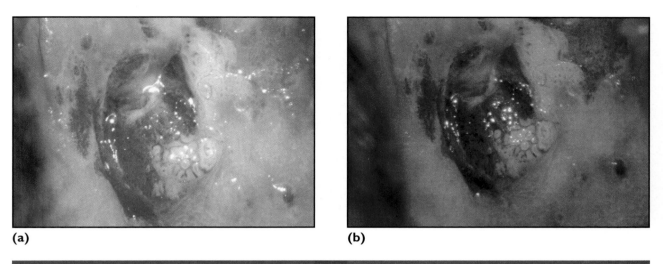

FIGURES 9.83a,b A macular CIN 3 is seen at 5 o'clock **(a)**. A coarse mosaic vessel pattern is seen using the green filter **(b)**.

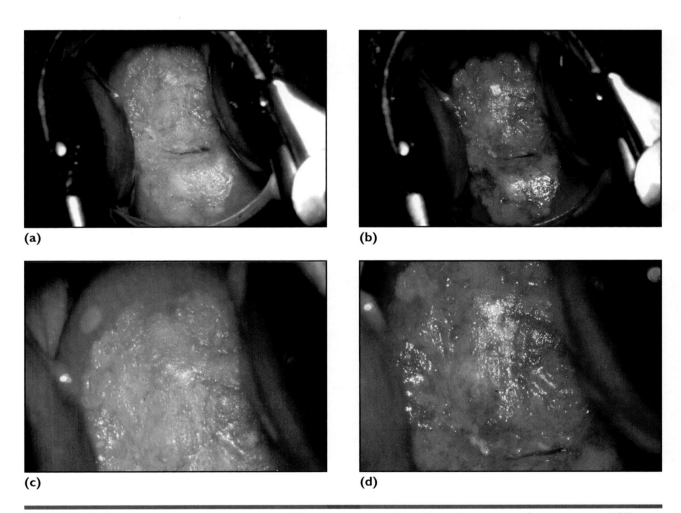

FIGURES 9.84a–d A thickened four-quadrant CIN 3 can be seen in this HIV positive woman after application of 5% acetic acid solution and Lugol's iodine solution **(a,b)**. No vessels are seen with higher magnification **(c,d)**.

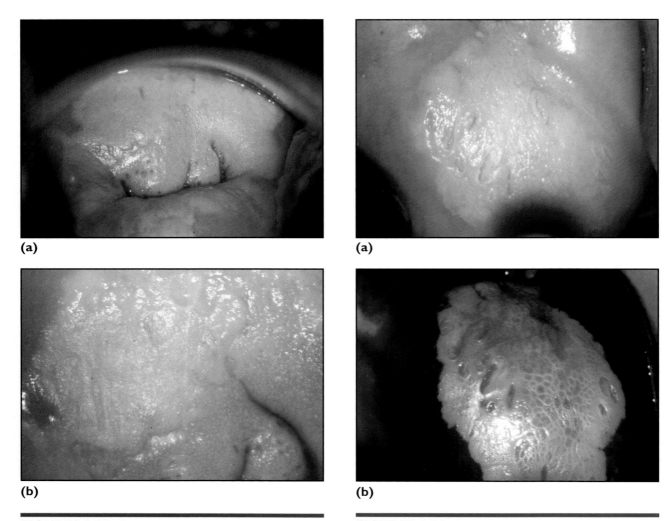

(a)

(b)

(a)

(b)

FIGURES 9.85a,b Another woman with HIV has a thickened CIN 3 lesion. The epithelium cannot be transilluminated by the white light of the colposcope. ▬

FIGURES 9.86a,b A thickened, elevated CIN 3 with gland cleft involvement is seen on the posterior cervix **(a)**. Application of Lugol's iodine solution results in an unusual, variegated staining pattern **(b)**. ▬

slightly elevated epithelium may be seen (Figures 9.86a,b; 9.87a,b,c,d), most CIN 3 is flat. Some severe CIN 3 lesions demonstrate topographic elevations seen simply as blood vessel protrusion above the surface of the epithelium. In these cases, the light of the colposcope will reflect tangentially from the edges of dilated vessels. If a similar, extremely dilated mosaic pattern is present, a scalloped, pockmarked epithelial surface will be seen. A nodular, papillary, papular, or exophytic contour noted within an area of CIN 3 lesions suggests the presence of cancer.

9.3.3.3 Margins of CIN 3

The lesion margins of CIN 3 are smooth, gently rounded, or straight, creating a distinct demarcation between normal epithelium and neoplastic epithe-

lium (Figures 9.88a,b; 9.89a-c). These straight margins are the most common presentation for CIN 3 lesions. However, CIN 3 may also have peeling edges or internal margins. "Peeling" margins imply extensive neoplasia within the acetowhite epithelium, and a confident diagnosis of CIN 3 can be made. The only exception would be if non-thickened, normal or minimally abnormal epithelium has been traumatized unintentionally, and was then mistaken for a peeling margin (Figure 9.90). The thickened epithelium of CIN can be sheared from the underlying stroma because the neoplastic process adversely affects the hemidesmosomes that bind the epithelium to the basement membrane and underlying stroma. A small ulceration will usually be seen in the area adjoining the avulsed epithelium. This area must be carefully inspected because cervical

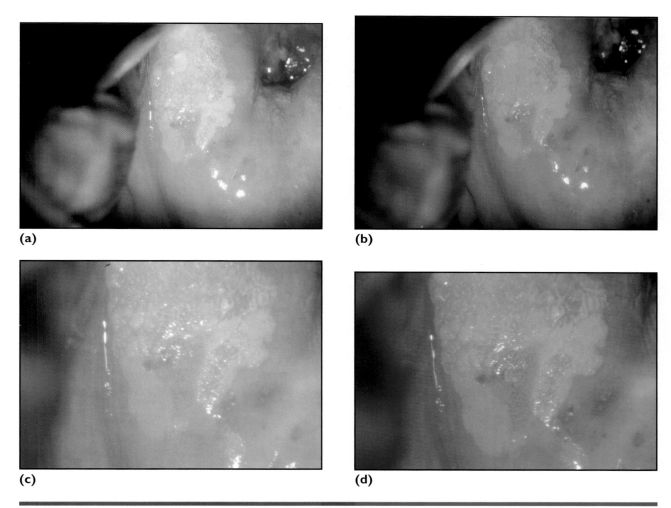

FIGURES 9.87a–d   An area of leukoplakia covers a CIN 3 at 9 o'clock **(a,b)**. However, with higher magnification, a coarse punctation can be seen along the posterior margin of the lesion **(c,d)**.

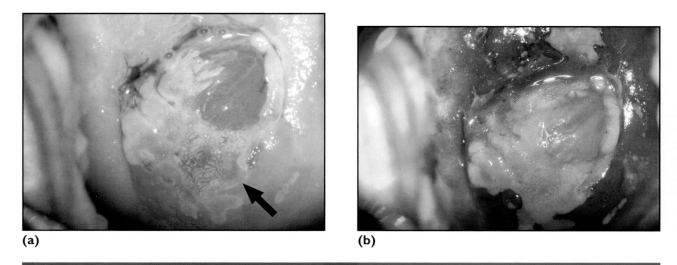

FIGURES 9.88a,b   A smooth margin is seen in CIN 3 **(a)**. This lesion (arrow) also has an opaque acetowhite color, and a coarse caliber punctation and mosaic. The rounded margin is nicely seen following application of Lugol's iodine solution **(b)**.

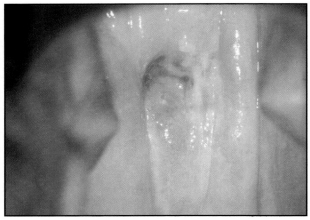

(a)

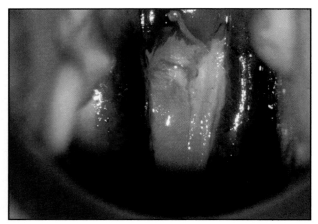

(b)

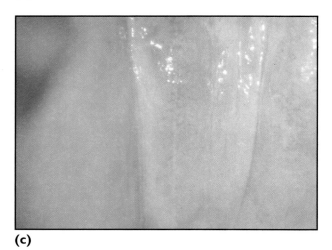

(c)

FIGURES 9.89a–c This CIN 3 on the posterior cervix has a straight, rounded margin **(a,b)**. A coarse mosaic vessel pattern is seen using higher magnification **(c)**. ━━━

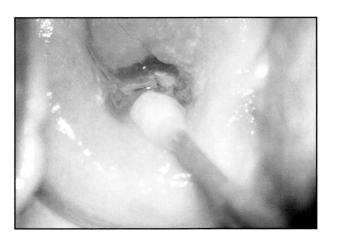

FIGURE 9.90 A CIN 3 with a peeling margin is seen within the endocervical canal. ━━━

ulcerations are also associated with invasive cancer. Biopsy is always indicated in this circumstance.

An internal border or margin that distinctly separates epithelia of differing levels of neoplasia may be noted (Figures 9.91a,b). To form an internal border, a very large low-grade lesion encompasses a more centrally located CIN 3 along the squamocolumnar junction (Figures 9.92a,b). Novice colposcopists tend to overlook internal margins unless taught to recognize this subtle change (Figures 9.93a-h). Once the complete circumference of any acetowhite lesion has been outlined, then the colposcopist should look from the margins toward the os. Abrupt contrasts in appearance of the epithelium or internal margins may be observed distinctly as one looks from the lateral border across a lesion towards the os. This process can be compared to observing the spokes of a bicycle wheel, from the outer rim to the center axle. The inner lesion will exhibit more opaque epithelium and a smooth, sometimes slightly elevated, margin can be observed demarcating the central high-grade lesion from the translucent low-grade lesion in the periphery (Figure 9.94). If this inspection process is adopted as routine, colposcopists will rarely fail to identify an internal margin and more centrally positioned CIN 3.

9.3.3.4 Color of CIN 3

Although "dull oyster-grey," and "dense white" have been used to describe the color of CIN 3 lesions, it actually may be better to consider the opacity of the epithelium (Figure 9.95). CIN 3 has a nuclear dense epithelium, with abundant protein and little water. As a result, the epithelium functions like a mirror after acetic acid application, reflecting the

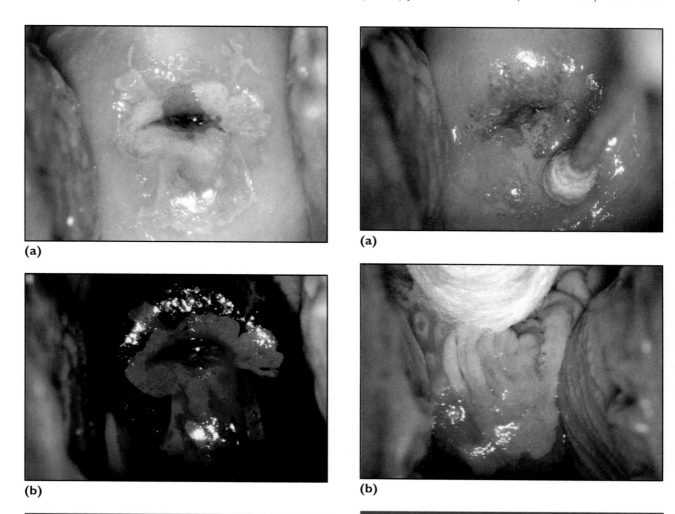

(a)

(b)

(a)

(b)

FIGURES 9.91a,b   A three-quadrant opaque CIN 3 is seen in **(a)**. A small, translucent CIN 1 can be seen at 6 o'clock. The border between these two lesions is called an internal margin. The demarcation is also seen following application of Lugol's iodine solution **(b)**. The low-grade lesion contains glycogen and appears both yellow and brown (variegated). The high-grade lesion does not contain glycogen and as a result appears yellow.

FIGURES 9.92a,b   An internal margin separates the area of CIN 3 from CIN 1 **(a)**. The CIN 3 has an opaque color and coarse vessels. The CIN 1 is translucent white with a fine punctation and mosaic pattern. An opaque CIN 3 without visible vessels adjoins a more translucent, larger CIN 1 in this pregnant patient **(b)**.

intense white light of the colposcope back to the colposcopist's eyes (Figure 9.96). This opaque white color characterizes CIN 3 (Figure 9.97). CIN 3 lesions are significantly more acetowhite than CIN 1 lesions (Figures 9.98a-d).[15] CIN 3 lesions resemble a wall that has been painted repeatedly with white latex paint. A CIN 1 lesion or immature metaplasia more closely resembles a wall that has only received an initial primer coat of white paint or several layers of translucent white watercolor. Moreover, the acetowhite effect persists longer in CIN 3 lesions than in CIN 1 lesions.[15] Therefore, when inspecting a large, complex lesion of the cervix, pro-

vided that 5% acetic acid solution was applied uniformly and at the same time to the cervix, the last area remaining acetowhite will likely be the area of most severe disease.

9.3.3.5 Vessels of CIN 3

Coarsely dilated blood vessels, in either punctation or mosaic patterns, are the classic vascular characteristics of a CIN 3 lesion (Figure 9.99). When these coarse vessels are noted, a diagnosis of CIN 3 must be considered (Figures 9.100a-d; 9.101a,b; 9.102; 9.103a-d). Furthermore, the intercapillary

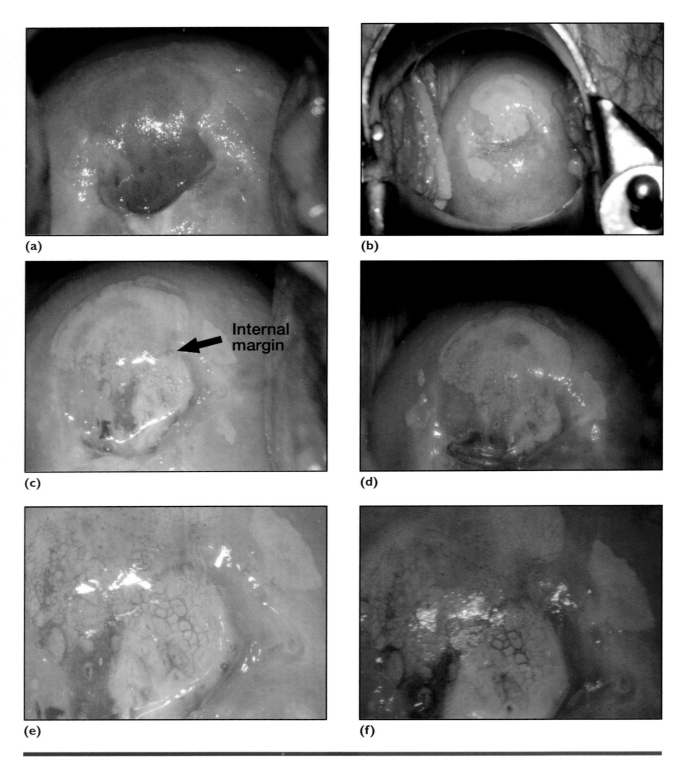

(a)

(b)

(c)   **Internal margin** ←

(d)

(e)

(f)

FIGURES 9.93a–h   No lesion is seen on the ectocervix following saline application **(a)**. Following application of acetic acid solution, acetowhite lesions are seen on the anterior and posterior cervix **(b)**. At greater magnification, an internal margin (arrow) is seen on the anterior cervix **(c,d)**. With even greater magnification, a coarse mosaic and punctation vessel pattern is seen **(e,f)**.

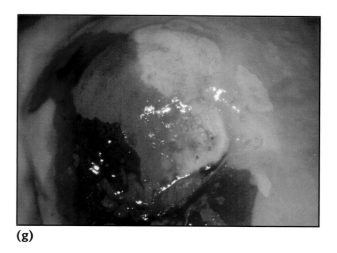

(g)

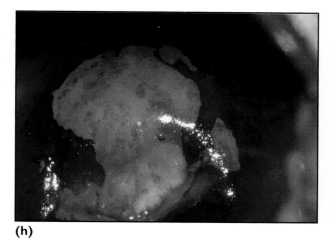

(h)

FIGURES 9.93a–h   Continued. The translucent and opaque epithelia of CIN 1 and CIN 3 are observed, respectively. The corresponding yellow color following application of Lugol's iodine solution is noted in **(g,h)**.

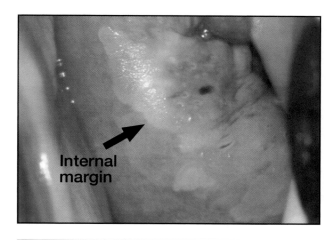

FIGURE 9.94   An elevated, opaque CIN 3 is demarcated from the surrounding CIN 1 by an internal margin (arrow). No blood vessels are seen.

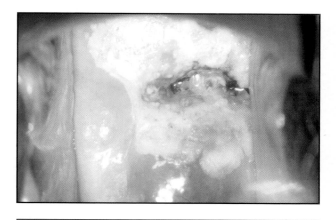

FIGURE 9.96   A thickened acetowhite CIN 3 involving three quadrants of the cervix. This epithelium cannot be transilluminated by the colposcope's white light; hence, most of the white light reflects off the surface.

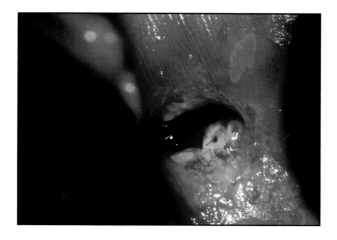

FIGURE 9.95   A very opaque acetowhite CIN 3 seen at the cervical os.

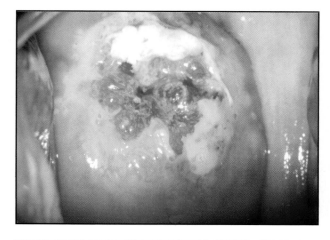

FIGURE 9.97   An opaque CIN 3 seen at 4 o'clock is contrasted with the translucent metaplastic epithelium.

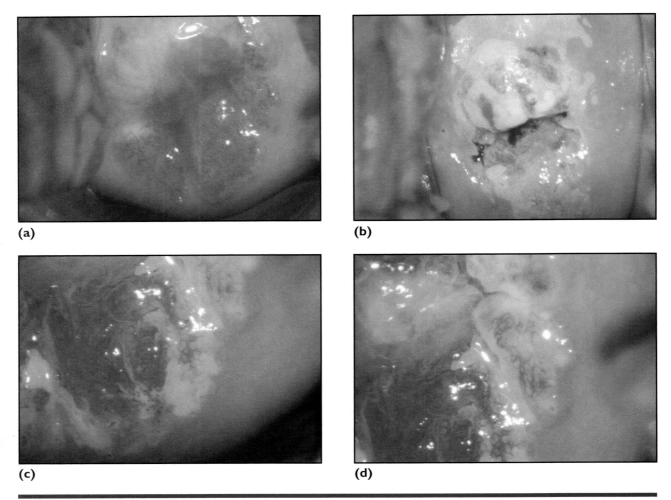

(a) (b)

(c) (d)

FIGURES 9.98a–d The cervix is seen in **(a)** following saline application. An opaque acetowhite lesion is seen on the anterior cervix after application of acetic acid solution **(b)**. An internal margin separates the CIN 3 from a large CIN 1. Less opaque epithelium of CIN 1 is also seen on the posterior cervix. Within the opaque acetowhite epithelium of the CIN 3, coarse caliber mosaic and punctation **(c,d)** are observed.

FIGURE 9.99 Coarse mosaic and punctation of CIN 3 is contrasted with the fine vessels of CIN 1 (Figure 9.43b). The intercapillary spacing is wider, the vessels are of greater diameter, and the vessel pattern is more random in CIN 3.

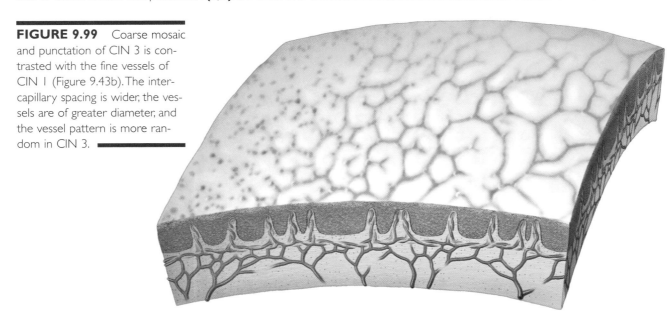

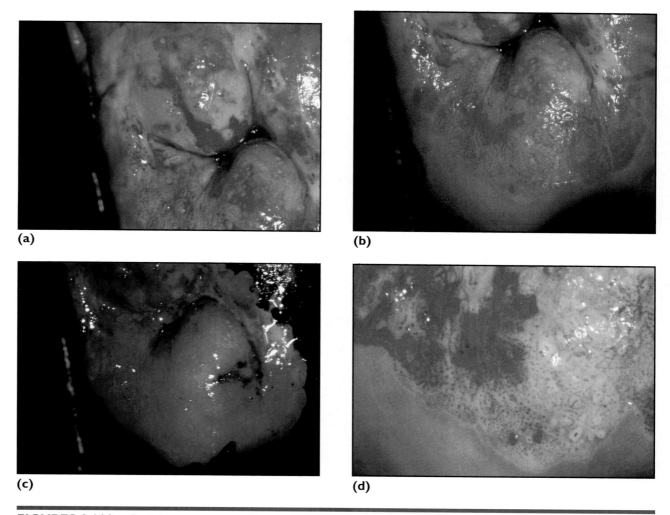

FIGURES 9.100a–d   A large, opaque, peeling acetowhite CIN 3 lesion with a coarse mosaic and punctation pattern **(a,b,d)**. This lesion contains no glycogen and rejects Lugol's iodine solution, assuming a yellow color **(c)**. Notice also the smooth margin characteristic of CIN 3.

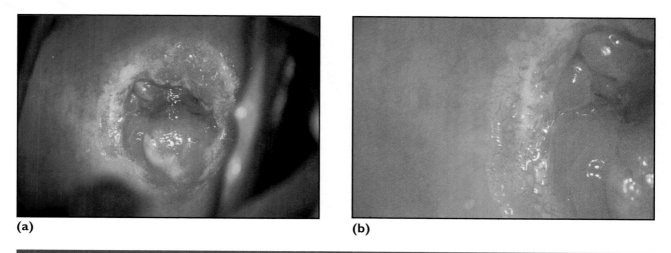

FIGURES 9.101a,b   A coarse mosaic and punctation pattern are seen at 9 o'clock. A biopsy of this tissue was diagnosed as CIN 3.

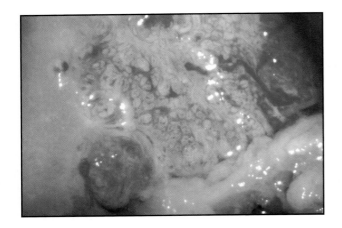

FIGURE 9.102 This CIN 3 has a coarse mosaic vessel pattern.

distances are greater in CIN 3 than in CIN 1 (Figures 9.104a-m). Vessel patterns and intercapillary distances also tend to be more random, disjointed, and less uniform than in CIN 1 (Figures 9.105a-c). However, it is unusual to see blood vessels in a thick, opaque CIN 3 lesion (Figures 9.106a-c). Physiologically, this can be explained by the fact that expanding blocks of dysplastic epithelium have occluded or pushed aside the afferent and efferent capillary loops normally present. A greater pressure is needed to obstruct the arterial side of the vascular system than the venous system. That may be why in very severe CIN 3 lesions, no vessels are noted. With other CIN 3, assuming less pressure is exerted by the blocks of neoplastic epithelium, only the venous return is occluded, allowing intense capillary dilatation

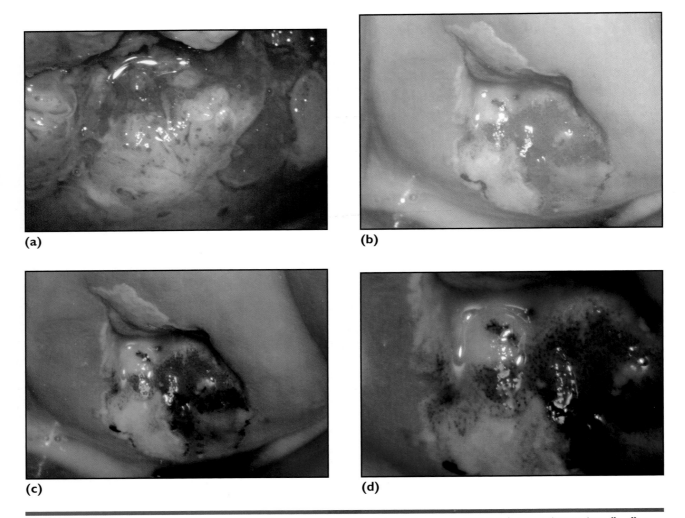

(a)

(b)

(c)

(d)

FIGURES 9.103a–d A coarse punctation pattern can be seen in this small, opaque CIN 3 **(a)**. In another patient **(b–d)** a thickened acetowhite lesion is seen on the anterior and posterior cervix. Coarse punctation is well seen using the green filter **(d)**.

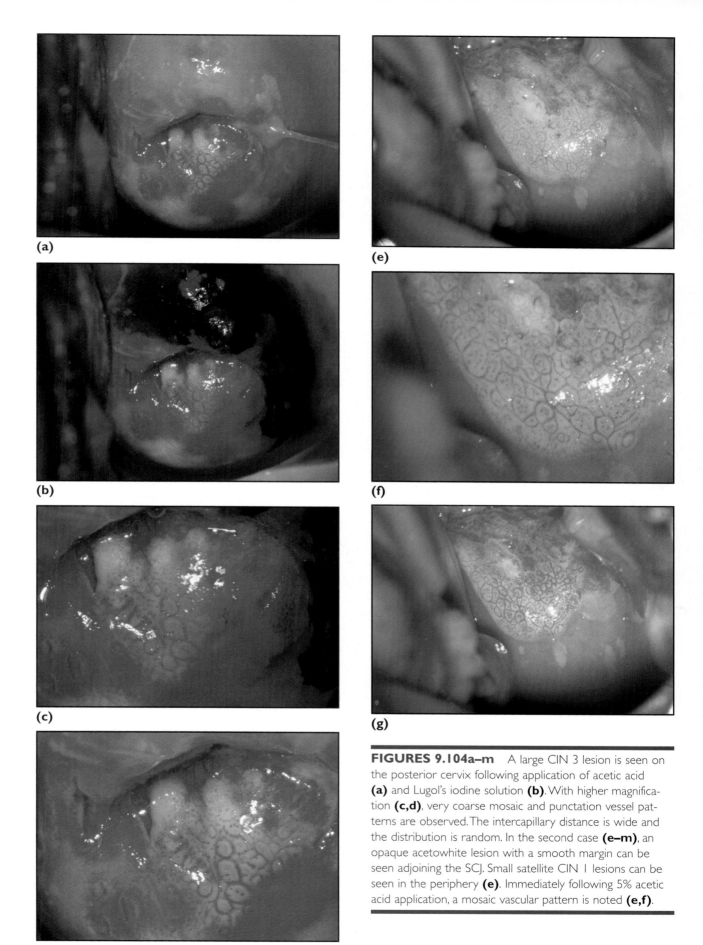

(a)

(b)

(c)

(d)

(e)

(f)

(g)

FIGURES 9.104a–m A large CIN 3 lesion is seen on the posterior cervix following application of acetic acid **(a)** and Lugol's iodine solution **(b)**. With higher magnification **(c,d)**, very coarse mosaic and punctation vessel patterns are observed. The intercapillary distance is wide and the distribution is random. In the second case **(e–m)**, an opaque acetowhite lesion with a smooth margin can be seen adjoining the SCJ. Small satellite CIN 1 lesions can be seen in the periphery **(e)**. Immediately following 5% acetic acid application, a mosaic vascular pattern is noted **(e,f)**.

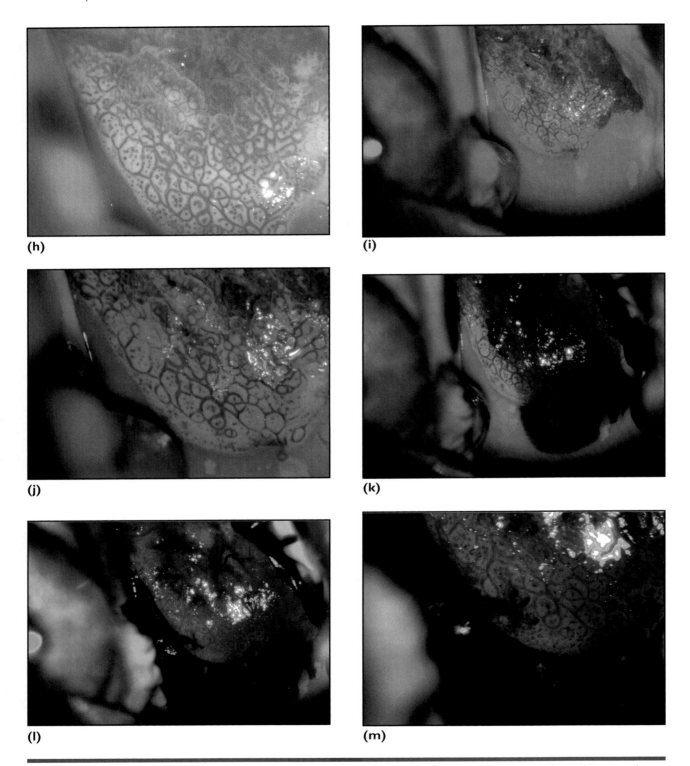

(h)

(i)

(j)

(k)

(l)

(m)

FIGURES 9.104a–m Continued. The intercapillary distances are wide and non-uniformly spaced. Later, these vessels dilate to resemble the coarse caliber vessels seen with CIN 3 **(g,h)**. The green filter examination **(i,j)** allows clear identification of the mosaic pattern. The next photo **(k)** was taken after Lugol's iodine was applied to half of the acetowhite CIN 3. The last two photographs **(l,m)** show that the CIN 3 now assumes a yellow (iodine negative) color and the surrounding normal squamous epithelium, still containing glycogen, appears mahogany brown.

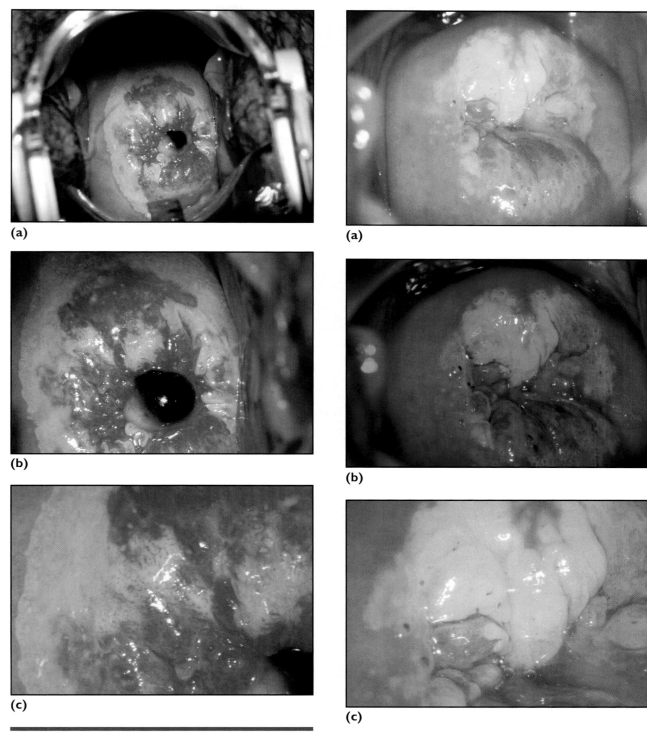

(a)

(b)

(c)

(a)

(b)

(c)

FIGURES 9.105a–c   A large 4-quadrant acetowhite area representing a congenital transformation zone is seen at low colposcopic magnification **(a)**. With increased magnification, the fine caliber mosaic of the congenital transformation zone is apparent against the translucent acetowhite epithelium **(b)**. However, 2 opaque acetowhite lesions between 9 o'clock and 10 o'clock are noted closer to the cervical os. At higher magnification **(c)**, a randomly distributed coarse punctation of CIN 3 is observed.

FIGURES 9.106a–c   An opaque CIN 3 lesion on the anterior cervix contrasts with the translucent acetowhite immature metaplastic epithelium on the posterior cervix **(a)**. No vessels are noted with the green filter **(b)**. Most CIN 3 lesions have no visible vessels as seen at this high magnification **(c)**.

(Figures 9.107a,b). Any evidence of atypical vessels suggests cancer, not CIN 3, even though approximately 2% to 6% of histologically confirmed CIN 3 lesions demonstrate atypical blood vessels.[17,18]

9.3.3.6 Iodine staining of CIN 3

There is no glycogen in CIN 3 lesions. Hence, a yellow, iodine–negative color appears following application of Lugol's iodine solution (Figures 9.108a-d). These iodine negative areas match the previously detected acetowhite lesions (Figures 9.109a-d). A variegated or speckled pattern is not usually found in CIN 3. Severe CIN 3 lesions may assume a pale, yellowish white, iodine-negative appearance that can be contrasted with the darker yellow, iodine-negative area seen in CIN 1 lesions.

9.3.3.7 Size and distribution of CIN 3

CIN 3 lesions tend to be confluent, and longer and wider than CIN 1 or CIN 2 lesions. The mean linear length of CIN 3 is approximately 7.5 mm.[16,19] The maximum linear length of CIN 3 does not usually exceed 15 mm.[19] The mean surface area of CIN 3 measures 63 mm,[2] contrasted with 46 mm [2] for CIN 1/2.[20] Therefore, it is not uncommon to see CIN 3 occupy 2 or 3 quadrants of the cervix (Figures 9.110a–f). Because CIN 3 is more confluent and expansive, many lesions will extend into the external os and beyond colposcopic view (Figure 9.111).

CIN 3 is usually located within the central portion of the cervix, inside the inner curve towards the external os (Figures 9.112a,b). In general, CIN 3 is found between 1 mm distal and 21 mm proximal to the most caudal point of the ectocervix.[19] This distribution varies as the SCJ advances within the endocervical canal as a woman ages. The distribution also may differ after cervical surgery. In these cases, the volume and/or normal rounded contour of the cervix may be reduced and the SCJ may be deep within the endocervical canal. It must be remembered that CIN 3 is nearly always found along the SCJ (Figure 9.113).

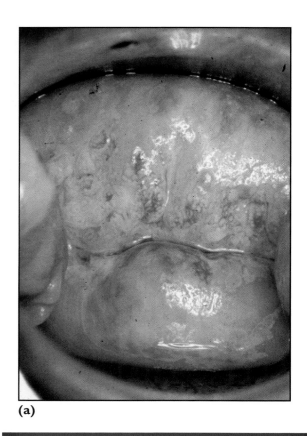

(a)

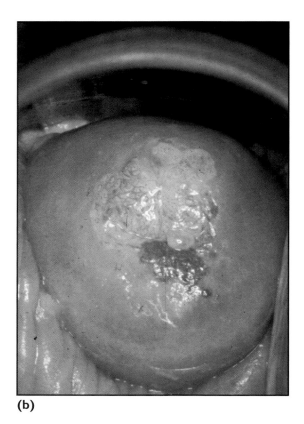

(b)

FIGURES 9.107a,b   Very dilated vessels are seen in these two patients with CIN 3. Photos courtesy of Dr. Vesna Kesic.

CIN 3 is rarely occult when present on the ecto-cervix. If CIN 3 has penetrated the epithelium surrounding and within a gland cleft, then a wide, opaque acetowhite band around a gland opening will be observed. The periglandular acetowhite cuffing can be contrasted with the narrow acetowhite rim of a normal gland opening surrounding a red central area that represents underlying columnar epithelium within the gland clefts (Figure 9.79b). Evidence of opaque white, wide, periglandular acetowhite cuffing is almost always pathognomonic of CIN 3. CIN 3 can

extend 4.8 mm into gland clefts, but the mean depth is less than 1.6 mm.[16,19,21] The depth of CIN 3 involvement in gland clefts also appears to correlate, in general, with advancing patient age. A small CIN 3 lesion positioned within a larger CIN 1 lesion may be overlooked, even if careful colposcopy is performed. Very large CIN 3 lesions may also extend into the vaginal fornices, producing VAIN 3 (Figure 9.114). When compared with CIN 1, CIN 3 is more likely to be solitary and not multifocal or diffuse in distribution.

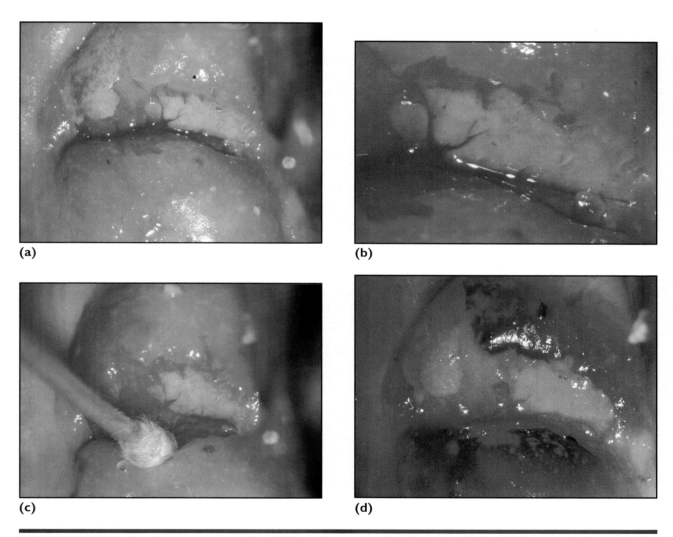

(a)

(b)

(c)

(d)

FIGURES 9.108a–d   An opaque acetowhite CIN 3 can be seen on the anterior cervix **(a,b)**. The examination must be considered unsatisfactory until the assistance provided by a cotton-tipped applicator is able to visualize the proximal extent of the lesion **(c)**. The CIN 3 assumes a transient yellow color following Lugol's iodine solution **(d)**. The surrounding normal squamous epithelium absorbs the iodine becoming a dark brown color.

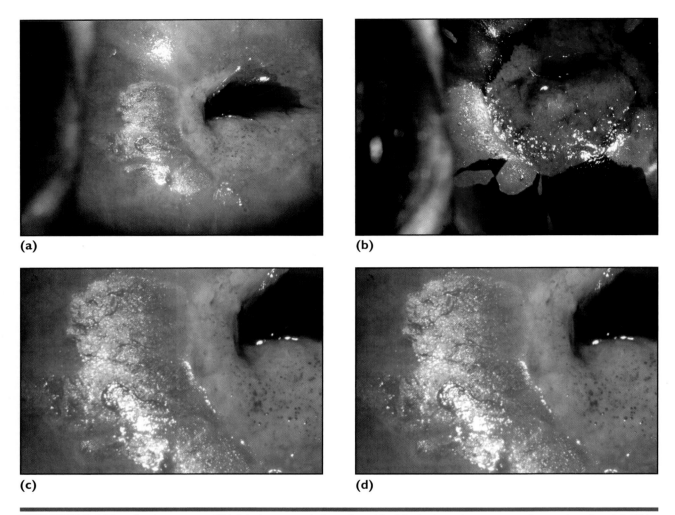

(a)

(b)

(c)

(d)

FIGURES 9.109a–d   An opaque CIN 3 lesion extends from 3 to 12 o'clock along the squamocolumnar junction **(a)**. This tissue rejects iodine application and appears yellow **(b)**. However, a larger yellow area is seen peripheral to the CIN 3. With closer inspection **(c,d)** an area of leukoplakia adjoins the CIN 3 and explains why this area also appears yellow. The CIN 3 has a very coarse, randomly distributed punctation.

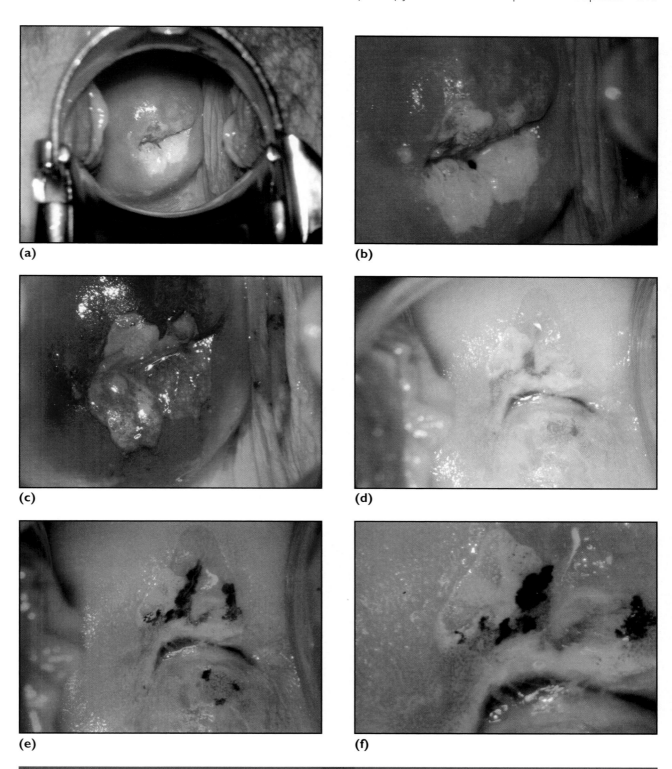

(a)

(b)

(c)

(d)

(e)

(f)

FIGURES 9.110a–f   A CIN 3 lesion involving two or more quadrants of the cervix is not uncommon **(a)**. This CIN 3 is on the anterior and posterior cervix. The margins are smooth, the color is an opaque white, and a coarse mosaic pattern is seen in the anterior lesion. No vessels are noted within the posterior cervical lesions **(b)**. The Lugol's iodine solution helps to determine the location of the most severe disease **(c)**. The anterior lesion has no glycogen, as evident by its pure yellow color. The lesion at 4 o'clock is variegated. In another patient **(d)**, CIN 3 lesions can be seen on the anterior and posterior cervix. With the green filter, a coarse mosaic pattern and punctation are seen **(e,f)**.

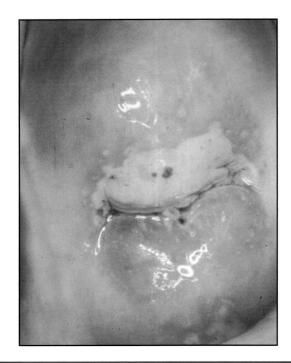

FIGURE 9.111   This CIN 3 lesion extends within the endocervical canal. ▬▬▬

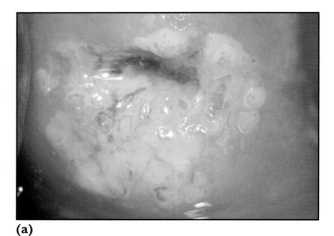

(a)

FIGURES 9.112a,b   Most CIN 3 lesions are found in the central portion of the ectocervix **(a)**. This CIN 3 has coarsely dilated blood vessels. ▬▬▬

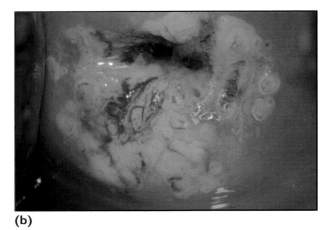

(b)

FIGURES 9.112a,b   Continued. (b), which are easily visualized by using the green filter. ▬▬▬

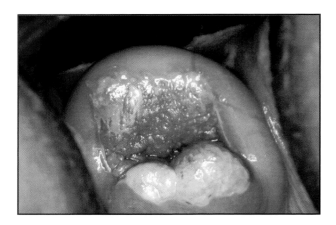

FIGURE 9.113   This CIN 3 lesion is located along the SCJ.

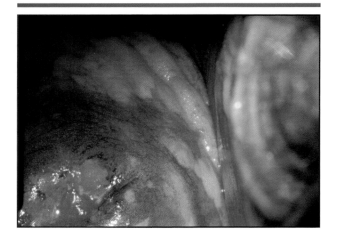

FIGURE 9.114   This woman with HIV has a VAIN 3 in the left anterior vaginal fornix. The lesion rejects Lugol's iodine solution and has a smooth margin. She also was found to have CIN 3. ▬▬▬

References

1. Hopman E H, Kenemans P, Helmerhorst T J M. Positive predictive rate of colposcopic examination of the cervix uteri: an overview of the literature. *Obstet Gynecol Survey.* 1998;53:97–106.

2. Solomon D, Davey D, Kurman R, Moriarty A, O'Connor D, Prez M, et al. The 2001 Bethesda System terminology for reporting results of cervical cytology. *JAMA* 2002;287:2114–9.

3. Stoler M H, Schiffman M. Interobserver reproducibility of cervical cytologic and histologic interpretations. Realistic estimates from the ASCUS-LSIL Triage Study. *JAMA* 2001;285:1500–5.

4. Marana H R, Andrade J M, Duarte G, Matthes A C, Taborda M F, Bighet S. Colposcopic scoring systems for biopsy decisions in different patient groups. *Eur J Gynaecol Oncol* 2000;21:368–70.

5. Stellato G, Paavonen J. A colposcopic scoring system for grading cervical lesions. *Eur J Gynaecol Oncol* 1995;16:296–300.

6. Ferris D G, Miller N M. Colposcopic accuracy in a residency training program: Defining competency and proficiency. *J Fam Pract* 1993;36:515–20.

7. Benedet J L, Anderson G H, Matisic J P, Miller D M. A quality control program for colposcopic practice. *Obstet Gynecol* 1991;78:873–5.

8. Ferris D G, Cox J T, Burke L, et al. Colposcopy quality control: establishing colposcopy criterion standards for the NCI ALTS trial using Cervigrams. *J Lower Genital Tract Dis* 1998;2:195–203.

9. Coppleson M. Colposcopic features of papillomaviral infection and premalignancy in the lower genital tract. *Obstet Gynecol Clin North Am* 1987;14:471–94.

10. Stafl A. Colposcopy. *Clin Obstet Gynecol* 1975;18:195–213.

11. Kolstad P. The development of the vascular bed in tumors as seen in squamous-cell carcinoma of the cervix uteri. *Br J Radiol* 1965;38:216–23.

12. Burke L, Antonioli D A, Ducatman B S. *Colposcopy Text and Atlas.* Norwalk, Connecticut: Appleton and Lange, 1991.

13. Reid R, Scalzi P. Genital warts and cervical cancer. VII An improved colposcopic index for differentiating benign papillomaviral infections from high grade cervical intraepithelial neoplasia. *Am J Obstet Gynecol* 1985;153:611–8.

14. Ferris D G, Greenberg M D. Reid's colposcopic index. *J Fam Prac.* 1994;39:65–70.

15. Sakuma T, Hasegawa T, Tsutsui F, Kurihara S. Quantitative analysis of the whiteness of the atypical cervical transformation zone. *J Reprod Med* 1985;30:773–6.

16. Abdul-Karim F W, Fu Y S, Reagan J W, Wentz W B. Morphometric study of intraepithelial neoplasia of the uterine cervix. *Obstet Gynecol* 1982;60:210–4.

17. Sillman F, Boyce J, Fruchter R. The significance of atypical vessels and neovascularization in cervical neoplasia. *Am J Obstet Gynecol* 1981;139:154–9.

18. Sugimori H, Matsuyama T, Kashimura M, Kashimura Y, Tsukamoto N, Taki I. Colposcopic findings in microinvasive carcinoma of the uterine cervix. *Obstet Gynecol Surv* 1979;34:804.

19. Boonstra H, Aalders J G, Koudstaal J, Oosterhuis J W, Janssens J. Minimum extension and appropriate topographic position of tissue destruction for treatment of cervical intraepithelial neoplasia. *Obstet Gynecol* 1990;75:227–31.

20. Rome R M, Urcuyo R, Nelson J H. Observations on the surface area of the abnormal transformation zone associated with intraepithelial and early invasive squamous cell lesions of the cervix. *Am J Obstet Gynecol* 1977;129:565–70.

21. Anderson M C, Hartley R B. Cervical involvement by intraepithelial neoplasia. *Obstet Gynecol* 1980;55:546–50.

CHAPTER 10

Colposcopic, Clinical, and Etiologic Predictors of Invasive Squamous Cell Carcinoma of the Uterine Cervix

Table of Contents

10.1 Introduction

The most fundamental purpose of colposcopy is to determine whether the patient being examined has a cancer. This determination is based on information from cervical cytologic screening, the colposcopic impression, and any subsequent histologic findings. Each parameter has equal importance, and when either of the first two suggests presence of a squamous cancer that is not confirmed on colposcopically directed biopsy, excision is required to either confirm the suspicion or rule it out.

Both microinvasive or frankly invasive squamous cell carcinoma is tissue that has proliferated and transformed, altering cervical surface configuration and causing the formation of exaggerated, contorted, and unusual blood vessels to support tumor growth. Because surface contour and blood vessel patterns are reliable indicators of disease progression, it is essential that all individuals practicing colposcopy on patients with abnormal cytology learn to recognize the colposcopic signs of microinvasive and more advanced disease. Additionally, it is important to be familiar with the clinical and etiologic predictors, such as age, cytology, and location of disease.

10.2 Differentiating Normal from Abnormal Metaplasia

In order to be able to determine whether findings are significant or insignificant, the colposcopist must be able to recognize the normal presentations of native, metaplastic, and neoplastic squamous epithelium. This includes familiarity with their various associated blood vessels, in an original cervix and in a developing and matured transformation zone (Figures 10.1, 10.2). The colposcopist studies vascular patterns and intercapillary distances before acetic acid, and then surface contours, color tone, and the lines of demarcation between normal and abnormal areas after acetic acid with or without iodine solution (the standard colposcopic criteria of Kolstad and Stafl).[1] There are: insignificant findings, such as benign polyps or inflammation; significant findings, such as an abnormal transformation zone; and, colpo-

scopic mimics of cancer, such as post-radiation changes, condylomata, traumatic ulcers, and microglandular hyperplasia that are insignificant with regard to cancer. With acetic acid, significant squamous lesions become densely acetowhite with sharp borders and exhibit punctation of coarse or unequal-caliber, coiled, or bizarrely branching vessels that vary in intercapillary distances and have irregular surfaces. Excessively abnormal vessels or irregular surfaces observed colposcopically are early indications of an imminent microinvasive or invasive squamous cell cancer.[1,2]

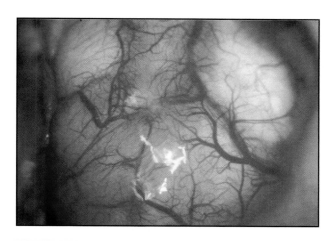

FIGURE 10.1   Large normal tapering and branching blood vessels coursing over a large Nabothian cyst. Reproduced with permission from Wright V C: *Color Atlas of Colposcopy—Cervix, Vagina and Vulva.* Houston: Biomedical Communications, 2000.

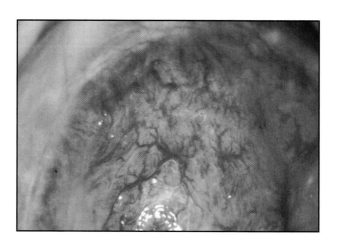

FIGURE 10.2   Matured transformation zone with blood vessels that taper off in a uniform manner and anastomose with similar blood vessels. Reproduced with permission from Wright V C: *Color Atlas of Colposcopy—Cervix, Vagina and Vulva.* Houston: Biomedical Communications, 2000.

10.3 Satisfactory vs. Unsatisfactory Colposcopic Examination

The second most important consideration is whether cancer can be reliably excluded when no suspicious lesion is seen. When the examination is unsatisfactory, the examiner cannot see the transformation zone for some reason, cannot see the entire lesion, cannot achieve exposure to evaluate the cervix, is faced with discharge or exudate, or is otherwise unable to assess the situation.

10.4 The Correlation Process after a Satisfactory Colposcopic Examination

Once there has been a satisfactory colposcopic examination and the biopsy report has been received, the practitioner can carry out the correlation process. This process determines whether the patient can be managed by observation in the absence of a high-grade lesion, by an ablative/cytodestructive treatment, such as cryosurgery or CO_2 laser ablation, or by excision to determine whether the patient has a malignancy. Excision is required when (1) any lesion intrudes on the endocervical canal; (2) the endocervical curettage (ECC) specimen is positive; (3) microinvasive or invasive disease is suspected colposcopically or cytologically but not proven histologically; (4) microinvasive squamous disease is detected by biopsy; (5) there is a failure to correlate (+/– one cervical intraepithelial neoplasia [CIN] grade between cytology, colposcopy and histology) unless histology is two or more grades less severe than cytology or colposcopy. (For example, if biopsy is CIN 2 but impression is metaplasia and Pap test is ASC, excision is not required for diagnosis); or (6) adenocarcinoma in situ is reported on biopsy or there are colposcopic indications of glandular disease that is not proven histologically.

10.5 When Excision Is Required Because of Suspected Cancer

Although monopolar electrosurgical loop excision is available and frequently used, especially in the presence of high-grade cytologic findings, colposcopic expertise is still required to identify the abnormal squamous disease location and extent. Colposcopy is also used to plan the surgical configuration of the specimen. In the presence of suspected or confirmed microinvasive squamous disease or a glandular lesion, the "loop" excision technique is inappropriate because electric current follows the path of least resistance, which is offered by mucus in the endocervical crypts. The electric current can produce excessive thermal burns with or without pseudostratification of glandular epithelium or fragmentation and denudation that make margins pathologically uninterpretable. These artifacts make it difficult or impossible to differentiate between microinvasive and invasive squamous cell carcinoma or between adenocarcinoma in situ and adenocarcinoma.[3-6] Additionally, artifacts in the intact cervix may interfere with follow-up assessment.

10.6 Why Cancer Is Missed

Missing a cervical cancer has serious ramifications, both for the patient and the clinician. It happens because of any of several potential inadequacies: (1) an inadequate case load (i.e., not enough patients to develop an adequate level of expertise), (2) a poor understanding of the disease processes, (3) deviation from or deficiencies in a diagnostic protocol, (4) insufficient biopsies (i.e., too small, no stroma, inadequate number) or samples from the wrong sites, (5) failure to perform an ECC when indicated, (6) failure to excise when ECC is positive, (7) cervical ablation without prior biopsy, (8) failure to correlate cytologic, colposcopic, and histologic findings, (9) failure to appreciate the indications for excision, (10) failure to refer in difficult cases, such as in the presence of exaggerated patterns of pregnancy; and, (11) miscommunication with the pathologist. Being aware of and avoiding these pitfalls will reduce the likelihood of missed cancers.[7]

10.7 Circumstances That Warrant Concern

10.7.1 Patient age

Cancer of the cervix is rare in patients younger than 25 years. The majority of high-grade squamous intraepithelial disease (specifically CIN 3) is found in women between 28 and 32 years of age. The incidence of microinvasive and occult invasive cancers increase as women grow older. For every 100 CIN 3 cases, 3 (3%) of the cases will be discovered to have cancer. Of these, one half will be microinvasive and one half will be more advanced disease.[8]

10.7.2 Cytology

Although cancer can be found with any grade of cytologic finding, more severe cytologic abnormalities correlate with a greater likelihood of cancer. Cytologic findings demonstrating squamous cell carcinoma will invariably be associated with a significant cervical or vaginal neoplasm. Only occasionally are malignant cells shed from an intraepithelial lesion, and those smears should not be repeated. Patients with malignant cells on cytologic testing require immediate colposcopic assessment with biopsy, ECC, and excision when biopsy does not confirm cancer.

A glandular lesion may be present together with a squamous lesion that is shedding abnormal squamous cells. Two percent to three percent of CIN 3 lesions will have a glandular component,[9,10] but cytologic testing often will not detect the glandular lesion.[11,12] Cytologic severity should be considered in connection with the patient's age. Markedly abnormal cells in an older patient (40 years or older) should suggest cancer to the colposcopist.

10.7.3 Linear length, surface area of lesions, and cervical diameter

The linear length of CIN 3 lesions, defined as the distance over the tissue surface between caudal and cephalad edges, varies between 2 mm and 22 mm (Figure 10.3).[13-16] Mean linear lengths range from 6 mm to 10 mm. Long linear lesions—those greater than 10 mm, particularly when there is endocervical involvement—are always suspicious for cancer (Figure 10.3). As the surface area of lesions increases to more than 40 sq mm, so should the suspicion for cancer. Since the size of the cervix itself increases due to tumor infiltration and proliferation in invasive cancer, an abnormally large cervix can also be indicative of cancer.

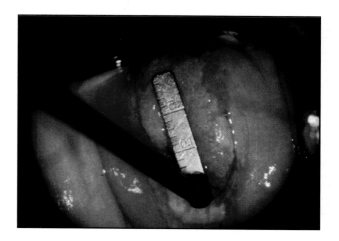

FIGURE 10.3 Measuring the linear length (greater than 20 mm) of the high-grade epithelial lesion on the ectocervical portion. The lesion however extends into the endocervical canal where most cancers are located. Reproduced with permission from Wright V C: *Color Atlas of Colposcopy— Cervix, Vagina and Vulva.* Houston: Biomedical Communications, 2000. ■

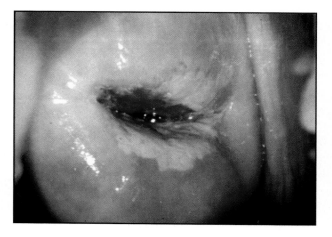

FIGURE 10.4 A high-grade squamous intraepithelial lesion, specifically CIN 3, located peripherally. The lesion extends into the endocervical canal. Potentially, the worst disease is located cephalad, which, in this case, is in the endocervical canal. Excision is required to exclude malignancy if not proven on biopsy. Reproduced with permission from Wright V C: *Color Atlas of Colposcopy—Cervix, Vagina and Vulva.* Houston: Biomedical Communications, 2000. ■

10.7.4 High-grade lesions with complete or partial canal involvement

Squamous disease develops and worsens in the wake of the atypical metaplastic process. As women grow older, atypical metaplasia starts peripherally and advances toward, into, and up the endocervical canal. Thus, disease on the periphery can be of lesser severity than that located more centrally (Figure 10.4). Low-grade disease is peripheral to coexisting high-grade disease, which is peripheral to any coexisting cancer.[17–19] Biopsies, therefore, should be taken from the leading edge of the lesion where the most severe histologic results will likely be found. At least 50% of CIN 3 lesions involve the endocervical canal (Figure 10.4).[14] The worst disease will always be located centrally.[15–20] Invasive cancer will be found at the inner/upper lesion border. When lesions are located high in the canal, the upper margin must be sampled, most often requiring a cylindrical excision (Figure 10.5).

Missing cancer—the most serious error made in colposcopy—usually can be attributed to inadequate evaluation of the endocervical canal. When a squamous cancer is found more peripherally on the cervix, it is more likely to be highly differentiated and, therefore, will have a better prognosis.[16] Cancers found within the canal can be of any degree of severity.

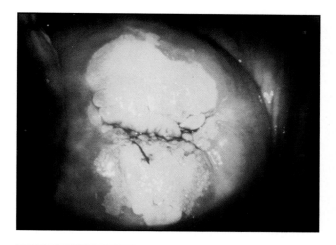

FIGURE 10.5 A large area of high-grade squamous intraepithelial lesion covers the ectocervix with canal extension. Some method of excision in the endocervical canal is necessary to exclude malignancy if not already proven on biopsy. Reproduced with permission from Wright V C: *Color Atlas of Colposcopy—Cervix, Vagina and Vulva.* Houston: Biomedical Communications, 2000. ■

10.7.5 Surface contour

Microinvasive and occult cancers can produce irregular surfaces, erosions, granular appearances or, in more advanced disease, necrosis (Figures 10.6 and 10.7).

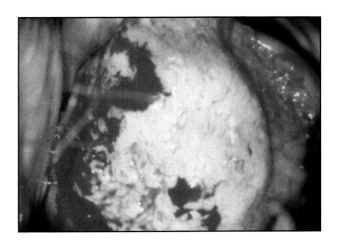

FIGURE 10.6   A large squamous cell cancer of the anterior cervical lip with an irregular ulcerative surface. A high-grade squamous intraepithelial lesion is noted peripherally from 7 o'clock to 12 o'clock. Reproduced with permission from Wright V C: *Color Atlas of Colposcopy—Cervix, Vagina and Vulva.* Houston: Biomedical Communications, 2000. ▬▬

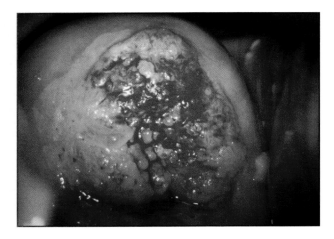

FIGURE 10.8   A large squamous cell cancer producing an enlarged cervix. It is dense white due to keratin and increased nuclear activity. Reproduced with permission from Wright V C: *Color Atlas of Colposcopy—Cervix, Vagina and Vulva.* Houston: Biomedical Communications, 2000. ▬▬

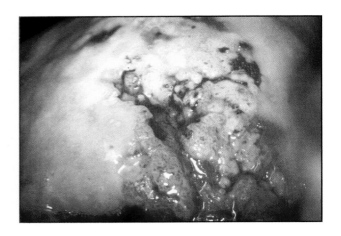

FIGURE 10.7   A large squamous cell cancer with surface irregularities and ulceration. Irregular punctation is seen and, in some areas, elongated irregular vessels are forming. Reproduced with permission from Wright V C: *Color Atlas of Colposcopy—Cervix, Vagina and Vulva.* Houston: Biomedical Communications, 2000. ▬▬

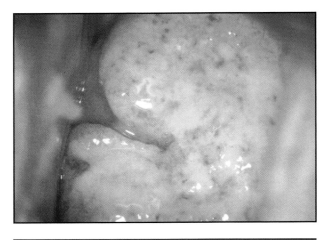

FIGURE 10.9   A large squamous cell cancer with necrosis, demonstrating a yellow hue. Reprinted with permission from Wright V C. *Principles of Cervical Colposcopy.* Houston: Biomedical Communications, in press. ▬▬

10.7.6 Color

Dense acetowhiteness is a distinct colposcopic feature of either high-grade squamous intraepithelial neoplasia or the presence of keratin. Keratin is associated with malignancy and is also seen in condylomata and in posttreatment states. One can differentiate between the two because keratin appears white before application of acetic acid, even to the naked eye. The degree of whiteness in neoplasia is a reflection of the amount of nuclear activity (Figure 10.8).[1-2] Visualization using a blue or green filter often reveals punctation or mosaicism and white epithelium after the application of acetic acid. High-grade squamous lesions are usually dense white from border to border, whereas glandular lesions often exhibit a variegated red and white coloration. Squamous cancers can be yellowish, a characteristic associated with necrosis (Figure 10.9). A red color reflects marked vascularity (Figure 10.10). These invasive

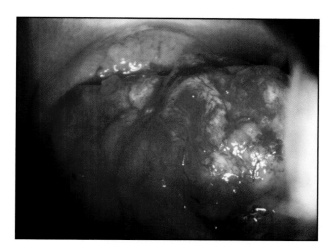

FIGURE 10.10   This very large squamous cell cancer appears red due to the abundance of long irregular angioarchitecture. Cancer bleeds easily with physical trauma. Reprinted with permission from Wright V C. *Principles of Cervical Colposcopy.* Houston: Biomedical Communications, in press.

lesions produce vaginal bleeding, most commonly postcoital, and a watery discharge as well.

10.7.7 Atypical vessels

Abnormality of angioarchitecture is an expression of stage of disease. Mosaicism and punctation, whether regular, irregular, fine, or coarse, are indicative of some grade of intraepithelial neoplasia. In microinvasive cancer, the punctate and mosaic patterns become degraded and disorganized as if the vessels are breaking out of the typical arrangements and transmuting into more atypical vessels (Figures 10.11–10.14).[1,2] These formations are commonly referred to as corkscrew, spaghetti, irregular coarse, irregular parallel, comma, tendril, and waste-thread depending on what they resemble (Figures 10.10, 10.15–10.19). Other atypical forms have non-branching vessels that bulge and constrict, exhibiting variable calibers (Figure 10.18). They sometimes appear within an area of uneven surface contour because these vessels are supporting active, proliferating tumors (Figure 10.19).

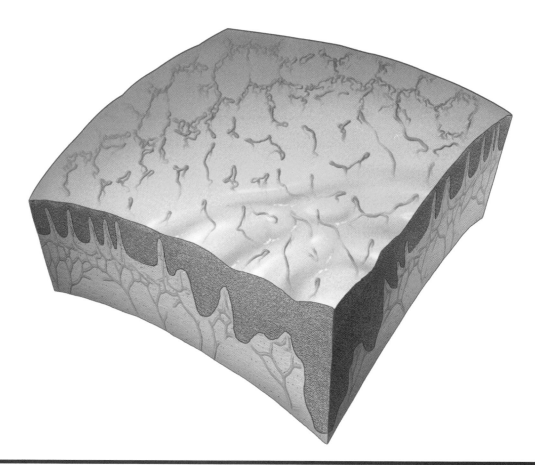

FIGURE 10.11   Schematics of the mosaic pattern breaking up, as seen in the beginning stages of squamous cell invasion.

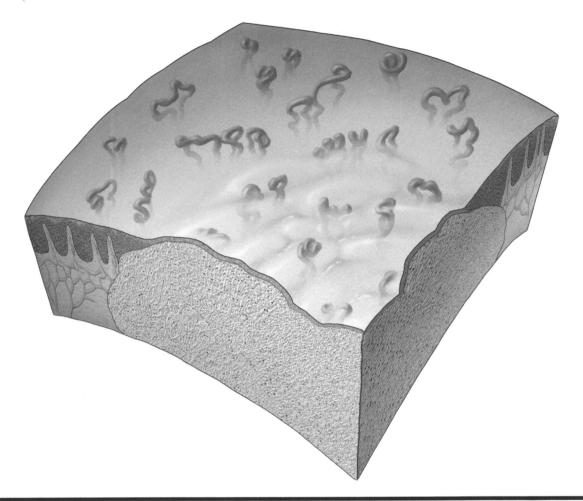

FIGURE 10.12 Schematics of irregular blood vessels of an invasive squamous cell carcinoma demonstrating corkscrew-like formations.

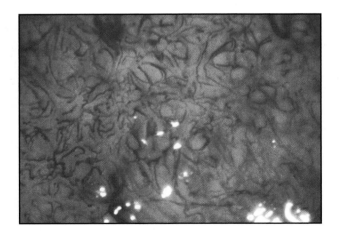

FIGURE 10.13 The mosaic pattern is becoming degraded and disorganized, a finding seen in early invasive squamous cell cancer. Reproduced with permission from Wright V C: *Color Atlas of Colposcopy—Cervix, Vagina and Vulva.* Houston: Biomedical Communications, 2000.

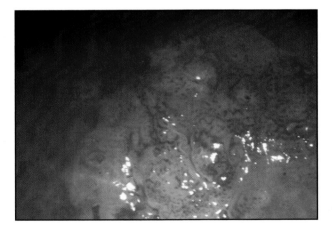

FIGURE 10.14 A microinvasive squamous cell cancer in which the punctate pattern is becoming disorderly and irregular elongated vessels are seen. Reproduced with permission from Wright V C: *Color Atlas of Colposcopy—Cervix, Vagina and Vulva.* Houston: Biomedical Communications, 2000.

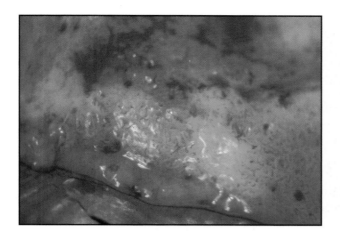

FIGURE 10.15   Irregular blood vessel formations over the surface of an invasive squamous cell cancer. Reproduced with permission from Wright V C: *Color Atlas of Colposcopy—Cervix, Vagina and Vulva—Cervix, Vagina and Vulva.* Houston: Biomedical Communications, 2000.   ▬

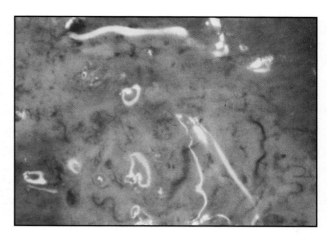

FIGURE 10.17   Numerous different blood vessel formations seen in squamous cell cancer. Reproduced with permission from Wright V C: *Color Atlas of Colposcopy—Cervix, Vagina and Vulva.* Houston: Biomedical Communications, 2000.   ▬

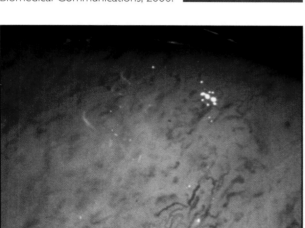

FIGURE 10.16   Irregular dilated (corkscrew) blood vessels of a squamous cell cancer. Reproduced with permission from Wright V C: *Color Atlas of Colposcopy—Cervix, Vagina and Vulva.* Houston: Biomedical Communications, 2000.   ▬

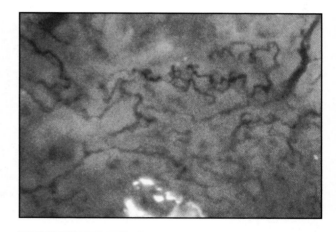

FIGURE 10.18   A high-power colposcopic view of irregular angioarchitecture seen in squamous cancer. Reproduced with permission from Wright V C: *Color Atlas of Colposcopy—Cervix, Vagina and Vulva.* Houston: Biomedical Communications, 2000.   ▬

10.7.8 Colposcopic grading systems

Different colposcopic grading schemes have been described.[2,21,22] They address squamous lesions' angioarchitecture, surface contour, acetowhiteness, and demarcation using acetic acid and iodine solutions. In all three, greater severity of disease correlates with more pronounced findings, and any area with atypical vessels is suspicious for malignancy. None of the grading schemes is applicable to glandular lesions and grading systems are not applicable to cancer staging.

10.7.9 Persistence or recurrence of high-grade lesions after treatment

When high-grade squamous disease persists or returns after treatment, colposcopy is frequently unsatisfactory because the remaining lesion looks very atypical or lies within the endocervical canal (Figures 10.20 and 10.21). Since this is where most cancers are located, there is a higher likelihood of cancer, warranting some method of excision.

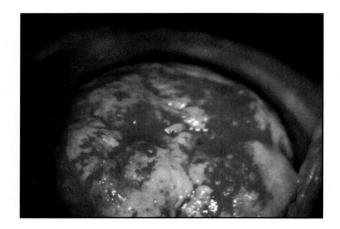

FIGURE 10.19 Advanced tumor growth and proliferation of blood vessels with bleeding associated with trauma. Reproduced with permission from Wright V C: *Color Atlas of Colposcopy—Cervix, Vagina and Vulva.* Houston: Biomedical Communications, 2000.

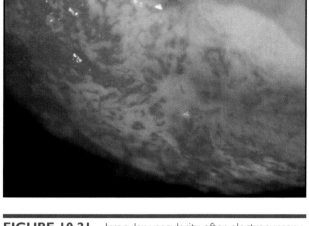

FIGURE 10.21 Irregular vascularity after electrosurgery for a high-grade squamous intraepithelial lesion. Such a formation requires excision to exclude malignancy. Reproduced with permission from Wright V C: *Color Atlas of Colposcopy—Cervix, Vagina and Vulva.* Houston: Biomedical Communications, 2000.

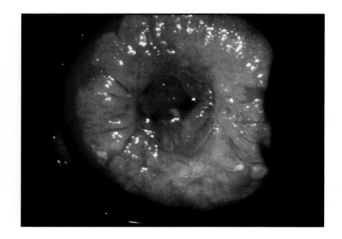

FIGURE 10.20 Recurrent/persistent disease after laser ablation for high-grade squamous intraepithelial lesion. This distribution is characteristic and resembles a white-walled tire. It is most likely related to activation of latent human papillomavirus during the healing phase. Reproduced with permission from Wright V C: *Color Atlas of Colposcopy—Cervix, Vagina and Vulva.* Houston: Biomedical Communications, 2000.

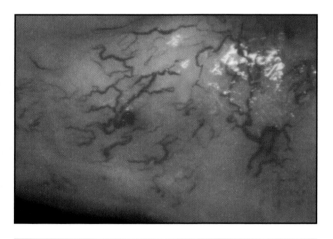

FIGURE 10.22 The angioarchitecture seen in normal cervical squamous epithelium after radiation for cancer of the cervix. The spatial distribution and corkscrew-like formations are characteristic. Reproduced with permission from Wright V C: *Color Atlas of Colposcopy—Cervix, Vagina and Vulva.* Houston: Biomedical Communications, 2000.

10.8 Colposcopic Mimics

More than one histologic diagnosis can exhibit the same colposcopic features, known as colposcopic mimics. Colposcopic mimics of malignancy relate to surface contours and atypical vessels. The enti-ties that produce cancer mimics are condyloma, post-radiation changes, polyps (cervical or endometrial), decidual tissue, and fibroids that have prolapsed into or through the endocervical canal unless colposcopic biopsy reveals invasive cancer (Figures 10.22–10.26).

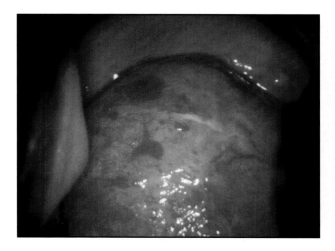

FIGURE 10.23   A prolapsed endocervical fibroid. Reproduced with permission from Wright V C: *Color Atlas of Colposcopy—Cervix, Vagina and Vulva.* Houston: Biomedical Communications, 2000.

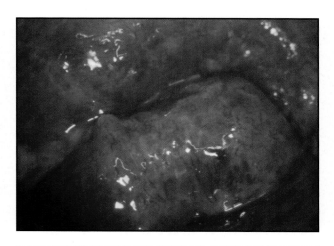

FIGURE 10.25   The characteristic distribution of blood vessels coursing over the surface of a large mass of decidual tissue, as seen in pregnancy. Reproduced with permission from Wright V C: *Color Atlas of Colposcopy—Cervix, Vagina and Vulva.* Houston: Biomedical Communications, 2000.

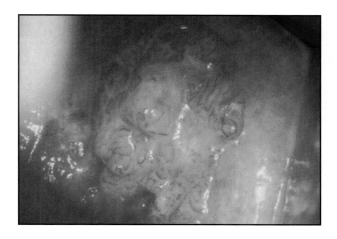

FIGURE 10.24   The irregular vascularity of a cervical condyloma resembling the angioarchitecture of malignancy. Reproduced with permission from Wright V C: *Color Atlas of Colposcopy—Cervix, Vagina and Vulva.* Houston: Biomedical Communications, 2000.

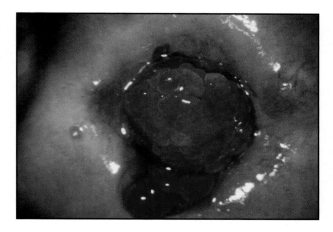

FIGURE 10.26   A large endocervical polypoid mass. Removal is necessary to exclude malignancy. In this case, the lesion was benign polyp. Reproduced with permission from Wright V C: *Color Atlas of Colposcopy—Cervix, Vagina and Vulva.* Houston: Biomedical Communications, 2000.

References

1. Kolstad P, Stafl A. Terminology and definition. In: Kolstad P, Stafl A: *Atlas of Colposcopy* (1st ed.). Oslo: Universitetsforlaget, 1972: 21–25.
2. Coppleson M, Pixley E C, Reid B L. *Colposcopy: A Scientific and Practical Approach to the Cervix, Vagina and Vulva in Health and Disease* (3rd ed.). Springfield, IL: Charles C. Thomas, 1986.
3. Dalrymple C, Russell P. Thermal artifact after diathermy loop excision cone biopsy. *Int J Gynecol Can* 1999;9:238–42.
4. Ioffe O B, Brooks S E, DeRezende R B, Silverberg S G. Artifact in cervical LLETZ specimens: Correlation with follow-up. *Int J Gynecol Pathol* 1999;18:115–21.
5. Missing M J, Otken L, King L A, Gallup D G. Large loop excision of the transformation zone (LLETZ): a pathologic evaluation. *Gynecol Oncol* 1994;52:207–11.
6. Montz F J, Holschneider C H, Thompson L D. Large loop excision of the transformation zone: Effect on the pathologic interpretation of resection margins. *Obstet Gynecol* 1993;81:976–82.

7. Powell J L. Pitfalls in cervical colposcopy. In: Wright V C, ed. *Contemporary Colposcopy*. Obstet Gynecol Clin NA. 1993;20:177–88.

8. Benedet J L, Anderson G H, Boyes D A. Colposcopic accuracy in the diagnosis of microinvasive and occult invasive carcinoma of the cervix. *Obstet Gynecol* 1985;65:557–62.

9. Christopherson W M, Nealson N, Gray L A. Noninvasive precursor lesions of adenocarcinoma and mixed adenosquamous carcinoma of the cervix uteri. *Cancer* 1979;44:975–83.

10. Boon M E, Baak J P A, Kurver P G H, et al. Adenocarcinoma in situ of the cervix. An underdiagnosed lesion. *Cancer* 1981;48:768–73.

11. Nguyen G-K, Jeannot A B. Exfoliative cytology of in situ and microadenocarcinoma of the uterine cervix. *Acta Cytol* 1984;28:461–7.

12. Östör A G, Duncan A, Quinn M, et al. Adenocarcinoma in situ of the uterine cervix: an experience with 100 cases. *Gynecol Oncol* 2000;79:207–10.

13. Przybora L A, Plutowa A. Histological topography of carcinoma in situ of the cervix uteri. *Cancer* 1959;12:268–73.

14. Abdul-Karim F W, Yao S F, Reagan J W et al. Morphometric study of intraepithelial neoplasia of the uterine cervix. *Obstet Gynecol* 1982;60:210–4.

15. Boonstra H, Aalders J G, Koudstaal J, et al. Minimum extension and appropriate topographic and position of tissue destruction for treatment of cervical intraepithelial neoplasia. *Obstet Gynecol* 1990;75:227–31.

16. Reagan J W, Hicks D J. A study of in situ and squamous-cell cancer of the uterine cervix. *Cancer* 1953;6:1200–14.

17. Holzner J H. Dysplasia of cervical epithelium—an intermediate or final stage in the development of epithelial atypia. In: Burghardt E, Holzer E, Jordan J A, eds.: *Cervical Pathology and Colposcopy*. Stuttgart: George Thieme Publishers, 1978:46–57.

18. Reagan J W, Patten F Jr. Dysplasia: a basic reaction to injury in the uterine cervix. *Ann NY Acad Sci* 1962;97:662–7.

19. Holzer E. Localization of dysplasic epithelium. In: Burghart E, Holzer E, Jordan J A, eds. *Cervical Pathology and Colposcopy*. Stuttgart: George Thieme Publishers, 1978:49–57.

20. Roman L D, Felix J C, Muderspach L I, et al. Risk of residual invasive disease in women with microinvasive squamous cancer in a conization specimen. *Obstet Gynecol* 1997;90:759–64.

21. Stafl A, Mattingly R F. Colposcopic diagnosis of cervical neoplasia. *Obstet Gynecol* 1973;41:168–72.

22. Reid R, Stanhope C R, Herschman B R, et al. Genital warts and cervical cancer IV. A colposcopic index for differentiating subclinical papillomaviral infection from cervical intraepithelial neoplasia. *Am J Obstet Gynecol* 1984;149:815–9.

Colposcopy of Adenocarcinoma In Situ and Adenocarcinoma of the Uterine Cervix

Table of Contents

11.1 Introduction

Historically, colposcopy was limited to the identification of squamous lesions. However, it is now beginning to be appreciated that there are valid and reliable colposcopic indications for the presence of a glandular lesion on the cervix. These lesions can develop by themselves or with a coexistent squamous abnormality. Colposcopists can learn when to suspect that an adenocarcinoma in situ (AIS) or adenocarcinoma exists and how to confirm or dismiss these suspicions.

11.2 The Columnar Epithelium

The columnar epithelium that lines the endocervical canal consists mostly of tall, cylindrical, single-layer, secretory cells with basally situated nuclei (Figure 11.1). Ciliary cells account for only 4% to 6% of the columnar epithelium. Reserve cells lie beneath the basal zone of the epithelium. The columnar cells lie over stroma in the form of ridges and clefts. The columnar epithelium can also demonstrate an ectocervical expression showing villous structures measuring 1.0 mm × 0.2 mm with a central core covered by a similar single layer of columnar cells (Figures 11.1, 11.2). The cervical columnar epithelium extends from the endometrium down the canal to the native squamous epithelium or to metaplastic epithelium.[1-3]

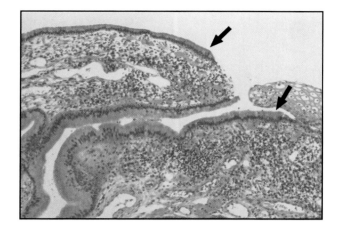

FIGURE 11.1 Histology of the villous structures of an ectopy demonstrating tall columnar epithelium with basally situated nuclei (see arrows). Hematoxylin and eosin stain, medium power magnification. Reprinted with permission from Wright V C: *Color Atlas of Colposcopy—Cervix, Vagina and Vulva.* Houston: Biomedical Communications, 2000. ▬

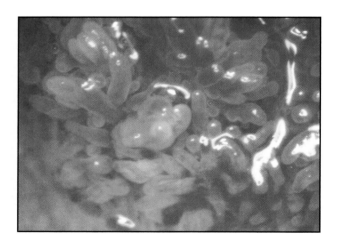

FIGURE 11.2 Colposcopic photo of the villous structures of an ectopy. They remain transparent after acetic acid is applied and blood vessels are not well defined. Reprinted with permission from Wright V C, Shier R M: *Colposcopy of Adenocarcinoma In Situ and Adenocarcinoma of the Cervix—Differentiation from other Cervical Lesions.* Houston: Biomedical Communications, 2000. ▬

11.3 The Fate of Columnar Epithelium

The glandular epithelium can present in many different ways. It can remain in its original form, be transformed into glandular neoplasia, undergo normal metaplasia to become normal squamous epithelium, or undergo an atypical metaplastic process producing squamous neoplasia. Furthermore, more than one process may occur at the same time. So, for example, a field of AIS may coexist with normal metaplasia or a glandular lesion may coexist with squamous disease. The latter is termed "mixed disease," and in about half of AIS cases there is an accompanying squamous lesion that is usually high grade. In about 2% of high-grade squamous intraepithelial neoplasia cases, a glandular lesion is also present.[4-8]

11.4 Neoplastic Transformation of Columnar Epithelium

The exact nature of the cytologic and histologic transformation from normal glandular cells to neoplastic cells is poorly understood. Controversy exists about whether the process is related to reserve cell hyperplasia, as in squamous disease. The undifferentiated bipotential reserve cell can differentiate into either a squamous or a glandular cell. The abnormal cells can exist in single or multiple layers and can be stratified or pseudostratified. The underlying villous structures in disease can remain as single structures (Figure 11.3) or colposcopically appear as coalescing or clumping masses (Figure 11.4). The result produces colposcopic findings that are different from those of squamous disease.

11.5 Stimulus of Disease Development

The human papillomavirus, particularly types 16 and 18, have been implicated in intraepithelial and malignant squamous as well as glandular disease.[9-12] This indicates that a common etiological factor (in association with trauma to columnar cells, alteration of vaginal pH or hormone stimulation) produces two types of abnormal histological findings by reserve cell stimulation that can occur either independently or simultaneously.[9-10] This is further supported by the fact that AIS can be seen histologically within superficial and deep endocervical crypts whose surface epithelium has been replaced by benign metaplastic or dysplastic epithelium in the same specimen (Figure 11.5).[4-6,13] Using PCR-based tests, 99.7% of cervical squamous cell cancers are

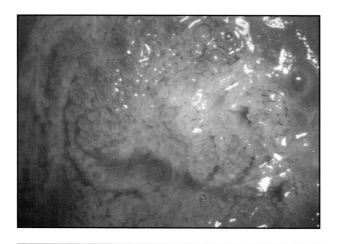

FIGURE 11.3   Adenocarcinoma in situ of the anterior cervical lip demonstrating simple villous structures that stain faintly acetowhite. The area is surrounded by typical, normal villi. Reprinted with permission from Wright VC, Shier RM: *Colposcopy of Adenocarcinoma In Situ and Adenocarcinoma of the Cervix—Differentiation from other Cervical Lesions.* Houston: Biomedical Communications, 2000. ▬▬▬

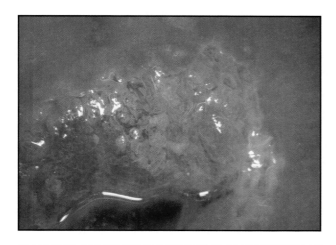

FIGURE 11.4   AIS after acetic acid extending from 12 o'clock to 4 o'clock. The glandular proliferative process gives the colposcopic appearance of coalescence or clumping. Reprinted with permission from Wright V C, Shier R M: *Colposcopy of Adenocarcinoma In Situ and Adenocarcinoma of the Cervix—Differentiation from other Cervical Lesions.* Houston: Biomedical Communications, 2000. ▬▬▬

HPV positive.[14-16] In cervical glandular disease (AIS and adenocarcinoma), the correlation is less strong with HPV DNA viral types being found in 64–88% of cases.[17-19] Viral types 16 and 18 predominate with type 18 being most common in adenocarcinoma and type 16 in AIS lesions. In women younger than age 40, HPV was identified in 89% of cases but only 43% of cases older than 60 (that is, the frequency of HPV DNA negative adenocarcinomas increased with age[19]).

Most cases of AIS occur in the company of squamous disease.[4,6] However, squamous metaplasia itself, either normal or abnormal, does not produce glandular disease. Glandular metaplasias do occur. Two types have been identified: tubal (ciliated cell) and intestinal (goblet cell) metaplasia. There is an association between these glandular metaplasias and cervical glandular and squamous neoplasias. Although 48% of these neoplasias contain glandular metaplasia, there is no clear evidence that the changes are precursors to AIS and adenocarcinoma.[20]

Another factor relating to increased incidence of adenocarcinoma of the cervix, particularly in young women, is long term use of oral contraceptives.[21-22] An epidemiological study by Brinton et al[22] reported a comparable risk (RR) of approximately 2 for both adenocarcinoma and squamous carcinoma for oral contraceptive users. Other authors have reported no significant differences in oral contraceptive use among cervical adenocarcinoma or squamous carcinoma cases versus controls.[23-24] Nonetheless, a potential association between adenocarcinoma and

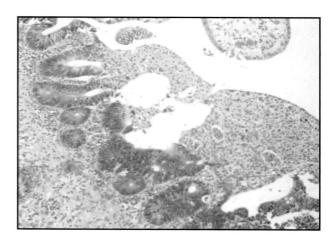

FIGURE 11.5   Histology of buried disease beneath dysplastic epithelium. It is obviously not visible colposcopically. Hematoxylin and eosin stain, medium power magnification.

contraceptive pill use has been advanced.[25] Obesity appears to be a risk factor for adenocarcinoma but not squamous cell cancer. This, in combination with contraceptive pill use, suggests a hormonally associated process for the development of glandular disease.[25]

11.6 Morphologic Spectrum of Glandular Intraepithelial Lesions

In 1953, Friedell and McKay[26] were the first to describe AIS. Intraepithelial glandular lesions of the cervix are now understood to have a morphologic spectrum (like squamous) from mild to severe. The entire range has been referred to as cervical intraepithelial glandular neoplasia and variably abbreviated as CIGN, CGIN or GIN. As with squamous changes, glandular changes have been divided into low- and high-grade classifications. Low-grade classification includes glandular atypia and glandular dysplasia. High-grade classification consists solely of AIS which appears to be increasing in incidence and today is found in women from 18 to 75 years of age (average age at diagnosis, 35.8 years).[27–30]

11.7 Problems Detecting Adenocarcinoma In Situ and Adenocarcinoma

Glandular disease often goes unnoticed because of imperfect cytologic findings, including inadequate sampling and failed screening. Another difficulty is colposcopic inexperience, i.e., so few cases encountered by a single colposcopist, resulting in failure to recognize the sometimes subtle indications, sizes, and locations of the lesion (skip/multifocal lesions, buried disease). Finally there is the challenge of mixed disease because the colposcopist is satisfied to have recognized a squamous lesion and does not search for a coexisting glandular one.

11.7.1 Cytologic difficulties

Cytologic smears, particularly from cervical scrapes, may not contain cells diagnostic of glandular disease. Atypical glandular cells are on cytologic reports in only 41% to 70% of cases of AIS.[27,31–34] Cytologic results often indicate a squamous abnormality because these are more proximal, more likely to be ectocervical, and more likely to be sampled, whereas glandular lesions are more likely to be in the canal or buried beneath squamous tissue, and so less likely to be sampled. A squamous cytologic report motivates the colposcopist to search for a squamous lesion and

be satisfied to have found it, rather than suspecting the presence of a glandular lesion as well.

Cullimore et al[27] noted that women with pure AIS were 4.8 years older than women with mixed disease. This finding suggests that cytologic studies are more accurate in identifying the squamous component than the glandular component. It also suggests that earlier diagnosis of mixed disease may be possible when colposcopists are motivated to search for and find the glandular lesions that can coexist with squamous ones.[27] Endocervical sampling, using an endocervical brush, may improve the detection of AIS existing either by itself or coexisting with a squamous lesion. Another potential problem with cytologic testing is that cells demonstrating AIS, even if present on the smear, may not be noticed.[32,34–36]

The Bethesda System 2001[37] assigned new subcategories for atypical glandular cells (AGC) replacing atypical glandular cells of undetermined significance (AGUS). Importantly, endocervical adenocarcinoma in situ now has its own category. Regardless, such smears cannot predict the final histologic results or differentiate between AIS and adenocarcinoma.[32,37] Cumulative studies of cases presenting with AGC cytologic findings qualified as favor neoplastic indicate that a pathologic component will be found in 42.0% of cases. Some grade of cervical intraepithelial neoplasia (CIN) will be found in 28.3%, AIS in 3.5%, endometrial hyperplasia in 4.7%, and cancer in 5.5% of cases.[38] Patients with squamous findings on cytologic smears may have a glandular as well as a squamous lesion.

For the colposcopist, the cytologic result may not always be entirely informative. In 98% of cases, an AIS smear indicates that a glandular lesion will be found.[39] However, in the AGC classification, AIS must be differentiated from the following: 1) reactive and regenerative changes in the columnar and squamous epithelium; 2) Arias-Stella changes in the cervix (a rare pregnancy change of endocervical crypts characterized by enlarged hyperchromatic nuclei of irregular shape with abundant cytoplasm ± increased secretory activity, however mitotic changes are not seen); 3) cervical polyp; 4) mesonephric duct hyperplasia; 5) tubal or serous metaplasia; 6) cervical endometriosis; 7) microglandular hyperplasia; 8) endocervical changes associated with an intrauterine device; 9) squamous dysplasia involving glandular epithelium; 10) cervical adenocarcinoma; and 11) invasive endometrial carcinoma.[40]

11.7.2 Colposcopic inexperience

Most colposcopists have found colposcopy to be of little value in recognizing AIS. The lack of firm criteria upon which to base a suspicion of glandular disease is due in part to the rarity of these cases and, hence, the inexperience of even the most "experienced" colposcopists. The ratio of AIS to CIN grade 3 (severe dysplasia/carcinoma in situ) varies from 1:26 to 1:239 (average 1:50 or 2% AIS[9]), but the ratio of adenocarcinoma to invasive squamous cell cancer is 1:14.[4,8] AIS is less commonly diagnosed than its malignant counterpart, which comprises 6% to 18% of all invasive cancers of the cervix.[4,41,42] The difference tells us that we are missing AIS and probably unknowingly destroying AIS when we treat squamous lesions. This is also why AIS comes as a surprise finding on biopsy reports and loop specimens. To make matters worse, the proportion of women with both AIS lesions and adenocarcinoma is increasing in a statistically significant manner.[43] Concerted efforts should be directed at finding these glandular lesions.

11.7.3 Lesion size and location

Studies indicate that most glandular lesions are located within the transformation zone. Specifically, Muntz et al[44] found AIS lesions to involve the ectocervical transformation zone in 53% of cases, the endocervical canal in 5%, and contiguous involvement in 38%, indicating that 95% of cases were available for partial or complete colposcopic scrutiny. Many of the lesions are small.[5,27,36] Forty-eight percent of AIS lesions involve only one cervical quadrant versus only 10% occupying four quadrants.[44] The linear length of AIS disease (the distance over the tissue surface between caudal and cephalad edges) usually does not exceed 15 mm.[5,27,36] Women younger than age 36 have a significantly lower disease volume than do women aged 36 years or older.[12] It is likely that the precursor lesion increases in extent and depth prior to becoming invasive. The largest lesions with the greatest linear length and underlying crypt involvement are found in older patients.[12] The worst histologic findings occur centrally, meaning that adenocarcinoma is more likely to be located toward or within the canal than widely out on the ectocervix, especially in older women.

Bertrand et al[13] studied the highest focus of cervical involvement of AIS measured from the maximal convexity of the cervix in hysterectomy specimens and from the resection margin in excisional specimens. Using these measurement parameters, the highest focus did not exceed 19.9 mm in 78.9% of cases. Just over 21% extended beyond 19.9 mm but none exceeded 29.9 mm. Such measurements do not reflect the true linear length of disease but rather provide guidelines for designing cylindrical excisional specimen measurements to encompass the disease.

11.7.4 Skip (multifocal) lesions

Skip glandular lesions are foci involving different portions of the endocervical mucosa. Multifocal AIS by definition is a complete normal radial histologic section separating two areas of AIS. The finding of normal and involved glands within the same slide is not accepted as multifocal.[13,36] Skip lesions occur in 6.5% to 15% of AIS lesions.[13,36] Skip lesions are uncommon, but when they do exist and are not far apart, they rarely interfere with colposcopic assessment.

11.7.5 Buried disease

Glandular disease can involve the superficial and deep crypts that are covered by benign metaplastic or dysplastic squamous epithelium (Figure 11.5).[4,6,13] Although the crypts open through such tissue, the glandular component may not be colposcopically visible. Buried disease occurs in 60% of cases.[12,13]

11.7.6 Mixed disease

A squamous lesion coexists with AIS in more than one half of AIS cases.[45] More than 80% of the squamous lesions will be CIN 3. Less than 3% to 4% of squamous disease cases are invasive, but when they are, they are usually microinvasive. The squamous component is usually colposcopically visible, whereas the glandular area can: 1) abut the squamous lesion (Figure 11.6); 2) be sandwiched between two squamous lesions (Figure 11.7); or 3) be cephalad to the squamous one (most common

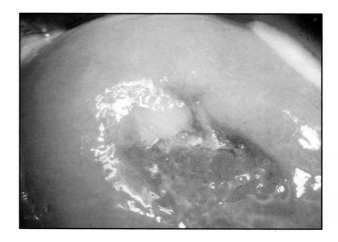

FIGURE 11.6 Adenocarcinoma in situ appearing like the villous structures of an ectopy on the posterior cervical lip. A well-defined afferent and efferent vessel can be seen. Abutting it anteriorly is a well defined densely acetowhite CIN 3 lesion. Photo courtesy of Dr. V. Cecil Wright. ▬

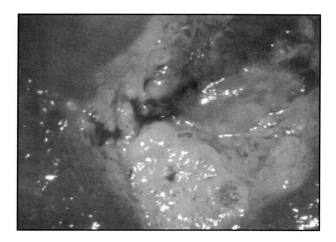

FIGURE 11.7 A well-defined adenocarcinoma in situ lesion from the 5 o'clock to 10 o'clock positions separates two high-grade squamous lesions. Reprinted with permission from Wright V C, Shier R M: *Colposcopy of Adenocarcinoma In Situ and Adenocarcinoma of the Cervix—Differentiation from other Cervical Lesions.* Houston: Biomedical Communications, 2000.

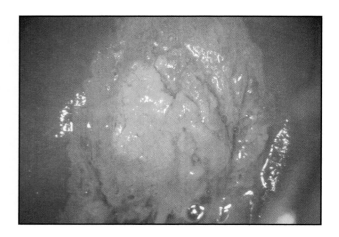

FIGURE 11.8 A densely acetowhite papillary adenocarcinoma in situ lesion lies centrally. Peripherally, it is surrounded by a high-grade squamous lesion. Reprinted with permission from Wright V C, Shier R M: *Colposcopy of Adenocarcinoma In Situ and Adenocarcinoma of the Cervix—Differentiation from other Cervical Lesions.* Houston: Biomedical Communications, 2000.

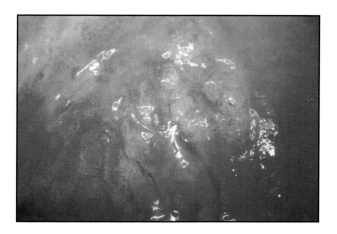

FIGURE 11.9 An adenocarcinoma in situ lesion after acetic acid application demonstrating discrete patches of budding, proliferating villi of different sizes. Single and multiple dots created by vessel loops within the growing projections are visible. The areas resemble the fused villous processes of early normal metaplasia. Reprinted with permission from Wright V C, Shier R M: *Colposcopy of Adenocarcinoma In Situ and Adenocarcinoma of the Cervix—Differentiation from other Cervical Lesions.* Houston: Biomedical Communications, 2000.

11.8 Three Colposcopic Presentations of Adenocarcinoma In Situ (AIS) and Adenocarcinoma

Three colposcopic appearances of glandular disease have been described.[47] The most common form is a papillary expression resembling an immature transformation zone. After acetic acid is applied, discrete patches of somewhat acetowhite, proliferating villi, varying in size, can be identified. They look like the fused villous processes of early, normal metaplasia (Figures 11.9 and 11.10), which is why these lesions are dismissed without sampling.[47,48] The second most common form is that of a flat, variegated red and white area resembling an immature transformation zone (Figure 11.11).[47] The least common presentation consists of one or more individual, isolated, elevated, densely acetowhite lesion overlying columnar epithelium (Figure 11.12).[47] The degree of acetowhiteness exhibited by glandular disease reflects the degree of the villous proliferative process and multiplication of the central villous core (the more, the whiter) and the histologic pseudostratification of columnar cells with their enlarged hyperchromatic nuclei (Figures 11.13–16).[47] In most cases, when glandular and squamous diseases coexist, the squamous component is more likely to be noted because it is more likely to be visible and distinct (Figure 11.6).

location, Figure 11.8). Studying the vascular patterns, intercapillary distance, surface contour, color tone and opacity, and clarity of demarcation (the latter three before and after the application of acetic acid) can enable the colposcopist to grade the squamous lesion(s).[46] The glandular component, when seen, often can be differentiated from other cervical lesions using the criteria described below.[47]

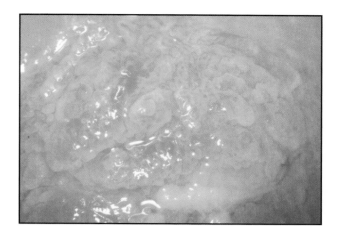

FIGURE 11.10   Benign metaplasia with formation of discreet patches of fused villi after the application of acetic acid. It easily could be confused with an adenocarcinoma in situ lesion (compare with Figure 11.9). Reprinted with permission from Wright V C: *Color Atlas of Colposcopy—Cervix, Vagina and Vulva.* Houston: Biomedical Communications, 2000. ▬

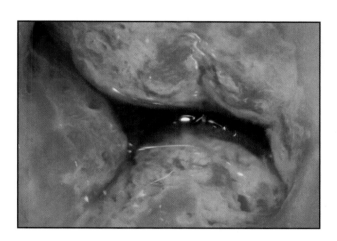

FIGURE 11.11   An adenocarcinoma in situ lesion displaying large crypt openings. The lesion occupies the endocervical canal and exhibits a patchy red and white color after acetic acid has been applied. Reprinted with permission from Wright V C, Shier R M: *Colposcopy of Adenocarcinoma In Situ and Adenocarcinoma of the Cervix—Differentiation from other Cervical Lesions.* Houston: Biomedical Communications, 2000.

11.9 Differentiating Glandular Disease from Other Entities

There is no single colposcopic appearance that characterizes glandular dysplasia, AIS, or adenocarcinoma. To complicate matters, colposcopic appearances of these entities often mimic other conditions. The generally accepted colposcopic criteria for grading squamous lesions do not apply to glandular lesions.[46,49,50]

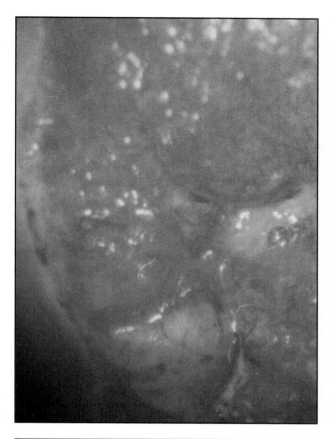

FIGURE 11.12   A well-defined adenocarcinoma in situ lesion overlying columnar epithelium and not in contact with the squamous border. It is elevated, well demarcated, and has a branching taproot blood vessel coursing over its surface. Reprinted with permission from Wright V C, Shier R M: *Colposcopy of Adenocarcinoma In Situ and Adenocarcinoma of the Cervix—Differentiation from other Cervical Lesions.* Houston: Biomedical Communications, 2000. ▬

Glandular lesions are to be suspected when any of the following colposcopic findings are observed: 1) a lesion overlying columnar epithelium not contiguous with the squamocolumnar junction; 2) large crypt openings; 3) papillary-like lesions; 4) epithelial budding; 5) variegated red and white lesions; 6) waste-thread-like vessels, 7) tendril-like vessels; 8) root-like vessels; 9) character-writing-like vessels, and 10) single- or multiple-dot formations as seen in the tips of the papillary excrescences.[47,51,52]

11.9.1 Surface patterns in glandular disease

11.9.1.1 Elevated lesions

When elevated lesions, particularly those exhibiting irregular surfaces, are lying over columnar epithelium, the differential diagnosis includes metaplasia

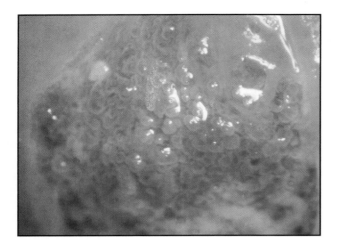

FIGURE 11.13 An adenocarcinoma in situ lesion after acetic acid exhibiting original, individual villi as well as proliferating villi. The colposcopic appearance is similar to the benign metaplastic process in which original, individual villi fuse together creating clumps or tongues in their transformation into squamous epithelium. Reprinted with permission from Wright V C, Shier R M: *Colposcopy of Adenocarcinoma In Situ and Adenocarcinoma of the Cervix—Differentiation from other Cervical Lesions.* Houston: Biomedical Communications, 2000.

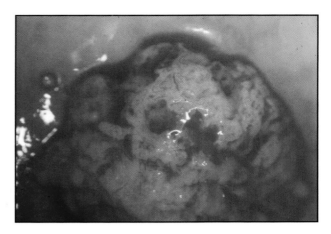

FIGURE 11.15 An invasive cervical adenocarcinoma after acetic acid application. It is papillary and more densely acetowhite than is the adenocarcinoma in situ lesion shown in Figure 11.13. Numerous atypical blood vessels are evident. Reprinted with permission from Wright V C, Shier R M: *Colposcopy of Adenocarcinoma In Situ and Adenocarcinoma of the Cervix—Differentiation from other Cervical Lesions.* Houston: Biomedical Communications, 2000.

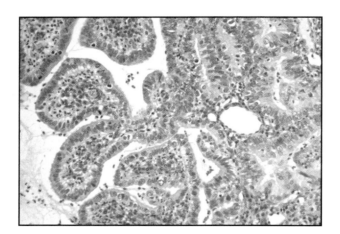

FIGURE 11.14 The histology of the adenocarcinoma in situ lesion in Figure 11.13 showing multiplication of the central villous core. The colposcopic impression is very similar to that caused by the fusing of villous structures that occurs in active metaplasia. Hematoxylin and eosin stain, medium power magnification. Reprinted with permission from Wright V C, Shier R M: *Colposcopy of Adenocarcinoma In Situ and Adenocarcinoma of the Cervix—Differentiation from other Cervical Lesions.* Houston: Biomedical Communications, 2000.

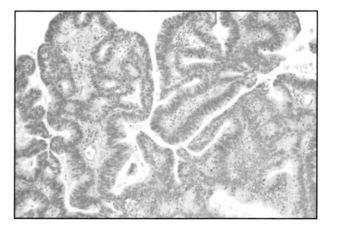

FIGURE 11.16 The histology of the lesion in Figure 11.15 revealing the proliferative process and multiplication of the central villous core that is responsible for the dense acetowhiteness. Hematoxylin and eosin stain, medium power magnification.

(Figure 11.17), condylomata, AIS (Figures 11.3, 11.4, 11.9, 11.12), adenocarcinoma and microglandular hyperplasia. In glandular disease, after the application of acetic acid, proliferating villi appear in discrete patches that vary in size resembling immature metaplasia. This is the most common colposcopic presentation of AIS.[48,49,52] Less commonly, a single, densely acetowhite lesion overlies columnar epithelium with no contact with the squamous border (Figure 11.12). Metaplastic-looking areas, particularly in the presence of a glandular smear, should be biopsied since this may be actually a glandular lesion.

11.9.1.2 Lesions with large crypt openings

Many AIS lesions occupy the endocervical canal in whole or in part. Some demonstrate a patchy red and white surface rather than the uniform dense acetowhiteness as seen in high-grade squamous intraepithelial neoplasia (Figures 11.11, 11.18, 11.19). Frequently, very large crypt openings are seen (Figure 11.11).

11.9.1.3 Papillary lesions

Papillary excrescences must be differentiated from normal papillary glandular mucosa (the villous structures of columnar epithelium constituting the ectopy [Figure 11.2]) and also from metaplasia (Figure 11.10), condylomata (Figure 11.20), adenocarcinoma in situ (Figures 11.3, 11.4, 11.9, 11.21–23),

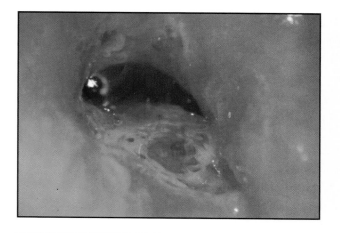

FIGURE 11.18   An adenocarcinoma in situ lesion occupies the endocervical canal. It is patchy red and white (variegated) after acetic acid. A large "gland"/crypt opening can be seen at the 11 o'clock position with glandular proliferation surrounding it. Reprinted with permission from Wright V C, Shier R M: *Colposcopy of Adenocarcinoma In Situ and Adenocarcinoma of the Cervix—Differentiation from other Cervical Lesions.* Houston: Biomedical Communications, 2000.

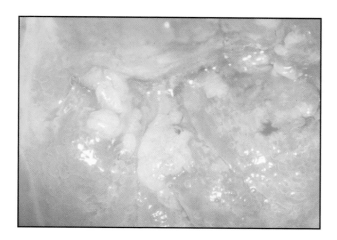

FIGURE 11.17   Metaplasia after acetic acid has been applied. Elevated, well-defined acetowhite areas lie over columnar epithelium. Biopsy is recommended to exclude glandular disease. Reprinted with permission from Wright V C: *Color Atlas of Colposcopy—Cervix, Vagina and Vulva.* Houston: Biomedical Communications, 2000.

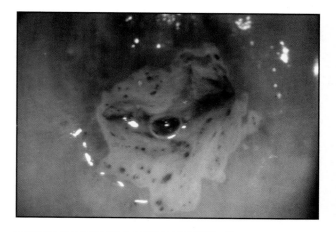

FIGURE 11.19   A high-grade cervical intraepithelial squamous neoplastic lesion (CIN 3) occupies the endocervical canal. After acetic acid, the lesion has become densely acetowhite from border to border and does not exhibit the red and white coloration seen with glandular lesions. Reprinted with permission from Wright V C: *Color Atlas of Colposcopy—Cervix, Vagina and Vulva.* Houston: Biomedical Communications, 2000.

adenocarcinoma (Figures 11.15, 11.24–27), squamous cell carcinoma, and microglandular hyperplasia (Figures 11.28, 11.29). In AIS, the papillary processes may appear colposcopically as single villi (Figures 11.3 and 11.6) or as proliferative villi, appearing clumped in a manner similar to that of a developing metaplastic transformation zone (Figures 11.4, 11.9, 11.10, 11.13, 11.15, 11.21, 11.22). Differentiating colposcopically between these entities may be impossible, hence the need for biopsies.

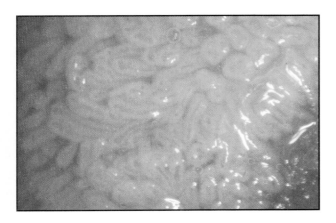

FIGURE 11.20 The papillary proliferations of a cervical condyloma. It is villous-appearing and each excrescence has a very well-defined afferent and efferent blood vessel. This angioarchitecture produces single or multiple dots in their tips. Reprinted with permission from Wright V C, Shier R M: *Colposcopy of Adenocarcinoma In Situ and Adenocarcinoma of the Cervix—Differentiation from other Cervical Lesions.* Houston: Biomedical Communications, 2000.

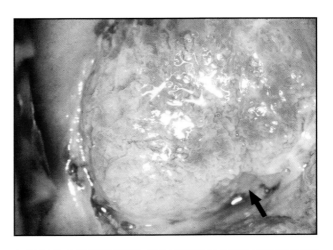

FIGURE 11.22 After acetic acid is applied, normal metaplastic epithelium can be identified between the 12 o'clock and 5 o'clock positions. In contrast, adenocarcinoma in situ exists between the 5 o'clock and 12 o'clock positions. Note that the two lesions look almost identical except that the adenocarcinoma in situ is slightly more papillary. The arrow depicts the external os. Reprinted with permission from Wright V C, Shier R M: *Colposcopy of Adenocarcinoma In Situ and Adenocarcinoma of the Cervix—Differentiation from other Cervical Lesions.* Houston: Biomedical Communications, 2000.

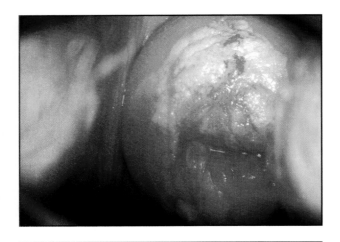

FIGURE 11.21 Extensive adenocarcinoma in situ of the cervix looking much like the fused, acetowhite excrescences of metaplasia. Small dots are created by internal vessel loops. Reprinted with permission from Wright V C, Shier R M: *Colposcopy of Adenocarcinoma In Situ and Adenocarcinoma of the Cervix—Differentiation from other Cervical Lesions.* Houston: Biomedical Communications, 2000.

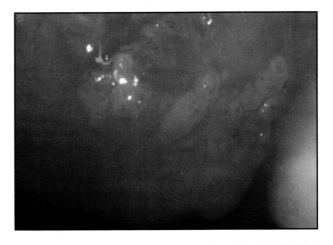

FIGURE 11.23 An adenocarcinoma in situ lesion appearing densely acetowhite and elevated is visible on the patient's left posterior cervical quadrant. Biopsy and excision proved adenocarcinoma in situ disease. Reprinted with permission from Wright V C: *Principles of Cervical Colposcopy.* Houston: Biomedical Communications, in press.

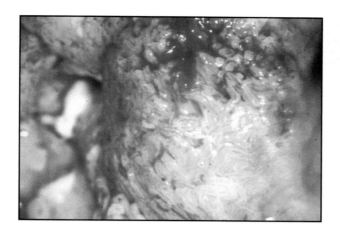

FIGURE 11.24   Papillary villous-like excrescences of an adenocarcinoma. Reprinted with permission from Wright V C, Shier R M: *Colposcopy of Adenocarcinoma In Situ and Adenocarcinoma of the Cervix—Differentiation from other Cervical Lesions.* Houston: Biomedical Communications, 2000. ▬▬

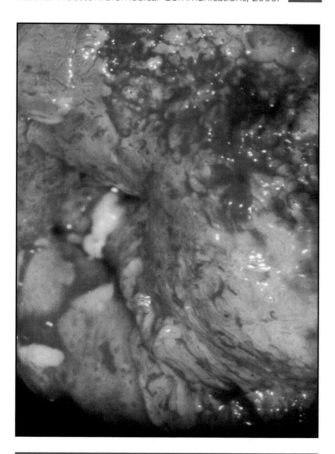

FIGURE 11.25   Higher magnification of Figure 11.24. The papillary structures resemble the villous structures of an ectopy. In some of the projections, afferent and efferent vessels can be identified. Reprinted with permission from Wright V C, Shier R M: *Colposcopy of Adenocarcinoma In Situ and Adenocarcinoma of the Cervix—Differentiation from other Cervical Lesions.* Houston: Biomedical Communications, 2000.

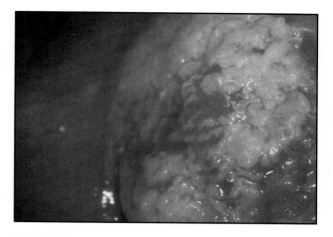

FIGURE 11.26   A large cervical adenocarcinoma after acetic acid has been applied. Dense white papillary masses that are created by proliferation look like agglutinated villi. Reprinted with permission from Wright V C, Shier R M: *Colposcopy of Adenocarcinoma In Situ and Adenocarcinoma of the Cervix—Differentiation from other Cervical Lesions.* Houston: Biomedical Communications, 2000. ▬▬

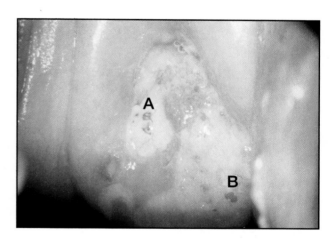

FIGURE 11.27   The smaller, densely acetowhite lesion is adenocarcinoma in situ (Site A). It is separated by normal tissue from a large acetowhite microinvasive squamous cell cancer (Site B). Reprinted with permission from Wright V C, Shier R M: *Colposcopy of Adenocarcinoma In Situ and Adenocarcinoma of the Cervix—Differentiation from other Cervical Lesions.* Houston: Biomedical Communications, 2000. ▬▬

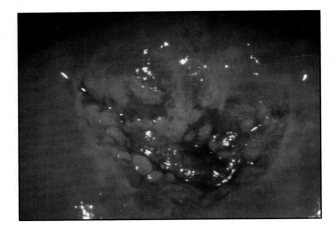

FIGURE 11.28 Microglandular hyperplasia. Large, yellow globular masses (with the color of chicken fat) lie over columnar epithelium. Reprinted with permission from Wright V C, Shier R M: *Colposcopy of Adenocarcinoma In Situ and Adenocarcinoma of the Cervix—Differentiation from other Cervical Lesions.* Houston: Biomedical Communications, 2000.

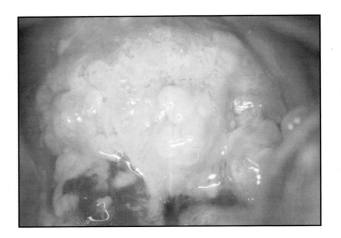

FIGURE 11.29 Extensive microglandular hyperplasia in a patient who is six weeks postpartum. Large papillary, globular masses having a whitish-yellow texture are noted. This mimics an adenocarcinoma (see Figure 11.26). Reprinted with permission from Wright V C, Shier R M: *Colposcopy of Adenocarcinoma In Situ and Adenocarcinoma of the Cervix— Differentiation from other Cervical Lesions.* Houston: Biomedical Communications, 2000.

11.9.1.4 Epithelial budding

AIS can cause villi to proliferate in a "budding" fashion (Figure 11.30). The proliferations have broad bases and many have serrated outer edges. In the case of budding, differentiation should be made between the budding of immature metaplastic epithelium (Figure 11.31), budding of immature condylomata (Figure 11.32) and that of adenocarcinoma in situ (Figure 11.30). Colposcopically directed biopsy may be necessary to differentiate.

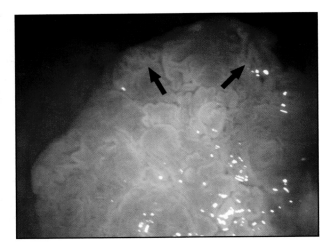

FIGURE 11.30 An adenocarcinoma in situ lesion demonstrating a papillary nature and scalloped-edged epithelial budding. Blood vessel patterns resembling character writing are noted in several peripheral locations (See arrows). Reprinted with permission from Wright V C, Shier R M: *Colposcopy of Adenocarcinoma In Situ and Adenocarcinoma of the Cervix—Differentiation from other Cervical Lesions.* Houston: Biomedical Communications, 2000.

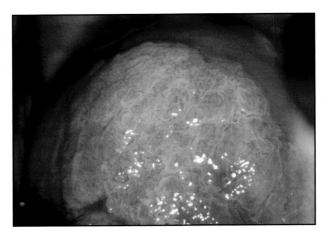

FIGURE 11.31 Metaplasia demonstrating epithelial budding similar to that in Figure 11.30. Reprinted with permission from Wright V C, Shier R M: *Colposcopy of Adenocarcinoma In Situ and Adenocarcinoma of the Cervix—Differentiation from other Cervical Lesions.* Houston: Biomedical Communications, 2000.

11.9.1.5 Lesions with a patchy (variegated) red and white surface

This is the second most common expression of glandular disease. The surface may be slightly uneven or rough (Figures 11.11, 11.18, 11.33, 11.34) or it can simply resemble an immature transformation zone. When a variegated coloration is seen after acetic acid

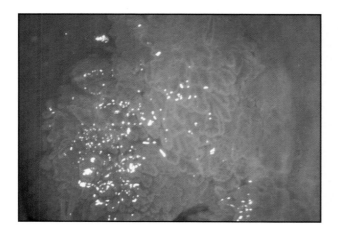

FIGURE 11.32   Epithelial budding structures in a cervical condyloma. Many of the structures contain proliferating angioarchitecture resembling character-writing. Reprinted with permission from Wright V C: *Color Atlas of Colposcopy—Cervix, Vagina and Vulva*. Houston: Biomedical Communications, 2000.

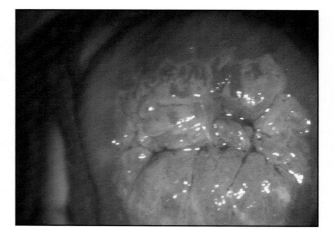

FIGURE 11.34   An extensive adenocarcinoma in situ lesion involving all cervical quadrants. It is patchy red and white after acetic acid. Reprinted with permission from Wright V C, Shier R M: *Colposcopy of Adenocarcinoma In Situ and Adenocarcinoma of the Cervix—Differentiation from other Cervical Lesions*. Houston: Biomedical Communications, 2000.

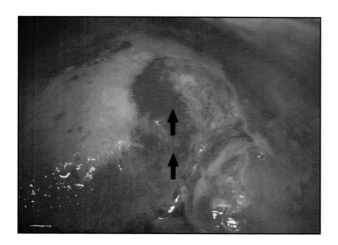

FIGURE 11.33   A variegated red and white adenocarcinoma in situ lesion splits two acetowhite epithelial lesions (see arrows). The indication that there is a glandular lesion is that squamous intraepithelial lesions are densely acetowhite from border to border. Photo courtesy of Dr. V. Cecil Wright.

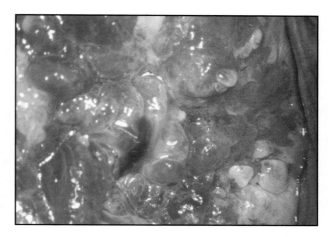

FIGURE 11.35   The variegated red and white acetowhite appearance of metaplasia. Metaplasia is forming glazed villi and bouquets of well-demarcated acetowhite epithelium overlying columnar epithelium. It mimics glandular disease. Reprinted with permission from Wright V C, Shier R M: *Colposcopy of Adenocarcinoma In Situ and Adenocarcinoma of the Cervix—Differentiation from other Cervical Lesions*. Houston: Biomedical Communications, 2000.

application, the colposcopist should differentiate between a developing normal transformation zone (Figure 11.35), AIS (Figures 11.11, 11.18, 11.33, 11.34), and adenocarcinoma (Figure 11.36). A biopsy may be necessary.

11.9.2 Atypical blood vessels

Glandular disease causes a variety of atypical blood vessels to form (Figures 11.37–39). The most common are the single and multiple dots that can be seen in the tips of single or proliferating excrescences (Figures 11.40, 11.41). Less common are waste-thread, tendril (Figures 11.15, 11.42, 11.43), tap and tuberous root shaped (Figures 11.44, 11.45), and character-writing blood vessels (Figures 11.46–49). Some of these configurations are also found in other cervical entities such as metaplasia (Figure 11.50),

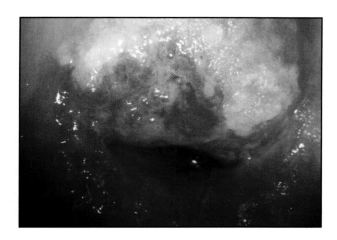

FIGURE 11.36   The densely acetowhite high-grade squamous intraepithelial lesion is easily identified peripherally. Beneath it and extending into the endocervical canal is a variegated red and white lesion with dilated blood vessels representing an adenocarcinoma. Reprinted with permission from Wright V C, Shier R M: *Colposcopy of Adenocarcinoma In Situ and Adenocarcinoma of the Cervix—Differentiation from other Cervical Lesions.* Houston: Biomedical Communications, 2000.

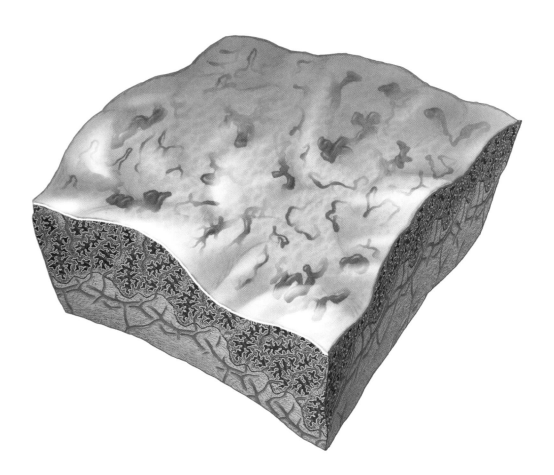

FIGURE 11.37   Schematics of waste-thread-like and dilated tuberous-root-like angioarchitecture.

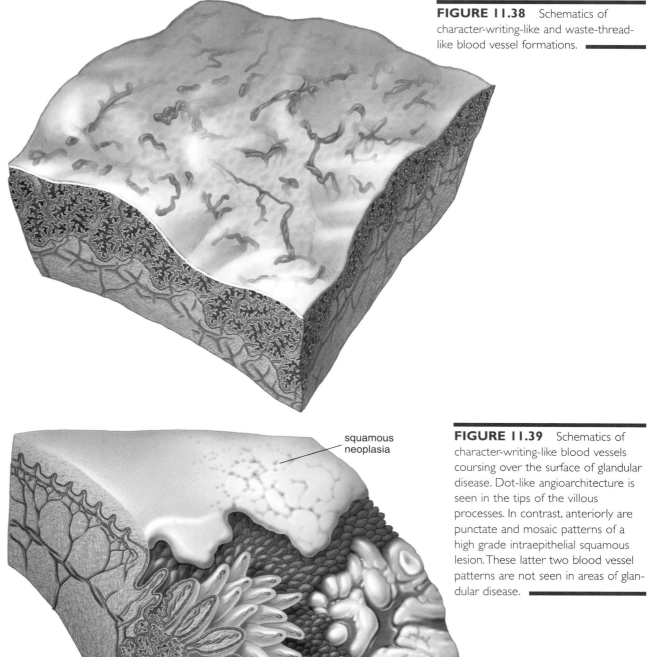

FIGURE 11.38 Schematics of character-writing-like and waste-thread-like blood vessel formations.

FIGURE 11.39 Schematics of character-writing-like blood vessels coursing over the surface of glandular disease. Dot-like angioarchitecture is seen in the tips of the villous processes. In contrast, anteriorly are punctate and mosaic patterns of a high grade intraepithelial squamous lesion. These latter two blood vessel patterns are not seen in areas of glandular disease.

squamous
neoplasia

variegated red
and white
glandular neoplasia

papillary
glandular
neoplasia

densely acetowhite
glandular neoplasia

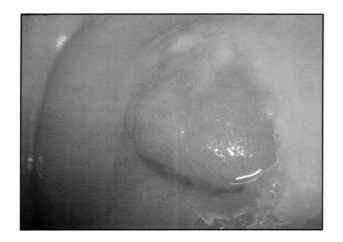

FIGURE 11.40 An adenocarcinoma in situ lesion demonstrating patches of multiple dots on the anterior cervical lip lies over columnar epithelium prior to the application of acetic acid. Reprinted with permission from Wright V C: *Principles of Cervical Colposcopy.* Houston: Biomedical Communications, in press.

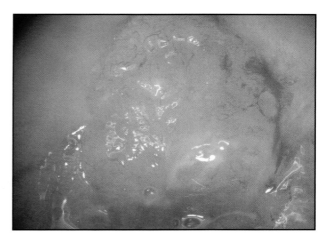

FIGURE 11.42 This adenocarcinoma demonstrates dense acetowhiteness with papillary excrescences. Note large irregular waste thread and other looped and tendril vessels. Reprinted with permission from Wright V C: *Principles of Cervical Colposcopy.* Houston: Biomedical Communications, in press.

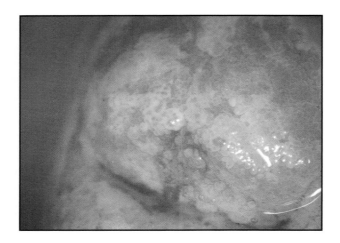

FIGURE 11.41 The lesion in Figure 11.40 after application of acetic acid. The adenocarcinoma in situ lesion contains proliferating excrescences that look like the fusing villi of metaplasia. Dots are seen in the tips. Reprinted with permission from Wright V C, Shier R M: *Colposcopy of Adenocarcinoma In Situ and Adenocarcinoma of the Cervix—Differentiation from other Cervical Lesions.* Houston: Biomedical Communications, 2000.

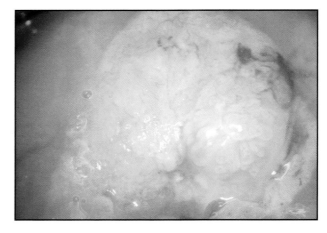

FIGURE 11.43 The lesion in Figure 11.42 after acetic acid. The vessels are obscured by the dense acetowhiteness. An irregular papillary proliferative process is evident. Reprinted with permission from Wright V C, Shier RM: *Colposcopy of Adenocarcinoma In Situ and Adenocarcinoma of the Cervix—Differentiation from other Cervical Lesions.* Houston: Biomedical Communications, 2000.

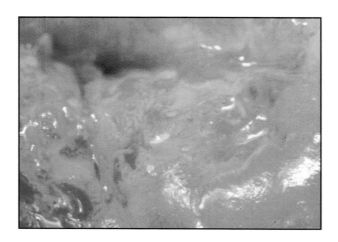

FIGURE 11.44   Large dilated, root-like and character-writing-like blood vessels in a cervical adenocarcinoma. Reprinted with permission from Wright V C, Shier R M: *Colposcopy of Adenocarcinoma In Situ and Adenocarcinoma of the Cervix—Differentiation from other Cervical Lesions.* Houston: Biomedical Communications, 2000.

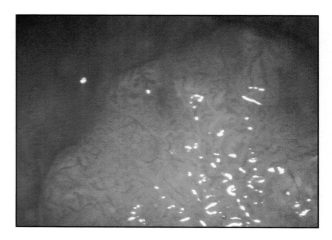

FIGURE 11.46   A variety of blood vessel patterns are contained in this adenocarcinoma in situ lesion. They are character-writing, taproot-like and tendril-like. Reprinted with permission from Wright V C, Shier R M: *Colposcopy of Adenocarcinoma In Situ and Adenocarcinoma of the Cervix—Differentiation from other Cervical Lesions.* Houston: Biomedical Communications, 2000.

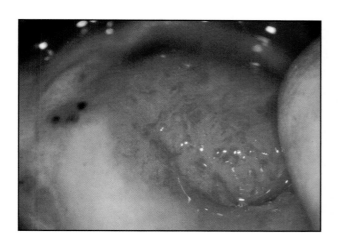

FIGURE 11.45   Large, dilated, tuberous root-like blood vessels in an adenocarcinoma. Reprinted with permission from Wright V C, Shier R M: *Colposcopy of Adenocarcinoma In Situ and Adenocarcinoma of the Cervix—Differentiation from other Cervical Lesions.* Houston: Biomedical Communications, 2000.

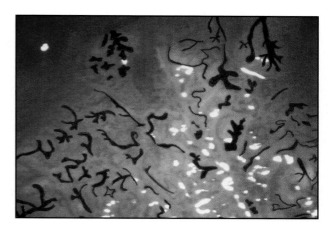

FIGURE 11.47   Vessels in the above lesion that have been "inked-in" for easier identification. Reprinted with permission from Wright V C, Shier R M: *Colposcopy of Adenocarcinoma In Situ and Adenocarcinoma of the Cervix—Differentiation from other Cervical Lesions.* Houston: Biomedical Communications, 2000.

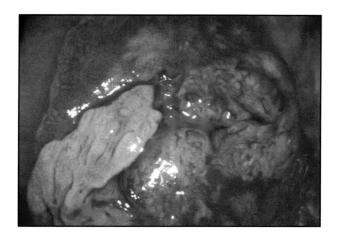

FIGURE 11.48 A mixed lesion. The very densely acetowhite, well demarcated high-grade squamous intraepithelial lesion is easily identified extending from the 7 o'clock to 10 o'clock positions. Centrally and also involving the endocervical canal is the adenocarcinoma in situ component exhibiting numerous root-like and character-writing-like patterns. Reprinted with permission from Wright V C, Shier R M: *Colposcopy of Adenocarcinoma In Situ and Adenocarcinoma of the Cervix—Differentiation from other Cervical Lesions.* Houston: Biomedical Communications, 2000. ▬▬

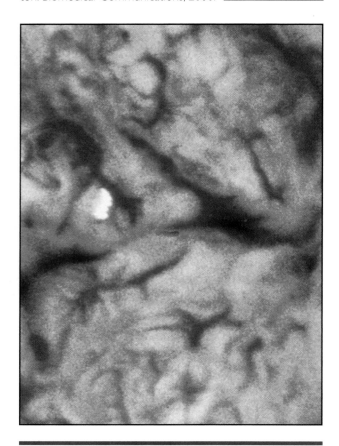

FIGURE 11.49 A higher magnification of the vessels in the lesion illustrated in Figure 11.48. Reprinted with permission from Wright V C, Shier R M: *Colposcopy of Adenocarcinoma In Situ and Adenocarcinoma of the Cervix—Differentiation from other Cervical Lesions.* Houston: Biomedical Communications, 2000. ▬▬

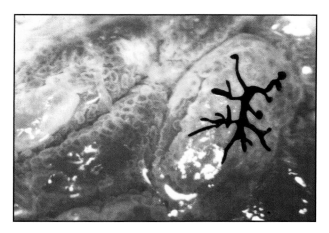

FIGURE 11.50 "Inked-in" character-writing vessels as seen in benign metaplasia similar to that seen in AIS. Differentiation cannot be made from AIS without a punch biopsy. Reprinted with permission from Wright V C, Shier R M: *Colposcopy of Adenocarcinoma In Situ and Adenocarcinoma of the Cervix—Differentiation from other Cervical Lesions.* Houston: Biomedical Communications, 2000. ▬▬

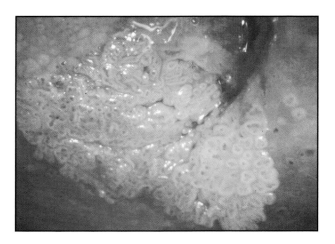

FIGURE 11.51 Single and multiple dots created by vessels in the tips of the proliferations of a cervical condyloma. Reprinted with permission from Wright V C: *Color Atlas of Colposcopy—Cervix, Vagina and Vulva.* Houston: Biomedical Communications, 2000. ▬▬

condylomata (Figures 11.20, 11.32, 11.51) and squamous cell cancer (Figure 11.52). Punctation, mosaicism, and corkscrew vessels, although common in squamous disease, do not appear in glandular disease (See Chapter 10).

11.10 Confirming the Diagnosis

When AIS is obtained on biopsy or is suspected cytologically or colposcopically, an excisional procedure producing negative margins is required to be sure no invasive disease is present. Some con-

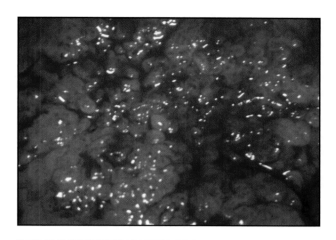

FIGURE 11.52   Single and multiple dots in a papillary squamous cell cancer. Reprinted with permission from Wright V C, Shier R M: *Colposcopy of Adenocarcinoma In Situ and Adenocarcinoma of the Cervix—Differentiation from other Cervical Lesions.* Houston: Biomedical Communications, 2000.

sideration should be given to the size and configuration (height and radius) of the specimen. Basically, it should be cylindrical and deep enough to account for the depth of crypt involvement and long enough to encompass the length of disease.[13,53] Both of these measurements are influenced by age as well as disease extent and location. The excision should be carried out under colposcopic guidance.[47,51] If the colposcopic biopsy or biopsies prove AIS, and the lesion was not predicted by colposcopy, the practitioner should re-examine the cervix with the colposcope, noting the lower border and, if possible, the upper margin (i.e., the entire linear extent). These measurements serve as a guide for determining the dimensions of the specimen to be produced by the excisional procedure.[51]

The cylindrical excision is best done with a high energy per pulse carbon dioxide laser using a scalpel to excise the apex or with a scalpel alone. Monopolar electrosurgical (loop excision) current follows the path of least resistance (into the glandular mucus) and thus can potentially distort the benign as well as diseased glandular epithelium making histologic interpretation difficult if not impossible.[51]

11.10.1 Management of the patient who desires to maintain fertility

The safe conservative management of the patient who desires to maintain fertility in most centers depends on the pathological reporting of negative surgical margins in the excised specimen. The adequacy and accuracy of screening and invasive detection methods are inadequate for reliable detection of persistent and recurrent disease.[32,34,54,55] Patients who choose conservative management for AIS must be counseled regarding the importance of compliance and the potential risks of undetected persistent and recurrent glandular disease despite negative screening methods.[54,55]

11.10.2 Significance of negative margins in the excised specimen

Most studies indicate that if the excised specimen's margins are negative, conservative management is permissible in women who desire future childbearing.[5,27,33,44,55,56] Negative margins are associated with persistent AIS in the extirpated uterus in 12.5% of cases.[5,7,13,36,44] On occasion, studies have identified adenocarcinoma even when specimens had negative margins.[35,54,57]

The follow-up should consist of cytologic sampling, colposcopic examination, and endocervical curettage every four months for one year and then every six months continuously.[7,51,57] Once reproduction is complete, hysterectomy has been advocated. It is not known whether this is necessary in the compliant patient with no evidence of persistent disease.

11.10.3 Significance of positive margins in the excised specimen

Cumulative studies indicate that positive margins in the excised specimen are of great significance because of the high risk of remaining AIS (46% of cases) and invasive adenocarcinoma (16.7% of cases).[27,36,44,54,57,58] Repeat excision is necessary to obtain negative margins for the conservatively managed patient who desires further childbearing. Repeat excision producing negative margins is also necessary before a simple hysterectomy is performed in the patient who desires no future childbearing. Failure to do so in the latter circumstance may result in inappropriate surgery (simple hysterectomy instead of radical hysterectomy) should invasive adenocarcinoma be found in the extirpated uterine cervix. When it is not possible to obtain negative margins, the next step is a modified radical hysterectomy, not a simple one.

References

1. Hafez ESE. Structural and ultrastructural parameters of the uterine cervix. *Obstet Gynecol Survey* 1982;37:507–16.

2. Philipp E. Normal endocervical epithelium. *J Reprod Med* 1975;14:188–91.

3. Fluhmann CF, Dickman Z. The basic pattern of glandular structures of the cervix uteri. *Obstet Gynecol* 1958;11:543–55.

4. Christopherson WM, Nealson N, Gray L, Sr. Noninvasive precursor lesions of adenocarcinoma and mixed adenosquamous carcinoma of the cervix uteri. *Cancer* 1979;44:975–83.

5. Anderson ES, Arfmann E. Adenocarcinoma in situ of the uterine cervix: A clinico-pathologic study of 36 cases. *Gynecol Oncol* 1989;35:1–7.

6. Colgan TJ, Lickrish GM. The topography and invasive potential of cervical adenocarcinoma in situ, with and without associated squamous dysplasia. *Gynecol Oncol* 1990;36:246–9.

7. Weisbrot IM, Stabinsky C, Davis AM. Adenocarcinoma in situ of the uterine cervix. *Cancer* 1972; 29:1179–87.

8. Boon ME, Baak JPA, Kurver PJH, et al. Adenocarcinoma in situ of the cervix: an underdiagnosed lesion. *Cancer* 1981;48:768–73.

9. Farnsworth A, Laverty C, Stoler MH. Human papilloma virus messenger RNA expression in adenocarcinoma in situ of the uterine cervix. *Int J Gynecol Path* 1989;8:321–30.

10. Tase T, Okagaki T, Clark BA, et al. Human papillomavirus DNA in glandular dysplasia and microglandular hyperplasia: presumed precursors of adenocarcinoma of the cervix uteri. *Obstet Gynecol* 1989;73:1005–8.

11. Smotkin D, Berek JS, Yao S, et al. Human papilloma virus desoxyribonucleic acid in adenocarcinoma and adenosquamous carcinoma of the uterine cervix. *Obstet Gynecol* 1986;68:241–4.

12. Nicklin JL, Wright RG, Bell JR, et al. A clinicopathological study of adenocarcinoma in situ of the cervix. The influence of HPV infection and other factors, and the role of conservative surgery. *Aust NZ Obstet Gynecol* 1991;31:179–83.

13. Bertrand M, Lickrish GM, Colgan TJ. The anatomical distribution of cervical adenocarcinoma in situ. *Am J Obstet Gynecol* 1987;1:21–6.

14. Rolon PA, Smith JS, Munoz J, et al. Human papillomavirus infection and cervical cancer in Paraguay. *Int J Cancer* 2000;85:486–91.

15. Bosch FX, Manos MM, Munoz N, et al. Prevalence of human papillomavirus in cervical cancer: A world wide perspective. *JNCI* 1995;87:796–802.

16. Walboomers JMM, Jacobs MV, Manos MM, et al. Human papillomavirus is a necessary cause of invasive cervical cancer worldwide. *J Pathol* 1999;189:12–9.

17. Kado S, Kawamata Y, Shono Y, et al. Detection of human papillomaviruses in cervical neoplasias using multiple sets of generic polymerase chain reaction primers. *Gynecol Oncol* 2001;81:47–52.

18. Riethdorf S, Riethdorf L, Milde-Langosch K, et al. Differences in HPV 16 and HPV 18 E6/E7 oncogenic expression between adenocarcinoma in situ and invasive adenocarcinomas of the cervix. *Virchows Arch* 2000;437:491–500.

19. Anderson S, Rylander E, Larsson B, et al. The role of human papillomavirus in cervical adenocarcinoma carcinogenesis. *Eur J Cancer* 2001;37:246–50.

20. Dlott JS, Dlott TR, Matthews TH, et al. Endocervical metaplasias and their association with squamous abnormalities. *J Lower Genital Tract Dis* 1999;3:77–82.

21. Jones MW, Silverberg SG. Cervical adenocarcinoma in young women: Possible relationship to microglandular hyperplasia and use of oral contraceptives. *Obstet Gynecol* 1989;73:984–8.

22. Brinton LA, Reeves WC, Herrero R, et al. Oral contraceptive use and risk of invasive cervical cancer. *Int J Epidemiol* 1990;19:4–11.

23. Silcox PBS, Thornton-Jones H, Murphy M. Squamous and adenocarcinoma of the uterine cervix: A comparison using routine data. *Br J Cancer* 1987;55:321–5.

24. Horowitz IR, Jacobson LP, Zucker PK, et al. Epidemiology of adenocarcinoma of the cervix. *Gynecol Oncol* 1988;31:25–31.

25. Parazzini F, La Vecchia C. Epidemiology of adenocarcinoma of the cervix. *Gynecol Oncol* 1990;39:40–6.

26. Friedell GH, McKay DG. Adenocarcinoma in situ of the endocervix. *Cancer* 1953;6:887–97.

27. Cullimore JE, Luesley DM, Rollason TP, et al. A prospective study of conization of the cervix in the management of cervical intraepithelial glandular neoplasia (CIGN)—a preliminary report. *Br J Obstet Gynecol* 1992;99:314–8.

28. Gloor E, Hurlimann J. Cervical intraepithelial neoplasia (adenocarcinoma in situ and glandular dysplasia). *Cancer* 1986; 58:1272–82.

29. Östör AG, Duncan A, Quinn M, et al. Adenocarcinoma in situ of the uterine cervix: An experience with 100 cases. *Gynecol Oncol* 2000;79:207–10.

30. Anderson MC. Glandular lesions of the cervix: diagnostic and therapeutic dilemmas. *Baillières Clin Obstet Gynecol* 1995;9:105–19.

31. Leusley DM, Jordan JA, Woodman CBJ, et al. A retrospective review of adenocarcinoma in situ and glandular atypia of the uterine cervix. *Br J Obstet Gynecol* 1987;94:699–703.

32. Laverty CR, Farnsworth A, Thurloe T, et al. The reliability of a cytological prediction of cervical adenocarcinoma in situ. *Aust NZ J Obstet Gynecol* 1998;28:307–12.

33. Ayer B, Pacey F, Greenberg M, et al. The cytological diagnosis of adenocarcinoma in situ of the cervix and related lesions 1. Adenocarcinoma in situ. Acta Cytol 1987;31:394–411.

34. Nguyen G-K, Jeannot A B. Exfoliative cytology of in situ and microadenocarcinoma of the uterine cervix. *Acta Cytol* 1984;28:461–7.

35. Widrich T, Kennedy A W, Myers T M, et al. Adenocarcinoma in situ of the uterine cervix: management and outcome. *Gynecol Oncol* 1996;61:304–8.

36. Östör A G, Paganor R, Davoran A M, et al. Adenocarcinoma in situ of the cervix. *Int J Obstet Gynecol Path* 1984;3:179–90.

37. Solomon D, Davey D, Kurman R, et al. The 2001 Bethesda System: Terminology for reporting results of cervical cytology. *JAMA* 2002;287:2114–9.

38. Veljovich D S, Stoler M H, Andersen W A, et al. Atypical glandular cells of undetermined significance. A five-year retrospective histopathologic study. *Am J Obstet Gynecol* 1990;179:382–90.

39. Nasu I, Meurer W, Fu Y S. Cytological features alone do not allow accurate distinction between in situ and invasive adenocarcinoma. *Int J Gynecol Pathol* 1993;12:208–18.

40. Lickrish G M, Colgan T. Management of adenocarcinoma in situ of the uterine cervix. In: Wright V C, Lickrish G M, Shier R M (eds.). *Basic and Advanced Colposcopy—A Practical Handbook for Treatment* (2nd edition). Houston: Biomedical Communications 1995;30-1–30-8.

41. Brinton L A, Herrero R, Reeves W C, et al. Risk factors for cervical cancer by histology. *Gynecol Oncol* 1993;51:301–6.

42. Leminen A, Paavonen J, Forss M, et al. Adenocarcinoma in situ of the uterine cervix. *Cancer* 1990;65:53–9.

43. Plaxe S C, Saltzstein S L. Estimation of the duration of the preclinical phase of cervical adenocarcinoma suggests there is ample opportunity for screening. *Gynecol Oncol* 1999;75:55–61.

44. Muntz H G, Bell D A, Lage J M, et al. Adenocarcinoma in situ of the uterine cervix. *Obstet Gynecol* 1992;80:935–9.

45. Jaworski R C, Pacey N F, Greenberg M L. The histologic diagnosis of adenocarcinoma in situ and related lesions of the cervix uteri. *Cancer* 1988;61:1171–81.

46. Kolstad P, Stafl A. Terminology and definition. In: Kolstad P, Stafl A: *Atlas of Colposcopy* (1st edition). Oslo: Universitetsforlaget, 1972:21–5.

47. Wright V C. Colposcopy of adenocarcinoma in situ and adenocarcinoma of the uterine cervix: differentiation from other cervical lesions. *J Lower Genital Tract Dis* 1999;2:83–97.

48. Coppleson M, Atkinson K H, Dalrymple J C. Cervical squamous and glandular neoplasia: clinical features and review of management. In: Coppleson M, (ed.) *Gynecologic Oncology.* Edinburgh: Churchill Livingston, 1992;571–607.

49. Coppleson M, Pixley E C, Reid B L. *Colposcopy: A Scientific and Practical Approach to the Cervix, Vagina and Vulva in Health and Disease* (3rd edition). Springfield, IL: Charles C Thomas, 1986.

50. Reid R, Stanhope C R, Herschman B R, et al. Genital warts and cervical cancer IV. A colposcopic index for differentiating subclinical papillomaviral infection from cervical intraepithelial neoplasia. *Am J Obstet Gynecol* 1984;149:815–9.

51. Wright V C, Dubue-Lissoir J, Ehlen T, et al. Guidelines on adenocarcinoma in situ of the cervix: Clinical features and review of management. *J Soc Obstet Gynaecol Can* 1999;21:699–706.

52. Wright V C, Shier R M. Differentiating Adenocarcinoma In Situ and Invasive Adenocarcinoma from Other Cervical lesions. In: Wright VC, Shier RM (eds.). *Colposcopic Features of Adenocarcinoma In Situ and Invasive Adenocarcinoma of the Cervix.* Houston: Biomedical Communications, 2000.

53. Wright V C, Davies E, Riopelle MA. Laser cylindrical conization to replace conization. Am J Obstet Gynecol 1983;145:181–5.

54. Poynor E A, Barakat R R, Hoskins W J. Management and follow-up of patients with adenocarcinoma in situ of the uterine cervix. *Gynecol Oncol* 1995;57:158–64.

55. Wolf J, Levenback C, Malpica A, et al. Adenocarcinoma in situ of the cervix: significance of cone biopsy margins. *Obstet Gynecol* 1996;88:82–6.

56. Im D I, Duska L R, Recension N B. Adequacy of conization margins of adenocarcinoma in situ of the cervix as a predictor of residual disease. *Gynecol Oncol* 1995;59:179–82.

57. Kennedy A W, Tabbakh G H, Biscotti C V, et al. Invasive adenocarcinoma of the cervix following LLETZ (Large Loop Excision of the Transformation Zone) for adenocarcinoma in situ. *Gynecol Oncol* 1995;58:274–7.

58. Hopkins M, Roberts J A, Schmidt R W. Cervical adenocarcinoma in situ. *Obstet Gynecol* 1988;7:842–4.

Table of Contents

12.1 Introduction

Precautions must be exercised when evaluating and treating any pregnant woman to avoid fetal compromise. This basic premise applies particularly to the diagnosis and management of pregnant women with cervical neoplasia. Because of the close proximity of the disease to the fetus, modified management strategies are required to maintain fetal viability and facilitate maturation, if possible. Pregnancy complications and failure to diagnose cancer may also jeopardize the welfare of the patient and fetus. Colposcopy remains the assessment method of choice for pregnant women found to have abnormal cervical cytologic findings. Many of the basic principles of colposcopy discussed previously apply in this special population. However, hampered visualization, altered vascularity, challenging assessment, and cautious, conservative sampling characterize the necessity for a unique approach to colposcopic evaluation during pregnancy. Consultation with colposcopic experts may be necessary in managing pregnant women with cervical neoplasia when prior experience is limited. This chapter includes a discussion about the basic principles of colposcopy during pregnancy to enhance the provision of safe and exemplary care by skilled, experienced colposcopists.

12.2 Human Papillomavirus (HPV) and Pregnancy

12.2.1 Epidemiology of HPV during pregnancy

Women may contract new or harbor previously acquired human papillomavirus infections of the lower genital tract during pregnancy (Figure 12.1). A state of pregnancy induced, temporarily impaired cell-mediated immunity facilitates the clinical expression and accelerates the rapid growth of HPV lesions. However, there are inconsistent data regarding whether HPV infections are more common during pregnancy than in the nonpregnant state. The incidence of HPV infection during pregnancy has been reported to be 11% to 16%,[1-3] a range similar to that reported for nonpregnant women. The incidence and prevalence of HPV may vary because of the specific population sampled and the type and sensitivity of the particular HPV DNA test used to detect infection. For example, studies that have used PCR-based HPV testing generally report greater rates of HPV because of their increased sensitivity.

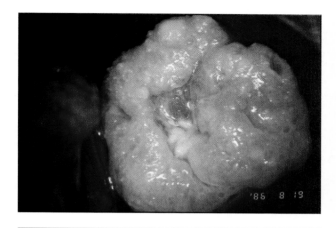

FIGURE 12.1 Condylomas on the cervix of a woman at 16 weeks' gestation.

Prevalence rates for HPV infection during pregnancy vary between 10% and 42%.[4-9] Several studies have shown greater prevalence rates of HPV during pregnancy,[1,8,10] but others have shown either a reduced prevalence[7] or no difference when compared with prevalence among nonpregnant women.[4,5,10] Some of the pregnant women who test positive for HPV have no obvious clinical evidence of HPV and no abnormal cytologic changes suggestive of HPV. In other pregnant women, merely subclinical changes are noted only during colposcopic examination. The remaining women have clinically detectible condylomas or cervical neoplasias.

Some evidence exists that pregnancy may be a risk factor for the presence of lower genital tract HPV. Hildesheim et al[11] found a positive association between current pregnancy and HPV prevalence in a study of inner city low-income women. Fife et al[10] demonstrated that pregnancy appeared to be an independent predictor for the presence of carcinogenic HPV when pregnant patients were compared with patients from sexually transmitted disease (STD) and gynecology clinics (odds ratio [OR]=1.79). This finding would not normally be anticipated, especially given the presumably higher risk expected for the STD group. The authors suggested that the increased rate of detection of carcinogenic HPV during pregnancy may be attributable to hormonal or immunologic factors associated with pregnancy. However, Tenti et al[9] found that the prevalence of carcinogenic HPV was lower in pregnant women compared with nonpregnant women. Others have shown no difference in prevalence for high-risk HPV or capsid antibodies in pregnant and nonpregnant women.[4,12]

The presence of HPV during specific intervals of pregnancy has also been evaluated. Findings differ regarding whether HPV positivity fluctuates during the course of pregnancy.[5,13] Rando and colleagues[13] demonstrated that HPV detection increased from the first to third trimesters, but then decreased postpartum. But Kemp et al[5] found no signification variation of HPV detection during pregnancy when using a more sensitive PCR assay. Obviously, further prospective studies are needed to determine the actual epidemiology of HPV infection during pregnancy.

12.2.2 Natural history of HPV during pregnancy

Little data are available concerning the natural history of HPV infections in pregnant women. Epidemiologic studies have not clearly substantiated whether pregnant women are more susceptible to acquiring or reactivating HPV. However, pregnant women are known to have fewer T lymphocytes, particularly a reduced level of CD4 + T lymphocytes, especially noted during the third trimester.[14] While insult to the immune system from changes associated with pregnancy may influence susceptibility to HPV, additional negative effects on the immune system, such as are posed by diabetes mellitus, do not appear to compound risk for harboring HPV during pregnancy.[15]

As in the general nonpregnant population, subclinical HPV disease is more common during pregnancy than is the actual clinical expression of condyloma acuminata.[5] Cell-mediated immunity normally limits the active expression of HPV infection in immunocompetent women. However, the transiently impaired immunity during pregnancy permits accelerated growth of lower genital tract condylomas. These warts may expand to very large, bulky lesions, though only rarely enlarge to a size that might obstruct vaginal delivery (Figure 12.2). Just as in nonpregnant women, condylomas may be distributed throughout the epithelium of the lower genital tract, affecting the cervix, vagina, vulva, and perianal regions.

Anecdotal reports seem to suggest that condylomas present during pregnancy are more recalcitrant to local treatment. However, there are little data concerning treatment failure rates of condylomas encountered during pregnancy. Many condylomas regress spontaneously in the postpartum period as immunity recovers. Regardless of the apparent clinical resolution, subclinical HPV infection may be observed to persist just as in nonpregnant women.

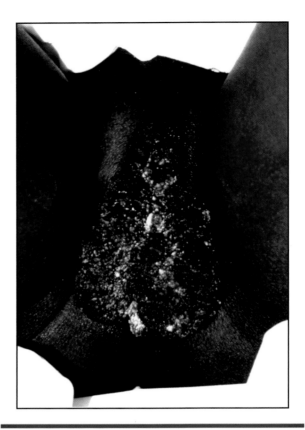

FIGURE 12.2 Extensive, bulky condylomas involving the vulva and also the vagina. This woman's baby was delivered by cesarean section because of significant outlet obstruction.

12.2.3 Potential complications from HPV infections during pregnancy

HPV infection during pregnancy affects the patient, potentially impairs the birth process, and may afflict the fetus. In most pregnant women, HPV infections are unnoticed as latent and subclinical disease. Routine Pap smear sampling performed during the first trimester may detect cytologic evidence of HPV. Young women with significant histories of multiple sexual partners are at greatest risk. Previous HPV exposure, as evidenced by HPV-16 seropositivity, does not increase the risk of an adverse obstetric outcome.[12] Likewise, subclinical and most clinical expressions of HPV pose no serious hazard to pregnant patients (Figure 12.3). Small condylomas of the cervix, vagina, vulva, or perianal regions are usually more of a nuisance than a threat. Even

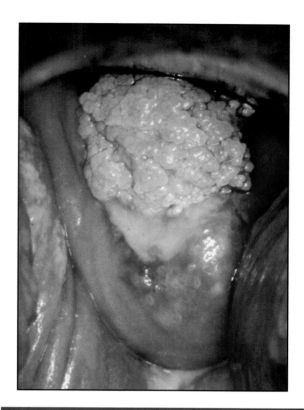

FIGURE 12.3 Large condyloma on the anterior cervix in a pregnant women (Photo courtesy of Dr. Vesna Kesic).

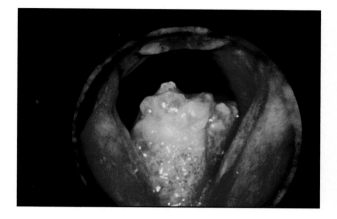

FIGURE 12.4 Recurrent respiratory papillomatosis of the larynx.

premalignant HPV-associated neoplasias rarely influence pregnancy outcomes. Only HPV-induced lower genital tract malignancies pose serious risk for the patient. Usual maternal psychological concerns about HPV may be amplified because of concern for the welfare of the fetus. Appropriate counseling helps to alleviate anxiety.

Several complications may ensue when condylomas, large or small, occupy space within the birth canal. Shearing forces generated by birth may tear condylomas and cause unexpected bleeding. Warts positioned on the perineum and in the midline may be problematic when an episiotomy must be done. Proper wound closure may be challenging because of relatively friable tissue and uneven, irregular epithelial surfaces. Wound dehiscence may be more likely when large warts are included within the suture line. More importantly, if large condylomas are present within the vagina or at the introitus, dystocia may occur. Consequently, when very large condylomas are encountered in pregnant women, aggressive treatment should be initiated early simply to minimize

the chance of mechanical outlet obstruction. However, such lesions rarely prevent a normal vaginal delivery, necessitating a cesarean delivery (Figure 12.2). In the absence of obstruction, the mere presence of lower genital tract condylomas is not an indication for cesarean section.

HPV also presents several real risks for the fetus and neonate. HPV, and perhaps other concomitant lower genital tract pathogens, may increase the risk for first-trimester spontaneous abortions.[16] This presumption is supported by a small case controlled study that demonstrated HPV E6 and E7 sequences in 60% of spontaneously aborted products of conception compared with only a 20% rate of HPV E6 and E7 found by PCR testing of electively aborted tissue. Whether HPV presence is causal or merely associated with spontaneous abortions remains unknown. However, a history of spontaneous abortion may predict the presence of HPV of the lower genital tract in women.

Of perhaps greater importance is the rare but potentially devastating development of condylomas in the upper respiratory tract of infants or young children born to mothers with a lower genital tract HPV infection. Known as recurrent respiratory papillomatosis (RRP), this condition challenges otolaryngologists, frustrates parents, and may severely impact the affected child (Figure 12.4).[17] The vast majority of cases of RRP are caused by HPV 6 or 11, considered to be noncarcinogenic types of HPV. Based on evidence from several studies,[18,19] vertical transmission of HPV from mother to offspring appears convincing. RRP is thought to be acquired by direct contact or aspiration during vaginal delivery in women with lower genital tract HPV. A recent study found that the concordance between specific HPV types in the mother and afflicted infant was 69%.[19] Although once thought to be acquired exclusively by direct exposure, infants born by cesarean section have been shown to harbor the same HPV type detected in the mother's lower genital tract.[19] The retrieval of HPV DNA in amniotic fluid aspirates of women with cervical HPV lesions appears to support theoretical transplacental transmission.[20] By testing fetal membranes, amniotic fluid, and neonatal pharyngeal swabs for the presence of HPV DNA and comparing the results with third trimester cervical HPV test results, researchers estimated a potential 50% maternal-fetal transmission rate for HPV by vaginal delivery and 33% rate for HPV transmission by cesarean section.[21] However, in another study in which 25% of the women tested positive for cervical HPV by Hybrid Capture® II testing, inability to detect the presence of HPV DNA in placental tissue by PCR testing failed to support antepartum transmission.[22]

Infants born to women with lower genital tract HPV rarely demonstrate a lower genital tract lesion at birth. Infants are more likely to develop upper respiratory condylomas. If warts infect the larynx and vocal cords (site of epithelial trauma), hoarseness will be noted. Because the larynx and trachea are narrow, airway compromise of variable severity may develop and may rarely lead to suffocation if rapid proliferation of therapy-resistant warts should ensue. The majority of cases of RRP are diagnosed prior to 5 years of age. The course of the disease is variable. Laryngeal HPV disease is best managed currently by laser excision and ablation. Some children may require repeated surgical procedures. Generally, the disease resolves spontaneously in adulthood, if not earlier.

Most infants born to mothers with lower genital tract condylomas do not contract RRP. While more than 50 percent of mothers whose offspring develop RRP have genital tract condylomas, a substantial number have only subclinical genital HPV infections (Figures 12.5a–e). Therefore, the absence of clinically obvious lower genital tract condylomas in the mother does not eliminate the risk of RRP in the infant. Because the incidence of RRP is less than 1 per 100,000 deliveries and direct transmission of HPV from mother to fetus may not be essential, universal screening of women for HPV DNA to prevent RRP would be neither helpful nor cost effective. Likewise, cesarean section as prophylaxis against RRP is not indicated for pregnant women with lower genital tract HPV.

12.3 Cervical Intraepithelial Neoplasia (CIN) and Pregnancy

12.3.1 Epidemiology of CIN during pregnancy

Pregnant women are as likely to harbor CIN as non-pregnant women of similar age. Thus, cervical cytologic sampling during the first trimester of pregnancy is considered routine care. The incidence of CIN in pregnancy varies among different populations, ranging from 3.4% to as high as 10%.[23,24] There is some evidence to suggest that CIN in pregnancy is becoming more common.[25] Generally, the majority of pregnant women with CIN have CIN 1 or other evidence of HPV infection. CIN 3 is much less common, occurring in only 0.1% to 1.8% of pregnant women (Figure 12.6).[23–26]

Because childbearing age is limited, the epidemiology of CIN during pregnancy is skewed toward younger women. The mean age of pregnant women with carcinoma in situ is 29.9 years, with an average parity of 4.0.[27] Less-severe CIN may be expected more frequently in younger pregnant women of lower parity. However, high-grade lesions (CIN 3) have been detected in the pregnant teenage population.

12.3.2 Natural history of CIN during pregnancy

Because little research is actually conducted on pregnant women, particularly for women who harbor neoplastic lesions of the cervix, the natural history of CIN during pregnancy remains poorly documented. In general, CIN does not progress to high grade disease or cancer more frequently during this relatively brief time frame than comparably severe levels of CIN do in nonpregnant women. However, such a minimal risk does not imply casual triage, evaluation or management. The risk of CIN 3 progressing to microinvasive or invasive carcinoma during pregnancy has been reported to be as high as 6.6% in a small study from Poland.[28] However, others studies have shown that CIN 3 is unlikely to progress to frankly invasive cancer during pregnancy.[29] In one, 68% of antepartum CIN 2 and 70% of CIN 3 regressed at the postpartum examination, and, 25% of CIN 2 and 30% of CIN 3 progressed. Regression or progression was not influenced by route of delivery.

Although of insufficient sample size to adequately portray the complete story, Patsner[30] demonstrated that 45% of pregnant women with cytologic and histologic evidence of CIN 1 had disease regression at a

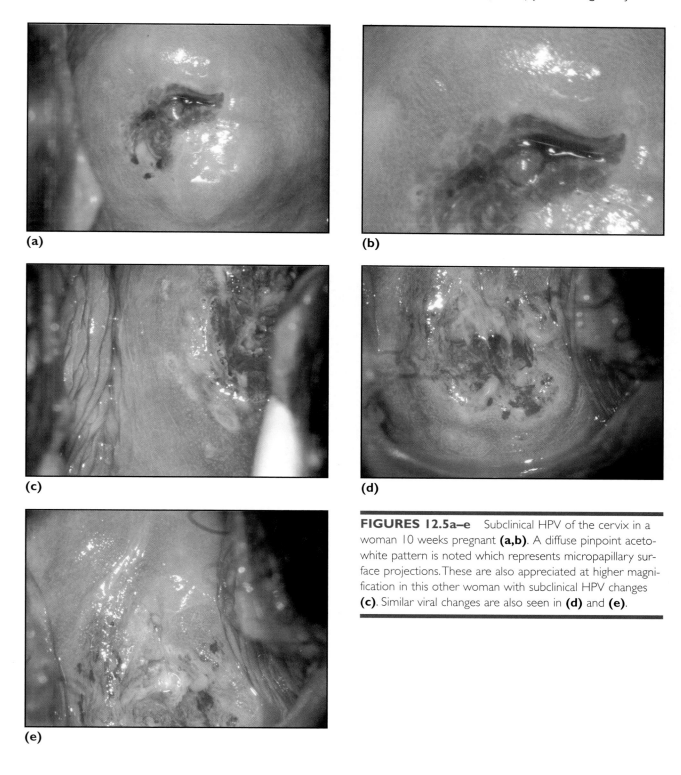

(a)

(b)

(c)

(d)

(e)

FIGURES 12.5a–e   Subclinical HPV of the cervix in a woman 10 weeks pregnant **(a,b)**. A diffuse pinpoint aceto-white pattern is noted which represents micropapillary surface projections. These are also appreciated at higher magnification in this other woman with subclinical HPV changes **(c)**. Similar viral changes are also seen in **(d)** and **(e)**.

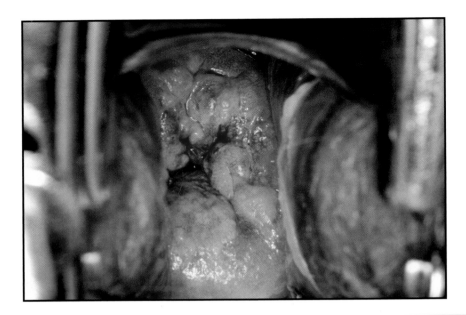

FIGURE 12.6   A large four-quadrant CIN 3 lesion in a pregnant woman with an estimated gestational age of 7 months. A dense acetowhite epithelium with a coarse mosaic vascular pattern is seen.

postpartum evaluation, the remainder (55%) had persistence of CIN 1, and none progressed. Palle[31] found that 25% of CIN regressed, 47% persisted, and 28% progressed during pregnancy. Of the women who progressed, fewer than 1% were found to have microinvasive cancer. Others have shown that CIN either regresses or persists at the same severity of disease for approximately 98% of pregnant women, and thus, rarely advances in severity.[32] Therefore, CIN generally regresses or remains stable throughout pregnancy (Figure 12.7). Only a minority may appear to have progressed at the postpartum examination. The fact that cervical cytologic findings may underestimate cervical neoplasia demands proper examination by means of colposcopy and biopsy for women with cytologic abnormalities.

12.3.3 Complications of CIN during pregnancy

CIN does not cause complications during pregnancy (Figures 12.8a–c). Yet, such a diagnosis may inflict psychological distress. Colposcopists must educate women about the potential implications of CIN during pregnancy, with careful optimism and appropriate reassurance. The noninvasive nature of CIN should be emphasized, while conveying the importance of serial evaluations and expectant postpartum therapy, when necessary.

Excellent expectant outcomes may be attributed almost entirely to contemporary colposcopic practice. The morbidity associated with the evaluation of CIN during pregnancy was drastically reduced when

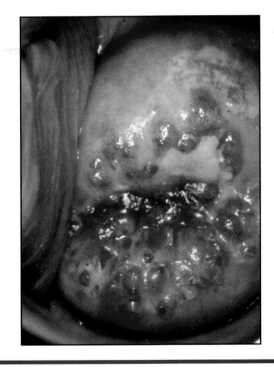

FIGURE 12.7   A large CIN 3 seen postpartum that did not progress during pregnancy (Photo courtesy of Dr. Vesna Kesic).

colposcopy and targeted biopsy supplanted cold-knife conization. Severe hemorrhage, postoperative infection, premature labor, and even fetal and maternal death are now practically nonexistent as a consequence of the more conservative colposcopic evalua-

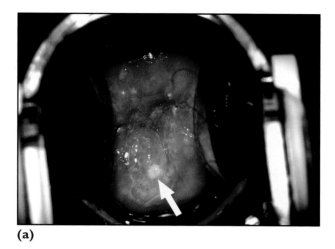

(a)

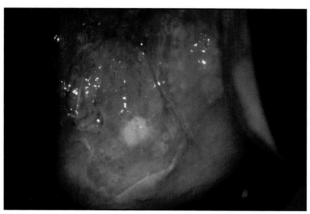

(b)

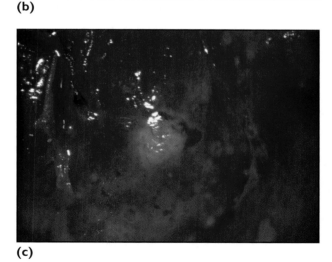

(c)

FIGURES 12.8a–c A small CIN 3 (arrow) within metaplastic epithelium in this pregnant patient. ■

tion of neoplasia during pregnancy. However, when a cervical conization is indicated because of a possible cervical malignancy, certain risks to the fetus and mother must be acknowledged.

In some cases during pregnancy, CIN 3 can appear colposcopically more severe than it is, prompting

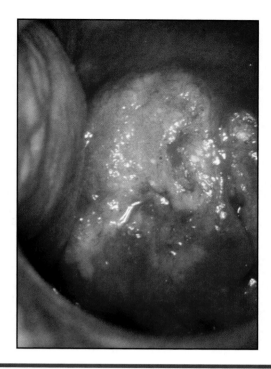

FIGURE 12.9 Cervical cancer in pregnant woman (Photo courtesy of Dr. Vesna Kesic). ■

aggressive evaluation. Large CIN 3 lesions may also contain smaller, focal areas of microinvasion that are not readily detected. Women who have advanced cervical cancer infrequently become pregnant. Therefore, most adverse outcomes as a consequence of cervical neoplasia in pregnancy occur in women with microinvasive or very early invasive cancer, not CIN.

The presence of CIN is also not an indication for a cesarean delivery. In fact, some authors have hypothesized that vaginal delivery may promote the regression of CIN based on the potential for debulking or a shearing, traumatic injury exerted upon cervical lesions. Clearly, a reduction of viral load has been thought partially responsible for effecting cure of premalignant neoplasia, especially low-grade disease. Because most pregnant women deliver vaginally with satisfactory outcomes, they experience problems similar to those encountered by nonpregnant women with cervical neoplasia.

12.4 Cervical Cancer and Pregnancy

12.4.1 Epidemiology of cervical cancer during pregnancy

Few clinicians will ever diagnose cervical cancer in pregnant women (Figure 12.9). The incidence of frankly invasive cervical cancer in pregnant women varies from 0.01% to 0.09%. The incidence of microinvasive cancer is similar but varies because of nonuniform diagnostic criteria.[25–27,33,34] Expressed differently, approximately 1 in 34 to 55 women with cervical cancer is pregnant at the time of diagnosis.[27,33] The mean age of pregnant women with cervical cancer is 33.8 years, with a range of 17 to 47 years,[27] approximately 15 years younger than the mean age in nonpregnant women. This difference is most likely attributable to the confounding effect of a younger expected age range for pregnancy.

The most common presenting symptom of cervical cancer in pregnancy is painless vaginal bleeding (41 % to 63 %).[27,33–35] The wide range in the percentage of women presenting with bleeding is probably a consequence of the variations in stage of disease at diagnosis and size of the cancer. Bleeding may be minor spotting, postcoital bleeding, or massive hemorrhage. Clinicians must remember that vaginal bleeding in pregnant women may result from cancer, as well as from more common pregnancy-related causes of placenta previa, abruption, ectopic pregnancy, abortion, or trophoblastic disease. Therefore, unexplained vaginal bleeding during pregnancy demands proper evaluation of the lower genital tract for malignancy by cytologic and colposcopic testing and if indicated, directed biopsy. Other, less-common presenting symptoms of cervical cancer during pregnancy include vaginal discharge, lower extremity edema, and pelvic pain. These symptoms are also very common in pregnant women without cervical cancer. However, 18% to 59% of pregnant women with cervical cancer will present with no symptoms, with absence of symptoms most likely reflecting earlier disease.[24,27,33–35] Almost all pregnant women with microinvasive cervical cancer are asymptomatic.

In pregnant women, cervical cancer types and stage at diagnosis are similar to those in nonpregnant women with cervical cancer. Squamous cell carcinoma predominates, followed by less-frequent cases of adenocarcinoma and adenosquamous carcinoma.[27,33–35] The majority of women with cervical cancer in pregnancy have stage IB (42%) or stage II disease (33 %).[27] Fortunately, fewer women (25%) who are pregnant at the time of diagnosis have Stage III or IV cervical cancer.[27–36] A similar distribution of cervical cancer is found primarily in nongravid populations in which cytologic screening programs have been implemented.

12.4.2 Natural history of cervical cancer during pregnancy

Once researchers confirmed that pregnancy downregulates the immune system, many oncologists presumed that pregnancy would accelerate disease in women diagnosed with invasive cervical cancer. This premise resulted in interventions that caused many cases of fetal demise in efforts to optimize maternal outcomes. However, careful studies have shown that the course of cervical cancer is not accelerated in pregnancy.[34,35] In fact, the 5-year and 30-year survival data for women with early cervical cancer demonstrate no survival difference between women diagnosed during pregnancy and nonpregnant women.[34–39] Furthermore, the purposeful delay of early-stage cervical cancer treatment during pregnancy to achieve fetal maturation appears to have minimal effect on maternal outcomes.[34,38] Knowing this can be helpful when determining appropriate management. When stage of disease is controlled for, there appears to be no difference in prognosis for pregnant and nonpregnant women with carcinoma of the cervix.[35] Age, parity, and trimester of pregnancy at the time of diagnosis also appear to have no effect on survival within a given stage of disease.[35,37,38] Nevertheless, the stage of disease at the time of diagnosis conveys important prognostic information.[27,35,37] Moreover, the gestational age at diagnosis influences survival, with first-trimester diagnosis conveying improved prognosis compared with third trimester and postpartum diagnoses.[27] Although early intervention frequently results in fetal demise, when pregnant women with cervical cancer are compared with controls without cancer, fetal outcomes are equivalent with respect to gestational age and preterm birth.[36] However, birthweight appears to be significantly lower for infants born to pregnant women with cancer compared with neonates of normal pregnant women.[36]

12.4.3 Potential complications from cervical cancer diagnosed during pregnancy

Adverse outcomes can be anticipated when caring for pregnant women who have cervical cancer. Maternal complications are similar to those expected for nonpregnant women. Because most cancers in pregnancy are early-stage disease, maternal deaths during pregnancy, independent of intervention, are extremely uncommon. Immediate adverse events usually result from diagnostic and therapeutic intervention. Colposcopic visualization, assessment and cervical biopsy may be complicated by bleeding since the tissue may be friable and necrotic. Cone biopsy during pregnancy poses increased risks for the patient with cervical cancer.[40] The main maternal complication is a greater risk for hemorrhage, frequently requiring transfusion. Fetal complications also result from conization, including spontaneous abortion, preterm labor, premature delivery, infection, and stillbirth.[36] Fetal demise is an inevitable complication of immediate cervical cancer therapy in the first two trimesters. Fetal complications resulting from preterm birth during the early third trimester may create additional hazards. Because of the potential for these rather common serious complications, gynecologic oncologists should be consulted as soon as pregnant women are found to have cervical cancer.

12.5 Lower Genital Tract Modifications of Pregnancy

12.5.1 Physiology

The cervix serves many functions during a woman's lifetime and undergoes certain alterations. The greatest modifications of the cervix occur during pregnancy. Shortly following fertilization, the cervix induces changes to preserve the pregnancy until shortly before delivery when very different characteristics are demanded of the tissue to facilitate birth. The vagina also prepares to permit delivery without associated trauma or obstruction. The degree of physiologic change varies depending on parity.[41]

Uterine blood flow increases during pregnancy to support fetal growth. The more rapid blood flow, a result of increased cardiac output and reduced vascular resistance, causes increased cervical vascularity and a bluish cervical hue (Chadwick's sign). Moreover, the cervix softens gradually throughout pregnancy (Goodell's sign) until the initiation of effacement. Endocervical epithelium proliferates and an abundance of thick mucus congeals to produce the mucus plug that seals the cervix from unwanted pathogens or other intrusion (Figures 12.10a,b). The voluminous production of tenacious mucus may make colposcopic visualization challenging.

Most significant changes are a result of the high estrogen levels during pregnancy. Cervical epithelium is highly sensitive to alterations in estrogen levels. Higher estrogen levels in early pregnancy increase cervical volume through hypertrophy of the fibromuscular stroma. Consequently, as the diameter of the cervix increases, the endocervical epithelium everts onto the ectocervix (Figures 12.11a,b).[42] Additionally, the external os dilates a small amount.[41,42] These events differ in extent depending on parity. Cervical eversion is more likely for the primiparous patient, while mild canal dilation or gaping is more typical in the multiparous woman (Figures 12.11c–e).[41] Eversion begins during the early weeks of pregnancy and usually will be apparent in the early second trimester. Eversion and mild canal dilation facilitate colposcopy when an unsatisfactory examination results from the inability to observe the entire squamocolumnar junction (SCJ) during early pregnancy. By reexamining the patient at approximately 20 weeks' gestation, when eversion and gaping are normally pronounced, a pre-

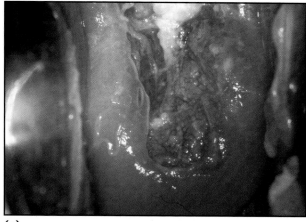

(a)

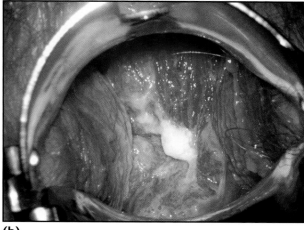

(b)

FIGURES 12.10a,b Proliferation of the columnar epithelium with mucus production during pregnancy in two women.

viously unsatisfactory colposcopic examination will often become satisfactory because the SCJ may be more readily seen in its entirety (Figure 12.12).

By the physiologic processes of eversion and dilation, columnar epithelium becomes exposed to the acidic vaginal environment mediated by *Lactobacillus acidophilus*. Through the process of squamous metaplasia, a traumatized columnar epithelium is transformed by metaplasia to a mature epithelium resembling squamous epithelium, including the addition of the morphologic remnants of the transformation process. During pregnancy, particularly in nulliparous women, everted epithelium enters a strikingly dynamic phase of squamous metaplasia that is progressive throughout pregnancy (Figure 12.13). The area of metaplasia is returned, partly or completely, to the canal in the puerperium. In subsequent pregnancies, the preexistent area of metaplasia may again evert. However, a gaping or widening of the endocervical

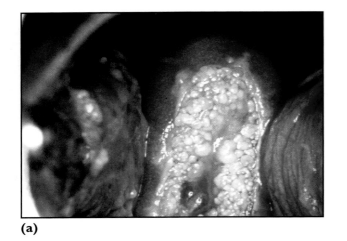
(a)

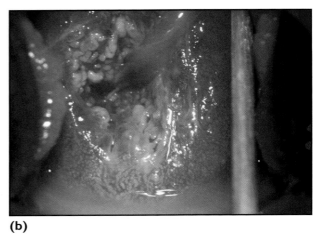
(b)

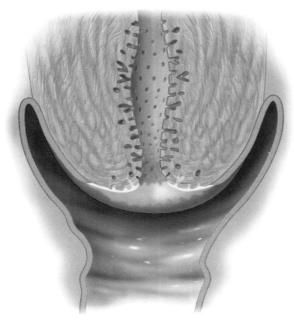
(c)

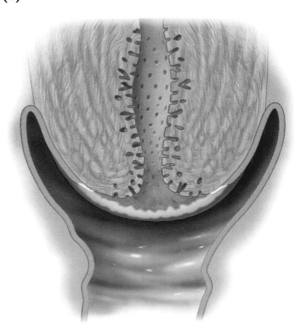
(d)

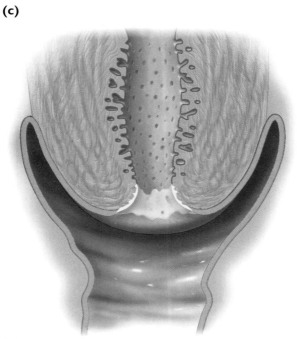
(e)

FIGURES 12.11a–e Eversion of columnar epithelium during pregnancy **(a,b)** (Photos courtesy of Dr. Vesna Kesic). Large villi covered by columnar epithelium are also seen in **(b)**. The cervix in early pregnancy **(c)** resembles the non pregnant cervix. In the nulliparous women, an active transformation zone with abundant immature metaplasia and eversion is noted in **(d)**. Note the os remains constant diameter and narrow. In contrast, the multiparous woman **(e)** has more gaping of the os along with active transformation.

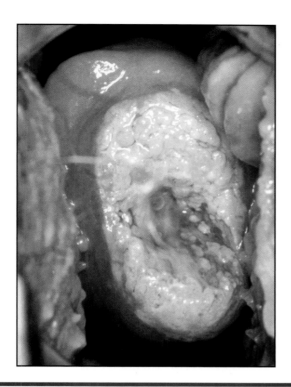

FIGURE 12.12   Maximum eversion of columnar epithelium at 20 weeks' estimated gestational age. ▬

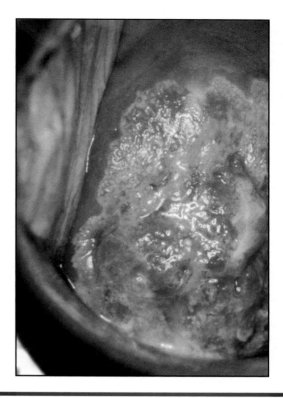

FIGURE 12.13   Active squamous metaplasia seen on the ectocervix of a woman at 14 weeks' gestation during her first pregnancy (Photo courtesy of Dr. Vesna Kesic).

canal predominates over eversion. The gaping is progressive through pregnancy, particularly during the third trimester. As a result, squamous metaplasia tends to occur predominantly in late pregnancy. Yet, great variability among women exists.

The appearance of the cervix in pregnancy is determined largely by gestational age. Toward the end of the first trimester, eversion of columnar epithelium and dynamic phase metaplasia produce areas of fusion of columnar villi and distinct islands of immature metaplastic epithelium. This process is rapidly progressive through the second trimester, producing a layer of smooth squamous metaplasia that will blanch acetowhite after application of acetic acid (Figures 12.14a–d). The acetic acid reaction of the immature metaplastic epithelium in pregnancy is exaggerated by the bluish hue caused by increased vascularity. In the third trimester, eversion and progressive metaplasia continue until about 36 weeks' gestation and then cease. The dimensions of the cervix at this time have significantly increased in varying proportions, with associated remodeling of surface contours. Increased vascularity and abundant mucus production are clearly evident.

Physiologic changes are not limited to the cervix. The vaginal squamous mucosa thickens and the vagina increases in length during pregnancy. As is true for the cervix, an increase in vascularity gives the vaginal epithelium a blue hue. A softening of the vaginal and cervical connective tissue is essential to accommodate birth. Therefore, the vaginal sidewalls develop some laxity and become redundant, prolapsing into the middle of the vagina. Prolapsing of the vaginal sidewalls may significantly hinder the colposcopic examination in late pregnancy (Figures 12.15a–c).

12.5.2 Cytology

Even though impressive physiologic changes in the cervix occur during pregnancy, these alterations do not appear to affect the diagnostic accuracy of cervical cytologic examinations.[43] Because cervical neoplasia prevalence rates are similar for pregnant and nonpregnant women, the Pap smear remains an important screening tool for this special population, despite its cost.[44] For many women, particularly those not using prescription dependent contraceptives, a first trimester Pap smear may be the only smear collected in the recent past.

For many years, Pap smears were collected from pregnant women using an Ayre spatula and a moistened cotton-tip applicator. However, researchers have found that cotton fibers tend to trap cervical cells, thus

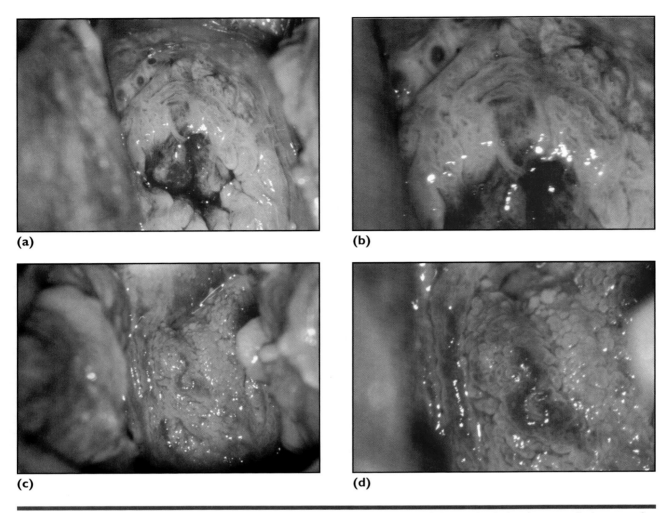

(a) **(b)** **(c)** **(d)**

FIGURES 12.14a–d Immature metaplasia on the anterior and posterior lip of the cervix during the second trimester of pregnancy **(a,b)**. Active metaplasia in a woman 7½ months pregnant **(c,d)**. Tongue-like projections of translucent acetowhite epithelium are seen along with focal changes on the tips of columnar villi.

significantly hindering cellular transfer to the glass slide. Newer sampling devices that increase the detection of neoplasia evolved, but these devices tend to cause excessive bleeding when used improperly.[45] Although some concerns were initially raised about their safe use during pregnancy, several studies have now documented the safety of the Cytobrush® and Cervex-Brush® during pregnancy, even though the former device does not carry a product indication for use in pregnancy.[46–48] Moreover, these endocervical sampling devices yield significantly more endocervical cells in pregnant women compared with use of the cotton or Dacron swabs.[46–49] As a result, fewer unsatisfactory Pap smears will be reported. Because of cervical eversion during pregnancy, a sufficient endocervical cellular yield is expected. Satisfactory Pap smears are significantly more common for pregnant women compared with those for nonpregnant women.[45]

Interpretation of Pap smears collected from pregnant women is similar to the analysis of cervical cytologic results for nonpregnant women. Because large areas of squamous metaplasia may be sampled, a shift in proportion of types of cervical cells may be encountered. Inflammatory cells may be commonly noted in association with immature metaplasia. Navicular and decidual cells (Figure 12.16) may be seen. The latter cells should not be confused with neoplasia or reparative change. They are large cells with a large nucleus and variably staining cytoplasm.

12.5.3 Histology

The evaluation of lower genital tract histology is similar for pregnant and nonpregnant women with few exceptions. However, squamous and columnar epithelium may be modified in pregnancy. Basal cell

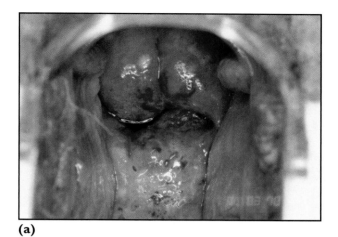

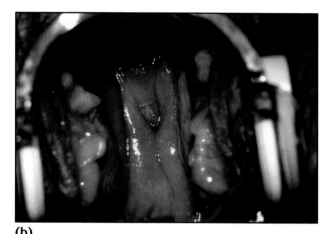

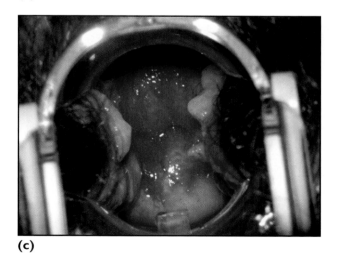

FIGURES 12.15a–c   Prolapsing vaginal sidewalls noted during pregnancy. In these cases, the prolapse is mild to moderate.

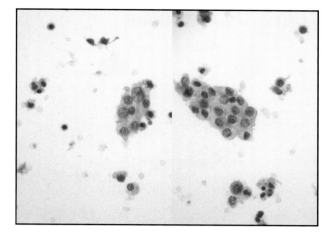

FIGURE 12.16   Decidual cells seen on the Pap smear from a pregnant woman (Papanicolaou stain, high power magnification).

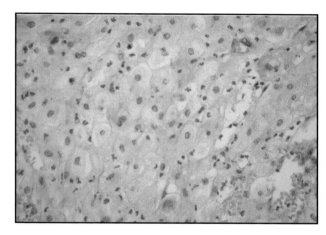

FIGURE 12.17   Histologic specimen demonstrating decidua (Hematoxylin-eosin stain; high power magnification).

and columnar cell hyperplasia may be noted. A greater percentage of mitotic figures may be detected in the basal layers. Evidence of immature metaplasia associated with a submucosal inflammatory process will be commonly seen. Stromal edema and an increased vascularity are also observed. None of these findings are pathognomonic for pregnancy, since they can be noted with other entities. However, the presence of decidua, endometrial cells of pregnancy derived from pluripotential mesenchymal stroma cells, implicates pregnancy in a histologic specimen (Figure 12.17). Decidual cells may exhibit cytoplasmic vacuolization and nuclear enlargement that suggest neoplasia. Occasionally, these specialized decidual cells, which are thought to help maintain

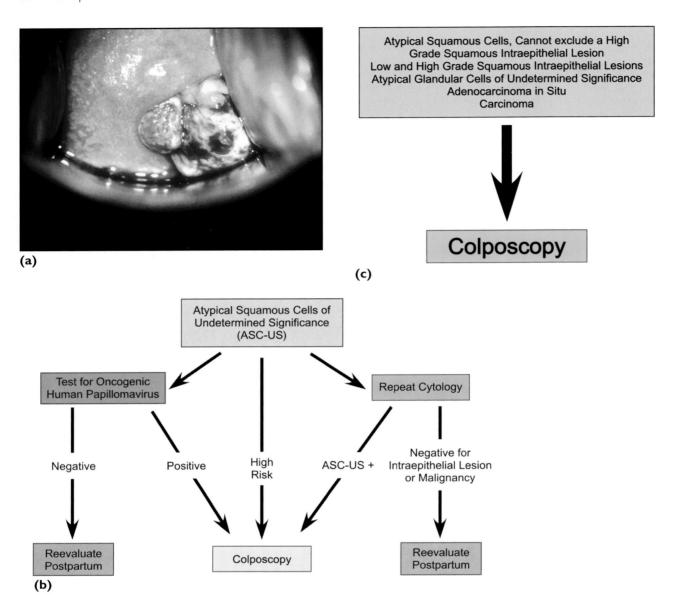

FIGURES 12.18a–c Decidua of the cervix that mimics an invasive cancer **(a)** (Photo courtesy of Burton Krumholz, M.D., Department of Obstetrics and Gynecology, Long Island Jewish Medical Center). Algorithms for cytologic and virologic triage to colposcopy **(b,c)**. Women with an ASC-US Pap smear result have three triage options: a test for high-risk HPV DNA, or repeat cytologic or colposcopic evaluation. If a liquid-based Pap test was collected, HPV testing is preferred **(b)**. Women with more severe cytologic changes should be examined by means of colposcopy **(c)**. Endocervical sampling is unacceptable during pregnancy.

pregnancy and initiate labor, will be positioned on the ectocervix because of cervical eversion and dilation of the external os. Stromal decidualization occurs in the second and third trimesters in about 30% of pregnant women. Decidual tissue can also mimic neoplasia colposcopically as an irregular exophytic projection from the surface of the cervix (Figure 12.18a). Prominent atypical-like blood vessels may also be seen with decidua. Therefore, if present, decidual tissue is biopsied frequently to rule out cervical cancer or condylomas.

12.6 Colposcopy of Pregnant Women

12.6.1 Indications for colposcopy during pregnancy

The indications for colposcopy are the same for pregnant and nonpregnant women. These include: (1) abnormal cervical cytologic findings indicating or suggestive of neoplasia (Figures 12.18b,c); (2) a cervical mass or clinically apparent abnormality observed or palpated during a pelvic exam; (3) a positive carcinogenic HPV result detected by DNA testing; (4) a positive cervigram or positive speculoscopic exam; (5) clinical or histologic evidence of lower genital tract HPV or neoplasia; or (6) any history of abnormal or otherwise unexplained vaginal bleeding or postcoital spotting. The latter indication may more frequently represent specific complications of pregnancy, such as abortion, placenta previa, and placental abruption, and these should be excluded prior to attempting colposcopy. It is important to be cautious in considering pregnancy-related bleeding problems to avoid overlooking the equally ominous dangers of cervical carcinoma.

When colposcopy is indicated, pregnant women should be scheduled for the examination as soon as possible. Early in pregnancy, the cervix and lower genital tract still assume features more similar to the nonpregnant anatomy. Therefore, an examination in the early first trimester will avoid late pregnancy changes that hinder the colposcopic exam. Some colposcopists caution against intervention in the first trimester because of medicolegal concerns that a harmless cervical biopsy may be followed closely by an unassociated spontaneous abortion. If pregnant patients are instructed initially about the harmless nature of colposcopy, the need for proper evaluation, and the unlikely probability of an unrelated spontaneous abortion, immediate intervention should present few emotional or legal difficulties. Immediate intervention also helps allay the psychological concerns of the pregnant woman regarding the potential for disease interfering with a positive outcome. Although colposcopic examinations can be performed throughout pregnancy, inspection during the first two trimesters is preferred. Women with previously detected cervical lesions are also monitored by colposcopic and cytologic examinations during the course of the pregnancy, including the postpartum phase.

12.6.2 Objectives of colposcopy during pregnancy

The main objective of colposcopy for pregnant women is to establish the presence, severity, and extent of neoplasia involving the lower genital tract. However, several unique colposcopic objectives should be recognized by any colposcopist providing care for pregnant women. First, colposcopic expertise for pregnant women must be assured. When not available, consultation is appropriate. Next, when possible, no harm should be inflicted upon the fetus. Consequently, endocervical curettage (ECC) is contraindicated during pregnancy because this procedure

could accidentally prematurely rupture the membranes. As previously mentioned, nonaggressive sampling of the endocervical canal using a cytobrush® will still permit assessment of the epithelium. Third-trimester hypotension from inferior vena cava compression during an examination can be prevented by selective patient positioning and abbreviated inspection. Cervical biopsy of the most severe area of colposcopic atypia, when indicated, provides a necessary histologic specimen. However, biopsy sampling should be representative but conservative and limited in number. Cervical conization should be considered only when invasive cancer is suspected.

In desired pregnancies, all attempts should be made to preserve the pregnancy to term, unless doing so would risk the life of the mother or the mother chooses not to maintain fetal viability. Colposcopy of pregnant women may be undertaken to diagnose and monitor disease status. Definitive treatment of CIN should be delayed until the postpartum. At that time, women with CIN should be reevaluated by colposcopic and cytologic examinations. Otherwise, except for not obtaining an ECC, the same colposcopic objectives utilized for nonpregnant women (Chapter 7) should be undertaken.

The identification of suspected areas of neoplasia does not differ during pregnancy. Determining the adequacy of the colposcopic examination may be more challenging late in pregnancy when increased cervical size, thick mucus, and prolapsing vaginal sidewalls complicate colposcopic inspection. As with nongravid women, the correlation of cytologic, histologic and colposcopic impressions should guide management strategy for pregnant women.

12.6.3 Colposcopic examination of pregnant women

The procedure of colposcopy is essentially identical for pregnant and nonpregnant women. Sequential colposcopic steps of visualization, assessment, sampling and correlation must be followed as usual. However, significant visualization problems, unique assessment challenges and certain sampling precautions can hinder proper colposcopic examination of the pregnant patient (Table 12.1). In a review of more than 1,000 pregnant women evaluated by means of colposcopy, the diagnostic accuracy was 99.5% and the complication rate merely 0.6%.[27] No cases of invasive cancer were missed and only 4% of women received a conization.[27] This low complication rate for evaluation by colposcopically directed biopsy is substantially less than that experienced with diagnostic conization in pregnant women. Clinical recognition of the unique situation and formal

Table 12.1 Physiologic Changes of Pregnancy and Colposcopic Consequences

Physiologic Changes	Colposcopic Consequences
Abundant cervical mucus Vaginal wall prolapse Stromal hypertrophy	Visualization hindered
Cervical eversion External os and endocervical canal dilation	Visualization enhanced
Presence of decidual tissue Increased blood volume and cardiac output, dilated blood vessels Active immature squamous metaplasia Epithelial cyanosis Edema and glandular hyperplasia	Assessment challenge
Cervical eversion External os and endocervical canal dilation	Assessment enhancement
Increased vascularity Intrauterine pregnancy	Sampling complication from bleeding Sampling of endocervix contraindicated
Decidua, immature metaplasia and glandular neoplasia	Correlation challenge

acknowledgment of the same to a typically nervous mother-to-be would be considered empathetic and appropriate. Consequently, additional precolposcopic counseling should be anticipated and provided for pregnant women.

12.6.3.1 Visualization

Colposcopic visualization of the lower genital tract may be difficult in pregnancy. Early on, the hormonally induced physiologic changes are less noticeable, but young women often experience a heightened degree of anxiety in relation to the pregnancy and the possible ramifications of clinical and colposcopic examinations on the fetus. Although colposcopic assessment of the cervix in pregnancy will not harm either the pregnancy or the fetus, the colposcopist must provide reassurance. In pregnancy, unobstructed visualization of the cervix is mandatory. As pregnancy progresses, however, increased laxity of the lateral vaginal walls may allow the lateral walls to prolapse through the vaginal speculum blades, impairing visualization (Figure 12.19). As the cervix enlarges during pregnancy, the vaginal walls prolapse more, progressively reducing the proportion of the ectocervix that can be visualized. A large speculum may be necessary, and the use of a lateral vaginal sidewall retractor will often permit unhindered access to the cervix. Use of condoms or a cut latex glove finger with the tip removed and rolled onto the speculum blades is an inexpensive way to achieve a

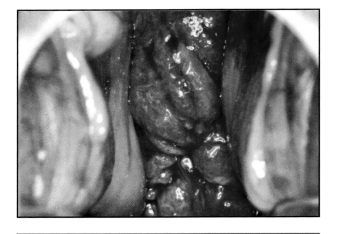

FIGURE 12.19 Prolapsing vaginal sidewalls hinder colposcopy during pregnancy. Decidual changes can be seen on the ectocervix.

similar level of visualization. These latex barriers also minimize the risk for painful, interspeculum blade pinching of prolapsed vaginal tissue that may be encountered with use of the lateral sidewall retractor. Otherwise, colposcopists can examine the entire ectocervix by inspecting smaller, visible portions of the ectocervix separately. This restricted examination requires repositioning the cervix so that all sections are within colposcopic view at the completion of the examination.

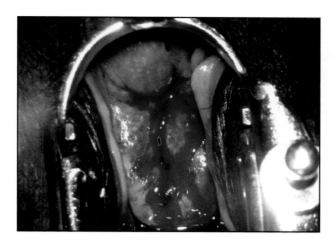

FIGURE 12.20   Bleeding during the third trimester of pregnancy obscures a CIN 3.

Tenacious endocervical mucus encountered in pregnancy can be a significant obstacle to adequate visualization (Figures 12.10a,b), although the deeply positioned mucus plug rarely interferes with visualization. Application of 5% acetic acid as a mucolytic will aid in mucus removal. Sponge-holding forceps or small tissue forceps may be used to carefully remove viscous mucus from the ectocervix or endocervical canal. If the mucus cannot be satisfactorily removed, it can be manipulated gently using moistened cotton-tipped applicators, allowing for a systematic examination of the cervix in quadrants. Finally, gently pushing the mucus a short distance back up the endocervical canal with a small cotton-tipped applicator will sometimes facilitate proper inspection.

Visualization may be impaired further if the vascular cervical epithelium is traumatized, causing bleeding (Figure 12.20). This is particularly true in the third trimester, when vascularity is most pronounced. Any associated inflammation accentuates tissue friability (Figures 12.21a,b). Bleeding can be easily controlled with gentle pressure exerted by a large cotton swab. Bleeding observed from the external os should be evaluated for more typical pregnancy-associated causes.

Regardless of these pregnancy-induced changes, the vast majority of pregnant women actually have satisfactory colposcopic examinations (Figures 12.22a,b).[50] Such a high rate of satisfactory examinations implies a reduced need for cervical conization in women who have cytologic evidence of significant neoplasia. Although abundant cervical mucus and vaginal wall prolapse hinder colposcopic visualization, cervical eversion and dilation of the external os enhance the exam-

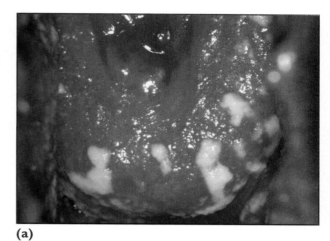

(a)

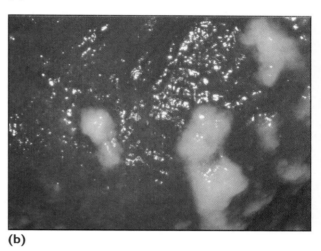

(b)

FIGURES 12.21a,b   An intense inflammatory response to vulvovaginal candidiasis of the cervix during pregnancy **(a)**. At higher magnification, dilated loop capillaries can be seen **(b)**.

ination, particularly if performed after the 20th week of gestation. Thus, when the previous examinations have been unsatisfactory early in pregnancy and the patient has an abnormal Pap smear report, it may be useful to reschedule a patient to return at that time (Figure 12.22c). Moreover, the cervical tissue gradually becomes softer and more amendable to gentle manipulation as the pregnancy progresses.

12.6.3.2 Assessment

Although colposcopic assessment of pregnant women may be difficult, particularly for the novice, most cervical lesions seen during pregnancy appear remarkably similar to those seen in nonpregnant women. The size of cervical lesions may vary during pregnancy. In one study, the mean surface area of

CIN 3 in nonpregnant women was larger than that in pregnant women with CIN 3 (61.0 mm^2 and 45.7 mm,^{2} respectively). However, for CIN 1 and CIN 2, the reverse was true: the mean surface area was greater for pregnant than for nonpregnant women (36.7 mm^2 and 24.0 mm,^{2} respectively).[51] Although these differences are small, in the latter case, CIN 1 lesions may be slightly larger during pregnancy because of the concomitant immunosup-

pression. The features of cervical neoplasia remain the same during pregnancy. Colposcopists should consider the margin, color, vessels, contour, and iodine-staining reaction. Critical appraisal of these colposcopic findings allows the derivation of a meaningful colposcopic impression.

Many of the colposcopic features seemingly suspicious for disease in the nonpregnant patient occur as physiologic variants in pregnancy. Acetowhite

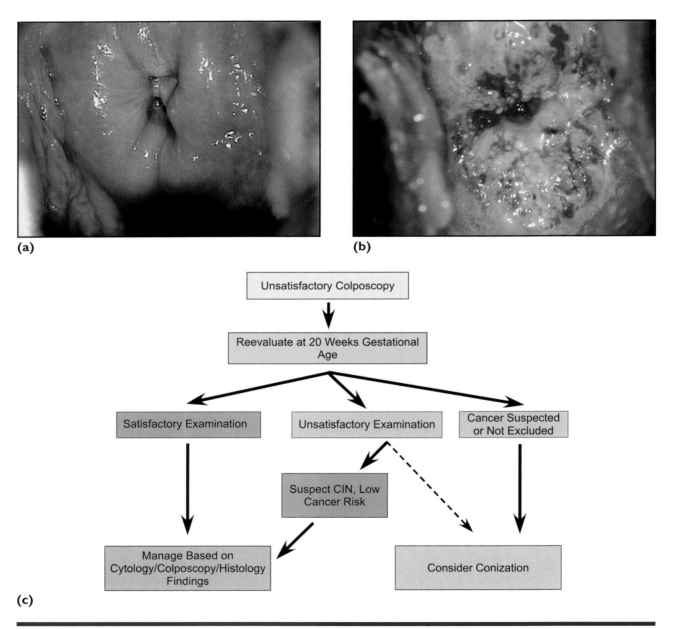

(a)

(b)

(c)

FIGURES 12.22a–c An unsatisfactory colposcopic examination **(a)** of this pregnant woman at 12 weeks' gestation. Her examination revealed parakeratosis secondary to prior loop conization. It is doubtful that her examination will be satisfactory at 20 weeks because of her postsurgical changes. A satisfactory colposcopic examination is seen in pregnant woman with CIN 1 **(b)**. Algorithm for first-trimester pregnancy with an unsatisfactory colposcopic examination **(c)**. Unless invasive cancer is identified, treatment is unacceptable during pregnancy.

areas of immature metaplastic epithelium are clearly visualized, most notably later during pregnancy. Experienced colposcopists will usually recognize these normal variants in pregnancy. Extensive immature metaplasia located on everted tissue frequently produces a prominent acetowhite epithelium that immediately draws attention. The acetowhite color is somewhat translucent and fades quickly following the application of 5% acetic acid. A fine punctation and mosaic vessel pattern may be noted within acetowhite areas of physiologic immature metaplasia (Figures 12.23a–c). These small-caliber vessels are closely and uniformly spaced. An associated cyanosis of pregnancy may alter the contrast between acetowhite epithelium and the normal epithelial background color. The prominent increased vascularity of the cervix during pregnancy may be exaggerated against acetowhite epithelium. Consequently, a confusing angioarchitecture may be observed. This appearance may lead to normal physiologic changes being misinterpreted as neoplasia, particularly low-grade lesions.

Excluding low-grade dysplasia in extensive areas of immature metaplasia may be difficult since the appearances are similar in pregnancy (Figures 12.24a–d). However, precise discrimination is not critical since low-grade CIN may require only observation (no biopsy) through pregnancy and reassessment in the puerperium. During the second and third trimesters, normally fine-caliber vessels change appearance secondary to increased blood volume, cardiac output, and vascular dilation.[52] Low-grade lesions may be colposcopically overestimated as high-grade lesions because of the physiologic dilation. If the colposcopist also considers other colposcopic signs, such as color, contour, and lesion margin (Figures 12.25a–d), however, proper discrimination is still possible.

In pregnancy, condylomas appear as exophytic growths, with a shiny acetowhite color and fine-caliber loop capillaries. They may be isolated on the cervix or distributed throughout the lower genital tract. Condylomas may vary in morphology among flat, raised, papular, papillary, cerebriform, inverted or micropapillary (Figures 12.26a,b). These lesions may proliferate rapidly during pregnancy. Low-grade (CIN 1) cervical lesions are flat, with irregular or geographic margins, mildly and transiently acetowhite epithelium, iodine-negative or -positive staining, and fine, closely spaced but evenly distributed blood vessels (Figures 12.24,12.27a,b). These lesions tend to be smaller than high-grade lesions but can at times occupy all four quadrants. They are usually located on the ectocervix, particularly in younger women.

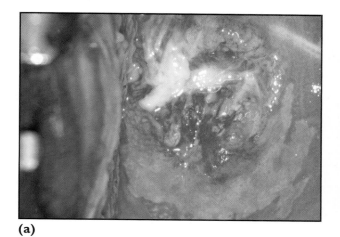

(a)

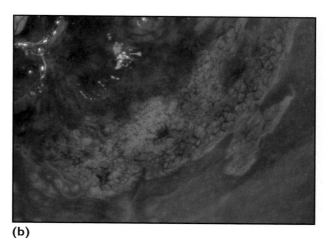

(b)

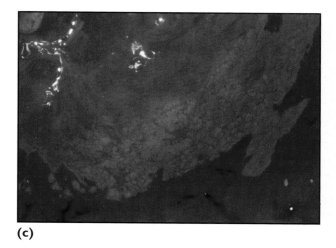

(c)

FIGURES 12.23a–c An area of faint acetowhite epithelium with irregular margins is noted in this pregnant woman with immature metaplasia **(a)**. A fine caliber, lacy mosaic pattern is seen with the green filter **(b)**. This same fine mosaic is also seen in iodine-negative epithelium of immature metaplasia following the application of dilute Lugol's iodine solution **(c)**.

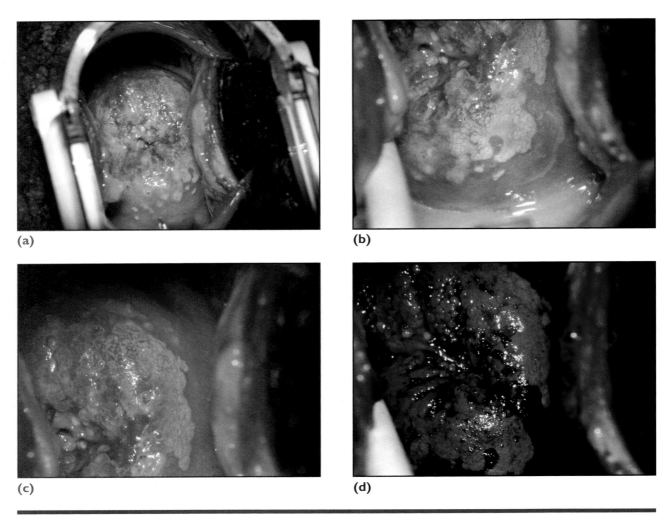

(a)

(b)

(c)

(d)

FIGURES 12.24a–d Acetowhite epithelium is noted in this pregnant woman with a satisfactory colposcopic examination **(a)**. At higher magnification, a fine mosaic and punctation vascular pattern can be seen **(b,c)**. Iodine-negative staining **(d)** confirms the colposcopic findings seen in Figure 12.24c. It is difficult to discriminate immature metaplasia from CIN 1 as seen. ■

The colposcopic features of high-grade CIN during pregnancy are usually obvious, but again must be discriminated from low-grade lesions and cancer (Figures 12.28a–c). High-grade lesions (CIN 2 or CIN 3) are characterized by smooth, straight margins, dense acetowhite epithelium that may be easily disrupted, iodine-negative staining, and rather coarsely dilated vessels that are widely spaced and nonuniformly distributed (Figures 12.29a,b). These lesions may be positioned within a larger low-grade lesion and an abrupt interface or internal margin may be delineated between the two types of lesions (Figures 12.30a,b). Some high-grade lesions are opaque acetowhite with no blood vessels observed on the surface. The acetowhite reaction will also persist longer in high-grade lesions, helping to isolate the area of most severe colposcopic atypia.

Cervical cancer, particularly of advanced stage, should be readily identifiable during pregnancy (Figure 12.9). Large exophytic tumors may demonstrate leukoplakia, yellow necrotic epithelium, or a dense acetowhite color. The margins are usually well defined, especially when adjoining normal epithelium. Atypical blood vessels may be particularly prominent, coarsely dilated, and nonbranching. Superficial erosions or ulcerations and tissue friability with necrosis may be seen when the rapidly expanding cancer exceeds its vascular supply.

Knowledge of the warning signs of early invasive cancer is critical in colposcopic assessment of the cervix in pregnancy. The presence of any finding suspicious for invasive disease requires biopsy at a minimum and the most conscientious colposcopic, histologic, and cytologic review. The surface contour

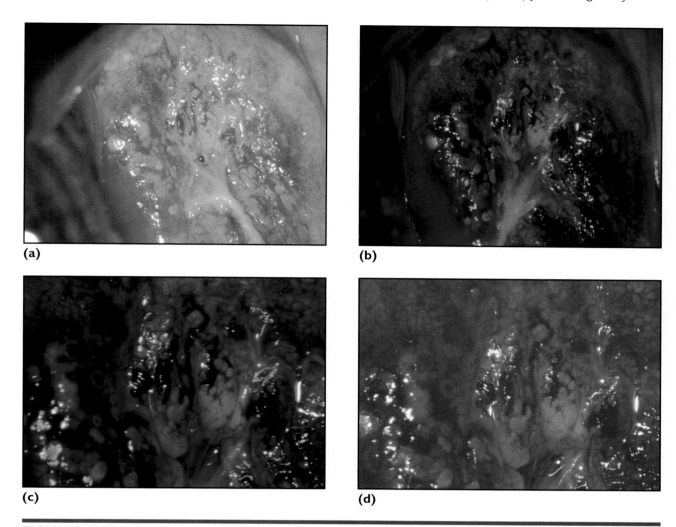

FIGURES 12.25a–d   A large CIN 3 lesion is seen in the pregnant woman **(a,b)**. With closer inspection **(c,d)**, a very coarsely dilated mosaic pattern is seen. These vessels mimic those associated with cancer.

changes associated with mucus-filled glands and decidual reaction may create diagnostic problems. Decidua frequently has a polypoid or exophytic appearance that can be confused with condylomas or cancer (Figures 12.31a–f). When prominent vascular changes accompany decidual reaction, the appearance may mimic an invasive cancer.

The ability of experienced colposcopists to formulate colposcopic impressions reliably in pregnant women supports this diagnostic form of triage for cervical neoplasia. In a study of more than 400 pregnant women, colposcopists' antepartum colposcopic diagnoses agreed with 87% of patient's postpartum histologic diagnoses within one degree of severity.[53] In the remaining women, 11% had a colposcopic impression more severe than the histologic impression, and colposcopic undercall was noted for merely

2% of women with significantly more-severe lesions diagnosed by means of histology. Of note, there is a small propensity to overdiagnose cervical neoplasia colposcopically during pregnancy.[50,54–56] However, underdiagnosis can be substantial. In one study of pregnant patients, 54% of women with a colposcopic impression of normal had CIN 1 or 2, and 14% of women with a colposcopic impression of CIN 1 had CIN 3 confirmed by biopsy.[55]

12.6.3.3 Sampling

As mentioned earlier, Pap smears can be obtained using a Cytobrush® or broom-like sampling device.[46–49] Of note, colposcopically directed brush cytology, relatively nontraumatic compared with biopsy, correlates well with biopsy (Kappa =0.73), able to detect 86% of CIN 2 or 3 in pregnant women.[57] Colposcopically

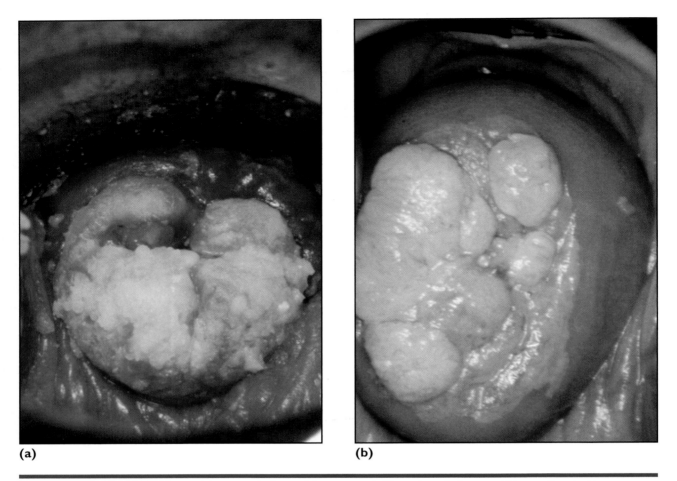

(a)   (b)

FIGURES 12.26a,b   Large condylomatous lesions of the ectocervix. These large lesions could be confused with an exophytic invasive cancer (Photo courtesy of Dr. Vesna Kesic).

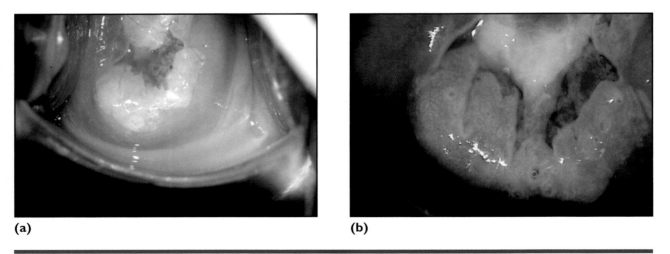

(a)   (b)

FIGURES 12.27a,b   A small CIN I on the posterior lip of the cervix **(a)**. Fine caliber vessels are seen at higher magnification using the green filter in this pregnant woman **(b)**.

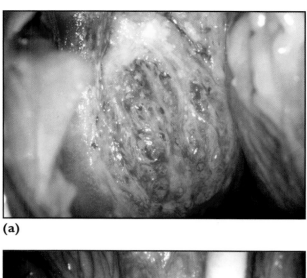

(a)

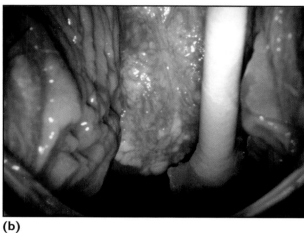

(b)

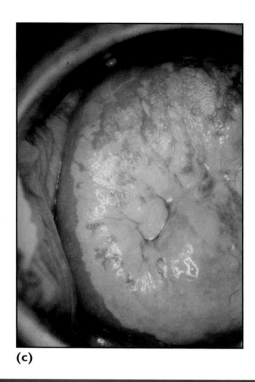

(c)

FIGURES 12.28a–c CIN 3 can vary in presentation during pregnancy. A subtle dense acetowhite area of epithelium with a coarse punctation within immature metaplasia is seen in a pregnant woman **(a)**. Visualization may be challenging to detect features of CIN 3 **(b)**. A more obvious CIN 3 with dense thickened acetowhite epithelium and no blood vessels is seen in **(c)**. (Latter photo courtesy of Dr. Vesna Kesic).

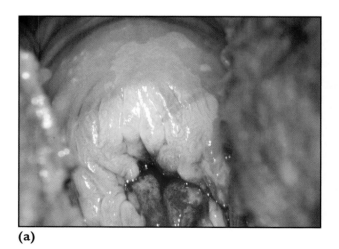

(a)

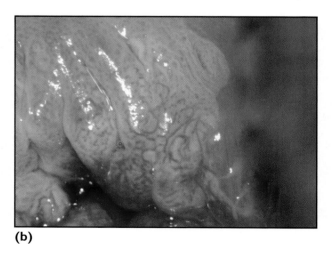

(b)

FIGURES 12.29a,b A high-grade lesion of the cervix in a pregnant woman **(a)**. An internal margin, dense acetowhite epithelium and a coarse mosaic pattern with punctation can be seen **(b)**.

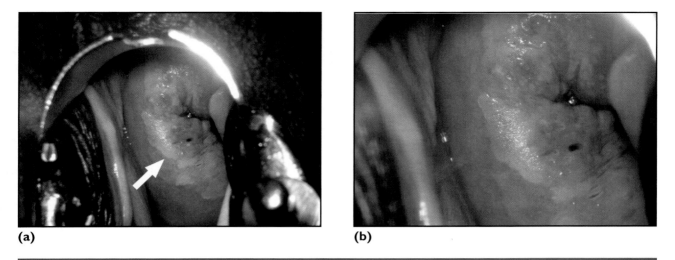

(a)

(b)

FIGURES 12.30a,b   A high-grade lesion is positioned within a low-grade lesion seen in this pregnant patient **(a)**. Some leuko-plakia precluded visualization of blood vessels **(b)**. An internal margin can be seen demarcating the low from high-grade lesion (arrow).

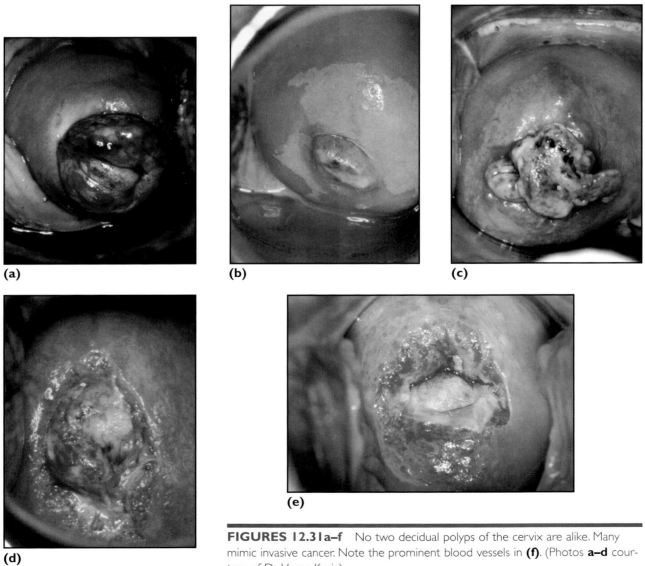

(a)

(b)

(c)

(d)

(e)

FIGURES 12.31a–f   No two decidual polyps of the cervix are alike. Many mimic invasive cancer. Note the prominent blood vessels in **(f)**. (Photos **a–d** cour-tesy of Dr. Vesna Kesic).

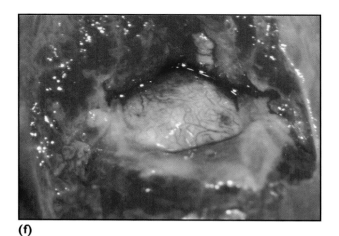

(f)

FIGURES 12.31a–f   Continued.

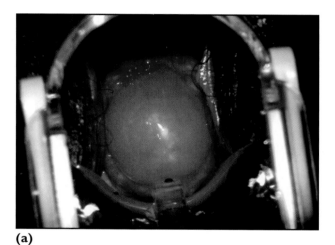

(a)

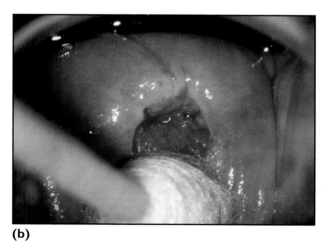

(b)

FIGURES 12.32a,b   Histologic sampling of this pregnant woman (24 weeks) with a LSIL Pap smear was delayed upon visual detection of amniotic membranes **(a)**. Her postpartum colposcopic examination was normal **(b)**.

directed cytologic evaluation, however, cannot be considered a replacement for histologic evaluation. Histologic sampling can be done safely during pregnancy, but it must be performed carefully (Figures 12.32a,b).[50] Selective biopsy of the most severe area(s) of colposcopic atypia minimizes potential complications from noncritically assessed sampling. Because potentially excessive bleeding may result after cervical biopsy during pregnancy, most colposcopists prefer to obtain biopsies from only cervical lesions suspicious for high-grade CIN or cancer.

Bleeding is the main concern when obtaining biopsies in pregnancy. Marked edema and vascularity of the cervix contribute to potentially significant bleeding after biopsy. Bleeding tends to be more brisk in late pregnancy compared with that noted during the first trimester. However, serious bleeding complications from biopsy are actually rare in pregnancy.[56] Hemostasis is usually readily secured. The risks of severe hemorrhage associated with biopsy are significantly less than those associated with conization or missed diagnosis of early invasive cancer.

Biopsy techniques for pregnant and nonpregnant women are the same. Small, sharp biopsy forceps of the clinician's choice should be used. Biopsy forceps that obtain a greater amount of tissue may provoke more bleeding if the jaws are filled to the maximum extent. After placing the forceps jaws over the lesion, a quick biopsy is obtained. Colposcopists must ascertain whether an adequate specimen has been obtained once the jaws are removed from the cervix. Because pregnant women may have increased bleeding after biopsy, the colposcopist should be prepared to rapidly administer hemostatic agents. Cotton-tipped applicators soaked in Monsel's paste or silver nitrate sticks should be readily available during biopsy for immediate placement on the wound, if needed. Once the biopsy is taken with one hand, the Monsel's-soaked cotton-tipped applicator or silver nitrate stick is pressed firmly onto the bleeding site with the other hand. The applicator should be held in place, covering the base of the wound and wound edges until hemostasis is achieved. Sutures are rarely necessary to secure hemostasis when other cautery methods fail, but an experienced colposcopist should have the required equipment available for the rare emergency. If necessary, a tampon or gauze packing can be inserted in the vagina to temporarily absorb cervical bleeding and the patient should rest in the office/clinic for 15 to 30 minutes. She should avoid vigorous activity for 48 hours afterward. Occasionally, some bright red spotting and serous vaginal discharge may continue for several days. However, the patient should be cautioned to seek care from her healthcare provider if bleeding becomes heavy.

Occasionally, high-grade disease may extend deep into the endocervical canal. Despite a gaping endocervical canal and cervical eversion, the extent of disease and tenacious endocervical mucus may render assessment of the upper extent of the lesion most difficult. A carefully placed endocervical speculum can improve assessment of the distal endocervical canal in some pregnant patients. If this approach fails to improve visualization, reevaluation at 20 weeks' gestation may permit an unencumbered view of the entire lesion and SCJ. The delay may be appropriate, provided no hint of invasive disease is present. However, endocervical curettage is contraindicated in pregnancy. As an alternative, a cytobrush® collection device may be inserted carefully within the lower endocervical canal to obtain cytologic samples to help exclude more significant disease further within the lower canal. Even this procedure must be performed with great care. After collection, the specimen should be sent separately in formalin for histologic diagnosis. It is important to keep in mind that a negative endocervical curettage using a cytobrush® may not eliminate the need for conization when the upper extent of a high-grade lesion cannot be determined, particularly if there is cytologic or histologic evidence of invasive cancer. Although cervical biopsy and limited canal sampling are relatively benign procedures, patients may be particularly frightened. Auscultation of fetal heart tones following histologic sampling may reassure the patient that on the procedure has not harmed the fetus.

12.6.3.4 Correlation

Finally, the correlation of cytologic, histologic, and colposcopic impressions determines proper management of pregnant women with cervical neoplasia. Agreement within one degree of severity should be expected, just as for nonpregnant women.[50,54–56] Discordance may prompt further diagnostic evaluation. A diagnostic cone is usually undertaken when suspicion of invasive cancer is warranted by cytologic, histologic, or colposcopic inspection. Provided cancer has been excluded, minor discordance will generally require only serial cytologic and colposcopic monitoring.

12.7 Antepartum Management of Pregnant Women with Cervical Neoplasia

The management of pregnant women with cytologic evidence of cervical neoplasia should be determined following comprehensive evaluation by means of colposcopy and directed biopsy, when necessary (Figures 12.33 and 12.34). In general, if there is no colposcopic finding suspicious for invasive disease, the patient is followed prospectively through the pregnancy, commonly without biopsy. This is particularly true for women with cytologic and colposcopic evidence of low-grade disease. If evaluated by an experienced colposcopist, obvious high-grade lesions without cytologic or colposcopic warning signs of cancer need not be biopsied. However, some women with high-grade lesions, particularly those exhibiting features suggestive of microinvasive or invasive cancer, require histologic sampling. Because cold-knife conization during pregnancy may cause serious complications, such as abortion, hemorrhage, cervical incompetence, cervical stenosis, infection, stillbirth, preterm labor, and maternal death, it is reserved for diagnosing cancer and, therefore, done infrequently. A diagnostic cone during pregnancy is simply for that purpose and should never be considered therapeutic.[56] Definitive diagnostic workup and treatment for CIN are delayed until the puerperium. Appropriate management of the distinct levels of neoplasia during pregnancy will be discussed in greater detail in the next sections.

12.7.1 Atypical squamous cells (ASC) and low-grade squamous intraepithelial lesions (LSIL)

12.7.1.1 Atypical squamous cells and low-grade SIL Pap smear reports

Pregnant women with an atypical squamous cell (ASC) or low grade squamous intraepithelial lesion Pap smear results are managed similar to nonpregnant women with the same cytologic findings (Chapter 18). Because ASC Pap smear results are the most common abnormality seen, many pregnant women will also present with ASC. Pregnant women with ASC-US can be managed by a repeat Pap smear, reflex HPV testing or colposcopy (Figure 12.18b). Pregnant women with two ASC-US Pap smears, one ASC-H Pap smear, or a positive high-risk HPV DNA test are managed as women with LSIL (Figures 12.18c and 12.34).

Low-grade SIL Pap smear reports are less frequently encountered in pregnant women. However, the rate of LSIL is similar for pregnant and nonpregnant women, primarily because the rate of HPV infection evidenced by HPV DNA detection is equivalent for pregnant and nonpregnant women (5.0% vs. 5.2%, respectively).[58] The rate of LSIL in HIV-infected pregnant women (17%) is much higher than that of the general population.[59] The same classic cytologic feature of HPV infection, koilocytotic

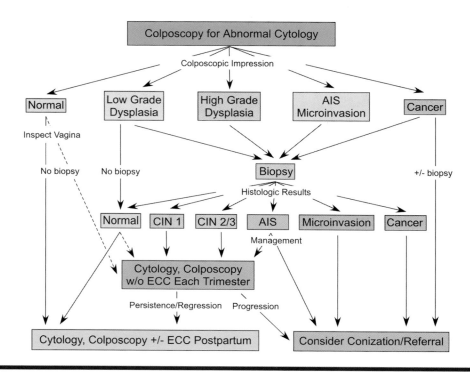

FIGURE 12.33   Algorithm for management of pregnant women with an abnormal Pap smear report. Biopsy of a low-grade dysplasia is acceptable, but biopsy of more severe dsyplasia is preferred.

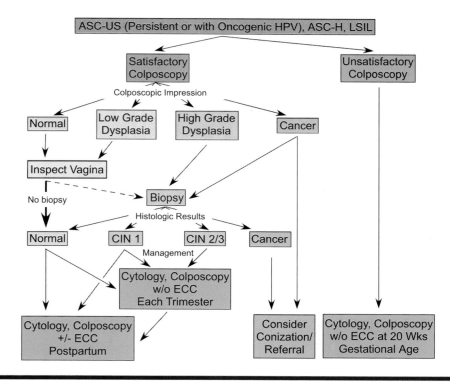

FIGURE 12.34   Algorithm for evaluation and management of women with two ASC-US or one ASC-H Pap smear report, a positive high-risk HPV DNA test or LSIL. Pregnant women with a colposcopic impression of cancer and a biopsy discordance should have a review of all specimens and a repeat colposcopic examination, as necessary. A cervical biopsy is also appropriate when the colposcopic impression is cancer.

atypia, is seen in pregnant patients irrespective of HIV infection. Colposcopic assessment should be performed in response to a LSIL Pap smear detected during pregnancy since cytologic follow-up alone may be insufficient and prone to underestimate the true disease state.[60]

The majority of women with a LSIL Pap smear report will be found to have a low-grade lesion, condylomas, or subclinical HPV detected by colposcopy. Occasionally, no lesion will be seen, particularly when there is a lengthy delay between Pap smear collection and colposcopic examination. High-grade lesions occur in as many as 27% of women reported to have a LSIL Pap smear.[61] Invasive cancer is very rare, but it can occur in association with only minor cytologic atypia, more commonly expected with an ASC-US Pap smear report than with LSIL.

12.7.1.2 Colposcopy

Colposcopy should be performed on pregnant women with two ASC-US, ASC-H, and LSIL Pap smear reports in order to define the etiology, distribution, and extent of disease in the lower genital tract. In general, low-grade lesions appear the same in pregnant and nonpregnant women (Figures 12.35a,b 12.36, 12.37a–c). Low-grade lesions noted during pregnancy may be exophytic or papular condylomas, or acetowhite macular lesions with irregular margins. The condyloma may be snowy white after acetic acid application or opaque white prior to acetic acid application, denoting the presence of HPV-related leukoplakia (Figures 12.26a,b). The macular lesions have a transient, faint acetowhite color. The blood vessels are fine caliber, closely spaced, and arranged in a uniform pattern. Later in pregnancy, these vessels may dilate as cardiac output and blood volume increase. However, intercapillary distances remain constant. These lesions may appear iodine-positive or -negative following application of Lugol's iodine, depending on the amount of glycogen in the tissue (Figure 12.24). Low-grade lesions may be seen inside or outside the transformation zone. Lesions positioned along the SCJ are potentially of greater risk. Small, diffuse micropapillary projections, known as asperities, may be noted on the cervix or in the proximal vagina. These subclinical changes may appear with a distinct unifocal or multifocal low-grade lesion(s) or they may exist independently (Figures 12.38a–c). When no discrete cervical lesion is noted, vaginal condylomas may be the source of a LSIL Pap smear (Figures 12.39, 12.40a,b).

If the colposcopic examination is satisfactory and entirely normal or demonstrates only low grade

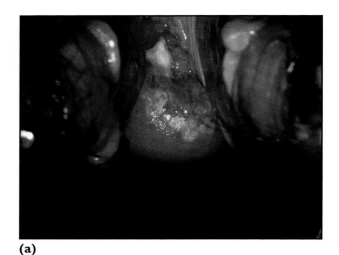

(a)

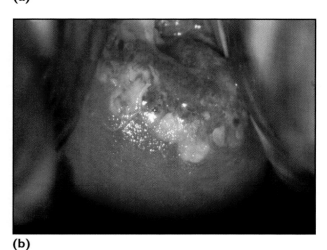

(b)

FIGURES 12.35a,b A CIN 1 on the posterior cervix in this pregnant woman. ▪

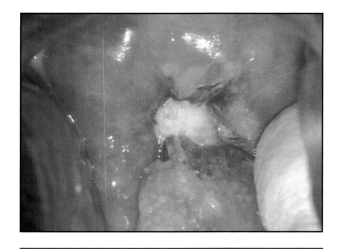

FIGURE 12.36 A faint acetowhite CIN 1 on the anterior cervix. ▪

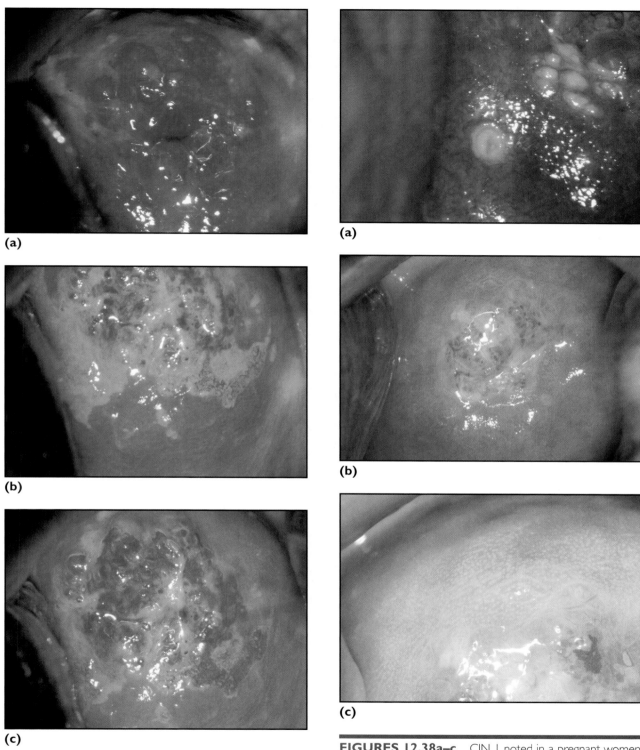

FIGURES 12.37a–c Nabothian follicles are seen on this pregnant woman's cervix prior to the application of acetic acid **(a)**. After acetic acid has been applied, a geographic acetowhite lesion can be seen **(b)**. The lesion is still apparent as the effects of the 5% acetic acid diminish **(c)**.

FIGURES 12.38a–c CIN 1 noted in a pregnant women with a LSIL Pap smear report **(a)**. Involvement of a gland cleft can also be appreciated by the wide acetowhite band of CIN 1 encompassing the gland opening. A small low grade lesion is seen at the 10 o'clock position in the next pregnant patient **(b)**. With closer inspection **(c)**, a faint acetowhite lesion is seen along the SCJ. In the periphery, a fine mosaic vessel pattern is noted. Nearby, the fine punctation appears to be consolidating into **(b)** the mosaic pattern.

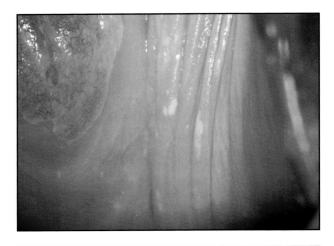

FIGURE 12.39 A vaginal condyloma is seen in this pregnant woman with CIN 3. ▬▬▬▬

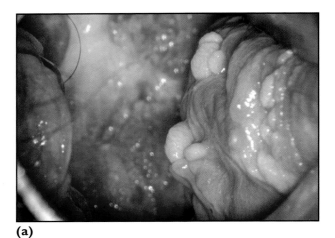

(a)

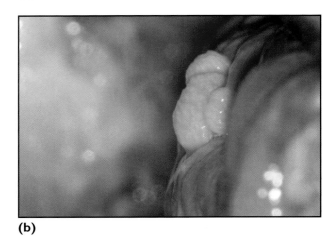

(b)

FIGURES 12.40a,b Condylomas are seen in this pregnant woman's vagina. ▬▬▬▬

or subclinical HPV changes of the cervix or vagina, no biopsy is necessary (Figure 12.33). However, even in the nongravid state and with colposcopic expertise, 5% to 10% of colposcopically suspected low-grade CIN will be diagnosed as high-grade disease by histologic review of a colposcopically directed biopsy. Thus, if a high grade lesion is seen and any uncertainty remains as to the severity, a directed biopsy is required. If no biopsy is obtained, cytologic and colposcopic surveillance once during each trimester is a reasonable alternative. Alternatively, some colposcopists may elect to defer further cytologic and colposcopic evaluation until the postpartum examination. If the colposcopic examination is unsatisfactory, reappraisal with Pap smear and colposcopic evaluation at approximately 20 weeks' gestational age may be beneficial (Figure 12.34).

12.7.1.3 Management

Low-grade SIL includes CIN 1 and subclinical HPV-induced changes on the cervix or occasionally of the proximal vagina. Such lesions are conservatively monitored because these minor changes will often regress spontaneously in the puerperium (Figure 12.34).[30,63] Some patients will have persistent low-grade lesions following delivery, but few lesions will progress in severity during this relatively brief interval.[62,63] The mother should be reassured that neither she nor the baby are at significant risk. Raised, exophytic condylomas of the cervix may be luxuriant in pregnancy. These lesions should raise the suspicion of cervical cancer, and careful colposcopy by an experienced colposcopist is indicated. If there is any doubt, a biopsy specimen should always be obtained.

Pregnant women with histologically confirmed low-grade cervical lesions should be monitored and not treated. A clinical diagnosis of a low-grade lesion is usually established in the first 12 to 18 weeks of pregnancy following an abnormal first-trimester Pap smear. In most cases, provided the Pap smear and colposcopic impression are low-grade and the examination is satisfactory, the patient may be reexamined during a postpartum visit. If necessary, the patient can also be cytologically and colposcopically reexamined at approximately 28 weeks' gestation. A biopsy should be obtained only if there is cytologic or histologic indication of progression.

Women with a low-grade cervical lesion will almost always have an uneventful pregnancy and deliver vaginally, unless other complications arise. Yet, condylomas in pregnancy may be associated with secondary dystocia, intrapartum and postpartum hemorrhage, and even soft-tissue disproportion. Lower genital tract (vulvar) condylomas are best treated conservatively during pregnancy using topical di- or trichloroacetic acid or an ablative modality, such as cryosurgery. Multiple treatments may be necessary to eliminate condylomas in pregnant women. Podophyllin arrests cells in mitosis, and thus, podophyllin and podophyllotoxin are contraindicated for use during pregnancy. Topical 5 fluorouracil cream (infrequently utilized today) is also contraindicated during pregnancy.

Large HPV lesions may increase the risk of vertical transmission of the virus to the fetus, conveying an attendant risk of recurrent respiratory papillomatosis, a rare condition. Cesarean section has been suggested by some to be indicated in the presence of cervical subclinical or clinical HPV-induced lesions to avoid the risk of neonatal HPV infection of the larynx during a vaginal delivery. Yet, there is no evidence that neonatal transmission is prevented by Cesarean section. In fact, there is evidence of transplacental HPV acquisition detected by amniocentesis.[20] Therefore, fetal exposure may occur prior to delivery. Hence, the increased risk of maternal morbidity and mortality associated with Cesarean section appears unjustified. Clinical or subclinical HPV-induced disease of the cervix is rarely, if ever, an indication for Cesarean section. Only very large vulvovaginal condylomas that obstruct the birth canal would precipitate a Cesarean delivery.

12.7.2 High-grade squamous intraepithelial lesions (HSIL)

12.7.2.1 High-grade SIL Pap smear report

High-grade SIL Pap smears are seen in approximately 1% to 2% of pregnant women, depending on the population studied. The cytologic changes of HSIL are the same for pregnant and nonpregnant women. If the Pap smear demonstrates abnormalities consistent with high-grade SIL, careful colposcopy is clearly mandated (Figure 12.41). Although the presence of pregnancy-induced cytologic changes, immature metaplasia, and an inflammatory infiltrate may be occasionally misinterpreted as HSIL, colposcopists are still obligated to examine these women. The majority will have high-grade cervical lesions detected during colposcopic examination. In some cases, the cytologic results may overestimate the severity of the cervical lesion, and rarely, they may underestimate the presence of a malignancy. However, the remote possibility of cytologic underestimation is the reason colposcopic evaluation is a necessity.

12.7.2.2 Colposcopy

High-grade lesions during pregnancy appear similar to the same lesions seen in nongravid women (Figures 12.42a,b). However, in many cases, these

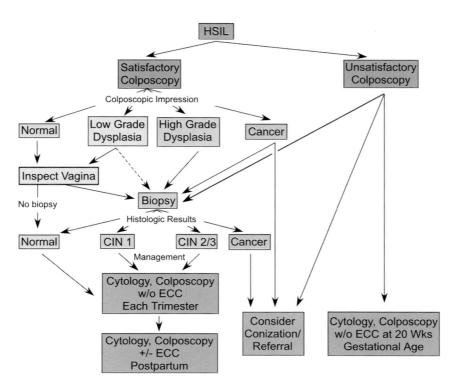

FIGURE 12.41 Algorithm for the management of pregnant women with HSIL cytology.

lesions are not as obvious during pregnancy (Figures 12.42c–g). They also may be large, involving multiple quadrants of the cervix. The margins are smooth, peeling, or may exhibit an internal border separating the high-grade lesion from a larger surrounding low-grade lesion (Figure 12.43). Epithelial

thickening may be observed. These lesions are an opaque dull acetowhite color that persists for a prolonged time following 5% acetic acid application (Figures 12.44a–d). Prominent coarsely dilated blood vessels with an irregular, nonuniform, and widely spaced capillary pattern (Figure 12.45) are

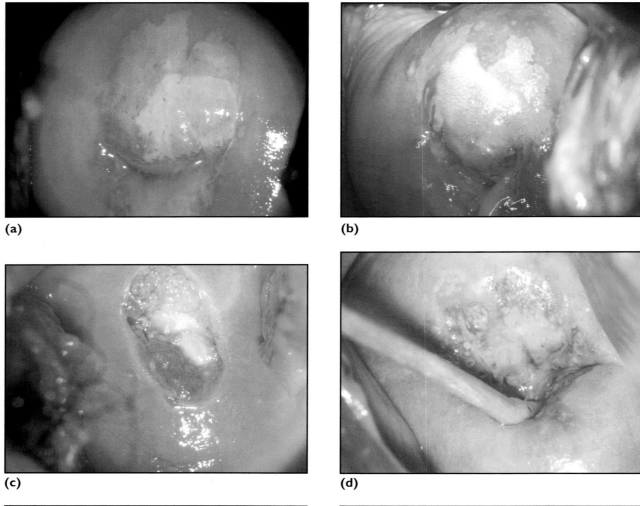

(a)

(b)

(c)

(d)

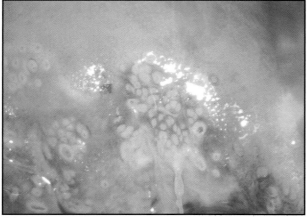

(e)

FIGURES 12.42a–g CIN 2 **(a)** and CIN 3 **(b)** seen in pregnant women. The CIN 2 is seen demarcated from immature metaplasia by an internal margin. The CIN 3 has an opaque acetowhite color with a coarse punctation and mosaic vascular pattern. Reprinted with permission from Wright VC. *Color Atlas of Colposcopy—Cervix, Vagina and Vulva.* Houston: Biomedical Communications, 2000. A less obvious CIN 3 is seen in **(c)**. There is a red, non-acetowhite lesion from the 6 o'clock to the 8 o'clock position along the SCJ; a faintly acetowhite lesion is seen in **(d)** and **(e)**. The wide opaque periglandular cuffing suggests a high-grade lesion.

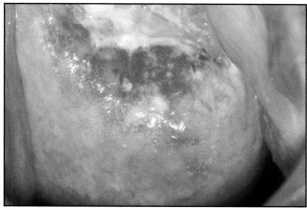

(f)

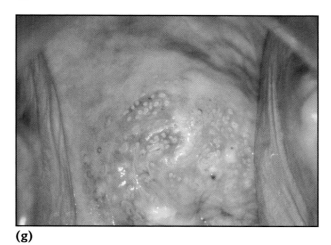

(g)

FIGURES 12.42a–g Continued. The other lesion in **(f)** and **(g)** is also similar, faintly acetowhite but with opaque periglandular cuffing.

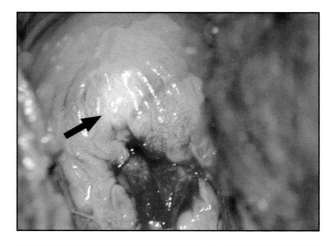

FIGURE 12.43 A high-grade lesion (arrow) is demarcated from a low-grade lesion by an internal margin in this pregnant woman.

seen, particularly later in pregnancy. However, many high-grade lesions contain no colposcopically observable blood vessels.

If a definite high-grade colposcopic lesion is present and consistent with the HSIL cytologic abnormality, a directed biopsy should probably be performed. Some very experienced colposcopists elect to merely monitor these lesions instead of confirming disease by biopsy. For most colposcopists, however, histologic sampling would be prudent. Moreover, histologic sampling would be generally advisable for older pregnant women, since they are at greater risk for occult cancer (Figure 12.9).[52] If the colposcopic impression is consistent with low-grade CIN, a directed biopsy may be taken and the original cytologic and histologic findings of the biopsy carefully reviewed by an expert gynecologic pathologist. If all tests are consistent, prospective surveillance is adequate. If the high-grade cytologic atypia is confirmed, but is not in concordance with more or less severe colposcopic and histologic diagnoses, consultation may be advisable. Patients with less severe colposcopic and histologic diagnoses should be cytologically and colposcopically reevaluated in 4 to 8 weeks, particularly if the colposcopy examination is unsatisfactory. If a colposcopic impression of early invasion is contemplated, a large, deep biopsy or wedge biopsy is mandatory. In this case, a gynecologic oncologist also should be consulted prior to diagnostic conization. When intervally monitoring women with cervical lesions during pregnancy, a rapid increase in the size of a lesion may denote the presence of a high-grade lesion,[64] or rarely, a cancer.

12.7.2.3 Management

Pregnant women with high-grade cervical lesions do not require treatment of the neoplasia during pregnancy. If high-grade CIN is confirmed by biopsy, patients should be seen at 8 to 10-week intervals throughout the pregnancy. Repeat cytologic and colposcopic evaluation should be performed at each visit to monitor for disease progression. Only in rare instances will a high-grade lesion progress to cancer by the postpartum period.[27,53] Approximately, 80% of CIN 3 will persist at the postpartum examination.[65] Complete disease regression occurs in approximately 12% to 30% of patients by the postpartum period.[59,65] Partial regression may occur in approximately 25% to 30% of patients.[64,56] Pregnant women with high-grade CIN should be permitted to deliver vaginally at term, if otherwise appropriate.

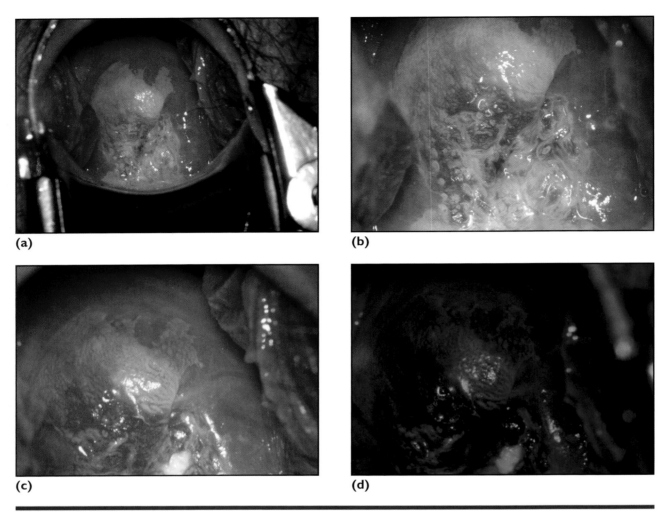

(a) **(b)**

(c) **(d)**

FIGURES 12.44a–d A high-grade lesion with opaque acetowhite epithelium and a coarse mosaic in this pregnant woman.

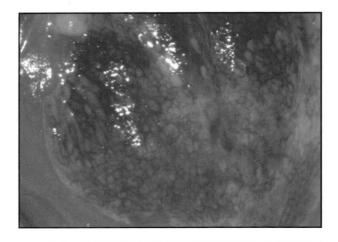

FIGURE 12.45 A CIN 3 with a smooth margin and a coarse, widely spaced mosaic vessel pattern in this pregnant woman.

12.7.3 Microinvasive carcinoma

12.7.3.1 Suspicious Pap smear report

Microinvasive cancer cannot be diagnosed specifically by cytologic examination. Cellular abnormalities indicative of cancer may be detected, but determination of the extent of invasion requires a histologic specimen. The presence of microinvasive carcinoma of the cervix is generally considered in pregnant women who have a particularly severe high-grade SIL Pap smear or a Pap smear suspicious for cancer. These women must have a colposcopic examination to further evaluate these suspicious cytologic findings.

12.7.3.2 Colposcopy

Microinvasive cancer is suspected when the colposcopic examination reveals a worrisome large high-grade lesion. Otherwise, a focal area of microinvasion may be hidden within a larger high-grade lesion. Colposcopists

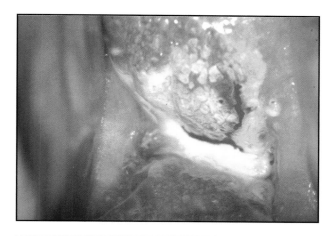

FIGURE 12.46 Microinvasive cervical cancer in a pregnant woman. Reprinted with permission from Wright V C. *Principles of Cervical Colposcopy.* Houston: Biomedical Communications, in press.

may not notice a focal contour change or the earliest vessel changes associated with an evolving lesion. The microinvasion may present as a small opaque, acetowhite lesion with short atypical vessels (Figure 12.46). Prominent, dilated vasculature noted during late pregnancy may make a severe high-grade lesion appear as a potential microinvasive lesion. Therefore, microinvasion can either be easily overlooked colposcopically or overdiagnosed. A low threshold for histologic sampling should be considered.

A simple cervical biopsy is usually insufficient to detect a microinvasive lesion. This is particularly true if the area of microinvasion is so focal in nature that the colposcopist may not sample the most severe area. Furthermore, a cervical biopsy will usually not obtain sufficient depth to allow a diagnosis of microinvasion. Thus, the diagnosis of microinvasive carcinoma can rarely be made only from histologic evaluation of a large biopsy specimen. In most cases, a large wedge biopsy or a cone biopsy is required. Consultation with a gynecologic oncologist for diagnostic and therapeutic assistance must be obtained, particularly for pregnant women. Conizations are best performed in the second trimester or following fetal maturity.

12.7.3.3 Management

The management of pregnant women with microinvasive cervical cancer should be undertaken with the expertise of a gynecologic oncologist. For most colposcopists, this means simply a referral for evaluation and perhaps joint management. Patients diagnosed with microinvasive carcinoma before the 24th week of gestation require careful evaluation and individualization of management. If invasive cancer is

excluded by cone biopsy and the pregnancy is wanted, the pregnancy may be allowed to continue.

The timing and route of delivery may be influenced by the depth of invasion and other prognostic features relating to microinvasive carcinoma, including lymphvascular space involvement, confluence of foci of invasion, and surface area of tumor. There is no convincing evidence that the route of delivery influences the management outcomes for microinvasive cervical carcinoma. Patients are usually permitted to deliver vaginally before definitive management of microinvasive carcinoma is begun. Antepartum therapy is generally not undertaken. Conization during pregnancy is diagnostic only and should not usually be considered therapeutic. Extrafascial hysterectomy is indicated for women not desiring to maintain fertility. A postpartum cone with negative margins, depth of invasion less than 3 mm, and no lymphvascular space involvement may suffice for women who wish to maintain fertility. Microinvasive carcinoma associated with high-risk features, particularly deep stromal invasive or lymphatic vascular space involvement, may require more radical management. A Cesarean section and radical hysterectomy may be the required management after close consultation with the patient. Following definitive treatment of microinvasive carcinoma of the cervix diagnosed during pregnancy, the patient should remain in close cytologic, colposcopic, and, if appropriate, histologic follow-up for at least 2 years after treatment.

12.7.4 Invasive carcinoma

12.7.4.1 Invasive cancer Pap smear report

Cytologic abnormalities of cervical cancer are the same in all women, irrespective of pregnancy. These cells exhibit an increased nuclear-to-cytoplasmic ratio, generally with a scant rim of cytoplasm surrounding a hyperchromatic, irregularly shaped nucleus. Cells may be elongated and spindle shaped, and a lack of uniform cellular shape may be appreciated. An associated tumor diathesis of blood, debris and inflammatory cells may signal the presence of cancer. The extent of invasion cannot be determined from a cytologic specimen. Therefore, these women must be examined by means of colposcopy, and suitable histologic specimens should be obtained (Figure 12.47).

12.7.4.2 Colposcopy

The changing clinical profile of cervical cancer mandates a high index of suspicion for symptoms and signs of cervical cancer in pregnant women. If there is no apparent pregnancy-related cause for bleeding, a colposcopic examination should be performed to exclude a rare occult invasive cancer. Also, if the cervix

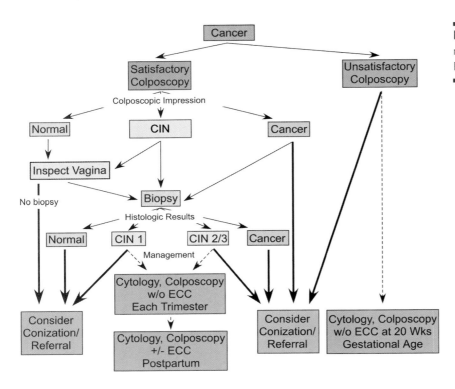

FIGURE 12.47 Algorithm for the management of pregnant women with a Pap smear suggestive of cervical cancer.

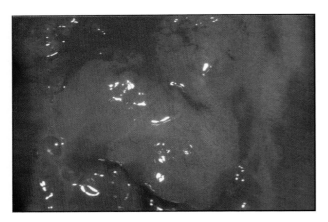

FIGURE 12.48 Cervical cancer in a pregnant woman. A yellow color and atypical blood vessels are seen. Reprinted with permission from Wright V C. *Color Atlas of Colposcopy—Cervix, Vagina and Vulva.* Houston: Biomedical Communications, 2000. ■

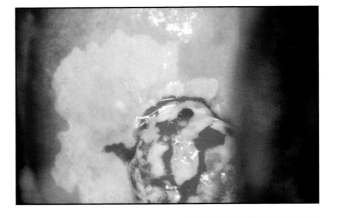

FIGURE 12.49 A macular acetowhite high-grade lesion can be seen alongside decidual tissue that mimics invasive cancer. Biopsy of both lesions is mandatory, given this women's HSIL Pap smear report (Photo courtesy of Burton Krumholz, M.D., Department of Obstetrics and Gynecology, Long Island Jewish Medical Center). ■

feels abnormally firm and indurated or demonstrates an unusual surface contour during pelvic examination in pregnancy, colposcopy is indicated to exclude cervical cancer. The same colposcopic warning signs for cervical cancer in nonpregnant women also apply for pregnant women (Chapter 10). Atypical blood vessels are the hallmark of cervical cancer. During pregnancy, these large-caliber vessels may be particularly engorged. Exophytic cancers may be readily

detected by an irregular contour change of the ecto-cervix (Figure 12.48). Decidual tissue of pregnancy may be confused easily with small exophytic tumors (Figure 12.49). Uncertainty of etiology always demands appropriate histologic sampling. Since cervical volume enlarges, both in pregnancy and invasive cancer, endophytic cancers may not be as easily noted. Ulcerations may indicate cancer in a necrotic area surrounded by yellow, friable epithelium. Large four-quadrant, opaque acetowhite lesions are likely to harbor cancer, as are the same lesions that extend deeply within the endocervical canal.

The colposcopic diagnosis of cervical cancer in pregnancy requires an appropriate biopsy for confirmation. If the histologic diagnosis of invasive cancer is in doubt, an additional pathologist's opinion should be obtained. If the tumor is clinically obvious, a directed biopsy may be adequate to establish the diagnosis. In some cases, however, a larger tissue sample, either a wedge or cone biopsy, is required to determine depth of invasion. Colposcopists must be prepared for the extensive bleeding that may be experienced after pregnant woman are biopsied or excisional procedures are performed. Therefore, histologic sampling of pregnant patients with lesions suggestive of cancer should be performed by experienced colposcopists or gynecologic oncologists.

12.7.4.3 Management

When determining proper management of pregnant women with cervical cancer, expert consultation must be obtained from a gynecologic oncologist. A gynecologic pathologist should also be consulted to review cytologic and histologic specimens prior to embarking on therapy. Treatment selection should be individualized and influenced by the length of gestation, cell type, tumor size, lymphvascular space involvement, cone margin status, disease stage, and patient preference.[67,68] Treatment of cervical cancer during pregnancy is similar to that for non-pregnant women. Therapy is based on clinical staging, along with ancillary studies that may include cystoscopy, intravenous urography, proctoscopy, chest radiography, and magnetic resonance imaging (MRI).[68]

If the diagnosis is made late in pregnancy, a few months' delay in definitive management to permit fetal viability should not negatively affect treatment outcome, particularly for stage I lesions.[34,38] Women with small stage I or IIA invasive cancers diagnosed in the late second or third trimester (more than 20 weeks' gestation) can be treated by Cesarean delivery and radical hysterectomy with pelvic lymphadenectomy at fetal viability. However, the combination of Cesarean section and radical hysterectomy increases risk of hemorrhage compared with the latter surgery alone. Women with advanced disease may also carry the pregnancy to term since earlier treatment would be unlikely to modify the poor prognosis.

If the pregnancy is not wanted and the fetus is not viable, immediate treatment may be undertaken. If early-stage invasive cancer is diagnosed during the first 2 trimesters (less than 20 weeks' gestation), a radical hysterectomy and pelvic lymphadenectomy with ovarian preservation is normally performed

immediately. Even though radiation therapy has been advocated by many, immediate radical surgery yields equivalent survival rates and low comparative morbidity for pregnant patients in the first or early second trimester with stage I or IIA cervical cancer.[69] Radiation therapy with concomitant chemotherapy (cisplatin) has become the treatment of choice for women with advanced stage cervical cancer.[27,70-72] External beam pelvic radiotherapy is combined with intracavitary brachytherapy.

Survival is primarily determined by the stage of disease at the time of treatment.[39] Prognosis is best when diagnosed in the first trimester (69%) compared with diagnoses in the postpartum period (47%).[27] A delay in diagnosis conveys an adverse prognosis and decreased survival. Furthermore, pregnancy does not modify the prognosis when controlling for age and disease stage as compared with the nonpregnant state.[38,39]

The method of delivery should also be carefully planned. Although, survival rates are equivalent for women with stage I cervical cancer who deliver vaginally as opposed to Cesarean section,[35,39] concerns in relation to intrapartum and postpartum hemorrhage from the cervical cancer may favor abdominal delivery. This approach may also decrease the risk of pulmonary embolism. Abdominal delivery will avoid the rare occurrence of tumor implants in an episiotomy site.[73-75] Abdominal delivery also is preferred for early stage disease. Vaginal delivery is a significant predictor of recurrence (OR = 6.9), as is increasing stage of disease (OR = 4.7).[76]

12.7.5 Complications experienced during the management of pregnant women with cervical neoplasia

12.7.5.1 Abortion

Certain complications unique to pregnant women may be encountered during the management of their cervical neoplasia. One risk is abortion, whether spontaneous or therapeutic. Spontaneous abortion does not appear to be more common for pregnant women with cervical neoplasia, but it may be erroneously blamed on the disease process. Generally, the greatest risk posed is from invasive rather than premalignant disease. Inadvertent trauma from the procedures required for proper evaluation may result rarely in an accidental iatrogenic abortion. If not carefully performed and modified for the pregnant patient, cervical conization may precipitate abortion. As many as 27% of pregnant women experience abortion following first trimester diagnostic conization.[40]

Table 12.2 Conization Induced Maternal Blood Loss in Pregnant Women

Study	Immediate hemorrhage	Delayed hemorrhage
Hannigan et al[77]	12.4%	3.7%
Daskal and Pitkin[80]	5.2%	5.2%
Averette et al[40]	7.2%	4.4%

In comparison, a mean abortion rate of 18% during the first trimester can normally be expected when reported series are considered collectively.[77] Abortion rates have been reported as high as 19% in women receiving second-trimester conization.[40] Therefore, first trimester conization may not be preferable to second trimester conization based only on the risk of abortion. Postcone cervical stenosis and cervical incompetence, although encountered infrequently, are always potential complications that should be recognized and discussed preoperatively with the patient. Aggressive endocervical curettage, although contraindicated during pregnancy, could contribute to abortion in women in the first trimester of pregnancy when both the patient and colposcopist are more likely to be unaware of the woman's status. This theoretical iatrogenic complication is probably also exceedingly rare. Otherwise, abortion resulting from radiation therapy or surgical treatment of women with invasive cervical cancer is an unfortunate but predictable outcome. Preterm labor and premature delivery also may result as consequences of necessary diagnostic interventions.

12.7.5.2 Hemorrhage

Hemorrhage during pregnancy is most commonly a result of pregnancy-related complications, such as placenta previa or abruption, particularly in the third trimester. However, unexplained cervical or vaginal bleeding during pregnancy must be evaluated by means of cytology and colposcopy with directed biopsy, when appropriate, to exclude a rare cervical cancer. Otherwise, when not caused by malignancy, bleeding complications during pregnancy most commonly occur as a consequence of biopsy or conization. Abnormal bleeding secondary to diagnostic procedures during pregnancy has been reported in as many as 12% of patients,[77] with 6% to 9% requiring transfusion following conization.[40,77] Clinicians should be cognizant of this potential serious complication (Table 12.2). Measures should be taken to minimize bleeding when diagnostic interventions such as wedge biopsy or conization are required. Hemostatic sutures, vasoconstrictive drugs and minimal, but sufficient excision of tissue should limit operative complications of hemorrhage. Operative bleeding complications are experienced most frequently during the third trimester.[40] Therefore, it is preferable to do conizations during the late first trimester or early second trimester.

12.7.5.3 Conization-related complications

Conization is rarely done during pregnancy, and only then for cases of suspected invasive or microinvasive cancer. As stated previously, cervical conizations during pregnancy may cause significant hemorrhage, premature delivery, or spontaneous abortion. Of note, pregnant women with CIN 3 treated by conization are more likely to deliver a premature and low-birthweight infant (OR = 1.6 and 1.8, respectively) than are women without CIN 3.[78] Cervical lacerations requiring repair at the time of spontaneous vaginal delivery may occur in as many as 18% of pregnant women who had a prior conization during pregnancy. Conizations are done during pregnancy when cytologic, histologic, or colposcopic suspicion of microinvasive cancer or frankly invasive cancer exists. Discordant histologic, cytologic, and colposcopic diagnosis may also prompt a conization. Conizations are also necessary when the entire transformation zone or proximal extent of a lesion are not visualized colposcopically. Unsatisfactory colposcopic examinations may occur because of visualization problems encountered during pregnancy. Unsatisfactory evaluation of the transformation zone in the case of preexisting cervical neoplasia may be less common during pregnancy. In one study, only 18% of pregnant women required a conization because of an unsatisfactory colposcopic examination.[77] It should be stressed that the usual indications for conization, inability to visualize the entire SCJ and proximal extent of a lesion extending up the endocervical canal, may not be independently sufficient criteria for conization during pregnancy. Additional criteria of cytologic, histologic or colposcopic suspicion of invasion also must be present.

Of greater importance is the fact that cervical conizations performed during pregnancy are rarely therapeutic. Such histologic specimens tend to be smaller and shallow for the purpose of minimizing complications for the patient and fetus. Postconization residual neoplasia (CIN 3) detected in postpartum hysterectomy specimens has been reported to be as high as 52% to 63%.[25,26,77] The majority of residual disease is located deep within the endocervical glands. Therefore, women who receive diagnostic conization during pregnancy should be reevaluated postpartum with cytologic, colposcopic, and histologic sampling, when appropriate. Residual disease may require retreatment. The use of loop excision instead of cold-knife conization during pregnancy appears to offer no additional benefits.[79] Positive margins, maternal and fetal morbidity, and nondiagnostic specimens are encountered with either approach.

12.7.5.4 Condyloma-related complications

Beyond its contribution to the development of cervical neoplasia, HPV is known to potentially contribute to several pregnancy-related complications. Dystocia secondary to massive condylomas of the lower genital tract is rare (Figure 12.2). However, the presence of disease of this magnitude that obstructs the birth canal will generally require delivery by cesarean section. The mere presence of lower genital tract condylomas without obstruction is never an indication for cesarean delivery. Another complication of HPV disease, recurrent respiratory papillomatosis (Figure 12.4), may potentially affect the fetus (Section 12.2.3). The virally induced condition of RRP is exceedingly rare but the potential affects on the child are significant and occasionally devastating. Children with RRP frequently require repeated laser treatments of laryngeal papilloma in order to maintain a patent airway and facilitate unencumbered speech.

12.8 Postpartum Management of Women with Cervical Neoplasia

Provided cancer has been excluded during pregnancy, treatment of cervical neoplasia is postponed until postpartum. In fact, treatment is not initiated based on antepartum findings. Instead, women with preinvasive disease are reevaluated with cervical cytology, colposcopy and histologic sampling, when indicated. Management is then determined with respect to these postpartum results.

Women are generally examined 8 to 16 weeks postpartum to allow time for the cervix to complete the reparative process. In some cases, no disease is detected in women who had a cervical lesion while pregnant. This is particularly true for women with low grade lesions or condylomas which are apt to resolve spontaneously. However, high grade lesions may also vanish without surgical intervention. Clinicians should obtain a Pap smear and then proceed with colposcopic examination. Significant cervical lesions should be biopsied and endocervical curettage performed as indicated. Clinicians should then follow the management guidelines outlined in Chapter 18. It is important to emphasize that women are usually managed based on postpartum findings.

Women who received a conization during pregnancy for high-grade disease should also undergo postpartum reevaluation because the rate of residual disease often exceeds 50%.[25,26] A repeat Pap smear and biopsy (when necessary) should be taken, then subsequent treatment decided. Occasionally, even with a high-grade lesion not treated during pregnancy, the physical trauma of labor and delivery may remove a large portion of the tumor load. Should this occur, the cervix may heal without cytologic or colposcopic evidence of residual disease. If the patient is a good follow-up candidate, treatment can be avoided. The patient should be assessed by means of cytology and colposcopy at 4- to 6-month intervals for 2 years before returning to a normal cytologic screening interval. A small but definite risk exists that new disease may evolve elsewhere within the transformation zone if treatment is not offered. Furthermore, small lesions, not apparent to initial postpartum colposcopic examination, may become colposcopically distinct thereafter. If the patient with postpartum regression of histologically proven antepartum high-grade CIN is not a good follow-up candidate, an argument can be made for empiric transformation zone treatment to prevent undetected disease recurrence. Otherwise, following a postpartum evaluation and biopsy, histologically confirmed high grade CIN should be treated 12 to 16 weeks postpartum by either indicated ablative or excisional modalities. Cytologic, histologic, or colposcopic findings of cancer may require further diagnostic evaluation prior to definitive treatment.

References

1. Fife KH, Rogers RE, Zwickl BW. Symptomatic and asymptomatic cervical infections with human papillomavirus during pregnancy. *J Inf Dis* 1987;156:904–11.

2. Lorincz AT, Temple GF, Patterson JA, Jensen AB, Kurman RJ, Lancaster VD. Correlation of cellular atypia and human papillomavirus deoxyribonucleic acid sequences in exfoliated cells of the uterine cavity. *Obstet Gynecol* 1986;68:508–12.

3. Wickenden C, Steele A, Malcolm ADB, Coleman DV. Screening for women with virus infections in normal and abnormal cervices by DNA hybridization of cervical scrapes. *Lancet* 1985;1:65–7.

4. deRoda Husman AM, Walboomers JM, Hopman E, et al. HPV prevalence in cytomorphologically normal cervical scrapes of pregnant women as determined by PCR: the age related pattern. *J Med Virol* 1995;46:97–102.

5. Kemp EA, Hakenewerth AM, Laurent SL, Gravitt PE, Stoerker J. Human papillomavirus prevalence in pregnancy. *Obstet Gynecol* 1992;79:649–56.

6. Patsner B, Baker DA, Jackman E. Human papillomavirus. In: Gonik B, ed. *Viral Diseases in Pregnancy.* Springer-Verlag, New York, NY, 1994.

7. Peng TC, Searle CP, Shah KV, Repke JT, Johnson TR. Prevalence of human papillomavirus infections in term pregnancy. *Am J Perinatol* 1990;7:189–92.

8. Schneider A, Hotz M, Gissmann L. Increased prevalence of human papillomavirus in the lower genital tract of pregnant women. *Int J Cancer* 1987;40:198–203.

9. Tenti P, Zappatore R, Migliora P, et al. Latent human papillomavirus infection in pregnant women at term: a case-control study. *J Inf Dis* 1997;176:277–80.

10. Fife KH, Katz BP, Roush J, Handy VD, Brown DR, Hansell R. Cancer-associated human papillomavirus types are selectively increased in the cervix of women in the first trimester of pregnancy. *Am J Obstet Gynecol* 1996; 174:1487–93.

11. Hildesheim A, Gravitt P, Schiffman MH, et al. Determinants of genital human papillomavirus infection in low income women in Washington, D.C. *Sex Trans Dis* 1993;20:279–85.

12. Hagensee ME, Slavinsky J III, Gaffga CM, Suros J, Kissinger P, Marti DH. Seroprevalence of human papillomavirus type 16 in pregnant women. *Obstet Gynecol* 1999; 94: 653–8.

13. Rando RF, Lindheim S, Hasty L, Sedlacek TV, Woodland M, Eder C. Increased frequency of detection of human papillomavirus DNA in exfoliated cervical cells during pregnancy. *Am J Obstet Gynecol* 1989;161:50–5.

14. Sridama V. Pacini F, Yang SL, Moawad A, Reilly M, Degroot LJ. Decreased levels of helper T cells: a possible cause of immunodeficiency in pregnancy. *NEJM* 1982;307:352–6.

15. Hietanen S, Ekblad A, Pellinieng TT, Syrjanen K, Helenius H, Syrjanen S. Type I diabetic pregnancy and subclinical human papillomavirus infection. *Clin Inf Dis* 1997;24:153–6.

16. Hermonat PL, Han L, Wendel PJ, et al. Human papillomavirus is more prevalent in first trimester spontaneously aborted products of conception compared to elective specimens. *Virus Genes* 1997;14:13–7.

17. Kashima HK, Shah K. Recurrent respiratory papillomatosis. *Obstet Gynecol Clin N Am* 1987;14:581–8.

18. Puranen M, Yliskoski M, Saarikoski S, Sydanen K, Syjanen S. Vertical transmission of human papillomavirus from infected mothers to their newborn babies and persistence of the virus in childhood. *Am J Obstet Gynecol* 1996;174:694–9.

19. Puranen MH, Yliskoski MIR, Saarikoski SV, Sydanen KJ, Syrjanen SM. Exposure of an infant to cervical human papillomavirus infection of the mother is common. *Am J Obstet Gynecol* 1997;176:1039–45.

20. Armbruster-Moraes E, Ioshimoto LM, Leao E, Zugaib M. Presence of human papillomavirus DNA in amniotic fluids of pregnant women with cervical lesions. *Gynecol Oncol* 1994;54:152–8.

21. Wang X, Zhu Q, Rao H. Maternal-fetal transmission of human papillomavirus. *Chin Med J* 1998; 111:726–7.

22. Eppel W, Worda C, Frigo P, Ulm M, Kucera E, Czerwenka K. Human papillomavirus in the cervix and placenta. *Obstet Gynecol* 2000; 96:337–41.

23. Bertini-Oliveira AM, Keppler MM, Luisi A, et al. Comparative evaluation of abnormal cytology, colposcopy and histopathology in preclinical cervical malignancy during pregnancy. *Acta Cytol* 1982;26:636–44.

24. Hannigan EV. Cervical cancer in pregnancy. *Clin Obstet Gynecol* 1990;33:837–45.

25. Boutselis JG, Ullery JC. Intraepithelial carcinoma of the cervix in pregnancy. *Am J Ostet Gynecol* 1964;90:593–609.

26. Dudan RC, Yon JL, Ford JH, Averette HE. Carcinoma of the cervix and pregnancy. *Gynecol Oncol* 1973;1:283–9.

27. Hacker NF, Berek JS, Lagasse LD, Charles EH, Savage EW, Moore JG. Carcinoma of the cervix associated with pregnancy. *Obstet Gynecol* 1982;59:735–46.

28. Madej JG. Colposcopy monitoring in pregnancy complicated by CIN and early cervical cancer. *Eur J Gynaecol Oncol* 1996;17:59–65.

29. Yost NP, Santoso JT, McIntire DD, Iliya FA. Postpartum regression rates of antepartum cervical intraepithelial neoplasia II and III lesions. *Obstet Gynecol* 1999; 93: 359–62.

30. Patsner B. Management of low-grade cervical dysplasia during pregnancy. *So Med J* 1990;83:1405–6.

31. Palle C, Bangsboll S, Andreasson B. Cervical intraepithelial neoplasia in pregnancy. *Acta Obstet Gynecol Scand* 2000; 79:306–10.

32. Talebian F, Krumholz B A, Shayan A, Mann L I. Colposcopic evaluation of patients with abnormal cytologic smears during pregnancy. *Obstet Gynecol* 1976;47:693–6.

33. Norstrom A, Jansson I, Andreasson H. Carcinoma of the uterine cervix in pregnancy. A study of the incidence and treatment in the western region of Sweden 1973 to 1992. *Acta Obstet Gynecol Scand* 1997;76:583–9.

34. Duggan B, Maderspach L L, Roman L D, Curtin J P, d'Ablaing G, Morrow C P. Cervical cancer in pregnancy: Reporting on planned delay in therapy. *Obstet Gynecol* 1993;82:598–602.

35. Creasman W T, Rutledge F N, Fletcher G H. Carcinoma of the cervix associated with pregnancy. *Obstet Gynecol* 1970–36:495–501.

36. Zemlickis D, Lishner M, Degendorfer P, Panzarella T. Sutcliffe S B, Koren G. Maternal and fetal outcome after invasive cervical cancer in pregnancy. *J Clin Oncol* 1991;9:1956–61.

37. Kinch R A. Factors affecting the prognosis of cancer of the cervix in pregnancy. *Am J Obstet Gynecol* 1961;82:45–51.

38. Hopkins N W, Morley G W. The prognosis and management of cervical cancer associated with pregnancy. *Obstet Gynecol* 1992;80:9–13.

39. Lee R B, Neglia W, Park R C. Cervical carcinoma in pregnancy. *Obstet Gynecol* 1981–58:584–9.

40. Averette B E, Nasser N, Yankow S L, Little W A. Cervical conization in pregnancy. *Am J Ostet Gynecol* 1970;106:543–9.

41. Singer A. The cervical epithelium during pregnancy and the puerperium. In: Jordan J A, Singer A, eds. *The Cervix*. London: W B Saunders Co., 1976.

42. Coppleson M, Reid B. A colposcopic study of the cervix during pregnancy and the puerperium. *J Obstet Gynecol Br Commonw* 1966;73:575–85.

43. Ueki M, Ueda M, Kumagai K, Okamoto Y, Noda S, Matsuoka M. Cervical cytology and conservative management of cervical neoplasia. *Int J Gynecol Path* 1995; 14:63–9.

44. Carter P M, Coburn T C, Luszczakm. Cost-effectiveness of cervical cytologic examination during pregnancy. *J Am Bd Fam Pract* 1993;6:537–45.

45. Ferris D G, Berrey M M, Ellis K E, Petry L J, Voxnaes J, Beatie R T. The optimal technique for obtaining a Papanicolaou smear with the Cervex-Brush. *J Fam Pract* 1992;34:276–80.

46. Rivlin M E, Woodliff J M, Bowlin R B, et al. Comparison of cytobrush and cotton swab for Papanicolaou smears in pregnancy. *J Reprod Med* 1993;38:147–50.

47. Orr J W, Barrett J M, Orr P F, Holloway R W, Holimon J L. The efficacy and safety of the cytobrush during pregnancy. *Gynecol Oncol* 1992;44:260–2.

48. Paraiso N T R, Brady K, Helmchen R, Roat T W. Evaluation of the endocervical cytobrush and Cervex-Brush in pregnant women. *Obstet Gynecol* 1994;84:539–43.

49. Stillson T, Knight A L, Elswick R K Jr. The effectiveness and safety of two cervical cytologic techniques during pregnancy. *J Fam Pract* 1997; 45:159–63.

50. Kohan S, Beckman E M, Bigelow B, Klein S A, Douglas G W. The role of colposcopy in the management of cervical intraepithelial neoplasia during pregnancy and postpartum. *J Reprod Med* 1980;25:279–84.

51. Rome R M, Urcuyo R, Nelson J H. Observations on the surface area of the abnormal transformation zone associated with intraepithelial and early invasive squamous cell lesions. *Am J Obstet Gynecol* 1977;129:565–70.

52. Benedet J L, Boyes D A, Nichols T M, Nfillner A. Colposcopic evaluation of pregnant patients with abnormal cervical smears. *Br J Obstet Gynecol* 1977;84:517–21.

53. Benedet J L, Selke P A, Nickerson K G. Colposcopic evaluation of abnormal Papanicolaou smears in pregnancy. *Am J Obstet Gynecol* 1987;157:932–7.

54. Ostergard D R, Nieberg R K. Evaluation of abnormal cervical cytology during pregnancy with colposcopy. *Am J Obstet Gynecol* 1979;134:756–8.

55. Economos K, Veridiano N P, Delke 1, Collado M L, Tancer M L. Abnormal cervical cytology in pregnancy: a 17-year experience. *Obstet Gynecol* 1993;81:915–8.

56. Baldauf J J, Dreyfus M, Ritter J, Phillippe E. Colposcopy and directed biopsy reliability during pregnancy: A cohort study. *Eur J Obstet Gynecol Reprod Biol* 1995;62:31–6.

57. Lieberman R W, Henry M R, Laskin W B, Walenga J, Buckner S B, O'Connor D M. Colposcopy in pregnancy: directed brush cytology compared with cervical biopsy. *Obstet Gynecol* 1999; 94:1054–5.

58. Chang-Claude J, Schneider A, Smith E, Blettner M, Wahrendorf J, Turek L. Longitudinal study of the effects of pregnancy and other factors on detection of HPV. *Gynecol Oncol* 1996;60:355–62.

59. Stratton P, Gupta P, Riester K, et al. Cervical dysplasia on cervicovaginal Papanicolaou smear among HIV-1-infected pregnant and nonpregnant women. Women and infants transmission study. *J Acquir Immune Defic Syndr Hum Retrovirol* 1999;20:300–7.

60. Hellberg D, Axelsson O, Gad A, Nilsson S. Conservative management of the abnormal smear during pregnancy. *Acta Obstet Gynecol Scand* 1987;66:195–9.

61. LaPolla J P, O'Neill C, Wetrich D. Colposcopic management of abnormal cervical cytology in pregnancy. *J Reprod Med* 1988;33:301–6.

62. Siddiqui G, Kurzel R B, Lampley E C, Kang H S, Blankstein J. Cervical dysplasia in pregnancy: progression versus regression postpartum. *Obstet Gynecol* 2001;97: S13.

63. Lurain JR, Gallup DG. Management of abnormal Papanicolaou smears in pregnancy. *Obstet Gynecol* 1979;53:484–8.

64. Mikhail MS, Anyaegbunam A, Romney SL. Computerized colposcopy and conservative management of cervical intraepithelial neoplasia in pregnancy. *Acta Obstet Gynecol Scand* 1995–74:376–8.

65. Coppola A, Sorosky J, Casper R, Anderson B, Buller RE. The clinical course of cervical carcinoma in situ diagnosed during pregnancy. *Gynecol Oncol* 1997; 67: 162–5.

66. Ortiz R, Newton M. Colposcopy in the management of abnormal cervical smears in pregnancy. *Am J Obstet Gynecol* 1971;109:46–9.

67. Thompson JD, Caputo TA, Franklin EW, Dale E. The surgical management of invasive cancer of the cervix in pregnancy. *Am J Obstet Gynecol* 1975;121:853–63.

68. Zanotti KM, Belinson JL, Kennedy AW. Treatment of gynecologic cancers in pregnancy. *Sem Oncol* 2000; 6:686–98.

69. Monk BJ, Montz FJ. Invasive cervical cancer complicating intrauterine pregnancy: Treatment with radical hysterectomy. *Obstet Gynecol* 1992;80:199–203.

70. Morris M, Eifel PJ, Lu J, et al. Pelvic radiation with concurrent chemotherapy compared with pelvic and para-aortic radiation for high-risk cervical cancer. *NEJM* 1999; 340:1137–43.

71. Rose PG, Bundy BN, Watkins EB, et al. Concurrent cisplatin-based radiotherapy and chemotherapy for locally advanced cervical cancer. *NEJM* 1999; 340: 1144–53.

72. Keys HM, Bundy BN, Stehman FB, et al. Cisplatin, radiation, and adjuvant hysterectomy compared with radiation and adjuvant hysterectomy for bulky stage 1B cervical carcinoma. *NEJM* 1999; 340:1154–61.

73. Copeland LJ, Saul PB, Sneige N. Cervical adenocarcinoma: tumor implantation in the episiotomy site of two patients. *Gynecol Oncol* 1987–28:230–5.

74. Gordon AN, Jensen R, Jones HW. Squamous carcinoma of the cervix complicating pregnancy: recurrence in episiotomy after vaginal delivery. *Obstet Gynecol* 1989;73:850–2.

75. Cliby WA, Dodson NM, Podratz KC. Cervical cancer complicated by pregnancy: episiotomy site recurrences following vaginal delivery. *Obstet Gynecol* 1994;84:179–82.

76. Sood AK, Sorosky JI, Mayr N, Anderson B, Buller RE, Niebyl J. Cervical cancer diagnosed shortly after pregnancy: prognostic variables and delivery routes. *Obstet Gynecol* 2000; 95:832–8.

77. Hannigan EV, Whitehouse HH, Atkinson WD, Becker SN. Cone biopsy during pregnancy. *Obstet Gynecol* 1982;60:450–5.

78. El-Bastawissi AY, Becker TM, Daling JR. Effect of cervical carcinoma in situ and its management on pregnancy outcome. *Obstet Gynecol* 1999; 93:207–12.

79. Robinson WR, Webb S, Tirpack J, Degefu S, O'Quinn AG. Management of cervical intraepithelial neoplasia during pregnancy with LOOP excision. *Gynecol Oncol* 1997; 64:153–5.

80. Daskal JL, Pitkin RM. Cone biopsy of the cervix during pregnancy. *Am J Obstet Gynecol* 1968;32:1–5.

Colposcopy in Special Situations

Table of Contents

13.1 Introduction

Nature is never static, and this adage applies to all areas of the human body. Age, hormones, intravaginal products, contraceptive agents and devices, and trauma from sexual relations, both consensual and otherwise, all influence the colposcopic appearance of the lower genital tract. Colposcopists must be able to recognize these modifications as the result of various external, natural, or developmental influences. For example, hormonal changes induced by oral contraceptive pills and other factors can cause benign pseudoneoplastic glandular lesions of the uterine cervix that may mimic glandular neoplasia.[1] Exposure to diethylstilbestrol (DES) in utero resulted in some women developing columnar epithelium in the vaginal mucosa (adenosis), having an increased risk of clear cell adenocarcinoma of the vagina, and developing structural changes in the cervix and other areas of the genital tract.[2–8] Loss of estrogen in menopausal and postmenopausal women results in structural changes to the cervical stroma, as well as epithelial alterations.

In addition to the myriad of changes that may be caused by hormones, the effects of foreign objects on the vaginal and cervical epithelium may result in confusing colposcopic findings. Tampons, vaginal spermicides and lubricants, diaphragms, cervical caps, and a host of sexually introduced objects may traumatize the epithelium. Consequently, erosions, tears, abra-

sions, and epithelial regeneration patterns may hamper the colposcopist's ability to identify and diagnose disease. Colposcopists must recognize these effects if underdiagnosis and overdiagnosis are to be avoided.

As society has moved towards greater protection of individuals from unwanted sexual contact, a new colposcopic subspecialty, the colposcopy of sexual assault victims, has become very important.[9,10] Well-trained sexual assault response teams have been established in many communities. Members of these teams are trained in the use of the colposcope, particularly for identification of normal anatomic and mucosal findings seen with consensual sexual relations and abnormal changes seen in victims of sexual assault. While it is not within the scope of *Modern Colposcopy* to provide a complete review of the forensics and major colposcopic findings associated with unwanted sexual advances, some familiarity with these issues is an important part of every colposcopist's training.

13.2 Hormonally Induced Changes

13.2.1 Changes due to oral contraceptive pills

Combination estrogen-progestin oral contraceptive pills (OCPs) can induce both stromal and epithelial changes. Hypertrophy of the stroma results in enlargement of the cervix that often causes the columnar epithelium to evert.[11] The size of such ectopy appears to be related to the duration of oral contraceptive use.[12] Increased vascularity may be noted colposcopically as hyperemia of the exposed columnar epithelium.[12] Abundant mucus may be observed, and the fusing of enlarged columnar villi may produce globular, hyperemic, polypoid shapes. Prior to the application of a 5% acetic acid solution, this hyperemic ectopy may appear to be eroded; hence, the misnomer "cervical erosion."[12] However, a typical, faint and transient acetowhitening of these polypoid villi clearly delineates the tissue as normal, frond-like columnar villi (Figures 13.1a, b). Particularly large, irregular villi may appear similar in shape to small condylomata.

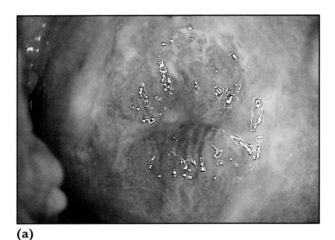

(a)

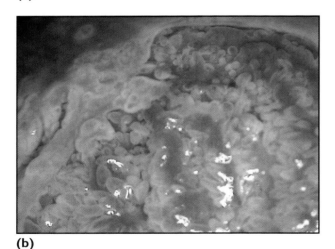

(b)

FIGURES 13.1a,b **(a)** Hyperemic ectopy accentuated by oral contraceptive use appears "eroded" because of the increased vascular congestion. **(b)** After the application of acetic acid, acetowhitening of these polypoid villi clearly delineates the area as normal columnar villi. ▬▬▬

Although these findings represent a normal physiologic event, their prominence can be confusing.

13.2.2 Microglandular hyperplasia

An exaggeration of tissue response to OCPs, called microglandular hyperplasia (MGH), is another example of lower genital tract epithelial alterations caused by hormones. Both progestins in oral contraceptive pills and the increased progesterone levels of pregnancy can stimulate columnar cellular changes that are difficult to reliably discriminate colposcopically from glandular neoplasia. For many years, it had been assumed that MGH of the cervix occurred almost exclusively in women with either endogenous or exogenous stimulation of the progestational phase of the menstrual cycle.[12] Although this concept has recently been challenged,[13] there is no question that hormonal influence can induce budding of the endocervical crypts. Proliferation of these crypts expands the columnar villi, producing polypoid excrescences (Figure 13.2a). Clumping of these structures produces irregular masses that may appear quite abnormal. Even if the vascular pattern is normal, a yellow hue in areas of microglandular hyperplasia should raise concern about the presence of occult cancer (Figure 13.2b).

Cervical biopsy reveals numerous gland crypts lined by cuboidal cells with regular nuclei. Mitotic figures can be found, but they are not abnormal. Budding of these endocervical crypts produces a microglandular pattern against a background of reserve cell hyperplasia. Maturing metaplasia within gland crypts that appears to be separate from the surface epithelium occasionally has been confused with carcinoma, and the atypical glandular cells sometimes seen in cytology of cells from women with MGH can be confused with adenocarcinoma in situ.[14] However, the normal appearance of the nuclei and the normal appearance and minimal number of mitotic figures should reassure the colposcopist that the lesion is benign.

13.2.3 Vaginal adenosis

Vaginal adenosis is simply the presence of glandular cells in the vaginal epithelium, thought to be derived from persistent paramesonephric epithelial islets in post-embryonic life.[15,16] Columnar epithelial cells have been detected in vaginal histologic specimens in approximately 10% to 15% of female infants under the age of 1 month and in a similar percent of women between the onset of puberty and 25 years of age.[15] Vaginal adenosis was initially considered an entirely benign process. However, in 1971, a link was identified between *in utero* exposure

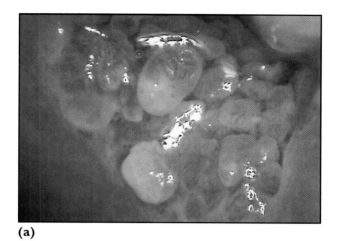

(a)

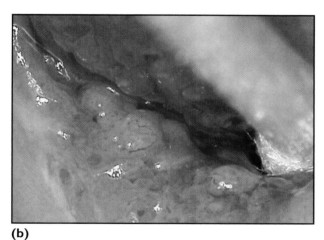

(b)

FIGURES 13.2a,b Colposcopy of microglandular hyperplasia. **(a)** Individually, the polypoid structures of microglandular hyperplasia may resemble small polyps **(b)**. Clumping of these polypoid structures produces irregular polypoid masses that are often cream to yellow in color.

to diethylstilbestrol (DES), vaginal adenosis , and an increased risk of vaginal and cervical adenocarcinoma.[4] Although subsequent long-term follow-up of women with vaginal adenosis has not documented a single case of transformation of clear cell adenocarcinoma directly from an area of benign adenosis[17–19], the relationship of DES with both vaginal adenosis and with clear cell adenocarcinoma is undeniable.[4] For several decades prior to 1971, the estrogen DES was given to pregnant women to prevent miscarriage. The National Diethylstilbestrol Screening Project evaluated 1,275 women exposed to DES *in utero*, documenting that 34% had evidence of adenosis or had areas of squamous metaplasia in the vagina or the byprod-

ucts of this activity, such as gland openings and Nabothian cysts.[8] The presence of these findings was associated with the gestational age at which DES exposure began, the length of exposure, and the dose. The risk of developing clear cell adenocarcinoma from birth through the fourth decade of life for individuals exposed to DES has been estimated to be approximately 1 in 1000.[17] The concern that DES exposure might place women at increased risk for developing other cancers so far has not been realized.[18,19] However, the increased risk these women have for developing estrogen-receptor positive breast cancers after the age of 40 years remains.[20]

For most DES-exposed women, the vaginal adenosis is replaced by benign squamous metaplasia that eventually transforms into mature squamous epithelium, which has no increased risk of developing into vaginal neoplasia. Adenosis has also been reported to develop after 5-fluorouracil (5-FU) treatment of HPV-induced vaginal lesions.[21,22] Although it had been presumed that adenosis developing in women secondary to treatment with 5-FU did not increase the risk of those patients developing glandular neoplasia, reports of clear cell adenocarcinoma detected in areas of iatrogenic adenosis have resulted in increased vigilance in evaluating these women.[23] Benign structural changes within the lower genital tract have also been reported more frequently in women exposed to DES *in utero*.[8] These changes include cervical pseudopolyps, grossly irregular cervix, rough or smooth anterior cervical protuberance ("cockscomb"), columnar ectopy completely covering the portio or beyond the cervical-vaginal margins, hypertrophy of tissue surrounding the cervical ectopy (cervical collar), and circular or irregular sulci on the portio (Figures 13.3a–g). While more commonly seen in DES-exposed women, each of these structural changes can also be found in women who have not been exposed to DES.

Women with vaginal adenosis are usually asymptomatic, although some may experience a greater than usual volume of mucoid vaginal discharge or have postcoital bleeding. Gross inspection of the vagina may reveal erythematous areas similar in color and texture to cervical ectopy. Rarely, eroded or ulcerated areas may be present. Colposcopic evaluation using high magnification will confirm the glandular nature of the red vaginal changes surrounded by the homogeneous appearance of normal, pink squamous epithelium. After application of acetic acid, the typical "grapelike" clusters of columnar epithelium can be seen. When vaginal adenosis is precipitated by in utero exposure to DES, the benign nature of similar findings that indicate an increased

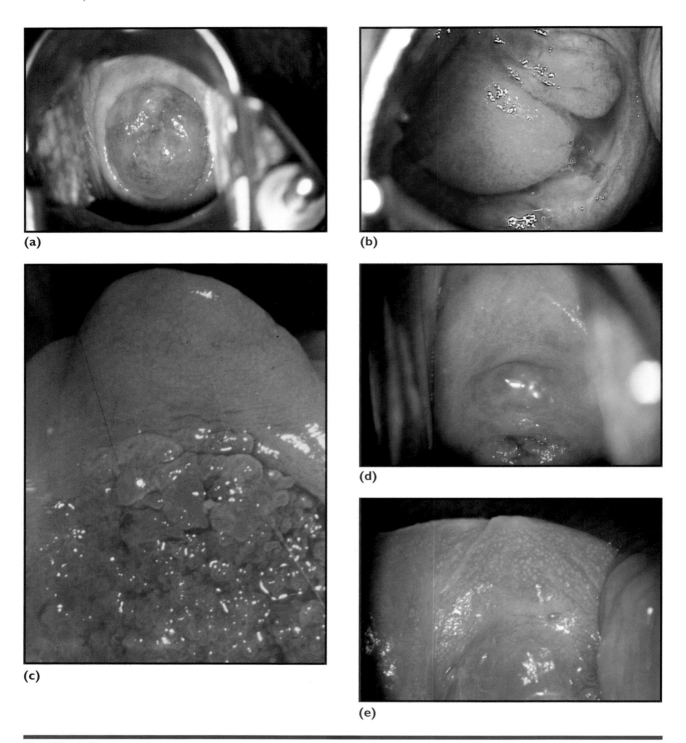

FIGURES 13.3a–g   Benign structural changes noted in women who were exposed to DES in utero: **(a)** Cervical pseudopolyp, **(b)** Grossly irregular cervix, **(c and d)** "Cockscomb", **(e)** complete covering of the portio beyond the cervical-vaginal margin with columnar epithelium undergoing metaplasia, and **(f and g continued on next page)** cervical collar. Figure 13.3c photo courtesy of Dr. Duane Townsend.

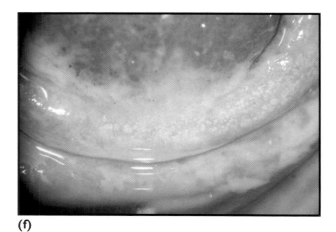

(f)

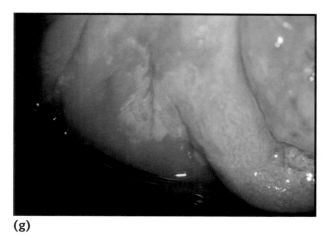

(g)

FIGURES 13.3a–g (continued) ▬▬▬

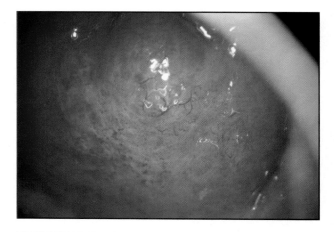

FIGURE 13.4 Large portio ectopy extending to the vaginal wall entirely around the circumference of the cervix is seen in this DES-exposed woman. ▬▬▬

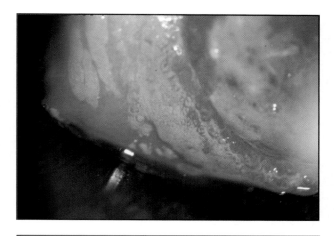

FIGURE 13.5 A large area of adenosis extends to the right posterior vaginal fornix in this DES-exposed woman.

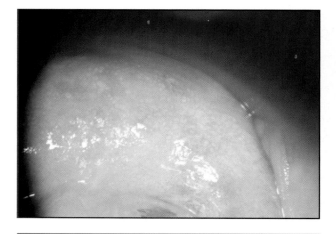

FIGURE 13.6 Fine mosaic is present in this area of adenosis that is undergoing metaplasia. Biopsy confirmed that this was normal immature metaplasia. ▬▬▬

glandular presence on the ectocervix, including irregularity, pseudopolyps, and sulci, can be confirmed colposcopically by the absence of atypical vessels and other warning signs of cancer. Adenosis is most commonly associated with large cervical ectopy that extend onto the vaginal wall (Figure 13.4). However, diffuse small patches of adenosis may be noted throughout the vagina, and larger isolated patches may be found within the vaginal fornices (Figure 13.5). Extensive immature metaplasia within the transforming adenosis often produces readily apparent acetowhite areas with striking fine-caliber vascular changes having mosaic and punctation (Figure 13.6). When viewed colposcopically, this dynamic physiologic metaplasia can appear to be very similar to intraepithelial neoplasia (Figures 13.7a,b). Detection of other suspicious-looking benign entities can be equally worrisome (Figures 13.8a,b). High-grade CIN can develop within large areas of ectopy and immature metaplasia (Figures 13.9a,b), which can complicate the diagnosis, just as it can when present within a

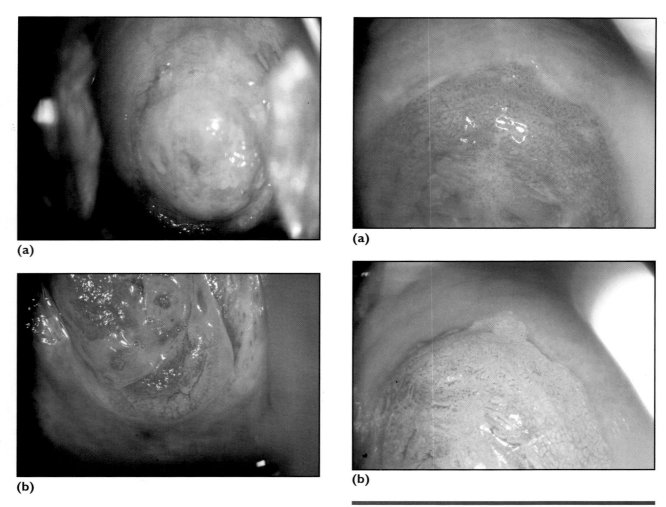

FIGURES 13.7a,b   DES-adenosis with extensive meta-plasia extends to the vagina. ▬▬▬▬▬▬

FIGURES 13.8a,b   DES-exposed woman with a minor cervical collar and a protuberant large area of columnar epithelium **(a)** pre-acetic acid and **(b)** post-acetic acid. Photos courtesy of Dr. Ken Hatch. ▬▬▬▬▬▬

large congenital transformation zone (Figure 13.10). Patches of adenosis can bleed on contact, heightening the colposcopist's concern that neoplasia is present, as can an irregular surface contour. Oral contraceptive pills can stimulate hyperplasia within areas of vaginal adenosis, in much the same way they affect areas of normal cervical columnar epithelium. The resulting microglandular hyperplasia can mimic adenocarcinoma. Additionally, palpation of the vagina may detect large Nabothian cysts in areas of adenosis that may be confused with tumors.[16] Puncturing these palpable cysts with a small needle will produce clear mucous as evidence of their benign nature. Previously, clear cell adenocarcinoma (CCA) had not been reported in women over the age of 40 years, and it was thought that by the year 2011 (40 years from the date DES was last administered to a woman during pregnancy) that DES-exposed women would no

longer be at increased risk of developing cancer. However, the DES Registry now has identified at least 6 cases in which clear cell adenocarcinoma has been detected in DES-exposed women over the age of 40 years (personal communication, Dr. Kenneth L. Noller). Furthermore, a bimodal curve noted for CCA for both women exposed to DES and for unexposed women raises concern that new cases could occur in the postmenopausal years.[24] Because clinicians had become less concerned about detecting clear cell adenocarcinoma in DES-exposed women, the DESAD Project has begun a national education campaign to alert clinicians that DES-exposed women continue to be at some risk. The original DESAD protocol called for obtaining 2 separate Pap smears, with one smear taken from the cervix and the other from the vaginal fornices; conducting a full colposcopic evaluation that included the application of

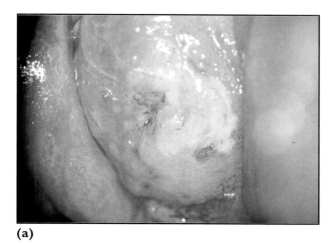

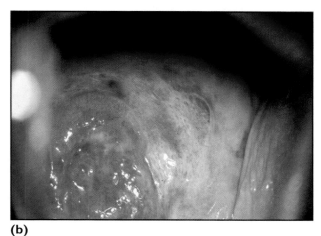

FIGURES 13.9a,b **(a)** CIN 2/3 within a pseudopolyp surrounded by a prominent cervical collar **(b)** same patient post-laser. Photos courtesy of Dr. Ken Hatch.

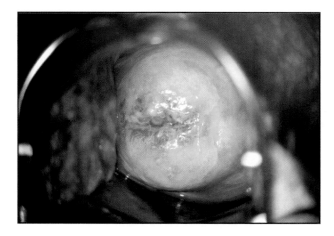

FIGURE 13.10 Large symmetrical acetowhite with fine mosaic in a young DES-exposed woman resembles the CTZ seen in 3% of non-DES exposed women.

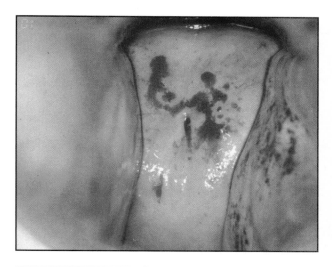

FIGURE 13.11 The classic thin, friable epithelium of the atrophic vagina and cervix. Note the subepithelial hemorrhagic appearance.

acetic acid and aqueous iodine to visualize areas of cell changes; and palpating the entire vagina and cervix after the speculum was removed.[25] Others have argued that adequate evaluation can be accomplished by conducting a gross inspection before and after applying Lugol's solution, and that conducting a full colposcopic examination is not necessary unless inspection and palpation of the vaginal wall raises concerns. Any patient in whom an abnormality is detected could then be referred for a more comprehensive colposcopic evaluation.

13.2.4 Estrogen deficiency

Up to 40 percent of postmenopausal women have symptoms of atrophic vaginitis, as do some non-menopausal women taking anti-estrogenic medications.[26] Vaginal epithelial integrity is highly dependent upon adequate estrogen. In its absence, the epithelium becomes thin and atrophic and capillary fragility may result in punctate hemorrhages into the mucosa and hemosiderin deposits. Cytologic smears can become quite difficult to interpret, as parabasal cells with an increased nuclear:cytoplasmic ratio predominate.[27-29] As a result, estrogen deficient women are commonly referred for colposcopic evaluation for such "atypical" smears.[28,29] Colposcopically, the vaginal epithelium appears thin, with enhancement of the underlying vasculature (Figure 13.11). The epithelium is friable, often bleeding upon contact with a cotton swab. Ulcerations, erosions or epithelial tears may result from minor trauma precipitated by intercourse, pessaries and even by the introduction of the vaginal speculum. Loss of the protective effect of full epithelial thickness often results in inflammation of the vaginal mucosa that produces a thin discharge with profuse numbers of WBC's noted on wet mount examination.[16,26,27] Lugol's uptake is minimal due to the lack of estrogen induced glycogen in the epithelium. Consequently, a diffusely light brown-to-yellow color results from the application of Lugol's. If the adequacy of the evaluation for the presence of a vaginal or cervical lesion is significantly diminished by vaginal atrophy, the patient should be treated with vaginal estrogen cream for three weeks and told to return for colposcopy following treatment.[30] Following estrogen replacement, parabasal cells will quickly mature into intermediate and superficial squamous cells that convey a normal colposcopic appearance. If a lesion is present, it is often not possible to detect it until this step is taken. It must also be remembered that occasionally a woman may be on adequate exogenous oral estrogen replacement, and yet have atrophic vaginal epithelium.[16] Additionally, premenopausal women on DepoProvera or Lupron may have similar atrophic findings from suppression of the production of endogenous estrogen.[27]

13.3 Radiation Induced Changes

Radiation of cervical, vaginal, or, in some cases, endometrial cancer may result in thinned, friable epithelium in the lower genital tract and atypical blood vessels. These radiation-induced changes may be extremely worrisome and difficult to interpret colposcopically. The majority of these women are also estrogen deficient because they are postmenopausal, either having gone through menopause prior to radiation treatment or having had radiation reduced menopause through ablation of ovarian function. In either case, atrophic vaginitis further complicates the colposcopic interpretation. Long-term cytologic changes caused by radiation are often seen in the Pap test. Benign post-radiation cytologic changes can range from mild to severe and may consist of cytoplasmic vacuolization, nuclear wrinkling and enlargement, and multinucleation (See Chapter 2).[31] These cytologic findings may be confused with dysplastic changes. The presence of large, bizarre, hyperchromatic nuclei should increase the colposcopist's concern and dictates the need for vigilance, especially since the patient has a history of genital tract cancer that may recur in the vagina.

Radiation-induced colposcopic findings may be difficult to discriminate from similar findings associated with cancer. The mucosa is pale and thin, often friable, with poor iodine uptake (Figure 13.12). Telangiectasias and atypical blood vessels are usually present (Figure 13.13).[16] Neovascularization resulting from the effects of radiation can be quite bizarre.

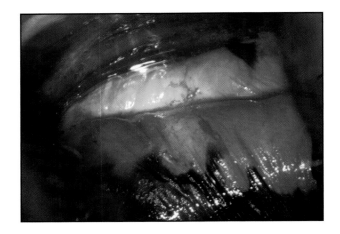

FIGURE 13.12   A sharply demarcated iodine-negative area is seen in this vaginal cuff post-radiation.

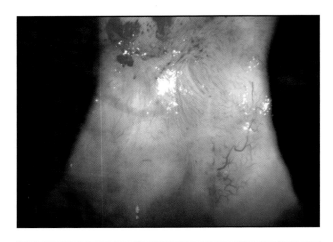

FIGURE 13.13   Friable thinned epithelium with atypical vessels can be seen in this woman treated previously by radiation for a vaginal sarcoma. Such findings are extremely difficult to interpret.

Dilated, tortuous, or elongated non-branching vessels may be seen. The thin epithelium is susceptible to trauma; hence, postcoital bleeding, petechiae or purpura, and leukorrhea are symptoms often reported by patients. If adhesions are not disrupted during the several weeks or months required for healing following radiation treatment, the vagina will become foreshortened and areas of the lower genital tract that are at risk for recurrent disease will become inaccessible to colposcopic evaluation. Atrophy secondary to estrogen deficiency further complicates the evaluation. The application of 1 g of vaginal estrogen cream daily for 3 to 4 weeks prior to the colposcopic examination will increase the thickness of the vaginal epithelium, resulting in less patient discomfort and minimizing the confusion caused by atrophic changes.[16,30] Frequent follow-up examinations and biopsy of suspicious areas are mandatory to ensure positive outcomes in these patients. Palpation of the vaginal wall prior to inserting a speculum also can be helpful, since areas of localized thickened epithelium found will need to be inspected visually during the subsequent colposcopic examination.

13.4 Cervical Polyps

Polyps that present at the cervical os are almost always benign extensions of endocervical or endometrial epithelium. They are usually asymptomatic findings noted during routine examination. Although women with polyps typically are asymptomatic, occasionally they may present with complaints of postcoital bleeding, or if the polyps are necrotic, with a foul-smelling yellow discharge. Virtually all cervical polyps arise from the columnar epithelium of the endocervix. Most evolve from a single enlarged endocervical villus.[32] Extension of the tip of the polyp into the acidic vaginal environment beyond the cervical os will initiate the metaplastic process. A single polyp may contain both immature and mature metaplasia, while columnar epithelium may cover the stalk (Figures 13.14a,b). This combination of immature metaplasia and inflammation may produce an acetowhite area with a mosaic vascular pattern that may be confused with neoplasia. Women with endocervical polyps may have abnormal Pap smear results that indicate the presence of inflammatory or atypical glandular cells.[33] The differential diagnosis for polyps presenting at the cervical os includes pseudopolyps, rare prolapsing submucosal fibroids, and polypoid endocervical or endometrial adenocarcinoma. Rarely, premalignant squamous neoplasia and adenocarcinoma may present exclusively on the tips of cervical polyps (Figure 13.15).

A pseudopolyp is an accentuated outfolding of the endocervical canal that appears to be a polyp, but on close inspection the colposcopist will see that it does not have a stalk. Rather, the apparent polypoid surface has a broad base (Figure 13.16). Differentiating pseudopolyps from true polyps is important because attempted removal of a pseudopolyp may cause excessive bleeding. Pseudopolyps are not an abnormality. Colposcopic identification of the broad base and healthy surface epithelium should reassure the colposcopist that this finding is normal. Iatrogenic pseudopolyps that develop following loop electrosurgical excision (LEEP) may be created by the button-like appearance of the cervical portio seen in many women who have undergone LEEP.

Submucosal fibroids can extrude through the external cervical os. Compromise of the vascular sup-

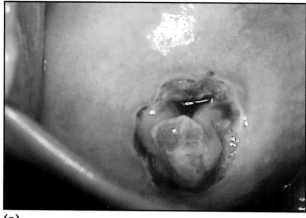

(a)

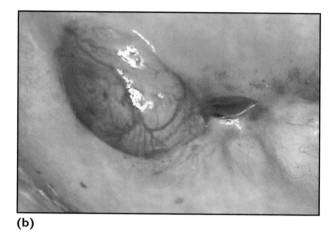

(b)

FIGURES 13.14a,b **(a)** Cervical polyps often demonstrate metaplasia in various stages of maturity on the tip of the polyp and columnar epithelium on the more protected stalk. **(b)** Polyp with prominent branching blood vessels. ▬

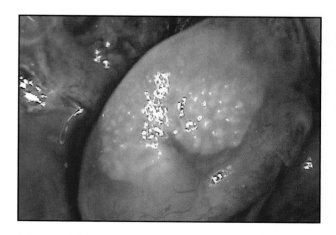

FIGURE 13.15 CIN I on the tip of a polyp. ▬

ply can cause necrosis that may colposcopically and histologically mimic carcinoma. Endocervical adenocarcinoma may occasionally present as a polypoid, necrotic lesion similar in appearance to necrotic submucosal fibroids, however; both are extremely uncommon.

Endocervical polyps will frequently recur if the stalks are not completely eliminated. However, polyps are common and pose little risk of becoming malignant. Therefore, extensive procedures to eliminate the entire stalk of a polyp by cautery or other measures are not necessary if neoplasia has been ruled out. Grasping the polyp with a ring forceps and repeatedly rotating the forceps 360° until the polyp "twists" off at the base is an easy way of removing most polyps with thin stalks. Polyps on thin stalks also can be removed by using biopsy forceps to either sever the stalk at the base, or if the polyp is small, simply by biopsying the entire polyp. Wire loop snares may also be used. Bleeding from polyps removed by these techniques is usually minimal.

Histologic examination of a cervical polyp will reveal normal, endocervical epithelium covering normal lamina propria. The presence of metaplasia of varying degrees of maturity and an inflammatory stromal infiltrate of predominantly plasma cells is typical. Necrosis results in loss of surface epithelium and granulation. Dilated endocervical crypts are also common. In rare cases, involvement of the surface epithelium with HPV-induced intraepithelial neoplasia or cancer can occur, sometimes without evidence of other cervical involvement.

13.5 Post-Treatment Findings

13.5.1 Mimics of cervical neoplasia

Cellular and tissue regeneration and repair within the cervix following surgical treatment often creates confusing cytologic, colposcopic, and histologic findings that may mimic residual intraepithelial neoplasia. The cervix generally heals more rapidly after excision than after ablation. This is because ablation leaves nonviable tissue that must first undergo necrosis and sloughing before repair and reepithelialization can occur. Therefore, cervical tissue treated by electrical loop excision, laser, or cold knife conization often appears colposcopically to have healed completely within 3 to 4 weeks (Figure 13.17). However, cytology will usually continue to show reparative changes for many more weeks, which although normal, may appear to be quite atypical. In contrast, a cervix that has undergone cryotherapy may continue to slough residual necrotic eschar for 4 to 6 weeks and may have colposcopically identifiable areas still undergoing regeneration for up to 6 months (Figure 13.18). Therefore, the ASCCP Guidelines recommend that the first post-treatment examination be delayed until 4 to 6 months after either ablation or excision.[34]

The most common colposcopic finding during the first post-treatment examination is an acetowhite reaction within the epithelium of the regenerating squamocolumnar junction following the application of an acetic acid solution. When the acetowhite effect is quite transient and the whitening appears more translucent than opaque, the area may be readily identified as normal immature metaplasia (Fig-

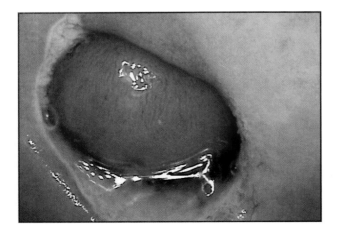

FIGURE 13.16 Pseudopolyp: An apparent cervical polyp is found to have a broad base, which is consistent with an outfolding of the stroma and columnar epithelium of the endocervical canal. This patient was not exposed to DES.

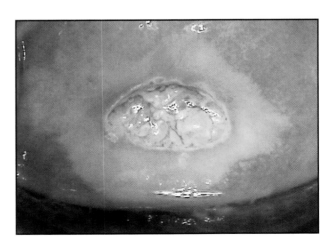

FIGURE 13.17 Four weeks after loop excision was performed, this cervix appears to be almost back to normal.

ure 13.19). However, areas in which the acetowhite effect persists and appears more opaque can be seen during epithelial regeneration within a cervix that is free of HPV-induced changes and residual intraepithelial neoplasia (Figures 13.20a,b). Often the colposcopic picture is further complicated by the presence of punctation. When this punctation assumes a

linear pattern radiating out from the os, it usually indicates the area is undergoing repair. Linear punctation may be found following cervical laser, loop excision, or conization, but occurs more commonly following cryotherapy. Linear punctation is usually fine in caliber and evenly spaced. The punctation may protrude slightly above the surface plane of the epithelium, commonly within a ridge of parakeratosis. Benign linear punctation can usually be discriminated from neoplasia-associated punctation by the absence of dense surrounding acetowhite epithelium as well as by the linear pattern. However, dilated punctation with variable intercapillary distances is occasionally present in areas histologically confirmed to be normal (Figure 13.21).

Hyperkeratotic epithelium may also be present as part of normal repair. Most commonly, these

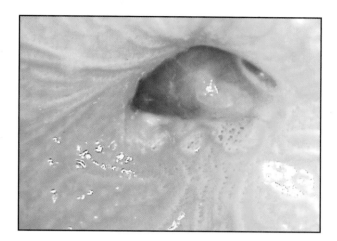

FIGURE 13.18   Four months after this patient underwent cryotherapy, a small dense acetowhite area with sharp margins and punctation is seen at the SCJ, a finding usually suspect for persistent CIN. However, a biopsy was performed and the histology interpreted as only metaplasia and inflammation. Leukoplakic ridges with fine punctation radiate out from the os, a common benign finding post-cryotherapy.

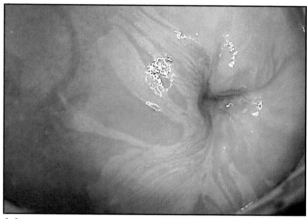

(a)

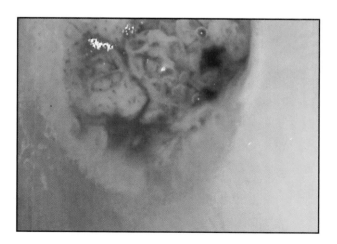

FIGURE 13.19   A regenerating area at the squamocolumnar junction and over the tips of villae is transiently acetowhite and appears more translucent than is usually seen with persistent CIN. Punctation and mosaic are also seen but the translucent and transient nature of the acetowhitening are more consistent with a diagnosis of normal regenerating immature metaplasia.

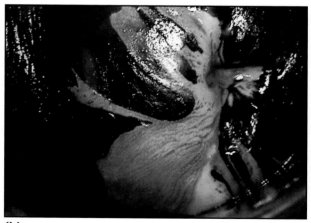

(b)

FIGURES 13.20a,b   Almost 4 months after cryotherapy was performed, an acetowhite geographic area is noted following acetic acid application **(a)** and post-Lugols application **(b)**. Biopsy read as metaplasia with mild atypia.

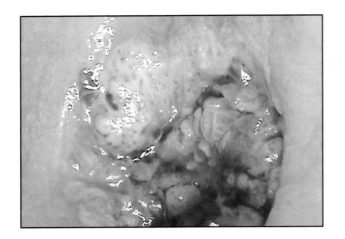

FIGURE 13.21   This area of dilated, worrisome punctation with variable intercapillary distance was noted on the first follow-up examination of a patient who had undergone cryotherapy. The colposcopic impression was high-grade CIN (CIN 2). However, the results of both the Pap smear and the biopsy were normal.

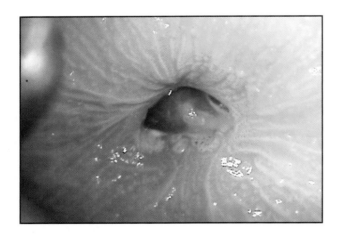

FIGURE 13.22   Radially distributed leukoplakic excrescences extending out as far as the tissue destruction of the cryoprobe are noted in the same patient as seen in Fig. 13.18 four months after cryotherapy. The radial distribution of these hyperkeratotic ridges can also be highlighted by the absence of iodine staining.

leukoplakic excrescences extend from the os in a radial pattern (Figure 13.22), but they also can have a random distribution. Since they are either hyperkeratotic or parakeratotic, they do not absorb iodine and appear as tiny yellow dots against a brown background when Lugol's solution is applied. Their appearance may be strikingly similar to that of HPV-induced colpitis, except that the

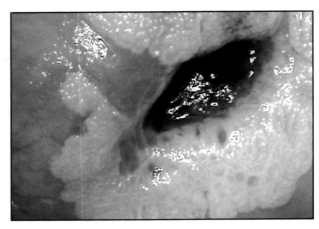

FIGURE 13.23   Extensive recurrence of CIN 1 post-cryotherapy.

HPV-induced changes are in a more random pattern. Many of these colposcopically identified minor changes will resolve spontaneously within 6 to 12 months after treatment. Major acetowhite lesions with or without punctation (Figure 13.23) should always be biopsied.

13.5.2 Other post-treatment findings

Other cervical findings include a "flush" cervix, coaptation of the external os following formation of occluding bands of tissue, or even complete stenosis and a completely distorted (knobby) cervix. Many post-treatment findings are fairly specific for the type of treatment that the patient received. For instance, a "puckered" appearance to the cervix is a typical effect of cryotherapy (Figure 13.24). A pronounced endocervical "button" may develop following laser or loop excision (Figure 13.25). Marked accentuation of a "button" may occur when a "groove" is sculpted into the cervical portio at the ectocervical margin of the ablated or excised area. The healing endocervical epithelium essentially everts onto the cervical portio, producing a red mushroom-like mass surrounding the endocervical os. The resulting "button" may look like a protruding endocervical polyp when present on only one side of the os (Figure 13.26). Such "pseudopolyps" can be differentiated from true polyps by gentle exploration of the broad base of the protruding columnar epithelium.

Any excisional or ablative treatment may narrow the cervical os and endocervical canal. The new squamocolumnar junction may assume an endocervical position beyond the field of colposcopic view. When this occurs, cytologic testing and colposcopy become less reliable follow-up procedures. Inade-

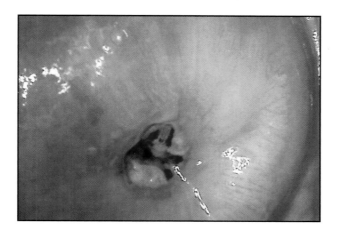

FIGURE 13.24   This "puckered" appearance is a typical finding in women who have undergone cryotherapy. Minor degrees of puckering can be seen after any ablative or excisional procedure. An area of recurrent CIN 2 is present at the new SCJ. ▬

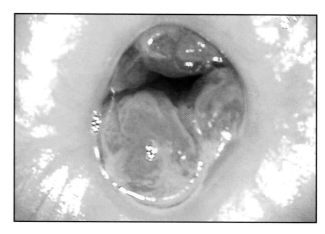

FIGURE 13.26   A groove at the edge of the treatment area during laser ablation of a high-grade lesion resulted in the appearance of several small polyps. These iatrogenically created pseudopolyps were recognized as not being true polyps because none were on a stalk. ▬

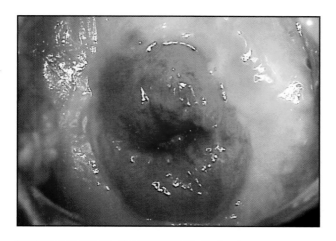

FIGURE 13.25   This pronounced endocervical "button" is typically seen following laser treatment and occurs when a "groove" is sculpted into the ectocervix to deliberately evert endocervical mucosa onto the portio. It may also occasionally be noted following LEEP. ▬

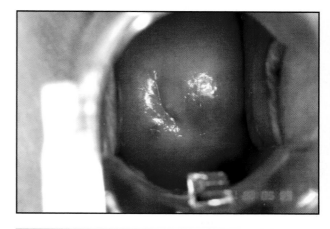

FIGURE 13.27   Cervical stenosis is seen in this premenopausal woman who began experiencing cyclic pain and amenorrhea after undergoing laser treatment for CIN.

quate sampling and poor visualization are less common problems in patients who undergo loop excision, laser ablation or excision, or cryotherapy in which a flat or very shallow cone probe is used.

Any surgical procedure performed within the lower genital tract can cause cervical stenosis, but it occurs most frequently (in 1% to 4% of cases) following laser or cold-knife conization (Figure 13.27).[35-37] Cervical stenosis can also occur after any ablative procedure, including laser ablation, diathermy, and cryotherapy when performed with a cryoprobe tip that extends more than 5 mm into the endocervical canal. The development of cervical stenosis following cryotherapy is rare when flat or minimally sculpted cryoprobes are used. Cervical stenosis resulting from a cervical procedure is more common in older women because of their lower estrogen levels and the increased incidence of disease within the endocervical canal requiring deeper excisional procedures. Post-treatment administration of vaginal estrogen during the healing phase may decrease the risk of stenosis in these women. Similarly, post-treatment stenosis may be more common in women who are using contraceptives containing only progestin during the post-treatment healing phase. Additionally, women who were exposed to DES in utero have been reported to have an increased risk for developing cervical stenosis of up to 75% following cervical treatment.[38,39] Cervical stenosis may be either complete, in which the os is closed, or incomplete, in which the cervix is narrowed, but still open. Usually therapeutic intervention is necessary only when a significant change in the menstrual history is reported. In a premenopausal woman, complete stenosis will result in entrapment of menstrual blood (hematometra), amenorrhea, severe cyclic dysmenorrhea, and infertility. In contrast, significant narrowing of the os may lead to diminished menstrual flow and increased dysmenorrhea. For the purpose of conducting a cervical examination in a patient with cervical stenosis, local anesthesia should be administered, and then a series of increasingly larger cervical dilators should be inserted one at a time to open the canal. The most effective treatments for complete cervical stenosis are carbon dioxide laser vaporization of a few millimeters of tissue at the proximal end of the stenosed os, or loop excision of the occluding tissue using a small (10 mm) loop electrode. Following either procedure, the patient should be rechecked weekly for the first several weeks to ensure that the os remains open. If the os begins to close, it should be gently reopened with a cervical dilator. Vaginal estrogen cream applied nightly for several weeks may decrease the risk of recurrent stenosis, as estrogen deficiency has been reported to increase the incidence of this problem post-laser ablation.[40]

13.6 Developmental Malformations

Several developmental anomalies of the cervix and vagina may contribute to difficulties in obtaining an adequate cytologic sample or to colposcopic evaluation of the cervix following an abnormal Pap smear. Vaginal malformations include transverse vaginal septa, complete and partial vaginal duplication, and Gartner's duct cysts derived from Wolffian duct remnants (discussed in Chapter 14). Vaginal agenesis and imperforate hymen are not discussed here since these conditions prohibit cervical screening and are therefore irrelevant to the colposcopist. Cervical malformations include a double cervical os and complete duplication of the cervix.

13.6.1 Transverse vaginal septum

Recanalization of the vaginal plate by the 20th week of gestation usually produces a completely patent vaginal canal.[16] However, in rare cases, failure to completely canalize the plate results in the formation of a transverse vaginal septum that can be located anywhere in the vagina.[41] Most commonly the septa

can be found in the cephalad or middle third of the vagina.[16] If the septum is completely imperforate, cyclic pain similar to that caused by an imperforate hymen will be felt at menarche, prompting the patient to seek medical help.[42] Often the presenting complaint will be mucocolpos or hematocolpos,[43,44] usually identifiable by ultrasound.[45,46] Degeneration of cells within the septum during vaginal recanalization will result in a perforated septum that often is not detected until the first attempt at sexual intercourse or vaginal speculum insertion. Increased canalization may leave only vaginal bands, rather than septa (Figure 13.28). Small openings in the septa may permit cervical evaluation. The most common complaint reported by patients who have incomplete transverse vaginal septa is dyspareunia. Significant vaginal discomfort may warrant surgical extirpation of the septum. When only vaginal bands are present, simple division of the bands using a surgical knife (a procedure that is easily accomplished in the office) usually suffices. Several incisions (such as at the 10 o'clock, 2 o'clock and 4 o'clock positions) may be necessary to remove more extensive septa.[16] Excision also may be necessary if the septum is fibrotic.

13.6.2 Vaginal and cervical duplication

When the paramesonephric ducts fail to fuse at their caudal end, duplication of the vagina, cervix, and uterus may occur.[16] Partial fusion at the extreme distal end of the paramesonephric ducts produces partial vaginal duplication. Partial or complete vaginal duplication is not extremely uncommon; therefore, colposcopists are likely to encounter this situation a

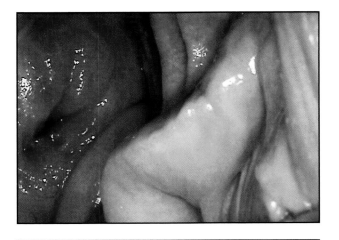

FIGURE 13.28 Large partial vaginal septum extends from near the hymen to the posterior cul de sac. ▬▬

number of times. The colposcopist is sometimes first alerted to the problem when colposcopy results do not correlate with cytologic results. This occurs when the Pap smear is taken from one cervix and the colposcopic evaluation is performed on the other cervix. A diligent search for the cause of a non-correlating colposcopy examination should lead to detection of the second vagina and cervix. When duplication is complete, the presence of an anterior-posterior septum and left and right vaginas adjacent to the hymeneal ring usually can be identified easily. However, vaginal duplication is often only partial and introduction of the speculum may displace the septum laterally. If this has occurred, the only finding upon colposcopic examination will be a lateral crease in the vaginal wall. Exploration of the crease with a cotton-tipped applicator will demonstrate either a patent canal, or in the case of partial duplication, a blind "pouch." The speculum can then be repositioned to evaluate the duplicated canal and cervix.

Alternatively, a longitudinal vaginal septum may be detected accidentally during bimanual examination of the cervix if one finger of the examiner's hand is inserted into one compartment and the other finger into the other compartment. In rare cases, duplication of the vagina causes dyspareunia; otherwise, most women with this condition are completely asymptomatic. Soft tissue damage may be noted during childbirth; however, the septum is usually able to stretch to accommodate the neonate. The finding of a duplicated vagina or cervix should instigate a thorough evaluation of the upper genital and urinary tracts to determine whether other areas of duplication exist. Complete duplication of the vagina is often associated with other anomalies within the genitourinary tract, whereas partial duplication is not.[16,46,47] If the patient is symptomatic, surgically separating the septum will eliminate dyspareunia.

13.6.3 Cervical anomalies

The most common cervical anomalies seen are the distorted shapes related to DES exposure in utero. These findings are discussed under "Vaginal Adenosis," in section 2.6 of this chapter. Duplication of the cervix is usually accompanied by complete or partial duplication of the vagina. However, occasionally a double os or a complete double cervix will be present without a vaginal septum. A false endocervical canal also may be present if a double os exists. This occurs when canalization of the cervical canal leaves a band of cervical tissue through the center of the cervical os. Exploration of each os with a small dilator or other probe will reveal a common endocervical canal.

13.7 Colposcopy of Sexual Assault Victims

13.7.1 Findings in consensual intercourse and non-intercourse-related trauma

Although the introital mucosa is quite elastic, even consensual sexual relations may produce traumatic microtears, superficial abrasions, and ecchymoses. The number and severity of injuries are usually less in women having consensual relations than in women sexually assaulted, but the sites where injuries occur are the same for women in both groups.[9,48] This is because the sites of tissue stress and the position of the male are usually the same. Most commonly, injuries sustained during consensual sexual relations occur because the female is not aroused adequately; thus, the introital mucosa is dry and not receptive to penetration except by force.[48] Since these characteristics differ from those of a woman being sexually assaulted only by the degree of force used during entry, it is not surprising that the locations of injuries in these 2 groups of patients are similar.[9,49]

Of women who sustained injuries while having consensual intercourse, 4% to 10% will have fissures in the posterior fourchette that can be identified without magnification (Figure 13.29).[9,49] Erythema in the mucosa of the hymen, introitus, and vagina secondary to vascular engorgement may also be seen in both women injured during consensual intercourse and those injured during sexual assault (Figure 13.30). When the trauma is minimal, the engorgement will

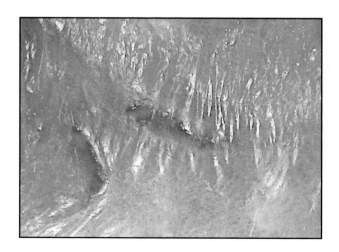

FIGURE 13.29 Minor fissures can be seen in the posterior fourchette of this woman who had consensual intercourse the prior evening. ■

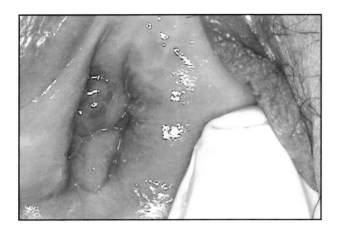

FIGURE 13.30   Erythema in the mucosa of the hymen, introitus, and vagina secondary to vascular engorgement is seen in this woman following consensual intercourse. These findings may be similar to erythema occurring with sexual assault, except that in rape cases other findings of genital trauma are likely. ▬

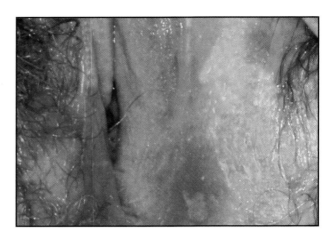

FIGURE 13.31   Introital abrasions are seen in a woman having consensual intercourse without adequate lubrication. Abrasions are usually very shallow and can sometimes be confused with herpes, particularly because they are often very sensitive to touch and to urine. ▬

be transitory, usually disappearing within minutes to hours after the sexual encounter occurs. However, with increasing friction and force against the dry mucosa, capillary walls rupture and ecchymoses appear. Prolonged, dry intercourse can occasionally cause abrasions at the introitus that can be quite painful, particularly during urination (Figure 13.31). Any decrease in normal mucosal thickness (i.e., atrophy) will enhance the potential for fissures, ecchymoses, or abrasions to occur.[50,51] Women with vulvovaginal candidiasis often present with introital fissures secondary to decreased elasticity resulting from inflammation-induced mucosal edema. Ecchymoses caused by sexual intercourse may be observed in the thinned epithelium of lichen sclerosus. Deep tears in the hymeneal ring have also been noted in women who have adjacent thick condyloma.

The second most common site of tears in a woman who has been injured during consensual sexual relations is in the lateral hymeneal ring at approximately the 3 o'clock and 9 o'clock positions (Figure 13.32).[9] The presenting complaint is either the sudden onset of coital-induced bleeding or localized searing pain. Once a laceration occurs, it will not heal until the woman abstains from intercourse for 2 to 4 weeks. The duration of healing depends upon the length of time that the laceration has been present. Any woman presenting with a history of introital dyspareunia should be asked whether the pain is generalized throughout the introitus or localized. Generalized discomfort is most commonly caused by vulvovaginal candidiasis, whereas localized pain is

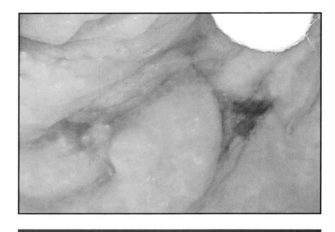

FIGURE 13.32   A tear is noted at the 3 o'clock position of the hymenal ring. This woman had consensual sexual relations before she was well lubricated. The presenting complaint was localized pain and bright red bleeding during intercourse. ▬

usually from an acute or chronically non-healing tear. A chronic tear will often have a yellow base of granulation tissue and hyperkeratotic ridges that are best identified through the colposcope (Figure 13.33).

Trauma may also result from nonsexual events. The examiner should ask the patient whether she has recently placed tampons or other foreign objects in the vagina. A fall onto the horizontal bar of a bicycle or a piece of gymnastic or playground equipment can cause injuries that range from minor tears and abra-

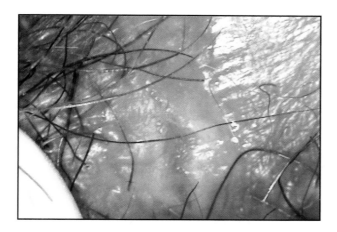

FIGURE 13.33   This 20-year-old woman presented with a complaint of localized dyspareunia of 2 months duration. A chronic tear was identified on the perineum. Note the elevated hyperkeratotic edges to the tear, indicating that this is not of an acute duration. Resolution occurred following 4 weeks of abstinence with lubrication once intercourse resumed.

sions to severe vulvar lacerations. In contrast to injuries sustained during sexual assault, these injuries are almost always located externally. Vigorous foreplay can also result in superficial mucosal trauma.

13.7.2 Findings in sexual assault

Sexual assault is not uncommon.[52] Thirteen percent of adolescent girls have been sexually assaulted, and 10% to 14% of women have been raped by a spouse.[9] Incest is also quite common, reported to happen to more than 25% of women. Unwanted sexual contact is the defining behavior that constitutes sexual assault.[9] Rape is sexual assault involving penetration, whereas sexual contact is sexual assault involving only external contact. In legal terms, sexual assault is considered rape if it meets the following criteria: (1) forced sexual intercourse occurred, (2) psychological coercion, verbal threats, and/or physical force were used, and (3) the person being assaulted did not consent to these actions.[52] Penile penetration is not required to satisfy the legal definition of rape, nor is penetration of the vagina. Any unwanted penetration by fingers, tongue, or foreign objects of the vagina, anus, or oral cavity is considered rape.[9] Also, by definition, rape can be committed by any individual, whether someone of the opposite sex or the same sex, and regardless of their relationship to the victim (eg, spouse, acquaintance, stranger).

While genital injury may not always occur during sexual assault, the majority (87%) of female rape victims will sustain one or more of the following injuries

(Figures 13.34a–d): (1) swelling, abrasions, and/or tears in the labia minora, posterior fourchette, fossa navicularis, and/or hymen, (2) abrasions, ecchymoses, and lacerations in the vagina, (3) ecchymoses and erosions on the cervix. These injuries have been given the acronym TEARS, which stands for: tears (T), ecchymoses (E), abrasions (A), redness (R), and swelling (S).[9,53] All of these injuries are more likely to occur during nonconsensual penetration rather than during consensual intercourse. In cases of sexual assault, the victim's vagina is not lubricated, physical constraints may place the pelvis in an awkward position, and insertion of the penis or other object into the vagina is usually by excessive force.[9,49] The anus is even more vulnerable to laceration during sexual assault because of the greater sphincter tone surrounding this orifice. Hence, forced anal copulation almost always causes perianal tears (Figure 13.35).[9]

When the perpetrator is in the superior position on top of a supine victim, the perpetrator exerts maximum force on the posterior fourchette during the rape. A woman who has been raped while in this position typically will have a combination of erythema, edema, ecchymoses, abrasions, and lacerations (tears) of the introitus from the 5 o'clock to the 7 o'clock position (Figure 13.36).[9,49,54] Forced penetration from any angle can result in abrasions and ecchymoses on the labia minora, and similar findings or lacerations in the hymen. Hymeneal swelling is often difficult to document at the time of the initial examination, but it can often be detected by comparing photographs taken at the follow-up examination with those taken initially.[55] Injuries are similar in adults and adolescents, except that hymeneal lacerations are more frequent in the latter.[54] In one study of adolescent victims of sexual assault the most common findings were tears in the posterior fourchette (36%); erythema of the labia minora, hymen, cervix, or posterior fourchette (18%–32%); and swelling of the hymen (19%).[54] More severe injuries are often seen in elderly female victims of sexual assault because of the increased mucosal atrophy and sexual abstinence in this population.[51] Abrasions and edema occur twice as frequently in sexual assault victims in this age group, and lacerations occur 4 times more frequently.

Other genital sites may be injured during sexual assault. Intense rubbing or sucking on the clitoris may produce swelling and ecchymoses. Cervical ecchymoses and erosions occur in approximately 13% of sexually assaulted women.[9] Vaginal lacerations are rare and found in only 1% of assault victims.[56] The elasticity of the vaginal walls protects against all but excessively violent thrusting or penetration with a sharp object. Forced oral copulation may traumatize the soft and hard palate, lips, gums

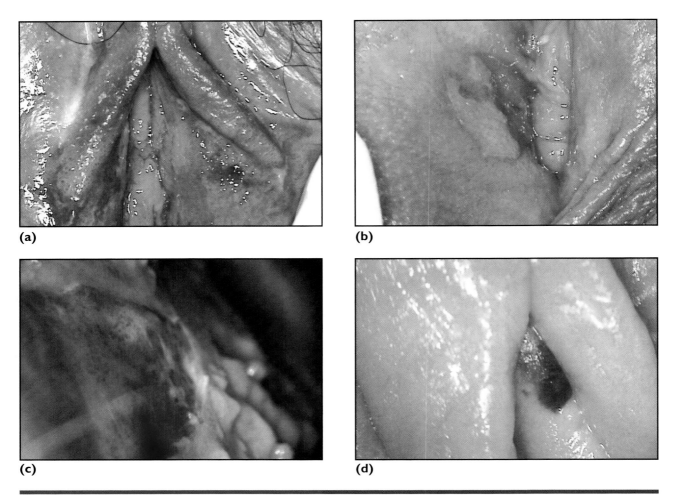

(a)

(b)

(c)

(d)

FIGURES 13.34a–d **(a)** Swelling and abrasions can be identified in the labia minora and introitus of this young assault victim, **(b)** abrasions 6 days post-rape reveal a yellow granulation to the base noted when the abrasion is several days old, **(c)** a vaginal abrasion was sustained when this woman was assaulted with a blunt object, **(d)** an ecchymotic area next to the clitoris is present post-assault.

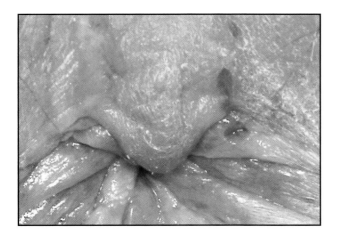

FIGURE 13.35 Perianal fissures are present in this individual who was sodomized. The ability of the anal sphincter to stretch usually prevents deep tears.

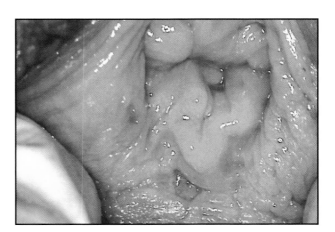

FIGURE 13.36 Introital tear several days post-sexual assault can be seen in consensual intercourse as well.

and uvula.[9] Oral trauma is manifested by erythema and ecchymoses, but swelling and petechiae have also been reported.

The 13% of women who do not have signs of physical injury following rape most commonly have been penetrated with less aggression, or have not fought back with as much resistance due to fear, than have women with injuries.[9] The importance of fully documenting injuries cannot be overstated. The examiner should be proficient in the colposcopic evaluation of the sexual assault victim. Examination without magnification can result in overlooking important occult findings. Whereas only 10% to 30% of genital injuries will be identified by the naked-eye examination, the detection rate increases to 87% when expert colposcopic evaluation is employed.[9,49,57] Special training in the colposcopic evaluation of the sexual assault victim is now available through many courses taught in the United States. These courses are becoming a prerequisite for those who serve as expert witnesses.

Another reason for not finding genital injuries following sexual assault is failure of the victim to seek medical care in a timely manner. Acute injuries almost always heal within 14 days, and shallow fissures and abrasions may be difficult to identify as early as 3 days after the assault.[9] Many victims are frightened, ashamed, or have other reasons for not seeking medical or legal attention immediately after the assault. Some women only seek medical evaluation after taking time to reflect on the events or at the urging of others. Additionally, whenever physical findings indicative of sexual assault are absent, the possibility that the alleged victim is making false allegations should be considered. False allegations are not common, but occasionally do occur, usually motivated by feelings of anger and/or guilt that are unrelated to the alleged assault.[9] Approximately 4% of sexual assault allegations are false.[9] Even when a false allegation is suspected, a comprehensive and completely nonjudgmental examination is mandatory.

References

1. Nucci M R. Symposium part III: tumor-like glandular lesions of the uterine cervix. *Int J Gynecol Pathol* 2002;21:347–59.
2. O'Brien P C, Noller K L, Robboy S J. Vaginal epithelial changes in young women enrolled in the National Cooperative Diethylstilbestrol Adenosis (DESAD) Project. *Obstet Gynecol* 1979;53:300–8.
3. Sherman A I. Cervical-vaginal adenosis after in utero exposure to synthetic estrogens. *Obstet Gynecol* 1974;44:531–45.
4. Herbst A L, Ulfelder H, Poskanzer D C. Adenocarcinoma of the vagina: Association of maternal stilbestrol therapy with tumor appearance in young women. *N Engl J Med* 1971;284:878–81.
5. Melnick S, Cole P, Anderson D, et al. Rates and risks of diethylstilbestrol-related clear cell adenocarcinoma of the vagina and cervix. *N Engl J Med* 1987;316:514–6.
6. Kaufman R H, Adam E. Findings in female offspring of women exposed in utero to diethylstilbestrol. *Obstet Gynecol* 2002;99:197–200.
7. Kaufman R H, Noller K, Adam E, Irwin J, Gray M, Jefferies J A, Hilton J. Upper genital tract abnormalities and pregnancy outcome in diethylstilbestrol-exposed progeny. *Am J Obstet Gynecol* 1984;148:973–84.
8. Jefferies J A, Robboy S J, O'Brien P C, Bergstralh E J, Labarthe D R, Barnes A B, Noller K L, Hatab P A, Kaufman R H, Townsend D E. Structural anomalies of the cervix and vagina in women enrolled in the Diethylstilbestrol Adenosis (DESAD) Project. *Am J Obstet Gynecol* 1984;148:59–66.
9. Girardin B W, Faugno D K, Seneski P C, Slaughter L, Whelan M. *Color Atlas of Sexual Assault.* St Louis, MO: Mosby Year Book, 1997.
10. Slaughter L, Brown C R V. Colposcopy to establish physical findings in rape victims. *Am J Obstet Gynecol* 1992;166:83.
11. Saunders N, Anderson D, Gilbert L, Sharp F. Unsatisfactory colposcopy and the response to orally administered oestrogen: a randomized double blind placebo controlled trial. *Br J Obstet Gynaecol* 1990;97:731–3.
12. Critchlow C W, Wolner-Hanssen P, Eschenbach D A, Kiviat N B, Koutsky L A, Stevens C E, Holmes K K. Determinants of cervical ectopia and of cervicitis: age, oral contraception, specific cervical infection, smoking, and douching. *Am J Obstet Gynecol* 1995;173:534–43.
13. Greeley C, Schroeder S, Silverberg S G. Microglandular hyperplasia of the cervix: a true "pill" lesion? *Int J Gynecol Pathol* 1995;14:50–4.
14. Selvaggi S M, Haefner H K. Microglandular endocervical hyperplasia and tubal metaplasia: pitfalls in the diagnosis of adenocarcinoma on cervical smears. *Diagn Cytopathol* 1997;16:168–73
15. Kranl C, Zelger B, Kofler H, Heim K, Sepp N, Fritsch P. Vulvar and vaginal adenosis. *Br J Dermatol* 1998;139:128–31.
16. Kaufman R H, Friedrich E G, Gardner H L. *Benign Diseases of the Vulva and Vagina.* Chicago, Ill: Year Book Medical Publishing; 1989.
17. Treffers P E, Hanselaar A G, Helmerhorst T J, Koster M E, van Leeuwen F E. [Consequences of diethylstilbestrol during pregnancy; 50 years later still a significant problem] *Ned Tijdschr Geneeskd* 2001;145:675–80.

18. Hatch E E, Palmer J R, Titus-Ernstoff L, et al. Cancer risk in women exposed to diethylstilbestrol in utero. *JAMA* 1998;280:630–4.

19. Titus-Ernstoff L, Hatch E E, Hoover R N, et al. Long-term cancer risk in women given diethylstilbestrol (DES) during pregnancy. *Br J Cancer* 2001;84:126–33.

20. Palmer J R, Hatch E E, Rosenberg C L, et al. Risk of breast cancer in women exposed to diethylstilbestrol in utero: preliminary results (United States). *Cancer Causes Control* 2002;13:753–8.

21. Dungar C F, Wilkinson E J. Vaginal columnar cell metaplasia. An acquired adenosis associated with topical 5-fluorouracil therapy. *J Reprod Med* 1995;40:361–6.

22. Bornstein J, Sova Y, Atad J, Lurie M, Abramovici H. Development of vaginal adenosis following combined 5-fluorouracil and carbon dioxide laser treatments for diffuse vaginal condylomatosis. *Obstet Gynecol* 1993;81:896–8.

23. Goodman A, Zukerberg L R, Nikrui N, Scully R E. Vaginal adenosis and clear cell carcinoma after 5-fluorouracil treatment for condylomas. *Cancer* 1991;68:1628–32.

24. Hanselaar A, van Loosbroek M, Schuurbiers O, Helmerhorst T, Bulten J, Bernhelm J. Clear cell adenocarcinoma of the vagina and cervix. An update of the central Netherlands registry showing twin age incidence peaks. *Cancer* 1997;79:2229–36.

25. Noller K L. Role of colposcopy in the examination of diethylstilbestrol-exposed women. In: Wright VC, ed. Contemporary Colposcopy. *Obstet Gynecol Clin* 1993;20:165–76.

26. Bachmann G A, Nevadunsky N S. Diagnosis and treatment of atrophic vaginitis. *Am Fam Physician* 2000;61:3090–6.

27. Miller L, Patton D L, Meier A, Thwin S S, Hooton T M, Eschenbach D A. Depomedroxyprogesterone-induced hypoestrogenism and changes in vaginal flora and epithelium. *Obstet Gynecol* 2000;96:431–9.

28. Selvaggi S M. Atrophic vaginitis versus invasive squamous cell carcinoma on ThinPrep® cytology: Can the background be reliably distinguished? *Diagn Cytopathol* 2002;27:362–4.

29. Acs G, Gupta P K, Baloch Z W. Glandular and squamous atypia and intraepithelial lesions in atrophic cervicovaginal smears. One institution's experience. *Acta Cytol* 2000;44:611–7.

30. Davis G D. Colposcopic examination of the vagina. *Obstet Gynecol Clinic N Amer* 1993;20:217.

31. Shield P W. Chronic radiation effects: a correlative study of smears and biopsies from the cervix and vagina. *Diagn Cytopathol* 1995;13:107–19.

32. Anderson M, Jordan J A, Morse A R, Sharp F. A *Text and Atlas of Integrated Colposcopy*. Mosby. London. 1991. p. 80.

33. Valdini A, Vaccaro C, Pechinsky G, Abernathy V. Incidence and evaluation of an AGUS Papanicolaou smear in primary care. *J Am Board Fam Pract* 2001;14:172–7.

34. Wright T C Jr, Cox J T, Massad L S, Twiggs L B, Carlson J, Wilkinson E J; 2001 ASCCP-Sponsored Consensus Conference. 2001 Consensus Guidelines for the management of women with cervical intraepithelial neoplasia. *J Low Gen Tract Dis.* 2003;7:154–67.

35. Mitchell M F, et al. A randomized clinical trial of cryotherapy, loop electrosurgical excision for treatment of squamous intraepithelial lesions of the cervix. *Obstet Gynecol* 1998;92:737–44.

36. A El-Toukhy S, Mahadevan A E, Davies T. Cold knife cone biopsy—a valid diagnostic tool and treatment option for lesions of the cervix. *J Obstet Gynaecol* 2001;21:175–8.

37. Diakomanolis E, Haidopoulos D, Rodolakis A, Messaris E, Sakellaropoulos G, Calpaktsoglou C, Michalas S. Treating intraepithelial lesions of the uterine cervix by laser CO_2. Evaluation of the past, appraisal for the future. *Eur J Gynaecol Oncol* 2002;23:463–8.

38. Schmidt G, Fowler W C Jr. Cervical stenosis following minor gynecologic procedures on DES-exposed women. *Obstet Gynecol* 1980;56:333–5.

39. Kalstone C. Cervical stenosis in pregnancy: a complication of cryotherapy in diethylstilbestrol-exposed women. *Am J Obstet Gynecol* 1992;166:502–3.

40. Spitzer M, Krumholz B A, Seltzer V L. Cervical os obliteration after laser surgery in patients with amenorrhea. *Obstet Gynecol* 1990 ;76:97–100.

41. Deppich L M. Transverse vaginal septum: histologic and embryologic considerations. *Obstet Gynecol* 1972;39:193.

42. Fritz E B, Carlan S J, Greenbaum L. Pregnancy and transvaginal septation. *J Matern Fetal Neonatal Med* 2002;11:414–6.

43. Ahmed S, Morris L L, Atkinson E. Distal mucocolpos and proximal hematocolpos secondary to concurrent imperforate hymen and transverse vaginal septum. *J Pediatr Surg* 1999;34:1555–6.

44. Rana A, Manandhar B, Amatya A, Baral J, Gurung G, Giri A, Giri K. Mucocolpos due to complete transverse septum in middle third of vagina in a 17-year-old girl. *Obstet Gynaecol Res* 2002;28:86–8.

45. Thabet S M, Thabet A S. Role of new sono-imaging technique 'sonocolpography' in the diagnosis and treatment of the complete transverse vaginal septum and other allied conditions. *J Obstet Gynaecol Res.* 2002;28:80-5.

46. Rosenburg H K, Udassin R, Howell C, et al. Duplication of the uterus and vagina, unilateral hydrometrocolpos, and ipsilateral renal agenesis: Sonographic aid to diagnosis. *J Ultrasound Med* 1982;1:289–91.

47. Balasch J, Moreno E, Martinez-Roman S, Molini J L, Torne A, Sanchez-Martin F, Vanrell J A. Septate uterus with cervical duplication and longitudinal vaginal septum: a report of three new cases. *Eur J Obstet Gynecol Reprod Biol* 1996;65:241–3.

48. Elam A L, Ray V G. Sexually related trauma: A review. *Ann Emerg Med.* 1986;15:576.

49. Slaughter L, Brown C R, Crowley S, Peck R. The pattern of genital injury in female sexual assault victims. *Am J Obstet Gynecol* 1997;176:609.

50. Cartwright P S. Factors that correlate with injury sustained by survivors of sexual assault. *Obstet Gynecol* 1987;70:44–6.

51. Cartwright P, Moore A. Elderly victims of rape. *South Med J* 1989;82:988.

52. US Bureau of Justice Statistics. *Violent Crime* (NCI-147486). US Dept of Justice, Washington, DC: US Bureau of Justice Statistics; 1995. 51

53. Slaughter L, Brown C R V. Cervical findings in rape victims. *Am J Obstet Gynecol* 1991;164:528.

54. Slaughter L, Shackelford S. Genital injury in rape. *Adolesc Pediatr Gynecol.* 1993;6:175.

55. Adams J A, Girardin B, Faugno D. Adolescent sexual assault: documentation of acute injuries using photo-colposcopy. *J Pediatr Adolesc Gynecol* 2001;14:175–80.

56. Geist R F. Sexually related trauma. *Emer Med Clin N Amer* 1988;6:439.

57. Lenahan L C, Ernst A, Johnson B. Colposcopy in evaluation of the adult sexual assault victim. *Am J Emerg Med* 1998;16:183–4.

Colposcopy of the Vagina

Table of Contents

14.1 Introduction to Vaginal Colposcopy

For many decades the colposcope was utilized almost exclusively to evaluate the cervix. Even when a Pap smear abnormality remained unexplained by colposcopy of the cervix, the vagina was rarely evaluated. The reasons for this oversight may lie in the rarity of vaginal cancer. Hence few colposcopists had training or experience in detecting vaginal neoplasia colposcopically. The recognition that recurrent or residual intraepithelial neoplasia may occur in the vagina post-hysterectomy and the link between diethylstilbestrol (DES) exposure and vaginal clear-cell adenocarcinoma led to an awareness that in many clinical situations it was important to evaluate the vagina as well as the cervix. While early texts on colposcopy did not mention evaluation of the vagina,[1] colposcopy of the vagina is now included in most colposcopy courses and textbooks. The first description of vaginal intraepithelial neoplasia (VAIN) was published in 1933.[2] However, because of the delay in inclusion of colposcopy of the vagina in traditional training, VAIN continued to be considered to be a rare entity. In 1981, Woodruff reported that only 300 cases of VAIN CIS of the vagina could be found in the world literature.[3]

Of course, once vaginal colposcopy became a routine procedure for the clinical situations listed below, it quickly became evident that VAIN, especially low-grade VAIN, is a very common finding.[4] Increasingly, evaluation of other perplexing clinical

Table 14.1 Indications for Performing Meticulous Vaginal Colposcopy

(1) An abnormal Papanicolaou (Pap) smear following hysterectomy
(2) An abnormal Pap smear after apparently successful treatment of cervical neoplasia
(3) Any Pap smear unexplained by cervical colposcopy or sampling of the endocervical canal
(4) Any palpable or unexplained grossly visible vaginal lesion
(5) All women with cervical, vulvar or perianal/anal HPV disease
(6) Confirmed cervical neoplasia in an immunosuppressed patient
(7) Monitoring all women with a history of in-utero DES exposure
(8) Any woman with abnormal, unexplained, recalcitrant vaginal discharge or bleeding
(9) All women with unexplained introital pain and/or dyspareunia
(10) Prior to cervical conization for non-correlating cytology, histology and colposcopic impression

problems such as introital pain, profuse chronic leukorrhea, unexplained post-coital spotting and non-correlating colposcopy all became less perplexing under the gaze of the expert colposcopist. In a short 30 years, vaginal colposcopy has become indispensable for the evaluation of diseases of the lower genital tract.

14.2 Indications for Vaginal Colposcopy

While some evaluate the vagina routinely whenever cervical colposcopy is indicated, most colposcopists reserve intensive vaginal colposcopic appraisal for women with a history of DES exposure, or with symptoms or abnormal cervical cytology that remain unexplained following cervical evaluation.[5,6] The amount of time and thoroughness spent during vaginal evaluation will depend on the clinical situation. The reason for this measured approach is the rarity of serious vaginal neoplasia and the tedious and time-consuming nature of a comprehensive vaginal colposcopic inspection. The specific indications that demand a more meticulous colposcopic assessment of the entire vagina are shown in (Table 14.1).

14.3 Technique of Vaginal Colposcopy

Careful gross assessment of the vagina can be easily performed during speculum removal after every cervical colposcopy exam; however, colposcopy permits a more accurate examination of the vaginal epithelium when a thorough clinical assessment is indicated. The vagina is much more difficult to evaluate than the cervix because it includes a much larger surface area; areas are hidden under speculum blades, between rugae, in the fornices, and in the vaginal

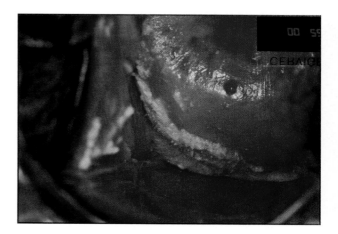

FIGURE 14.1 Vaginal lesions in the cul de sac and posterior vaginal wall can be most difficult to detect because the posterior blade of the speculum will cover this area, and the cervix will usually drop back into the cul de sac as the speculum is removed. Adequate visualization often requires manipulation of the cervix anteriorly with an Ayre spatula or other instrument as the speculum is rotated to expose the posterior vaginal wall. Patience and dexterity are often required. Here the speculum has been manipulated to expose condylomas in the cul de sac.

reflection proximal of the cul de sac (Figure 14.1).[5] Furthermore, the majority of the epithelium is parallel to the plane of visual inspection. Thus, a greater degree of manual dexterity and patience are demanded of the colposcopist. Full colposcopic evaluation of the vagina may add some discomfort in comparison with that of the cervix only. However, sedation and anesthesia are rarely necessary even when the patient is extremely anxious and the likelihood exists of an extensive, prolonged examination and multiple biopsies.

Vaginal colposcopy is usually performed on completion of the cervical examination unless the cervix is absent from previous hysterectomy. However, evaluation of the vestibule is often warranted and is best done prior to application of Lugol's solution to the vagina. Hence, prior to insertion of the speculum, a quick inspection of the hymen, the proximal mucosa, the minor and major vestibular gland openings and urethral meatus will usually suffice to assure normalcy or to indicate the need for more detailed assessment. Once this is completed, if the vagina is not atrophic or particularly small, a medium Grave's or larger speculum may be inserted. The cervix or vaginal vault is visualized prior to the application of acetic acid. If there have been any symptoms attributable to the vagina or an abnormal discharge is noted, a sample of this discharge should be collected first for microscopic examination and appropriate cultures. The cervix should then be evaluated in the manner described in Chapter 7. Following completion of the cervical evaluation, if a pool of acetic acid is not already present, it is best to first apply a saline-soaked cotton-ball or large swab to the vaginal walls to remove discharge. The vagina can then be visualized prior to the application of acetic acid, which may obscure abnormal vaginal vessels, just as it may similarly obscure cervical vasculature. The looser connective tissue of the vagina is more richly vascularized than that of the cervix. Consequently, somewhat more enhanced punctation and atypical vessels are found grade-for-grade in lesions in the vagina compared with cervical lesions. However, mosaic vascular changes are uncommon in the vagina. The normal vaginal epithelium has a fine terminal capillary network that is similar to that seen on the cervix (Figure 14.2). The vascular pattern may be diffusely enhanced by inflammation (Figure 14.3), whereas

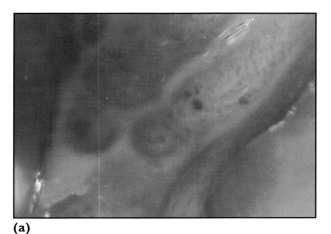

(a)

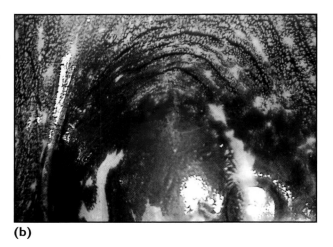

(b)

FIGURE 14.2   Typical network capillaries within the native squamous epithelium of the vagina resemble those seen in similar epithelium of the cervix. The diffuse nature of the vessels and the uniform caliber and shape reassure that the vessels are normal. However, vessels on the ridges of rugae can be accentuated by trauma such as is seen here with overuse of tampons. ■

FIGURES 14.3a,b   **(a)** Diffuse punctation as demonstrated in this woman with vaginal streptococcal infection is seen only in inflammatory conditions. In contrast, punctation due to neoplasia is localized within the margins of the lesion. **(b)** Application of Lugol's iodine to the vagina of the patient in **(a)** demonstrates diffuse spotty non-staining. ■

vascular changes in neoplasia will be localized to a circumscribed lesion. Atrophy may also diffusely enhance the appearance of the vascular pattern by thinning the overlying epithelium through which the vessels are seen (Figure 14.4).

Once the vagina has been evaluated in this manner for vaginal discharge and vascular changes, a cotton ball soaked in 3% to 5% acetic acid is applied gently to the upper vagina using a large cotton swab. A further acetic acid application then follows. A dry cotton ball is used to remove the excess acetic acid and mucus. The vaginal fornices and vault are then assessed. Because these areas are often difficult to view, manipulation of the cervix with small or large cotton tipped applicators can aid in visualization. To assess the right lateral fornix, press the cotton tip carefully but firmly in the left lateral fornix (Figures 7.6a,b). This moves the cervix to the left and stretches the rugous folds in the right fornix. After examining the right fornix, transfer the cotton tipped applicator to the opposite side and press firmly to examine the left fornix. Similarly, anterior and posterior fornices can be assessed by raising or depressing the cervix by firm pressure with the cotton tipped applicator in the fornix opposite the one to be studied. If these maneuvers are unsuccessful, a wooden spatula may be pressed directly against the cervix to gently coax it away from each fornix.

If the patient has had a hysterectomy, the folds (corners) or "dog ears" in the lateral aspects of the vault can be difficult to assess. This is occasionally problematic since recurrent neoplasia may be hidden in these folds. A hook or mirror can help gain access to these important sites. However, the hook may be uncomfortable and will frequently cause bleeding. The Campion endocervical forcep (modified deJardin's gallbladder forceps, discussed in Chapter 6) or a narrow endocervical speculum may also be used to gain access to these hidden areas. It is wise to apply acetic acid deep into the fold using a small cotton-tipped applicator, since the initial application with a larger swab or cotton-ball may not have penetrated into these areas.

The vaginal sidewalls will have been exposed to the acetic acid at the time of application to the vaginal vault or fornices. After examination of these areas, the middle and proximal sidewalls should be evaluated colposcopically, with reapplication of acetic acid as necessary. Once completed, the speculum can be collapsed, then gently rotated to the lateral position to expose the anterior and posterior vaginal walls. Significant vaginal atypia is often more common on anterior and posterior walls, which are sheltered by the blades of the examining speculum, so it is very important to examine these more

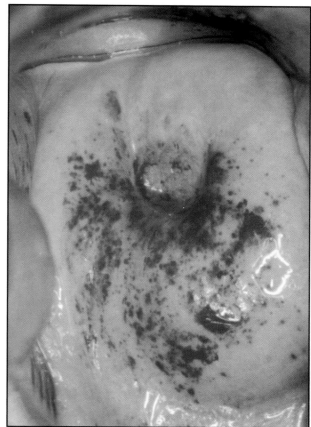

(a)

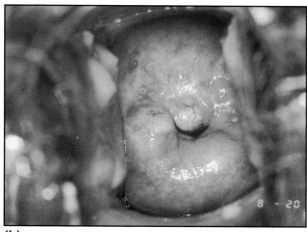

(b)

FIGURES 14.4a,b **(a)** This post-menopausal woman demonstrates classic findings secondary to the effects of estrogen loss on the vaginal epithelium including ecchymosis secondary to capillary fragility, and pale, thin epithelium. **(b)**. Significant atrophic changes and multiple Nabothian cysts are noted in this 36-year-old woman on Depo-Provera®.

inaccessible areas. Sufficient time must be taken to permit the acetic acid reaction to occur and a degree of dexterity is required in manipulating the speculum and reapplying the acetic acid. During this time the exposed areas can be inspected with the colposcope. This can be the most uncomfortable part of the exam, so rotation should be accomplished with care and should not be rushed. Before returning the speculum to the standard anterior-posterior position, stain the anterior and posterior vaginal walls with ½ strength Lugol's solution and inspect fully for non-staining yellow areas, and then do the same for the lateral vaginal walls. Rotation of the speculum after Lugol's application can be difficult as the dehydrating effect of Lugol's solution on the epithelium often results in significant resistance to manipulation of the speculum. This problem can be avoided by covering the external surface of the speculum blades with a thin film of lubricating jelly prior to insertion.[6]

An alternative to the approach discussed above is to complete the entire vaginal exam with acetic acid and also visualize the anterior and posterior vaginal walls as they fold into view during speculum removal, then reinsert a lubricated speculum. After application of Lugol's solution to the lateral side-walls, Lugol's can be applied to the anterior and posterior vaginal walls as the speculum is slowly withdrawn for the second time. When possible, however, most women prefer that the speculum be introduced only a single time.

Except for the indications listed in (Table 14.1), such comprehensive evaluation of the vagina is not standard. For the majority of colposcopy examinations performed for the evaluation of an abnormal Pap smear, a more cursory evaluation may be appropriate. The vagina can be evaluated reasonably for these women at lower risk of having vaginal lesions by closely observing the vaginal walls through the colposcope as the speculum is slowly withdrawn. The speculum can be gently rotated as it is withdrawn and Lugol's solution can be applied to the vaginal walls as they fold into view. Sharply demarcated non-staining areas, if of significant concern, may be further evaluated by withdrawing the speculum and reinserting in 5 to 10 minutes. The Lugol's effect does not persist beyond this time interval, so the area in question can be more completely evaluated after the staining has dissipated. A non staining yellow pattern that identifies sharply demarcated lesion(s) is the most reliable and accurate predictor of the presence of premalignant vaginal epithelium. However, once located, the severity of the disease process cannot be carefully appraised without full evaluation of the non-staining areas before and after acetic acid. Many

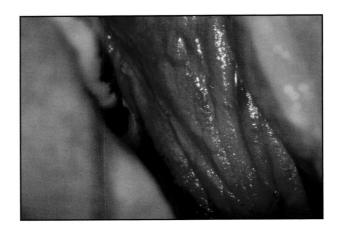

FIGURE 14.5   Diffuse non-staining of the vaginal epithelium occurs in women with inadequate estrogen priming of the vaginal epithelium and compromises evaluation of the vagina for significant lesions. This occurs most frequently in women who are post-menopausal, but is also frequently seen in women on Depo-Provera. Diffuse non-staining can also occur with excessive tampon use such as seen in this young well-estrogenized woman. ■

non-staining areas will be obvious low-grade flat HPV lesions, often with small asperites that help to confirm the diagnosis without the need to perform this extra step. At completion of the exam, excess iodine should be removed and the patient given a pad to wear to catch residual iodine that could permanently stain clothes.

In patients on progestin-only contraception and in women in the postmenopause, significant vaginal mucosal atrophy may prohibit adequate colposcopic evaluation of the vagina. Since inadequate estrogen results in loss of the normal glycogen storage in the vaginal cells, Lugol's uptake may be minimal and landmarks between normal and neoplastic epithelium may be lost (Figure 14.5). When the patient is found during colposcopy to have inadequate estrogen to exclude significant vaginal neoplasia, repeat colposcopy after a course of vaginal estrogen cream may appropriate.[6] Vaginal atrophic changes may even be present in up to 10% of post-menopausal women on oral estrogen replacement therapy regardless of the dose, and in younger women who use Depo-Provera® for contraception or Lupron for treatment of endometriosis or uterine myoma. Under these circumstances a course of one gram of topical vaginal estrogen is prescribed for daily insertion for 3 weeks, followed soon thereafter by repeat colposcopy. It is unlikely that any of the usual medical contraindications to estrogen use would place the patient at risk in the use of such a short course of minimally absorbed estrogen. Therefore, there are few situations where such a short course of topical estrogen is contraindicated in the interest of excluding or detecting significant vaginal neoplasia.

14.4 Vaginal Biopsy

Because the colposcopic findings of neoplasia are less specific in the vagina than on the cervix, colposcopists are far less accurate in the evaluation of vaginal findings. Therefore, biopsy is necessary in all but obvious low-grade lesions. Prior to the advent of colposcopy, strip biopsies under anesthesia were often utilized in an attempt to determine the size and distribution of VAIN.[3] Colposcopically directed punch biopsies are more accurate and can be taken from most areas of the vagina without injection of local anesthetic. A sharp biopsy forceps is mandatory. The Burke or Tischler biopsy forceps are superior in this setting. If disease extends well into the lateral fornices, or into the corners of the vaginal cuff commonly present following hysterectomy, these lateral folds may need to be everted as far as possible using a skin hook or tenaculum. Biopsy of posthysterectomy folds may be more sensitive and may require injection with a local anesthetic. The absence of glandular structures or skin appendages in most vaginal mucosa allows biopsy specimens to be only 1.5 mm–3.0 mm in depth, while still adequately sampling the mucosa and underlying stromal tissue.

The biopsy should be taken quickly and accurately after warning the patient of a possible "twinge of discomfort." Because the upper two-thirds of the vagina has little to no nerve supply, vaginal biopsy of these areas usually results in little to no discomfort. Therefore, injection with a local anesthetic is rarely required except for biopsy in the lower one-third of the vagina. If multiple biopsies are required in the presence of extensive disease, consideration may be given to examination under general or regional anesthesia, but the need for this is rare. Biopsies should be taken as perpendicular to the vaginal mucosa as possible to ensure an adequate sample. Bleeding is usually minimal and is readily stopped by application of Monsel's solution or silver nitrate (Figures 14.6a,b).

14.5 Colposcopy of Benign Vaginal Epithelial Changes

The vagina hosts a complex ecosystem and is commonly subjected to trauma from tampon insertion, intercourse, lubricants, creams, diaphragms, and

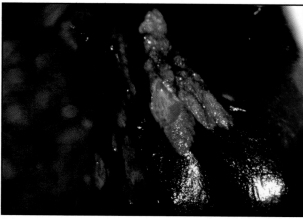

(a)

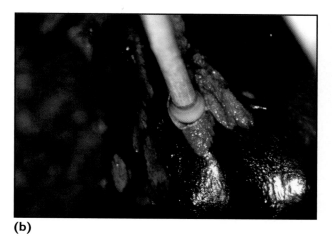

(b)

FIGURES 14.6a,b **(a)** Vaginal biopsies usually bleed very little but when bleeding does occur, **(b)** Hemostasis can be obtained by application of either Monsel's solution or with a silver nitrate stick such as seen here.

other items. It is, therefore, common that many factors unrelated to neoplasia may significantly alter the vaginal appearance and either obscure otherwise normal colposcopic findings, or mimic neoplasia. The colposcopist must become familiar with the colposcopic patterns presented by these entities; failure to do so will diminish the ability to accurately diagnose both benign and neoplastic vaginal changes. Mastering the following colposcopic appearances will help bridge the gap of diagnostic capability between the "cervical" colposcopist and the expert in diagnosis of all lower genital tract diseases. Several colposcopic appearances may be found in the vagina that are not related to neoplastic disease and may obscure the usual colposcopic findings when neoplasia is present (Table 14.2).

Table 14.2 Colposcopic Appearances That May Obscure or Mimic Neoplasia

Inflammation
   Trichomonas
   Candida
   Bacteria induced desquamative disorders
   Erosive lichen planus
   Atrophic "vaginitis"
   Radiation induced atrophy
Congenital transformation zone
Vaginal adenosis
Vaginal ulcers
Granulation tissue
Endometriosis

14.5.1 Inflammation

Inflammatory conditions may hamper colposcopic evaluation of the vagina by enhancing vascularity, by thinning or denuding epithelium, and by decreasing glycogen storage in the epithelium. This may hamper evaluation for neoplasia or DES sequelae. Therefore, specifically identified inflammatory conditions should be treated and the patient should return for reevaluation after the vaginal mucosa has had time for epithelial regeneration and healing prior to final colposcopic evaluation. These inflammatory conditions include infections caused by Candida, Trichomonas vaginalis and bacteria-induced desquamative disorders.

14.5.1.1 Candida

Vaginal candidiasis is the most common cause of non-neoplastic vaginal colposcopic changes in premenopausal women. Although Candida is often present without an associated inflammatory response, when inflammation occurs, it may result in excessive desquamation of the vaginal epithelium, producing thickened areas interspersed with thinned epithelium (Figure 14.7). These thickened pseudomembranous areas are called "thrush patches" and if localized, may at first glance mimic hyperkeratotic patches secondary to neoplasia or to diaphragm use. When these patches are removed, the underlying mucosa is frequently denuded, unroofing inflammation-induced increased vascularity. The resulting shallow erosions and bleeding may cause diagnostic confusion.

More commonly, "thrush patches" are not present with vaginal candidiasis. Instead, the vaginal epithelium may vary in appearance from normal to diffusely or patchy mild erythema. Application of acetic acid will highlight epithelial regeneration and repair, which will appear as various degrees of enhanced acetowhite epithelium due to the increased nuclear density of epithelial cells undergoing repair and the associated stromal inflammatory process. Lugol's iodine uptake may range from diffuse to patchy yellow, to normal brown interspersed with a background of tiny non-staining spots. Such spots, also termed "reverse punctation," may also be seen with minimal HPV expression and are, therefore, non-specific (Figures 14.8a,b). When Candida causes patchy uptake of Lugol's iodine, the borders of the iodine positive areas are usually vague and diffuse (Figure 14.9a), unlike the sharper borders noted in high-grade VAIN (Figure 14.9b). However, low grade VAIN may have either sharp borders or the ill defined borders observed with Candida. In general, however, Candida induced vaginal changes are more commonly diffuse and lack the increased epithelial thickness noted with VAIN.

Some patients will not have symptoms related to Candida yet will be found during colposcopy to have findings suggestive of Candida vaginitis. Confirmation of yeast may be compromised by acetic acid and aqueous iodine already applied to the vaginal walls. When this occurs, vaginal scrapings may often be obtained from behind the anterior speculum blade for pH, KOH and saline wet-mount microscopic evaluation. If yeast is confirmed and the colposcopic evaluation of the vagina is compromised by this infection, then the patient will require antifungal treatment before returning for a repeat colposcopy exam. Vulvovaginal Candidiasis may be treated with either topical or oral antifungal medication. The exam should not

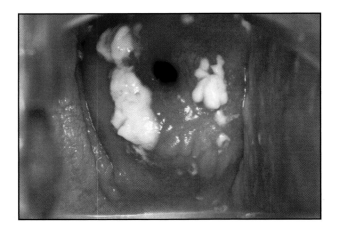

FIGURE 14.7 Thickened areas of adherent desquamated vaginal cells and mycelia "thrush patches" interspersed with thinned inflamed areas are seen in some women with vulvovaginal candidiasis.

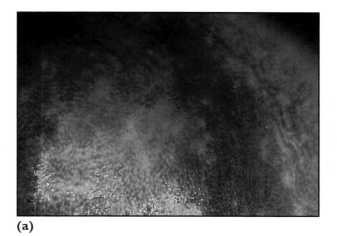

(a)

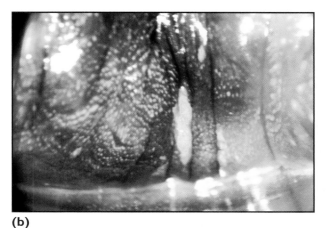

(b)

FIGURES 14.8a,b "Reverse punctation" may be seen in several inflammatory conditions as well as in women with minimal vaginal HPV expression. **(a)** this colpo-photograph demonstrates these tiny nonstaining punctate areas in a woman with vaginal candidiasis. **(b)** the likely HPV etiology of "reverse punctation" seen on the cervix and in the left vaginal fornix in this patient is strengthened by the well-circumscribed adjacent VAIN 1. Photos courtesy of Dr. Ken Hatch.

be repeated for at least two weeks following completion of the treatment in order to allow adequate time for vaginal epithelial regeneration.

14.5.1.2 Trichomonas

Although many women with Trichomonas vaginitis have only diffuse vaginal erythema, small hemorrhagic papules termed "strawberry spots" frequently dot the vagina (Figures 14.10a,b). Each of these red spots consists of the tips of a cluster of greatly dilated sub-epithelial capillaries that reach almost to the surface and are enhanced by desquamation of the overlying vaginal epithelium. Because these papules are denuded of much of the overlying epithelium, only

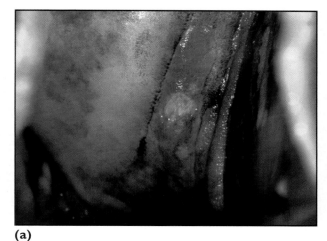

(a)

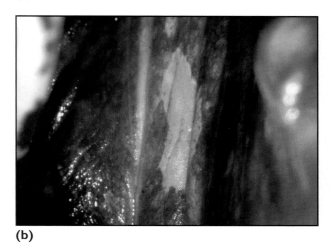

(b)

FIGURES 14.9a,b **(a)** Diffuse borders to nonstaining areas are seen with inflammatory conditions such as the vaginal candidiasis this woman has. Biopsy (site shown here) demonstrated only inflammation. **(b)** Contrast with the sharply nonstaining areas of this VAIN.

immature, non-glycogenated squamous cells are present. Lugol staining will, therefore, show a multitude of minute to large non-staining yellow spots. The larger spots are characteristically so denuded that they do not even stain yellow, but instead appear pink on the mahogany background (Figure 14.11).

The colposcopic appearance of "strawberry spots" has been termed colpitis macularis and is virtually classic for trichomonas cervicitis/vaginitis.[7,8] In one study, colpitis macularis was detected by colposcopy in 52 of 118 trichomonas infected women. Women with colpitis macularis had more trichomonas on wet mount (mean 18 +/− 20 Trichomonas vaginalis organisms/field × 400 magnification) compared with women with Trichomonas but without colpitis macularis (7 +/− 17).[7] However,

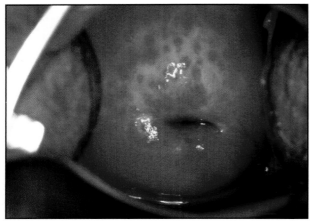

(a)

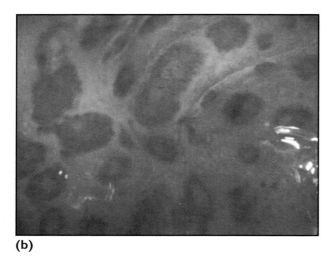

(b)

FIGURES 14.10a,b **(a)** Classic "strawberry spots" of vaginal trichomonal infection represent terminal capillary dilation. Similar spots can occasionally be seen in desquamative inflammatory vaginitis and in vaginal streptococcal infection. **(b)** Terminal capillaries are clearly seen at higher magnification. Fig. 14.10b Photo courtesy of Dr. VC Wright, Biomedical Communications, Houston, Texas. ▬

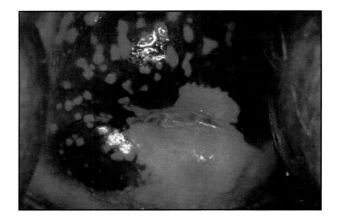

FIGURE 14.11 Loss of surface epithelium over dilated terminal capillaries leaves these areas devoid of squamous cells that would normally stain yellow in the absence of glycogen. This results in complete rejection of aqueous iodine stain and a glistening, pink, almost raw appearance to these "spots" post-Lugols. ▬

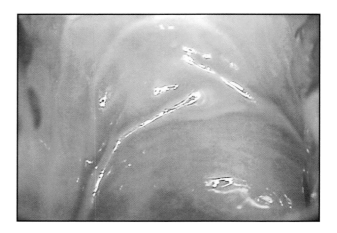

FIGURE 14.12 Frothy, greenish-yellow, watery vaginal discharge commonly seen in trichomonas infections. Many women with this disease will not have such classic findings. Digitalization artifact over areas of glare. ▬

two other entities may occasionally mimic trichomonas.[9] Some women with desquamative inflammatory vaginitis (see below) have a vaginal inflammatory appearance similar to trichomonas induced "strawberry spots". Additionally, extensive erosion of the vaginal epithelium often noted during treatment of vaginal HPV induced lesions with 5-fluorouracil (5-FU) causes small diffuse "papules" of vaginal adenosis that may be challenging to discriminate from a trichomonas infection (see below).

More often, "strawberry spots" are caused by Trichomonas vaginalis. Since they can normally be seen prior to application of acetic acid and aqueous iodine, vaginal secretions for saline and KOH wet mounts and vaginal pH testing can be collected without compromising the specimen. Classic trichomonal discharge is usually described as thin and watery, with a frothy (Figure 14.12), greenish-yellow tint and a pH of >4.5. However, the discharge may be minimal or creamy yellow in color and without a frothy appearance.[8] Other than recognizing the cause of this unusual colposcopic appearance and treating the infection, the primary importance of this finding during the colposcopic exam is that appropriate evaluation may be prohibited until the inflammation is treated and the epithelium healed. However, in most cases, this infection does not significantly interfere with a diagnostic evaluation for neoplasia. Trichomonas is treated effectively with a single 2-gram oral dose of oral metronidazole.

14.5.1.3 Bacterial induced desquamative disorders

Both excessive Lactobacillus acidophilus and the presence of Leptothrix, an extremely long anaerobic Lactobacillus, have been described as causative agents of cytolysis and desquamation of vaginal epithelium. Cibley named the presence of excessive Lactobacillus in symptomatic women cytolytic vaginosis.[10] The patient usually complains of an excessive vaginal discharge during the last 1 to 2 weeks before menses, accompanied by mild introital irritation. The nature of the symptoms is similar to yeast and since the symptoms are cyclic, resolution after menses, and after treatment with antifungal medications, may misleadingly reassure the woman that the origin is indeed caused by Candida. The non-odorous discharge is white and homogeneous with a pH below 4.0. An excessive number of Lactobacilli, nuclei denuded of their cytoplasm ("naked nuclei"), and other cellular debris from degeneration of squames are noted in the wet prep exam. Yeast and other pathogenic organisms are not present. Treatment consists of suppression of the acid-producing Lactobacillus by alkalinizing the vagina by douching with 1-tsp. baking soda in one pint of water as needed. If the condition should interfere with the adequacy of examination of the vagina, the patient may be treated as outlined and brought back for repeat colposcopy. However, this is not usually necessary.

Vaginal lactobacillosis presents with similar symptoms of increased vaginal discharge and introital irritation occurring in the second half of the menstrual cycle. Horowitz attributed these symptoms to the presence of an excessively long (60–70 millimicron) gram-positive anaerobic Lactobacillus which has previously been named Leptothrix.[11] Leptothrix has long been considered either a harmless commensal or an organism found in the presence of Trichomonas, perhaps as a co-pathogen. Some symptoms, when present, may be related to co-infection with this known pathogen. This organism has been described in 1% of women of reproductive age, but 78% are asymptomatic. However, when cyclic introital irritation and dyspareunia occur and no pathogenic organism can be identified other than these long organisms, treatment with a course of oral tetracycline or amoxicillin/clavulinic acid, is indicated. As in cytolytic vaginosis, inflammatory erythema is absent, but diffuse acetowhitening and

patchy Lugol's iodine uptake may obscure colposcopic findings of vaginal neoplasia.

14.5.2 Non-bacterial desquamative disorders

14.5.2.1 Desquamative inflammatory vaginitis

Desquamative inflammatory vaginitis (DIV) is an erosive, inflammatory vaginitis of uncertain etiology first described by Herman Gardner in 1969.[12] DIV has been considered by some to be a form of lichen planus.[13] Others designate it a separate entity that most commonly occurs in perimenopausal women who are not yet estrogen deficient. The presenting complaint is usually excessive vaginal discharge, sometimes with postcoital bleeding.[13–15] The introitus may be slightly sensitive with mild burning or pruritus suggestive of a candidal infection. Mild dyspareunia may also occur.

A profuse seropurulent discharge is present, with a very alkaline pH in the range of 6–7.[14] Wet-mount microscopic examination will reveal only sheets of leukocytes, parabasal cells and absence of lactobacillus or other bacteria (Figure 14.13). No specific infectious etiology can be documented, but an absence of lactobacilli and an overall increase in prevalence of group B streptococci has been demonstrated.[15] Colposcopic evaluation of the vagina may reveal either diffuse or localized patches of erythema or erosion (Figure 14.14). Other women may present with erythematous spots resembling the "strawberry spots"

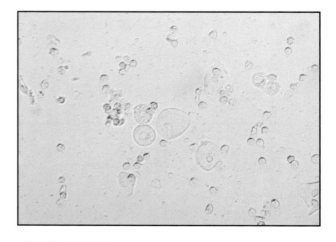

FIGURE 14.13   Wet mount of profuse vaginal discharge in a woman with DIV shows numerous WBCs and parabasal cells. More commonly evaluation of the discharge will reveal inflammatory findings more dramatic than seen here. ■

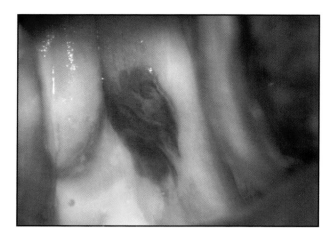

FIGURE 14.14 Shallow erosions are commonly seen in DIV and may present as erythematous patches. ▬▬▬

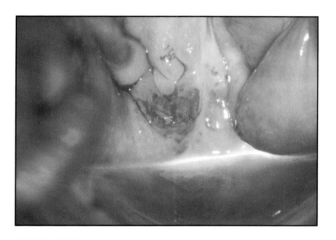

FIGURE 14.15 Deeper erosions resembling ulcers may occasionally be seen in women with DIV. Secondary infection of shallow erosions may be responsible for these deeper lesions. Differentiation from similar erosions seen in lichen planus can only be made if the more classic introital and buccal lesions of LP are also present. This cul de sac presentation is most common. Photo courtesy of Dr. Gordon Davis. ▬▬▬

of a trichomonas infection. Areas of involvement often appear denuded of epithelium, and these areas are occasionally covered by a gray pseudomembrane. Eroded areas are usually shallow, but may occasionally present as deep ulcers (Figure 14.15). Application of acetic acid will often cause a diffuse or patchy acetowhite color in areas of involvement that are not eroded, reflecting high-cellular turnover. Lugol's iodine will not stain these areas but the margins with staining areas are not sharp. As with any process involving erosion, biopsy should extend across non-eroded to adjacent eroded epithelium. Histology will

reveal only a dense infiltrate of PMNs, loss of surface epithelium, and thinning and immaturity of adjacent epithelium.[15] Not present are the more classic histological findings of vulvar lichen planus, particularly histology obtained from vulvar biopsies through a reticulated area of Wickham's striae.[16]

The most successful treatment has been the intravaginal application of 2% clindamycin suppositories or vaginal cream for a minimum of 2 weeks.[15] This results in clinical improvement in > 95% of patients, although relapse may occur in 30%.[15] Post-menopausal patients with desquamative inflammatory vaginitis also may need vaginal or oral estrogen therapy to maintain remission.[14]

14.5.2.2 Erosive lichen planus

Women with "pure" DIV have only vaginal involvement. However, some women with lichen planus present initially with vaginal involvement only, developing erosion of the vestibule and labia minora, Wickham's striae, or manifestations at other anatomic sites months or years after presentation.

Although lichen planus is most commonly a disease of the skin, about 15% to 25% of patients will have only mucosal involvement.[17] The diagnosis of erosive lichen planus can be easily established when erosion of the vestibule and/or vagina is accompanied by the characteristic buccal and gingival plaques. However, when it only involves the genital mucosa, the diagnosis often depends on eliminating other possible erosive disorders (Figure 14.16). The finding of vestibular erosion makes atrophic vaginitis unlikely since this most commonly affects the vagina only. Otherwise, these two entities can be clinically similar in that they both may cause an excessive seropurulent exudate that is quite alkaline and lacking in lactobacillus. With lichen planus, however, the mucosa is usually more denuded, may have a gray pseudomembrane, and may be gradually obliterated by adhesions, especially in the absence of sexual activity. If the vestibular mucosa is eroded as well, irritation and dyspareunia may be severe. Pemphigus and Behcet's may also present with an eroded vestibular area but usually do not involve the vagina.[14] Behcet's ulcers are usually deep and destructive in comparison with the shallow erosion of lichen planus. For more complete discussion of lichen planus see Chapter 15.

14.5.3 Vaginal papillomatosis

Localized or diffusely enlarged vaginal papillae are occasionally encountered which may be confused with neoplasia. In DES exposed women, these are most frequently encountered superior and lateral to

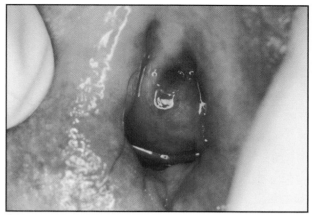

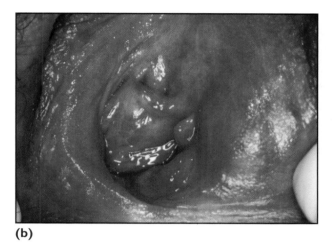

FIGURES 14.16a,b Occasionally introital erosions are present without classic signs of lichen planus and the vaginal findings are most consistent with DIV. These findings suggest that the two may be closely related, as seen in these two women with vaginal erosions and minor vestibular erosions **(a)** and **(b)**. Photos courtesy of Dr. Gordon Davis. ▬▬▬

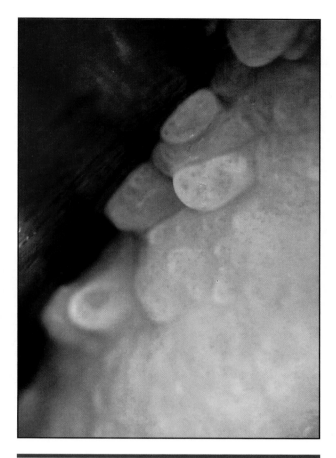

FIGURE 14.17 A papillary appearance is noted superior and lateral to the cervix in this woman who was not exposed to DES in utero. ▬▬▬

the cervix.[18] However, most women with these findings have not been exposed to DES in utero and may have prominent vaginal papillae anywhere in the vagina (Figure 14.17). Often these papillae may be identified just cephalad to the hymen in the proximal vagina and may be confused with HPV-induced lesions.[19] Although these papillary projections may feel like a mass (or masses) during digital exam, the benign nature of these findings can be easily confirmed by simple inspection after application of aqueous iodine. Since the epithelium covering these papillary structures is normal, application of Lugol's iodine should result in a mahogany-brown staining (Figure 14.18). Colposcopically, these structures are homogeneously pink, just as the surrounding mucosa, with no remarkable vascular structure present. Biopsy is generally not required to establish a diagnosis. In fact, because of the potential for misclassification of normal glycogen containing cells as koilocytes, biopsy may be incorrectly interpreted as condyloma when it simply represents a normal benign anatomic variant.

14.5.4 Congenital transformation zone

Approximately 3% to 4% of women have metaplastic epithelium that is persistently arrested in a nonglycogenated, acanthotic phase. Although the congenital transformation zone (CTZ) is often confined to the cervix, it is mentioned here because this finding extends onto the vaginal wall in some women.[20] Although the exact etiology of the CTZ is not well established, it is speculated that some female fetuses that have columnar epithelium everted onto the ectocervix, and occasionally onto the upper vagina,

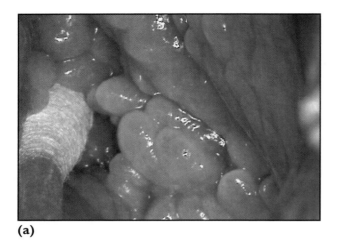

(a)

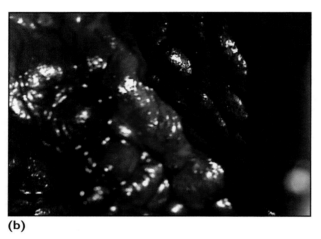

(b)

FIGURES 14.18a,b Benign vaginal papillae as they appear **(a)** before and **(b)** after application of Lugol's solution. The mahogany-brown staining assures the colposcopist of the normalcy of these papillae.

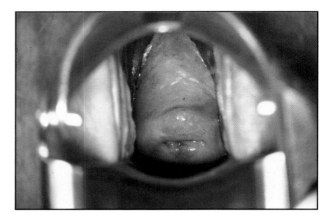

FIGURE 14.19 Extension of arrested metaplasia (congenital transformation zone) onto the anterior vaginal wall.

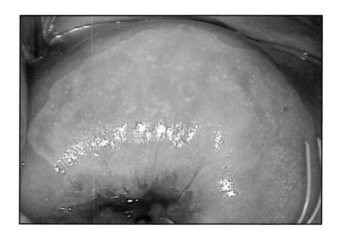

FIGURE 14.20 Before application of acetic acid a translucent pale and waxy CTZ can be seen to extend over much of the anterior cervix.

proceed into a metaplastic process before birth and in the prepubertal years when cervical transformation is usually quiescent.[21] This process may be initiated by the influence of maternal estrogen during the third trimester of fetal life. If this association with timing of the metaplastic process is correct, then the timing must be responsible for the arresting of this process in a perpetual state of non-maturation.

This benign finding may be localized to the cervix, but when it extends to the vagina, it most commonly extends anteriorly or posteriorly (Figure 14.19),[21] although occasionally extension may be found lateral to the cervix. Colposcopically the CTZ may have a waxy, pale appearance prior to application of acetic acid (Figure 14.20). The acetowhite response is generally slow to develop, then lingers for some time before fading. A fine, regular-to-irregular mosaic and fine punctation are usually present. The

appearance is quite homogeneous throughout, unless a HPV induced lesion is present within the CTZ. Because the epithelium remains non-glycogenated, Lugol's iodine application is either rejected entirely (yellow staining) or irregularly stained (variegated) (Figure 14.21). The margin is definite but often slightly feathery.

When a large area of cervical atypia extends to the vaginal wall, considerable colposcopic experience is required to differentiate HPV-infected epithelium in the upper vagina from the normal congenital transformation zone (CTZ) extending into the anterior and posterior vaginal fornices. The primary colposcopic dilemma with vaginal extension of the CTZ is the same dilemma encountered with evaluation of the cervical portion. Because the CTZ has colposcopic features similar to those encountered with

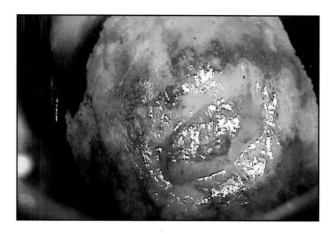

FIGURE 14.21 The CTZ after application of Lugol's solution demonstrates a relatively homogeneous lack of iodine uptake, although some mosaic plates partially stain.

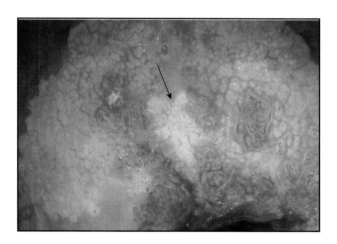

FIGURE 14.22 An internal margin (arrow) within an area of immature metaplasia resembling a CTZ defines an area of CIN 1.

intraepithelial neoplasia, [particularly a fine mosaic pattern] histologic sampling may be warranted. The large, uniform nature of the process, symmetry, somewhat smooth margins, and the unusually slow development of the acetowhite effect commonly enable the colposcopist to predict the benign, acanthotic nature of the process. Unfortunately, the occurrence of HPV-induced intraepithelial neoplasia within a benign CTZ, may increase the difficulty of detecting the lesion. In this situation, however, a margin, or internal border, with a more prominent colposcopic finding in the lesion should direct the biopsy placement (Figure 14.22).

Colposcopic biopsies from a CTZ can be very difficult to interpret.[20] The characteristic histologic find-

ings are acanthosis, which is frequently misdiagnosed as HPV infection, and subepithelial pearling, which has even been over-called as indicative of early invasion. The caudal margin of this acanthotic epithelium is sharply demarcated from adjacent normal mature squamous epithelium.

14.5.5 Vaginal adenosis

Vaginal adenosis is the presence of glandular cells in the vagina.[22] Vaginal adenosis was initially considered an entirely benign process until the 1971 report on the finding of clear cell adenocarcinoma in a number of women exposed in utero to diethylstilbestrol (DES).[23] Because DES exposure during fetal life also resulted in structural changes to the cervix and other areas in the genital tract, the complete discussion on DES and vaginal adenosis is located in Chapter 13: Colposcopy in Special Situations.

14.5.6 Traumatic vaginal lesions

Several effects of vaginal tampons may make vaginal colposcopic evaluation more difficult and may actually mimic changes associated with neoplasia. Recent tampon use, even when not prolonged, causes dehydration of the superficial layers of mucosa and may result in microulcerations and peeling of affected epithelium.[14] The resulting regeneration and repair appear colposcopically as patchy acetowhite areas that stain only mustard-yellow after Lugol's iodine application. These areas may be virtually indistinguishable from low-grade HPV induced vaginal lesions (VAIN 1). Occasionally the tampon-induced nature of the changes can be surmised by a history of recent tampon use and a linear lineup of nonstaining patches on the prominent folds of the vaginal rugae (Figures 14.23a,b). If differentiation is considered important, the patient can be advised to not put any tampon into the vagina for the ensuing two weeks and return for repeat staining of the vagina with Lugol's solution. At that time, epithelial regeneration will usually be complete and a mahogany brown color of the vaginal epithelium will provide reassurance of the non-HPV related nature of the previous findings.

Tampons, first reported to cause vaginal ulcers in 1977,[24] are now recognized as the most common cause of such ulcers.[14,25,26] Excessive or prolonged tampon use may first lead colposcopically to minor vaginal erosions. These erosions may present as erythematous, superficially denuded areas or as deep ulcers with atypical vessels resembling invasive cancer (Figure 14.24).[25,26] Because these lesions may bleed, women often continue to use tampons with the mistaken belief that the bleeding is menstrual in

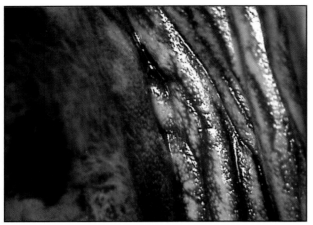

(a)

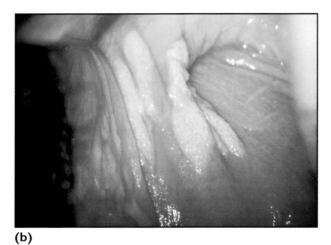

(b)

FIGURES 14.23a,b **(a)** A linear lineup of nonstaining iodine-negative areas is suggestive of tampon-induced epithelial trauma rather than intraepithelial neoplasia. **(b)** contrast to this linear line-up of flat vaginal warts/VAIN 1. Figure 14.23b photo courtesy of Dr. Ken Hatch.

nature, thus prolonging exposure of the denuded area to further irritation. Tampon ulcers have a clean base of granulation tissue and are usually surrounded by a prominent rolled edge. If the history is compatible with excessive tampon use, if the patient may be relied upon to return for re-evaluation, and if the patient is willing to refrain from using tampons for at least the next 4 weeks, biopsy may not be necessary until a return visit for repeat examination. Since these ulcers most often disappear within 2 to 3 weeks of removal of the offending agent,[14] any persistent lesion should be biopsied. Any patient considered to be at-risk for not returning for evaluation should have biopsy of the ulcerated area and adjacent rolled edge at the initial visit. The differential diagnosis includes vaginal carcinoma, chancroid, syphilis, and granuloma inguinale. Iatrogenic or sexual blunt trauma and use of a pessary are other possible causes.

Diaphragms will occasionally produce a thickened, hyperplastic epithelium around the margins of contact with the vaginal mucosa that will appear somewhat acetowhite, but then rarely cause ulceration. If the diaphragm has been used particularly frequently or had been incorrectly inserted or improperly fitted, an area of leukoplakia may be noted prior to the application of acetic acid (Figure 14.25). Even though diaphragm use may be suspected in the etiology of such leukoplakia, a biopsy is usually indicated, particularly after abnormal cervical cytology. Additional abnormal colposcopic findings may be noted with recent use of spermacides, which may induce inflammatory changes in the vagina in women sensitive to non-oxynol 9. The inflamed tissue may appear erythematous following saline application and very patchy mustard yellow following Lugol's iodine application.

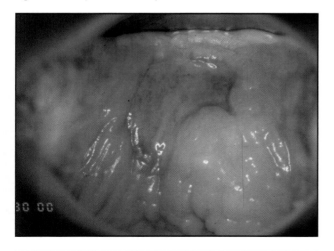

FIGURE 14.24 A deep ulcer on the anterior vaginal wall secondary to chronic tampon use.

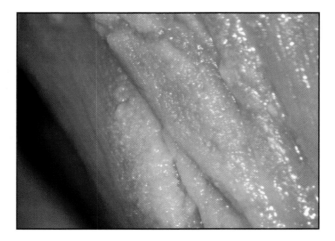

FIGURE 14.25 An area of leukoplakia caused by frequent diaphragm use can be seen on the left vaginal wall into the cul de sac.

14.5.7 Miscellaneous vaginal findings

14.5.7.1 Vaginitis emphysematous

One of the more dramatic, but very rare, colposcopic findings is emphysematous vaginitis, also called Vaginitis emphysematosa.[14]. In this disorder, the vagina and the cervix present with diffuse gas filled "blebs" or cystoid cavities that are most likely caused by bacteria or trichomonas infections. The name "vaginitis emphysematosa" was first given by Zweiful in 1877 following two earlier reports on the subject.[27] Most of these cases have been reported in pregnant or immunosuppressed individuals,[28] although occasionally they appear to be random. The cysts are usually microscopic to a few millimeters in diameter, but some cysts may be as large as 2 cm. Affected patients rarely have symptoms other than an increased vaginal discharge and other symptoms specific for the etiologic agent. Occasionally, the patient will report a "popping" sound during intercourse secondary to rupture of these cysts. Postcoital bleeding has also been reported. The process is self-limited following appropriate treatment of the etiologic agent.

The vagina has been described colposcopically as rough, or "pebbly" (Figure 14.26). The findings are usually most pronounced over the ectocervix and distal vagina.[14] Pressure from a vaginal speculum or examining hand will often rupture some of these tense blebs, with mild bleeding secondarily. Often the diagnosis can be made clinically without biopsy, but when performed, the histology reveals cystoid spaces in the lamina propria, with acute and chronic inflammatory cells, and normal squamous epithe-

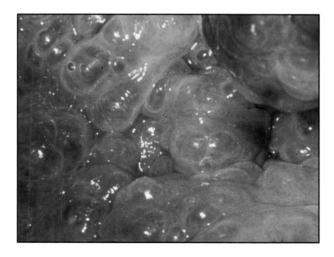

FIGURE 14.26 Extensive gas-filled blebs consistent with a diagnosis of vaginitis emphysematosa are apparent in this woman with a trichomonas infection. Photo provided courtesy of Duane E. Townsend, MD.

lium. Hyperkeratosis and acanthosis, however, may occur in the epithelium. These histologic changes resolve with treatment of the infectious agent responsible for the findings.[14]

14.5.7.2 Gartner's duct cysts

The most common vaginal cysts found incidentally during examination of the vagina are called Gartner's duct cysts. While originally believed to be of common mesonephric (Wolffian) duct origin, many are derived from the paramesonephric (Mullerian) ducts or remnants of the urogenital sinus.[14,29] These cysts usually occur on the lateral to anterolateral vaginal walls. Most cysts do not have a distinctive colposcopic appearance and, unless quite large, are not usually noticed during routine speculum examination. The majority of Gartner's duct cysts are small (1 to 2 cm.). However, cysts as large as 2 to 10 cm. in diameter are occasionally seen. Large cysts are clinically obvious, with epithelium tensely stretched over the cyst. This results in an almost translucent epithelium, displaying fine but prominent branching blood vessels (Figures 14.27a,b). Large cysts located in the anterolateral vagina may cause urinary urgency during intercourse. Most women with Gartner's duct cysts, however, are asymptomatic.

Most Gartner's duct cysts are incidental findings noted during palpation of the vaginal walls during bimanual exam. The cysts are round, soft and smooth. These palpable cysts should be easily differentiated from neoplastic nodules. Since the overlying epithelium is normal, application of Lugol's iodine solution will stain the overlying epithelium a mahogany brown, confirming the benign nature of the mass or masses. Large cysts that stretch the overlying epithelium thinly, however, may demonstrate decreased Lugol's iodine uptake without sharp borders. Evaluation of Gartner's duct cysts can usually be accomplished without a colposcope, although magnification may help provide better visualization of the area of concern.

14.5.7.3 Endometriosis

Endometriosis is not commonly found in the vagina, but when present is most often found in the cul-de-sac. As with cervical endometriosis, vaginal endometriosis may arise from implantation of endometrial fragments shed during childbirth or menstruation that implant into traumatic breaks in the vaginal epithelium.[30,31] However, primary extension of pelvic endometriosis through the cul-de-sac is the more common etiology of vaginal endometriotic implants.[14] When endometriosis is this extensive, women most commonly present with symptoms of severe dysmenorrhea and deep dyspareunia. Vaginal

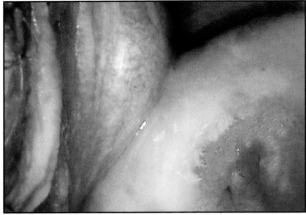

(a)

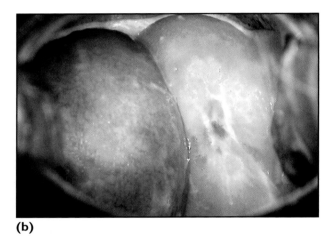

(b)

FIGURES 14.27a,b **(a)** A large vaginal cyst can be seen anterolateral arrow to the cervix. **(b)** Marked stretching of the overlying vaginal wall results in thinning of the epithelium and increased visualization of the normal branching vasculature.

endometriosis usually appears colposcopically as brown to blue colored spots (Figures 14.28a,b) similar to the "powder burns" visualized laparoscopically on the peritoneum. Occasionally, extension of peritoneal implants through the cul-de-sac will present as larger nodules that may be palpable during bimanual exam. Biopsy will confirm the diagnosis. Excision or destruction with cryotherapy or laser vaporization can effectively treat all but large nodules in the cul-de-sac. However, treatment of pelvic endometriosis, when present, will also be necessary. When nodularity in the recto-vaginal septum is pronounced, erosion through the vaginal wall may mimic cancer. Biopsy is important to secure the diagnosis and to exclude the possibility of adenocarcinoma arising in endometrial implants.

14.5.7.4 Vaginal melanosis

Any pigmentation in the vagina is of concern, since the vaginal epithelium is not derived from ectoderm and neural crest tissue does not migrate to this area.[14] Nevertheless, benign pigmented epithelium may occasionally be identified in the vaginal mucosa.[32] More commonly, dark areas in the vagina are due to either endometriotic implants or to neoplasia. Any melanotic lesion can mimic a vaginal melanoma, and vaginal melanoma has been demonstrated to arise in a large area of melanosis.[33] (see below, Vaginal melanoma). Therefore, biopsy is always advised to establish the correct diagnosis. If the area of pigmentation is large, multiple biopsies taken from the most darkly pigmented areas will be necessary. If histological interpretation documents

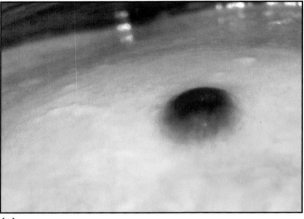

(a)

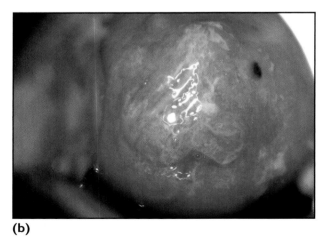

(b)

FIGURES 14.28a,b **(a)** A "powder burn" brown spot is noted near the cervicovaginal margin of this woman with pelvic endometriosis. **(b)** Trauma-induced heme deposited at the edge of this large ectopy resembles an endometriotic implant.

only benign appearing melanocytes in the basal epithelium, annual colposcopic evaluation may still be prudent despite the unlikelihood of malignant degeneration.[34]

14.5.7.5 Vaginal hemangioma and telangiectasia

Benign vascular changes may be seen during colposcopy of the vagina. These changes are not alarming when found on external skin but are of concern when visualized in the vagina, where their presence is less common. Both hemangiomas and telangiectasias are occasionally noted and have the same etiology as their external counterparts. Most women are asymptomatic, but if present within the rich nerve supply of the introitus, dyspareunia may result. Colposcopically, the vessels may appear atypical, but they are not found within an identifiable lesion (Figures 14.29a,b). Capillary (or "strawberry") hemangiomas are commonly located in the external anogenital region, usually appearing at birth or in the first few months of life.[14] Spontaneous involution, usually by 7 years of age, is common. However, most vaginal hemangiomas, when not accompanied by such external anogenital involvement, are discovered as an incidental finding in the vagina during colposcopic evaluation for other indications. They are most commonly small, less than 1 to 2 cm. in diameter, and have the erythematous vascular appearance of those seen externally. Although the overlying epithelium will usually stain brown with aqueous iodine, biopsy may be appropriate to confirm the benign nature of the findings. Histology will show normal epithelium overlying prolific vascular channels. Telangiectasias are tiny vascular changes of a similar benign nature. Some may be of congenital origin, although the etiology of most is not clear. Cavernous hemagiomas are occasionally seen on the external genitalia and may extend into the vagina, where they may be palpated beneath the vaginal mucosa (Figures 14.30a,b).[14] They are larger vascular spaces that usually appear in the first few months of life, then may spontaneously involute. Because cavernous hemagiomas may result in severe hemorrhage if torn during childbirth, their presence on the vulva or vagina frequently requires delivery by cesarean section.

14.5.7.6 Granulation tissue

Granulation tissue may be visible along the vaginal cuff in some patients following hysterectomy (Figure 14.31). The reddish brown mass may be friable, raising concern for cancer. Biopsy readily establishes the diagnosis. While most women are asymptomatic, some may notice vaginal bleeding or spotting. Cau-

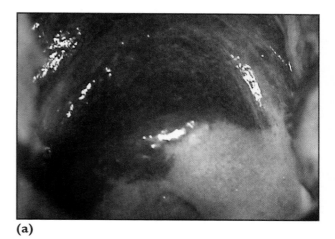

(a)

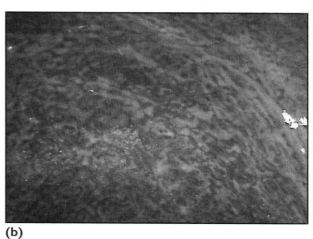

(b)

FIGURES 14.29a,b   **(a)** A hemangioma extends from the mid-right vagina nearly to the cervical os **(b)**. Higher magnification shows the rich vascularity of a vaginal hemangioma. Biopsy was taken at the edge (to reduce the degree of bleeding) to confirm that their was no element of neoplasia present. Normal epithelium with enhanced vascularity on biopsy confirmed clinical diagnosis of hemagioma. ▬

terization with silver nitrate will most commonly result in resolution, but occasionally excision or laser vaporization may be necessary.

14.6 Vaginal Neoplasia

More than 95% of primary vaginal cancers are of squamous cell origin, and the remainder is most commonly clear cell or other adenocarcinomas. More rarely, sarcomas and melanomas are encountered. During the last 40 years, the majority of vaginal adenocarcinomas have been found in young women who were exposed to DES in utero,[35]

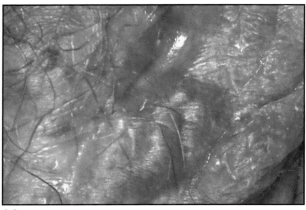

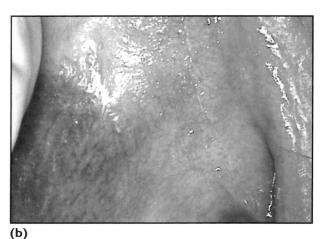

(a)

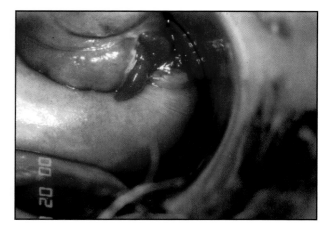

(b)

FIGURES 14.30a,b   **(a)** A hemangioma extends from the groin to the labia minora **(b)** and into the right vestibule. Patient had always had some degree of insertion dyspareunia, which may have been secondary to the vascular abnormality. ■

FIGURE 14.31   Granulation tissue at the vagina cuff is noted 6 months post-hysterectomy. ■

whereas adenocarcinomas of the vagina found in non-DES exposed women have been primarily in women over the age of 60–70.[36] Primary vaginal malignancies are among the rarest of cancers in women, affecting only 6 women per million annually, or 1–4% of all gynecologic malignancies.[37] Secondary vaginal cancers occur occasionally, usually arising from direct spread from the cervix, or less commonly, from the endometrium, ovary, and rectum. Metastasis from cancers distant to the vagina has been reported, but is exceedingly rare.

HPV-induced vaginal intraepithelial neoplasia (VAIN), which is relatively common, is the primary vaginal disease evaluated by colposcopists. During the past decade, the diagnosis of VAIN has been made with increasing frequency. Women with VAIN are asymptomatic, and therefore the presence of VAIN is detected only by colposcopic examination, usually following referral for abnormal cervical cytology. The increased number of women with VAIN is likely to be the result of both increased awareness of the need to evaluate the vagina colposcopically and of an absolute increase in incidence. VAIN is most commonly detected in young women in whom recent infection with HPV may produce proliferative lesions in the vagina, as well as on the cervix and vulva. However, the median age for squamous vaginal cancer is 71,[37] indicating that a very long time between the initial exposure to HPV and oncogenesis is required in the etiology of vaginal squamous cancer. Additionally, because vaginal HPV lesions are common and vaginal squamous cell cancer is rare, most women with low-grade vaginal lesions are at minimal risk for cancer. However, as will be discussed subsequently, very little is known about the natural history of VAIN, and high-grade lesions definitely increase risk for vaginal squamous cancer.

The true incidence of VAIN is not known, but it is significantly less than the incidence of CIN. Women with VAIN 1 or 2 are, on average, 15 years younger than women with VAIN 3.[38] However, rarely VAIN 3 can be found in very young women. VAIN is frequently associated with CIN, since as many as 65% of women with VAIN have either concomitant or prior CIN.[39,40] Approximately 3% of high-grade cervical lesions (CIN 3) will extend into the vagina[41] and between 85% and 92% of VAIN is found in the upper 1/3 of the vagina.[42] Fifty percent of VAIN is multifocal, and the remainder solitary.[2]

While up to 25% of women with VAIN 3 have had a prior hysterectomy for CIN, the risk of developing high-grade VAIN after hysterectomy for high-grade CIN is only 1%. Additionally, VAIN may be found in women after hysterectomy for benign conditions.[39] Nevertheless, when VAIN presents following hysterectomy, it may be difficult to detect since it may be mostly hidden within the vaginal cuff or in the recessed areas of the lateral vaginal corners.[43] Since it is much easier to monitor women for post-treatment recurrence of disease when the cervix is left intact, treatment of CIN by means other than hysterectomy is preferable. Women with CIN who require hysterectomy for other coexistent gynecologic problems should have colposcopic verification of the distal margin of cervical disease or negative cone margins prior to surgery. This should reduce the possibility that extension of a cervical lesion into the vaginal cuff will be overlooked.

Previous radiation therapy to the cervix or vagina, and immunosuppression, increase the risk of acquiring high-grade VAIN.[44,45] Immunosuppressed women are more likely to have persistent, multifocal lesions. Risk factors for persistence or progression of VAIN include multifocal lesions within the vagina or throughout the lower genital tract, which has been termed "anogenital neoplasia syndrome."

Pathology

As with cervical intraepithelial neoplasia, VAIN is divided into three grades: VAIN 1, VAIN 2, and VAIN 3. VAIN 1 and 2 are diagnosed when histologic atypia occupies only the bottom one-third to two-thirds of the epithelium respectively.[43] If dysplastic cells occupy more than two-thirds of the vaginal epithelium, a diagnosis of VAIN 3 is established. Except for the absence of glandular elements, the histologic features of nuclear pleomorphism, abnormal mitoses, and loss of polarity are identical with that seen in CIN. Recently, many pathologists have adopted nomenclature for VAIN that is consistent with the Bethesda System for cervical cytology, with VAIN 1 reported as low-grade VAIN/SIL and VAIN 2 and 3 as high-grade VAIN/SIL. Vaginal cancer is diagnosed when histology reveals atypical cells beneath the basement membrane.

14.6.1 Epidemiology and natural history of VAIN and vaginal cancer

The natural history of VAIN has not been well defined, but the majority of VAIN 1 and 2 appears to regress spontaneously.[46–49] The rate of progression is probably far less than for CIN. As with CIN 3, VAIN 3 may be a true cancer precursor. Spontaneous regression of various degrees VAIN has been reported in 78% of women followed for 5 years, although 13% had persistent VAIN and 9% developed invasive vaginal cancer.[47] Progression from documented VAIN 3

to vaginal cancer has been reported in 20% of women with high-grade VAIN not treated and in 5% of women treated for VAIN 3.[48] Reported risk factors for persistence or progression include multifocal lesions and anogenital neoplastic syndrome, but not grade of vaginal intraepithelial neoplasia, associated cervical neoplasia or immunosuppression.[48] Most squamous vaginal cancers (up to 76%) are positive for oncogenic HPV by PCR.[50] Another 5% are HPV negative adenocarcinomas, most being secondary to DES exposure.[50] The remaining 19% test HPV negative and have no obvious etiology. Smoking does not appear to be an influence in vaginal oncogenesis.

14.6.2 Colposcopy of vaginal intraepithelial neoplasia

Because VAIN is usually subtle, colposcopy with application of acetic acid and Lugol's solution are necessary for the detection of these lesions. An abnormal cervical cytologic smear generally initiates the discovery process. However, simple use of the colposcope does not insure recognition of VAIN, for even with the use of the colposcope and these contrast solutions, VAIN may not be recognized readily. Women with various inflammatory conditions of the vagina lack consistent glycogen storage in the vaginal epithelium that is necessary for Lugol's iodine uptake. Therefore, as discussed previously, treatment of inflammatory conditions such as yeast, trichomonas, or atrophic changes is most often necessary prior to colposcopic evaluation. Once potentially obscuring inflammation is cleared, the following colposcopic features associated with various neoplastic manifestations will become evident.

14.6.2.1 VAIN 1/low-grade HPV expression

HPV infection of the vagina is very common. The majority of infection is located in either the proximal or distal one-third portions of the vagina. The moist, rugose, mucosal surfaces of the vagina readily permit acquisition and expression of HPV. Frequently, extensive HPV induced changes affect the entire vagina. Although HPV infection of the vagina may pose minimal clinical consequences, it represents a significant reservoir of infection for HPV types associated with condylomata acuminata, subclinical HPV infection and genital neoplasia in both sexes.

The colposcopic features of low-grade vaginal intraepithelial neoplasia are in most cases identical to those of low-grade disease of the native epithelium of the cervix. The colposcopic signs include punctation, acetowhite epithelium, leukoplakia, changes in the contour of the vaginal wall and iodine negative epithelium.[42] Mosaic vessels are not normally seen in the vagina unless a congenital transformation zone or cervical neoplasia extends into the vagina or in areas of active metaplasia within vaginal adenosis. Low-grade vaginal HPV lesions may have varied morphologic appearances including: condyloma acuminata, tiny diffuse punctate spots, small non-staining asperites and flat warts or VAIN1.

14.6.2.1.1 Vaginal condylomata acuminata

As many as 30% of women presenting with vulvar condylomata acuminata will have similar lesions in the vagina. Although many vaginal condylomata will be large and clinically apparent, many are small and thus best detected using the magnified illumination of the colposcope after application of acetic acid. Occasionally the lateral vaginal walls will be devoid of HPV lesions, yet extensive and large condylomata acuminata on the anterior and posterior vaginal walls may be hidden by the examining speculum blades (Figure 14.32). Careful assessment of the vaginal fornices and the rugose vaginal anterior, posterior and lateral walls, as discussed previously, is required for detection and accurate diagnosis.

Condylomata acuminata may be exuberant in the vagina, even in women with normal immune systems. However, extensive condylomata are particularly common in immunosuppressed patients and in pregnant women. Women who have extensive condylomas may have a particularly thick white vaginal discharge and pruritus that mimics yeast vaginitis (Figure 14.33). Occasionally, postcoital bleeding may occur as a result of trauma to large vaginal warts. Pregnant women with massive vaginal condylomata acuminata notably risk hemorrhage secondary to

tearing of these lesions, and the high quantitative HPV level may place the baby at-risk for developing laryngeal papillomatosis (Chapter 12).[51,52]

Vaginal condylomata acuminata are similar in appearance to condylomata seen elsewhere in the lower genital tract. They usually present as raised, papillary structures with central capillaries in each papilla (Figures 14.34a,b). Application of 5% acetic acid will usually produce a dense, snow-white response. Following Lugol's iodine application, condylomata assume a yellow color if significant hyperkeratosis is present. Hyperkeratosis will also result in a rougher surface and will obscure the vessels. It is not unusual for multiple condylomata acuminata to be in the vagina. Similar HPV induced lesions may be present on the cervix.

Vaginal condylomata acuminata are usually caused by low-risk HPV types 6 and 11, as are similar lesions elsewhere in the genital tract. The natural history tends to be one of spontaneous regression, but the length of time over which regression occurs is extremely variable. Women are presumed to be contagious to a susceptible consort when clinical lesions are present. Successful treatment of cervical or vulvar HPV induced disease may be followed by spontaneous regression of vaginal HPV lesions, which may in part be due to an increase in the effectiveness of the immune response secondary to decreasing HPV viral load.

Although vaginal condylomata acuminata are normally caused by low-risk HPV types, their presence indicates an increased risk of concomitant exposure to high-risk HPV types as well. Also, 20% of women with vaginal condyloma have cervical condyloma. There-

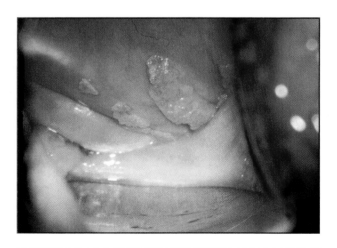

FIGURE 14.32 Extensive low-grade lesions are seen in the cul-de-sac only when the cervix is elevated and the speculum retracted slightly. ■

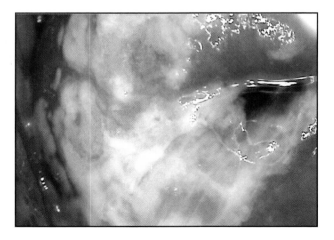

FIGURE 14.33 Extensive low-grade HPV lesions often exfoliate excessive squamous epithelial cells that create a profuse, thick vaginal discharge resembling yeast. Wet mount was negative for fungal elements. ■

fore, some colposcopists consider that detection of lower genital tract condyloma acuminata is an indication for colposcopy, regardless of the results of other screening tests such as cervical cytology. Vaginal intraepithelial neoplasia (VAIN), including VAIN 3 (severe dysplasia/carcinoma in situ), has been reported in association with vaginal condylomata. Although extremely rare, vaginal cancers with a papillary appearance do occur. Therefore, any unusual appearing vaginal papillary lesion or any lesion that fails to respond to therapy must be biopsied.

14.6.2.1.2 Subclinical HPV infection of the vagina
Both cervical and vaginal HPV infections are most frequently subclinical and are, therefore, not easily detected nor diagnosed. Except for the STD implications of vaginal subclinical HPV disease, this

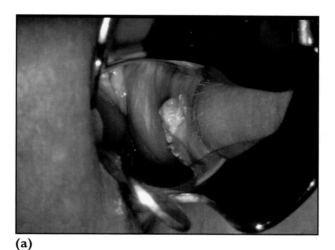

(a)

(b)

FIGURES 14.34a,b Typical exophytic condylomas on the right vaginal wall are seen at **(a)** low and **(b)** high power. Note the typical vascular pattern of condyloma.

disease is of minimal importance from a cancer perspective. Therefore, the aggressive management of subclinical vaginal HPV lesions must be tempered by the realization that these lesions pose little risk for cancer. The following discussion is a comprehensive review of the clinical profile of vaginal colposcopic atypia secondary to HPV, but is not intended to suggest that such atypia requires aggressive approaches to diagnosis and treatment. Nonetheless, the frequent association of minor vaginal HPV infection with low grade SIL Pap smear abnormalities does foster anxiety for both the patient and her clinician that demands knowledge about the various colposcopic appearances of subclinical HPV infection. Subclinical HPV infection of the vagina may be manifested in different ways. Some lesions are completely inapparent to the naked eye and are detected only by colposcopy after application of 5% acetic acid (Figure 14.35). These lesions may appear as flat acetowhite epithelium or as small acetowhite spots. Other lesions consist of tiny micropapillary asperites.

14.6.2.1.2.1 Condylomatous vaginitis Both micropapillary asperites, which are tiny epithelial projections from the vaginal walls, and punctate acetowhite spots that do not stain with Lugol's solution, may diffusely cover the entire vaginal vault. These manifestations have been termed "condylomatous vaginitis".[53,54] Similar involvement of the cervix is called "condylomatous colpitis." Micropapillary asperites are virtually diagnostic of HPV infection, but the tiny punctate dots, which have been called "reverse punctation", are much more nonspecific and should not be considered a definitive finding of the presence of this virus. However, it would seem prudent to include this possible HPV manifestation in this discussion, with the caveat that the etiology of "reverse punctation" may be multifactorial and not pathognomonic of HPV expression.

These vaginal entities may be responsible for LSIL Pap smear abnormalities in the absence of an obvious cervical lesion. The dilemma of an inability to explain the source of a HPV positive ASCUS or a LSIL Pap smear result at colposcopy will often be resolved when the colposcopist looks for these subtle vaginal manifestations of HPV infection. Tall spiked papillary projections may occasionally be detected without the aid of the colposcope, whereas detection of reverse punctation requires magnification and epithelial contrast agents. Reverse punctation has also been called minimally expressed papillomavirus infection (MEPI). Colposcopically, MEPI, or reverse punctation, presents as a myriad of tiny, acetowhite pinpoint dots on the cervix and vagina, highlighted against the flat pink vaginal mucosa. The name

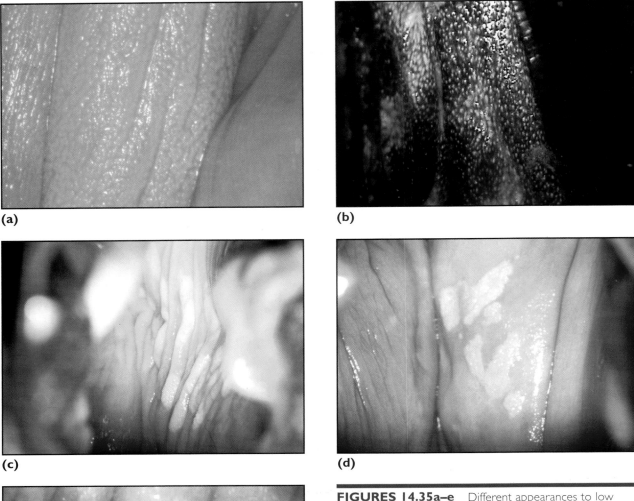

(a)

(b)

(c)

(d)

(e)

FIGURES 14.35a–e Different appearances to low grade subclinical HPV manifestations are seen in these five images. **(a)** A myriad of tiny acetowhite spots are found in the right vaginal fornix in this woman with low-grade cytologic changes and a positive HPV test as seen here after application of acetic acid and **(b)** after staining with Lugol's solution. In this situation, the "reverse punctation" changes are presumed to be secondary to HPV, but the etiology is difficult to establish with certainty. **(c)** and **(d)** flat acetowhite lesions also noted in the follow-up to LSIL Paps, each with normal cervical findings. **(e)** Flat vaginal low-grade HPV changes with asperities are seen in the right vaginal fornix only after the cervix is pushed to the right. ▬▬

"reverse punctation" comes from the resemblance of these tiny round dots to vascular punctation in size and random distribution, but their dissimilarity in being white rather than red. Each of these white dots corresponds to a pinpoint elevation of parakeratotic epithelium capping a prominent intraepithelial capillary. Even after application of 5% acetic acid and inspection using the colposcope, these dots can be

quite subtle. They are better visualized as yellow dots against the normal mahogany brown squamous epithelium following the staining of the vagina and cervix with Lugol's iodine. MEPI is simply a transient manifestation of HPV infection and does not require treatment. Additionally, it is a very non-specific finding, as other inflammatory conditions of the vagina, such as vulvovaginal candidiasis, may produce a similar colposcopic appearance. Therefore, "reverse punctation" should not be considered definitive proof of HPV infection unless other more specific HPV findings are also present.

Abnormal histologic findings are extremely focal as they are limited to the tiny pinpoint areas of parakeratosis. Histologic interpretations, therefore, may range from normal to "condyloma" depending upon whether any of these tiny areas of abnormality are noted in the histologic sections. When abnormalities are found, focal areas of minimal basal hyperplasia, mild koilocytosis, variable dyskeratosis, parakeratosis and prominent intraepithelial capillary growth can be identified.

Micropapillary asperites are the more definitive manifestation of condylomatous vaginitis. Prior to application of acetic acid, multiple small pink micropapillary asperites may be seen projecting from the vaginal mucosa. These small lesions are usually multiple and diffuse, but may be confined to smaller areas. Most commonly, the micropapillae arise from completely normal surrounding vaginal mucosa (Figures 14.36a,b), but occasionally they may be found atop slightly hyperkeratotic, acetowhite epithelium that individually do not stain with Lugol's. When viewed through a colposcope, a fine caliber central capillary loop is usually identified in each papilla. If the papillae are poorly developed, they will appear short and blunt with a granular surface contour.

Histologic evaluation of colposcopically directed biopsies may reveal cytopathic effects of HPV infection, but the manifestations are so tiny that they are often not histologically documented. When present, the histologic features may vary from more subtle changes such as basal hyperplasia and dyskeratosis to florid koilocytotic atypia. A central capillary will be found within each papillary excrescence.

14.6.2.1.2.2 Flat vaginal warts/VAIN 1
Subclinical vaginal warts and VAIN 1 are flat to slightly raised, moderately well circumscribed lesions of a few millimeters to several centimeters in diameter. Flat vaginal warts are often difficult to identify even following application of 5% acetic acid and colposcopic evaluation. However, following Lugol's iodine application, these lesions are usually readily detected. The margins may be distinct or indistinct, and sharply circumscribed or irregular and feathered. The surface of a flat vaginal wart is either smooth, slightly elevated and plaque-like, or slightly "spiky" with fine overlying asperites. Usually no vascular patterns are apparent, but if present, the vessels are usually fine, non-dilated punctation of uniform caliber. The intercapillary distance is narrow but regular, in contrast to

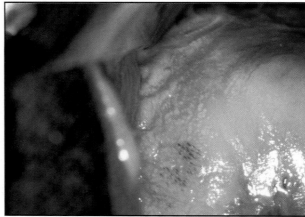

(a)

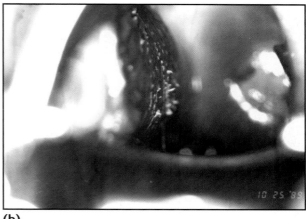

(b)

FIGURES 14.36a,b Micropapillary asperities in which **(a)** diffuse epithelial "spikes" are seen surrounded by normal mucosa. **(b)** Here isolated diffuse non-staining micropapillary aspirates arise from normal glycogen-rich mucosa. ▄▄▄▄

the more widely irregularly spaced punctation that may be seen in some high-grade VAIN.

Flat acetowhite lesions are most frequently detected in the upper one-third of the vagina (Figures 14.37a,b). These lesions may be a direct extension from cervical atypia onto the vaginal fornix or they may arise de novo within the vagina. Lugol's iodine stains the surrounding uninvolved vaginal epithelium a dark mahogany brown, usually contrasting sharply with the lesion, which may appear yellow in color. The lesions may also appear a mixed yellow brown variegated color.

Histology of colposcopically directed biopsies will show classic cytopathic effects of HPV infection, including basal hyperplasia and nuclear atypia in the bottom one-third of the epithelium and koilocytes in the upper layers. Flat vaginal warts and VAIN 1 are the

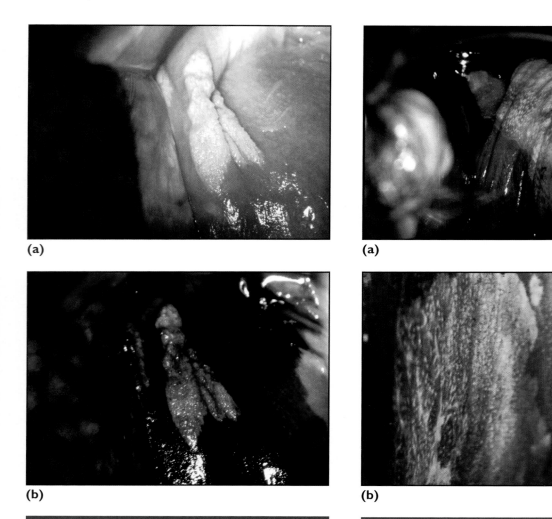

(a)

(b)

FIGURES 14.37a,b Multiple flat vaginal warts/VAIN 1 as seen **(a)** after application of acetic acid and **(b)** after staining with Lugol's solution.

(a)

(b)

FIGURES 14.38a,b The "tortoise shell" variegated staining pattern noted in lesions **(a)** and **(b)** is indicative of low-grade vaginal HPV lesions.

same entity; however, some pathologists require the presence of abnormal mitotic figures for the latter diagnosis. From the therapeutic standpoint, there is no true cytologic, histologic or biologic difference between "flat vaginal warts" and VAIN 1 (mild dysplasia).

Acetowhite HPV-induced lesions of the vagina are often multifocal. The lesions may be present diffusely within the vagina and may extend to the cervix and vulva. If application of aqueous iodine solution results in variegated staining, the lesion is likely to be low-grade (Figures 14.38a,b). However, since both low- and high-grade lesions may stain a mustard yellow color, Lugol's application is most useful to identify and locate lesions and evaluate their margins. Liberal use of colposcopically directed biopsy is required to exclude high-grade disease if either cytology or colposcopy suggests a higher grade lesion. The most frequently

detected HPV types associated with flat vaginal warts and VAIN 1 are the "high-risk" types 16, 31, 33 and 35.

Because most vaginal low-grade HPV lesions are the manifestations of benign, transitory HPV infections, treatment options should always weigh potential benefit against the potential for treatment complications. The natural history of flat vaginal warts/VAIN 1 has not been studied prospectively. However, vaginal low grade SIL is significantly less of a risk for cancer than cervical low-grade disease, which itself carries little risk. Eventually, in most cases, these lesions resolve spontaneously provided the host has a competent immune system. Based upon the relatively uncommon diagnosis of high-grade VAIN and vaginal cancer, it can be deduced that progression of VAIN 1 is extremely infrequent. A histologic continuum of epithelial neoplasia from HPV infection to high-grade dysplasia exists. However, as with the cervix, development of high-grade vaginal intraepithelial neoplasia (VAIN 3) is most likely a monoclonal event and a distinct disease process from VAIN 1. The natural history of VAIN 2 is even more obscure, and many have suggested that VAIN 2 should be considered a low-grade lesion. The relative rarity of high-grade vaginal neoplasia suggests that the occurrence of these monoclonal events in the mature epithelium of the vagina is uncommon.

The major significance of vaginal low-grade lesions is the potential for transmission of HPV to others and the association with minor atypia detected on a cervical or vaginal vault smear. A major concern is the belief that all vaginal papillae, acetowhite patches and iodine-positive areas are HPV-related. Benign papillations of congenital origin are commonly found in the vagina of many women. They may mimic the papillae of HPV-induced condylomatous vaginitis except that normal non-HPV related papillae stain brown when exposed to Lugol's iodine solution. Histology can also be misleading, as papillary features and the clinical impression of "rule out HPV" often places the pathologist in the difficult position of discerning whether minor cellular changes, otherwise not diagnostic, are sufficient to support a diagnosis of HPV-related change. Subjectivity in histologic diagnosis may result in over-diagnosis but also in under-diagnosis. Over-diagnosis may prompt therapy that is not otherwise indicated. Expert colposcopic assessment is critical if over-diagnosis of normal papillae and other potential low-grade changes are to be avoided.

14.6.3 Vaginal high-grade intraepithelial neoplasia (VAIN 2–3)

Because the vaginal mucosa usually appears clinically normal to the unaided eye, colposcopic examination with application of acetic acid and aqueous iodine are essential for detecting VAIN of any grade. Vaginal high grade SIL has essentially the same colposcopic characteristics as cervical high-grade SIL except that a mosaic vascular pattern is not usually seen unless the lesion arises in vaginal epithelium that was initially an extension of a congenital transformation zone or in an area of adenosis. Vaginal high-grade SIL is usually flat, with varying degrees of surface irregularity that cannot be well appreciated without colposcopic magnification (Figure 14.39).[46] When hyperkeratosis is present, raised white leukoplakic lesions may be seen during colposcopic examination prior to the application of 5% acetic acid, or rarely may be palpated during vaginal examination. More rarely,

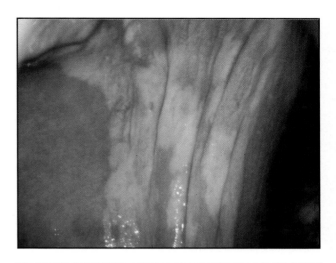

FIGURE 14.39   These diffuse flat vaginal HPV-induced lesions appear to be low-grade. However, the acetowhite effect is very prominent. Biopsy revealed VAIN 2/3, illustrating the value of histologic sampling prior to treatment decisions. From Wright, VC. Biomedical Communications, Houston, TX. With permission.

slightly raised pink lesions may be found. As with cervical high-grade SIL, intercellular desmosomes in VAIN 3 are loosened, diminishing intercellular cohesion. Therefore, peeling or abrasions of the epithelium may occur within high-grade VAIN lesions, particularly in the peri- or postmenopausal women. The margins of VAIN 3 tend to be well circumscribed and regular or smooth. Furthermore, these lesions may be elevated above the surrounding normal epithelium.

After application of 5% acetic acid, VAIN of all grades becomes acetowhite. The acetic acid reaction that accompanies VAIN is often more subtle and less easily detected than with cervical intraepithelial neoplasia. The reaction takes longer to develop and the contrast with normal vaginal epithelium is less vivid. Additionally, the rugose nature of the vaginal epithelium may compromise detection of the changes. An acetowhite color may predominate as the major colposcopic finding in most high-grade VAIN, as the epithelium is often fairly opaque, preventing transillumination of the underlying vasculature (Figure 14.40). However, even with dense acetowhitening, a fine to coarse capillary punctation may be detected at greater colposcopic magnification when the acetic acid reaction fades. The more prominent vascular patterns associated with VAIN 3 develop late in the neoplastic process (Figures 14.41a–c). A well developed, varicose, widely spaced capillary punctation or, more rarely, a mosaic pattern in an area of high-grade VAIN, may be seen. An exaggeration of the coarse caliber vessel arrangement is highly suspicious for invasive cancer.

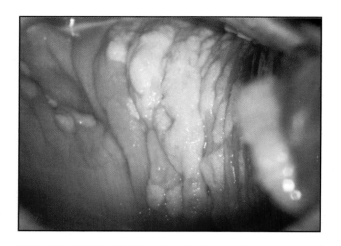

FIGURE 14.40 Dense acetowhite vaginal intraepithelial lesion (VAIN 2).

Vaginal high grade intraepithelial neoplasia may be unifocal or multifocal. VAIN 3 is usually unifocal, although it may be found in association with multifocal lesions of lesser grade. VAIN 1 and VAIN 2 lesions are often multifocal, as they are more likely to represent a diffuse "field effect" of HPV infection. Sometimes lesions appear clinically to be condyloma acuminata, but reveal high-grade dysplastic morphology by biopsy. These occasional nonspecific colposcopic features, and the difficulty of gaining visual access to the entire vagina, make colposcopy of the vagina a challenge. The need for thorough expert examination and liberal biopsy of any lesion suspected to be high-grade VAIN is critical if significant lesions, including rare cancers, are to be detected and treated appropriately. Examination by colposcopy under regional or general anesthesia may be necessary if disease is very extensive, or if the patient is not able to relax enough for adequate evaluation of the vagina and symptoms or cytology are of concern.

The subtle acetic acid reaction of VAIN coupled with the technical difficulties in colposcopic assessment of the vagina render examination after application of aqueous iodine solution invaluable in vaginal colposcopy. Half- or quarter-strength Lugol's iodine will provide adequate staining and minimize the patient discomfort often noted with the full-strength solution. Poorly differentiated vaginal epithelium does not contain glycogen. Therefore, high-grade vaginal intraepithelial neoplasia rejects iodine, resulting in a mustard yellow color that is in sharp contrast with the mahogany brown staining of the normal vaginal mucosa or the variegated, partial uptake of iodine noted in some partially glycogenated low-grade VAIN. This simple test permits clear demarcation of areas of high-grade epithelial

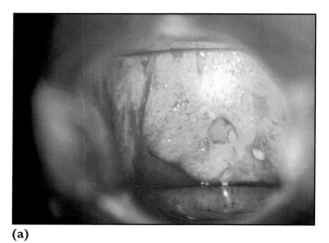

(a)

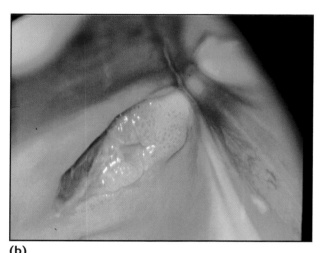

(b)

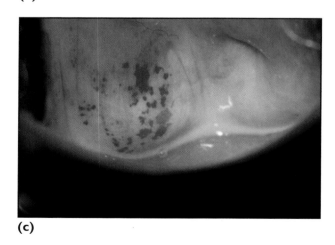

(c)

FIGURES 14.41a–c **(a)** Atypical vessels and erosion within a sharply defined lesion are seen in this VAIN 3 raising concern for invasion. **(b)** VAIN 3 is seen with the green filter enhancement of abnormal vascular findings. **(c)** VAIN 3 with atypical vascular findings and adjacent acetowhite.

atypia, allows for accurate colposcopically directed biopsy and helps determine disease extent and distribution. The use of Lugol's iodine solution is mandatory for delineation of treatment margins. Iodine staining will not compromise histologic assessment of the biopsy specimen.

14.6.4 Invasive vaginal cancer

Vaginal cancers constitute only 1% to 4% of all gynecologic cancers. Squamous cell carcinoma is the most common of the vaginal cancers. Adenocarcinoma, melanoma, and sarcomas are extremely rare. The age of the patient helps predict the cancer cell-type. Endodermal sinus tumor and botryoid embryonal rhabodomyosarcoma are the most commonly seen vaginal cancers of infancy.[55,56] Botryoid cancers and adenocarcinomas may appear during adolescence. Leiomyosarcoma is the most common vaginal cancer in late reproductive years. Squamous carcinoma and melanoma are most common in the 7th and 8th decades of life.[57]

These cancers have colposcopic features similar to those seen in cervical squamous cancers; namely, atypical vessels, papillary excrescences, ulcerations, irregular topography, and friability (Figures 14.42a,b). As with early invasive carcinoma of the cervix, tumor angiogenesis factor (TAF) produced by the neoplastic process stimulates vascular proliferation that presents as bizarre, varicose blood vessels. Wide intercapillary distances occur secondary to expanding tumor volume.

14.6.4.1 Squamous cell carcinoma of the vagina

Approximately 40% of squamous cell carcinomas of the vagina arise from the upper vagina, often in the posterior fornix where the cervix obscures the lesion. Invasive squamous cell carcinoma of the vagina most commonly presents in older women (average age 62 years), however it has been reported as early as the fourth decade of life. Approximately 10% of vaginal squamous cancers are found in women with a previous history of invasive squamous cell cancer of the cervix. Some of these lesions arise from cervical cancer that has extended into the vagina. Some distal lesions near the introitus evolve secondary to metastasis from cervical lesions. However, vaginal cancers may develop as asynchronous primary lesions initiated by oncogenic HPV. Advanced lesions involving the full vagina are seen in about 30% of cases. Approximately 40% occur on the anterior wall, 30% on the posterior, and 28% on the lateral walls. Early primary spread is local, however the abundant lymphatics of the vagina allow metastatic spread to the inguinal nodes (for lesions near the introitus) and to the pelvic nodes (for lesions in the upper vagina).

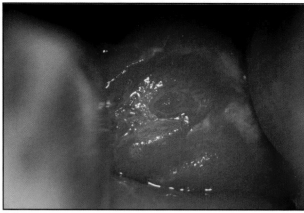

(a)

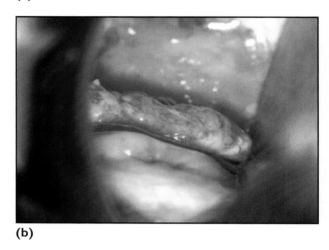

(b)

FIGURES 14.42a,b   (a) Anterior vaginal wall cancer. **(b)** This primary squamous cell carcinoma of the vagina displays bizarre atypical vessels, and irregular topography. Upon examination, the lesion was noted to be friable. ■

Women with vaginal cancer most commonly present with bleeding or a vaginal discharge that is malodorous, blood tinged and foul-smelling. Urinary distress and pain have also been reported. However, flat, infiltrating, superficially spreading or ulcerating carcinomas have been reported. A rectovaginal exam is often helpful in delineating submucosal extension, paravaginal infiltration, and rectal involvement. Deep involvement of the anterior vaginal wall can spread to the bladder and produce urinary symptoms.

14.6.4.2 Adenocarcinoma

Adenocarcinoma of the vagina may be either primary, or metastatic from glandular tumors of the endocervix, endometrium, or from distant sites, particularly from the breast, ovary, or bowel. Primary adenocarcinomas of the vagina are far less frequent than metastatic spread from local or distant glandular tumors. Therefore, the diagnosis of adenocarcinoma in the vagina should always raise suspicion of the possibility of a primary elsewhere. Treatment of vaginal adenocarcinoma is similar to treatment of squamous cell types.

14.6.4.2.1 Primary clear cell adenocarcinoma

Primary clear cell adenocarcinoma has been found primarily in women [between the ages of 7 and 40] who were exposed in utero to diethylstilbestrol (DES).[23,58] In non-DES exposed women, this is a very rare cancer that usually occurs in women over the age of 50. Clear cell adenocarcinomas most likely arise from glandular elements of mullerian origin in the vaginal wall. These foci of glandular cells, or adenosis, are most commonly found in women exposed to DES in utero. For the past several decades, this has been the most common vaginal adenocarcinoma of young women. Because of the aging of the population of women exposed to DES, adenocarcinoma of this cell-type is becoming less common. Both polypoid and ulcerative clear cell adenocarcinomas occur. Atypical vessels predominate as the most identifiable sign in lesions that are less developed. Extremely rare clear-cell adenocarcinomas in elderly women probably also arise in areas of adenosis,[59] or in vaginal endometriosis.[60]

14.6.4.2.2 Metastatic adenocarcinoma to the vagina

Adenocarcinoma metastatic to the vagina is uncommon but has been reported from primary cancers of the endocervix, ovary, fallopian tube, endometrium, breast, kidney, pancreas, colon and other distant sites. Metastatic adenocarcinoma cannot be differentiated colposcopically from primary adenocarcinoma since it does not have any distinguishing features that would differentiate it from a primary invasive malignancy.

14.6.4.3 Malignant melanoma

Malignant melanoma is an extremely rare cancer in the vagina. However, any pigmented vaginal lesion should be suspect and biopsied. Until recently, melanocytes were not considered to occur in the vagina, and therefore, vaginal melanoma was considered a metastatic lesion. However, many cases of primary vaginal melanomas have now been reported[57,61,62] and primary melanocytes have now been documented to occur in this area.[32–34] Melanomas of the vagina have been reported in women between the ages of 22 and 83, with an average age of 55. Most vaginal melanomas are detected after the onset of postcoital bleeding or with light blood-tinged vaginal discharge that is often purulent and foul smelling.

Colposcopically, vaginal melanomas are similar to melanomas occurring externally, except that their hidden location often results in much larger lesions before they are recognized. Vaginal melanomas are commonly described as polypoid, pedunculated, papillary or fungating. Ulceration and necrosis are common. Most vaginal melanomas are brown or black, although red and yellow (necrotic), and amelanotic types (5%) have been reported. Adjacent spread of pigment is less common than with external lesions. Women with vaginal melanoma have a very poor prognosis because the lesion is aggressive and detection late.

14.6.5 Treatment of vaginal neoplasia

14.6.5.1 Low-grade VAIN and condyloma

Realization that most low-grade vaginal HPV-related lesions spontaneously resolve without medical intervention has influenced most clinicians to take a less aggressive approach to treatment. Observation has become accepted practice in many cases.[46] Lesions reported as VAIN 1 are almost invariably HPV-induced, with little potential of progression to high-grade VAIN or vaginal squamous cell cancer.[47] In fact, the progressive potential of VAIN 1 to high-grade precursors has not been established, nor has a cancer potential been definitively documented. Therefore, from a cancer perspective, treatment is unnecessary. However, many women may desire some sort of active medical intervention under the premise that these lesions nevertheless represent a sexually transmittable disease. Although reducing viral load by eliminating some lesions may theoretically reduce the potential for sexual transmission, in reality the possibility of eliminating all low-grade vaginal lesions with presently available therapies is virtually non-existent. If explanation of this reality does not dissuade the patient's desire to "do something," then selection of the most benign and safe treatment approach may be warranted. This would include conservative use of appropriate topical agents such as trichloracetic acid (TCA) or, rarely, 5-fluorouracil. Follow-up to such treatment must be conservative, usually by observation only, or gingerly reapplication of trichloracetic acid.

The reduction of endogenous estrogen in postmenopausal women may cause confusing cellular changes that mimic atypia, and the general lack of glycogen storage makes colposcopy difficult. Therefore, before embarking on treatment of vaginal lesions in women with vaginal mucosal atrophy, it is wise to first treat the vagina as previously described with topical estrogen therapy.[46,63] Re-evaluation following estrogen therapy will often reveal resolution of the vaginal cytologic and colposcopic changes and clarify their non-HPV related origins.

Treatment of vaginal lesions with TCA is best accomplished under colposcopic guidance. In order to minimize the amount of TCA introduced in the vagina, many clinicians will apply 50%–85% TCA on the wooden end of a cotton-tip applicator to each lesion. Broad lesions may be treated more efficiently using a TCA-soaked cotton-tipped applicator. However caution must be taken to prevent excess TCA from running off the treated areas and damaging normal adjoining tissue. TCA treatment of VAIN 1 may accelerate lesion regression. The primary difficulties of this therapeutic modality are the imprecise depth of tissue destruction, the diffuse nature of vaginal low-grade lesions, and the occurrence of new lesions between patient visits.

The diffuse nature of low-grade vaginal HPV disease prompted widespread use of vaginal 5-fluorouracil (5-FU) in the late 1980s.[64] Many treatment protocols were developed for both low- and high-grade VAIN and vaginal condylomata. However, because of significant complications, including the common occurrence of extensive vaginal ulcerations and the difficulty in subsequent healing of these lesions, this treatment approach is now rarely taken and generally should be discouraged.[65]

Extensive vaginal condylomata acuminata can be a cosmetic and aesthetic nuisance. They are infectious to an unexposed host, and most women desire adequate and prompt eradication. Eradication can be usually achieved by observation or simple chemotherapeutic regimens. Extensive recalcitrant disease may require more aggressive treatment. However, the patient must be advised that even laser surgery is no guarantee against recurrence. A rescue strategy of topical chemotherapy, systemic interferon or repeat ablative treatment may be necessary to control disease. Excision of pedunculated condyloma may also be an appropriate form of therapy.

14.6.5.2 High-grade VAIN

VAIN 2 and VAIN 3 are grouped as high-grade intraepithelial neoplasia of the vagina. VAIN 3 is a potential cancer precursor, yet the transit time is greater and the progressive potential reduced compared to that for CIN 3. Regardless, this progressive potential still dictates that treatment is indicated. Three treatment options are presently available for high-grade VAIN; vaginal 5-FU, CO_2 laser, and surgical excision.[66] Other investigational topical agents, such as immune response modifiers, may be used in the future.

Vaginal 5-FU As discussed above, 5-FU is now rarely used to treat genital HPV lesions. However, there may be an occasional indication for its use in the treatment of extensive, multifocal VAIN 2 or 3. Clearance had been reported in approximately 50–80% of high-grade VAIN treated by 5-FU.[66,67] Because severe chemical vulvovaginitis may develop as a consequence of 5FU use, the enthusiasm for this approach decreased dramatically. However, more conservative, less frequent application regimens have proven to be effective, yet less prone to complications. The safest regimen has been application of 1/4 to 1/3 of an applicator of 5-FU cream, equivalent to 1 to 1.5 grams, vaginally once per week before bedtime, and rinsing the medication out in the morning.[68] To prevent introital irritation, application of zinc oxide or petroleum jelly to the vulva is advised before 5-FU insertion. When lesions are present only in the upper vagina, insertion of a small tampon into the lower vagina may further reduce the risk of introital symptoms. Because of marked variability in patient response and potential for serious complications, frequent colposcopic monitoring of the vagina every 3 to 4 weeks is required. Any erosion or excessive erythema should serve as a warning. Treatment should be stopped if erosions are noted. If frequent monitoring provides reassurance that vaginal 5-FU application may safely continue, then treatment does not usually extend beyond 10 weeks. Because 5-FU is contraindicated during pregnancy, women of child bearing age should use an appropriate contraceptive.

Vaginal lesions may be treated without significant discomfort because of the absence of certain sensory receptors in most of the vagina. Nevertheless, introital irritation and burning are not uncommon side effects, and vestibulitis has been reported (Figure 14.43). Significant vaginal erosion and ulceration may result in dyspareunia and postcoital bleeding.[65] However, using a once-a-week regimen, such symptoms are rarely significant enough to stop treatment. In a follow-up study 2 to 4 weeks after a single 5 daily vaginal 5-FU therapy, 42% of women were found to have signs of a chemical vaginitis and/or cervicitis and 11.4% had an acute ulcer. Most vaginal 5-FU ulcers occur in the apex of the vagina secondary to pooling of the medication in this area. Women treated with one-time weekly 5-FU had fewer complications, with only 5.7% developing ulcers. Unfortunately, 5-FU induced ulcers may persist chronically for more that 6 months in many women.[65] These ulcers vary in size from 0.5 to 7 cm in diameter with a mean diameter of 2.5 cm. Eighty percent of women with 5-FU induced ulcers have symptoms, which include serosanguinous or watery vaginal discharge,

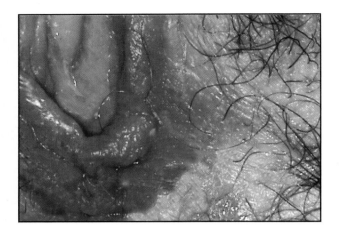

FIGURE 14.43 Erythematous mucosa with shallow erosions can be seen in the vestibule in this young woman treated vigorously with 5-FU. Symptoms of severe dyspareunia persisted after healing of the erosions. The patient was subsequently diagnosed with vulvar vestibulitis syndrome, probably secondary to treatment with 5-FU. ▬▬▬

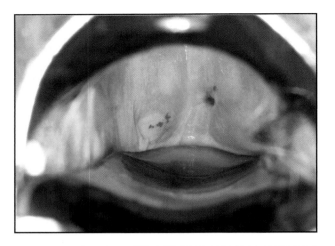

FIGURE 14.44 This patient presented with a HSIL Pap one year post-LEEP for CIN2. In the right vaginal fornix adjacent to the colposcopically normal but now diminished cervix is a small VAIN 3. This lesion would be easily vaporized with the CO_2 laser. ▬▬▬

postcoital or irregular bleeding or dyspareunia. These ulcers only rarely (<50%) heal without treatment.[65] Vaginal erosions or ulcers usually heal more quickly following vaginal acidification for 3 to 6 weeks with an acid-based gel. 5-FU treatment may also induce adenosis in the vagina.

CO_2 laser ablation The use of carbon-dioxide (CO_2) laser for treatment of lower genital tract intraepithelial neoplasia has steadily declined during the past 10 years. However, the inaccessibility of vaginal lesions and the need for exact control of the depth of destruction, support the continued use of CO_2 laser as the modality of choice for treating high-grade VAIN.[69-72] Physicians skilled in the use of the CO_2 laser can safely and effectively treat high-grade lesions. Healing is generally excellent and laser surgery is usually accepted very well by patients. However, a greater degree of operator skill is required by the vaginal laser surgeon than for laser surgery in most other lower genital tract locations.

Even with the introduction of efficient, modern electrosurgical equipment (electrosurgical loop excision procedure, or LEEP), the CO_2 laser still remains the treatment of choice for most cases of VAIN. The vaginal wall is thinner relative to other genital sites and vital organs are in close proximity. Surgical access is more difficult. Misdirected electrosurgical excision may place adjacent organs at risk, and delayed healing responses occur more commonly.

Despite the inevitable impact of modern electrosurgical techniques in the management of CIN, the wise clinician will ensure laser skills are maintained to manage challenging high-grade vulvar and vaginal disease (Figure 14.44).

The first report of the use of the CO_2 laser to treat VAIN was by Stafl in 1977.[69] Although the vaginal wall is relatively thin, maintaining a vaporization depth of 1 to 3 mm will successfully eliminate most VAIN with low risk of adjacent injury. The absence of gland ducts in the vaginal mucosa allows for such shallow vaporization. Generally, the lateral margin of the vaporization should extend 5–10 mm beyond disease margins.[46] Cure rates for CO_2 vaporization of VAIN range from 43% to 100%.[46,73] Extension of VAIN into the corners of the vaginal cuff increases the risk of persistent disease. Higher failure rates are also reported for multifocal and widespread low- and high-grade HPV disease (Figures 14.45a,b).

When a hysterectomy is performed and the patient is known to have CIN or VAIN, it is imperative that the entire extent of the intraepithelial neoplasia be treated. The cuff is usually best visualized from below in order to determine the extent of removal of the CIN and any remaining vaginal extension. Multifocal disease present at the time of hysterectomy should be treated by laser vaporization, or if localized, by excision. If the vaginal lesion is small and contiguous with, or in close proximity to, the

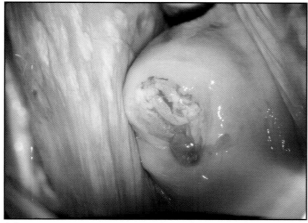

(a)

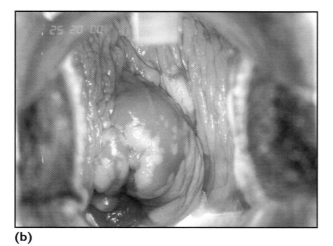

(b)

FIGURES 14.45a,b **(a)** Vaginal HPV-induced lesions can often be found with cervical lesions, such as is seen in this woman with both CIN1 and VAIN1. **(b)** and in another patient with CIN 2 and with VAIN 2 on the left anterolateral vaginal wall. CO_2 laser vaporization would be an ideal treatment option for extensive high-grade cervical and vaginal intraepithelial neoplasia such as seen here. ▬▬

cervical disease, extending the vaginal cuff to remove the vaginal lesion may be possible. If the vaginal lesion is more extensive, surgical excision will inevitably shorten the vagina. Vaporizing the vaginal part of the lesion and proceeding to hysterectomy is possible in this situation. The vaginal vault closure must leave the vault and angles available for adequate post-operative assessment and accessible to treatment if VAIN were to recur at this site.

Skilled application of conservative laser surgery is imperative in the treatment of high-grade VAIN. Delayed healing and scarring of the vagina may occur following unskilled or overenthusiastic destruction of vaginal mucosa, and post-operative vesicovaginal fistulas have been reported. Post-treatment complications can have serious implications for sexuality and post-operative monitoring.

Excisional and other surgical methods Because the depth of tissue destruction has been more difficult to control when cryotherapy and electrocautery have been used to treat VAIN, these modalities have been less commonly used for this purpose. The surrounding tissue damage may be excessive and risk of bowel or bladder damage may increase. The potential for iatrogenic injury has become particularly relevant as loop electrosurgical excision procedures have gained more widespread acceptance for management of CIN and other genital HPV induced lesions. Although VAIN is most commonly treated by laser ablation, surgical excision is indicated when VAIN recurs at the vaginal cuff following hysterectomy for high-grade CIN, and when invasive cancer within an area of high-grade VAIN cannot be ruled out.

Recurrence of VAIN at the vaginal cuff Laser treatment of VAIN in the vaginal vault in women who have had a hysterectomy was considered initially a very satisfactory treatment. However, studies with longer follow-up intervals have documented 75% recurrence rates. There is also an increased risk of subsequent development of invasive cancer in the vault[74] secondary to dysplastic epithelium buried in the suture line during hysterectomy. Because of this risk, high grade VAIN detected in the vaginal vault post-hysterectomy is usually best excised.[75,76]

Local excision to rule out invasion Excision of vaginal lesions may be performed either by scalpel or by CO_2 laser. CO_2 laser has the advan-tage of securing hemostasis at the time of the excision and reduction in the amount of tissue removed, but does require skill in using the CO_2 laser in order to prevent damage to underlying organs such as bladder and bowel. Sherman reported that injecting fluid under a high-grade VAIN lesion, thereby elevating the lesion and providing a buffer from underlying organs, increased the safety of CO_2 laser excision of these lesions.[73] Scalpel excision of VAIN has most often been in the form of a partial vaginectomy of the area involved when the possibility of occult invasive cancer is of concern. Depending upon the size of the area removed, split-thickness skin grafts may be used to restore normal vaginal length.[42]

References

1. Coppleson M, Pixley E, Reid B. *Colposcopy: A Scientific and Practical Approach to the Cervix in Health and Disease.* Springfield, IL: Charles Thomas, Publ. 1971

2. Hummer W K, Mussey E, Decker D G, Docherty M B. Carcinoma in situ of the vagina. *Am J Obstet Gynecol* 1970;108:1109–16.

3. Woodruff J D. Carcinoma in situ of the vagina. *Clin Obstet Gynecol* 1981;24:485–99.

4. Micheletti L, Zanotto Valentino M C, Barbero M, Preti M, Nicolaci P, Canni M. Current knowledge about the natural history of intraepithelial neoplasms of the vagina. *Minerva Ginecol* 1994 46:195–204.

5. Townsend G E. Colposcopy: How to examine the vulva and vagina. *Cont Obstet Gyn.* 1984;23:161.

6. Davis G D. Colposcopic examination of the vagina. *Obstet Gynecol Clinic N Amer.*1993;20:217–29.

7. Krieger J N, Wolner-Hanssen P, Stevens C, Holmes K K. Characteristics of Trichomonas vaginalis isolates from women with and without colpitis macularis. *J Infect Dis* 1990;161:307–11.

8. Wolner-Hanssen P, Krieger J N, Stevens C E, Kiviat N B, Koutsky L, Critchlow C, DeRouen T, Hillier S, Holmes K K. Clinical manifestations of vaginal trichomoniasis. *JAMA* 1989 27;261:571–6.

9. Sonnex C. Colpitis macularis and macular vaginitis unrelated to Trichomonas vaginalis infection. *Int J STD AIDS* 1997;8:589–91.

10. Cibley L J, Cibley L J. Cytolytic vaginosis. *Am J Obstet Gynecol* 1991;165:1245–9.

11. Horowitz B J, Mardh P A, Nagy E, Rank E L. Vaginal lactobacillosis. *Am J Obstet Gynecol* 1994;170:857–61.

12. Gardner H L, Desquamative inflammatory vaginitis. *Am J Obstet Gynecol* 1969 15;1041224–5.

13. Oates J K, Rowen D. Desquamative inflammatory vaginitis. A review. *Genitourin Med* 1990;66:275–9.

14. Kaufman R H, Friedrich E G, Gardner H L. *Benign Diseases of the Vulva and Vagina.* Chicago: Year Book Medical Publ. 1989.

15. Sobel J D. Desquamative inflammatory vaginitis: a new subgroup of purulent vaginitis responsive to topical 2% clindamycin therapy. *Am J Obstet Gynecol* 1994;171:1215–20.

16. Wilkinson E J, Stone I K. *Atlas of Vulvar Disease.* Williams and Wilkins, Baltimore, MD. 1995.

17. Ridley C M. Chronic erosive vulval disease. *Clin Exp Dermatol* 1990;15:245–52.

18. Jefferies J A, Robboy S J, O'Brien P C, Bergstralh E J, Labarthe D R, Barnes A B, Noller K L, Hatab P A, Kaufman R H, Townsend D E. Structural anomalies of the cervix and vagina in women enrolled in the Diethylstilbestrol Adenosis (DESAD) Project. *Am J Obstet Gynecol* 1984;148:59–66.

19. Garzetti G G, Ciavattini A, Goteri G, Menzo S, De Nictolis M, Clementi M, Brugia M, Romanini C. Vaginal micropapillary lesions are not related to human papillomavirus infection: in situ hybridization and polymerase chain reaction detection techniques. *Gynecol Obstet Invest* 1994;38:134–9.

20. Jordan J. Colposcopy of the abnormal transformation zone. *Obstet Gynecol Clinic N Amer.* 1993;20:69–81.

21. McDonnell J M, Emens J M, Jordan J A. The congenital cervicovaginal transformation zone in sexually active young women. *Br J Obstet Gynaecol* 1984;91:580–4.

22. Kranl C, Zelger B, Kofler H, Heim K, Sepp N, Fritsch P. Vulval and vaginal adenosis. *Br J Dermatol* 1998;139:128–31.

23. Herbst A L, Ulfelder H, Poskanzer D C. Adenocarcinoma of the vagina: Association of maternal stilbestrol therapy with tumor appearance in young women. *N Engl J Med* 1971;284:878–81.

24. Barrett K F, Bledsoe S, Greer B E, et al. Tampon induced vaginal or cervical ulceration. *Am J Obstet Gynecol* 1977;127:332–3.

25. Friedrich E G. Tampon effects on vaginal health. *Clin Obstet Gynecol* 1981;24:395–406.

26. Friedrich E G, Siegesmund K A. Tampon-induced vaginal ulcerations. *Obstet Gynecol* 1980;55:149–56.

27. Zweiful P. Die vaginitis emphasematosa, oder colpohyperplasia cystica nach Winlel. *Arch Gynekol* 1977;12:39.

28. Tjugum J, Jonassen F, Olsson J H. Vaginitis emphasematosa in a renal transplant patient. *Acta Obstet Gynecol Scan* 1986;65–377–8.

29. Evans D M D, Hughes H. Cysts of the vaginal wall. *Br J Obstet Gynecol* 1947;53:335.

30. Gardner H L. Cervical and vaginal endometriosis. *Clin Obstet Gynecol* 1966;9:358–72.

31. Gardner H L. Cervical endometriosis, a lesion of increasing importance. *Am J Obstet Gynecol* 1962;84:170–3.

32. Tsukada Y. Benign melanosis of the vagina and cervix. *Am J Obstet Gynecol* 1976;124:211–2.

33. Kerley S W, Blute M L, Keeney G L. Multifocal malignant melanoma arising in vesicovaginal melanosis. *Arch Pathol Lab Med* 1991;115:950–2.

34. Karney M Y, Cassidy M S, Zahn C M, Snyder R R. Melanosis of the vagina. A case report. *J Reprod Med* 2001;46:389–91.

35. O'Brien P C, Noller K L, Robboy S J. Vaginal epithelial changes in young women enrolled in the National Cooperative Diethylstilbestrol Adenosis (DESAD) Project. *Obstet Gynecol* 1979;53:300–8.

36. Trimble E L, Rubinstein L V, Menck H R, Hankey B F, Kosary C, Giusti R M. Vaginal clear cell adenocarcinoma in the United States. *Gynecol Oncol* 1996;61:113–5.

37. Di Saia P, Creaseman W T. Invasive cancer of the vagina and urethra. In: DiSaia P and Creaseman W. Eds, *Clinical Gynecologic Oncology*, St Louis, MO: C V Mosby and Co. p. 33.

38. Audet-Lapointe P, Body G, Vauclair R, Drouin P, Ayoub J. Vaginal intraepithelial neoplasia. *Gynecol Oncol* 1990;36:232–9.

39. Lenehan P M, Meffe F, Lickrish G M. Vaginal intraepithelial neoplasia: Biologic aspects and management. *Gynecol Oncol* 1986;68:333–7.

40. Mao C C, Chao K C, Lian Y C, Ng H T. Vaginal intraepithelial neoplasia: Diagnosis and management. *Chung Hua I Hsueh Tsa Chih* 1990;46:35–42.

41. Nwabineli N J, Monaghan J M. Vaginal epithelial abnormality in patients with CIN: clinical and pathological features and management. *Br J Obstet Gynecol* 1991;98:25.

42. Singer A, Monaghan J M. Vaginal intraepithelial neoplasia. In: *Lower Genital Tract Precancer: Colposcopy, Pathology and Treatment*. Oxford: Blackwell Science, 2000.

43. Hoffman M S, de Cesare S L, Roberts W S. Upper vaginectomy for in situ and occult superficially invasive carcinoma of the vagina. *Am J Obstet Gynecol* 1992;166:30–3.

44. Bowen-Simpkins P B, Hull M G. Intraepithelial vaginal neoplasia following immunosuppressive therapy treated with topical 5-FU. *Obstet Gynecol* 1975:46:360–2.

45. Townsend D E. Intraepithelial neoplasia of the vagina. In: Coppleson M (ed) Gynecologic Oncology. Churchill Livingston, Edinburgh. 1991, p. 493.

46. Lopes A, Monaghan J M, Robertson G. Vaginal intraepithelial neoplasia. In: Luesley D, Jordan J, Richart R, Eds. *Intraepithelial Neoplasia of the Lower Genital Tract*. New York: Churchill Livingston, 1995.

47. Aho M, Vesterinen E, Meyer B, et al. Natural history of vaginal intraepithelial neoplasia. *Cancer* 1991;68:195–7.

48. Sillman F H, Fructer R C, Chen Y-C et al. Vaginal intraepithelial neoplasia: Risk factors for persistence, recurrence, and invasion and its management. *Am J Obstet Gynecol* 1997;176:93–9.

49. Micheletti L, Zanotto Valentino M C, Barbero M, Preti M, Nicolaci P, Canni M. Current knowledge about the natural history of intraepithelial neoplasms of the vagina. *Minerva Ginecol* 1994;46:195–204.

50. Dahling J R, Madeleine M M, Sherman K J, et al. Anogenital tumors associated with human papillomavirus. In: Fortner J G, Rhoads J E, eds. Accomplishments in Cancer Research. Philadelphia: J B Lippincott, 1993.

51. Aaltonen L M, Rihkanen H, Vaheri A. Human papillomavirus in larynx. *Laryngoscope* 2002;112:700–7.

52. Syrjanen S, Puranen M. Human papillomavirus infections in children: the potential role of maternal transmission. *Crit Rev Oral Biol Med* 2000;11:259–74.

53. Rylander E, Eriksson A, von Schoultz B. Wart virus infection of cervix uteri and vagina in women with atypical cervical cytology. *Scand J Urol Nephrol Suppl* 1984;86:223–6.

54. Schneider A, de Villiers E M, Schneider V. Multifocal squamous neoplasia of the female genital tract: significance of human papillomavirus infection of the vagina after hysterectomy. *Obstet Gynecol* 1987;70:294–8.

55. Hilgers R D, Malkasian G D Jr, Soule E H. Embryonal rhabdomyosarcoma (botryoid type) of the vagina. A clinicopathologic review. *Am J Obstet Gynecol* 1970;107:484–502.

56. Leuschner I, Harms D, Mattke A, Koscielniak E, Treuner J. Rhabdomyosarcoma of the urinary bladder and vagina: a clinicopathologic study with emphasis on recurrent disease: a report from the Kiel Pediatric Tumor Registry and the German CWS Study. *Am J Surg Pathol* 2001;25:856–64.

57. Gupta D, Malpica A, Deavers M T, Silva E G. Vaginal melanoma: a clinicopathologic and immunohistochemical study of 26 cases. *Am J Surg Pathol* 2002;26:1450–7.

58. Melnick S, Cole P, Anderson D, et al. Rates and risks of diethylstilbestrol-related clear cell adenocarcinoma of the vagina and cervix. *N Engl J Med* 1987;316:514–6.

59. Stafl A, Mattingly R F. Vaginal adenosis: a precancerous lesion? *Am J Obstet Gynecol* 1974;120:666–77.

60. Grainai C O, Walters M D, Safaii H et al. Malignant transformation of vaginal endometriosis. *Obstet Gynecol* 1984;64:592–5.

61. Saito T, Takehara M, Tanaka R, Sato K, Fujita M, Kudo R. Usefulness of silver intensification of immunostaining for cytologic diagnosis of primary melanoma of the female genital organs. *Acta Cytol* 2002;46:1075–80.

62. Liu L Y, Hou Y J, Li J Z. Primary malignant melanoma of the vagina: a report of seven cases. *Obstet Gynecol* 1987;70:569–72.

63. Kaminski P F, Sorosky J I, Wheelock J B, Stevens C W Jr. The significance of atypical cervical cytology in an older population. *Obstet Gynecol* 1989;73:13–5.

64. Kirwin P, Naftalin N J. Topical 5-fluorouracil in the treatment of vaginal intraepithelial neoplasia. *Br J Obstet Gynecol* 1985;92:287–91.

65. Krebs H B, Helmkamp F. Chronic ulcerations following topical therapy with 5-fluorouracil therapy for vaginal human papillomavirus associated lesions. *Obstet Gynecol* 1991;78:205–8.

66. Rome R M, England P G. Management of vaginal intraepithelial neoplasia: A series of 132 cases with long-term follow-up. *Int J Gynecol Cancer* 2000;10:382–90.

67. Petrilli E S, Townsend D E, Morrow C P, Nakao C Y. Vaginal intraepithelial neoplasia: Biologic aspects and treatment with topical 5-fluorouracil and the carbon dioxide laser. *Am J Obstet Gynecol* 1980 1;138:321–8.

68. Krebs H B. Treatment of vaginal condylomata acuminata by weekly topical application of 5-fluorouracil. *Obstet Gynecol* 1987;70:68–71.

69. Stafl A, Wilkinson E J, Mattingly R F. Laser treatment of cervical and vaginal neoplasia. *Am J Obstet Gynecol* 1977;128–36.

70. Jobson V W, Homesley H D. Treatment of vaginal intraepithelial neoplasia with the carbon dioxide laser. *Obstet Gynecol* 1983;62:90–3.

71. Stuart G C E, Flagler E A, Nation J G et al. Laser vaporization of vaginal intraepithelial neoplasia. *Am J Obstet Gynecol* 1988;158:240–3.

72. Diakomanolis E, Rodolakis A, Boulgaris Z, Blachos G, Michalas S. Treatment of vaginal intraepithelial neoplasia with laser ablation and upper vaginectomy. *Gynecol Obstet Invest* 2002;54:17–20.

73. Sherman A I. Laser therapy for vaginal intraepithelial neoplasia after hysterectomy. *J Reprod Med* 1990;35:941–4.

74. Woodman C B, Jordan J A, Wade-Evans T. The management of vaginal intraepithelial neoplasia after hysterectomy. *Br J Obstet Gynaecol* 1984;91:707–11.

75. Monaghan J M. Vaginal Cancer. In: Burghardt E, Ed. Surgical gynecologic oncology. Stuttgart: George Thieme Verlag, 1993.

76. Hoffman M S, DeCesare S L, Roberts W S, Fiorica J V, Finan M A, Cavanagh D. Upper vaginectomy for in situ and occult, superficially invasive carcinoma of the vagina. *Am J Obstet Gynecol* 1992;166:30–3.

Vulvar Abnormalities

Table of Contents

15.1 Normal Anatomy and Histology

A detailed description of vulvar embryology, normal anatomy and histology is discussed in chapter 2. Some pertinent comments are reiterated here for correlation with the different pathophysiologies, clinical presentations and histopathologies of the various vulvar disorders. The vulva encompasses an area between the genitocrural folds laterally and between the mons pubis anteriorly and the anus posteriorly. This area includes the mons pubis, the labia minora and majora, the clitoris, and vestibule, Skene's glands and ducts, the hymen, Bartholin's glands and ducts, the urethral meatus and vestibulovaginal bulbs. The *vestibule* is defined as that portion medial to the labia minora extending from the clitoral region to the posterior fourchette (Figure 15.1).[1,2] The majority of the vulva is covered by keratinized skin. The exception is the vestibule, which is partially covered by a nonkeratinized surface that is flush with the vagina. The junction of keratinized squamous epithelium on the posterior fourchette and labia minora with the mucosa of the vestibule is known as *Hart's line*. Hart's line reflects the derivation of these 2 structures during embryonic development, as the vulva arises from ectoderm and the inner vestibule arises from the endodermally derived urogenital sinus.[2]

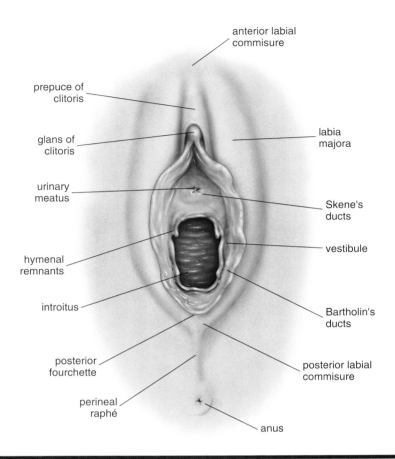

anterior labial
commisure

prepuce of
clitoris

glans of
clitoris

urinary
meatus

hymenal
remnants

introitus

posterior
fourchette

perineal
raphé

labia
majora

Skene's
ducts

vestibule

Bartholin's
ducts

posterior labial
commisure

anus

FIGURE 15.1   Illustration of a normal vulva. The labia minora are opened to reveal the vestibule.

The vestibule has numerous gland openings. Skene's ducts are directly inferior and lateral to the urethra. Bartholin's glands and ducts (the major vestibular glands and ducts) are located along the inferior lateral portion of the vulva, near the junction of the labia minora and labia majora. The minor vestibular glands are located in a semicircular area near Hart's line. The vestibule can also contain numerous micropapillary structures. These small papillomas have been previously confused with vulvar condylomas or subclinical human papillomavirus (HPV) infections; however, HPV has not been consistently identified in these structures.[3]

The hymeneal ring represents the boundary between the vulvar vestibule and the vagina. Prior to intercourse, the hymen is a plate-like structure with some degree of perforation. An imperforate hymen, in which the hymenal plate is solid, can lead to an accumulation of menstrual efflux and vaginal material known as a *hematocolpos.*

Histologically, the keratinized squamous epithelial surface or epidermis is divided into layers or strata. The entire epidermis is known as the *stratum malpighi.* The keratinized surface is the *stratum*

corneum epidermidis. The epithelial cells containing basophilic keratohyaline granules are located directly beneath the keratin layer and compose the *stratum granulosum epidermidis.* The *stratum spinosum epidermidis* represents the majority of the squamous cells. The *stratum basale epidermidis* is made up of the least mature squamous cells and is located adjacent to the basement membrane. The individual squamous cells that compose the keratinized surface are also known as *keratinocytes* (Figure 15.2).[2] The epidermis has undulating extensions into the underlying dermis, which are known as *rete pegs.* The superficial, loose dermis located between the rete pegs is known as the *papillary dermis.* The dense collagenous dermis below the papillary layer is the *reticular dermis.* The deepest layer beneath the dermis is the subcutaneous fat.

The adnexal structures found in the reticular dermis include eccrine (sweat) glands, apocrine glands that produce pheromones, specialized nerve receptors, and hair structures or pilosebaceous units. The free nerve endings, sensory structures that register itching and pain, are located in the superficial dermis directly beneath the stratum basalis. In older women who have a thin epidermis, there is increased poten-

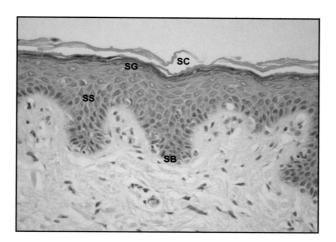

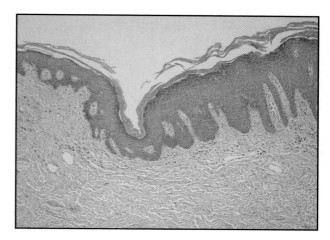

FIGURE 15.2 Photomicrograph of vulvar skin. The entire epidermal surface of the vulva is known as the stratum malpighi. SC: stratum corneum epidermidis (keratin layer). SG: stratum granulosum epidermidis. SS: stratum spinosum epidermidis or *prickle cell layer.* SB: stratum basale epidermidis or *germinativum.* (Hematoxylin-eosin stain; high power magnification). ▬

FIGURE 15.3 Photomicrograph of epidermal acanthosis. The epidermis at the right of the microscopic field is thickened. In addition, the rete pegs are lengthened and focally confluent (Hematoxylin-eosin stain; medium power magnification). ▬

tial for receptor exposure, which can lead to symptomatic burning and itching.

The keratinized portion of the vulva is subject to numerous dermatological diseases, and therefore is an area of interest to gynecologists, dermatologists, and gynecological, dermatological, and general surgical pathologists. The diverse diagnostic verbiage used by the different specialties has resulted in confusion among clinicians that treat vulvar diseases. In addition, many pathologists will often substitute descriptive terms for vulvar microscopic diagnoses, and it is important that the colposcopist understand these terms and their definitions as well.

The term *acantholysis* refers to the abrupt separation of epidermal cells resulting from dissolution of the intercellular cement substance, which leads to loss of cellular cohesion. There is localized clearing and bullous formation, with detached cells within the cavity. The term *acanthosis* is used to describe thickening in the epidermal layer, predominately though enlargement of the rete pegs. (Figure 15.3). *Dyskeratosis* is faulty and premature keratinization of individual squamous cells. When seen in vulvar dysplasia, individual dyskeratocytes are also known as *corps rondes* (Figure 15.4). *Exocytosis* is a condition in which inflammatory cells are present in the epidermis. *Hyperkeratosis* refers to an increase in the thickness of the stratum corneum or keratin layer. This is a subjective observation made by comparing the skin surface in question to skin that is considered to have

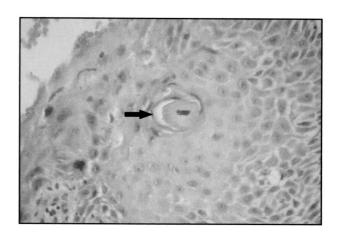

FIGURE 15.4 Photomicrograph of dyskeratocytosis. A single orangeophilic dyskeratocyte (arrow) is present (Hematoxylin-eosin stain, high power magnification). ▬

a normal keratin thickness. Lentiginous or *lentigo formation* is a linear pattern of melanocytic cell proliferation within the basal layer (Figure 15.5). A *lichenoid change* refers to the development of a plaque-like lesion with a flattened appearance of the epidermis or adjacent chronic inflammatory cells. *Parakeratosis* is the presence of nuclei within the keratin layer that, along with hyperkeratosis and dyskeratosis, implies that squamous epithelial cells are undergoing rapid and excessive keratinization (Figure 15.6). *Papillomatosis* refers to elongation of the papillary dermis and the associated extension of the adjacent epidermis. *Spongiosis* is intercellular edema that results in

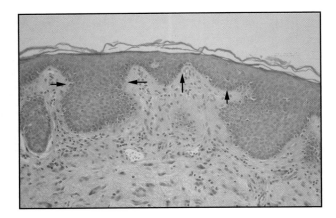

FIGURE 15.5 Photomicrograph of epidermal lentigo. Note the increase in the number of melanocytes and basal pigmentation (arrows). (Hematoxylin-eosin stain; medium power magnification.)

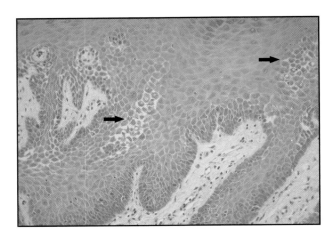

FIGURE 15.7 Photomicrograph of spongiosis. Individual keratinocytes are separated from each other (arrows) (Hematoxylin-eosin stain; medium power magnification).

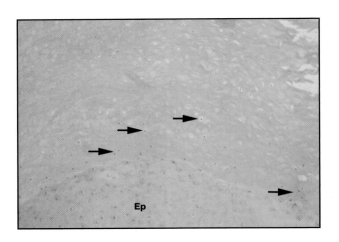

FIGURE 15.6 Photomicrograph of parakeratosis. Note the pyknotic nuclei scattered throughout the keratin layer (arrows). In addition, the keratin layer is markedly thickened (hyperkeratosis) (Ep=epidermis). (Hematoxylin-eosin stain; high power magnification.)

separation of individual epithelial cells. A mononuclear infiltrate is typically present when this condition occurs (Figure 15.7).[4]

15.2 Examination and Biopsy Techniques

The vulva is best examined using a good source of white light and a magnification device. The latter can be as simple as a handheld magnifying lens or as sophisticated as a colposcope. If a colposcope is used, the lower magnification levels of a fixed mag-

nification system or the wide-angle zoom on a variable magnification system is recommended to aid in identification of vulvar landmarks. Examination should be systematic and deliberate, incorporating all aspects of the vulvar surface. Any abnormal or ambiguous areas should undergo biopsy before any treatment is instituted.[5]

The vulvar examination can be aided by the application of various agents, including toluidine blue, dilute acetic acid and Lugol's solution (potassium iodide). Toluidine blue is a nuclear stain. When applied over vulvar tissue that contains increased nuclear material, a blue coloration is retained after washing the area with a saline or acetic acid solution (Figures 15.8a,b). Although commonly used in the past, toluidine blue has been generally abandoned because of its lack of sensitivity (areas of keratinized dysplasia would not stain) and specificity (retention of stain in cracks and fissures).

Dilute acetic acid functions as a contrast agent in examining the vulva and affects the tissues in much the same way as it affects tissues of the cervix and vagina. The majority of vulvar skin is keratinized; however, the amount of acetic acid solution and the length of exposure time required to achieve a reasonable effect are greater than those needed to evaluate cervicovaginal mucosa. To accomplish this, the vulva is covered with gauze that has been soaked in a 3% to 5% acetic acid solution, which is left in place for at least 5 minutes before the examination is started. Liberal amounts of acetic acid are then reapplied as the inspection continues. The ability of Lugol's solution to stain glycogenated squamous epithelial cells is of little use when applied to a keratinized epidermal surface. Nevertheless, a dilute iodide solution

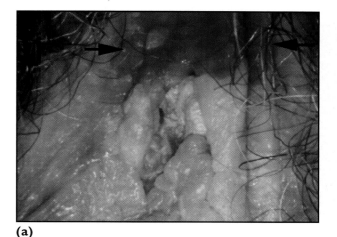

(a)

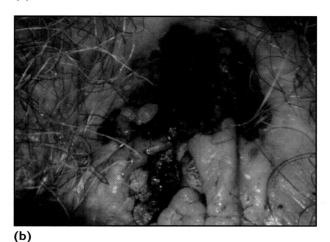

(b)

FIGURES 15.8a,b   The clinical application of toluidine blue dye. **(a)** The vulvar surface demonstrates an area that is slightly raised and hyperemic ("red lesion") (arrows), along with an area of leukoplakia in the vestibule. **(b)** Following the application of toluidene blue, the large anterior red area and the leukoplakia retain the blue stain after washing with acetic acid (Photos courtesy Wright V C. *Color Atlas of Colposcopy—Cervix, Vagina, Vulva.* Houston: Biomedical Communications, 2000, used with permission).

can enhance topographic changes, such as the micropapillary features of small condylomas.

The choice of a biopsy instrument is dependent on the type of abnormality or area to be sampled. Kevorkian or Tischler forceps can be used to easily sample raised or warty lesions. Macular lesions are best sampled by making an elliptical excision using a small knife blade or a Keyes punch. The latter, when twisted into the skin, creates a circular cookie-cutter incision. The central portion can then be raised and the specimen cut off at the base (Figure 15.9). A punch with a diameter of at least 4 mm is recom-

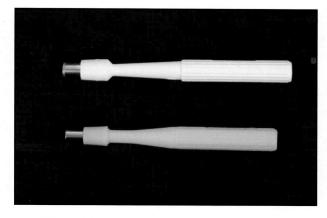

FIGURE 15.9   Keyes punch biopsy instruments. The round sharp end at the base is rotated into the skin and superficial dermis.

mended to remove an adequate cylinder. Areas of ulceration should be sampled along the edge in order to remove an area of surface epithelium; biopsies at the center will only demonstrate necrosis, granulation tissue, fibrin, and inflammation.

As with any skin biopsy, applying local anesthesia is necessary. This is easily accomplished by injecting a 1% lidocaine solution under the area to be sampled. A tuberculin syringe with a 30-gauge needle is ideal for this purpose. Particularly sensitive areas may require the application of an additional topical anesthetic. Lidocaine with epinephrine can be useful in reducing the bleeding that occurs after the biopsy. This anesthetic should not be injected into the clitoral region, however. Once the biopsy is accomplished, small defects at the biopsy site can be cauterized using silver nitrate sticks or Monsel's solution; larger defects can be approximated with interrupted absorbable suture.

15.3 Differentiation of Definite Disease from Normal

The extension of colposcopy to the management of vulvar diseases has opened up for many an unfamiliar area in which the clinician must guard against overdiagnosis and overreaction. Significant morbidity has resulted from overly aggressive treatment of both bona fide low-grade disease and of equivocal colposcopic changes that may be seen in many women. The two most important decisions facing any colposcopist in evaluating the vulva is, first to define whether there is definite disease present, and second to decide whether treatment intervention will provide specific and definable benefits that are greater than the risk of the procedure. The most common normal vulvar findings that have been misdiagnosed as disease are micropapillations, acetowhitening, vascular ectasia and sebaceous hyperplasia.

15.3.1 Micropapillations

Micropapillae of the inner labia minora, and acetowhite changes anywhere in the lower genital tract have commonly been misinterpreted as being secondary to human papillomavirus (HPV).[6] It was the presumed association of these findings with HPV that led the erroneous theory that vulvodynia was secondary to HPV.[7] *Micropapillomatosis* is a condition in which the vestibular papillae are prominent.[8] The papillae are usually small (1–3 mm) and are best detected with magnification, but can be seen with the naked eye. The papillae may be single or cover the majority of the mucosal surface of the labia minora. Visualization is enhanced with the use of three to five percent acetic acid, which results in a non-specific acetowhitening of these papillae. Biopsies of micropapillae have often been reported as having koilocytes, but up to 90% of such diagnoses have been re-read as normal when reevaluated by a panel of pathologists expert in HPV changes. Although such biopsy specimens contain papillomatosis, acanthosis, and sometimes, parakeratosis, they uniformly lack true koilocytes with nuclear atypia, multinucleated cells, or dyskeratosis necessary to make a firm diagnosis of HPV-related disease.[8,9] Instead, these equivocal diagnoses are made on the basis of papillomatosis and a misinterpretation of glycogen within the cytoplasm as koilocytotic vacuoles. More importantly, HPV-DNA is routinely not found in these specimens in excess of women not having micropapillations.[10,11] It is incumbent upon the modern colposcopist to be able to differentiate these normal findings from those that are due to expressed HPV disease without relying upon biopsy to make the diagnosis, as avoidance of biopsy in these equivocal situations offers the best chance of avoiding over-diagnosis and over-treatment. If biopsy must be done in equivocal vulvar situations, then it may be ideal to do an in-situ hybridization (ISH) as well as hematoxylin-eosin stains to definitively diagnose HPV involvement. Three patterns of normal and abnormal vulvar papillary changes may be found: normal micropapillae, vestibular papillomatosis, and papillary HPV disease.

Normal micropapillae are tiny fibrillary vestibular growths that are most commonly posterior, usually symmetrical, and may turn acetowhite. These are probably congenital in origin but may be accentuated by any inflammatory condition (Figure 15.10).

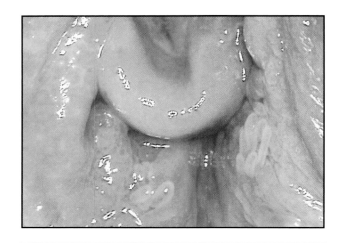

FIGURE 15.10   The normal micropapillae seen here are patchy, prominent, fairly symmetrical and they are single papillae not originating from a broad base.

Vestibular papillomatosis is the term applied when multiple papillae are present over the entire inner labia (Figures 15.11a,b). These papillae are often more clubbed and can be found in association with HPV although this association is not consistent and is felt to be casual rather than causal.[12] Acetowhitening may be more intense but is also non-specific. In some cases, these may be normal micropapillae, accentuated by inflammation.

Papillary HPV disease, in contrast, is more likely to be patchy with more starkly acetowhite papillae on a background of normal. The suspected association with HPV is often confirmed by the presence of definite HPV disease elsewhere and by the difference in morphology. Whereas each HPV lesion has multiple papillae on a single base, normal vestibular papillae originate individually directly from the epithelium. (Figure 15.12).

15.3.2 Acetowhitening

Areas of acetowhitening may also be found in the absence of micropapillations in the fossa navicularis and at the junction of this inferior part of the vestibule with the perineum. (Figure 15.13). Acetowhite changes are also frequently misdiagnosed as being secondary to HPV. Vulvar acetowhite changes may occur from the trauma of intercourse, from yeast infections, from other inflammatory conditions of the vulva, and from subclinical HPV changes[6], and therefore should always be considered to be non-specific. Acetowhite from trauma or inflammation is more likely to be diffuse and flat and may be either symptomatic or asymptomatic. In contrast, acetowhite from HPV is more likely to be slightly raised

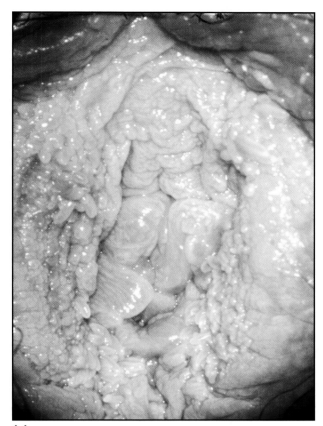

(a)

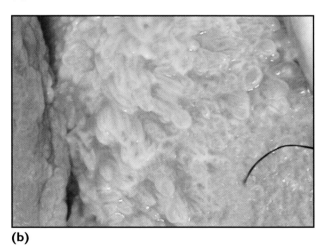

(b)

FIGURES 15.11a,b   The micropapillae in these examples of vestibular papillomatosis are diffuse, symmetrical, and cover the majority of the mucosal surface of the labia minora. Even though these micropapillae are not due to HPV, they turned significantly acetowhite with the application of acetic acid. The key to differentiating normal micropapillae from papillae of condyloma is the presence of a single base on each papillae for normal micropapillae in contrast to a broader base with multiple papillae for condyloma. Figure 15.11a Photo courtesy of Richard Reid, M.D.

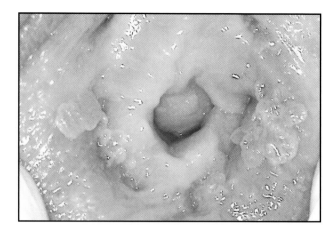

FIGURE 15.12   The papillae of these HPV lesions in this photomicrograph are patchy and more starkly acetowhite on a background of normal tissue.

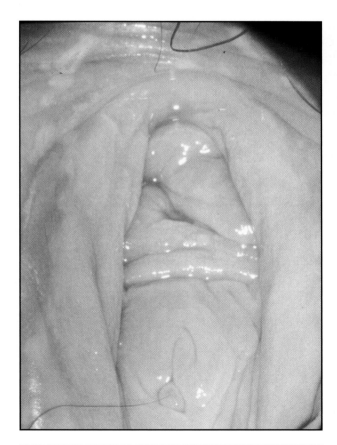

FIGURE 15.13   Acetowhite changes are seen here in the absence of micropapillations in the fossa navicularis and at the junction of this inferior part of the vestibule with the perineum. This represents a normal finding most likely seen in this patient because of increased cell turnover secondary to friction from intercourse. Photo courtesy of Richard Reid, M.D.

and may have colposcopically visible asperities (small papillations), or satellite lesions (Figure 15.14). Such areas may be slightly pruritic or may be asymptomatic. Colposcopic visualization prior to application of acetic acid will often reveal punctation or other vessel changes classic for condyloma (Figure 15.15).

15.3.3 Vascular ectasia

Depending upon the thickness of the mucosal epithelium, the vestibule may normally exhibit various degrees of erythema as the color of the underlying vasculature transmits through the non-keratinized epithelium. While vestibulitis is typically manifest by increased erythema in the vestibule (Figure 15.16),

marked individual variation in normal color makes this a difficult sign to interpret (Figure 15.17). In contrast, erythema of the labia majora usually signifies an enhancement of the underlying vasculature by inflammation or neoplasia (Figure 15.18).

15.3.4 Sebaceous hyperplasia

The area from Hart's line to the junction of the hair-bearing skin is particularly endowed with sebaceous glands. These glands may be more visible with the colposcope and may create a cobblestone appearance (Figure 15.19), or may be enlarged enough to be seen without magnification (Figure 15.20). Age and inflammation may both result in hypertrophy of

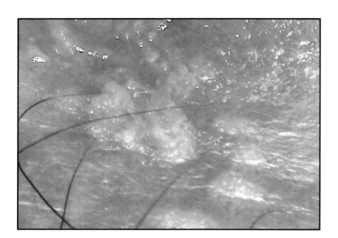

FIGURE 15.14   Here the acetowhite changes are typical of HPV induced lesions as they are raised from the surrounding skin with colposcopically visible asperities. ▬

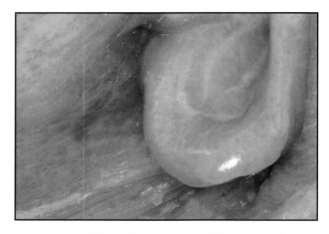

FIGURE 15.16   Localized erythema in this patient with vestibulitis is seen particularly in the area of the right major vestibular gland opening. ▬

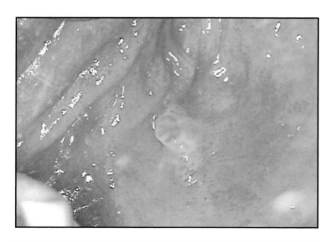

FIGURE 15.15   Another clue that the acetowhitening represents HPV changes is the colposcopic detection of localized punctation prior to application of acetic acid. ▬

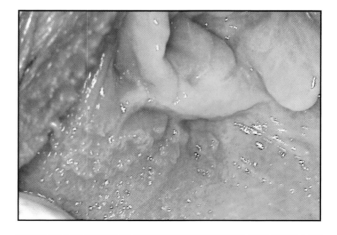

FIGURE 15.17   This woman has severe symptoms of VVS yet has no increased erythema and outwardly appears to be entirely normal. ▬

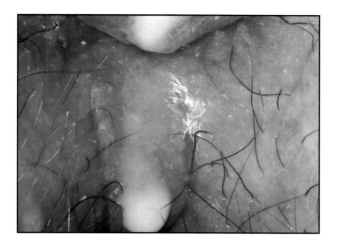

FIGURE 15.18   In contrast to erythema of the vestibule, seen in VVS, erythema of the labia majora and perineum, along with perineal fissuring and discharge as seen in this patient with candida vulvovaginitis, is characteristic of inflammation or neoplasia. ▬▬

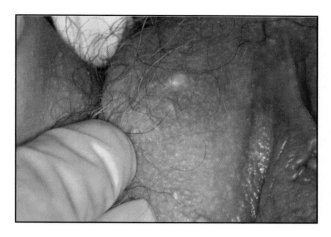

FIGURE 15.20   Several significantly enlarged sebaceous epidermal cysts are seen in the right inner labia majora. Photo courtesy of Richard Reid, M.D. With permission. ▬▬

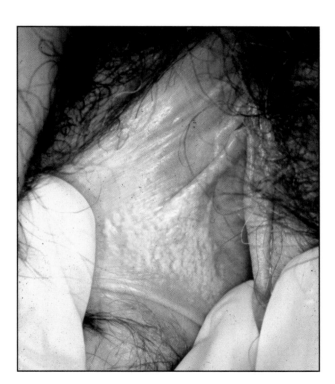

FIGURE 15.19   These fine to moderately coarse sebaceous glands are seen on the inner labia. ▬▬

these glands, but such hypertrophy should never be interpreted as a primary disease process.[5] Biopsy may be read as "sebaceous hyperplasia" and should be considered a variant of normal.

15.4 Vulvar Infections

The vulva is susceptible to a number of infectious agents including viral, bacterial, fungal, and chlamydial organisms. These organisms can result in discharge, surface irritations, and ulcerations. A complete description of the wide variety of vulvar infections is beyond the scope of this chapter, and the reader should refer to more detailed sources for additional information.[1,5,13–15] The web site for the Centers for Disease Control and Prevention (www.cdc.gov/std/treatment/default.htm) contains the most recent information on various antibiotic regimens, dosages and treatment durations for these infections. Brief discussions of the more common and unique abnormalities are included here.

15.4.1 Viral

15.4.1.1 Herpes simplex virus

The herpes viruses are double-stranded DNA viruses. There are two types of herpes viruses that affect the vulva. Herpes simplex virus (HSV) 2 is associated with genital lesions, and is usually contracted through sexual contact. Although HSV 1 is more commonly associated with oral lesions, it can be transmitted to the vulva by oral contact. The manifestations of herpes simplex occur approximately one week after incubation and usually present with initial burning, followed by the formation of small serpentine vesicles. These vesicles rupture to form ulcers that are extremely tender (Figure 15.21). Microscopically, epithelial cells with multiple, opaque

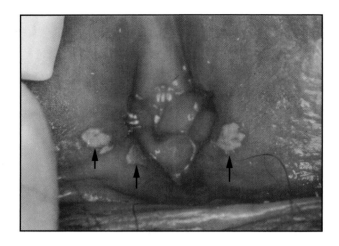

FIGURE 15.21   Herpes vulvitis. Three plaque-like ulcerations are located near the introitus (arrows) (Photo courtesy Dr. Gordon Davis, used with permission).

"ground glass" nuclei are present. These changes are best seen in exfoliated material using a Tzanck stain. A culture should be obtained to confirm the diagnosis. The culture should be taken from lesions in the vesicular or early ulcerative stage, which contain the highest concentration of viral particles. Treatment is symptomatic, e.g., sitz baths to relieve burning. The use of antiviral agents such as acyclovir can reduce the duration and intensity of the infection.[5,16]

15.4.1.2 Molluscum contagiosum

Caused by a brick-shaped DNA poxvirus, molluscum contagiosum is usually transmitted sexually in the adult population. The lesions are found on the perineum and inner thighs. They appear as small papules with central umbilicated cores that contain a cheesy material. As seen on microscopic examination, the papule consists of focally hyperplastic squamous cells. The squamous cells near the center are filled with numerous eosinophilic inclusions known as molluscum bodies (Figures 15.22a,b). These cells, containing large numbers of viral particles, lyse as they enter the center and move upwards. No treatment is necessary, although resolution may be accelerated in some cases by removing the central cores from the larger papules with a dermal curette or needle or destruction of lesions with liquid nitrogen or caustic agents.[16]

15.4.1.3 Condyloma

Human papilloma virus (HPV) is consistently identified in condylomata acuminata (genital condylomas). Although the most prevalent is HPV type 6, approximately one fourth of all condylomas contain

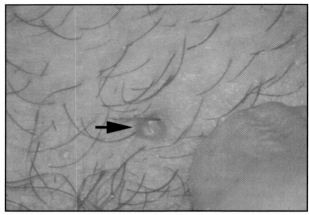

(a)

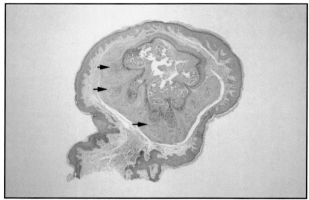

(b)

FIGURES 15.22a,b   Vulvar molluscum contagiosum. **(a)** Grossly, there is a small raised nodule with a central umbilicated dimple (arrow) (Photo courtesy Dr. Gordon Davis, used with permission). **(b)** Microscopically, there is acanthosis of the epidermis. Note the eosinophilic molluscum bodies that contain the viral particles (arrows). (Hematoxylin-eosin stain; low power magnification).

HPV 11. It is unclear whether there has been an increase in the incidence of these lesions. The association of HPV with condylomas has probably resulted in an increased awareness of their presence and subsequently increased reporting. They are commonly associated with vaginitis, pregnancy, oral contraceptive use, poor perineal hygiene, and sexual activity beginning at an early age with multiple partners. Approximately one third to one half of women with vulvar condylomas have associated cervical intraepithelial neoplasia.[1,5]

Vulvar condylomas consist of two types, flat and exophytic. Exophytic condylomas (genital warts) are typically papillary or verrucous in appearance (Figure 15.23). Although they can arise singly, condylomas usually occur in clusters and in many

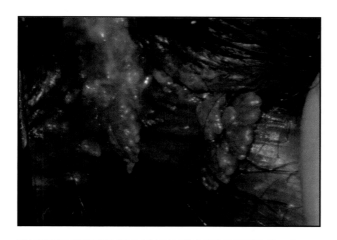

FIGURE 15.23   Vulvar condyloma. Grossly, there are multiple raised nodules. The larger ones demonstrate numerous micropapillary spikes (Photo courtesy Dr. Gordon Davis, used with permission).

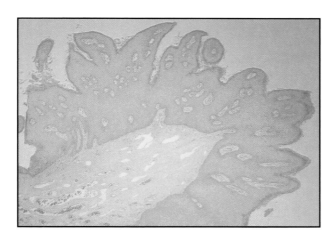

FIGURE 15.24   Photomicrograph of a vulvar condyloma. There is acanthosis and extension of the papillary dermis (papillomatosis), which forms small spikes. Hyperkeratosis is also present. (Hematoxylin-eosin stain; low power magnification.)

instances are confluent. These lesions can be found at any site along the vulvar surface, including inside the urethra and anus. Clinical identification of these lesions is usually straightforward because of their characteristic appearance. Soaking the affected area with a 5% acetic acid solution can identify small lesions.

Histologically, exophytic condylomas demonstrate papillomatosis, acanthosis, and hyperkeratosis (Figure 15.24). The granular cell layer is prominent (granulosis). Occasional dyskeratocytes are seen. Multinucleation and the presence of koilocytes (cells with hyperchromasia, irregular nuclear borders, and perinuclear clearing) differentiate condylomas from other benign papillary skin tumors.[5]

Flat condylomas are indistinguishable from low-grade vulvar intraepithelial neoplasia. Histologically, they demonstrate some basal epithelial hyperplasia and cells with features consistent with koilocytosis. Mitotic activity and multinucleation also are present. These lesions are treated with local ablation using astringents such as bichloracetic or trichloracetic acid. Podofilox, which can be self-administered, is a safer alternative to podophyllin, which has mutagenic and systemic side effects. Interferon has been used to reduce intractable condylomas; however, the long-term success from the use of this agent is not well established. Surgical excision, wire loop excision, and laser can also be used for larger lesions. Vigilant long-term observation is also acceptable for managing small isolated lesions. Nevertheless, lesions that enlarge, persist, or fail to respond to treatment require biopsy to exclude vulvar intraepithelial neoplasia or carcinoma.[5]

15.4.2 Bacterial

15.4.2.1 Syphilis

Syphilis is associated with the spirochete organism *Treponema pallidum*. Primary syphilis usually appears three weeks after inoculation, and is characterized by the formation of a single ulcer, which is indurated ("hard chancre") and non-tender. Inguinal adenopathy may be present. The ulcer regresses after one to two months, followed by a variable interval (weeks to months) before the appearance of the gray plaque-like lesions (condyloma lata) seen in secondary syphilis (Figures 15.25a,b). A biopsy of a syphilitic lesion will demonstrate numerous perivascular and dermal plasma cells. The diagnosis of syphilis can be confirmed by scraping the lesions and examining the collected material under darkfield microscopy for the presence of spirochetes. These organisms can also be identified on biopsy material by applying silver stains. Effective treatment consists of intramuscular injections of penicillin G or oral administration of tetracycline. Additional screening for coinfection with *Neisseria gonorrhea* and *Chlamydia trachomatis* is prudent.[1,5]

15.4.2.2 Granuloma inguinale

Granuloma inguinale, also known as *donovanosis*, is caused by *Calymmatobacterium granulomatis*, a gram-negative bacillus. This condition is seen in tropical and subtropical regions. Approximately 100 cases are reported annually in the southeastern United States. Clinically, small red lesions appear from 3 weeks to three months after inoculation. These evolve into

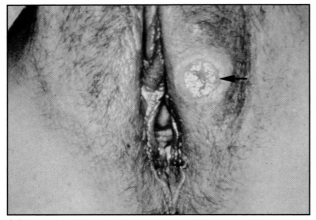

(a)

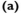

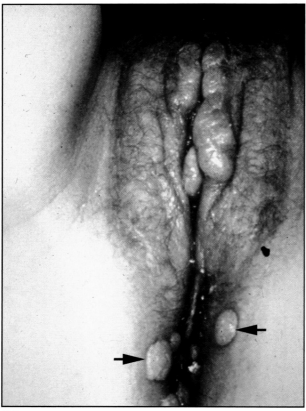

(b)

erosive ulcerations resulting in fibrosis and loss of superficial labial structures. Due to the extent of damage, fistula formation often occurs. Inguinal lymphadenopathy also develops, but the degree is less than that seen with lymphogranuloma venereum and chancroid. Identification of the causative organisms, known as Donovan bodies, in macrophages by silver stains confirms the diagnosis (Figures 15.26a,b). Treatment is oral doxycycline or trimethoprim-sulfamethoxazole. Alternative regimens consist of ciprofloxacin, erythromycin base or azithromycin. Treatment duration is a minimum of three weeks.[17]

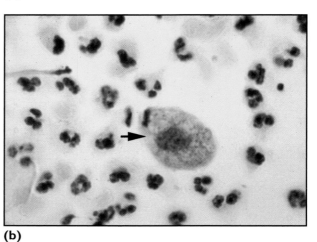

(a)

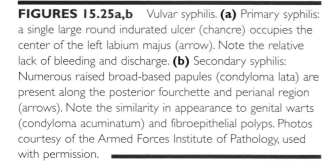

(b)

FIGURES 15.25a,b Vulvar syphilis. **(a)** Primary syphilis: a single large round indurated ulcer (chancre) occupies the center of the left labium majus (arrow). Note the relative lack of bleeding and discharge. **(b)** Secondary syphilis: Numerous raised broad-based papules (condyloma lata) are present along the posterior fourchette and perianal region (arrows). Note the similarity in appearance to genital warts (condyloma acuminatum) and fibroepithelial polyps. Photos courtesy of the Armed Forces Institute of Pathology, used with permission.

FIGURES 15.26a,b Vulvar granuloma inguinale. **(a)** Grossly large, irregularly shaped ulcerations erode the labia majora bilaterally and the perianal region (photo courtesy of the Armed Forces Institute of Pathology, used with permission). **(b)** Photomicrograph of Donovan bodies. A large macrophage (arrow) contains numerous small organisms, many of which show a characteristic halo. (Giemsa stain high power magnification.)

15.4.2.3 Chancroid

Chancroid is caused by *Hemophilus ducreyi*, a gram-negative anaerobic facultative bacillus. After an incubation period of 3 to 5 days, infected women will develop small papules that evolve into ulcers. These ulcers enlarge over time and become tender, yet do not indurate ("soft chancres") (Figure 15.27). Sinus tracts may develop. Adenopathy also occurs and may eventually enlarge to form a bubo. In its late stage, a chancroid resembles other erosive vulvar conditions such as Crohn's disease, granuloma inguinale, and lymphogranuloma venereum. In Crohn's disease, however, ulcerations occur along labial or inguinal skin folds and involve the bowel. In cases of lymphogranuloma venereum, the ulcers rapidly resolve into inguinal adenopathy with large draining buboes. The diagnosis is confirmed by a culture positive for *H. ducreyi*. The preferred treatment is oral administration of azithromycin, ceftriaxone, ciprofloxacin or erythromycin base.[5]

15.4.3 Chlamydia
15.4.3.1 Lymphogranuloma venereum

Lymphogranuloma *venereum* (LGV) is an ulcerative vulvar lesion that is associated with the Chlamydial organism. *Chlamydia trachomatis* are intracellular bodies that are associated with a number of mucosal abnormalities (trachoma, genital lesions), depending on the serotype. Serotypes L1, L2, and L3 are associated with LGV. LGV is characterized clinically by small painless ulcers on the vulva and perineum that appear 1 to 3 days after inoculation. These ulcers quickly heal, and a lymphangitis develops over the ensuing months. The disease extends bilaterally into multiple inguinal nodes, which enlarge, coalesce, and form draining abscesses or buboes (Figures 15.28a,b). These buboes can be found above and below the inguinal ligament. Due to obstructed lymphatic drainage, elephantiasis of the vulva has been observed. The microscopic features are nonspecific but can include a mixed inflammatory response and severe fibrosis. A culture or a compliment fixation assay using a titer greater than 1:64 can confirm the presence of chlamydial organisms. The recommended treatment for LGV is oral administration of doxycycline or erythromycin base for 3 weeks. Fluctuant buboes should be aspirated to prevent rupture. Incision or biopsy of buboes is not recommended, as sinus tracts may form.[5]

15.4.4 Fungi
15.4.4.1 Candidiasis

Candida is one of the more common skin infections involving the vulva and is usually caused by the organism *Candida albicans*. More resistant Candida infections often are caused by the organism *Candida glabrata*. Clinically, these infections are often associated with antibiotic use, but also are seen in women who are diabetic or immunosuppressed. Patients clinically present with vulvar itching and burning. On inspection, the skin surface is red and may demonstrate small satellite macules. Continuous rubbing of the area may cause excoriation. A white "cottage cheese" discharge may also be present (Figure 15.29). Microscopic examination of scrapings from the lesion edge or the surface discharge will demonstrate hyphal and budding forms consistent with *C. albicans*. In biopsy specimens, special stains such as periodic acid-Schiff stain or Gomori's stain are necessary to localize these organisms.[1,5]

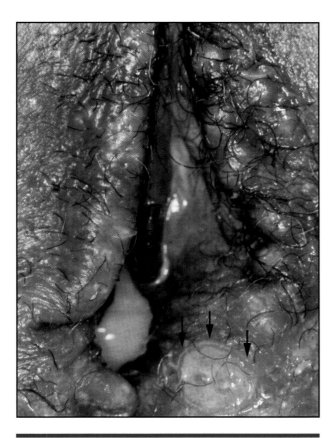

FIGURE 15.27   Vulvar chancroid. An ulcer is present on the left posterior labium majus (arrows). In contrast to a syphilitic chancre, the shape is less round and symmetrical. There is also less induration and a purulent discharge. Photo courtesy Wilkinson E J, Stone I K. *Atlas of Vulvar Diseases*, Baltimore, Williams and Wilkins, 1995, used with permission. ■

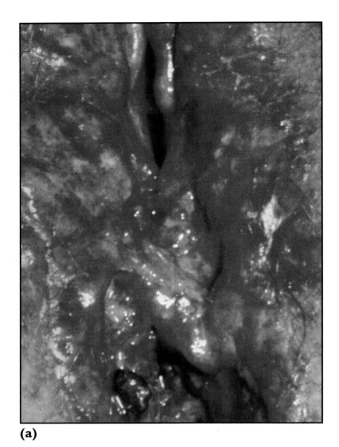

(a)

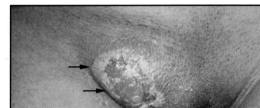

(b)

FIGURES 15.28a,b Vulvar lymphogranuloma venereum. **(a)** Large erosive areas replace a portion of the mons and the labia majora. Surface hemorrhage is present. **(b)** A large bubo (arrows) is located in the right inguinal region. Photos courtesy of the Armed Forces Institute of Pathology, used with permission.

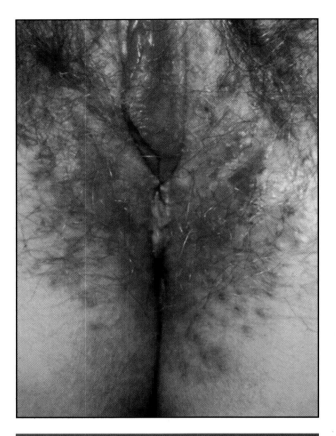

FIGURE 15.29 Vulvar candidiasis. A pink-red macular area covers the posterior fourchette and perianal region. Note the numerous red satellite lesions. Photo courtesy Wright V C. *Color Atlas of Colposcopy—Cervix, Vagina, Vulva.* Houston: Biomedical Communications, 2000, used with permission.

Treatment involves the application of a topical antifungal cream. If initial treatment with these creams is unsuccessful, then microscopic reexamination may be helpful. The presence of persistent budding forms may indicate the presence of *C. glabrata,* which may require treatment with terazol, intravaginal 5-flucytosine, boric acid, or oral antifungal medications. As women with resistant infections may have diabetes or be immunosuppressed, testing for these abnormalities may be worthwhile.[5] Weekly or monthly suppressive therapy may be useful in women with chronic recurrent candidal infections.

15.4.4.2 Tinea cruris

Tinea infections are caused by a variety of dermatophytes. These infections can occur at a number of sites, including the hands and feet, face and scalp, and trunk and perineum. Tinea cruris occurs along the inner aspect of the thigh and often extends into the perianal and perineal region. The organisms

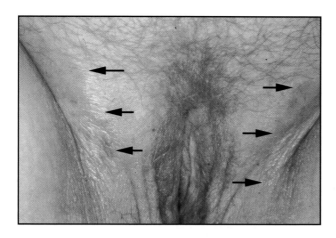

FIGURE 15.30   Vulvar tinea. Glistening slightly raised pink macular areas are located in the right and left inguinal regions (arrows) (photo courtesy Dr. Gordon Davis, used with permission).

responsible for this type of tinea are the dermatophytes, *Trichophyton rubrum*, *Trichophyton mentagrophytes* and *Epidermophyton floccosum*. Clinically, tinea cruris presents as a reddened area with raised sharp borders (Figure 15.30). Often these sites are asymptomatic, but itching may occur. The fungal organisms can be identified on wet mounts by scraping the lesion edge or in biopsy material in the region of the keratin or granular cell layer using special stains such as periodic acid—Schiff or Gomori's stain. Treatment involves application of topical antifungal creams or powders.[13]

15.5 Vulvodynia

One of the most challenging diagnostic and therapeutic dilemmas facing clinicians responsible for the care of women is the dilemma of idiopathic vulvar pain. The term applied to idiopathic vulvar pain is vulvodynia, derived from combining the word for vulva with the Greek word dynos, for pain. Over the last thirty years the entity of idiopathic vulvar pain has received various names, including "burning vulva syndrome," "focal vulvitis," "vestibular adenitis," "minor vestibular gland syndrome," "vulvar vestibulitis syndrome," vestibulodynia, "dysesthetic vulvodynia," and vulvar dysesthesia (generalized or localized). When no infection, injury, dermatoses or neoplasia can be identified as the cause of vulvar pain, the pain is likely to be idiopathic and to fit into one of the subsets of the pain syndrome known as *vulvodynia*. The 1984 ISSVD task force on vulvar pain defined vulvodynia as "chronic vulvar discomfort, especially that characterized by the patient's com-

plaint of burning, stinging, irritation or rawness".[18] To be considered chronic, the pain should be present for a minimum of three to six months. By 1988 the terminology of *vulvar vestibulitis syndrome* and *dysesthetic (essential) vulvodynia* were in common use[19] and continue despite the 1999 ISSVD proposal for a new classification system for vulvodynia with new definitions.[20] In the 1999 ISSVD proposal vulvar vestibulitis syndrome was renamed *vestibulodynia* and included with *clitorodynia* (pain localized to the clitoris) under a new category termed *localized vulvar dysesthesia*. Localized vulvar dysesthesia refers to pain usually present only with contact to the area, and can be localized by point-pressure mapping with a cotton-tipped applicator. Dysesthetic vulvodynia was renamed generalized *vulvar dysesthesia*, to refer to women with vulvar pain or burning that cannot be consistently localized by point-pressure mapping. Women with vulvar dysesthesia have pain that may occur with or without contact to the affected area and the pain may not be limited to the vestibule. In the 2001 meeting of the ISSVD the change in terminology to generalized vulvar dysesthesia and localized vulvar dysesthesia were accepted but the concept of provoked vs. unprovoked pain remained controversial and acceptance of the new terminology was suspended. The subsets of vulvodynia are not absolute groupings with known etiologies, but rather are based upon groupings of symptoms and clinical findings that enable the clinician to better approach treatment. Many women have combinations of symptoms that overlap these subgroups, or with time, may have a constellation of symptoms that transfer the patient from one subgroup to another. Therefore, a discussion of the subsets of vulvodynia will continue to include the subsets first defined by the ISSVD in the late 1980s. The two subsets most commonly described are vulvar vestibulitis syndrome and dysesthetic vulvodynia.

15.5.1 Vulvar vestibulitis

Vulvar vestibulitis is a subset of vulvodynia characterized by: 1) severe pain produced by touching the vestibule or by attempting vaginal penetration, 2) tenderness to pressure localized within the vulvar vestibule, and 3) physical findings confined to vestibular erythema of various degrees.[1,21] Tampon use and wiping the area post-urination may also be quite painful. Although erythema in the posterior part of the vestibule, especially at 4 and 8:00 near the major vestibular gland openings, is felt to be classic for vulvar vestibulitis, erythema in the vestibule is quite variable (Figures 15.31a,b). The syndrome is

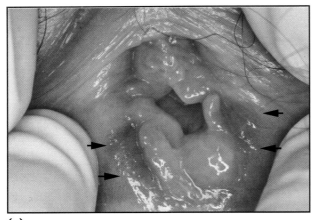

(a)

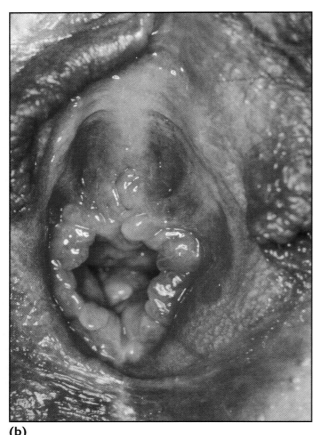

(b)

FIGURES 15.31a,b **(a)** Marked vestibular erythema in the posterior vestibule at 4:00 and 8:00 o'clock are classic for VVS. Photo courtesy of Dr. Gordon Davis. **(b)** Intense erythema around the hymen may occasionally extend to the anterior vestibule. Photo courtesy of Dr. Richard Reid.

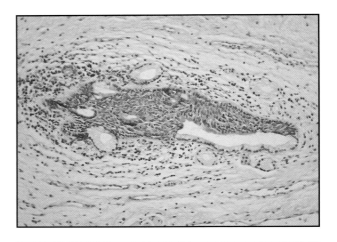

FIGURE 15.32 Photomicrograph of vulvar vestibulitis. Chronic inflammatory cells surround a cluster of minor vestibular glands. There is also focal squamous metaplasia. (Hematoxylin-eosin stain; medium power magnification.)

chronic and must have been present for a minimum of three to six months for the diagnosis to be made.

On microscopic examination, inflammatory cells occupy the surrounding stroma and only rarely are found within the vestibular gland lumen or disrupting the glandular epithelium (Figure 15.32).[1,22] Immunohistochemistry for immunoglobulins IgG, IgA, and IgM detects IgG-positive plasma cells in approximately 75% of patients suggesting chronic irritation, but an autoimmune etiology cannot be excluded or confirmed.[23] The pain associated with this abnormality may be related to increased serotonin secretion by neuroendocrine cells within the vestibular glands.[24]

Many have proposed a steroidal etiology for VVS.[25,26] An increased risk of VVS has been reported amongst women using oral contraceptive pills OCPs.[25,27] A significant increased risk has been noted for women using OCPs before age 17 (RR 11.0) and for women having their first intercourse at age 15 or earlier (RR 3.3).[25] When OCPs were first used before the age of 16 years, the relative risk of vulvar vestibulitis reached 9.3 and increased when the duration of OCP use was 2–4 years or longer. Additionally, the relative risk was higher when the pill used was of high progestogenic, high androgenic, and low estrogenic potency. It was suggested that these events occurring early in a woman's reproductive life may be important determinants of risk for developing VVS secondary to changes in the mucous producing glands of the vulvar vestibule. The authors proposed that mucous produced from these glands protects the fragile epithelium of the vestibule from the low pH of physiologic vaginal secretions of the reproductive years.

Because unprotected introital epithelium could be chronically irritated, this low level noxious stimulus could be one mechanism leading to dysfunction of the sensory nerves to this area. Such a theory, if confirmed, could explain the apparent marked increase in this syndrome beginning in the late 1970s as a result of increasing use of oral contraceptives.

One possible etiology that has been widely discussed is that vulvodynia represents a sympathetically maintained pain that occurs secondary to chronic irritation, such as candidiasis, contact irritants, alkaline vaginal secretions, destructive treatments for HPV, including TCA, 5-FU and CO2 laser, or urinary calcium oxalates.[28,29] Others have documented increased introital sensitivity to both hot and cold, results that are compatible with the hypothesis that patients with VVS have either increased enervation and/or sensitization of thermoreceptors and nociceptors in their vestibular mucosa.[30,31] A significant increase in the number of intraepithelial nerve endings has also been shown to be present in women with VVS, indicating another difference in the nerve supply of the afflicted area.[30]

Several papers have noted the association of interstitial cystitis and vulvar vestibulitis[32,33] and proposed a link between the two entities due to the common development of the bladder and the vulva from the urogenital sinus.[33,34] The frequent association of interstitial cystitis and VVS lends support to the theory that VVS is a primary neurological malfunction in epithelium of urogenital sinus origin.[33] In fact, VVS often begins with symptoms suggestive of a urinary tract infection, which may eventually resolve but leave introital dyspareunia as the primary symptom. The frequent association of interstitial cystitis and vulvar vestibulitis, and the presence of sterile inflammatory changes dominated by an increase in mast cells in both, further the theory that the inflammatory changes seen are secondary to neurogenic inflammation.[35,36] Additionally, both interstitial cystitis and VVS share positive immunofluorescence findings that are associated with vascular injury considered to be secondary to altered central neuronal processing.[32]

Human papillomavirus has been a suspect in the etiology of vulvodynia[37–41], but studies employing the most reliable of the HPV DNA tests have not found an association.[23,25,41–44] Conflicting results appear to have occurred for several reasons. First, the type of HPV test used in various studies has varied greatly, resulting in significant differences in the sensitivity for detection of HPV. Second, the ability of certain tests to detect unclassified types has continued to raise the question whether some "undiscovered" types not associated with usual HPV expression might be involved in vulvar pain syndromes. Third,

entry criteria for various studies have varied greatly, as well as the histologic parameters for diagnosing HPV. Although the exact cause, or causes, remains elusive, it can be clearly stated that vulvodynia is not a sexually transmitted disease.

15.5.1.1 Treatment of Vulvar Vestibulitis (VVS)

Treatment of any disorder of unknown etiology is always difficult and treatment of idiopathic vulvar pain is no exception. No single treatment has been uniformly successful. Initial treatment for acute vulvar vestibulitis should always be medical, with surgery reserved as a last-resort for treatment failures. Potential irritants and allergens should be eliminated, vulvovaginal infections should be treated, oral antifungal treatment should be considered if there is a possibility of yeast hypersensitivity, tricyclic antidepressants can be helpful. Biofeedback and physical therapy to the pelvic floor muscles have proven to be a mainstay in the treatment armamentarium.[45] Immunotherapy with interferon has been tried with mixed success in recalcitrant cases. If nonsurgical management fails, vestibulectomy and vaginal advancement provide symptomatic relief in many of these patients.[1]

15.5.2 Dysesthetic vulvodynia

A burning or rawness that is limited to the vulvar vestibule and is usually not accompanied by erythema, or even sensitivity to evaluation with a Q-tip, is most frequently termed dysesthetic vulvodynia.[46,47] The pain of dysesthetic vulvodynia is most often continuously present, not dependent upon touch or other stimuli to be triggered. When discomfort is associated with intercourse it is usually not one of increased pain at the time, but discomfort may be accentuated for prolonged period of time post-intercourse. Most commonly the discomfort extends beyond the vulvar vestibule to include the interlabial sulcus bilaterally, and often the labia majora. Dysesthetic vulvodynia and pudendal neuralgia may overlap in situations in which no obvious nerve injury may be elicited.[48] The description of burning pain in dysesthetic vulvodynia is similar to that of post-herpetic neuralgia (post-zoster neuralgia) and glossodynia (burning tongue), suggesting a problem with cutaneous perception either centrally or at the nerve root.[49]

15.5.2.1 Treatment of dysesthetic vulvodynia

Increasing recognition that VVS and dysesthetic vulvodynia represent primarily neuropathic disorders has fostered evaluation of tricyclic antidepressants (SSRIs),[46] and more recently, neuroleptics such as gabapentin.[50] Dysesthetic vulvodynia, as with pudendal neuralgia, has primarily been managed with tricyclic anti-depressants such as amitriptyline, or despiramine. However, neuroleptics, such as gabapentin, have demonstrated efficacy in treatment of post-herpetic neuralgia, diabetic neuropathy, trigeminal neuralgia, vulvodynia and interstitial cystitis.[50-53] When first initiated, gabapentin, as with the other neuroleptics, should be gradually increased in dose from 300 mg po qd × 3 days, to 300 mg bid × 3 days, 300 mg tid for one month, then gradually increasing the dose as tolerated, but not to exceed a total of 3600 mg per day.

Since this disorder most frequently occurs in postmenopausal women, it is imperative that atrophic vaginitis and vulvitis secondary to estrogen loss is eliminated as a possible etiology.

15.6 Vulvar Nonneoplastic Abnormalities

Longstanding uncertainty exists regarding the classification of the so-called "nonneoplastic" and "preneoplastic" vulvar lesions. In the past, various specialties have had an interest in identifying and categorizing vulvar abnormalities. In some cases this led to an overlapping of terms to represent the same clinical entity and considerable confusion among clinicians regarding the significance and management of these lesions.

In 1976, the International Society for the Study of Vulvar Diseases (ISSVD) proposed a categorization of the newly described *vulvar dystrophies* (defined as tissue degeneration from abnormal nutrition), dividing them into 2 general categories. The first encompassed those dystrophies having no premalignant potential and included lichen sclerosus or "atrophic dystrophy." The second category, termed hyperplastic dystrophy, included those dystrophies that could undergo atypical change and progress to invasive carcinoma. Table 15.1 summarizes this classification.[54]

Nevertheless, continued misunderstanding regarding terminology and definitions persisted as new terms were introduced to describe vulvar premalignant lesions. In 1986 the ISSVD, in conjunction with the International Society for Gynecologic Pathologists (ISGP) modified the original terminology into two categories. The first category representing little or no malignant potential was renamed, "Vulvar Nonneoplastic Abnormalities." The second category representing intraepithelial lesions was renamed, "Vulvar Noninvasive Neoplastic Abnormalities." Table 15.2 lists the Vulvar Nonneoplastic Abnormalities.[54] Treatment regimens for the nonneoplastic abnormalities usually include topical

Table 15.1   New Nomenclature for Vulvar Disease (1976)

Lichen sclerosus
Hyperplastic dystrophy
  Without atypia
  With atypia (graded as mild, moderate, marked)
Mixed (lichen sclerosus and hyperplastic) dystrophy
  Without atypia
  With atypia (graded as mild, moderate, marked)
Carcinoma in situ
Paget's disease

Table 15.2   Vulvar Nonneoplastic Abnormalities

Lichen sclerosus
Squamous hyperplasia
Other dermatoses

steroid creams or ointments. Table 15.3 lists the different steroid potency levels, and lists examples for each category.

15.6.1 Lichen sclerosus

In the dermatologic literature, lichen sclerosus is formally referred to as *lichen sclerosus et atrophicus*. Vulvar lichen sclerosus also has been labeled *kraurosis vulvae*. The lichen sclerosus that occurs in the male genital region is known as *balanitis xerotica obliterans*.[13] Gynecologists tend to prefer the term *lichen sclerosus* because the surface epithelial cells are metabolically active and not truly "atrophic."[55] In addition, the term *kraurosis vulvae* (shrinkage of the vulva) represents more of a clinical change than a distinct clinicopathologic diagnosis.[13] The prevalence and incidence of lichen sclerosus are unknown. The disorder tends to occur in infants and postmenopausal women. The etiology is likewise unknown, although there is some indication that the disease represents an autoimmune phenomenon. Lichen sclerosus can be histologically similar to morphea (circumferential or localized scleroderma). Various autoantibodies such as antithyroid, gastric parietal cell, intrinsic factor, and antinuclear and antismooth-muscle antibodies have been identified in patients with lichen sclerosus. An analysis of 84 patients with lichen sclerosus found an increase in the HLA antigens DQ7, DQ8, and DQ9.[56] Other etiologies that have been considered include familial associations and hypoestrogenism.

Table 15.3   Classification of Steroids by Potency

I (Super High Potency)	Clobetasol (0.05% cream/ointment) Betamethasone dipropionate (0.05% cream/ointment) Diflorasone diacetate (0.05% cream/ointment)
II	Amcinonide (0.1% cream/ointment) Fluocinonide (0.05% cream/ointment) Desoximetasone (0.25% cream/ointment)
III	Triamcinolone acetonide (0.5% cream) Fluticasone propionate (0.05% ointment) Betamethasone valerate (0.1% ointment)
IV	Flurandrenolide (0.05% ointment) Triamcinolone acetonide (0.1% ointment) Desoximetasone (0.05% cream)
V	Hydrocortisone butyrate (0.1% cream) Betamethasone benzoate (0.025% cream) Hydrocortisone valerate (0.2% cream/ointment)
VI	Alclometasone dipropionate (0.05% cream/ointment) Desonide (0.05% cream)
VII (Low Potency)	Dexamethasone Hydrocortisone Methylprednisolone

The clinical appearance and pathology of lichen sclerosus are very characteristic. Grossly, these lesions present as white patch-like areas overlying both labia and eventually, the perineum (Figure 15.33). In some cases, this may resemble a butterfly wing or an hourglass pattern. As the disease progresses, there may be a shrinkage and fusion of the labia minora and clitoris. The overlying skin becomes thinned and has a "cigarette paper" appearance. (Figures 15.34a,b). Areas of ecchymoses and erosion may be present from chronic rubbing and scratching and the skin splits easily due to loss of elasticity (Figure 15.35). Microscopically, the surface demonstrates hyperkeratosis. The epithelial surface is thinned. There is disruption of the basal layer and the rete pegs are lost. Directly beneath the epithelial surface, the superficial dermis is transformed into a homogenous, collagenized hypocellular matrix. Beneath this matrix is a band of chronic inflammatory cells. These histologic changes (hyperkeratosis, epithelial thinning with loss of rete pegs, sclerotic homogenization of the superficial dermis, and infiltration by a band of inflammatory cells) are diagnostic of lichen sclerosus (Figure 15.36). However, only minimal changes such as mild epithelial thinning and superficial chronic inflammation may be visible in the early transformation of the epithelium in lichen sclerosus. Focal hemorrhage and spongiosis may be seen in the epidermal/dermal

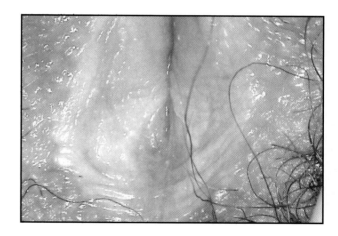

FIGURE 15.33 This 19-year-old woman presented with dyspareunia and mild vulvar pruritis. The white areas were felt to be classic for lichen sclerosus, and biopsy confirmed.

border. With advanced lesions, marked sclerosus is present within the underlying dermis.[13]

The number of lichen sclerosus cases associated with squamous cell carcinoma ranges between 3% and 6%. Nevertheless, patients with lichen sclerosus can have associated epithelial hyperplasia. In a series of 33 women with a mixture of lichen sclerosus and squamous hyperplasia (previously classified as "mixed

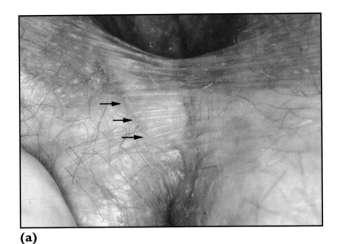

(a)

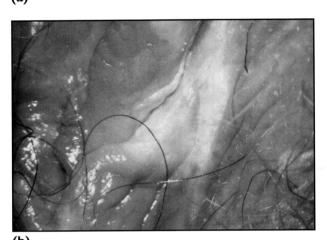

(b)

FIGURES 15.34a,b Vulvar lichen sclerosus. **(a)** The perineal body skin surface is thinned and contracted (arrows) (photo courtesy of Dr. Gordon Davis, used with permission). **(b)** The labial surface has a broad of leukoplakia. Photo courtesy Wright V C. *Color Atlas of Colposcopy—Cervix, Vagina, Vulva.* Houston: Biomedical Communications, 2000, used with permission.

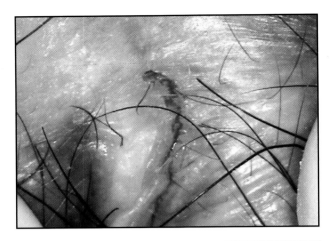

FIGURE 15.35 22-year-old woman with lichen sclerosus and chronic splitting of the perineum during intercourse secondary to the decreased elasticity of the skin with this disease process.

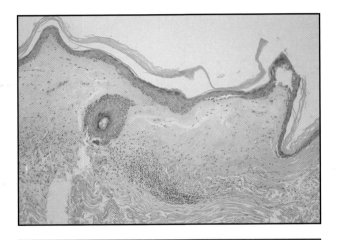

FIGURE 15.36 Photomicrograph of lichen sclerosus. There is hyperkeratosis, epidermal thinning with loss of the rete pegs, superficial dermal sclerosis, and a lichenoid band of chronic inflammatory cells. (Hematoxylin-eosin stain; medium power magnification).

dystrophy"), 3 (10%) developed squamous cell carcinoma of the vulva.[57] Thus, patients with a combination of lichen sclerosus and squamous hyperplasia need to be followed carefully. The carcinoma associated with these lesions is usually keratinizing and not commonly associated with human papillomavirus.

In the past, lichen sclerosus was treated with limited success with the topical application of testosterone cream.[58] Currently, the treatment of choice is topical fluorinated steroids such as clobetasol 0.05%. Treatment of non-lichen sclerosis affected genital skin with high-potency corticosteriods, such as clobetasol, may rather quickly result in steroid-induced epithelial atrophy. However, skin affected by lichen sclerosis is far less susceptible to the adverse effects of high-potency corticosteriods.[59] Nevertheless, adjacent normal skin may be particularly susceptible to repeated application over a prolonged period of time. Therefore, treatment should be limited to the areas involved with lichen sclerosis, and application should be tapered as the disease process improves.

15.6.2 Squamous hyperplasia

Formerly classified as a nonatypical hyperplastic dystrophy, squamous hyperplasia is considered a diagnosis of exclusion. It is characterized by epithelial hyperplasia that cannot be placed into other distinct

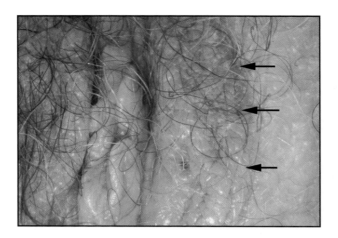

FIGURE 15.37   Vulvar squamous hyperplasia. Grossly, the labial surface is raised, roughened, and slightly erythematous (arrows). Photo courtesy of Dr. Gordon Davis. ■■■

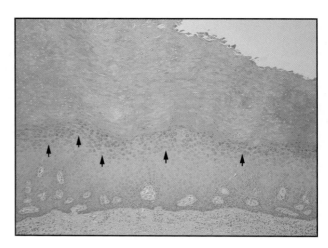

FIGURE 15.38   Photomicrograph of squamous hyperplasia. There is acanthosis with marked broadening and confluence of the rete pegs. There is also hyperkeratosis and an increase in the granular cell layer, or granulocytosis (arrows). The individual keratinocytes, however, are not atypical. (Hematoxylin-eosin stain; medium power magnification.) ■

dermatologic categories, and represents a compensatory surface thickening from constant rubbing and scratching of an irritated area of vulvar skin. The degree to which this diagnosis is made depends on the experience of the surgical pathologist with dermatopathologic conditions. A large number of cases diagnosed as squamous hyperplasia probably represent lichen simplex chronicus.[50] In a dermatopathologic review of 114 non-neoplastic vulvar lesions, all were categorized as specific dermatopathologic diagnoses; none was identified as squamous hyperplasia.[61]

The pathology of squamous cell hyperplasia is noncharacteristic. On gross physical examination, these lesions present as areas of hypopigmentation and surface thickening (Figure 15.37). These features are not distinct for squamous hyperplasia, and biopsy is necessary for definitive diagnosis. Histologically, mild to moderate hyperkeratosis and parakeratosis may be present. There is acanthosis with deepening of the rete pegs. The rete pegs are also broadened and the papillary dermis is narrowed. The squamous epithelial cells are not atypical and show normal maturation. Mitotic figures are infrequent but can be present. A mild superficial perivascular inflammation is present (Figure 15.38).[5]

As a distinct entity, vulvar squamous cell hyperplasia is not associated with human papillomavirus or the development of squamous cell carcinoma. Nevertheless, the squamous alterations adjacent to invasive cancers often encompass a form of squamous cell hyperplasia that reflects a reactive change to chronic irritation.[57,62] The recommended treatment for squamous hyperplasia is application of topical corticosteroids and antipruritics and avoidance of agents that cause surface irritation.[5,63]

15.6.3 Other dermatoses

This category encompasses a wide range of dermatopathologic conditions. They include psoriasis and other licheniformin changes such as lichen planus and lichen simplex chronicus. Depending on the experience of the pathologist, many of these lesions will be given descriptive interpretations ("hyperkeratosis," "acanthosis," "superficial perivascular inflammation") or misdiagnosed as squamous hyperplasia. The pathologist must be careful to identify the histopathologic changes unique to these dermatoses so that proper categorization is accomplished.

15.6.3.1 Lichen planus

Lichen planus is an inflammatory dermatosis of unknown etiology, but an autoimmune condition may be a factor. Gynecologically, the organ most commonly affected is the vagina, which undergoes marked erosion and desquamation, which may extend onto the vestibule. The vulvar vestibule will show reticular striae. Over time the vestibule and vagina will undergo scarring and retraction. Microscopically, lichen planus demonstrates marked destruction of the basal cells and erosion of the rete pegs by an underlying band-like chronic inflammatory infiltrate (Figures 15.39a,b). The rete pegs often contain apoptotic bodies (Civatte bodies). The initial treatment is application of topical corticosteroids. For advanced lichen planus, oral tacrolimus (an immunosuppressive medication) can be added.[5,13]

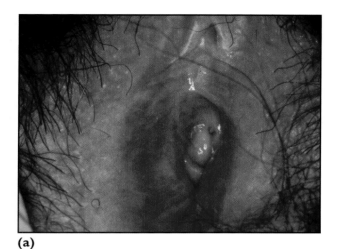

(a)

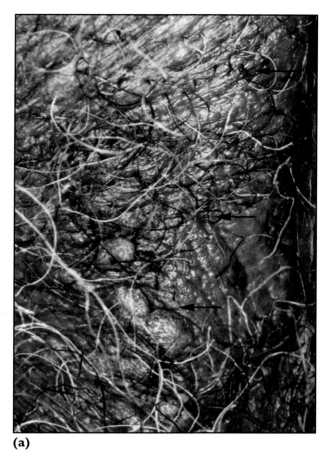

(a)

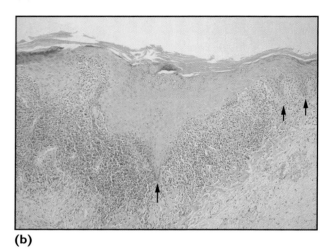

(b)

FIGURES 15.39a,b Vulvar lichen planus. **(a)** Grossly, there is marked erythema involving the vestibule extending to the introitus. In contrast, vestibulitis is generally more localized. Photo courtesy of Dr. Gordon Davis. **(b)** Microscopically, a band-like inflammatory infiltrate erodes and blunts the rete pegs, which become pointed (arrows). (Hematoxylin-eosin stain; medium power magnification.)

15.6.3.2 Lichen simplex chronicus

The etiology and clinical features of lichen simplex chronicus are similar to squamous hyperplasia, and it is likely that these abnormalities represent the same process.[60,61] The hallmark clinical feature is marked thickening of the skin that may excoriate from constant scratching. Histologically, lichen simplex chronicus demonstrates acanthosis and deepening of the rete pegs. The superficial dermis contains a band-like inflammatory infiltrate (Figures 15.40a,b). The treatment is application of topical corticosteroids to disrupt the itch-scratch cycle. White cotton gloves and a

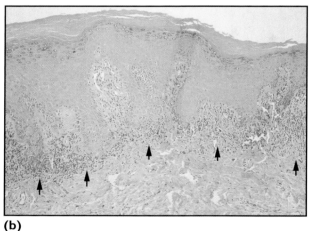

(b)

FIGURES 15.40a,b Vulvar lichen simplex chronicus. **(a)** Grossly, the involved area is slightly raised and roughened (arrows). Photo courtesy Wilkinson E J, Stone I K. *Atlas of Vulvar Diseases*. Baltimore: Williams and Wilkins, 1995, used with permission. **(b)** Microscopically, the histologic features are similar to squamous hyperplasia, with the exception of a more pronounced lichenoid (band-like) inflammatory infiltrate (arrows) (Hematoxylin-eosin stain; medium power magnification.)

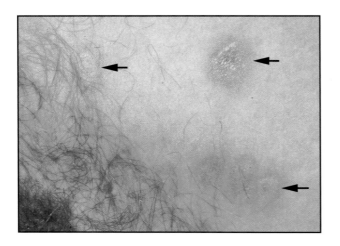

FIGURE 15.41   Vulvar psoriasis. Grossly, multiple macular, slightly raised patches are present (arrows). The larger areas have the characteristic silver coloration (photo courtesy Dr. Gordon Davis, used with permission). ▬

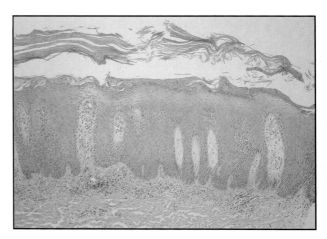

FIGURE 15.42   Photomicrograph of vulvar psoriasis. The rete pegs are uniformly elongated. There is hyperkeratosis and superficial dermal inflammation. (Hematoxylin-eosin stain; medium power magnification). ▬

pharmacologic agent to aid in sleeping are often required to prevent reflex scratching at night.[5]

15.6.3.3 Psoriasis

Psoriasis is a plaque-like dermatosis of unknown etiology. Clinically, the condition consists of pink or silver-white plaques that commonly cover the elbows, knees, scalp, and back. Nevertheless, other sites can be involved, including the vulva (Figure 15.41). Associated findings that help confirm the presence of psoriasis include the *Koebner phenomenon*, which is the occurrence of new lesions at a site of skin injury, and *Auspitz's sign*, which is the presence of small bleeding sites on the underside of an area where a plaque has been removed. Microscopically, there is hyperkeratosis and exocytosis. Acute inflammatory cells will aggregate in the surface (Munro abscess). There is acanthosis and deepening of the rete pegs. Mitoses are commonly seen; however, there is no cytologic atypia. The superficial dermis will contain scattered foci of inflammatory cells (Figure 15.42). Treatment includes washing the area with tar shampoo and, for more severe lesions, applying anthralin and corticosteroid creams. For intractable lesions, systemic agents such as retinoids, methotrexate and cyclosporine can be considered.[5,13]

15.7 Vulvar Noninvasive Neoplastic Abnormalities

In order to standardize the numerous terms used to describe intraepithelial squamous lesions of the vulva, including terms such as *Bowen's disease,*

Table 15.4   Vulvar Noninvasive Neoplastic Abnormalities

Squamous
   Mild dysplasia or vulvar intraepithelial
      neoplasia (VIN) 1
      basaloid type
      warty type
   Moderate dysplasia or VIN 2
      basaloid type
      warty type
   Severe dysplasia/carcinoma in situ or VIN 3
      basaloid type
      warty type
      differentiated type
Nonsquamous
   Paget's disease
   Melanocytic lesions
   Other

Bowenoid papulosis or *Bowenoid dysplasia, atypical hyperplastic dystrophy,* and *carcinoma simplex,* the ISSVD and ISGP introduced the category of Vulvar Noninvasive Neoplastic Abnormalities in 1986. This new grouping includes all premalignant abnormalities of the vulva, and is subdivided into squamous and nonsquamous lesions. All dysplastic squamous abnormalities are grouped into one category known as vulvar intraepithelial neoplasia (VIN). The other nonsquamous conditions include Paget's disease and intraepithelial melanocytic proliferations. Table 15.4 summarizes this classification.[54]

15.7.1 Vulvar intraepithelial neoplasia

The incidence of *vulvar intraepithelial neoplasia* (VIN) is difficult to determine because it depends on the persistence with which colposcopists search for and biopsy these lesions in asymptomatic patients so that a definitive diagnosis can be made. It is generally assumed, however, that the incidence of vulvar dysplasia has increased in recent decades and is now more common in younger women. Specifically, the incidence in women under age 35 years has nearly tripled in the past 20 years.[64,65]

15.7.1.1 Clinical appearance

The lesions associated with VIN often appear as raised plaques and papules on the surface of the vulva and perineum. Approximately one quarter of

these lesions are pigmented (brown). Although the remainder do not demonstrate pigment, 50% of all VINs are typically white (leukoplakia) or become acetowhite after soaking the vulva and perineum with dilute acetic acid. A few lesions may be red, corresponding to the older term *erythroplasia of Queyrat*. VIN can appear warty; therefore, it is prudent to perform a biopsy on any lesion originally diagnosed as a condyloma that does not respond to conservative therapy (Figures 15.43a–g).[5,14,15] The lesions are often multifocal and can be located throughout the vulvar surface, anus, and surrounding perineum.

15.7.1.2 Histology

Although most pathologists can agree on the histologic features of VIN 3, there is considerable disagreement over how one should grade the less severe vulvar lesions. Criteria used for grading the mild and

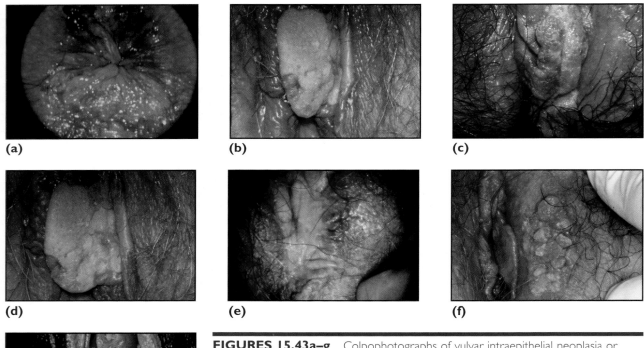

(a) **(b)** **(c)**

(d) **(e)** **(f)**

(g)

FIGURES 15.43a–g Colpophotographs of vulvar intraepithelial neoplasia or VIN. **(a)** A macular pigmented and white lesion surrounds the anus. **(b)** A broad based plaque covers the labium minus. Note the thickened area of leukoplakia. **(c)** A raised lesion replaces an area encompassing the left labium. Some areas have papillomatous features, similar in appearance to a condyloma acuminatum. This lesion, however, is more broad based and has focal leukoplakia. **(d)** A thickened area of leukoplakia replaces a large portion of the labium minus. Small areas of surface erosion are also present. **(e)** A brown pigmented lesion that could be mistaken for a benign lentigo **(f)** and **(g)** raised papillary lesions that could be mistaken for condylomas. VIN will often have less micropapillary spikes and broader bases. Photo courtesy Wright V C. *Color Atlas of Colposcopy—Cervix, Vagina, Vulva.* Houston: Biomedical Communications, 2000, used with permission. Photos b, c and d courtesy of Dr. Gordon Davis, used with permission.

moderate vulvar dysplasias are somewhat subjective, and incorporate the degree of atypia as well as the proportion of cells that demonstrate the atypia. When the degree of morphologic abnormality is "minimal" and appears confined to the lower one third of the epidermis, the diagnosis of VIN 1 should be rendered (Figure 15.44). Lesions with widely scattered koilocytes and minimal basal atypia ("flat condylomas") are included in this category, as the biologic behavior of these lesions is similar to that of VIN 1. A lesion is categorized as VIN 2 or moderate dysplasia if the degree of cytologic atypia is greater than that seen in a mildly dysplastic vulvar lesion and the proliferation of the atypical cells encompass one half to two thirds of the epidermis (Figure 15.45).[14,66]

VIN will contain variable numbers of mitotic figures. In VIN 1, the mitotic activity is usually sparse and confined to the lower one third of the vulvar epithelium. In VIN 2, the mitotic activity is more abundant and occupies the lower two thirds of the epithelial surface. Abnormal mitoses are also more consistent with a VIN 2 or worse lesion. However, mitotic figures are not unique to VIN, as they can also be seen in reactive processes such as squamous hyperplasia. Increased keratin production results in hyperkeratosis, parakeratosis, and dyskeratocytosis. The latter is represented histologically by isolated orangeophilic oval bodies *(corps ronds)* and probably represents irritated tonofilaments generated during abnormal cell division.[14,15]

The diagnostic reproducibility of VIN 1 and 2 is poor. In a review of 21 cases of previously diagnosed mild vulvar atypia, only 4 specimens were confirmed to be VIN when reevaluated by a surgical pathologist and a dermatopathologist.[67] In addition, the premalignant potential of these mildly to moderately dysplastic vulvar lesions is not well known, because studies that examine the cancer risk and presence of HPV in vulvar dysplasias do not differentiate between degrees of VIN. Nevertheless, the colposcopist must assume that any abnormal cell formation has premalignant potential.

The histologic features seen in Figure 15.46 are characteristic of VIN 3. There is an increase in cell number extending from the basal layer to a point at least

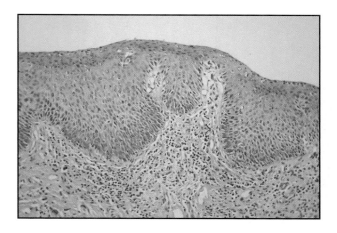

FIGURE 15.45 Moderate vulvar dysplasia (vulvar intraepithelial neoplasia or VIN 2). In some areas, the atypical basaloid cells extend through one half of the epidermal surface. (Hematoxylin-eosin stain; medium power magnification.)

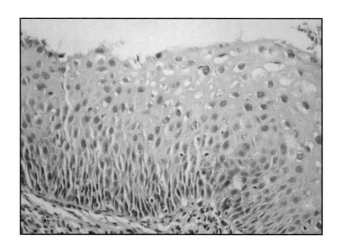

FIGURE 15.44 Mild vulvar dysplasia (vulvar intraepithelial neoplasia or VIN 1). As with mild cervical and vaginal dysplasia, there is proliferation of atypical basal cells over as much as one third of the epidermal surface. Koilocytes are present near the surface. (Hematoxylin-eosin stain; high power magnification.)

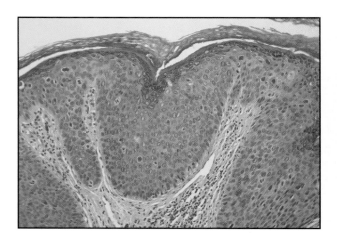

FIGURE 15.46 Severe vulvar dysplasia/squamous carcinoma in situ (vulvar intraepithelial neoplasia or VIN 3). There is proliferation of atypical basaloid cells over as much as two thirds of the epidermal surface. Mitotic figures are also present. The basement membrane, however, remains intact. (Hematoxylin-eosin stain; low power magnification.)

two thirds above the basement membrane, and usually to the surface. The cells lose their orderly arrangement and show a lack of maturation. The nuclei vary in size, shape, and chromatin distribution. Mitotic activity is abundant and this activity can be seen throughout the epithelium. Abnormal mitotic figures are common and are the result of aneuploidy and polyploidy.[14,15]

Commonly, VIN can involve the skin appendages. Although acanthosis, broadening of the rete pegs, and adnexal involvement are common, the basement membrane remains intact. VIN can also be subcategorized into different histologic types. The most common are basaloid and warty VINs (Figures 15.47a,b). The basaloid type of VIN consists of cells similar in appearance

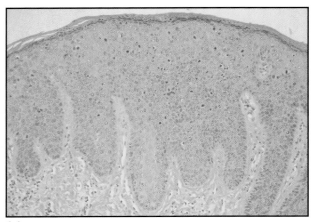

(a)

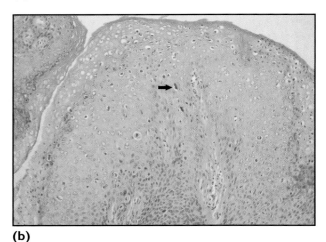

(b)

FIGURES 15.47a,b **(a)** Basaloid vulvar intraepithelial neoplasia. The predominant dysplastic cells are similar in appearance to the basaloid cells from the stratum germinativum (hematoxylin and eosin, medium power magnification.) **(b)** Warty vulvar intraepithelial neoplasia. In this case, there are large numbers of koilocytotic cells. Multinucleation is also seen (arrow). (Hematoxylin-eosin stain; medium power magnification.)

to epidermal basal cells, which are found throughout the epithelial surface. Total lack of maturation is present. The warty type of VIN contains mature squamous cells with large nuclei and peripheral chromatin clumping. Multinucleation and perinuclear cytoplasmic clearing reminiscent of koilocytes are present. The warty and basaloid VINs are related to HPV infection, most commonly type 16, and are often seen in younger women who are sexually active and smoke. The risk of invasive carcinoma of the vulva with basaloid and warty VIN is low to moderate. The least common is the differentiated (well differentiated) or simplex type of VIN.[14,68,69] The differentiated type of VIN occurs in older women, usually at a site that has been chronically irritated. There is generally no association with HPV exposure or tobacco use. (Figure 15.48). Differentiated VIN has an epidermis with squamous cells that have markedly pleomorphic nuclei. The chromatin is peripherally clumped and there are large nucleoli present. Keratin pearls are prominent within the rete pegs. In the past, this lesion has been labeled *carcinoma simplex* (Figure 15.49). The differentiated VIN has an extremely high association with vulvar squamous cell cancer. Because of this, differentiated VIN is always considered grade 3. Table 15.5 summarizes the features of the different morphologic types of VIN.[68]

15.7.1.3 Behavior and treatment

The association of invasive carcinoma with VIN is reported to range from 2% to 20% for the basaloid and warty types, and greater than 95% for the differentiated types.[14,68–71] Immunocompromised women also appear to have a greater risk of VIN progressing

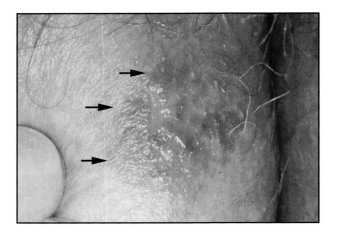

FIGURE 15.48 Differentiated (simplex) vulvar intraepithelial neoplasia. The area is broad, slightly raised with alternating red and white coloration (arrows), consistent with chronic irritation. Photo courtesy of Dr. Gordon Davis.

to invasive carcinoma. Patients with VIN 1 can be followed by close observation. Patients with high grade VIN (2 and 3) should have their lesions removed. This has traditionally been accomplished surgically (wide local excision or laser), but more recently the treatment has included administration of topical interferon agents.[71,72] While it is acceptable to treat the basaloid and warty VINs with ablation, the differentiated VINs should always be excised. Additionally, lesions in hair bearing areas are generally treated with a wide local excision. Resected VIN specimens should be examined closely by the pathologist for completeness of excision and potential areas of superficial squamous cell carcinoma. Reporting microscopic diagnoses of VIN should include not only the grade, but also the histologic type.

15.7.2 Paget's disease

In 1874, Sir James Paget originally observed that excoriation of the areola could represent "a chronic affliction of the nipple succeeded by scirrhous carci-

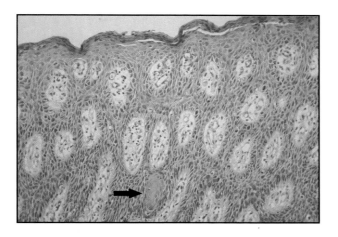

FIGURE 15.49 Photomicrograph of differentiated (simplex) vulvar intraepithelial neoplasia. The keratinocytes are atypical, but they continue to resemble mature squamous cells. A squamous pearl is present in a rete peg (arrow). (Hematoxylin-eosin stain; medium power magnification.)

nomas of the breast." He also suggested that this characteristic change could result in a "similar sequence of events in other sites." Dubreuilh described the first case of extramammary Paget's disease of the vulva in 1901 in a 51-year-old woman.[73] The significance of Paget's disease of the nipple is well known, in that it represents the surface extension of an underlying ductal carcinoma of the breast. The association of vulvar Paget's disease and other neoplastic processes is less clear. The most common is apocrine gland neoplasia; however, it can involve other sites, including the bladder and colorectal region.[5,74] Rarely, Paget's disease may present as surface extension of a ductal carcinoma arising from vulvar ectopic breast tissue that forms along the mammary ridge. The frequency of malignancy in extramammary Paget's disease also is less common than that in Paget's disease of the nipple. Quoted incidences range from 20% to 30%, but are probably lower.[75] Paget's disease of the nipple also has been known to occur in women with extramammary Paget's disease.

Clinically, the lesions will present on the vulva as geographic red macular areas that can appear excoriated. Often small white patches will overlay this region. The area may be asymptomatic, but can be pruritic or burn (Figure 15.50). The diagnosis is made by identification of the so-called "pagetoid" cells that occupy the epidermis. These cells are round in shape and considerably larger than the surrounding keratinocytes or melanocytes. The cytoplasm is pink but often retracts; the nuclei are large, round, and have prominent nucleoli. The pagetoid cells tend to cluster and form small nests in the rete pegs. Single cells spread into the superficial epidermis (Figure 15.51). The appearance is similar to superficial melanoma. In some cases, stains using markers that separate malignant melanocytes from adenocarcinoma in situ (Pagetoid) cells may be necessary to identify the correct tumor.[1,5,76]

Once diagnosed, a patient with vulvar Paget's disease should undergo a work-up to identify any associated invasive carcinoma. The evaluation

Table 15.5   Comparison of the Three Morphologic Types of Vulvar Intraepithelial Neoplasia (VIN)

Morphologic Type	Age	Smoking History	Association with Human Papillomavirus	Invasive Cancer Risk
Basaloid VIN	Younger	Smoker	Common	Low-Intermediate
Warty VIN	Younger	Smoker	Common	Low-Intermediate
Differentiated (Simplex) VIN	Older	Non-smoker	Uncommon	High

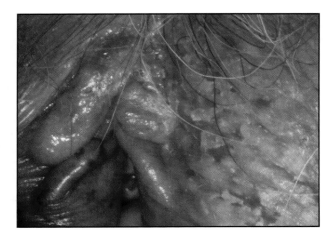

FIGURE 15.50 Extramammary Paget's disease of the vulva. Grossly, there is a broad erythematous area covered by white patches that extends from the left lateral vulva to the anterior clitoral hood. Note the indistinct lateral borders. Photo courtesy Wright V C. *Color Atlas of Colposcopy—Cervix, Vagina, Vulva.* Houston: Biomedical Communications, 2000, used with permission.

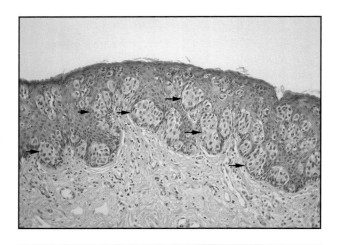

FIGURE 15.51 Vulvar Paget's disease. As viewed microscopically, nests and individual Pagetoid cells are scattered throughout the epidermis (arrows). (Hematoxylin-eosin stain; medium power magnification.)

should include cystoscopy, proctosigmoidoscopy, breast examination, and mammography. The treatment is wide local excision. Depending on the size of the lesion, simple vulvectomy may be necessary. The tissue excised should include the reticular dermis so that adnexal structures, particularly apocrine glands, can by examined microscopically. Complete excision of Paget's disease can be difficult. Examination of frozen sections of the margin is often frustrating, as the lesion usually extends beyond any recognizable

border. If no invasive carcinoma is found, the patient should be followed closely for any recurrence.[1,5]

15.7.3 Melanocytic lesions, melanoma in situ

Superficial melanoma consists of melanocarcinoma cells that spread along the epidermis but do not extend into the papillary dermis. As such, this lesion is considered a "melanoma in situ" and is included in the noninvasive neoplastic abnormalities. Nevertheless, many melanoma specialists consider melanoma in situ a true cancer.

Clinically, these lesions present as pigmented areas that are usually flat or slightly raised. Their appearance is similar to other benign pigmented lesions, and excision is necessary for a definitive diagnosis to be made. Nevertheless, features that suggest melanoma are large pigmented areas with irregular borders and satellite lesions. Microscopically, malignant melanocytes spread across the superficial epidermis in a "scattered buckshot" pattern and occupy the rete pegs (Figures 15.52a,b). As the pattern may resemble extramammary Paget's disease, special stains may be necessary to confirm the melanocytic origin of these cells.[66,77] The treatment for superficial melanoma is wide local excision, including enough lateral skin and subcutaneous tissue to ensure the entire lesion is removed.[5]

15.7.4 Other

Although not listed under vulvar noninvasive neoplastic abnormalities, numerous additional benign vulvar neoplasms occasionally are found on routine examination. These lesions rarely develop a subsequent carcinoma; however, excision is usually necessary for a definitive diagnosis. The following represent examples of the more common abnormalities seen by the colposcopist.

15.7.4.1 Papillary hidradenoma

Also known as *hidradenoma papilliferum*, a *papillary hidradenoma* is a benign neoplasm thought to arise in specialized sweat glands. While its exact origin is unknown, evidence of derivation from an apocrine-type cell includes the presence of occasional hidradenomas in the areola and the ability to identify apocrine gland proteins in these neoplasms. Interestingly, papillary hidradenomas occur almost exclusively in Caucasian-American women, who commonly have fewer apocrine glands than women of other races, including African-American women.[5] Clinically, these tumors present as small dermal nodules, usually in the labial sulci. They can, how-

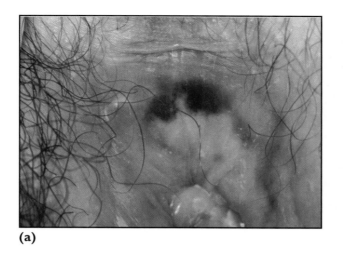

(a)

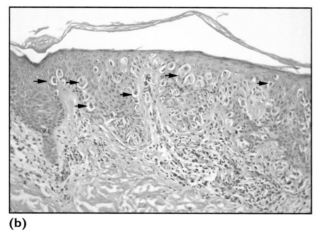

(b)

FIGURES 15.52a,b Superficial melanoma of the vulva. **(a)** An irregularly pigmented lesion is present on the anterior vulva. Lesions such as this must be sampled to differentiate a benign lentigo or melanosis (increased numbers of basal melanocytes) from a superficial melanoma. Photo courtesy of Dr. Gordon Davis. **(b)** Microscopically, malignant melanocytic cells are scattered throughout the epidermis in a "scattered buckshot" pattern (arrows). Melanin pigment is present in the superficial dermis, which helps differentiate this entity from Paget's disease. (Hematoxylin-eosin stain; medium power magnification.)

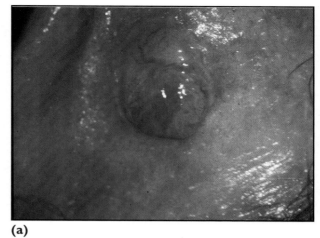

(a)

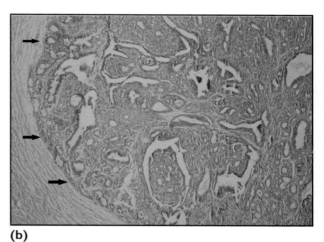

(b)

FIGURES 15.53a,b Papillary hidradenoma of the vulva. **(a)** Grossly, a round, raised intradermal lesion is present. Note the dilated superficial vessels, which branch normally. Photo courtesy Wright V C. *Color Atlas of Colposcopy— Cervix, Vagina, Vulva.* Houston: Biomedical Communications, 2000, used with permission. **(b)** Microscopically, the tumor contains numerous irregularly shaped gland-like cystic spaces. Note the pushing border between the tumor and surrounding dermis (arrows) (Hematoxylin-eosin stain; medium power magnification.)

ever, occur in any site including the mons. They are hard, mobile, nontender, and about 0.5 cm to 1.0 cm in size. Ulceration is uncommon. Histologically, the neoplasm is circumscribed with a pushing border. The gland pattern is complex and suggests an adenocarcinoma; however, there is no cytologic atypia and mitoses are absent (Figures 15.53a,b). On high-power microscopic examination, 2 cell lay-

ers are seen: an inner layer of acinar cells surrounded by contractile myoepithelial cells. The treatment is surgical removal.

15.7.4.2 Granular cell tumor

Formerly known as *granular cell myoblastomas, granular cell tumors* are benign neoplasms that originate from the peripheral nerve sheath. While they commonly occur on the vulva, these tumors also have been reported in the tongue and gall bladder. The etiology is probably related to a proliferation of malformed lysosomes in Schwann cells. The most common vulvar site is the labia majora and the initial presentation is a local swelling. Granular cell tumors are intradermal, although thickening or ulceration of the overlying skin can sometimes occur. Microscopically the reticular dermis is infiltrated by large round cells with eosinophilic granular cytoplasm. The nuclei are small, dark, and have few mitoses (Figure 15.54). The tumor margins are indistinct. The granular cells' origin from the peripheral nerve sheath can be confirmed by the presence of cytoplasmic neural markers. The treatment is wide local excision. Although granular cell tumors at other sites have shown malignant potential, recurrences and metastases from vulvar neoplasms are extremely rare.[78]

15.7.4.3 Nevi

Nevi are skin tumors that arise from melanocytic-type cells derived from the neural crest that are located in the epidermis and superficial dermis. Although occasionally congenital, they are more often seen in sun-exposed areas of the skin after birth. Nevi are divided into 3 types. *Junctional nevi* are characterized by nevus cells in the dermal epidermal junction; microscopically, the nevus cells cluster in the rete pegs. A *compound nevus* has nevus cells along the basal epidermis as well as the superficial dermis. The *intradermal nevus* contains nevus cells located exclusively in the superficial dermis. The evolution of these lesions starts with junctional activity. Over time, the nevus cells start to migrate into the superficial dermis. Continued migration results in loss of the epidermal nevus cells, resulting in the mature, intradermal nevus.

Nevi are pigmented tumors. Colors range from tan to black, although the most common are different shades of brown. The border is usually distinct. Junctional nevi are flat, while compound and intradermal nevi may be raised (papules) (Figure 15.55). The latter can be rubbed and become irritated. The major differential diagnosis is melanoma, although the latter have irregular contours and variegated coloration. Nevertheless, it is best to remove any vulvar pigmented lesion as the characteristics of nevi and melanomas often overlap. Microscopically, nevus cells are somewhat larger than melanocytes; the cells contain large oval nuclei and little cytoplasm. They can occasionally elongate and resemble neural elements. Melanin pigment may or may not be present. The location of the nevus cell in the epidermis of superficial dermis dictates the type of tumor (junctional, compound, or intradermal) (Figure 15.56).

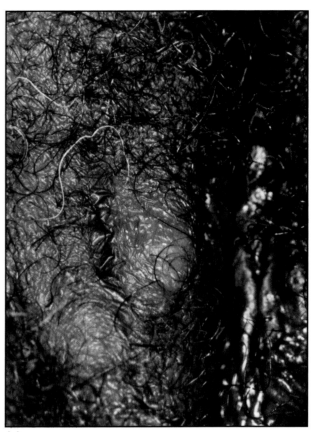

(a)

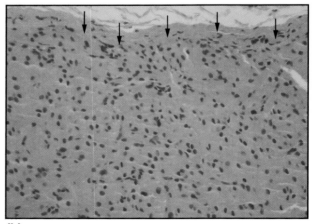

(b)

FIGURES 15.54a,b Granular cell tumor of the vulva. **(a)** Grossly, a slightly raised area of dermal expansion is present. Although occasionally pigmented, the epidermis in this case is normal. Photo courtesy of Wilkinson EJ, Stone IK. *Atlas of Vulvar Diseases.* Baltimore: Williams and Wilkins, 1995, used with permission. **(b)** Microscopically, sheets of pink neoplastic cells are present (arrows). The cytoplasm demonstrates a fine granular appearance. (Hematoxylin-eosin stain; high power magnification.)

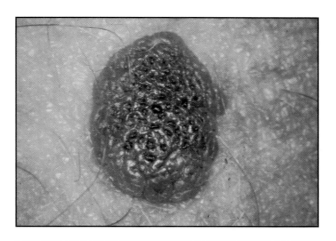

FIGURE 15.55 Vulvar melanocytic nevus. Grossly, a symmetrical, slightly raised tan-brown macule is present. Photo courtesy Wright V C. *Color Atlas of Colposcopy—Cervix, Vagina, Vulva.* Houston: Biomedical Communications, 2000, used with permission. ■■■■■■■

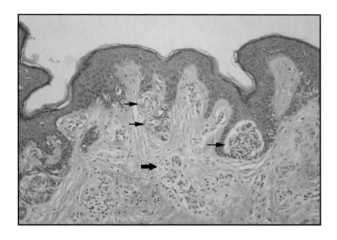

FIGURE 15.56 Photomicrograph of a vulvar nevus. Nests of nevus cells are present in the rete pegs (small arrows), indicating junctional activity, as well as in the superficial dermis (large arrow). These changes are diagnostic of a compound nevus. (Hematoxylin-eosin stain; medium power magnification.) ■■■■■■

Nevi are benign and excision is usually all the treatment that is needed. Malignant degeneration into a melanoma is rare and difficult to document but can occur. Differentiating a melanoma from a benign or dysplastic nevus can require careful microscopic examination. Melanomas will have atypical melanocytic cells that extend into the middle and superficial epidermis, while nevus cells tend to remain at the base of the epidermis.[5]

15.8 Vulvar Invasive Carcinoma

Nearly all vulvar invasive carcinomas are either squamous cell or melanocytic in origin, which reflects a strong dermatologic impact. In contrast to other sites in the female lower genital tract, primary vulvar adenocarcinomas are rare.

15.8.1 Squamous cell

Vulvar squamous cell carcinomas are similar in appearance and histology to squamous cell cancers that occur in the vagina and cervix. The most common histologic type is a well-differentiated keratinizing squamous carcinoma, although variants such as non-keratinizing squamous, warty (condylomatous), verrucous, and basaloid carcinomas can occur in the vulva.[66] Although the incidence of VIN has been rising in recent decades, the incidence of invasive keratinizing squamous carcinoma has remained relatively stable.[64] The cause for this may be related to the unique histologic types and the disparate etiologies of VIN and vulvar keratinizing squamous cell carcinoma. Squamous cell carcinoma of the vulva occurs in older women at a site that has been chronically irritated because of prolonged itching or burning. Antecedent or adjacent lesions include squamous hyperplasia variants or differentiated VIN. HPV is generally not found in these cancers. The common VINs (basaloid and warty) occur in younger women who are sexually active and often use tobacco. The cancers associated with these VINs are also basaloid and warty and are seen less frequently. HPV, usually type 16, is consistently identified in these basaloid and warty intraepithelial lesions and cancers.[70,79,80]

After discovering a tumor, patients often allow a significant amount of time to pass before seeking medical evaluation. By the time care is sought, these tumors are often quite large and may be exophytic or ulcerative (Figure 15.57). Enlarged inguinal or femoral lymph nodes may be identified. Ideally, regular examinations will result in early recognition of vulvar cancers. In 1984, the ISSVD defined *superficially invasive carcinoma of the vulva* as a unifocal lesion measuring 2 cm or less in diameter with a depth of invasion no greater than 1 mm.[66] The term "microinvasive carcinoma of the vulva" should not be used since this term refers to early invasive carcinomas of the cervix that have specific diagnostic criteria. The clinical appearance of lesions that represent early or superficially invasive carcinoma of the vulva is similar to that of vulvar intraepithelial neoplasia. They often present as red and white plaques or as small ulcers (Figures 15.58a–c). Extremely small lesions may only appear after the application

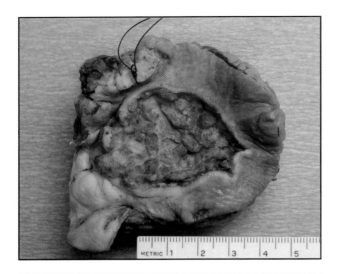

FIGURE 15.57 Invasive squamous cell carcinoma of the vulva. This pathologic specimen represents a radical resection of a large ulcerative lesion. Residual labial structures are difficult to identify, but are towards the left.

of acetic acid. In contrast to cervical colposcopic abnormalities, different degrees of whiteness or vascular patterns are not useful criteria to differentiate early carcinomas from intraepithelial lesions. Because of this, tissue samples for histologic examination should be taken of any unexplained lesion on the vulva. Solid lesions can be sampled centrally, while ulcers should have tissue removed along the lesion edge. The biopsy should extend far enough into the reticular dermis to document invasion.

Histologically, invasive squamous cell carcinomas of the vulva are similar to squamous cancers of the vagina and cervix (Figures 15.59a,b). Pushing or infiltrating nests of malignant squamous cells extend beyond the basement membrane into the surrounding dermis and subcutaneous tissues. A desmoplastic response, characterized by fibrosis and inflammation, usually occurs around these nests and can help in identifying them. Histologically, the keratinocytic malignant cells are characterized by large irregularly shaped nuclei, prominent nucleoli, and abundant eosinophilic cytoplasm. Mitoses, including abnormal forms, are present. The keratinizing squamous cancers will contain squamous pearls. Extension into lymphatic or vascular spaces can occur. Although the significance of this finding is not clear in vulvar cancers, its presence or absence should be reported.[16,66]

The depth of invasion is an important prognostic variable and it should be measured on all excisional specimens. Information that should be included in the final report is the tumor's thickness, lateral dimensions, and depth of invasion as measured from the nearest papillary dermis basement membrane. By convention, the tumor thickness is determined by

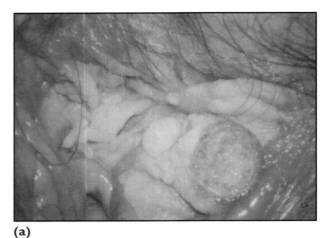

(a)

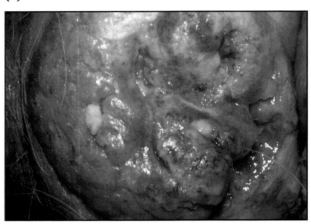

(b)

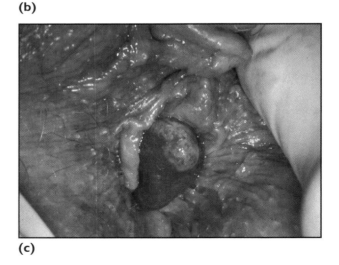

(c)

FIGURES 15.58a–c Colpophotographs of vulvar invasive squamous cell carcinoma. **(a)** There is an exophytic, round, pink lesion present in the periphery of a large area of leukoplakia. **(b)** A broad-based, raised lesion. Note the irregular (undulating) surface and the root-like atypical vessels. **(c)** A discrete raised hemorrhagic lesion. Numerous small coiled atypical vessels are present. Photos courtesy Wright V C. *Color Atlas of Colposcopy—Cervix, Vagina, Vulva.* Houston: Biomedical Communications, 2000, used with permission.

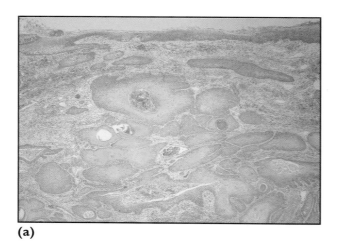

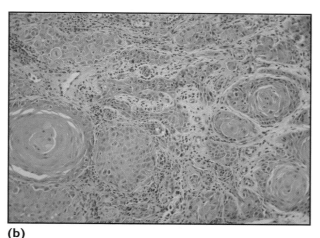

FIGURES 15.59a,b   Photomicrographs of vulvar invasive keratinizing squamous cell carcinoma. **(a)** Irregular nests of malignant squamous cells are present beneath the epidermis, surrounded by a fibrotic response (desmoplasia). (Hematoxylin-eosin stain; medium power magnification.) **(b)** Nests of malignant squamous cells are seen infiltrating throughout the dermis. Numerous keratin pearls are present. (Hematoxylin-eosin stain; medium power magnification.)

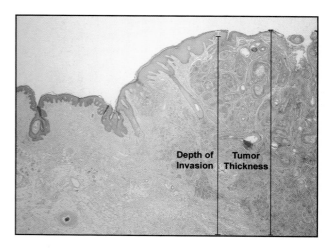

FIGURE 15.60   Measuring the depth of invasion in a squamous cell carcinoma of the vulva. The tumor invasion depth is determined by measuring from the nearest normal dermal papilla to the deepest invasion point. It can also be determined by subtracting the normal epidermal thickness (white bracket) from the tumor thickness. The latter is measured from the tumor surface to the deepest point of invasion. (Hematoxylin-eosin stain; medium power magnification.)

measuring from the surface of the squamous epithelium if nonkeratinized, or the stratum granulosum (granular cell layer) if keratinized, to the deepest extent of tumor invasion. The depth of invasion is determined by subtracting the normal epidermal thickness, which is measured from the surface or stratum granulosum to the papillary dermal junction, from the tumor thickness. When reporting the various measurements of tumor size and depth, it is important that the method by which these measurements were determined be described (Figure 15.60).[1]

The present treatment for vulvar squamous cell cancer includes wide and deep resection of the primary tumor with unilateral regional (inguinal and femoral) lymph node dissection; bilateral regional nodes are removed for midline lesions. Pelvic node dissection or treatment of this area by radiation may be necessary if the tumor is identified in the sentinal inguinal node (Cloquet's node).[81] Recently, sentinal node mapping has been used to more accurately identify this node.[81] Patients who have tumors of less than 1 mm have minimal risk for regional lymph node metastasis, and local excision may be all that is necessary.[82,83] The outlook for women with vulvar squamous cell carcinoma is dependent on the tumor's size, depth of invasion, and extension into regional lymph nodes or surrounding structures.[15,84]

Verrucous carcinomas are squamous cell carcinoma variants that make up approximately 1% of vulvar carcinomas. Verrucous carcinomas occur as large exophytic wart-like tumors that occupy considerable surface area. In the past, they have been classified as giant condylomas or Buschke-Lowenstein condylomas (Figure 15.61). Histologically, these neoplasms are composed of large papillae containing bland keratinocytes. The invasive component, consisting of nests of invading tumor cells, can only be noted at the broad tumor base. These tumors are associated with HPV, particularly subsets of type 6. Verrucous carcinomas are locally erosive tumors that grow into surrounding structures, including bone. The treatment is wide and deep excision. Microscopic

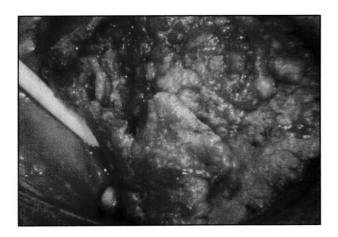

FIGURE 15.61 Verrucous carcinoma of the vulva. A broad-based, raised, exophytic, warty lesion partially obscures the labia and vestibule. A white Foley catheter identifies the urethral meatus. Photo courtesy of the Armed Forces Institute of Pathology, used with permission. ▬

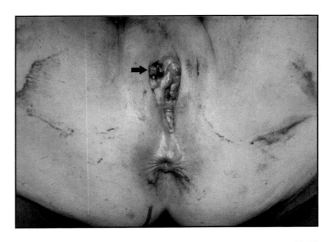

FIGURE 15.62 Malignant melanoma of the vulva. Grossly, there is a raised asymmetric blue-black lesion along the right labial sulcus (arrow). Photo courtesy Wright V C. *Color Atlas of Colposcopy—Cervix, Vagina, Vulva.* Houston: Biomedical Communications, 2000, used with permission. ▬

examination should pay particular attention to the base where the small invasive foci will be found.[1,66]

Condylomatous or warty carcinomas are also squamous cell variants that histologically will show cytologic features of HPV (koilocytosis, multinucleation). These tumors probably represent the invasive counterpart of warty VIN. Basaloid carcinomas consist of small, immature cells similar to abnormal basal cells and probably represent the invasive counterpart to basaloid VIN. Condylomatous and basaloid carcinomas both contain HPV, usually type 16.[1,66,79]

15.8.2 Melanocytic carcinoma (melanoma)

Melanomas make up approximately 5% of vulvar malignancies. They occur in older women and are more common in Caucasian-Americans than African-Americans. Their clinical appearance can be nonspecific and resemble other pigmented lesions such as nevi, benign lentigo, or melanosis. Features that suggest melanoma are large size, variegated coloration, irregular borders, and satellite lesions (Figure 15.62). Nevertheless, any pigmented lesion of questionable etiology should be removed for histologic examination, especially if it is new or it recently changed in appearance.[14,15]

Histologically, melanomas demonstrate three growth patterns: (1) superficial spreading, with a predominant lateral spread; (2) nodular, with a predominant vertical spread; and (3) acral lentiginous, with mixed lateral and vertical spread patterns. The hallmark cell is the malignant melanocyte, which is

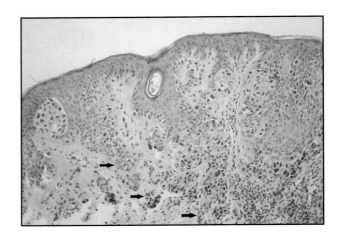

FIGURE 15.63 Photomicrograph of malignant melanoma. Nests of malignant melanocytes, many of which contain brown pigment, are found in the epidermis and the superficial dermis (arrows). (Hematoxylin-eosin stain; medium power magnification.) ▬

typically round with large, round to oval nuclei and prominent nucleoli. The presence of melanin pigment varies. Initial tumors will have malignant cells scattered throughout the epidermis in a "buckshot" pattern; however, continued growth will result in extension into the superficial (papillary) dermis and eventually into the subcutaneous tissues (Figure 15.63). The distribution of nonpigmented malignant melanocytes in the epidermis may resemble the intraepithelial adenocarcinoma cells of Paget's disease. Those arising in large tumors can resemble epithelioid cells seen in poorly differentiated carcinomas. Markers are occasionally required to document a melanocytic origin.[15] Determining the depth of invasion is extremely important, as this is a valuable prognostic tool and will dictate the method of treatment. Because of this, it is better to excise a pigmented lesion suspicious for melanoma, rather than remove a small biopsy. The resultant crush artifact and scarring may render measurements inaccurate. Traditionally, Clark's levels were used to classify these tumors, but these could be highly variable due to the background morphology of the epidermis and dermis. Precise measurements extending from the stratum granulosum into the underlying dermis (Breslow's depth) are the presently preferred method (Figure 15.64).[84]

Treatment for melanomas is similar to that for other invasive carcinomas. Wide, local excision is usually undertaken to remove the primary lesion. The extent of the excision is dependent on the size of the tumor and the depth of invasion. Small tumors that are minimally invasive can be treated by local excision with a 1 to 2-cm wide margin. Large tumors and those that invade into the reticular dermis or subcutaneous fat are usually treated by radical excision and regional lymphadenectomy.[1,15]

15.8.3 Adenocarcinoma

Vulvar adenocarcinomas can be metastatic or arise from glandular structures that comprise the skin adnexa and the vestibular glands, the most common site being Bartholin's glands. Clinically, these carcinomas often present as raised irregular firm nodules or erosive ulcerations. Microscopically, the histology is typical of other glandular cancers, with nests of malignant cells that form irregular gland lumens. The

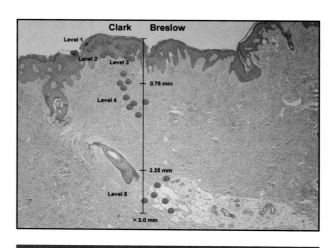

FIGURE 15.64   Measuring the depth of invasion in malignant melanoma of the vulva (reference 44, p 582). Traditionally, the depth was marked by different levels (Clark): I indicates confinement to the epidermis, II indicates extension into the papillary dermis, III indicates malignant cells filling the dermal papillae, IV indicates extension into the reticular dermis, V indicates extension into the subcutaneous fat. Because the actual depths of these levels vary depending on the skin morphology, absolute measurements are now used (Breslow). (Hematoxylin-eosin stain; medium power magnification.)

degree of differentiation is dependent on the ability of the adenocarcinoma cells to recapitulate gland structures. Poorly differentiated neoplasms consist mostly of solid sheets of malignant cells with only an occasional gland structure.[14] The recommended treatment for adenocarcinoma is similar to that for squamous carcinomas of the vulva, and includes radical excision of the tumor and regional lymph node sampling.

References

1. Wilkinson E J. Benign diseases of the vulva. In: Kurman R J, ed. *Blaustein's Pathology of the Female Genital Tract*. 4th ed. New York, NY: Springer-Verlag; 1994:31–87; 93–108.

2. Wilkinson E J, Hart N S. Vulva. In: Sternberg S S, ed. *Histology for Pathologists*. New York: Raven Press; 1992:865–81.

3. Bergeron C, Ferenczy A, Richart R M, Guralnick M. Micropapillomatosis labialis appears unrelated to human papillomavirus. *Obstet Gynecol* 1990; 76:281–6.

4. Murphy G M, Mihm M C. The skin. In: Cotran R S, Kumar V, Collins T, eds. *Robbins Pathologic Basis of Disease*. 6th ed. Philadelphia, PA: W B Saunders Co; 1999:1172–3.

5. Wilkinson E J, Stone I K. *Atlas of Vulvar Disease*. Baltimore, Md: Williams and Wilkins; 1995:5–8; 27–29; 60–8; 77–8; 82–3; 91–3; 98–9; 122–4; 137–8;141–3; 154–5; 171–6; 183–6.

6. Cone R, Beckmann A, Aho M, et al. Subclinical manifestations of vulvar human papillomavirus infection. *Int J Gynecol Pathol* 1991;10:26.

7. di Paola G R, Rueda N G. Deceptive vulvar papillomavirus infection. A possible explanation for certain cases of vulvodynia. *J Reprod Med* 1986; 31:966–70.

8. Bergeron C, Ferenczy A, Richart R M and Guralnick M (1990) Micropapillomatosis labialis appears unrelated to human papillomavirus. *Obstet Gynecol* 76:281–85.

9. Julian T M. Vulvar pain: diagnosis, evaluation and management. *J Lower Gen Tract Dis* 1997;1:185–94.

10. Wilkinson E J, Guerrero E, Daniel R, Shah K, Stone I K, Hardt N S, Friedrich E G Jr. Vulvar vestibulitis is rarely associated with human papillomavirus infection types 6, 11, 16, or 18. *Int J Gynecol Pathol* 1993;12:344–9.

11. Origoni M, Rossi M, Ferrari D, Lillo F, Ferrari A G. Human papillomavirus with co-existing vulvar vestibulitis syndrome and vestibular papillomatosis. *Int J Gynecol Obstet* 1999;64:259–63.

12. Micheletti L, Preti M, Bogliatto F, Chieppa P. Vestibular papillomatosis. *Minerva Ginecol* 2000;52(Suppl 1):87–91.

13. Lever W F, Schaumburg-Lever G. *Histopathology of the Skin.* 6th ed. Philadelphia, PA: Lippencott, 1990:156–61; 168–74; 308–12; 364–8.

14. Wilkinson E J. Premalignant and malignant tumors of the vulva in Kurman R J, ed. In: *Blaustein's Pathology of the Female Genital Tract.* 4th ed. New York: Springer-Verlag, 1994:87–93. 117–121.

15. Kurman R J, Norris H J, Wilkinson E. *Tumors of the Cervix, Vagina and Vulva. Atlas of Tumor Pathology* (Third Series: Fascicle 4) Washington, DC: American Registry of Pathology, Armed Forces Institute of Pathology 1992;191–202.

16. Reed R J, Parkinson R P. The histogenesis of molluscum contagiosum. *Am J Surg Pathol* 1977;1:161–6.

17. Wysoki R S, Majmudar B, Willis D. Granuloma inguinale (donovanosis) in women. *J Reprod Med* 1988;33:709–13.

18. Report of the ISSVD task force. *J Reprod Med* 1984;457–9.

19. MacKay M. Subsets of vulvodynia. *J Reprod Med* 1988;33:695–98.

20. Edwards L, Lynch P J. The terminology and classification of vulvodynia: past, present and future. *www.behavioural-medicine.com/womenshealth/info/terminology.htm*

21. Marinoff S C, Turner M L. Vulvar vestibulitis syndrome: an overview. Am J *Obstet Gynecol* 1991;165(Pt 2):1228–33.

22. Bazin S, Bouchard C, Brisson J, et al. Vulvar vestibulitis syndrome: an exploratory case control study. *Obstet Gynecol* 1994;83:47–50.

23. Chadha S, Gianotten W L, Drogendijk A C, Weijmar Schultz W C, Blindeman L A, van der Meijden W I. Histopathologic features of vulvar vestibulitis. *Int J Gynecol Pathol* 1998;17:7–11.

24. Slone S, Reynolds L, Gall S, et al. Localization of chromogranin, synaptophysin, serotonin, and CXCR2 in neuroendocrine cells of the minor vestibular glands: an immunohistochemical study. *Int J Gynecol Pathol* 1999; 18:360–5.

25. Bazin S, Bouchard C, Brisson J, Morin C, Meisels A, Fortier M. Vulvar vestibulitis syndrome: an exploratory case-control study. *Obstet Gynecol* 1994;83:47–50.

26. Sjoberg I, Nylander Lundqvist E N. Vulvar vestibulitis in the north of Sweden. An epidemiologic case-control study. *J Reprod Med* 1997;42:166–8.

27. Bouchard C, Brisson J, Fortier M, Morin C, Blanchette C. Use of oral contraceptive pills and vulvar vestibulitis: a case-control study. *Am J Epidemiol* 2002;156:254–61.

28. Cox J T. Deconstructing vulval pain. *Lancet* 1995;345:53.

29. Reid R, Omoto K H, Precop S L, Berman N R, Rutledge L H, Dean S M, Pleatman M. Flashlamp-excited dye laser therapy of idiopathic vulvodynia is safe and efficacious. *Am J Obstet Gynecol* 1995;172:1684–96; discussion 1696–701.

30. Bohm-Starke N, Hilliges M, Falconer C, Rylander E. Increased intraepithelial innervation in women with vulvar vestibulitis syndrome. *Gynecol Obstet Invest* 1998;46:256–60.

31. Bohm-Starke N, Hilliges M, Brodda-Jansen G, Rylander E, Torebjork E. Psychophysical evidence of nociceptor sensitization in vulvar vestibulitis syndrome. *Pain* 2001;94:177–83.

32. Stewart E G, Berger B M. Parallel pathologies? Vulvar vestibulitis and interstitial cystitis. *J Reprod Med* 1997;42:131–4.

33. Fitzpatrick C C, DeLancey J O, Elkins T E, McGuire E J. Vulvar vestibulitis and interstitial cystitis: a disorder of urogenital sinus-derived epithelium? *Obstet Gynecol* 1993;81:860–2.

34. Parsons C L, Dell J, Stanford J, Bullen M. The prevalence of interstitial cystitis in gynecologic patients with pelvic pain, as detected by intravesical potassium sensitivity. *Am J Obstet Gynecol* 2002;187:1395–1400.

35. Chaim W, Meriwether C, Gonik B, Qureshi F, Sobel J D. Vulvar vestibulitis subjects undergoing surgical intervention: a descriptive analysis and histopathological correlates. *Eur J Obstet Gynecol Reprod Biol* 1996;68:165–8.

36. Wesselmann U. Neurogenic inflammation and chronic pelvic pain. *World J Urol* 2001;19:180–85.

37. Turner M L, Marinoff S C. Association of human papillomavirus with vulvodynia and the vulvar vestibulitis syndrome. *J Reprod Med* 1988;33:533–7.

38. Umpierre S A, Kaufman R H, Adam E, Woods K V, Adler-Storthz K. Human papillomavirus DNA in tissue biopsy specimens of vulvar vestibulitis patients treated with interferon. *Obstet Gynecol* 1991;78:693–5.

39. Sonnendecker E W, Sonnendecker H E, Wright C A, Simon G B. Recalcitrant vulvodynia. A clinicopathological study. *S Afr Med J* 1993;83:730–3.

40. Bornstein J, Shapiro S, Goldshmid N, Goldik Z, Lahat N, Abramovici H. Severe vulvar vestibulitis. Relation to HPV infection. *J Reprod Med* 1997;42:514–8.

41. Wilkinson E J, Guerrero E, Daniel R, et al. Vulvar vestibulitis is rarely associated with human papillomavirus infection types 6,11,16 or 18. *Int J Gynec Pathol* 1993;12:344–49.

42. Bergeron C, Moyal-Barracco M, Pelisse M, Lewin P. Vulvar vestibulitis. Lack of evidence for a human papillomavirus etiology. *J Reprod Med* 1994;39:936–8.

43. Prayson R A, Stoler M H and Hart W R. Vulvar vestibulitis: a histopathologic study of 36 cases including human papillomavirus in situ hybridization analysis. *Amer J Cervical Path* 1995;19:154–160.

44. Morin C, Bouchard C, Brisson J, Fortier M, Blanchette C, Meisels A. Human papillomaviruses and vulvar vestibulitis. *Obstet Gynecol* 2000;95:683–7.

45. Glazer H I. Dysesthetic vulvodynia. Long-term follow-up after treatment with surface electromyography-assisted pelvic floor muscle rehabilitation. *J Reprod Med* 2000;45:798–802.

46. MacKay M. Dysthetic ("essential") vulvodynia: Treatment with amitriptyline. *J Reprod Med* 1993;38:9–13.

47. MacKay M, Frankman O, Horowitz B J, et al. Vulvar vestibulitis and vestibular papillomatosis: Report of the ISSVD Committee on Vulvodynia. *J Reprod Med* 1991;36:413–15.

48. Turner M L, Marinoff S C. Pudendal neuralgia. *Am J Obstet Gynecol* 1991;165:1233–6.

49. Gaitonde P, Rostron J, Longman L, Field E A. Burning mouth syndrome and vulvodynia coexisting in the same patient: a case report. *Dent Update* 2002;29:75–6.

50. Bates C M, Timmins D J. Vulvodynia—new and more effective approaches to therapy. *Int J STD AIDS* 2002;13:210–2.

51. Hansen H C. Interstitial cystitis and the potential role of gabapentin. *South Med J* 2000;93:238–42.

52. Magnus L. Nonepileptic uses of gabapentin *Epilepsia* 1999;40:Suppl 6:S66–72; discussion S73–4.

53. Ben-David B, Friedman M. Gabapentin therapy for vulvodynia. *Anesth Analg* 1999;89(6):1459–60.

54. Wilkinson E J. The 1989 Presidential Address: International Society for the Study of Vulvar Disease. *J Reprod Med* 1990;35:981–91.

55. van Hoeven K H, Kovatich A J. Immunohistochemical staining for proliferating cell nuclear antigen, BCL-2, and Ki-67 in vulvar tissues. *Int J Gynecol Pathol* 1996;15:10–6.

56. Marren P, Yell F, Charnock M, et al. The association between lichen sclerosus and antigens of the HLA system. *Br J Derm* 1995;132:197–203.

57. Rodke G, Friedrich E G, Wilkinson E J. Malignant potential of mixed vulvar dystrophy. (Lichen sclerosus associated with squamous cell hyperplasia.) *J Reprod Med* 1988;33:545–50.

58. Paslin D. Treatment of lichen sclerosus with topical dihydrotestosterone. *Obstet Gynecol* 1991;78:1046–9.

59. Dalziel K L, Wojnarowska F. Long-term control of vulval lichen sclerosus after treatment with a potent topical steroid cream. *J Reprod Med* 1993; 38:25–7.

60. Ambros R A, Malfetano J H, Carlson J A, Mihm M C. Non-neoplastic epithelial alterations of the vulva: Recognition and comparisons terminologies used among the various specialties. *Mod Pathol* 1997;10:401–8.

61. O'Keefe R J, Scurry J P, Dennerstein G, et al. Audit of 114 non-neoplastic vulvar biopsies. *Br J Obstet Gynaecol* 1995;102:780–6.

62. Toki T, Kurman R J, Park J S, Kessis T, et al. Probable nonpapillomavirus etiology of squamous cell carcinoma of the vulva in older women; a clinicopathologic study using in situ hybridization and polymerase chain reaction. *Int J Gynecol Pathol* 1991;10:107–25.

63. Cattaneo A, Bracco G L, Maestrini G, Carli G, Colafranceschi M, Marchionini M. Lichen sclerosus and squamous hyperplasia: A clinical study of medical treatment. *J Reprod Med* 1991;36:301–5.

64. Sturgeon S R, Brinton L A, Devesa S S, Kurman R J. In situ and invasive vulvar cancer incidence trends (1973 to 1987). *Am J Obstet Gynecol* 1992;166:1482–5.

65. Hart W R. Vulvar intraepithelial Neoplasia: Historical aspects and current status. *Int J Gynecol Pathol.* 2001;20:16–30.

66. Scully R E, Bonfiglio T A, Silverberg S G. *Histologic Typing of Female Genital Tract Tumours. World Health Organization International Histological Classification of Tumours.* 2nd ed. New York: Springer-Verlag; 1994: 64–70; 74–5.

67. Micheletti L, Barbero M, Zanotto V, Preti M, et al. Vulvar intraepithelial neoplasia of low grade: a challenging diagnosis. *Euro J Gynaecol Oncol* 1994;15:70–4.

68. Yang B, Hart W R. Vulvar intraepithelial neoplasia of the simplex (differentiated) type: a clinicopathological study including analysis of HPV and p53 alterations. *Am J Surg Pathol* 2000;24:429–41.

69. Park B S, Jones R W, McLean M R, Currie J L, Woodruff J D, Shah K V, Kurman R J. Possible etiologic heterogeneity of vulvar intraepithelial neoplasia: a correlation of pathologic characteristics with human papillomavirus detection by in situ hybridization and polymerase chain reaction. *Cancer* 1991;67:1599–1697.

70. Rouzier R, Haie-Meder C, Lhomme C, Avril M F, Duvillard P, Castaigne D. Prognostic significance of epithelial disorders adjacent to invasive vulvar carcinomas. *Gynecol Oncol* 2001;81:414–6.

71. Barbero M, Micheletti L, Preti M, et al. Biologic behavior of vulvar intraepithelial neoplasia. Histologic and clinical parameters. *J Reprod Med* 1993;38:108–12.

72. Davis G, Wentworth J, Richard J. Self-administered topical imiquimod treatment of vulvar intraepithelial Neoplasia. *J Reprod Med* 2000; 45:619–23.

73. Basket B F. *On the Shoulders of Giants. Eponyms and Names in Obstetrics and Gynaecology.* London: RCOG Press; 1998:166–7.

74. Turner A G. Pagetoid lesions associated with carcinoma of the bladder. *J Urol* 1980;123–6.

75. Fanning J, Lambert H C L, Hale T M, Morris P C, Schuerch C. Paget's disease of the vulva: prevalence of associated vulvar adenocarcinoma, invasive Paget's disease, and recurrence after surgical excision. *Am J Obstet Gynecol* 1999;180:24–7.

76. Roth L M, Lee S C, Ehrlich C E. Paget's disease of the vulva: A histogenetic study of five cases including ultrastructural observations and review of the literature. *Am J Surg Pathol* 1977;1:193–206.

77. Estrada R, Kaufman R. Benign vulvar melanosis. *J Reprod Med* 1993; 38:5–8.

78. Majmudar B, Castellano P Z, Wilson R W, Siegel R J. Granular cell tumors of the vulva. *J Reprod Me.* 1990;35:1008–14.

79. Anderson W A, Franquemont D W, Williams J, Taylor P T, Crum C P. Vulvar squamous cell carcinoma and papillomavirus: two separate entities? *Am J Obstet Gynecol* 1991;165:329–35.

80. Rusk D, Sutton G P, Look K Y, Roman A. Analysis of invasive squamous cell carcinoma of the vulva and vulvar intraepithelial neoplasia for the presence of human papillomavirus DNA. *Obstet Gynecol* 1991;77:918–22.

81. Levenback C, Coleman R L, Burke T W et al. Intraoperative lymphatic mapping and sentinel node identification with blue dye in patients with vulvar cancer. *Gynecol Oncol* 2001; 83:276–81.

82. Hicks M L, Hempling R E, Piver M S. Vulvar carcinoma with 0.5 mm of invasion in associated inguinal lymph node metastasis. *J Surg Oncol* 1993;54:271–3.

83. Atamdede F, Hoogerland D. Regional lymph node recurrence following local excision for microinvasive vulvar carcinoma. *Gynecol Oncol* 1989; 34:125–8.

84. Hacker N F. Vulvar cancer. In: Berek J S, Hacker N F, eds. *Practical Gynecologic Oncology.* 3rd ed. Philadelphia: Williams and Wilkins, 2000: 563–76.

Colposcopy of Men

Table of Contents

16.1 Expanded Role of Colposcopy

The colposcope was invented specifically and has been used primarily as an instrument to examine the lower genital tract of women. Along with several epithelial contrast solutions, the colposcope enables clinical inspection of neoplastic alterations not always appreciated by naked-eye exam. Colposcopy has been particularly beneficial for assessing asymptomatic women with cellular abnormalities detected by a previous cervical cytologic screening test. The magnification and intense light source of the colposcope allow a detailed examination of epithelium that is remotely positioned and, hence, not otherwise seen with natural ambient light.

Colposcopy has also been touted, by some, as a method to help examine the external genitalia and anorectal area of men. However, because genital neoplasia is less common in men and no screening test for premalignant disease is available, the colposcope is used less frequently for this purpose. Furthermore, most male anatomy is comparatively easier to access

than female genital mucosae and adequately illuminated by ambient light. Gross lesions are readily detected by naked-eye inspection unless positioned deeply within the urethra or anus. Furthermore, a less-expensive handheld magnifying lens or low-power loupes often suffice for visualization of small lesions. Regardless, just as for women, the colposcope may have a great value in facilitating identification, assessment, and sampling of otherwise undetected anogenital epithelial neoplasias in men.

16.1.1 Colposcopy of men—purpose

The purpose of colposcopy for men is to examine the external genitalia and anorectal area for human papillomavirus (HPV)-associated lesions that include condylomas, penile, urethral and perianal intraepithelial neoplasia, and invasive cancer of the penis, urethra, scrotum, or anus (Figure 16.1). A detailed colposcopic inspection helps to discriminate normal anatomic variants and other mimics of anogenital neoplasia from significant neoplastic lesions. Following comprehensive colposcopic visualization of the entire anogenital region and critical assessment of

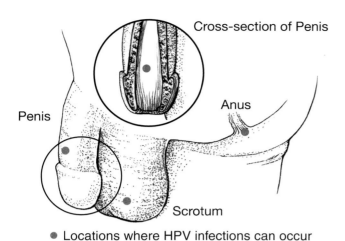

Cross-section of Penis

Penis

Anus

Scrotum

● Locations where HPV infections can occur

FIGURE 16.1   Anatomical sites of the male genitalia affected by HPV-induced neoplasia.

suspicious lesions, selective targeted biopsy enables histologic confirmation of the clinical diagnosis, when indicated. Colposcopic appraisal also assists the determination of disease distribution, which is necessary to selection of proper management.

16.2 Epidemiology of HPV-Related Disease in Men

16.2.1 Risk factors for penile cancer

The vast majority of penile cancers (>95%) are derived from squamous cells. In the United States, the incidence of squamous cell carcinoma of the penis is approximately 1 per 100,000 men.[1] During the past 30 years, the incidence of penile cancer has not fluctuated in the United States. This rare cancer accounts for 1,000 cases per year, representing less than 1% of all cancers in men.[2] In developed nations, the incidence of penile cancer is similar to that in the United States. However, the incidence is six-fold greater in some African and South American countries.[1] The reason for these widely varied rates may be explained by certain factors that place some men at increased risk for developing penile cancer.

Carcinoma of the scrotum is even more rare (0.132/100,000). Occupational exposure of chimney sweeps to hydrocarbons in soot and tar has been shown to be a significant risk factor for scrotal cancer. Awareness of this risk has helped to make scrotal cancer an uncommon disease.

16.2.1.1 Age

The incidence of penile cancer increases with age.[1] Penile cancer rarely occurs prior to 35 years of age

and is most common in men older than 75 years (6.5/100,000). The majority of cases occur between the ages of 40 and 70,[2] with a mean age at diagnosis of 58 years.[3] This mean age of penile cancer in men is at least a decade greater than the mean age of cervical cancer in women. One possible explanation for the difference in the mean age of cancer between the sexes is a lack of susceptible immature metaplastic epithelium on the penis.

16.2.1.2 Race

Although data vary depending on other factors, penile cancer may be more prevalent in African-American men than in White men[1]. Socioeconomic or environmental factors, rather than race factors, may account for the small difference in observed incidence. While the peak age incidence of penile cancer for the White population is past 75 years, the peak incidence among African-American men is noted a decade earlier in life.

16.2.1.3 Circumcision

In populations where male infants are circumcised shortly following birth, penile cancer is exceedingly rare.[3] Therefore, the malignancy is rarely reported in Jewish men, and is only slightly more common in Muslims, who delay circumcision until young childhood.[4] The timing of circumcision during life appears critically important since circumcision performed on adults conveys no added protection from development of penile cancer.[5] In a U.S.-based study, of 89 men with reported penile cancer, only 2.3% had been circumcised as newborns.[6] Furthermore, 15.7% of men with carcinoma in situ (CIS) of the penis were circumcised as newborns. Although the incidence of penile cancer is far greater for uncircumcised (Hindu) men,[5] circumcision alone is not universally preventive. Circumcision improves hygiene, prevents phimosis, and may reduce sexually transmitted disease acquisition. Additionally, exposure to many of these risk factors conveys an increased risk of penile cancer among men circumcised as adults.

16.2.1.4 Phimosis

Phimosis, or stricture of the foreskin preventing retraction around the glans, is noted in half of the men who develop penile cancer.[1] In the majority of these cases, phimosis is congenital and is not usually a consequence of the development of penile cancer. Epithelial atypia, a potential precursor lesion, has been noted in the foreskin of 35% of men with phimosis, compared with no cases noted in the foreskin of men without phimosis.[7] Thus, phimosis may foster the pathogenesis of epithelial precursor lesions by limiting personal hygiene, promoting accumulation of smegma, and providing a sheltered microenvironment that is more conducive to carcinogenic factors. For uncircumcised men, the presence of phimosis has been found to be a significant risk factor (RR=37.2) for penile cancer.[8] Although considered to be an important risk factor, not all men with phimosis develop penile cancer. Penile cancer may be prevented by surgical correction of a congenital or acquired phimosis.

16.2.1.5 Hygiene

Early researchers postulated that hygiene may play an important role in the acquisition of penile cancer. However, poor personal hygiene has not been shown to be an independent cause of penile cancer. Rather, poor hygiene may be more commonly seen in men with penile cancer. Alternatively, good hygiene does not prevent the occurrence of penile cancer.[2] Poor hygiene is more often seen in uncircumcised men and in men with phimosis. When neglectful, these men may allow the accumulation of smegma beneath the foreskin, which has also been postulated to promote the development of penile cancer.

16.2.1.6 Smegma

Smegma is defined as the accumulation of desquamated squamous epithelial cells between the glans penis and foreskin. Although some studies clearly implicate smegma as an oncogenic agent, most studies do not. Therefore, the role of smegma in carcinogenesis is controversial. Brinton found smegma to be associated with an eleven-fold increased risk for penile cancer, although its presence may have been only a consequence of the disease.[8] Smegma, or hydrocarbon and sterol byproducts, may act as a local irritant, facilitating malignant transformation of normal squamous epithelium.[1]

16.2.1.7 Human papillomavirus

The most compelling evidence for an etiologic agent for penile cancer is derived from studies evaluating the role of human papillomavirus (HPV) in this process (Figure 16.2). In the general population, the prevalence of HPV of the penis varies from 6% to 11% based on DNA hybridization tests.[9,10] Just as with women, oncogenic HPV 16 and 18 are the most commonly detected HPV types in penile cancer, with the former seen more frequently.[2] Yet, HPV 16 and 18 are not detected in all types of penile cancer.

High-grade penile intraepithelial neoplasia (PIN) is considered a potential penile cancer precursor lesion. There is evidence that as the severity of

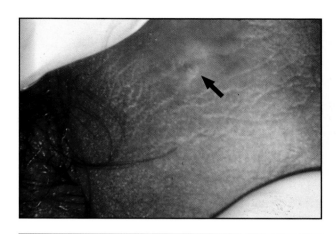

FIGURE 16.2 HPV-induced condyloma of the penile shaft (arrow) in a young man. The wart is not easily recognized.

PIN increases, so does the percentage of HPV DNA detected. HPV DNA had been detected in 75% of cases of PIN 1, 93% of PIN 2 and 100% of cases of PIN 3.[11] In one study, using a PCR amplification test, HPV DNA was detected in 71% of invasive squamous cell cancers, and in 83% of mild and 86% of severe intraepithelial neoplasias.[2] However, in a more recent study, HPV DNA was detected in only 22.2% of penile cancers.[12] These data may reflect the wide variety of different penile cancers considered. Of these various cancers, HPV DNA was detected in 75% of basaloid squamous cell cancers.[12] Another study using a PCR HPV test, detected HPV in 55% of invasive squamous cell cancers, 92% of carcinoma in situ (CIS), and 92% of PIN.[13] Selective testing for various HPV types may also account for the wide range of HPV detected in penile cancers.

The prevalence of genital HPV in men varies by age and specimen type. Genital HPV is nearly 2.5 times more common in young men (ages 16 to 35) than in older men (ages 36 to 85).[9] Just as with women, there is a bimodal age distribution for HPV in men, with the greatest peak from ages 16 to 35 and a second, much smaller peak in men older than 75 years.[9] The increased number in the older population may reflect active re-expression of HPV from a latent stage.

Testing results may also vary by the site sampled and specimen type. The yield of HPV is apt to be greatest where HPV is most likely to cause lesions, the glans and penile shaft. Although the majority of researchers have focused on detecting HPV within the epithelium, several studies have also shown that HPV may be found within semen.[14,15] Since HPV is a sexually transmitted disease, some of the best epidemiologic evidence supporting certain types of HPV as significant risk factors for penile cancer is derived from studies of mutual sexual partners with concomitant neoplasias of the lower genital tract.

16.2.1.8 The role of sexual partner(s)

Male sexual partners of women who have condylomas and CIN are at increased risk for having or developing penile condylomas or PIN.[16-18] When male partners of women with genital condylomas were evaluated, 41% to 69% were found to also have genital condylomas.[17,18] If only women with CIN were considered, 33% of their male consorts had penile intraepithelial lesions.[18] When women with genital condylomas or CIN were considered, 53% to 64% of their male sexual partners had genital lesions,[16,18] the majority of which were located on the glans or penile shaft. These lesions were detected either by naked-eye examination or through the use of a colposcope.

Furthermore, in a study by Barrasso,[18] 61 of 65 (about 94%) men with PIN were sexual partners of women who had CIN. Schneider et al[19] demonstrated that 65% of men who were sexual partners of genital HPV DNA positive women were found to harbor HPV. Oncogenic HPV types 16 and 18 were detected in 27% of both partners, and in nearly half of the couples, the same type of HPV was detected. These data are similar to those of Hippelainen et al, who, in examining male sexual partners of women with abnormal Pap smears, found HPV in 24.4% of both sexual partners and 22.7% of them had the same HPV type.[20] These data clearly demonstrate the role of sexually transmitted oncogenic HPV in the acquisition and development of genital neoplasias in both men and women.

Further evidence supporting the importance of oncogenic HPV and genital neoplasia can be found by examining the common link between spouses with genital malignancies. When the death rate of wives of men who died with penile cancer were compared with matched controls, a significantly greater percentage of women were found to have died from cervical cancer (11 deaths vs. 3.9 expected, p=0.002).[21] In a similar study, Graham et al[22] found that, when wives of men with penile cancer were analyzed, three times as many cases of cervical cancer were detected compared with controls. Martinez demonstrated an eight-fold increased rate of cervical cancer in wives of Puerto Rican men with penile cancer when compared with normal controls.[23]

The risk of "sharing" genital cancer with a spouse extends further. Not only is the primary spouse at increased risk, but when second wives of men whose first wife had cervical cancer were compared with normal controls, there was a 3.5-fold greater risk that the second wife also developed cervical cancer.[24] These

epidemiologic data denote what has been referred to previously as "the high-risk male."[25,26] This terminology was derived and spread by clinicians who viewed the association from a single perspective, even though this high risk status is not associated solely with a single sex. Rather than being gender related, the issue is rather the presence of oncogenic HPV that is shared sexually in both directions.

In many cases, male partners of women with histologically confirmed CIN 3 or cervical cancer harbor oncogenic HPV of the penis. On most occasions, clinical inspection reveals only subclinical evidence of HPV following colposcopic evaluation of epithelium that has been soaked with 5% acetic acid. A small percentage (8%) of these men have PIN 3.[27] Conversely, Campion et al[28] demonstrated that 76% of women who were sexual consorts of men with penile condyloma acuminata also had HPV-related lesions of the lower genital tract. Of these women, 36% had abnormal cervical pathology. Hence, sexual intercourse should be viewed only as facilitating the spread of a potentially dangerous virus.

16.2.1.9 Human Immunodeficiency Virus (HIV)

There are limited data on the risk of penile cancer in men infected with HIV. However, one study has determined that there appears to be an association between penile cancer (RR=3.9) and HIV/AIDS.[29] Males infected with HIV are also at increased risk for PIN 3 (RR=6.9).[30] More is understood about the risk of anal cancer in HIV-positive men (See section 16.2.2). For example, HIV-positive males are at greater risk for anal intraepithelial neoplasia (RR=60.1) and anal cancer (RR=37.9) than the comparative grades of penile neoplasia.[30]

16.2.1.10 Tobacco

Smoking tobacco products has previously been shown to increase the risk of developing cancers of various organ systems. The role of tobacco in penile cancer is not well established and the precise mechanism not understood. However, one study has determined that penile cancer appeared to be associated with smoking (p=0.002), chewing tobacco (p=0.001), and the use of snuff (p=0.004).[31] Furthermore, there was a significant dose response noted for smoking and chewing tobacco: the greater the use, the greater the rate of penile cancer. Another epidemiologic study of anogenital cancers determined that both former and current smokers (OR=1.5 and OR=2.9, respectively) are at increased risk for developing penile cancer when compared with nonsmoking controls.[32] The risk appeared to be significantly age related. For men between the ages of 40 and 59, the odds ratios for developing penile cancer in former and current smokers were OR=27.5 and OR=54.9, respectively. These rates differed for men more than 60 years old (OR=52.6 and OR=36.8, respectively).[32] For reasons that are not clear, a history of current smoking conveyed a greater risk for young men than for older men.

16.2.2 Risk factors for anal cancer

Anal cancer is not common in the general population, accounting for only 1.5% of digestive system cancers.[33] However, risks are significantly greater for certain population groups. Men with a history of anal receptive intercourse are considered at high risk (RR=33.1).[34] Furthermore, men with a history of anal condylomas are more prone to develop anal cancer.[34,35]

As with the cervix, anal cancers may require a precipitating event, that being infection with high-risk HPV. The condylomas likely serve as a surrogate marker for infection with multiple HPV types, both low and high risk. When anal cancers of men have been examined for HPV, researchers detected HPV 16 in 84% of the specimens.[36] Anal cancers in homosexual men are more likely to be associated with high-risk HPV types (P<0.01) than are the same cancers in heterosexual men.[37] Given ready access and trauma to the anal transformation zone, located at the interface of anal squamous epithelium and rectal columnar epithelium, high-risk HPV is able to initiate the neoplastic process within immature metaplastic cells. Provided the conditions are suitable, high-risk HPV may cause cellular transformation and the development of anal high-grade squamous intraepithelial lesions (ASIL). It is likely that ASILs are cancer precursors.

Behaviors that place men at risk for HIV amplify the risk for co-acquisistion of HPV. Consequently, their chance of developing anal neoplasia is increased. As such, anal cytologic screening has been advocated as a test for select populations. Anal HSIL is more likely to be found in HIV-seropositive men when compared with HIV-seronegative men (RR=3.7).[38,39] In one study, the 4-year incidence of anal HSIL was 49% among HIV-positive men and 17% among HIV-negative men.[38] Furthermore, those with low CD4 (P=0.007) counts or persistent HPV infection were more likely to develop anal HSIL (P=0.007 and P=0.0001, respectively).[38]

The progressive potential of low-grade anal lesions is presumed but not fully understood. However, men with less-severe anal cytologic changes may also be predisposed to developing more severe disease. According to one study, men with anal ASCUS or LSIL were more likely to develop HSIL (57%) compared with HIV-positive men (38%) without prior minor cytologic changes (P=0.001). In addition, HIV-negative men with ASCUS or LSIL (33%) are more likely to develop HSIL when compared with HIV-negative men (14%) without cytologic abnormalities (P=0.001).[38] In another prospective study comparing HIV-positive and HIV-negative men for nearly 2 years, 15% of HIV-positive and 5% of HIV-negative men developed anal HSIL. Identified risk factors included infection with HPV 16 or 18, persistent high HPV DNA loads, and a CD4 level less than 500/mμ.[39]

Other types of immunosuppressive and sexual exposure place men at a greater risk for developing anogenital neoplasia. A persistent HPV infection in renal transplant patients is associated with a 100-fold increased risk for anogenital cancer.[40] Therefore, just as with cervical neoplasia, infection of the anal transformation zone by a high-risk HPV type, particularly in an immunosuppressed patient, places the individual at great risk for developing an anal SIL or anal cancer. The sexual nature of anogenital neoplasia in men is also suggested by greater standard incidence ratios for anal cancer in husbands of women with CIN 3 (SIR=1.75) and cervical cancer (SIR-1.92).[41]

The effect of tobacco as a risk factor for anal cancer is less certain. In one study, smoking was not a statistically significant risk for anal cancer in men.[30] However, in another, current smoking was a significant risk for anal cancer in men (RR=9.4).[32] Further study of tobacco's influence on the development of anal cancer appears warranted.

16.3 Clinical Findings of HPV-Related Disease in Men

16.3.1 Condyloma acuminata

HPV can affect any epithelium of the male anogenital area. Low-risk (nononcogenic) HPV infection (HPV 6,11) may produce warty, epithelial proliferations known as condyloma acuminata. High-risk HPV types may also be detected in a minority of these lesions. The majority of condylomas are located on the foreskin, glans, or shaft of the penis, which are susceptible to abrasive-type superficial trauma (Figures 16.3a,b).[16] Disease can also extend to the scrotum, perianal, and pubic regions (Figure 16.4). In uncircumcised men, condylomas are frequently found on or beneath the foreskin (Figures 16.5a,b).[42] Lesions may also be noted on the glans or shaft of the penis. Mucosal epithelium is particularly prone to trauma, the portal for HPV infection. On occasion

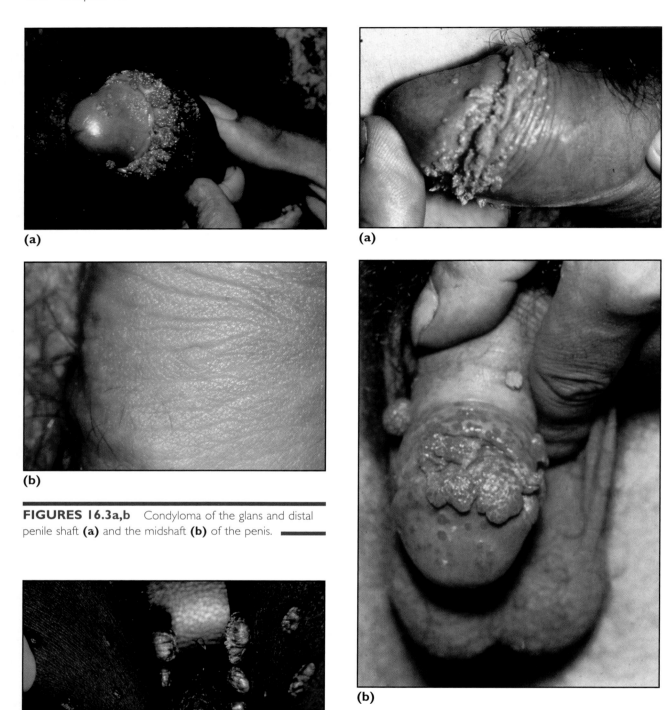

FIGURES 16.3a,b Condyloma of the glans and distal penile shaft **(a)** and the midshaft **(b)** of the penis.

FIGURE 16.4 Diffuse condyloma of the medial thighs, near the scrotum in this 19-year-old.

FIGURES 16.5a,b Condyloma located beneath the foreskin **(a)** and involving the glans **(b)**.

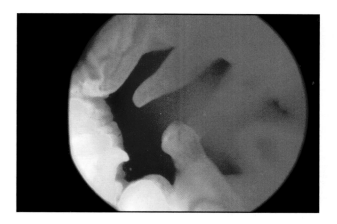

FIGURE 16.6 Condyloma of the penile urethra seen through a cystoscope.

(10% to 28%), condylomas may be seen at the urethral meatus or within the urethra (Figure 16.6).[18] If present, urethral involvement is limited mainly to the distal 20 mm to 25 mm of the urethra. Similarly, perianal condylomas may be observed, sometimes extending into the distal anus (Figures 16.7a–c). The patient's sexual history, particularly in regard to sexual practices, will help guide clinicians to potential sites of disease. Men with a history of anal receptive intercourse are very susceptible to anal condylomas.

Condylomas may be distributed widely on keratinized and mucosal anogenital epithelium in men. Condylomas may reside in more than one anatomic site, as solitary or multiple condylomas. Mucosal sites include the urethra and glans/inner foreskin in uncircumcised men. Keratinized sites include the shaft of the penis and scrotum in all men and glans in circumcised men. Condylomas can also present with varied frequency and size. In a study of male sexual partners of women with CIN, between 0 to 50 condylomas (median 3) were detected in men.[43] Most individuals have fewer than 10 condylomas, but this number varies according to many factors. HPV lesions vary in size from several centimeters in diameter to small lesions visible only using magnification. The median size of condylomas in men is 3mm.[43] Therefore, although naked-eye inspection may detect large condylomas in men with multiple lesions, only assisted visualization using magnification and contrast agents is apt to detect all lesions.

Condylomas present in a multitude of shapes and color. These lesions may have papillary, frond-like epithelial projections that sometimes resemble a large cauliflower-like mass. However, HPV-related penile lesions are more likely to be papular, flat, spiked, or a mixed type (85%) than a papillary condyloma (15%) (Figures 16.8a–f).[43] Flat condylomas

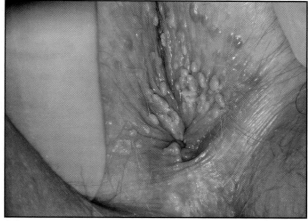

(a)

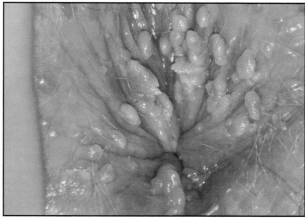

(b)

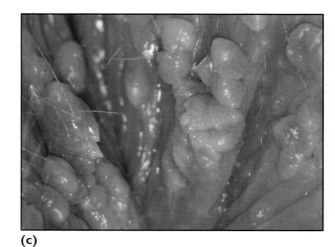

(c)

FIGURES 16.7a–c Perianal condyloma

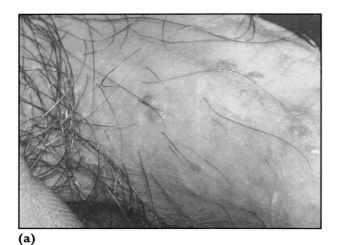

(a)

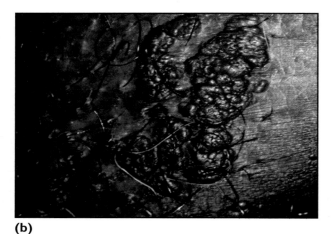

(b)

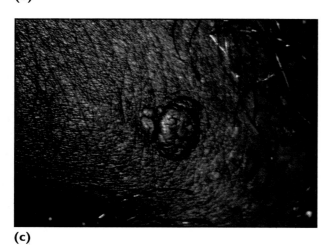

(c)

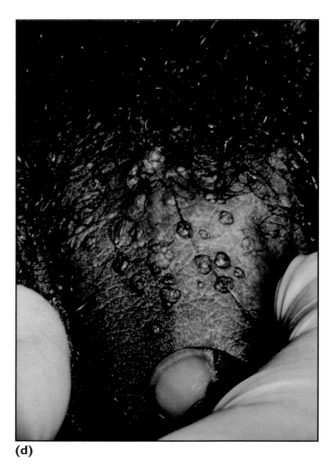

(d)

FIGURES 16.8a–f Multiple papular HPV-related lesions on the shaft of the penis **(a)** and pigmented papular condyloma on the base of the penis **(b,c,d)**.

tend to convey greater risk for the patient and are difficult to discriminate from PIN. Lesion color depends on the amount and location of vascularization, extent and color of pigmentation and presence of keratinization. Exophytic condylomas are usually a natural skin tone color, and therefore, some very small condylomas may not be seen by casual inspec-

tion (Figure 16.9). Pigmented condylomas, which comprise only about one third of all condylomas,[44] may contrast with the surrounding epithelium and consequently may be more easily detected (Figures 16.10a–c). Following 5% acetic acid application, many condylomas, particularly those located on moist mucosal surfaces, will temporarily blanch acetowhite. The importance of acetic acid application is verified by the fact that 22% of HPV-associated lesions of the penis would not otherwise be detected.[43] Warts with hyperkeratinized epithelium may not assume a transient white color after an application of 5% acetic acid. These condylomas may have a silver or "dried" appearance. Hence, some condylomas may appear white prior to the application of 5% acetic acid. Central afferent and efferent capillary loops may be seen within the long papillary projections when inspected using high-power colposcopic

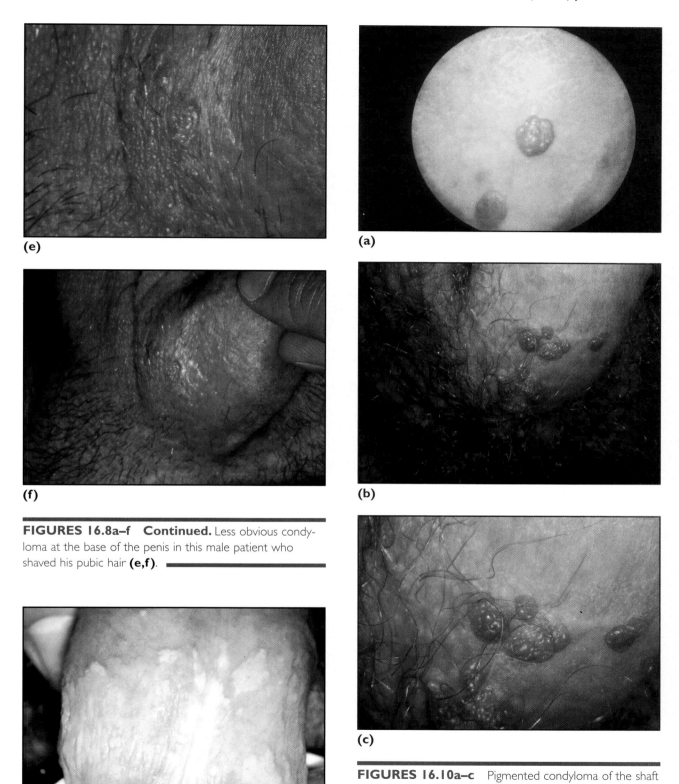

(e)

(f)

FIGURES 16.8a–f   Continued. Less obvious condyloma at the base of the penis in this male patient who shaved his pubic hair **(e,f)**.

FIGURE 16.9   Maculopapular, flesh-colored acetowhite lesion visible only following application of 5% acetic acid and magnified inspection.

(a)

(b)

(c)

FIGURES 16.10a–c   Pigmented condyloma of the shaft of the penis.

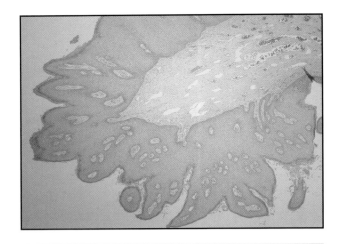

FIGURE 16.11 Histology of penile condyloma (Hematoxylin-eosin stain; medium power magnification). ▬

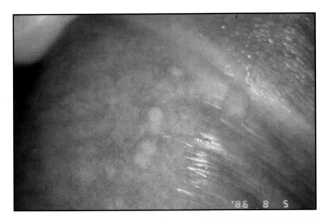

FIGURE 16.12 Subclinical HPV infection of the penile skin seen as multifocal acetowhite lesions. HPV 16 was detected by DNA hybridization testing. ▬

magnification. When viewed from above or down the length of the condyloma, a red punctate or loop vascular pattern may be noted. The histologic features of penile condylomas are the same as those also seen in genital condylomas of women (Figure 16.11).

As in women, HPV is not apt to cause symptoms in men. The majority of men (76%) with genital condylomas are asymptomatic.[43] The most common symptom reported is pruritus. Trauma occasionally may cause minor bleeding and pain if the warts are avulsed. Urethral lesions may produce a deviated urinary stream, and cause obstruction when enlarged, or rarely, hematuria.

16.3.2 Penile intraepithelial neoplasia (PIN)

Penile intraepithelial neoplasia (PIN) is a lesion that is analogous to VIN in women. As such, most of these lesions (92%) are associated with different HPV types.[13] PIN grade 1 is associated predominately with nononcogenic types of HPV (HPV 6,11).[44] However, HPV 16 (an oncogenic HPV type) has been detected in as many as 36% of PIN 1 lesions.[11] In contrast, most PIN 3 lesions are caused by oncogenic HPV types, such as HPV 16 (Figure 16.12).[44,11] Oncogenic HPV can be found in 80% to 90% of PIN 3 lesions. As with CIN, HPV does not integrate into the nucleus of PIN 3 lesions, but remains as an episomal viral genome.[44] PIN is considered a precursor of penile cancer, although only a minority of these lesions develops into cancer.

The mean age of men with PIN 3 is 37 years, 7 years greater than the mean age of men with PIN 1.[11] This age differential for PIN stages suggests that PIN 1 may progress sequentially to PIN 3 just as progres-

sion may occur along the continuum of CIN. PIN 3 may progress to penile cancer less rapidly, based on the fact that the mean age of men with penile cancer is approximately 20 years greater than that for men with PIN 3.[45] Circumcision appears to provide some level of protection against PIN. A greater percent of men with PIN are uncircumcised than circumcised.[11]

PIN is the modern term that describes precancerous lesions of the penis (Figures 16.13a,b). The term PIN encompasses older terminology of Bowen's disease, erythroplasia of Queyrat, Bowenoid papulosis, and carcinoma in situ.[46] Confusion arises from persistent use of the older terminology. Because many clinicians continue to use these archaic names, it may be beneficial to review them from the historical perspective. Bowen's disease refers to small, dull, erythematous plaques on the glans of the penis. These nonpainful plaques may ooze and become crusted and may also be found in other nongenital areas of the body. Some believe that men with Bowen's disease have an increased risk for gastrointestinal cancer, but this assumption has not been substantiated by further study. However, Bowen's disease is a true precursor of penile cancer. Because of the red, plaque-like appearance, psoriasis and eczema may mimic Bowen's disease. Oncogenic HPV 16 is almost always detected within these lesions when tested. Bowen's disease is actually a carcinoma in situ or PIN 3 of dermis containing hair follicles. Histologically, these lesions demonstrate cellular atypia and mitotic figures (Figure 16.14) of high-grade neoplasia.

In contrast, erythroplasia of Queyrat is a PIN 3 of mucocutaneous epithelium. These papular or plaque-like lesions are erythematous, well demarcated, with a "velvet"-like texture. They are generally located on the glans or prepuce and may be solitary

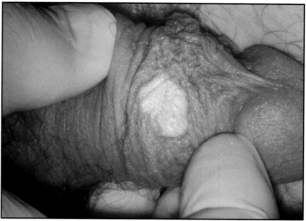

(a)

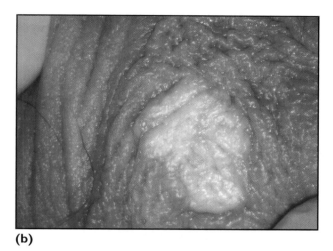

(b)

FIGURES 16.13a,b   A large dense acetowhite lesion of the penis diagnosed as PIN 2 by biopsy.

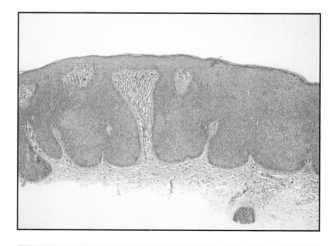

FIGURE 16.14   Histology of Bowen's disease of the penis (Hematoxylin-eosin stain; medium power magnification).

or multifocal. Just like with Bowen's disease, these lesions may ulcerate but most patients remain asymptomatic. Erythroplasia of Queyrat may be confused with syphilis, tinea, psoriasis, and monilia. Histologically, these lesions have atypical epithelial cells with hyperchromatic nuclei and loss of normal cellular polarity. Atypical mitoses may be seen. Many pathologists consider the histologic findings of erythroplasia of Queyrat and Bowen's disease the same. Most men with either of these two conditions are approximately 50 years of age or older and uncircumcised. Both lesions have been shown to progress to invasive penile cancer.

Bowenoid papulosis, another PIN 3, is described classically as multiple, small, violaceous or reddish-brown papules involving the shaft of the penis or glans. Consequently, these lesions may mimic lichen planus, seborrheic keratosis, psoriasis, and condylomas. In contrast with men who have Bowen's disease or erythroplasia of Queyrat, men with Bowenoid papulosis are generally younger (20 to 30 years old) and circumcised. Although most pathologists consider Bowenoid papulosis and PIN 3 histologically indistinguishable, these lesions are not known to progress to invasive cancer. Bowenoid papulosis is thought to be a transient and self-limiting process. These lesions have histologic evidence of hyperkeratosis, atypical cells with hyperchromatic and pleomorphic nuclei, some mitotic figures, and an associated dermal inflammatory response. Oncogenic HPV 16 has been identified frequently in these lesions.

The clinical diagnosis of PIN can be very challenging. Because PIN lesions are difficult to distinguish from condylomas or other benign dermatologic conditions,[44] a low biopsy threshold may be advisable. These lesions may be macular, papular, or slightly elevated. Although PIN is more likely to be pigmented than condyloma, only 57% of PIN 3 lesions are pigmented (Figures 16.15 and 16.16).[44] A well-demarcated, sometimes raised lesion margin delineates PIN 3 from the surrounding normal epithelium (Figures 16.17–16.19). According to Barrasso and colleagues,[11] most (53%) PIN lesions are macular, and therefore, are detected only after application of 5% acetic acid. These lesions may appear red prior to acetic acid application, and fine punctation may be noted with colposcopic magnification. Dilated, large-caliber vessels also may be seen. Other PIN lesions are papular and pigmented brown or black. Some PINs exhibit leukoplakia with thickened, white epithelium and an irregular, micropapillary surface. Otherwise, condylomas, which equate histologically to PIN 1, appear as exophytic, nodular, or papular lesions that also appear transiently white following the application of 5% acetic acid.

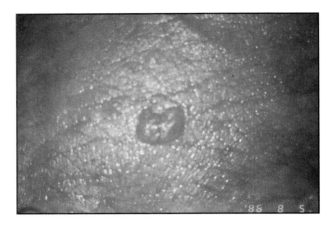

FIGURE 16.15 A pigmented, papular lesion of the penis.

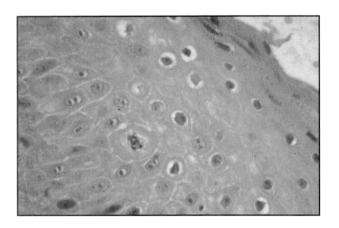

FIGURE 16.16 Histology from a biopsy of the lesion seen in Figure 16.15 (Hematoxylin-eosin stain; high power magnification). Prominent cytopathic effects of HPV and basal atypia are seen in this low-grade penile lesion.

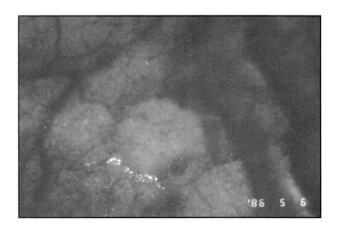

FIGURE 16.17 A solitary acetowhite penile lesion with varicose punctation in a sexual partner of a woman with CIN 3.

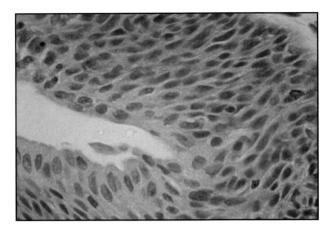

FIGURE 16.18 Histology from a biopsy of the penile lesion seen in Figure 16.17 demonstrating penile carcinoma in situ (Hematoxylin-eosin stain; high power magnification).

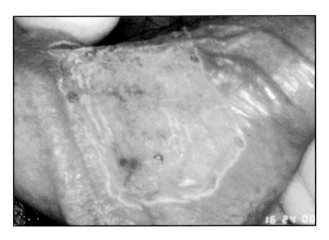

FIGURE 16.19 The lesion seen in Figure 16.17 following treatment by CO$_2$ laser. The surrounding epithelium (containing subclinical HPV) was also treated to reduce the possibility of recurrent disease.

16.3.3 Penile cancer

Some penile cancer appears to evolve from precancerous PIN.[13] Clinically, this is evidenced by the fact that PIN 3 may be seen surrounding a central malignant process. The complex process of carcinogenesis requires integration of oncogenic HPV, which is thought to initiate malignant transformation. Other various risk factors (See Section 16.2.1) contribute to the slow evolution of PIN 3 to cancer (an average of 20 years).[45] Men averaging age 60 years may first notice a small papule, nodule, or ulceration usually on the glans or prepuce (Figure 16.20). The prepuce may be phimotic and hiding an underlying small

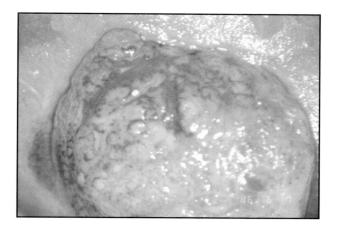

FIGURE 16.20   Invasive cancer of the glans.

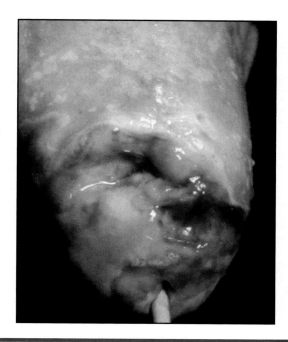

FIGURE 16.21   Cancer of the penis with associated bleeding and urinary obstruction.

mass. In this case, the cancer may become quite enlarged prior to being detected. Advanced penile cancers frequently ulcerate once tumor growth has exceeded the vascular supply. Tissue necrosis then ensues along with secondary infection. The tumor may grow outward from the epithelium (exophytic) as a nodular or papillary lesion. Otherwise, it may infiltrate tissues (endophytic), leaving a flat or indurated lesion that may not be easily identified. Penile cancer metastasizes via the lymphatics to regional lymph nodes. In addition to a mass, ulceration, and purulent drainage, patients may present with bleeding, pain, or urinary obstruction (Figure 16.21). In general, colposcopy is not required to diagnose penile cancer. Most lesions are readily apparent on naked-eye inspection. Although most penile cancer is of squamous origin, other types of penile cancers also may be seen. Melanomas are darkly pigmented, irregular, and often raised, aggressive malignant tumors. Basal cell carcinomas are also rare tumors, usually appearing on the shaft of the penis. They are nodular or papular with a rolled border.

16.3.4 Penile cancer mimics

Giant condyloma

Giant condyloma or Buschke-Lowenstein tumor can mimic penile cancer. The lesions are exophytic, papillary growths that resemble extremely large warts. They are caused by HPV 6 or 11. These tumors are usually considered benign but they can destroy local tissues without metastasizing. The growths appear most commonly on the glans or prepuce. Biopsy is necessary to confirm the diagnosis. These lesions are now thought to be distinct from verrucous carcinoma, although the two entities appear quite similar clinically. In the case of a positive biopsy, an oncolo-

gist or urologist should be consulted to help determine management.

Condyloma acuminata

Large, exophytic condylomas may be difficult to discriminate from cancer. Both may be papillary or exhibit an irregular, raised surface. These lesions can occur anywhere in the anogenital region. Each growth may appear acetowhite or have overlying leukoplakia. A biopsy is often required to establish a definitive diagnosis, but empiric therapy can follow a confident clinical diagnosis. However, condyloma lata, a lesion of syphilis, may closely resemble condyloma acuminata. Serologic testing is necessary to confirm the diagnosis of syphilis. Condylomas treated without an initial biopsy should be biopsied if not responding appropriately after a reasonable course of conservative therapy.

Molluscum contagiosum

Molluscum contagiosum are smooth, flesh colored, papular lesions with a slightly depressed central core (Figures 16.22a,b). A white cheesy substance containing molluscum bodies may be expressed from this central depression. These lesions are benign and may also involve the axilla, mons, and groin. If not inflamed by an unrelated process, the papules do not turn acetowhite following 5% acetic acid application. Biopsies are not generally required to establish the diagnosis. Various therapeutic options exist for these lesions.

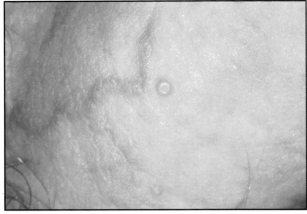

(a)

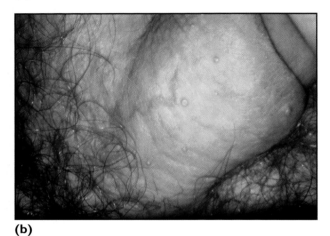

(b)

FIGURES 16.22a,b   Molluscum contagiosum can be confused with condyloma. These smooth pearly papules with central depression on the shaft of the penis may also be seen in the axillary areas.

Pearly penile papules

Pearly penile papules are normal, small, round or filiform papules of the corona of the glans (Figures 16.23a–c). They may represent a male arratomic variant of micropapillomatosis labials seen in some women. Several linear rows of fleshy papules may surround the glans or there may only be a small cluster of these papillary projections. These tiny growths do not change color following 5% acetic acid application provided there is no coexisting inflammatory condition. Pearly penile papules are sometimes confused with HPV-related disease (Figure 16.24). However, because they are a normal anatomic variant, no treatment is required.

16.3.5 Anal intraepithelial neoplasia (AIN)

Anal intraepithelial neoplasia (AIN) are premalignant epithelial lesions of the anus. They are graded histologically, much like CIN and PIN, from AIN 1 to AIN 3. The latter entity represents a potential anal cancer precursor. As such, histologic confirmation mandates appropriate therapy. These lesions are usually found within the anal transformation zone, analogous to the transformation zone of the cervix. Consequently, detection usually involves full appraisal of this anatomical site. Anal intraepithelial lesions usually are not visible without the use of a colposcope and 5% acetic acid. Some anal condyloma can be detected by naked-eye examination, but most AIN are macular and of normal epithelial color prior to the use of 5% acetic acid. Therefore, most AIN cannot be detected by palpation or inspection. These lesions have many of the same colposcopic features of CIN, such as acetowhite epithelium, leukoplakia, punctation, mosaic vessels, and various types of lesion margins. However, in contrast with the cervix, coarse vessels are more commonly found than are fine-caliber blood vessels (Figures 16.25a–c).[47] Just as on the cervix, atypical blood vessels denote the likely presence of an invasive process.

Although intraepithelial neoplasia of the anus and cervix appear to have similar colposcopic features, the accuracy of colposcopists to diagnose AIN was initially suspect. However, in evaluating the ability of colposcopists to diagnose anal HSIL, colposcopists achieved a 49% positive predictive value when using the same colposcopic features used to evaluate CIN.[47] Therefore, the colposcopic approach to AIN is very similar to that for CIN.

16.4 Colposcopy of Men

Although colposcopy has been used primarily to evaluate women following abnormal Pap smear results, the colposcope also may be used to examine the anogenital area of men. The purpose of colposcopy is to identify epithelial lesions consistent with condyloma acuminata, PIN, AIN, penile cancer and anal cancer.

16.4.1 Objectives and indications

Although some epithelial lesions in men are quite apparent to naked-eye inspection, other occult macular lesions are unrecognized without the application of an epithelial contrast solution and magnification of the colposcope. Careful inspection by

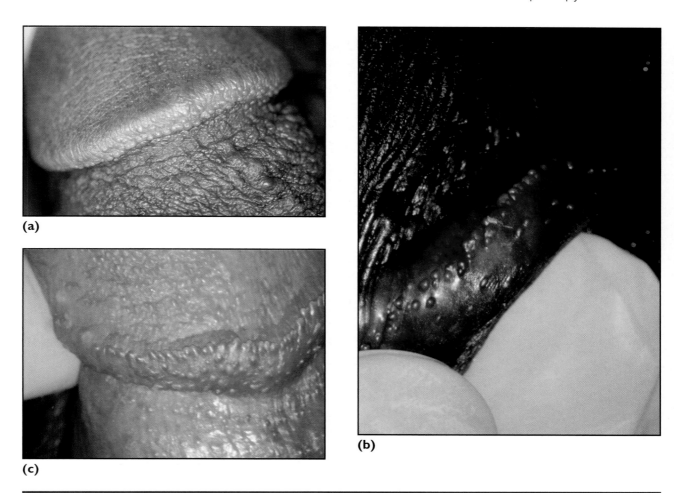

FIGURES 16.23a–c   Pearly penile papules of the glans coronal ridge **(a,b,c)** are a benign finding seen in some men.

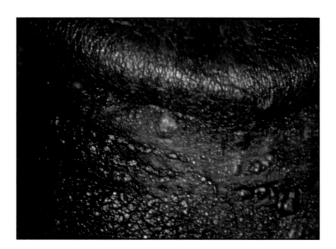

FIGURE 16.24   Pearly penile papules are sometimes confused with condyloma acuminata and therefore are treated inappropriately. However, these penile papules near the glans are caused by HPV.

colposcopy allows detailed assessment and colposcopically directed sampling, if necessary. The colposcope also may be used to direct treatment of the genital tract using laser equipment.

The objectives of colposcopy of men are to: 1) visualize the epithelium of the penis, distal urethra, scrotum, perianal and anal areas; 2) in the case of anal colposcopy, identify the anal transformation zone in its entirety; 3) identify and then assess suspected potential neoplastic lesions with regard to size, extent, and severity of disease; and 4) sample anogenital lesions for histologic evaluation, when appropriate.

Although men are rarely examined colposcopically by most healthcare providers, certain clinical scenarios may merit colposcopy. Sexual partners of women with cervical, vaginal, or vulvar cancer, or high-grade squamous intraepithelial lesions, are at increased risk for harboring penile intraepithelial neoplasia or penile cancer. Although the practice of

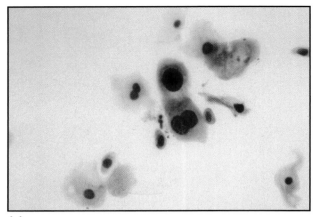

(a)

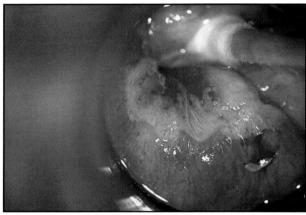

(b)

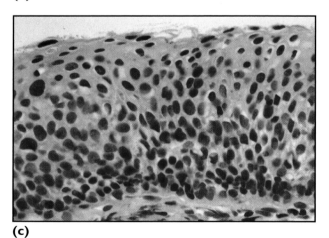

(c)

FIGURES 16.25a–c A liquid-based cytology smear **(a)** demonstrating AIN 3 (Papanicolaou stain; High power magnification). The corresponding AIN 3 seen by colposcopy **(b)**. Note the dense acetowhite epithelium along the SCJ. The margin is smooth and regular and a coarse punctation is seen. A biopsy of this lesion **(c)** also revealed AIN 3 (Hematoxylin-eosin stain; medium power magnification). Photos courtesy of Drs. Joel Palefsky and Teresa Darragh.

examining male sexual partners is somewhat controversial, some colposcopists consider these sexual partners deserving of careful examination. Because the majority of penile lesions are not detected by naked-eye examination,[48,49] a comprehensive examination of male partners should include colposcopy. Men with clinically apparent anogenital growths, ulcerations, or other lesions may benefit from colposcopy to direct biopsy and detect concomitant abnormalities. This is particularly true for men who have urinary tract symptoms. Human papillomavirus-induced lesions of the meatus and distal urethra may be best evaluated by colposcopy. Men with a positive anal cytologic result indicating ASIL or cancer should undergo a colposcopic examination. Colposcopy may be particularly useful for patients following successful treatment of genital lesions when recurrence is suspected but the initial clinical examination discloses no visible lesions. Finally, although rarely used for this purpose, colposcopy may help to allay real fears of men who harbor a concern that they have HPV-related diseases of the genitalia.

16.4.2 Patient preparation

Some men with HPV-induced anogenital lesions seek thorough examination of the anogenital area that may include colposcopy. In other cases, asymptomatic men who are sexual partners of men or women with HPV-induced lesions may present for colposcopic evaluation. Because many of these men are not well informed about the disease process or the procedure, patient education prior to the examination is very helpful to minimize needless anxiety. The benign nature of the examination should be disclosed to the patient. A brief overview of the procedure, including application of 5% acetic acid, careful inspection using the colposcope or magnifying lens, visualization of the genitalia, distal urethra, and anus (if appropriate), and possible biopsies should be explained to the patient. Colposcopy can be scheduled without prior patient preparation or screening. However, because 5% acetic acid is moderately irritating, colposcopy of the male anogenital region should be avoided if the patient has an acute inflammatory dermal condition. These inflammatory conditions also may obscure neoplastic changes and mimic or accentuate low-grade PIN or AIN.

16.4.3 Equipment, instruments, and supplies

The equipment, instruments, and supplies necessary to perform colposcopy on men are the same as that required for colposcopy of women (See Chapter 6). The exceptions are that a small nasal speculum may be useful for evaluating the distal urethra and an anoscope is required to examine the anus. An otoscope with a suitable sized ear speculum may be substituted to examine the distal urethra.[50] Additional supplies include: 5% acetic acid, 4×4 gauze pads, cotton-tipped applicators or cotton balls, an endocervical speculum, cervical biopsy forceps or Keyes dermal punch biopsy instruments, and hemostatic agents.

16.4.4 Technique

Because the majority of colposcopic examinations of males involve inspection of externally positioned epithelium, it is considerably easier than colposcopy of females. The one exception is examination of the anus. Colposcopy of men consists of three steps: visualization, assessment, and sampling. After explaining the procedure to the patient, exam preparations may begin. Patients may sit or recline during the examination so that the clinician can obtain ample exposure of the genitalia, perianal area, and anus, if necessary. Men can also be examined, much like women are, in stirrups.

Initially, the external genitalia, including the penis, scrotum, and perianal area can be inspected with the naked eye for growths or ulcers. Some clinicians may perform a cursory low-magnification colposcopic examination at this point prior to application of 5% acetic acid. Naked-eye or colposcopic visualization ensures that all the epithelium is surveyed for gross lesions. A 5% solution of acetic acid is applied to cover the penis, scrotum, and perianal area. In uncircumcised men, the foreskin should be retracted to ensure full coverage of acetic acid to the glans and mucosal surface of the prepuce. Although 5% acetic acid may be sprayed onto the patient using a misting bottle, a more commonly performed technique is to wrap the glans and penile shaft with a 4×4 gauze pad soaked in 5% acetic acid. A second soaked gauze pad should be placed overlying the scrotum and perianal areas. Because this epithelium is heavily keratinized, colposcopists must wait 3 to 5 minutes to detect potential acetowhite changes. Following sufficient time to soak the epithelial structures, the gauze is removed for assessment. Reapplication of 5% acetic acid may be required if the examination extends for more than 5 minutes.

Next, the genitalia are assessed using the colposcope at 2× to 4× magnification, with closer inspection of discrete lesions at 10× to 16×. Some practitioners may prefer to use a hand-held magnifying device or low-power loupes instead. The fossa navicularis, glans, prepuce, and penile shaft are inspected

systematically. A careful examination of the entire scrotum, followed by perianal colposcopic inspection, concludes the external examination.

Anoscopy (See chapter 7) may be indicated in certain circumstances: a high-risk patient, a positive anal cytologic report, a lesion that extends within the anus, or perianal neoplasia associated with lower gastrointestinal lesions (Figures 16.26 and 16.27). If meatal HPV-induced lesions are apparent, a careful inspection of the distal urethra may be appropriate.[17,51] The majority of HPV-related disease of the male urethra will be confined to the distal several centimeters. Therefore, adequate visualization can be

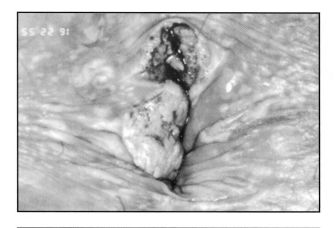

FIGURE 16.26 An anorectal squamous carcinoma that extends into the rectum above the dentate line. High-grade perianal intraepithelial neoplasia and subclinical HPV infection surround this lesion. ■

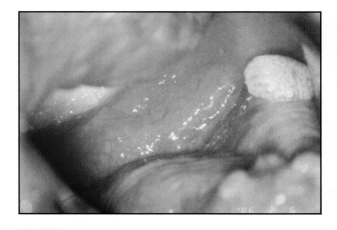

FIGURE 16.27 Anorectal region of a 27-year-old homosexual male with dense acetowhite epithelium extending into the lower rectum consistent with squamous rectal carcinoma in situ. A large condyloma is seen above the area of intraepithelial neoplasia. ■

obtained with gentle retraction at the meatus or use of an endocervical or nasal speculum for tissue retraction. If sentinel meatal or perimeatal lesions are not seen during the colposcopic examination, urethroscopy is unnecessary. Some clinicians avoid urethroscopy in these men because of concern that insertion of the scope may introduce (or seed) HPV into the upper urethra and bladder. To reduce this risk, urethroscopy is commenced only when meatal lesions have been treated successfully (Figure 16.6).

Suspect lesions vary in color from acetowhite, red, brown, or black (Figure 16.28). Many acetowhite changes in the male are nonspecific and may be caused by trauma, candidiasis, inflammation, or conditions other than HPV-related lesions. The anterior surface of the scrotum may blanch a mild acetowhite color, which is considered a variant of normal. The faint white color also may represent subclinical HPV infection or nonspecific inflammation. Although solitary lesions are frequently encountered, multiple lesions may be detected. These multiple lesions are often multifocal in location, involving different anogenital areas. In uncircumcised men, most neoplastic lesions are located in the moist mucosal areas beneath the prepuce and on the glans. In circumcised men, the lesions are usually found on the glans or penile shaft. Phimosis may preclude adequate evaluation of the distal penis. However, attempts should be made to inspect this high-risk area, particularly if surface irregularities of underlying tissue or penile bleeding are noted in elderly men.

Most high-grade lesions have well-circumscribed borders (Figure 16.29). Other low-grade lesions have irregular margins with or without satellite lesions. Penile lesions can assume a macular, papular, nodular, papillary, raised, or ulcerated contour. Areas of leukoplakia and parakeratosis secondary to trauma, infection, or neoplasia may also be observed. Blood vessels and specific vessel patterns are not usually seen during colposcopic assessment. Occasionally, a fine capillary punctation vessel pattern may be observed with high-power colposcopic magnification. The accuracy of colposcopist's evaluation of penile lesions is reasonably good. In one study, the positive predictive value of colposcopy was high (72%) when correlated with histologic results from the penis.[52] However, 19% of the specimens collected from an acetowhite area simply demonstrated an inflammatory response.[52] Other dermatoses were detected in the remaining 9% of cases.

Consequently, genital lesions may require biopsy for definitive diagnostic purposes. A biopsy should always be taken of high-grade intraepithelial neoplasia or lesions suspicious for invasive cancer. Condylomatous lesions suggestive of HPV do not always require biopsy. However, these lesions may be confused with other more ominous neoplastic lesions. After cleaning the site with alcohol, a small 27- to 30-gauge needle should be used to obtain local anesthesia with 1% to 2% xylocaine. Once a sufficiently large dermal wheal is achieved, the biopsy can be collected. Cervical biopsy forceps or a Keyes biopsy punch may be used to biopsy lesions. A small pair of scissors or a shave excision using a surgical knife blade may be used to excise small lesions superficially. Care should be exercised when biopsying lesions of the glans, the periurethral area, and scrotum. Following biopsy, hemostasis can be obtained using aluminum chloride, silver nitrate or Monsel's solution. Keyes punch biopsies and wide local excisions are generally closed with a soft, nonabsorbable

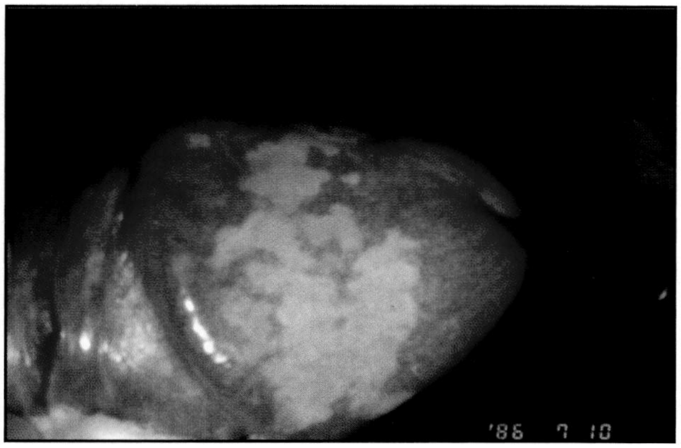

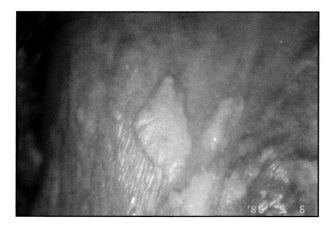

FIGURE 16.28 Dense multifocal acetowhite epithelium of the glans consistent with high grade penile intraepithelial neoplasia.

FIGURE 16.29 Nonpigmented, acetowhite papular lesion on the shaft of the penis. Note the well-circumscribed borders of this high-grade penile intraepithelial neoplasia.

suture. Biopsies should be obtained from all significant lesions. These specimens are then submitted in formalin for histologic diagnosis.

16.4.5 Documentation

The findings of the colposcopic examination should be documented in the medical record. A hand-drawn diagram assists localizing sites of lesions for followup purposes and conveying important information to other healthcare providers. A photo may best document areas of concern.

16.4.6 Patient education

Postbiopsy patients may need to take nonsteroidal antiinflammatory drugs for discomfort, but those who have colposcopy of the genitalia without biopsy require no medications. Postexamination written instructions or educational pamphlets may be useful. Men may notice a small amount of spotting, bleeding or serous drainage from the biopsy site. Although rather unlikely, extensive bleeding may require a followup office visit for cauterization. Patients should be instructed to keep the site clean and dry for a minimum of several days. Men who have had penile biopsies should refrain from sexual activity to allow sufficient time for the wound to heal. If applicable, the patient may need to return in a week for suture removal. It is important to explain to the patient that the histology report, when necessary, may not be immediately available. Finally, physicians should disclose to their patients what was found on examination. Follow-up management plans also may be shared with patients and family members at this time.

16.5 Treatment of Condylomas and PIN

The treatment of genital condylomas in men is very similar to that for women. Multiple treatment options exist including: the self-applied agents, podophyllotoxin and imiquimod, and clinician-rendered treatment by trichloroacetic acid and cryotherapy. Surgical treatment options include electrosurgery, laser therapy and simple excision.[53] 5-fluorouracil (5-FU) may be used to treat meatal condylomas provided particular caution is exercised. A detailed description of these types of therapy is included in Chapter 19.

Penile intraepithelial neoplasia is generally treated using surgical techniques. Excision provides for further histologic appraisal of lesion severity and margin status. This approach is also recommended in cases suspicious for invasion. Otherwise, laser abla-

tion of PIN provides good cure rates and acceptable cosmetic results.

16.6 Implications

Colposcopy of men may be an infrequent procedure compared with colposcopy of women. Men who harbor excessive or unrealistic psychological worries may benefit from colposcopic examination for reassurance purposes. However, reassurance that men are free from HPV infection and related disease is probably not guaranteed following naked-eye or even colposcopic examination. At best, when reasonable, clinicians could share there that is no obvious evidence of disease at the subclinical or more severe level.

For sexually transmitted infections, decreasing the viral load of HPV-related lesions in men by rapid detection and appropriate treatment may be beneficial for both men and women. Eradicating disease or volume of viral load may make it less likely that affected individuals will transmit disease to other sexual partners of either gender (Figure 16.30). Furthermore, reasonable appraisal and efficacious treatment of men with precancerous changes may actually prevent the development of penile and anal cancer. Unfortunately, many men who develop these anogenital malignancies do not seek medical care until advanced levels of change are noted. Whether sexual partners of women with HPV, CIN, or cervical cancer deserve colposcopic examination is debatable. Clearly, the majority of these men harbor some type of virally mediated epithelial change. Yet, couples must understand that treatment of a male partner's

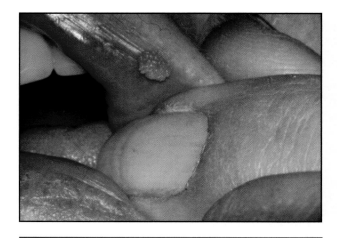

FIGURE 16.30   A small condyloma of the left upper lip is seen in a young woman whose sexual partner had penile condyloma.

penile intraepithelial neoplasia does not alter the course of coexisting cervical neoplasia in his female partner.[54,55] Furthermore, partners do not share HPV-related disease in a "ping pong" fashion. Once infection is established, these individuals retain, and perhaps resolve, these infections without necessarily passing them back and forth on repeated occasions. As can be seen, the role of colposcopy in men is perhaps limited and may be of marginal utility when compared with colposcopy of women. However, colposcopy greatly assists the diagnosis and management PIN and AIN in men.

References

1. Sufrin G, Huben R. Benign and malignant lesions of the penis. In: Gillenwater J Y, Grayhack J T, Howards S S, Duckett T W, eds. *Adult and Pediatric Urology,* 3rd ed. St. Louis: Mosby-Yearbook, Inc., 1996.
2. Malek R S, Goellner J R, Smith T F, Espy M J, Cupp M R. Human papillomavirus infection and intraepithelial, in situ, and invasive carcinoma of the penis. *Urol* 1993;42159–70.
3. Hoppmann H J, Fraley E E. Squamous cell carcinoma of the penis. *J Urol* 1978;120:393–8.
4. Owor R. Carcinoma of the penis in Uganda. *IARC Sci Publ* 1984;63:493–7.
5. Boon M E, Susanti I, Tasche M J A, Kok L P. Human papillomavirus (HPV)—associated male and female genital carcinomas in a Hindu population. *Cancer* 1989;64:559–65.
6. Schoen E J, Oehrli M, Colby C D, Machin G. The highly protective effect of newborn circumcision against invasive penile cancer. *Pediatrics* 2000;105:E36.
7. Reddy C R R M, Devendranath V, Pratap S. Carcinoma of penis—role of phimosis. *Urol* 1984;24:85–8.
8. Brinton L A, Jun-Yao L, Shou-De R, et al. Risk factors for penile cancer: results from a case-control study in China. *Int J Cancer* 1991;47:504–9.
9. Grussendorf-Conen E I, deVilliers E M, Gissmann L. Human papillomavirus genomes in penile smears of healthy men. *Lancet* 1986;2:1092.
10. Fried J J, Steinberg B, Leadbetter G, Nuovo G. Identification of human papillomavirus in penile smears of university students. *J Urol* 1989;141:251A.
11. Aynaud O, Ionesco M, Barrasso R. Penile intraepithelial neoplasia. Specific clinical features correlate with histologic and virologic findings. *Cancer* 1994:74:1762–7.
12. Gregoire L, Cubilla A L, Reuter V E, Hass G P, Lancaster W D. Preferential association of human papillomavirus with high-grade histologic variants of penile-invasive squamous cell carcinoma. *J Natl Cancer Inst* 1995;87:1705–9.
13. Cupp M R, Malek R S, Goellner J R, Smith T F, Espy M J. The detection of human papillomavirus deoxyribonucleic acid in intraepithelial, in situ, verrucous and invasive carcinoma of the penis. *J Urol* 1995;154:1024–9.
14. Ostrow R S, Zachow K R, Niimura M, et al. Detection of papillomavirus DNA in human semen. *Science* 1986;231:731–3.
15. Green J, Monteiro E, Bolton V N, Sanders P, Gibson P E. Detection of human papillomavirus DNA by PCR in semen from patients with and without penile warts. *Genitourin Med* 1991;67:207–10.
16. Levine R U, Crum C P, Herman E, Silvers D, Ferenczy A, Richart R M. Cervical papillomavirus infection and intraepithelial neoplasia: a study of male sexual partners. *Obstet Gynecol* 1984;64:16–20.
17. Sand P K, Bowen L W, Blischke S O, Ostergard D R. Evaluation of male consorts of women with genital human papillomavirus infection. *Obstet Gynecol* 1986;68 679–81.
18. Barrasso R, De Brux J, Croissant O, Orth G. High prevalence of papillomavirus-associated penile intraepithelial neoplasia in sexual partners of women with cervical intraepithelial neoplasia. *N Engl J Med* 1987;317:916–23.
19. Schneider A, Sawada E, Gissmann L, Shah K. Human papillomaviruses in women with a history of abnormal Papanicolaou smears and in their male partners. *Obstet Gynecol* 1987;69:554–62.
20. Hippelainen M I, Yliskoski M, Syrjanen S, et al. Low concordance of genital human papillomavirus (HPV) lesions and viral types in HPV-infected women and their male sexual partners. *Sex Trans Dis* 1994:21:76–82.
21. Smith P G, Kinlen L J, White G C, Adelstein A M, Fox A J. Mortality of wives of men dying with cancer of the penis. *Br J Cancer* 1980;41:422–8.
22. Graham S, Priore R, Graham M, Browne R, Burnett W, West D. Genital cancer in wives of penile cancer patients. *Cancer* 1979;44:1870–4.
23. Martinez I. Relationship of squamous cell carcinoma of the cervix uteri to squamous cell carcinoma of the penis. *Cancer* 1969;24:777–80.
24. Kessler II. Human cervical cancer as a venereal disease. *Cancer Res* 1976;36:783–91.
25. Singer A, Reid B L, Coppleson M. A hypothesis: the role of a high-risk male in the etiology of cervical carcinoma. *Am J Obstet Gynecol* 1976;126:110–5.
26. Brinton L A, Reeves W C, Brenes M M, et al. The male factor in the etiology of cervical cancer among sexually monogamous women. *Int J Cancer* 1989;44:199–203.
27. Campion M J, McCance D J, Mitchell H S, Jenkins D, Singer A, Oriel J D. Subclinical penile human papillomavirus infection and dysplasia in consorts of women with cervical neoplasia. *Genitourin Med* 1988;64:90–9.

28. Campion M J, Singer A, Clarkson P K. Increased risk of cervical neoplasia in consorts of men with penile condylomata acuminata. *Lancet* 1985;943–6.

29. Frisch M, Biggar R J, Engels E A, Goedert J J: AIDS-Cancer match registry study group. Association of cancer with AIDS-related immunosuppression in adults. *JAMA* 2001;285: 1736–45.

30. Frisch M, Biggar R J, Goedert J J. Human papillomavirus-associated cancer in patients with human immunodeficiency virus infection and acquired immunodeficiency syndrome. *J Natl Cancer Inst* 2000;92:1500–10.

31. Harish K, Ravi R. The role of tobacco in penile carcinoma. *B J Urol* 1995;75:375–7.

32. Daling J R, Sherman K J, Hislop T G, et al. Cigarette smoking and the risk of anogenital cancer. *Am J Epidemiol* 1992;135:180–9.

33. Greenlee R T, Murray T, Bolden S, et al. Cancer statistics, 1999. *CA Cancer J Clin* 2000;50:7–33.

34. Daling J R, Weiss N S, Hislop T G, et al. Sexual practices, sexually transmitted diseases, and the incidence of anal cancer. *N Engl J Med* 1987; 317:973–7.

35. Wexner S D, Milson J W, Dailey T H. The demographics of anal cancers are changing. Identification of a high-risk population. *Dis Colon Rectum* 1987;30:942–6.

36. Frisch M, Glimelius B, van den Brule A J, et al. Sexually transmitted infection as a cause of anal cancer. *N Engl J Med* 1997; 337:1350–8.

37. Frisch M, Fenger C, van den Brule A J, et al. Variants of squamous cell carcinoma of the anal canal and perianal skin and their relation to human papillomaviruses. *Cancer Res* 1999; 59:753–7.

38. Palefsky J M, Holly E A, Ralston M L, Jay N, Berry J M, Darragh T M. High incidence of anal high-grade squamous intraepithelial lesions among HIV-positive and HIV-negative homosexual and bisexual men. *AIDS* 1998;12:495–503.

39. Critchlow C W, Surawicz C M, Holmes K K, et al. Prospective study of high-grade anal squamous intraepithelial neoplasia in a cohort of homosexual men: influence of HIV infection, immunosuppression and human papillomavirus infection. *AIDS* 1995;9:1255–62.

40. Arends M J, Benton E C, McLaren K M, Stark L A, Hunter J A, Bird C C. Renal allograft recipients with high susceptibility to cutaneous malignancy have an increased prevalence of human papillomavirus DNA in skin tumors and a great risk of anogenital malignancy. *Br J Cancer* 1997;75:722–8.

41. Hemminki K, Dong C. Cancer in husbands of cervical cancer patients. *Epidemiology* 2000; 11:347–9.

42. Katelaris P M, Cossart Y E, Rose B R, et al. Human papillomavirus: the untreated male reservoir. *J Urol* 1988;140:300–5.

43. Krebs H B, Schneider V. Human papillomavirus-associated lesions of the penis: colposcopy, cytology, and histology. *Obstet Gynecol* 1987;70:299–304.

44. Demeter L M, Stoler M H, Bonners W, et al. Penile intraepithelial neoplasia: clinical presentation and an analysis of the physical state of human papillomavirus DNA. *J Infect Dis* 1993;168:38–46.

45. McCance D J, Karlache A, Ashdown K. HPV type 16 and 18 in carcinoma of the penis from Brazil. *Int J Cancer* 1986;37:55–9.

46. Gerber G S. Carcinoma in situ of the penis. *J Urol* 1994;151:829–33.

47. Jay N, Berry M, Hogeboorn C J, Holly E A, Darragh T M, Palefsky J M. Colposcopic appearance of anal squamous intraepithelial lesions. *Dis Colon Rectum* 1997;40:919–28.

48. Hippelainen M, Yliskoski M, Saarikoski S, Syrjanen S, Syrjanen K. Genital human papillomavirus lesions of the male sexual partners: the diagnostic accuracy of peniscopy. *Genitourin Med* 1991;67:291–6.

49. Carpiniello V, Sedlacek T V, Cunnane M. Magnified penile surface scanning in diagnosis of penile condyloma. *Urology* 1986;28:190–2.

50. O'Brien T S, Luzzi G A. Improving visualization of intrameatal warts: use of the otoscope. *Br J Urol* 1995;75:793.

51. Fralich R A, Malek R S, Goellner J R, Hyland K M. Urethroscopy and urethral cytology in men with external genital condyloma. *Urology* 1994;43:361–4.

52. Wikstrom A, Hedblad M A, Johansson B, et al. The acetic acid test in evaluation of subclinical genital papillomavirus infection; a comparative study on peniscopy, histopathology, virology, and scanning electron microscopy findings. *Genitourin Med* 1992;68:90–9.

53. von Krogh G, Horenblas S. The management and prevention of premalignant penile lesions. *Scand J Urol Nephrol Suppl* 2000;205:220–9.

54. Krebs H B, Helmkamp B F. Does the treatment of genital condyloma in men decrease the treatment of genital condylomata acuminata in women: role of the male sexual partner. *Obstet Gynecol* 1990;76:660–3.

55. Krebs H B, Helmkamp B F. Treatment failure of genital condylomata acuminata in women: role of the male sexual partner. *Obstet Gynecol* 1991;165:337–40.

Cervical Neoplasia Optical Screening Adjuncts

Table of Contents

17.1 Reason for Adjunct Optical Screening Tests

Cervical cancer surveillance programs are designed to detect premalignant disease by serial screening or case finding. When successful, cervical cancer can be prevented by treatment of preinvasive disease that preserves fertility and reproductive capacity.[1] However, the success of the Pap smear may be overstated, even for women who receive routine screening. No test is perfect and the Pap smear is no exception. Despite the widespread clinical acceptance and utilization of the Pap smear, cervical cancer has not been prevented nor eradicated entirely. The Pap smear dilemma stems from a suboptimal test sensitivity, most recently estimated at 51%.[2] For the woman who develops cervical cancer despite regular screening, a 70% decrease in population mortality from cervical cancer offers little solace. The occur-

rence of cervical cancer in screened women is viewed increasingly as an avoidable failure. Consequently, the cervical cancer screening process has become one of the most litigious areas in medicine.

Cytologic examination of a sample of exfoliated cervical cells can significantly decrease the incidence and mortality of cervical cancer. However, the Pap smear has a substantial false negative rate for invasive cervical cancer and precursor lesions. Only when Pap smears are considered normal for three consecutive samples can a woman be reassured with approximately 95% confidence that her cervix was free of cancer at the time of her last Pap smear.[3] Yet, when a woman presents for a screening procedure, her expectation is that invasive cancer or a significant precancer will likely be detected at that screening visit, rather than by serial screening. If the medical community were blatantly honest in reporting a recent normal Pap smear result to women by written correspondence, the letter would actually convey "your recent results show that you have a 50% to 80% chance of having a normal Pap smear." However, this realistic statement would likely generate unnecessary anxiety for the majority of women with truly normal Pap smear results, let alone countless telephone calls to your medical practice.

Women still perceive the Pap smear as an almost infallible screening test despite media attention suggesting otherwise.[4] The medical community's reliance on the Pap smear reinforces this former notion. The modern challenge in screening for cervical neoplasia is to improve the sensitivity of cervical screening to fulfill women's expectations of preventing the only truly preventable gynecologic cancer.

17.2 Pap Smear Adjunct Tests

Much attention has been focused on optical adjunctive tests to be used in conjunction with Pap smears for cervical screening. Several adjunctive tests maximize the sensitivity of ectocervical screening while depending on cytologic examinations to provide suitable endocervical canal disease detection. Some optical adjunct tests are being developed to assess both the endocervix and ectocervix. If truly complementary, an adjunct test enhances the sensitivity of cervical cytologic testing. Adjunct tests provide unique visual, biomolecular, or electromagnetic evidence of cervical neoplasia rather than microscopic appraisal of cytologic specimens. Many of these tests are intended to be used in conjunction with the Pap smear, rather than independently. Adjunctive human papillomavirus (HPV) DNA tests designed to detect high risk HPV are discussed in Chapter 18.

17.2.1 Colposcopy: a less-than-ideal screening test

Colposcopic examination has been used primarily as a diagnostic test following detection of an abnormal cytologic result. In some countries, colposcopy is also used for screening purposes because of limited resources to do cervical cytologic testing. However, the financial and time constraints, increased patient discomfort, widespread unavailability of colposcopes and the expertise required to do screening colposcopy make this impractical in most settings. Screening by means of colposcopy is problematic for older women or women who have had prior cervical surgery because the active transformation zone, which is the area at greatest risk for harboring neoplasia, is likely to be hidden from view within the endocervical canal. Colposcopic testing is better reserved for the additional investigation of abnormalities detected by more cost-effective and relatively noninvasive cervical screening methods. Furthermore, colposcopy is an effective technique to evaluate the ectocervix but not necessarily the endocervical canal for which the Pap smear is better suited. Yet, the combination of cervical cytologic and colposcopic evaluation is more effective in detecting cervical neoplasia than either test alone.[5,6]

17.2.2 Naked-eye cervical inspection after acetic acid wash
17.2.2.1 Concept of acetic acid wash

The most rudimentary Pap smear adjunct depends on a nonmagnified, contrast solution-enhanced inspection of the ectocervix immediately following collection of a conventional Pap smear. In resource-poor settings, the inspection may be done without an accompanying Pap smear.[7–10] Known by various terms (acetic acid wash, direct visual inspection, naked-eye examination, "slosh and see"), naked-eye inspection of the cervix following an acetic acid wash can be performed by clinicians who have no colposcopic training or expertise. No expensive medical equipment is required—only relatively inexpensive 5% acetic acid and cotton swabs. The 5% acetic acid solution creates a transient visual contrast of white, nuclear-dense epithelium from completely normal pink or red epithelium. However, reliance on only the nonspecific staining color of nuclear dense epithelium in a nonselected population contributes to the inherent weakness of this test.

17.2.2.2 Acetic acid wash procedure

After identifying the cervix using a vaginal speculum, the clinician applies 5% (or other more dilute concentrations) acetic acid to the fully visualized ectocervix for approximately 60 seconds. A standard examination room incandescent light source (i.e., 100-watt lamp) facilitates illumination of the cervix. No instrument is used to magnify the tissue. Clinicians inspect the cervix for changes in color of the epithelium. A positive test is indicated by the visual detection of a transient acetowhite area (Figure 17.1). Absence of an acetowhite lesion denotes a negative test result. The naked-eye examination lacks an adequacy parameter assessment, equivalent to identification of the entire squamocolumnar junction (SCJ) with colposcopy. Blood vessels, the shape, size, and margin of the lesion, and contour are not considered. Similarly, the opacity of the acetowhite change is not appraised.

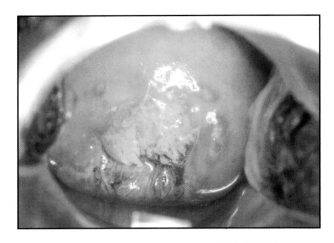

FIGURE 17.1 A positive naked-eye acetic acid wash test result indicated by an acetowhite lesion on the ectocervix.

17.2.2.3 Attributes of acetic acid wash examinations

Certain attributes of this crude test may be of benefit to financially deprived cervical cancer surveillance programs. For example, the performance of naked-eye inspection was compared with a simultaneously collected Pap smear in a large study in South Africa. The sensitivity and specificity of naked-eye examination were 75% and 81%, and the Pap smear were 82% and 93%, respectively.[10] In another report by the same authors, the respective test results were 67% and 85% for the naked-eye examination, and 78% and 97% for the Pap smear (using a low-grade squamous intraepithelial [LSIL] positive threshold) to detect CIN 2 and 3.[7] Although the Pap smear performed better, even in this rural setting, naked-eye inspection was able to identify two thirds of the women with high-grade cervical lesions.

Slawson and colleagues[11] reported that the acetic acid wash test improved the detection of cervical neoplasia by 30% when used in conjunction with the Pap smear. The positive predictive value for the acetic acid wash test alone was 55%. In a similar study, Van Le[12] reported that gross cervical visualization following acetic acid application detected 15% more cases of CIN than Pap smear testing. It would appear that acetic acid wash used in tandem with cervical cytologic testing is a more sensitive screen for detecting CIN in women. In the former study, the overall increased sensitivity was likely inflated above that expected for the general population since women older than 45 years of age, pregnant women, and women who had received prior ablative or excisional

cervical therapy were excluded. Many of these women will have lesions, if present, positioned along the SCJ and hidden within the endocervical canal. Therefore, a naked-eye ectocervical inspection may not be suitable for women who have the equivalent of an unsatisfactory colposcopy examination. Unfortunately, a determination of examination adequacy is not part of acetic acid inspection. Only an adequate inspection of the entire transformation zone, particularly the immature component, will allow maximum test sensitivity. Therefore, in this respect, women younger than 40 years are likely the best candidates for naked-eye inspection.

Frisch et al[13] also observed that naked-eye inspection increased the detection of CIN nearly threefold when compared with the Pap smear. Of greater importance was the fact that the combination of a negative Pap smear and negative naked-eye inspection had a 91% negative predictive value for detection of CIN, versus 67% for cytology alone. Surprisingly, the negative predictive value of only the naked eye inspection was 88%. This figure might have been greater had the study population reflected the general screening population and not an enriched sample of young women with cervical abnormalities.

17.2.2.4 Weaknesses of acetic acid wash examinations

The nonspecific nature of the naked-eye exam contributes to the major weakness of the noncritical test. The most disconcerting fact noted by Slawson et al[11] was that 45% of women with a positive acetic acid wash had no cervical abnormality detected by subsequent colposcopic examination. Similarly, 40% of women with a positive acetic acid screen had a normal colposcopic examination in the study by Van Le.[12] Furthermore, 80% of women with a positive naked-eye examination in the South Africa study had no cervical neoplasia.[7] In most settings, this yields an unacceptable rate of referral (approximately 15%) for colposcopy. In the same study, 21% of women with a normal naked-eye examination had cervical neoplasia. Ten percent of these women were found to have high-grade lesions.

An excessively high false-positive screening test rate means that many women would be inappropriately referred for colposcopic examination. The majority of these false-positive acetic acid wash cases probably result from observed acetowhite areas of normal immature metaplasia and congenital transformation zones, incorrectly interpreted as abnormal (Figure 17.2). These abnormal mimics would be detected more commonly in young women with

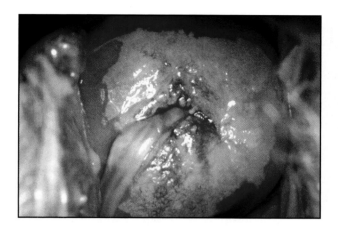

FIGURE 17.2 A false-positive naked-eye acetic acid wash examination. In this case, an acetowhite lesion is noted, but this area represents normal immature metaplasia, not neoplasia.

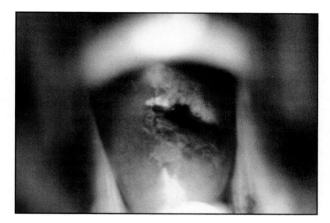

FIGURE 17.3 A positive speculoscopic test demonstrated by an acetowhite lesion seen on the cervix.

evolving transformation zones. Ideally, from the perspective of minimizing false-positive test results and excessive referral for colposcopy, women with fully mature transformation zones would be the more favorably screened population. However, selective screening of a more mature group of women will miss endocervical lesions previously discussed. If the acetic acid wash test were applied exclusively to an older population, one could expect an appealing lower false-positive rate accompanied by a greater false-negative rate. Although naked-eye inspection following acetic acid wash includes a visualization element similar in some aspects to a colposcopic examination, further critical assessment of acetowhite areas is not possible without sufficient magnification and proper education. For these reasons, naked-eye examination is not suitable for use outside developing countries or research trials.

17.2.3 Magnified chemiluminescent screening

17.2.3.1 Concept of magnified chemiluminescent screening

Magnified chemiluminescent screening represents a technologic modification of the naked-eye acetic acid wash test. The commercially available adjunct test, PapSure® (Watson Diagnostics, Corona, CA), provides a unique light source and low-power magnification to improve screening performance. Use of chemiluminescent illumination has been shown to be superior to incandescent light for detecting cervical neoplasia.[14] The blue-white light, produced by a nontoxic peroxyoxalate chemical reaction, is thought

to be seen reflected better from nuclear dense tissue as an intense fluorescent-like acetowhite color. Normal squamous epithelium absorbs the blue-white light and a bluish hue is seen. This intense blue-white contrast is touted to be more easily recognized by the observer than a white-red contrast provided by incandescent light. Detail is provided by 5× magnifying loupes worn by the examiner.

17.2.3.2 Speculoscopy equipment and technique

The speculoscopy equipment consists of a chemiluminescent light capsule and 5× magnifying loupes. Speculoscopic examination can be performed following brief training. After collecting the Pap smear and other necessary microbiologic tests, the cervix is moistened carefully with 5% acetic acid. Next, the small proprietary light source capsule is flexed to initiate the necessary chemiluminescent reaction and then attached to the inner surface of the upper vaginal speculum blade. Once the room lights are dimmed, the cervix is observed through the 5× magnifying loupes. Findings are described as either positive or negative. A positive test is indicated by the presence of chemiluminescent acetowhite areas (Figure 17.3). The absence of chemiluminescent acetowhite areas denotes a negative test.

17.2.3.3 Critical assessment of speculoscopy

Speculoscopy has been evaluated by a limited number of studies. One large multicenter clinical trial, conducted at primarily academic units and by clinicians with colposcopy experience, appears to have contributed the majority of manuscripts to the literature. The first report demonstrated that speculoscopic examination combined with Pap smear results detected 83% of women with cervical neoplasia compared with 31% detected by Pap smear alone.[15] Even though the sensitivity of the Pap smear is not ideal, one must question its exceedingly high false-negative rate reported in this trial. Furthermore, provided both tests were interpreted as negative, merely 1% of women with CIN were incorrectly diagnosed. Combination of the speculoscopic finding with the Pap smear result reduced the positive predictive value from 90% to 47%. The overall reduction can be attributed directly to a high false-positive rate tendency associated with speculoscopy. Moreover, most women with positive cytologic and negative speculoscopic findings actually had positive histologic results. Speculoscopic evaluation enhanced Pap smear sensitivity in detection of ectocervical neoplasia but cannot be used independently because the nonvisualized endocervical canal cannot be assessed properly.

In another study, colposcopic evaluation was found to be more sensitive than speculoscopic evaluation in detecting cervical neoplasia (97% vs 82%, $P<.001$).[16] The greater magnification provided by colposcopic examination permits critical analysis essential to derive accurate diagnoses. Since all speculoscopy evaluators in this trial were also trained colposcopists, the sensitivity dichotomy between the two tests appears to be strictly an inherent, functional limitation of speculoscopy and not attributable to the skill of clinicians. The function of speculoscopic examination is to identify abnormal and confirm normal, not to grade cervical lesions to derive a clinical impression. Manipulation of the cervix to view the SCJ and endocervical canal would be expected during a careful colposcopic examination prompted by abnormal cytologic findings. Such diligent probing to fully visualize the entire transformation zone will greatly enhance the detection of cervical neoplasia. The speculoscopic screening test, in contrast, consists of a brief cursory examination of the ectocervix, without extensive or instrument-assisted cervical manipulation. Thus speculoscopy cannot be substituted for colposcopy in the evaluation of abnormal cytology.

In an attempt to address the criticism that PapSure® would normally be performed by noncolposcopists in a typical outpatient clinic, nurse practitioners and nurse midwives assessed 689 women by Pap smear, followed by PapSure®.[17] Low-grade CIN was detected by means of Pap smear in 26% of cases and by speculoscopic examination in 84% of women. Clearly, significant colposcopic expertise is not required to perform PapSure® well, which makes the test amenable for screening the general population. These authors also considered the cost effectiveness of speculoscopic evaluation for cervical cancer screening.

Using a positive-test threshold to detect all cases of neoplasia, speculoscopic evaluation was found to be twice as cost effective per case of disease detection than was the Pap smear. However, when the case detection threshold was raised to include only women with CIN 3 or cancer, the reverse was true: the Pap smear was twice as cost effective per case detected compared with the addition of speculoscopic evaluation. It should be remembered that high case-detection thresholds also risk the failure to detect all cases of cancer. Moreover, speculoscopic evaluation has not been adequately assessed as a method of detecting cervical cancer.

The use of speculoscopic evaluation for intermediate triage of women with atypical squamous cells of undetermined significance (ASCUS) was evaluated by Massad et al.[18] In determining ideal schemes for referring for colposcopic examination, triage by means of speculoscopy was found to be more cost effective than triage by serial Pap smears (persistent ASCUS or more severe), when all women with ASCUS were referred for immediate colposcopic evaluation. Furthermore, the speculoscopy intermediate triage scheme was more efficacious than serial Pap smears in detecting women with cervical neoplasia.

Because speculoscopic evaluation is an adjunct screening and intermediate triage test, it does not replace colposcopic evaluation, nor can it be used independently for screening purposes. Larger, independent, prospective clinical trials are needed to determine whether speculoscopic examination can be recommended universally as an adjunct to Pap smear.

17.2.4 Cervicography

Cervicography™ is a static, photographic examination of the ectocervix.[19] Cervicography does not supplant either the Pap smear or colposcopic evaluation but is an adjunct test to be used in conjunction with the Pap smear for screening purposes, like speculoscopy and naked-eye examination. The two tests are complementary. The endocervical canal cannot be evaluated by means of cervicography, which is an ectocervical test. Hence, a Pap smear must always be used in conjunction with cervicographic evaluation. Cervicographic evaluation also provides reasonably good sensitivity for detecting cervical neoplasia, particularly when used as required with the Pap smear, which is conversely a test with high specificity.

Cervicography™ combines aspects of colposcopic evaluation with interpretation by experienced colposcopists and special quality assurance. The training program and examination process for cervicography evaluators, the evaluation form and technique, and the camera equipment and film processing are all standardized.

17.2.4.1 Cervicography equipment

Cervicography™ equipment and supplies (National Testing Laboratories Worldwide, Fenton, Mo.) include a Cerviscope™ and power unit, 5% acetic acid, a vaginal speculum, large cotton swabs or cotton balls, and ring forceps. The Cerviscope™ is a proprietary 35-mm camera with a fixed focal-length telephoto macrolens, illumination source, and strobe flash mounted on a hand-held platform (Figure 17.4). The camera design permits a panoramic view and photograph of the cervix and proximal vagina. A shutter-release button is located on the handle to permit index finger activation. The fast film (ASA 200) and maximal depth of field minimize the likelihood of blurred Cervigrams™ (2″ by 2″ slides and 3 ″ × 5″ color photographs). On-site cervicography training, technical manuals, and an educational videotape are provided with equipment purchase.

17.2.4.2 Cervicography technique

Cervicographic evaluation may be performed by either physicians or paraprofessionals. Prior colposcopic experience and techniques are not required. There are no absolute contraindications for cervicographic evaluation. Yet, because the procedure is limited in its ability to detect endocervical lesions, the benefit may be limited for older women, some women following cervical therapy, or for other women whose complete transformation zone cannot be visualized. Cervicographic evaluation may be compromised by menstruation. Relevant patient demographic information, pertinent history, and a serially unique cervigram identification number are entered on a patient log sheet. Appropriate cytologic and microbiologic sampling of the cervix and vagina must precede the procedure because the acetic acid used may distort cellular morphology and reduce cellular retrieval.

Certain precautions must be taken to ensure an adequate cervigram. The vaginal speculum should be positioned to visualize the entire cervix. Next, 5% acetic acid on a cotton ball or swab should be applied gently to the cervix for at least 30 seconds and the cervix then completely observed through the cerviscope (Figure 17.5). Any visual obstructions caused by mucus, blood, vaginal wall prolapse, pubic hair, or acetic acid pooling should be cleared. A second generous application of acetic acid is then completed prior to taking the cervigrams. Finally, once the cervix is clearly focused through the cerviscope, two cervigrams, or photographs, are taken within 30 seconds of the second application of acetic acid.

17.2.4.3 Cervigram processing and evaluation

When images from 10 patients have been taken, the roll of film is mailed to the cervicography laboratory, where the cervigrams are processed as 2″ × 2″ Kodachrome slides. The slides, along with a copy of the patient log, are evaluated critically by colposcopists with training and certification in cervicographic evaluation. Each slide is loaded into a slide projector, then projected individually onto a screen for interpretation. The cervigram is assessed for location of the SCJ and transformation zone, presence of lesion(s), morphologic findings and severity of lesions visualized, and technical quality. The cervigram is then interpreted as negative, atypical, or positive, and an evaluation report for each patient (Figure 17.6) is returned to the clinician, along with a 3″ × 5 ″ color cervigram print.

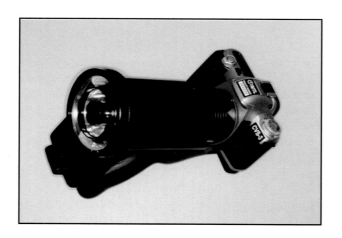

FIGURE 17.4   The cerviscope used for cervicography.

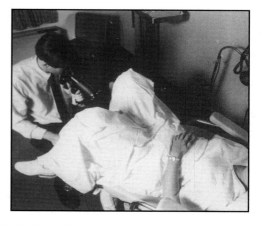

FIGURE 17.5   The cerviscope in clinical use.

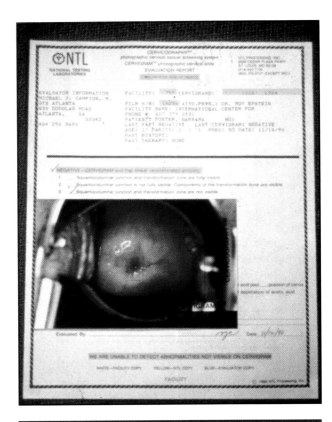

FIGURE 17.6 The Cervicography™ report form. A 3" × 5" color cervigram print would be attached to the report.

17.2.4.4 Cervigram™ interpretation and suggested management

A negative Cervigram™ (Figure 17.7) indicates that no premalignant or malignant lesions were noted on the ectocervix. Negative interpretation subcategories also describe the location of the SCJ and the transformation zone. When the SCJ and transformation zone are not visualized, a negative cervigram means no ectocervical disease was detected and any abnormal tissue is likely to be limited to the endocervical canal or vagina. The response to a negative cervigram evaluation, if the cytologic sample does not indicate a squamous intraepithelial lesion or invasive cancer, is to repeat screening at an appropriate interval.

An atypical Cervigram™ (Figure 17.8) indicates that an insignificant acetowhite lesion is visible. Such lesions commonly represent atypical immature squamous metaplasia or minor virally induced epithelial changes. Occasionally, atypical cervigrams represent low-grade or high-grade lesions. Based on the location of the lesion and its perceived severity, the cervigram interpreter would suggest that colposcopic evaluation is not currently recommended. In this

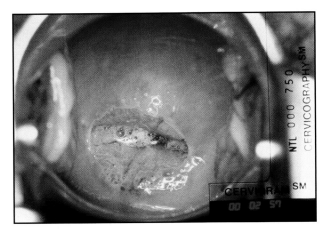

FIGURE 17.7 Negative cervigram, showing a normal cervix with an ectropion or eversion of columnar cells on the ectocervix.

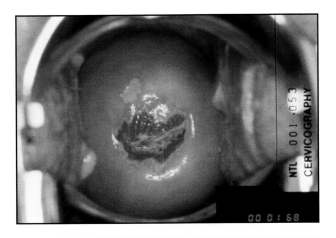

FIGURE 17.8 Atypical cervigram, showing a faint acetowhite change located at the 11-o'clock position outside the transformation zone.

situation, the typical recommendation would be to repeat the cervigram in 6 to 12 months, since approximately 25% of women with atypical cervigrams are considered to be at risk for developing a more significant lesion.[20]

A positive cervigram indicates morphologic changes consistent with premalignant or malignant lesions. Positive subcategorizations include low-grade disease (Figure 17.9), high-grade disease (Figure 17.10), and cancer (Figure 17.11). In such cases, colposcopic examination would be recommended to further evaluate the cervical lesion(s) identified by the positive cervigram.

Occasionally, despite attempts at careful preparation, the cervix may be obscured by mucus, blood,

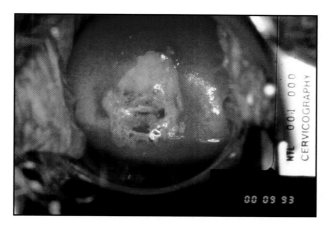

FIGURE 17.9 Positive cervigram, indicating low-grade premalignant disease. An acetowhite lesion with a fine mosaic vascular pattern is seen on the anterior cervix.

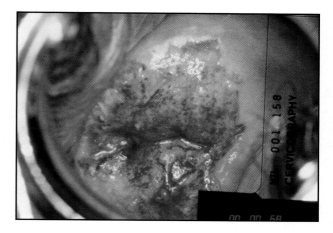

FIGURE 17.11 A positive cervigram, reported as suspicious for invasive cancer. Colposcopic examination confirmed a colposcopically overt invasive cancer of the cervix. The diagnosis was confirmed on histologic examination of a punch biopsy. The patient's Pap smear taken at the time of the cervigram was evaluated as showing a non-specific inflammatory reaction.

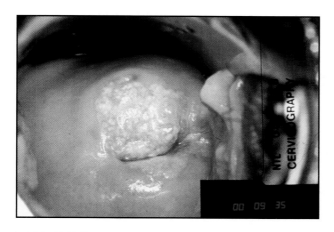

FIGURE 17.10 Positive cervigram, indicating high-grade premalignant disease. A dense acetowhite lesion with a rolled, peeling margin is located on the anterior cervical lip. The lesion extends within the endocervical canal. The histology from a conization confirmed CIN 3.

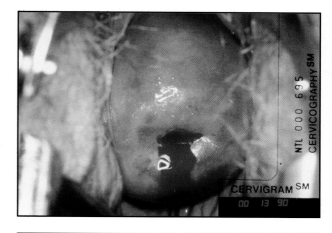

FIGURE 17.12 Technically defective cervigram, showing a cervix obscured by blood.

hair, vaginal walls, the vaginal speculum, a polyp, or acetic acid pooling. This type of cervigram, although infrequent (approximately 3% of cervigrams),[21] is reported as technically uninterpretable (Figure 17.12). If an image is taken too long after the application of acetic acid, causing the acetic acid reaction to fade, the cervigram is also reported as technically defective. Similarly, processing problems and focus difficulties may lead to technically defective reports. In these situations, a repeat cervigram would be recommended. Although the definition of an unsatisfactory Pap smear is controversial,[22,23] a technically uninterpretable cervigram is unequivocal.

17.2.4.5 Critical assessment of Cervicography™

There are two potential uses for cervicographic evaluation: an adjunct test to the Pap smear or an intermediate triage test.[24] Cervicography™ has been evaluated as an adjunct to the Pap smear in numerous studies.[25-30] Tawa et al,[25] in a study of 3271 patients screened for cervical intraepithelial neoplasia with cervical cytologic and cervicographic examination, demonstrated cervicography to be a more sensitive method of testing but less specific than the Pap smear. Evaluation by means of cervicography detected 88.9% of patients with biopsy proven CIN and the Pap smear correctly identified only 17.3% of patients. In a comparative study of 1449 women, Ferris et al[21] demonstrated that evaluation by means of Pap smear identified 25.6% of women with neoplasia and 37.5% of women with CIN 3. In contrast, evaluation by means of cervicography detected 50.5% of women with neoplasia and 77.8% of patients with CIN 3. However, when both tests were combined, 62.9% of women with neoplasia and 86.3% of patients with CIN 3 were appropriately detected. In the Guanacaste[30] study conducted by the National Cancer Institute, evaluation by means of cervicography had an overall sensitivity of 49% and specificity of 95% to detect women with CIN 2 and 3. The Pap smears collected from those same women had a sensitivity and specificity of 77% and 94%, respectively, to detect CIN 2 and 3. This large population-based study demonstrated that cervicographic evaluation actually had a poorer sensitivity than did the Pap smear. The overall performance of cervicographic evaluation was also age dependent, influenced by the ability to visualize the cervical transformation zone on the cervigram. The sensitivity of cervicographic evaluation was 55% for women less than 50 years of age and 27% for women older than 50 years. The Pap smear sensitivity was much better (76% and 85%, respectively) for those two age groups.

Cervicographic evaluation was not included as a triage test in the 2001 ASCCP Guidelines for the Management of Women with Cervical Cytological Abnormalities. HPV DNA testing and colposcopic examination are recommended for triage of women with an initial atypical squamous cell Pap smear result. Colposcopic evaluation is advocated for women with one or more Pap smears demonstrating atypia, since 15% to 25% of these women actually have more severe premalignant disease.[31] However, cervicographic evaluation may be a more sensitive intermediate triage test for identifying women with the greatest probability of having CIN who would be most likely to benefit from referral for colposcopic evaluation. August[32] demonstrated a sensitivity of 82% for cervicographic evaluation but only 26% for a repeat Pap smear when women with atypical cytologic changes were further examined for evidence of CIN. Jones et al[32] similarly evaluated 236 patients with an atypical Pap smear report by means of repeat Pap smear, cervicography™ and colposcopy. Cervical intraepithelial neoplasia was histologically detected in 58 women and a second repeat Pap smear demonstrated CIN in only 17% of these women. In contrast, 81% of the patients with CIN were identified by means of cervicography. Spitzer et al[33] evaluated 97 patients with an initial atypical Pap smear by means of repeat Pap smear, cer-

vicography and colposcopy. The repeat Pap smear correctly identified 58% of patients with colposcopically detected lesions, compared with 89% identified by means of cervicography. Ferris and colleagues[34] also evaluated the potential of intermediate triage of women with ASCUS Pap smears using cervicography. Of 166 women with histologic evidence of cervical neoplasia, 74.7% of women with CIN 1, 87.5% with CIN 2 and 75% of women with CIN 3 were detected by means of cervicography.™

Cervicography™ was also examined during the enrollment phase of the National Cancer Institute's ASCUS/LSIL triage study (ALTS).[35] Using a triage threshold of atypical or more significant changes, cervicographic evaluation had a sensitivity and specificity of 79% and 61%, respectively, for detecting CIN 3 or more severe disease. Sensitivity was greater (86%) for a repeat Pap smear collected on the same women. However, the positive and negative predictive values for cervicographic evaluation (8% and 99%, respectively) and a single repeat Pap smear (9% and 98%, respectively) were quite similar.

17.2.4.6 Cervicography limitations

No screening test is perfect. Cervicographic evaluation has been shown to be both more and less sensitive than the Pap smear. It is also less specific than the Pap smear. The higher false-positive rate for cervicography, reported to be 39% to 82%,[33,36] and a sensitivity lower than cytology in two large trials (Guanacaste and ALTS) have made it a controversial test.[37,38] Frequently, the false-positive cervigram represents atypical squamous metaplasia or subclinical HPV-induced changes in epithelium at high risk for evolving into significant disease. A false-positive cervigram increases the expense involved in evaluating potential pathologic findings. Consequently, when used on an annual basis for cervical cancer screening, evaluation by means of cervicography may not be cost effective,[33] although some studies have demonstrated cost effectiveness.[25,32] Future studies may determine an optimal cost-effective interval (non-annual) for adjunct screening by means of Cervicography™. Additional well-designed prospective trials are also necessary to determine the role and potential for this procedure in cervical neoplasia screening.[39] Presently, it has not been adopted as a standard of care, either as an adjunct or immediate triage test.

Finally, just as with unsatisfactory Pap smears, a certain number of cervigrams are reported to be technically uninterpretable.[31,40] The quality-assurance program that provides critical feedback of technically uninterpretable cervigrams to the clinicians limits the uninterpretable rate to approximately 2% to

3%.[34] If a cervigram™ is found to be defective, a repeat cervigram™ may be taken at no additional charge to the patient.

17.2.5 In vivo scanning devices for cervical neoplasia

Perhaps the most intriguing recent development in cervical neoplasia screening and management may evolve from currently experimental in-vivo scanning devices. Historically, the acquisition of cytologic and histologic specimens, in addition to findings from a colposcopic examination, has been considered an essential requirement for establishing proper management of women with cervical neoplasia. Hence, diagnosis and management of cervical neoplasia have been based entirely on macro- or microscopic findings. The traditional approach requires significant clinical skill, demands expert pathologic diagnosis, causes patient discomfort, invokes diagnostic interval anxiety, generates significant cost, and risks sampling complications or errors. Researchers have sought to create rapid, reliable noninvasive techniques for evaluating the epithelium of the lower genital tract that may circumvent these demands, insults, and disadvantages. Several companies are now in the process of developing and testing equipment that has the potential to provide accurate mechanisms to noninvasively assess for cervical neoplasia.

17.2.5.1 Optical spectroscopy equipment

For the past half century, scientists have known that nonmalignant and malignant cervical tissues react differently to electrical impulses.[41] Moreover, we are aware that the white light beam of the colposcope is absorbed and then emitted from and/or reflected off epithelia in varying color and intensity, to help guide our visual discrimination of normal epithelium from neoplasia. Various types of tissue respond differently to electromagnetic (light) energy. When a certain wavelength of light strikes epithelium, the energy may dissipate or be absorbed. If absorbed, converted wavelengths of light (energy) are subsequently emitted from the epithelium (Figures 17.13a,b). These unique wavelengths are seen as a reduced amount of a different color of light. The intensity of the emitted wavelengths differs depending upon interaction with specific types and concentrations of biological molecules (NADH, FAD, tryptophan, collagen, etc.) present. Some of these molecules fluoresce, particularly when excited by certain wavelengths of light. Light may also reflect or scatter from the surface in specific patterns that are characteristic for certain tissue types (Figures 17.14a,b). The intensity of reflected light also varies based on the inherent nature of the tissue. Hence, energy/tissue interaction determines characteristically unique emitted and reflected responses that vary in wavelength and intensity of light. Both the emitted and reflected light can be measured with special sensors. The wavelengths and intensities can be plotted on a graph as curves. Each curve represents a unique type of normal or abnormal tissue interrogated by specific wavelengths of light. As tissue of increasing abnormality is interrogated, the intensity of the fluorescence decreases and peak emission wavelengths shift to longer wavelengths. Hence, the

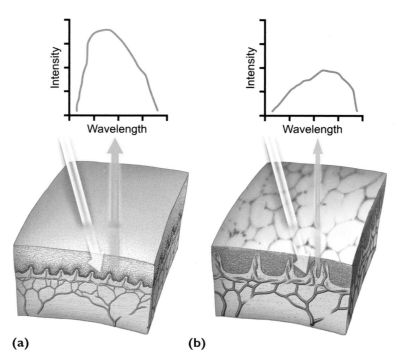

(a)   **(b)**

FIGURES 17.13a,b Light can be either absorbed and emitted, or reflected from epithelium. When tissue absorbs wavelengths of light, it is emitted from the epithelium as a reduced amount of a different color of light. The resulting light can be analyzed to estimate the type of tissue interrogated. The emitted light from normal squamous epithelium **(a)** differs from the emitted light from the CIN 3 seen in **(b)**. ▬▬▬

curve becomes flatter and the peak amplitude changes to a longer wavelength.

The standardized illumination of tissue using varied wavelengths of light (energy) is called optical spectroscopy. By capturing the electromagnetic spectra emitted by tissue, one can determine biomolecular characteristics of the epithelium examined or interrogated. These data can then provide objective information about the physical characteristics of the tissue examined. Each type of tissue responds with a unique curve or "signature," synonymous with a "tissue fingerprint." If the curves from an unknown tissue type are compared with a variety of previously documented template curves obtained from known histologic types, then a curve "match" should indicate the specific type of unknown histology. This principle of subjecting tissue to known wavelengths of energy, measuring the emitted energy, and comparing the wavelength/intensity patterns with templates to derive a histologic diagnosis forms the basis for the various in vivo cervical neoplasia detection devices. The instruments, currently under development by several companies, differ in the types of energy used, but still rely on the same principle of energy/tissue interaction. All of these instruments essentially provide an electromagnetic "biopsy" report, potentially obviating the need for a traditional biopsy-confirmed diagnosis.

17.2.5.1.1 Potential applications
Noninvasive optical biopsy tests designed to detect cervical neoplasia may have numerous potential applications.

Such a test could complement the Pap smear for general screening purposes provided a significantly better detection of neoplasia (sensitivity) was afforded while simultaneously limiting false positive (specificity) results. Ectocervical interrogation alone may suffice if optical biopsy tests were used simply as an adjunct to the Pap smear. Endocervical canal interrogation may present a significant technical challenge that could be accommodated by relying instead upon cytologic sampling of the endocervix. The techniques hold promise for immediate results and simplicity for nonskilled operator use. If screening sensitivity were improved dramatically by using an adjunct in vivo detection device, then a lengthened screening interval might be justified. Such a prolonged screening interval would help to financially offset the equipment expenditure and procedural costs. Although universal availability would be ideal, specialized cancer screening centers for women could evolve to offer one-stop testing for diagnostic procedures, such as mammograms, noninvasive cervical screening, and sigmoidoscopy.

Intermediate triage of women with minor cytologic abnormalities (i.e., ASC, LSIL) also may someday be accomplished with a reliable noninvasive test. If widely available, noncolposcopists could effectively triage women who are optical-biopsy positive to colposcopy while sparing women with little probability of harboring a significant neoplasia (i.e., HSIL or more severe) from having an extensive colposcopic examination. If noninvasive equipment and

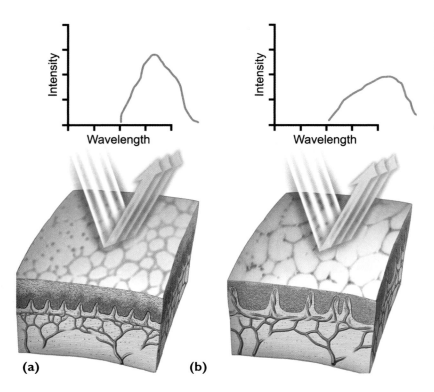

(a)   (b)

FIGURES 17.14a,b Light can also reflect off the surface of epithelium without being absorbed and then emitted (Figure 17.13). This response can help predict the type of tissue examined. Less light is reflected from CIN 1 **(a)** than CIN 3 **(b)**.

procedures were priced reasonably, then this triage test approach may be cost effective. Studies will be needed to compare and contrast intermediate triage tests (e.g., HPV DNA tests, biomarkers), including in vivo optical scanning devices.

Colposcopic assessment is a challenge for many colposcopists. Identifying the most severe area of abnormality also presents difficulty, particularly when large, seemingly homogenous lesions or four-quadrant complex lesions, are being assessed. A non-invasive tool could potentially be used by novice col-poscopists or noncolposcopists to assess the cervix and accurately pinpoint the area of greatest concern. In this scenario, multiple biopsies may be unneces-sary, resulting in less patient discomfort, lower cost, and less pathologic review. More importantly, replica-tive or nonessential biopsies may be eliminated. This may be particularly pertinent for the pregnant patient or difficult colposcopic evaluation of minor changes that could easily represent normal atypical metaplasia or perhaps CIN 1. If every colposcopist always provided a reliable evaluation, the application of noninvasive detection equipment to isolate biopsy sites would appear limited. However, if the noninva-sive test were combined with an automated stereotac-tic biopsy instrument that noncolposcopists could operate easily, the number of traditional colposcopy examinations may be reduced. Such an automated assessment/sampling device could possibly supplant colposcopy in the future.

How well does this new technology compare with colposcopy? A prototype of a fluorescent spectroscope developed at the University of Texas was able to differ-entiate histologically normal epithelium from abnor-mal epithelium with a sensitivity of 92%, specificity 90% and positive predictive value of 88%.[42] A more critical discrimination of nonneoplastic abnormal epithelium from neoplastic epithelium provided a 87% sensitivity, 73% specificity, and 74% positive predictive value. When compared with colposcopy, the prototype was 10% less sensitive but 20% more specific.[43]

Finally, noninvasive detection equipment could potentially replace cervical cytologic screening. Sev-eral obligatory provisions would be required before discarding a trusted, entrenched cytologic surveil-lance system. The noninvasive test would have to per-form better than the Pap smear, as documented by large prospective clinical trials. Second, the new tech-nology must be able to adequately assess the endo-cervical canal, not just the ectocervix. A method of determining scan adequacy would need to be devel-oped since this innovative technique could suffer from nonrepresentative assessment just as cervical cytologic testing suffers from unsatisfactory sam-pling. And lastly, the noninvasive system would need to be universally available, more cost effective than

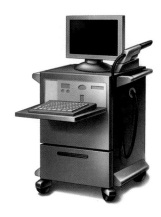

FIGURE 17.15 Basic components of a noninvasive opti-cal biopsy detection system for cervical neoplasia.

the Pap smear, rapidly performed, safe, and simplis-tic enough for all healthcare providers to use. Because the noninvasive test may not require highly skilled clinicians and laboratorians, tedious process-ing, and professional interpretation ability, the in vivo test could have greatest utility in countries lack-ing these skilled resources. Whether a novel high-tech detection system could displace exfoliative cyto-logic sampling is currently highly speculative and seemingly improbable. However, the robust test devised by Drs. Papanicolaou and Traut more than 50 years ago also was met initially with much skepti-cism. Whether the Pap smear will persevere as the screening test of the next millennium remains unknown, but in the near future it will persist as the gold standard. Of the potential applications dis-cussed thus far, this use of a high-tech detection sys-tem seems least likely to become standard of care.

17.2.5.1.2 Components and operation
All non-invasive detection systems for cervical neoplasia share basic design features (Figure 17.15): a light, laser or electrical source to generate unique energy wavelengths, a probe to transmit the light/electrical impulses, sensors to detect the modified waveforms emitted or reflected from the tissue, and a computer-based analyzer to interpret the signals and provide a report to the clinician. Although subject to change, at least five in vivo detection systems are currently under development. Several systems differ suffi-ciently to warrant a brief overview of their unique components and operation.

17.2.5.1.3 TruScreen®
The TruScreen®, formerly known as Polarprobe, unit (Polartechnics Ltd., Sydney, Australia) (Figure 17.16) can be distinguished from the other noninvasive detection devices by its use of

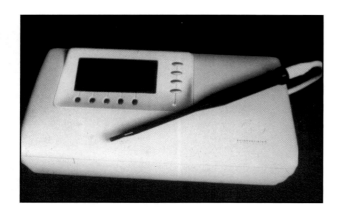

FIGURE 17.16   The TruScreen® (Polartechnics Ltd, Sydney, Australia) optoelectronic instrument used to detect cervical neoplasia. It consists of the probe, flexible cable, and console.

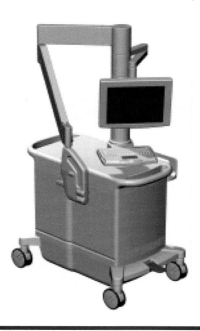

FIGURE 17.17   The Colpoprobe (MediSpectra, Cambridge, Massachusetts), designed to noninvasively detect cervical neoplasia. This device does not require tissue contact.

both light and electrical (optoelectronic) impulses to discriminate epithelial types.[44] The scanning probe is pencil sized and attached to the console by a cable. The distal tip of the probe, 5 mm in diameter, contains light emission and detection fibers and electrodes. The probe generates in rapid succession red, green, and infrared wavelengths and a low voltage pulse. Tissue responses are processed in the console computer and compared algorithmically with known waveform templates. Diagnostic categories are reported on a small LCD screen and include: (1) cancer and HSIL, (2) LSIL, and (3) normal. A disposable probe sheath to accommodate sterile technique and narrow side-view probe to permit endocervical canal assessment are essential components of the completed package currently under development.

Following unit calibration and sterilization, the probe is placed on the anterior cervix and small circular movements initiated while maintaining gentle probe tip/epithelial contact. The entire surface of the cervix is slowly scanned, taking an average of several minutes. While probing, the LCD screen displays a diagnosis for the tissue being interrogated. An "error" diagnosis occurs when the probe fails to achieve sufficient epithelial contact. A nondiagnostic reading, indicating failure to match emitted waveforms with known template curves, results if the probe bridges two distinctly different tissue types. A positive scan response can be confirmed by temporarily lifting the probe tip off the area of concern, and then reapplying the tip to the identical location, noting another positive result.

Preliminary results from initial testing of the TruScreen® appear encouraging.[44] Test sensitivities for LSIL, HSIL, and cancer were 85%, 90%, and 99%, respectively. False-positive rates were 3% for columnar epithelium and 14% for metaplasia. Larger prospective clinical trials are in progress to clarify and validate the attributes of TruScreen®.

17.2.5.1.4 Colpoprobe   The prototype Colpoprobe (MediSpectra, Cambridge, Massachusetts) was designed to measure tissue autofluorescence and spectral backscatter using equipment that does not require tissue contact. The instrument design permits indirect qualitative identification of neoplasia using quantitative measurements. The Colpoprobe (Figure 17.17) examines cervical epithelium by measuring and analyzing tissue autofluorescence and spectral backscatter following exposure to 337-nm UV and broadband 5,300 K light. The initial prototype equipment components consist of an optical head attached to a colposcope head, optical fibers, light sources, a fluorescence measurement device, computer, and software for analysis.

The prototype Colpoprobe operates in an aiming mode following calibration against a fluorescent target. A joystick controls a visible marking beam to select "sampling" foci on the epithelial surface. Once the beam is centered directly over the intended site of interest, the measurement mode is selected. Two different wavelengths of light, generated by light sources in the equipment, are used to excite tissue fluorescence. Emitted light is then measured and analyzed by the computer. Clinically relevant data are subsequently displayed for the clinician.

Results from a small clinical trial of 36 patients demonstrated test sensitivity, specificity, positive, and negative predictive values of 96%, 71%, 71% and 93%, respectively, when discriminating normal from abnormal epithelium.[45] Another study examined use of the Colpoprobe as a potential adjunct to colposcopy.[46] The sensitivity and specificity for the presence of CIN were 93% and 94%, respectively, and the positive and negative predictive values were 90% and 96%, respectively.

A second prototype using UV-excitation fluorescence spectroscopy and diffuse-reflectance spectroscopy was used to examine the cervix of 41 women referred for colposcopy.[47] Fluorescence spectroscopy alone had difficulty discriminating metaplasia from CIN. However, reflectance spectroscopy was better able to discriminate these two tissue types. Hence, the two types of spectroscopy were thought to be complementary.

17.2.5.1.5 Hyperspectral diagnostic imaging (HSDI)

The hyperspectral diagnostic imaging device (U.S. Army) is another noncontact instrument designed to detect cervical neoplasia by using tissue fluorescence. HSDI creates an image of the cervix to permit detection and localization of CIN. The aceticacid soaked surface of the cervix is interrogated by a 1.2 mm-wide beam of 365 mm UV light. The fluorescence is measured by a spectrometer. A small study of 35 women who had a colposcopically directed biopsy demonstrated that HSDI discriminated 80% of high-grade lesions from normal tissue.[48] However, HSDI was unable to distinguish low-grade lesions from normal metaplasia.

17.2.5.1.6 Multimodal hyperspectral imaging (MHI)

Multimodal hyperspectral imaging (MHI) is a device (Spect Rx, Norcross, Georgia) based on both tissue fluorescence and reflected light measurements (Figure 17.18). The prototype MHI system consisted of a light source and computer-controlled monochromator device for projecting certain wavelengths of light onto the cervix through a fiber optic probe. The multichannel spectrograph had a hyperspectral resolution of 5 mm and a spatial resolution of 1 mm. A change coupled device (CCD) camera, filter wheel and the spectrograph collected the emitted and reflected light.

At the completion of one study, receiver operating characteristic (ROC) curves were generated to determine MHI performance relative to a simultaneously collected Pap smear. At an equal specificity for each test, the Pap smear and MHI sensitivities were 72% and 97%, respectively.[49] When a disease threshold of $\geq$ CIN 2 was established, the area under the ROC curve was 78% for the Pap smear and 95% for MHI. These preliminary data demonstrated that MHI outperformed the conventional Pap smear.

A recent evaluation of fluorescence spectroscopy and other techniques for detecting cervical neoplasia

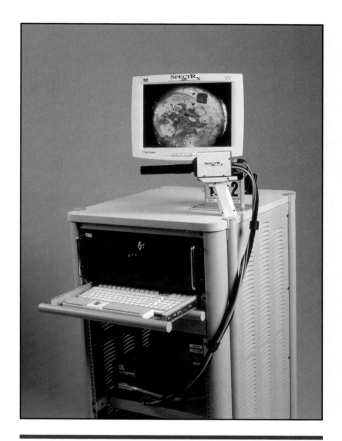

FIGURE 17.18 Multimodal Hyperspectral Imaging (MHI) (Spect Rx, Norcross, Georgia) prototype device designed to detect cervical neoplasia noninvasively. ▬

(Cervicography™, Pap smear, HPV testing, speculoscopy, and colposcopy) demonstrated that fluorescence spectroscopy performed better than colposcopy and the other diagnostic modalities based on calculations of ROC curves for each technique.[50] The cost effectiveness of fluorescence spectroscopy when used alone or in combination with colposcopy, including see-and-treat variations, has been examined.[51] See-and-treat spectroscopy was the least expensive but also least effective approach to detecting cervical neoplasia. The most expensive strategy was colposcopy. However, a combined spectroscopy/colposcopy see-and-treat approach was slightly more effective and less expensive than colposcopy alone. This adjunct scheme avoids histopathologic and patient recall costs. A great deal more research will be needed to confirm whether this type of management can actually be superior to our present system.

17.2.5.2 Computer-based colposcopy

Modern computers can now interface with various video devices to capture, digitize, and store static or dynamic images. Optical colposcopes with an attached CCD camera or video colposcopes can transfer images to computers equipped with video frame grabber cards. Once these colposcopic images are acquired and digitized, they can be manipulated and analyzed critically. This process encompasses the various functions of what is called computer-based colposcopy.

Computer-based colposcopy has been used for many purposes. The main application is that of an enhanced medical record for colposcopy (See Chapter 6). Many colposcope manufacturers market computer-based colposcopy systems designed to capture and store demographic information, colposcopically related results and colposcopic images. These systems operate as essentially independent electronic medical records. Colposcopists can modify, measure, and annotate the colposcopic images using accompanying software. Separate patient tracking or recall software programs can also be installed to interface with the colposcopic software.

Some of the computer-based colposcopy systems have integrated software to accommodate telemedicine, through which colposcopic images can be transmitted from a distant non-expert colposcopist to an off-site expert colposcopist for consultative purposes.[52] Some computer-based systems use static or "store and forward" technology. In this case, digitized colposcopic images can be transferred to another compatible computer. Other systems provide synchronous interaction between colposcopists through audio and video image annotation. At the present time, no computer-based systems provide either high-resolution video streaming in short segments or video images as a continuous function (real time). The latter type of telecolposcopy can be provided through established telemedicine networks that use dedicated fiberoptic broadband connections.

One study has compared telemedicine network telecolposcopy and computer-based telecolposcopy with on-site colposcopy.[52] On-site colposcopy provided a greater rate of satisfactory colposcopic examinations (74.9%) compared with telemedicine network (66.1%) and computer-based (43.6%) telecolposcopy. As a consequence, endocervical curettage was considered necessary less frequently by on-site colposcopists compared with the two types of telecolposcopy, but there were no significant differences noted for biopsy necessity among the three methods. Most importantly, the sensitivity and specificity for on-site, telemedicine network, and computer-based colposcopy at the ≥ CIN 2 or 3 threshold were not significantly different (47.7% and 58.5%, 43.2% and 55.3%, and 34.1% and 59.4%, respectively). These data indicate that telecolposcopy may be a reasonable alternative to on-site colposcopy for women in medically underserved areas.

A third application for computer-based colposcopy emanates from mathematical software designed to precisely calculate dimensions of digitized objects. Serially monitoring the presence and size of cervical lesions may be beneficial when following women with CIN 1 or observing cervical lesions in pregnant women. Computers enable precise measurement of lesion size when previously calibrated to colposcopic magnification settings. In a 12-month study using computer-based colposcopy that followed 68 women with biopsy-confirmed CIN 1, 6% of the lesions increased in size, 32% decreased in size, 13% remained unchanged, 21% resolved, and 28% changed to a completely different location.[53] Studies of the natural history of CIN based on precise measurement of size and location are limited, particularly as correlated with virologic and cytologic data. This attribute of computer-based colposcopy may also be of utility documenting therapeutic response of lower genital tract neoplasia in clinical trials.

Computer-based colposcopy may eventually be able to provide meaningful diagnostic assistance.[54–56] Automated evaluation of Pap smears using computer-based neural networks is now a reality. These systems analyze certain morphologic features on a microscopic level to render reliable diagnoses. These same principles could be applied to colposcopy. One such European computerized colposcopy system had greater concordance rates with histologic findings (85%, k=0.77) than did colposcopists' impressions (66%, k=0.40). Such a system could potentially improve the diagnostic accuracy of colposcopy.

Another experimental computer-based diagnostic system (GTV, Georgia Tech, Atlanta, Georgia) attempts to replicate, or exceed, human vision and cortical function by incorporating a multimodular approach (front-end, attentive processing, preattentive processing, selective attention, and performance). These modules consist of a series of unique

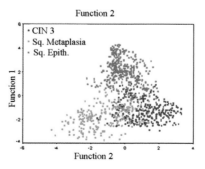

FIGURE 17.19 Computer-based colposcopy may assist the evaluation of cervical neoplasia in the future. The figure depicts a computer's discrimination of CIN 3 from normal squamous epithelium and immature metaplasia using artificial vision (Georgia Tech, Atlanta, Georgia).

algorithms that are designed to simulate various visual functions. An image of the cervix is introduced to the system and the computer-based algorithms assess the image in much the same fashion as humans do. A computer-based diagnosis is then generated. This system has been able to readily discriminate CIN 3 from normal squamous epithelium and immature metaplasia (Figure 17.19).[56]

It is conceivable that computers may someday augment or actually replace our current practice of colposcopy. Further advancement in computer technology is expected. Additional ways that computers can improve the management of women with lower genital tract disease will be discovered. These prospects hold great promise for both clinicians and women affected with cervical neoplasia.

References

1. Devesa S S, Young J L Jr, Brinton L A, Fraumeni J F Jr. Recent trends in cervix uteri cancer. *Cancer* 1989;64:2184–90.
2. Agency for Health Care Policy and Research. *Evidence report/technology assessment No 5: evaluation of cervical cytology.* Rockville, MD: Agency for Health Care Policy and Research; 1999. U.S. Department of Health and Human Services. AHCPR publication No. 99–E010.
3. Giles J A, Hudson E, Crow J, Williams D, Walker P. Colposcopic assessment of the accuracy of cervical cytology screening. *BMJ* 1988;296:1099–102.
4. *Wall Street Journal,* November 2,1987:1.
5. Navratil E, Burghardt E, Bajardi F, Nash W. Simultaneous colposcopy and cytology used in screening for carcinoma of the cervix. *Am J Obstet Gynecol* 1958;75:1292–7.
6. Limburg H. Comparison between cytology and colposcopy in the diagnosis of early cervical carcinoma. *Am J Obstet Gynecol* 1958;75:1298–1301.
7. Denny L, Kuhn L, Pollack A, Wainwright H, Wright T C Jr. Evaluation of alternative methods of cervical cancer screening for resource-poor settings. *Cancer* 2000;89:826–33.
8. Visual inspection with acetic acid for cervical cancer screening: test qualities in a primary care setting. University of Zimbabwe/JHPIEGO cervical cancer project. *Lancet* 1999;353:869–73.
9. Megavand E, Denny L, Dehaeck K, Soeters R, Bloch B. Acetic acid visualization of the cervix: an alternative to cytologic screening. *Obstet Gynecol* 1996;88:383–6.
10. Denny L, Kuhn L, Risi L, et al. Two-stage cervical cancer screening: an alternative for resource-poor settings. *Am J Obstet Gynecol* 2000;183:383–8.
11. Slawson D C, Bennett J H, Herman J M. Are Papanicolaou smears enough? Acetic acid washes of the cervix as adjunctive therapy: a Harnet study. *J Fam Pract* 1992;35(3):271–7.
12. Van Le L, Broekhuizen F F, Janzer-Steele R, Behar M, Samter T. Acetic acid visualization of the cervix to detect cervical dysplasia. *Obstet Gynecol* 1993;81:293–5.
13. Frisch L E, Milner F H, Ferris D G. Naked-eye inspection of the cervix after acetic acid application may improve the predictive value of negative cytologic screening. *J Fam Pract* 1994;39:457–60.

14. Lonky N M, Edwards G. Comparison of chemiluminescent light versus incandescent light in the visualization of acetowhite epithelium. *Am J Gynecol Health* 1992;6:11–5.
15. Mann W, Lonky N, Massad S, Scotti R, Blanco J. Vasilev S. Papanicolaou smear screening augmented by a magnified chemiluminescent exam. *Int J Gynecol Obstet* 1993;43:289–96.
16. Lonky N M, Mann W J, Massad L S, et al. Ability of visual tests to predict underlying cervical neoplasia: colposcopy and speculoscopy. *J Reprod Med* 1995;40:530–6.
17. Edwards G, Rutkowski C, Palmer C. Cervical cancer screening with Papanicolaou smear plus speculoscopy by nurse practitioners in a health maintenance organization. *J Lower Genital Tract Dis* 1997;1:141–7.
18. Massad L S, Lonky N M, Mutch D G, et al. Use of speculoscopy in the evaluation of women with atypical Papanicolaou smears: improved cost effectiveness by selective colposcopy. *J Reprod Med* 1993;38:163–9.
19. Stafl A. Cervicography: a new method for cervical cancer detection. *Am J Obstet Gynecol* 1981;139:815–25.
20. Campion M J, McCance D J, Cuzick J, Singer A. Progressive potential of mild cervical atypia: prospective cytological, colposcopic and virological study. *Lancet* 1986;2(8501):237–40.
21. Ferris D G, Payne P, Frisch L E, Milner F H, diPaola F M, Petry L J. Cervicography: adjunctive cervical cancer screening by primary care clinicians. *J Fam Pract* 1993;37(2):158–64.
22. Macgregor J E. What constitutes an adequate cervical smear? *Br J Obstet Gynaecol* 1991;98:6–7.
23. Campion M J. The adequate cervical smear: a modern dilemma. *J Fam Pract* 1992;34(3):273–5.
24. Reid R, Greenberg N M, Lorincz A, et al. Should cervical cytologic testing be augmented by cervicography or human papillomavirus deoxyribonucleic acid detection? *Am J Obstet Gynecol* 1991;164:1461–9.
25. Tawa K, Forsythe A, Cove J K, Saltz A, Peters H W, Watring W G. A comparison of the Papanicolaou smear and the Cervigram: sensitivity, specificity, and cost analysis. *Obstet Gynecol* 1988;71:229–35.
26. Gundersen J H, Schauberger C W, Rowe N R. The Papanicolaou smear and the Cervigram: a preliminary report. *J Reprod Med* 1988;33:46–8.

27. Spitzer M, Krumholz B A, Seltzer V L, Molho L. Cervical cancer detected by Cervicography in a patient with negative cervical cytology. *Obstet Gynecol* 1986;68:68S–70S.

28. Blythe J G. Cervicography: a preliminary report. *Am J Obstet Gynecol* 1985;152:192–7.

29. Ferris D G. Cervical carcinoma in situ undetected by Papanicolaou smear but identified by cervicography. A case report. *J Fam Pract* 1994;38(1):74–7.

30. Schneider A, Zahn D M, Kirchmayr R, Schneider V L. Screening for cervical intraepithelial neoplasia grade 2/3: validity of cytologic study, cervicography, and human papillomavirus detection. *Am J Obstet Gynecol* 1996;174:1534–41.

31. Jones D E, Creasman W T, Dombroski R A, Lentz S S, Waeltz J L. Evaluation of the atypical Pap smear. *Am J Obstet Gynecol* 1987;157:544–9.

32. August N. Cervicography for evaluating the "atypical" Papanicolaou smear. *J Reprod Med* 1991;36:89–94.

33. Spitzer M, Krumholz B A, Chernys A E, Seltzer V, Lightman A R. Comparative utility of repeat Papanicolaou smears, cervicography, and colposcopy in the evaluation of atypical Papanicolaou smears. *Obstet Gynecol* 1987;69:731–5.

34. Ferris D C, Payne P, Frisch L E. Cervicography: an intermediate triage test for the evaluation of cervical atypia. *J Fam Pract* 1993;37(5):463–8.

35. Ferris D G, Schiffman M, Litaker M S, the ALTS group. Cervicography for triage of women with mildly abnormal cervical cytology results. *Am J Obstet Gynecol* 2001;85:939–43.

36. Mould T A, Singer A, Mansell M E, Gallivan S. Cervicography to triage women with borderline or mild dyskaryotic cervical Pap smears. *Eur J Gynecol Oncol* 2000;21:264–6.

37. Solomon D, Wied G L. Cervicography: an assessment. *J Reprod Med* 1989;34:321–3.

38. Ferenczy A, Hilgarth M, Jenny J, Koss L G, Masubuchi K, Noda K. The place of colposcopy and related systems in gynecologic practice and research. *J Reprod Med* 1988;33:737–8.

39. Nuovo J, Melnikow J, Hutchison B, Paliescheskey M. Is Cervicography a useful diagnostic test? A systematic overview of the literature. *J Am Board Fam Pract* 1997;10:390–7.

40. Szarewski A, Cuzick J, Edwards R, Butler B, Singer A. The use of cervicography in a primary screening service. *Br J Obstet Gynaecol* 1991;98:313–7.

41. Langman L J, Burr H S. A technique to aid the detection of malignancy of the female genital tract. *Am J Obstet Gynecol* 1949;57:274–81.

42. Ramanujam N, Mitchell N E, Mahadevan A, et al. In vivo diagnosis of cervical intraepithelial neoplasia using 337-nm-excited laser-induced fluorescence. *Proc Natl Acad Sci USA* 1994;91:10193–7.

43. Ramanujam N, Mitchell N W, Mahadevan-Jansen A, et al. Cervical precancer detection using a multivariate statistical algorithm based on laser-induced fluorescence spectra at multiple excitation wavelengths. *Photochem Photobiol* 1996;64:720–35.

44. Coppelson M, Reid B L, Skladner V N, Dalyrmple J C. An electronic approach to the detection of pre-cancer and cancer of the uterine cervix: a preliminary evaluation of polarprobe. *Int J Cancer* 1994;4:79–83.

45. Burke L, Nilhoff J, Kobelin M, Abu-Jawdeh G, Zelenchuk A, Modell M. Use of Auto fluorescence of cells to evaluate cervical neoplasia. *J Gynecol Techniques* 1996;2:187–90.

46. Burke L, Modell M, Niloff J, Kobelin M, Abu-Jawdeh G, Zelenchuk A. Identification of squamous intraepithelial lesions: fluorescence of cervical tissue during colposcopy. *J Lower Genital Tract Dis* 1999;3:159–62.

47. Nordstrom R J, Burke L, Niloff J M, Myrtle J F. Identification of cervical intraepithelial neoplasia (CIN) using UV-excited fluorescence and diffuse-reflectance tissue spectroscopy. *Laser Surg Med* 2001;29:118–27.

48. Parker M F, Mooradian G C, Karins J P, et al. Hyperspectral diagnostic imaging of the cervix: report on a new investigational device. *J Lower Genital Tract Dis* 2000;4:119–24.

49. Ferris D G, Lawhead R A, Dickman E D, et al. Multimodal hyperspectral imaging for the noninvasive diagnosis of cervical neoplasia. *J Lower Genital Tract Dis* 2001;5:65–72.

50. Mitchell M F, Cantor S B, Ramanujam N, Tortolero-Luna G, Richards-Kortum R. Fluorescence spectroscopy for diagnosis of squamous intraepithelial lesions of the cervix. *Obstet Gynecol* 1999;93:462–70.

51. Cantor S B, Mitchell M F, Tortolero-Luna G, Bratka C S, Bodurka D C, Richards-Kortum R. Cost-effectiveness analysis of diagnosis and management of cervical squamous intraepithelial lesions. *Obstet Gynecol* 1998;91:270–7.

52. Ferris D G, Macfee M S, Litaker M S, Dickman E D, Miller J A. Telemedicine network telecolposcopy compared with computer-based telecolposcopy. *J Lower Genital Tract Disease (in press)*.

53. Mikhail M S, Merkatz I R, Romney S L. Clinical usefulness of computerized colposcopy; Image analysis and conservative management of dysplasia. *Obstet Gynecol* 1992;80:5–8.

54. Cristoforoni P M, Gerbaldo D, Perino A, Piccoli R, Montz F J, Capitanio G L. Computerized colposcopy: results of a pilot study and analysis of its clinical relevance. *Obstet Gynecol* 1995;85:1001–6.

55. Pogue B W, Mycek M A, Harper D M. Image analysis for discrimination of cervical neoplasia. *J Biomed Optics* 2000;5:75–82.

56. Dickman E D, Doll T J, Chiu C K, Ferris D G. Identification of cervical neoplasia using a simulation of human vision. *J Lower Genital Tract Dis* 2001;3:144–52.

Cervical Screening and Management of the Abnormal Pap

Table of Contents

18.1 Introduction

Prior to the late 1940s cervical cancer was the second most common malignancy in women in the US in both incidence and in mortality. In 2002 incidence had fallen to 10th and mortality to 13th, accounting for approximately 12,900 reported cervical cancers and 4400 deaths.[1] This is a 75% reduction from the estimated equivalent of nearly 50,000 cervical cancers that would have occurred in the US at this time in the absence of cervical screening.[2] Approximately 8000 women died of cervical cancer in 1950, which would be the equivalent of over 16,000 deaths today.[3] The decrease in both incidence and mortality began prior to the introduction of widespread Papanicolaou (Pap) screening in the 1950s and 1960s. However, the majority has been attributed to the diagnosis and treatment of intraepithelial neoplasia, which only became possible following the implementation of cervical cancer screening with the Pap smear.[4] Women treated for preinvasive squamous and glandular lesions have a five-year survival rate of nearly 100%, and even when invasion has occurred, cervical cancers detected at an early stage (1A) have a five-year survival rate of approximately 92 percent.[1] This ability to detect and treat precursor lesions before progression to invasion is responsible for the continuing decline in cervical cancer rates from 14 per 100,000 women in 1973 to 8 per 100,000 in 1994.[5] This decline has continued, albeit less significantly, into the early 21st century. In contrast, cervical cancer continues to rank first or second amongst all cancers in women in countries without cervical cancer screening, dramatizing the impact of screening where introduced.[6]

Within the last 20 years the confirmation of human papillomavirus (HPV) as a necessary cause of high-grade CIN and cervical cancer[7] has led to the development and evaluation of sensitive tests for HPV that may be utilized in primary cervical screening and in management of women with abnormal cervical cytology.[8,9,10] Natural history studies have shown that persistent high-risk HPV is required for the development of CIN3[11,12,13] and that persistence of both high-risk HPV and CIN3 is necessary for the accumulation of random mutations that eventually lead to the capability of the infected cell to invade below the basement membrane.[14] Although cervical screening with the Pap has been very successful in lowering the rate of cervical cancer, 40–50% of women who get cervical cancer have had cervical screening and some have had regular annual Paps. Additionally, concern has been increased following recognition of the relatively greater risk of missing significant glandular lesions on cytology.[15–18] These statistics have driven annual screening in the US and have highlighted the need to look for screening methods with increased sensitivity and predictive value to provide better protection and, at the same time, allow less frequent screening. However, an increase in sensitivity of a screening test usually results in decreased specificity that may raise costs and patient anxiety. The 2003 Food and Drug Administration (FDA) approval of HPV testing [Hybrid Capture 2 High-risk HPV DNA Test™, Digene, Gaithersburg, MD] as an adjunct to the Pap for primary cervical screening of women age 30 and over acknowledges the potential that HPV testing with the Pap may provide better screening. The inclusion of HPV testing with the Pap for women ≥30 in the primary screening guidelines issued in 2002 by the American Cancer Society (ACS)[19] and in 2003 by the American College of Obstetricians and Gynecologists (ACOG)[20], suggests that cervical cancer screening will likely change significantly over the next decade from that we have known for the past half century.

The understanding of the relationship between HPV and abnormal cervical cytology,[21,22] CIN and cervical cancer[23] has promoted a wealth of data on the clinical utility of testing for HPV in a variety of clinical settings.[24–26] In particular, the 1995–2001 commitment of the National Cancer Institute (NCI) to study the best management strategies for women with equivocal and low-grade Pap abnormalities (the ASCUS/LSIL Triage study or ALTS)[26] provided extensive data, which was utilized in management recommendations put forth by the 2001 ASCCP Consensus Conference for the Management of Women with Cervical Cytological Abnormalities and Cervical Cancer Precursors.[8,9] This chapter will discuss the screening and management issues related to both the Pap and to HPV testing and provides a comprehensive overview of the new 2002–2003 guidelines from the ACS, ACOG and the ASCCP.

18.2 Cervical Screening Technologies

18.2.1 The conventional Pap smear

The dramatic reduction in cervical cancer incidence and mortality following the introduction of cervical cytologic screening[27] provided indirect proof of the value of the Pap smear despite the absence of any randomized trial on its effectiveness. However, implementation of the Clinical Laboratory Improvement Act (CLIA '88),[28] the Bethesda System,[29] and the CDC's National Breast and Cervical Cancer Early Detection Program[30] were all, to some degree, secondary to recognition of problems with the cervical cancer screening system.[31–33] All of these activities added to the continued reduction of cervical cancer incidence and mortality through the 1990s, as shown by the National Cancer Institute's (NCI) Surveillance, Epidemiology, and End Results (SEER) program and other NCI data.[34-36] However, until recently the sensitivity of the conventional Pap smear was significantly overestimated. In 1999 the Agency for Health Care Policy Research (AHCPR) sponsored an analysis of the best 85 studies evaluating Pap sensitivity.[37] That review concluded that a single conventional Pap had detected cervical cancer precursor lesions with only 51% sensitivity, overturning the conventional wisdom that the sensitivity of the Pap smear was approximately 80%.[38] Similar poor sensitivity of cervical cytology has been repeated in other meta-analyses.[39] Therefore, conventional Pap smears are not particularly sensitive, but their use has resulted in the dramatic reduction in cervical cancer incidence and mortality discussed previously because the natural history of the development of cervical cancer is one that take many years to decades. This long precursor phase provides much room for missed significant lesions that are most commonly detected at some point prior to invasion.

18.2.2 Liquid-based cytology

During the 1990's several technological innovations revolutionized cervical cytologic screening, particularly the development of improved sampling devices, liquid-based collection systems, and computer-assisted screening.[40] Following the 1996 FDA-approval of the first liquid-based Pap (ThinPrep®, CYTYC Corporation, Boxborough, MA) and the second in 1999 (SurePath™, TriPath, Burlington, NC) there have been two very different modalities used to prepare cervical cytology slides: conventional dry slide Pap smears and liquid-based Paps (LBPs). Although liquid-based cytology has been available for less than a decade, it is now the more common Pap modality chosen in the US.

LBPs have a number of theoretical advantages over the conventional Pap smear. These include more complete collection of exfoliated cells, random and presumably more representative transfer of exfoliated cells to slides, and improved microscopic visualization attributable to reduced overlapping, obscuring blood and inflammation.[41-44] Liquid-based cytology also provides residual cells for testing for HPV, Chlamydia and gonorrhea. Two meta-analyses have concluded that liquid-based cytology is more sensitive, but possibly less specific than smears.[44-46] Increases in detection of all levels of Pap abnormalities are seen, including ASC-US, and some increase in the proportion of samples lacking an endocervical component has been reported, but rates of biopsy-proven detection of CIN also have increased.[41,42,47-51] Of these studies, three have shown an increase in ASC-US,[42,49,51] and four have shown either similar or

slightly decreased detection of ASC-US.[41,47,48,50] Five studies have also evaluated specificity, with two demonstrating slightly decreased specificity when compared to conventional cytology,[42,51] two showing no difference,[48,50] and one equivocal.[49] While specimen adequacy of LBPs is generally improved,[50] identification of endocervical cells as a marker for sampling of the transformation zone is often more difficult than with conventional Paps.[41,47,48] Only one study has found no significant difference in sensitivity between LBPs and conventional smears and in this study sampling was optimized for the conventional Pap by use of a specialized collection device, removal of mucus and cellular debris from the cervical surface prior to sampling, and colposcopically-guided sampling to verify collection of cells from the transformation zone.[19,48]

Three studies have shown that detection of glandular lesions by LBPs is significantly improved compared to detection rates noted with conventional smears[43,52,53] and specificity for glandular abnormality is also increased.[43] One study reported a 50% decline in the AGC rate with LBPs, yet a five-fold increase in the positive predictive value for AIS.[52] With the increased rate of cervical adenocarcinoma reported in the last two decades, the importance of more precisely detecting AIS and cervical adenocarcinoma could not be more evident. While the majority of data to date on LBPs is for the ThinPrep® technology, available studies on the SurePath™ method suggest equivalent performance. However, the absence of studies directly comparing the two methods precludes definitive statements on relative performance.[19]

The 2002 ACS Guidelines recognized the increased sensitivity of liquid-based cytology by recommending that women under the age of 30 can have either annual conventional Paps or a monolayer Pap every 2 years.[19] The gain in sensitivity and the logistical advantage of having a representative specimen for ancillary testing support the use of LBPs.[44] Despite these apparent advantages, the higher cost of LBPs has delayed universal conversion to this technique.

18.2.3 Automated screening

The development of automated screening devices has been driven more by the need to reduce the labor required for manual screening than by improvement in sensitivity.[54] Automated devices classify a set percentage of Paps as being so normal (negative) that they do not need to be reviewed by human eyes. One study of automated screening used a slide set highly enriched with abnormal thin-layer Paps, yet the automated screener was able to sort out 837/1275 (66%) as being so normal that they did not need human review and still detect 98% of the slides classified as

HSIL.[55] In contrast, 100% manual reading by cytopathologists of the same set of 1,275 slides detected only 91% of the slides classified as HSIL. Such data suggests that automated cytology may provide more rapid, accurate, standardized screening, while reducing labor and costs.[44] Automated screening instruments are presently being evaluated that save digital images of cells appearing to be most abnormal. Although these devices have not yet been shown to provide computer images that always agreed well with the microscopic classification, it is expected that the technology will eventually permit expert cytologic reviews without microscopic re-examination of glass slides.[44]

18.2.4 HPV DNA testing

18.2.4.1 Overview of the clinical utility

The first HPV test that became clinically available was the ViraPap™, which was Food and Drug Administration (FDA)-approved in 1988 [Life Technologies, Silver Spring, MD]. This was followed in 1991 by FDA approval of an expanded ViraPap set, called ViraType®, and in 1995 by approval of the first hybrid capture test [Hybrid Capture 1®, Digene Corporation, Gaithersburg, MD]. The HPV test presently in use clinically is a solution hybridization test called Hybrid Capture 2 (HC2)® [Digene Corporation, Gaithersburg, MD], which was FDA-approved in 1999. Two other methods commonly in use are polymerase chain reaction (PCR) and in situ hybridization (ISH). The clinical utility of HC2 will be discussed extensively in the section on Pap management, whereas description will follow here of the characteristics of a number of HPV tests that either are presently available for clinical use or are expected to become available in the future.

The primary role of HPV testing initially was in the study of the etiology and natural history of HPV and cervical cancer. Once these studies provided evidence of the involvement of HPV in the etiology of CIN and cervical cancer, attention turned to how to use this new technology to improve cervical screening and abnormal Pap management. Three main clinical uses of HPV testing have been delineated:

Primary screening with the Pap: Numerous studies have documented that combining a HPV test with the Pap in the primary population screening of women increases sensitivity for detection of CIN 2,3 and cancer to 96–100%.[56-63] The very high sensitivity of the HPV test alone suggests that this test may eventually be used as a stand-alone primary screen, perhaps with the less sensitive Pap as a secondary triage for women found to be HPV positive.[64] The high rate of HPV positivity in women below the age of 30 and the low rate of cervical cancer in this age group would appear at

this time to restrict the use of HPV testing in primary screening to those age 30 and over.[10,19,20]

Secondary triage: The high proportion of normal women noted in the follow-up of ASCUS cytology, amongst a smaller number with CIN 2,3 and rarer cancers, suggested that HPV testing might sort out those at-risk (HPV positive) from those not (HPV-negative). A number of studies documented that this assumption was correct,[24-26,65,66] with the ultimate confirmation of the clinical utility of HPV testing in the management of ASCUS coming from the National Cancer Institute sponsored ASCUS/LSIL Triage Study (ALTS).[26]

Follow-up of treated cases: Confirmation that the majority of women successfully treated for CIN become negative for HPV and that sensitivity of a HPV test for recurrent or persistent CIN post-treatment is comparable to the high sensitivity of the test for CIN 2,3 in screening and triage has promoted HPV testing as an alternative to repeat cytology in the follow-up of women treated for CIN. HPV negative women post-treatment are followed annually with cytology and women HPV-positive are referred for colposcopy.[9] HPV testing in the management of women post-treatment is discussed in depth in Chapter 19.

18.2.4.2 Specific HPV tests

At present only HC2 is FDA-approved for clinical use in both the management of ASC-US and in primary screening in combination with the Pap. However, there are a number of HPV tests that have played an important part in defining the epidemiology and natural history of HPV and in evaluation of the clinical utility of HPV tests, and some PCR and ISH methods are available for clinical use from laboratories that have internally validated the test (Table 18.1). The most used HPV tests include the various polymerase chain reaction tests (real-time PCR, the PGMY09/11 system, SPF-PCR system, Shorty-PCR [Roche Molecular Diagnostics]) and the hybrid capture systems (Hybrid Capture 2 and Hybrid Capture 3 [Digene]) and Amplicor MWP. New novel methods for HPV-detection include HPV genotyping chips and HPV serological assays. The HPV DNA tests validated to date in large clinical trials and epidemiological studies are HC2 and the PCR-based methods employing either MY09/11 or GP5/6 consensus primers.[67]

18.2.4.2.1 Hybrid capture systems for detecting HPV HC2® is the only HPV test evaluated to date in large clinical studies that has achieved FDA approval for clinical use. Hence, it is the only test at present routinely used for triage and follow-up in the ASCCP Guidelines[8,9] and in the new Interim Recommendations for primary screening with the Pap.[10] The

Table 18.1 Established HPV Test Technologies

The most common established HPV test technologies include hybridization techniques, PCR-protocols and PCR plus hybridization.

Hybridization-techniques	HC2® HPV DNA assay (Digene FDA-approved)
PCR-protocols	MY09/11
	GP5+/GP6+
	SPF-PCR
	PGMY09/11
PCR plus Hybridization	GP5+/6+ EIA ELISA-system
	GP5+/6+ RLB reverse line blot assay
	MY09/11 Dot Blot non-radioactive dot blot assay
	SPF-LiPA reverse line blot assay
	PGMY09/11 LBA reverse line blot assay

From: Iftner T, Villa L L. Chapter 12: Human papillomavirus technologies. *J Natl Cancer Inst Monogr.* 2003;31:80–8 with permission, Oxford University Press.

hybrid capture system is based on hybridization in solution of RNA probes complementary to the DNA of common, clinically relevant HPV types. HC2® has RNA probes containing the genomic sequences of 13 high-risk (16, 18, 31, 33, 35, 39, 45, 51, 52, 56, 58, 59 and 68) and of 5 low-risk (6, 11, 42, 43, 44) HPV types divided into two panels, called the high-risk panel and the low-risk panel. This division allows the ordering of only the high-risk panel, which minimizes cost and is recommended in all the new guidelines, since low-risk types are not involved in oncogenesis.[8–10] If one of these 13 high-risk HPV types is present in the clinical specimen, the RNA probe that corresponds to that type will hybridise in solution and will then be captured by antibodies specific for the RNA:DNA hybrid. The "captured" hybrid is then detected by a series of reactions that give rise to a luminescence that can be measured in a luminometer.[67] The intensity of light emitted is proportional to the number of viral genomes present in the sample, providing a semi-quantitative measure of the HPV viral load expressed as relative light units (RLU). The test is only semi-quantitative for viral load because it is not standardized for the cellularity of the sample being tested. A large number of HC-2 tests can be run at one time in its present 96-well microplate format. A significant advantage of the hybrid capture system over PCR is its ability to detect clinically relevant HPV DNA (detection threshold is set at 5000 genomes per test sample) without the amplification required for PCR. This decreases the potential for cross contamination that has been so problematic for clinical use of PCR tests.

The FDA-recommended cut-off value for test-positive results is 1.0 RLU (equiv. to 1pg/ml HPV DNA or 5000 genomes), which is similar in sensitiv-

ity to that of the various PCR consensus primer tests. Labs should report the results of a HC2® test as either positive (≥1 RLU) or negative (<1RLU). Some labs report weak positive signals just below or above the cut-off value of 1 RLU as "borderline" or as "equivocal" for HPV. This must be discouraged, for even though very low levels of HPV may be present, all clinical validation studies have set the threshold for a positive test at 1 RLU with no equivocal zone and have missed very little significant disease. Lowering the threshold brings in many more women for evaluation that are most likely to be normal and to remain so, greatly reducing the positive predictive value of the test and creating a dilemma for HC2 testing similar to the ASCUS problem with cytology.

Cross-reactivity between the high-risk HPV probe and types not represented in this 13-probe mix has been noted with HC2®.[67] Although the HC2 high-risk probe set was found in one study to cross-react with types 53, 66, 67 and 73 as well as with other undefined types, the effect of this cross-reactivity on the clinical performance of the test has been shown to be minimal.[68] In a primary screening mode with the Pap, cross-reactivity of HC2® significantly improved the accuracy of identifying CIN2+ in women with normal cytology, but decreased the accuracy somewhat in women triaged with ASC-US by HC2®.[68]

The HC2 test can be taken directly from the liquid-based cytology sample, as is most commonly done for "reflex HPV testing" in ASC-US management, or it can be obtained by taking a separate sample in Digene's proprietary transport media (STM)™. Laboratory workload in running the HC2 test is greater when the test is run out of the LBP sample than when run from the STM. Therefore, the use of

HC2 in primary screening with the Pap for women over the age of 30 may be best done from a separate STM sample taken at the same time as the Pap. In contrast, for women under 30 having LBPs, the only initial use for HPV testing is in ASC-US management. Hence taking a HPV specimen separately on every woman has not been necessary, as the smaller numbers of HPV tests performed for reflex testing have not overwhelmed laboratory resources.

18.2.4.2.2 PCR systems for detecting HPV

HPV DNA can be selectively amplified by a series of reactions that lead to an exponential and reproducible increase in the viral sequences present in the biological specimen.[69] Amplification can theoretically produce unlimited numbers of copies from a single HPV genome. It is this power to amplify that has until recently restricted PCR to highly controlled research settings where limiting cross-contamination of specimens is most successful. A number of different formats can be used to analyze the amplified product created by the chain reaction. These include gel electrophoresis, dot or line strip hybridization, direct DNA sequencing and capture methods that employ biotin-labeled PCR products.

Two main types of PCR primer sets are most commonly used; "consensus" and "general" primers. Consensus primers are generic primers that detect a region of the HPV L1 gene that is highly conserved between various HPV types. Almost all HPV types can be detected with consensus primers in a single PCR reaction. Specific types are then identified in the sample by analyzing the resulting PCR products by one of the methods listed above.[70] The most commonly used primer sets are the consensus primer sets MY09/11 and its recent modification PGMY09/11[71,72] and the GP5/6 and extended version GP5+/6+ general primer sets.[73,74] An advantage of PCR over the present hybrid capture method is the ability to distinguish nearly 40 different HPV types by hybridizing with type-specific probes in either strip line assays or in microtiter plates.[75] Another potential advantage is somewhat increased sensitivity and specificity and the potential for directly measuring viral load standardized to the cellular content of the sample.[67] However, HC2 has performed well in routine clinical settings and the clinical importance of viral load has yet to be determined.[76–79] Therefore it is not clear whether these potential advantages of PCR translate to superior clinical performance. While high viral load has been shown to be predictive of an increased risk for CIN3 in women with normal cytology,[76] the true clinical relevance of viral load measurement may continue to be problematic due to the inherent variability of sampling in the collection of cervical spec-

imens.[67] Additionally, viral load measurements are affected by lesion size and the proportion of infected to normal cells, which will always be very difficult to normalize to a cellular control.[67]

In general, there is an excellent concordance in numerous worldwide studies between these PCR testing modalities and HC2® with regard to sensitivity and specificity.[67] However, performance characteristics of the PCR tests are much more vulnerable to laboratory expertise and protocols for running the test than is HC2®. This problem has delayed the appearance of PCR tests for detection of HPV in clinical settings.

18.2.4.2.3 In situ hybridization (ISH)

ISH tests for HPV DNA within cells, either individually as in cytology, or in histology sections. Its primary use is in clarification of equivocal histology. Additionally, ISH could be used on cytology specimens to clarify equivocal (ASC-US) Paps, but is not yet FDA-approved for this function. ISH uses HPV DNA or RNA probes that are typically labeled with small molecules that can be detected by a variety of methods that hybridize to specific HPV DNA if present in the specimen. Because the morphology of the cytology or histology is not disrupted by the testing procedure, ISH allows documentation that one or more specific HPV types are actually responsible for the morphologic changes seen.

18.2.4.2.4 New HPV tests with potential clinical utility

There are a number of new HPV testing technologies that are presently vying for inclusion in the armamentarium of clinically useful tests. These include Hybrid Capture 3 (Digene Corporation, Gaithersburg, MD), the Taqman quantitative real-time PCR test, and the SPF-PCR system (Shorty-PCR, Roche Molecular Diagnostics, Pleasanton, CA).

Hybrid Capture 3 (HC3) (Digene Corporation, Gaithersburg, MD): HC3 is a new version of the hybrid capture method in which RNA probes in combination with biotinylated oligonucleotides capture target sequences specific for various HPV types onto streptavidin-coated wells of a microtiter plate.[67] Signals are generated by type-specific RNA probes that hybridize to other regions of the captured sequences. The problem of cross-hybridization noted with HC2® is reduced through the use of "blocker oligonucleotides", which are unlabelled DNA molecules that are complementary to the biotinylated capture oligonucleotides.[67] Other advantages of HC3 include the ability to use the same assay to test for either DNA or RNA targets and the capability to test for molecular variants of specific HPV types.[67] A new automated system for hybrid capture tests (HC2® and HC3) called the Rapid Capture System™ has also been developed (Digene Corporation, Gaithersburg, MD). This system runs off an automated platform that allows robotic handling of the 96 well microplate.[67] One step in the process (denaturation of the specimens) is still done manually, but the incubations, shakings and washings are all done robotically. This new technology will allow a single technician in a high-volume lab to perform 450 HPV tests during an 8-hour shift.

AMPLICOR MWP: This PCR HPV test is a generic reverse line blot test based on the PGMY09/11 consensus primers.[67] AMPLICOR MWP is a fully automated PCR detection system already available in many labs for the detection several microorganisms, and can be used for the detection of HPV. The automated system (COBAS AMPLICOR™) (Roche Molecular Diagnostics, Pleasanton, CA) has the capacity to run 96 samples a day.

SPF-PCR system or "Shorty-PCR": Shorty-PCR uses SPF1/2 consensus primers that target only a very small 65bp region of the HPV L1 gene and is designed to improve sensitivity of the test.[75] This short segment is contrasted to the 150bp segment for the GP primers and 450bp segment for MY09/11. The SPF-PCR system, Shorty-PCR (Roche Molecular Diagnostics, Pleasanton, CA) detects a broad spectrum of HPVs by reverse line blot hybridization. A recent report documented the ability to discriminate 43 HPV types despite concern that the small size of the genome targeted would reduce the ability to differentiate between viral types.[80] An advantage of this system over other PCR tests is the use of a more stable Taq DNA polymerase that provides shelf-life stability at room temperature, precluding the need for refrigeration. A recent report indicated that the increase in sensitivity of this test detected 13% more HPV in cervical smears than detected with the PGMY primers.[67] Shorty PCR tests for only high-risk types.

HPV genotyping chips: A new PCR HPV detection method [Biomedlab Co., Seoul, Korea] is based on immobilization of 22 HPV type-specific oligonucleotide probes and a control (β-globin probe) on an aldehyde-derivatized glass slide.[67] The test contains 15 high risk HPV probes (16, 18, 31, 33, 35, 39, 45, 51, 52, 56, 58, 59, 66, 68, 69; BG, β-globin) and 7 low risk HPV probes (6, 11, 34, 40, 42, 43, 44). The clinical specimen DNA is submitted to a standard PCR in the presence of fluoresceinated nucleotides (Cy5 or Cy3) that use primers for both the beta-globin (PC03/04) and for the L1 region of the HPV types in the cocktail using modified Gp5/6 primers.[67] The PCR products tagged by this method are then hybridized onto the chip and scanned by laser fluorescence. The method is in early development but is expected to have significant potential for clinical utility.

18.2.5 Using new technologies for cervical screening: pros and cons

The concerns expressed about using new technologies relate to specificity of the tests and to cost. Sensitivity of any test is improved by lowering the threshold for calling a test "positive". However, because lowered thresholds also bring more normals in for evaluation, specificity almost always suffers. Improvement in sensitivity will result in detection of only small numbers of missed significant lesions in a well-screened population with a very low prevalence of disease, but to achieve this success may require evaluation of many more women. In a normal screening population even small changes in specificity may require further evaluation large numbers of women.[19] Whether maximizing sensitivity at the expense of specificity is most valued depends on many societal and economic issues, not the least of which are societal expectations and medico-legal risks.[81,82]

Although sensitivity of the Pap has not been optimal, multiple screenings throughout life are quite effective in preventing most cervical cancers. In contrast to poor sensitivity, conventional Pap specificity is high, particularly for Paps read as LSIL or HSIL, while specificity for Paps read as "atypical" is less due to the large number of normal women having this finding. Specificity for both conventional and for monolayer cytology is reported to be in the range of 76–98%[33,51,63] but rates below 94% are rarely reported in studies in the US. Liquid-based cytologies do detect more ASC, LSIL and HSIL Paps, which are reflected in the increased sensitivity of this screening modality. However, it is not clear that liquid-based Paps decrease specificity, as noted in the conflicting studies discussed previously. It is clear that increased sensitivity does detect more high-grade CIN. In a large HMO screening study, about 25% of patients with CIN2 and CIN3 were detected in the follow-up of LSIL Paps, and 39% had ASCUS as their antecedent cytology.[83] Therefore, increased detection of ASC-US and LSIL, as well as HSIL, should significantly increase the detection of CIN 2,3. However, the natural history of progression of HPV infection to high-grade CIN to invasive cervical cancer generally occurs over many years to decades. Therefore, for the majority of women with high-grade CIN who get adequate screening, earlier detection of these lesions may make little difference. Unfortunately, many women do not participate in regular screening. About half of the women with cervical cancer have never had a Pap, and another 10% have had a least one Pap but have not participated in adequate screening. In order to have a major impact on cervical cancer rates, it is therefore necessary to get these

Table 18.2 Predicted Cancer Cases, Mortality and Hysterectomies

At various screening intervals per 100,000 women screened from age 15 through age 85. Based on AHCPR projections for technologies with increased sensitivity to 80%.

	Conventional Pap Smear	Increased Sensitivity to 80%	Change
Every 3 years			
Death	116	50	–57%
Cancer Cases	506	246	–51%
Hysterectomies	179	101	–44%
Every 2 years			
Death	65	25	–62%
Cancer Cases	305	25	–57%
Hysterectomies	118	59	–50%
Every year			
Death	21	10	–52%
Cancer Cases	14	4	–71%
Hysterectomies	47	16	–66%

From: Braly P, Kinney W, Sheet, E, Walton L, Farber F, Cox J T. Reporting the potential benefits of new technologies for cervical cancer screening. *J Low Gen Tract Dis* 2000;5:73–81. With permission.

women in for screening, and because they are at highest risk if significant disease is missed, and at highest risk for continued inadequate screening, use of the test with the highest sensitivity would seem to have clear benefit. Unfortunately, many underscreened women are indigent and underinsured, so the higher cost of more sensitive tests can be a substantial barrier.

The International Agency for Research on Cancer (IARC) estimated projected cervical cancer incidence based on what is known about the natural history of the disease and the sensitivity of the Pap smear. This analysis demonstrated that cervical cancer rates are explained by Pap smear sensitivity between 37% and 60%, which is in line with the AHCPR finding that the sensitivity of the Pap smear is 51%.[37,84] Therefore, any new screening approach that would reduce the false negative rate by 60% or more should improve clinical outcomes significantly. The AHCPR report projected improvement in outcomes with improved sensitivities of various levels and different screening intervals (Table 18.2)[33,37]. The new American Cancer screening guidelines that recommend annual conventional Pap smears or biennial liquid-based Paps for women between the onset of screening and age 30 reflect confidence in the increased reassurance provided by this modality.[19] However, other organizations recommend that screening should continue annually irrespective of the modality of Pap used.[20]

The potential for increased cost of the cervical cancer screening program secondary to the added cost of new technologies has been widely discussed, and continues to be of some concern, particularly among public funded programs with limited resources.[85,86] However, societal expectations of having a "perfect" test will likely continue to drive the use of tests with highest sensitivity. Several evaluations have determined that the actual cost of cervical screening with the new technologies is likely to decrease over that spent with conventional Paps performed annually, but only if clinicians and the public accept prolonged screening intervals that are recommended with the use of these tests. For example, one cost-modeling study demonstrated that a strategy of biennial LBPs and "reflex HPV testing" for ASC-US management was significantly more cost-efficient and somewhat more protective than annual conventional cytology with routine follow-up of ASC-US by repeat cytology.[87] The projected cost-savings of such a strategy was 15 billion dollars over the lifetime of a cohort of 16–24 year old women. Therefore, if screening and management recommendations for the new technologies are followed, the initial increased cost of these technologies appears to be more than made up by the savings accrued. However, excessive costs will accrue if the recommendations are not followed and women are over-screened.

18.3 Impediments to Screening

It is clear that getting women in for screening, and making sure that they have been adequately screened whenever they access health care, is imperative if the rate of cervical cancer incidence is to improve further.

Several public health studies addressing access to cervical screening concluded that cultural and social barriers and time-restraints have been more important impediments to access than cost and transportation.[88–90] Others, however, have concluded that economic barriers are also a significant barrier to access[91,92] These are difficult barriers to resolve and indicate why further significant reduction in the incidence of cervical cancer has been difficult to achieve. A number of projects are currently evaluating these issues, with the prospect that improved understanding of how to overcome these barriers will result in increased access to cervical screening amongst groups hither fore underscreened.[93,94]

18.4 Primary Cervical Screening Guidelines

In 2002 the ACS issued new primary cervical screening guidelines.[19] The United States Preventive Services Task Force (USPSTF) also issued new recommendations in early 2003[5] that differed significantly in some areas both with the ACS and with the ACOG recommendations that followed later that year.[20] These guidelines supplanted recommendations put in place in the late 1970s and updated in 1987 that have provided the basis for practice patterns for nearly 25 years. An understanding of the rationale behind each recommendation is imperative since many are dramatic departures from standards of practice established for over a quarter of a century and widely accepted by providers and by the public. Guidelines from each organization that are identical will be discussed together, and where they differ, each guideline will be discussed individually along with the differences in rationale.

18.4.1 When to begin screening

In 1987 the ACS issued guidelines that recommended that screening begin at the onset of vaginal intercourse or at age 18, whichever came first.[95] Improved understanding of the natural history of HPV and cervical cancer has now provided a far better appraisal of the most appropriate time to begin screening. There is almost no risk of developing cervical cancer within five years of first sexual exposure and very little risk during the subsequent five years. For this reason, cervical cancer is almost non-existent in adolescents, and there continues to be very low risk through the early 20's. The cervical cancer incidence rate reported by the National Cancer Institute's Surveillance, Epidemiology, and End Results (SEER) program for the years 1995–1999 was 0/100,000 per year for all females less than 20 years of age and only

1.7/100,000 per year for those ages 20 to 24.[96] Therefore, if screening were not to begin until after adolescence, based on this SEER data, the risk of not detecting and treating all high-grade lesions prior to the age of 24 would at most be 1.7 cases of cervical cancer per 100,000/year and many of these would likely be prevented by detection of high-grade lesions prior to invasion by screening in the late teens (for women beginning intercourse by age 16) and early 20's.[19] Additionally, reduction in cervical cancer incidence by cervical cytologic screening has not been demonstrated for women under the age of 30 (Figure 18.1).[97] This may partially reflect an increasing incidence in women under 30 of adenocarcinomas, whose precursor lesion is not as well detected by cytology,[44] or to other factors related to the natural history of cervical cancer and the host immune response that may differ when women get cervical cancer at an unusually young age.

Cervical screening in adolescents has also been shown to subject a significant percentage of these young women to diagnostic and treatment procedures that are most often unnecessary. This is because most HPV infections in women aged 13 to 22 results in only low-grade CIN, and most high-risk HPV infection and CIN 1 lesions are transient. The estimated rate for spontaneous resolution over a period of 2 to 3 years of high-risk HPV in young women ranges from 70[98] to over 90 percent[99] and approximately 90 percent of LSIL in females between 13 and 21 years of age will regress.[100] Host immunity appears to be most successful in clearing HPV lesions in young women and adolescents and less so as women age, for CIN 1 only clears in 58% of adult women.[101–103] There are two very important messages in this data. First, screening women within the first few years of intercourse offers almost no benefit and may create harm. Second, most low-grade lesions are caused by known oncogenic HPV types and yet spontaneously regress. For instance, 81 percent of low-grade lesions in young women caused by high-risk HPV types regressed and only 6% were shown to progress.[100] Therefore it is very important to not needlessly diagnose and treat lesions destined to resolve spontaneously. The best way to manage this potential for overdiagnosis and excessive treatment is to not screen women in this age group in the first place. Beginning screening at a later age places very little increased risk of missing significant lesions that would place women at increased risk for cervical cancer since CIN 2,3 that develops at this young age will almost invariably continue to be present and detectable when screening begins.

The ACS also took into account the cost-effectiveness of beginning screening at different ages. The most cost-effective strategy for when to begin

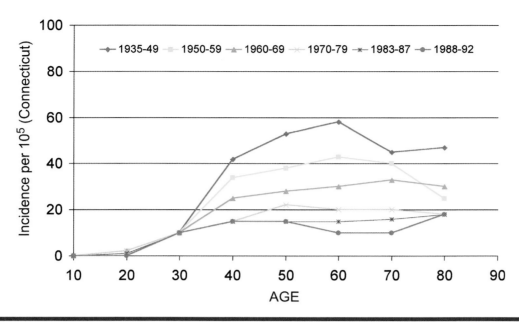

FIGURE 18.1   Gustaffson evaluated cervical cancer rates in Connecticut from the period prior to the onset of cervical screening in 1949 to 1992. Dramatic decreases in cervical cancer incidence occurred in all age groups except for women under age 30. For this latter group, no change in cervical cancer incidence could be demonstrated during the 43 years of screening. From: Gustafsson L, Ponten J, Zack M, Adami H O. International incidence rates of invasive cervical cancer after introduction of cytological screening. *Cancer Causes Control* 1997;8:755–63. With permission.

cytology-only screening of women under the age of 30 has been demonstrated by mathematical modeling to start three years after age of onset of vaginal intercourse, with an age cap at 25.[104] However, there was concern that beginning screening at age 25 would inevitably result in some women not getting screened until their late 20's, which could result in a more significant excess of missed cancers.[19] An age cap of 21 was also demonstrated to be cost-effective, particularly when compared to the onset of screening strategy of age 18 that has been advised for the past 25 years. The recommendation is also careful not to designate an exact date that screening should begin in order to avoid potential denial of health insurance coverage for teens and young women who have their first Pap before the suggested "three years from first intercourse".[19] As will be seen from the language of the recommendation, the onset of sexual activity was defined as the onset of intercourse because the risk of HPV transmission to the cervix is low for other types of sexual activity.[19] The upper age limit of 21 was set regardless of whether onset of sexual activity is documented in order to protect women unwilling to disclose, or unable to remember, prior sexual activity. However, provider discretion and patient choice following counseling should be used to guide the initiation of cervical cytology screening in young women aged 21 and older who have never had vaginal inter-

course and for whom the absence of a history of sexual abuse is certain.[19]

The data reviewed by the ACS also failed to demonstrate that women abused in childhood were at increased risk for cervical cancer at an early age. Therefore, there was no indication that women with a history of prepubescent sexual abuse required screening within 3 years of the abuse.[19] However, it was felt that pre-puberty victims having vaginal intercourse should be referred for screening post-puberty once they are psychologically and physically ready and that post-pubescent sexually abused girls should begin screening approximately 3 years from the event. In all cases of known abuse, great care must be taken not to add to the distress of the individual who may find the prospect of a vaginal exam to be difficult to separate from the pain of the abuse. Such screening must therefore be by a provider who has experience and sensitivity for working with abused adolescents.[19]

US Public Health Service Guidelines apply to the onset of cervical screening for women with HIV, as well as for women immunocompromised for other reasons.[105] These guidelines stress that immunocompromised women should obtain a Pap test twice in the first year after diagnosis of HIV or other reason for immune suppression. Annual screening can then proceed for women having normal reports on both initial screens. All of these considerations led the

Table 18.3 When to Begin Screening

Recommendation on when to begin screening from the ACS, USPSTF, and ACOG[5,19,20]
- Cervical cancer screening should begin approximately three years after the onset of vaginal intercourse.
- Screening should begin no later than 21 years of age.

Additionally ACS and ACOG recommend:
- Adolescents who may not need a cervical cytology test should obtain appropriate preventive health care, including assessment of health risks, contraception, and prevention counseling, screening and treatment of sexually transmitted diseases.
- The need for cervical cancer screening should not be the basis for the onset of gynecologic care.

ACS, the USPSTF and ACOG to make the recommendations listed in (Table 18.3) regarding the onset of cervical screening.

18.4.2 When to discontinue screening

Most cervical cancer that occurs in women over the age of 70 is almost entirely in the underscreened and unscreened portion of the population or in women who have not had three consecutive normal cytology results.[106-109] Therefore, screening women in this age group that have a history of having several recent normal Paps would not appear to offer much additional protection. Additionally, the epithelial effects of aging and of declining estrogen often produce cellular changes that are difficult to differentiate from those related to HPV and neoplasia.[44] These "misclassified" Paps often result in overevaluation, anxiety and increased costs with minimal benefit. Guidelines on when to discontinue cervical screening from the ACS, the USPSTF and ACOG all differ. For instance the USPSTF recommends discontinuing screening at age 65 for "women who have had adequate screening with normal Paps" and the ACS at age 70 for women with at least 3 normal Paps in the past 10 years.[5,19] Both are probably reasonable ages to cease screening once these parameters are met. In contrast, ACOG does not recommend an age at which to end screening.[20] The recommendations on when to cease screening are listed in (Table 18.4).

18.4.2.1 Screening after hysterecotmy

Vaginal cancer is one of the rarest of gynecologic malignancies, with an incidence of 1 to 2/100,000 per year.[1] However, abnormal Paps in women having hysterectomy with removal of the cervix are fairly common, primarily due to minor cytologic changes secondary to estrogen deficiency. Significantly abnormal Paps are uncommon and rarely identify a clinically important lesion. For example, of nearly 6000 women having a hysterectomy, of which 862 were for benign reasons, 1.1% had an abnormal Pap and none had vaginal cancer, resulting in a positive predictive value of zero.[110] Another retrospective study following for an average of 89 months 220 women who had a hysterectomy for benign conditions determined that there was no benefit in patient outcomes despite detection of 7 vaginal dysplasias, three of which spontaneously regressed.[111] Most studies of women previously having a hysterectomy for high-grade CIN also do not show statistically significant increased risk for subsequent detection of vaginal neoplasia.[111,112] However, concern that there is not enough data to validate that these women are definitely at the same low risk as women having a hysterectomy for benign disease has promoted increased surveillance for these women. In contrast, women with a history of DES-exposure may be at risk for clear cell adenocarcinoma throughout their lives. With these considerations in mind the ACS made the recommendations in (Table 18.5), with general concurrence from ACOG and the USPSTF.

18.4.3 Screening interval

The major departure in screening recommendations between the three organizations were in the area of screening intervals and whether to consider increased sensitivity for CIN 2,3 reported for both liquid-based cytology and for HPV testing in making screening interval recommendations. Only the recommendations from the ACS reflect recognition that increased sensitivity of liquid-based cytology could be the basis for lengthening the screening interval.[19] Both ACS and ACOG recognized the very high sensitivity of HPV testing and cytology combined as providing increased reassurance of the absence of significant disease that would allow lengthening of the screening interval.[19,20] The USPSTF essentially recommended

Table 18.4   When to Cease Screening

Recommendations on when to cease screening from the ACS, USPSTF, and ACOG

Recommendation from the ACS:[19]
- Women who are age 70 and older with an intact cervix and who have had three or more documented, consecutive, technically satisfactory normal/negative cervical cytology tests, and no abnormal/positive cytology tests within the 10-year period prior to age 70 may elect to cease cervical cancer screening.
- Screening is recommended for women who have not been previously screened, women for whom information about previous screening is unavailable, and for whom past screening is unlikely.
- Women who have a history of cervical cancer, in utero exposure to diethylstilbestrol (DES), and/or are immunocompromised should continue cervical cancer screening for as long as they are in reasonably good health and do not have a life-limiting chronic condition.
- Until more data are available, women aged 70 and older who have tested positive for HPV DNA should continue screening at the discretion of their health care provider.
- Women over the age of 70 should discuss their need for cervical cancer screening with their health care provider based on their individual circumstances (including the potential benefits, harms, and limitations of screening) and make informed decisions about whether to continue screening. Women with severe co-morbid or life-threatening illnesses may forego cervical cancer screening.

Recommendation from the USPSTF:[5]
- The USPSTF recommends against routinely screening women older than age 65 if they have had adequate recent screening with normal Pap smears and are not otherwise at increased risk for cervical cancer.

Recommendation from the ACOG:[20]
- Physicians can determine on an individual basis when an older woman can stop having cervical cancer screening, based on such factors as her medical history and the physician's ability to monitor the patient in the future. ACOG noted that there were limited studies evaluating cervical cancer screening older women and they felt that there was inadequate information to enable setting an across-the-board upper age limit for cervical cancer screening.

no change in screening interval based on any of the new technologies.[5] The rationale for these decisions follows.

Most of the data on conventional cytology comparing one-, two-, and three-year screening intervals comes from countries with organized screening programs, which increase attendance at recommended screening intervals. These studies show little difference in cervical cancer rates for women screened at each of these intervals.[113,114] However, there is a significant difference in the relative risk of a CIN 3 progressing to cervical cancer between two- and three-year screening intervals when compared with a one-year interval. Most of the data indicate that the relative risk is doubled with a two-year screening interval and tripled with a three-year screening interval when compared to annual screening.[115–117] However, the number of cancers occurring with 3 year intervals is still quite small.[19] Data from the National Breast and Cervical Cancer Prevention Program of the CDC from a prospective cohort study of 128,805 women in the US determined the age-adjusted incidence rate of CIN 2,3, CIS or invasive carcinoma

within three years of a normal Pap to be 25 per 10,000 for women screened at 9 to 12 months, 29 per 10,000 for women screened at 13 to 24 months, and 33 per 10,000 for women screened at 25 to 36 months.[106] Although the differences in incidence were not statistically significant, there was a definite trend upward with increasing intervals. Absolute risk for cervical cancer between two and three year intervals of women followed over 13 years was not shown to be great in a well screened HMO population, whereas the relative risk of being diagnosed with invasive cancer was doubled.[118] While the absolute risk of invasive squamous cell cancer within three years following three or more normal Paps was estimated to be <5 per 100,000 women per year, in a large population of women being screened, such as this HMO, this accounted for 53 cases of invasive cervical cancer. Estimating the cost of screening must take into account the costs in both human and economic terms of cervical cancers occurring in women who follow screening recommendations, as well as the costs related to overdiagnosis and over-treatment that often occurs with annual screening.[19]

Table 18.5 Screening After Hysterectomy

Recommendations on screening after hysterectomy from the ACS, USPSTF, and ACOG

ACS Recommendations:[19]
- Screening with vaginal cytology tests following total hysterectomy (with removal of the cervix) for benign gynecologic disease is not indicated.
- Efforts should be made to confirm and/or document via physical exam and review of the pathology report (when available) that the hysterectomy was performed for benign reasons (the presence of CIN2/3 is not considered benign) and that the cervix was completely removed.
- Women who have had a subtotal hysterectomy should continue cervical cancer screening as per current guidelines.
- Women with a history of CIN2/3 or for whom it is not possible to document the absence of CIN2/3 prior to/or as the indication for the hysterectomy should be screened until three documented, consecutive, technically satisfactory normal/negative cervical cytology tests and no abnormal/positive cytology tests within a 10-year period are achieved.
- Women with a history of in utero DES exposure and/or with a history of cervical carcinoma should continue screening after hysterectomy for as long as they are in reasonably good health and do not have a life-limiting chronic condition.
- Women having a hysterectomy for CIN2/3 should have follow-up cytology every four to six months until three documented, consecutive, technically satisfactory normal/negative vaginal cytology tests are obtained. No abnormal/positive cytology tests should be achieved within an 18- to 24-month period following hysterectomy before discontinuing cytology screening.

USPSTF and ACOG:[5, 20]
- Women who have had a total hysterectomy for benign disease should cease cervical screening.
- ACOG also recommended annual screening for women having had a hysterectomy for benign disease but also having had a history of CIN 2 or 3, until they have had three consecutive negative Pap, following which routine screening can be discontinued.

The problem in the US with 3 year recommended intervals for conventional cytology is compounded by the fact that Pap screening in this country is opportunistic, which means that there is no organized system to bring women in for screening at guaranteed intervals and many women would likely not get screening for 4 or 5 or more years. The number of cases of CIN3 progressing to invasion during an interval longer than three years is likely to be unacceptably high in the US,[19] and numerous studies have documented significant increases in risk for screening intervals of 4 to 10 years.[115-119] Additionally, many are concerned that the increasing incidence of cervical adenocarcinoma, already missed by cervical cytologic screening in increased proportion to squamous lesions, would miss an increasing proportion of more easily treatable precursor glandular lesions were the interval to be prolonged beyond annually.

It is important to note that screening all women in the US annually with conventional cytology would still miss some cancers, as an estimated 1.5 cases of cervical cancer per 100,000 women having a negative Pap result and at least three prior normal Paps would be detected within 0 to 18 months of their last Pap.[120] This risk might be reduced some by screening with newer technologies having higher sensitivity than conventional cytology, but it is unlikely to ever achieve 100% protection. Increasing the frequency of cervical cytologic screening for women in routine screening to less than every 12 months might pick up a few of these "missed cancers" before they occur but would result in huge expenditures monetarily, emotionally, and physically. Hence routine screening more frequently than every 12 months has never been recommended. Of course, women in a program of abnormal Pap management are in a much higher risk status and may be managed by accelerated Paps every 4 to 6 months. Increased screening intervals are only recommended for women having satisfactory Paps with endocervical cells or other evidence of transformation zone sampling.[121]

The risk of CIN 3 increases through the 20's and peaks at age 29. Hence, screening at annual intervals from the onset of screening until age 30 was considered optimal by both ACOG and the ACS, although ACS took into account the increased sensitivity of liquid-based Paps in making the recommendation that women in this age group screened with this technology could be screened every two years.[19,20] Both organizations considered women age 30 and over

Table 18.6 Screening Intervals

Recommendations on screening intervals from the ACS, USPSTF, and ACOG

ACS: Recommendation for intervals[19]
- After initiation of screening, cervical screening should be performed annually with conventional cervical cytology smears *or* every two years using liquid-based cytology.
- At or after age 30, women who have had three consecutive, technically satisfactory normal/negative cytology results may be screened every two to three years (unless they have a history of in utero DES exposure, are HIV+, or are immunocompromised by organ transplantation, chemotherapy, or chronic corticosteriod treatment).

ACOG: Recommendation for intervals[20]
- ***Women up to age 30***—Women this age should undergo annual cervical cytology screening.
- ***Women age 30 and older***—Similar to ACS recommendation that women having 3 consecutive normal Paps may not need annual screening and therefore may be screened at 2 to 3 year intervals depending upon clinician and patient preference.

USPSTF: Recommendation for intervals[5]
- The Task Force concludes that screening should be done at least every 3 years.

and having three consecutive satisfactory negative/normal Paps to be at less risk for subsequent detection of high-grade intraepithelial neoplasia and cancer and recommended that the interval for these women could be increased to 2 to 3 years.[19,20] Extensive data indicated that three or more consecutive normal Paps reduced the risk of missed significant cervical lesions to a level acceptable in the arena of public health.[114,120] Risk reduction of 90% is predicted in one analysis,[114] and another demonstrated a reduction in absolute risk of developing cervical cancer within 18 months of a single normal Pap to be 3.09/100,000 women, decreasing to 2.56 for 2 consecutive normals and 1.43 for three.[120] However, these screening recommendations apply only to women with normal immunity. Women with HIV should be followed at intervals recommended by the CDC[105] and women with DES should be screened annually.[19] No other risk factors are considered important because routine screening recommendations will detect most important lesions irrespective of risk factors previously used to determine screening intervals. These include recent acquisition of a new partner(s), numerous sexual partners, early age of onset of sexual intercourse or smoking.[84] The recommendations for screening intervals from ACS, ACOG and USPSTF are in (Table 18.6).

18.4.4 Screening with combined cytology and HPV testing

Prior to the 2002 ACS and 2003 ACOG recommendations, increased screening intervals were recommended only for women with three consecutive normal Paps who were considered at low-risk for cervical neoplasia on the basis of mostly non-verifiable patient history variables such as age of onset of intercourse, number of partners, number of her partner's partners, and history of smoking, amongst others.[84] However, most women had one or more of these "high-risk" factors. Additionally, the partner's history could almost never be verified. The result was that most clinicians did not feel comfortable increasing the screening interval for any but virginal women. Hence, many women have been overscreened by annual screening throughout their lives. The strict association of HPV with CIN 3 and cervical cancer, and numerous evaluations of HPV testing as an adjunct to the Pap, provided the basis for recommendations by both the ACS and ACOG that included HPV testing as an adjunct to cervical cytology for women age 30 and over. The rationale for these recommendations and for the use of HPV testing as the first objective marker for risk stratification follow.

HPV testing is, on average, 25–40% more sensitive than a single conventional Pap for the detection of CIN 3+, and 10–25% more sensitive than a single liquid-based Pap.[49,122-125] Overall, the sensitivity of HPV testing averages 25% greater than the Pap in these studies. Additionally, it is relatively easy to standardize the procedure of testing for HPV, such that interlaboratory variation is minimal. (Table 18.7) lists the series of large clinical trials that served as the basis for FDA approval of HPV testing with HC2 in conjunction with the Pap in the primary cervical screening of women ≥30. The data clearly demonstrates significant variation in the sensitivity of cytology from country-to-country and laboratory-to-laboratory when compared to the consistently high-sensitivity of the HPV test. Combining the Pap

Table 18.7   Performance of Cytology and HPV Testing (HC2) Alone and in Combination for Identifying CIN2+

A number of large clinical trials conducted in several countries on combined HPV testing and cytology and totaling over 44,000 patients provided the basis for FDA approval of the HC2 High-risk HPV DNA™ test to be used with the Pap in the primary screening of women ≥30.

| Population | n | CIN2+ | Sensitivity | | | Specificity | | NPV | |
			Pap	HPV	Combo	Pap	HPV	Combo	Combo
Germany	7592	1.01%	33.8	85.7	93.5	98.7	96.7	95.7	0.999
UK	10538	0.95%	72.2	96.9	100.0	98.7	93.4	94.2	1.000
Mexico	6115	1.41%	57.0	94.2	97.7	98.8	94.0	93.5	1.000
Costa Rica	6176	1.75%	80.4	86.3	92.2	94.5	94.4	90.3	0.998
South Africa	2925	3.56%	74.0	84.9	87.0	87.9	81.8	78.1	0.998
China	1936	4.34%	94.0	97.6	100.0	77.8	84.8	69.5	1.000
Baltimore	1040	0.48%	60.0	100.0	100.0	97.8	96.5	95.8	1.000

with HPV testing only increases the sensitivity slightly because the HPV test is so highly sensitive. All of the studies demonstrate sensitivity for the combination screen of greater than 92% except for the study from South Africa,[60] and 4 of the 8 have sensitivities from 95–100%. The compelling advantage of combining HPV testing with the Pap is the extremely high negative predictive value (NPV) of the combined test, with all studies reporting NPVs of 98 to 100%. In two of the studies, the HPV test sensitivity was 100% without the Pap, obviously suggesting that combining the two tests may not be necessary if screening paradigms were to utilize the most sensitive test first (HPV testing), followed by the more specific test (the Pap) as the triage test. One concern was that the NCI data from Portland was the only large data set from a US population.[126] However, despite the older, less sensitive collection technique used in this study for HPV testing (vaginal lavage), the results confirmed the universality of the findings across all studies. This high negative predictive value indicates that women with a concurrent normal Pap and a negative HPV test result are at exceedingly low risk for CIN 2,3 or cancer in comparison to women having only a normal conventional cytology result. This very high protective value of the combined test extends not only for present disease, but also predicts low risk for a number of years in the future,[11,12] providing the rationale for screening no more frequently than every 3 years. The advantage of this approach over the similar recommendation of screening every 2 to 3 years for women having 3 consecutive negative/normal Paps is that the reassurance provided is not subject to the significant variability in test sensitivity noted with the Pap, which requires serial screening to achieve high sensitivity. Rather it, is almost totally secondary to consistently high single test sensitivity.

This is particularly important because the women at highest risk are those who are screened infrequently and so are unlikely to obtain the three negative/normal tests required for extended screening. Both the ACS and ACOG guidelines strongly recommend that combined screening be done no more frequently than every 3 years for women testing negative/normal on both the Pap and the HPV test,[19,20] for screening more frequently would detect only new transient infections or early persistent lesions destined to be detected on the next 3 year screening interval (Table 18.8). Such overscreening would greatly increase cost without benefit and potentially result in the overtreatment of many women having only transient HPV infections.[127]

However, most women with a positive test for high-risk HPV and a normal Pap do not have significant cervical neoplasia. Combining the HPV test with the Pap results in further degradation of specificity of 0.5–4.1% in five of the studies, with an increase in specificity of 0.5% in the UK study and a decrease of 15% in the China study.[57,63,128–132] The aberration in the latter study was due to excessive overcall on the Pap and not to poor specificity for the HPV test[129]. In order to decrease the decrement in specificity of the HPV test, it is best to begin using this combination testing only for women age 30 and over, as the likelihood of being HPV positive in the absence of disease decreases with increasing age. Even women in this age group have a relatively low likelihood of having high-grade CIN when they have a positive HPV test/normal Pap result and have been previously screened. In the Portland NCI prospective study the risk of detection of a high-grade lesion over the 3–5 years following a positive HPV test/negative Pap was 4.4% but only 0.24% for women testing HPV negative/normal Pap.[126] It is this nearly 20-fold increased

Table 18.8   HPV Testing with the Pap in Primary Screening

Recommendations from the ACS and ACOG on the use of HPV testing with the Pap in primary screening

ACS Recommendation:[19]
- The ACS guideline review panel found HPV DNA testing with cytology for primary cervical cancer screening to be promising.
- For women aged 30 and over, as an alternative to cervical cytology testing alone, cervical screening may be performed every three years using conventional or liquid-based cytology combined with a test for DNA from high-risk HPV types.
- Frequency of combined cytology and HPV DNA testing should NOT be more often than every three years.
- Counseling and education related to HPV infection is a critical need.

ACOG Recommendation:[20]
- ***The combined use of a cervical cytology test and an FDA-approved test for high-risk types of HPV***—Under this option, women receive both a cervical cytology test and a genetic test that looks for certain high-risk types of HPV known to cause cancer (HPV DNA test).
- Once women test negative on both tests they should be rescreened with the combined tests no more frequently than every 3 years.
- If only one of the tests is negative, however, more frequent screening will be necessary.
- The combined testing is not appropriate for women under age 30, since they frequently test positive for HPV that will clear up on its own.

Table 18.9   Interim Guidance on the Use of HPV DNA Testing with Cytology in Primary Cervical Screening[10]

General considerations:
- HPV DNA testing may be added to cervical cytology for screening in women 30 years of age and older.
- Use of the combination of HPV DNA testing and cervical cytology should be discontinued at the same age and under the same circumstances, as cervical cytology screening.
- HPV DNA testing should not be added to cervical cytology for screening in women under the age of 30, or for women who are immunosuppressed for any reason, and following hysterectomy.

Management:
- Women negative by both cytology and HPV testing should not be rescreened before 3 years.
- Women negative by cytology but HPV DNA positive should not undergo colposcopy. Instead HPV testing and cytology should be repeated at 6–12 months.
- Other combinations of test results are covered in the 2001 ASCCP Consensus Guidelines.

risk with a positive HPV test that confirms the need for increased surveillance and the very low risk over 3–5 years for detection of a significant lesion in HPV-negative women that verifies the safety of 3-year extended screening intervals. Additionally, the level of risk with a positive HPV test is not dissimilar to that of an unscreened population and is below the level of risk of women referred to colposcopy for abnormal cervical cytology. For example, the positive predictive value for CIN 2,3 for referral to colposcopy of a woman with a single ASCUS Pap is 6–12% and for a HPV positive ASC-US is 15–20%.[24–26] Therefore, restricting referral to colposcopy to those women testing positive for high-risk HPV at a defined interval that documents persistence for at least 6–12 months has been proposed by the interim guidance committee on HPV testing in primary screening.[10] As with testing for HPV in the management of abnormal cervical cytology, only the high-risk HPV test panel should be done, as this is a cervical cancer screening test and low risk types are not involved in oncogenesis.[8,9,10] Recommendations on the use of HPV testing with cervical cytology in the screening of women over the age of 30 are outlined in (Table 18.9).

Table 18.10   HPV Testing and Patient Education: Key Counseling Points

Key counseling points for women having HPV testing
• Genital HPV infections are almost always acquired through sexual contact.
• The use of condoms gives minimal protection from getting HPV.
• Long-term persistent infection with certain types of HPV, called "high-risk" HPV, is necessary for cervical cancer to occur.
• HPV infections are so common that almost all sexually active people become infected at some point in their lifetime.
• Most HPV positive women become HPV negative within 1–2 years due to their immune response.
• HPV positive tests are much less common in women over the age of 30 than in younger women.
• Approximately 10% of women 30 years and older will be positive for "high-risk" types of HPV.
• Most HPV positive women do not have CIN 2,3 or cancer and most will not develop cervical disease.
• Women who are persistently infected with "high-risk" HPV types are at greater risk for having cervical disease, most of which is easily treated.

18.4.4.1 When HPV testing and the Pap should not be used in primary screening

There are several areas in which HPV testing and the Pap should not be used in combined primary cervical screening. Most importantly, combining HPV testing with cytology as a primary screen for women under the age of 30 is not recommended because the prevalence of high-risk HPV at this age is very high (15–46%) and most women testing positive have only transient infections.[99,133] Additionally, cervical cancer is uncommon in women under the age of 30, although it does begin to rise between 25–30.[1,97] In contrast, the prevalence of high-risk HPV in women age 40 and over is approximately 5%.

The prevalence of HPV in immunosuppressed women is also too high (up to 60% in some studies) to utilize combined HPV testing and cytology in the screening of women with HIV and other immunosuppression.[10] Also, the natural history of emergence and progression of high-grade lesions is shortened by immunosuppression and the incidence of CIN is increased.[134] Extended screening intervals based upon estimates derived from women with normal immunity may be unsafe.

Women having had a hysterectomy for benign disease, with no evidence of high-grade CIN or cervical cancer at the time of the hysterectomy do not need cervical screening as per the ACS and ACOG guidelines, and therefore are not candidates for combined HPV testing and cytology.[5,10,19]

18.4.4.2 Unknowns and cautions regarding HPV testing in primary screening

Clinicians using HPV testing in both primary cervical screening and in abnormal Pap management must thoroughly understand the natural history of HPV and cervical cancer. Otherwise there is significant concern that a number of problems will occur, particularly with combined screening.[135] While a double negative test gives great reassurance that a 3 year screening interval is quite safe, a positive test provides much more complex information. Clinicians must understand that 5–15% of women in this age range will test positive for high-risk HPV and only 0.5%–1.0% in an already well-screened population will have CIN 2,3 or an extremely rare cancer at the time of the initial positive HPV test.[126] Therefore it is imperative that the medical community not respond aggressively to a single positive test in the absence of an abnormal Pap. Because most HPV is transient, even in women over the age of 30, and only persistent high-risk HPV is at-risk for development of high-grade CIN and cancer, testing for persistence of HPV no sooner than 6 to 12 months will be necessary in order to minimize over-evaluation and overtreatment. This should capture most significant lesions within a reasonable time frame, while allowing non-persistent HPV (45–60% will become HPV negative within 6–12 months)[126,128] to resolve, thereby reducing the colposcopic referral load to a manageable level. It will also be imperative that clinicians understand that treating a woman with a positive HPV test in the absence of documented disease is not acceptable.

Educating women about the nature of a positive HPV test, including what is known about the risk of HPV transmission to a new partner, risk of developing a treatable cervical lesion, and the source of infection, is imperative if women are to not be made exceedingly anxious about testing positive for "high-risk" HPV (Table 18.10). Discuss the reason that high-risk HPV is given this name—that despite the association of certain HPV types with high-grade CIN and cervical cancer the risk of development of either of these

Table 18.11   Key Points for Clinicians Regarding HPV Testing

- Understand the natural history of HPV infections and be able to appropriately counsel patients before using the test.
- Reassure HPV positive patients that it is usually not possible to determine when or where they became infected.
- Reassure HPV DNA positive patients that most "high-risk" HPV DNA positive women do not have CIN 2,3 or cancer.
- Test only for "high-risk" HPV types.
- Utilize only well-characterized, highly sensitive testing methods.
- Focus on identifying women with persistent HPV infections, not transient infections.
- Do not utilize HPV DNA testing for primary screening of women under the age of 30.
- Do not perform loop excision, cryotherapy or conization simply on the basis of a positive "high-risk" HPV test in the absence of documented CIN.

lesions is relatively low and that only persistent HPV infections indicate enough potential for a treatable lesion to warrant colposcopy. Counseling and educating patients is made even more difficult by an incomplete understanding of viral latency and whether most HPV is eventually cleared completely or just suppressed by immunity to levels below the threshold for detection by very sensitive HPV tests. Reassure that even if it is not possible to know whether HPV is completely cleared, or just suppressed, once the HPV test becomes negative the individual is not likely to continue to be infective to a new partner. It is also imperative to reassure the patient that detectable HPV probably indicates that she shares this virus with her partner and that successful clearance or suppression of HPV by either partner is only dependent upon one's own immunity and is not affected by possible re-exposure to the same HPV type through continued sexual activity with their partner. These messages are complex and take time to discuss, but the importance of providing such education cannot be overstated. If clinicians do not feel equipped to provide this education, or do not feel that they have the time, then the anxiety generated in women testing positive will far outweigh any benefit derived by combined testing. There are several key points regarding the clinical use of HPV tests that must be understood by clinicians utilizing HPV testing (Table 18.11). Understanding these issues will ensure that primary screening with HPV testing is a success.

18.5 Guidelines for Specimen Adequacy

Recommendations on the clinical management of women with Paps reporting qualifiers to the adequacy of the specimen were not actually developed at the 2001 ASCCP Consensus Conference, but the committee that developed "specimen adequacy guidelines" was appointed at this conference and given the task of creating the guidelines in the following discussion.[121] In all cases adequacy issues only apply when no abnormal cells are identified, for by definition, the finding of abnormal cells designates the Pap as "Satisfactory for evaluation".[121] Table 18.12 lists the final adequacy recommendations, and the following text provides the rationale.

18.5.1 Management of women with a Pap lacking an endocervical/transformation zone (EC/TZ) component

A number of studies found that Paps were more likely to have abnormal cells identified when endocervical cells were present on the slide.[125,136,137] However, this association has not been shown in other studies,[123,138,139] nor have women lacking an EC/TZ component been shown to have increased detection of CIN in follow-up.[140,141] Additionally, retrospective case-control studies have failed to show an association between absence of an EC/TZ and false negative Paps.[142,143] Although improved sampling technique and the use of better sampling devices tend to increase the collection of EC/TZ cells,[137,138,144,145] it is not always possible to obtain these cells. Interobserver variability in the interpretation of EC/TZ cells[146,147] and the less frequent identification of these cells in women on oral contraceptives, or women pregnant or postmenopausal,[137,148,149] all prohibit consistent finding of these cells on the Pap despite good clinician technique and the use of appropriate endocervical sampling devices.[150] With all of these considerations in mind, the preferred option for most women lacking an EC/TZ component is to repeat the Pap in 12 months or postpartum

Table 18.12   Specimen Adequacy Guidelines[121]

ASCCP Guidelines on Issues Related to the Quality of the Pap Test

Issue 1.0: What is the appropriate follow-up for women with a negative/normal Pap lacking and endocervical/transformation zone (EC/TZ) component?

Recommendation: The preferred option for most women is an annual repeat Pap. A postpartum repeat is preferred for pregnant patients. An early repeat (6 months) may be beneficial for some women. Indications for considering an early repeat include: (1) a previous squamous abnormality (ASC-US or worse) without 3 consecutive negative Paps with at least one containing EC/TZ component, (2) a previous Pap with unexplained glandular atypia (AGC) or glandular neoplasia, (3) a positive high-risk/oncogenic HPV test within 12 months, (4) the clinician's inability to clearly visualize the cervix or sample the endocervical canal, or (5) insufficient previous screening (no prior Pap within 3 years or less than 3 in last 10 years).

Issue 2.0: What is the appropriate follow-up for women with a negative (for intraepithelial lesion or malignancy) Pap that has partially obscuring blood, inflammation, other partial obscuring factors or partial air-drying?

Recommendation: The preferred option for most women is an annual repeat Pap. A postpartum repeat is preferred for pregnant patients. Clinical correlation is suggested when there is partially obscuring blood or inflammation, especially if these findings persist in more than one Pap, or if there are other suspicious patient signs and symptoms. An early repeat (6–12 months) is acceptable and may be beneficial for some women. Indications for considering an early repeat include: (1) a previous squamous abnormality (ASC-US or worse) without 3 consecutive negative Paps with at least one containing EC/TZ component, (2) a previous Pap with unexplained glandular atypia (AGC) or glandular neoplasis, (3) positive high-risk/oncogenic HPV test within 12 months, (4) the clinician's inability to clearly visualize the cervix or sample the endocervical canal, or (5) insufficient previous screening (no prior Pap within 3 years or less than 3 in last 10 years).

Issue 3.0: What is the appropriate follow-up for women with an unsatisfactory Pap test?

Recommendation: The preferred management for most women with unsatisfactory Pap tests is a repeat Pap test within a short interval, generally within 2–4 months. Clinical correlation is suggested as some women may benefit from additional clinical evaluation that could include colposcopy and/or histologic studies where appropriate. Women with an unsatisfactory Pap test that is obscured by inflammation and have an identified organism should receive specific treatment prior to repeating the Pap. An exception to an early repeat Pap is when the current unsatisfactory Pap was unnecessary, and this Pap was either not processed or did not contain findings that are possible signs of a pathologic process (i.e. no excessive blood, inflammation, or necrosis).

Adapted from: Davey DD, Austin RM, Birdsong G, Buck HW, Cox JT, Darragh TM, Elgert PA, Hanson V, Henry MR, Waldman J; American Society for Colposcopy and Cervical Pathology. ASCCP patient management guidelines: Pap test specimen adequacy and quality indicators. *J Lower Gen Track Dis* 2002;6(3):195–9.

when the patient is pregnant.[121] However, if the patient has one of the following factors that increase risk, an early repeat at 6 months may be beneficial. Indications for considering an early repeat include:[121] (1) a previous squamous abnormality (ASC-US or worse) without 3 follow-up consecutive negative Paps with at least one containing EC/TZ component, (2) a previous Pap with unexplained glandular atypia (AGC) or glandular neoplasia, (3) a positive high-risk/oncogenic HPV test within 12 months, (4) the clinician's inability to clearly visualize the cervix or sample the endocervical canal, or (5) insufficient

previous screening (no prior Pap within 3 years or less than 3 in last 10 years).

18.5.2 Management of women with a Pap that has partially obscuring blood, inflammation, other partial obscuring factors or partial air-drying

Data on the significance of partially obscuring blood and inflammation is very limited, with only two retrospective case-control studies on the subject. Both found no difference in the rate of detection of CIN 3 between Paps partially obscured by these factors than those that were not.[142,143] However, despite the lack of information on the importance of partially obscuring factors, it was felt that providing this information on the Pap report was important and recognized the potential significance of conflicting data and increasing concern over the rising incidence of adenocarcinoma.[121] The recommendation that Paps with partially limiting factors should be repeated annually, rather than return to routine screening (which could be longer intervals) reflected the need to balance the potential for over-evaluation with the desire to protect women from the possibility of missed disease.

As with Paps lacking an EC/TZ component, Paps partially obscured by blood, inflammation or other factors may be repeated in 6 months in selected patients having one of the following: insufficient prior screening, women with incomplete visualization of the cervix, women with a history of abnormalities lacking 3 recent negative Paps, and women with a recent positive high-risk HPV test.[121] Liquid based Paps (LBP) may be considered when the Pap is repeated, as liquid sampling generally decreases obscuring problems. In contrast, a recent negative high-risk HPV test suggests a low risk for cervical pathology and would support a regular screening interval. Detection of CIN 3 or glandular abnormality on previous Paps or histology should increase concern for Paps partially obscured by these factors. Use of either LBP or more careful attention to fixation of a conventional Pap should be considered when air drying problems are responsible for the limiting factor.[121,151] Additionally, if partially obscuring blood or inflammation persist in more than one Pap or if there are patient symptoms or findings of increased concern, early repeat or colposcopy may be appropriate depending upon the clinical indications.

18.5.3 Management of women with an unsatisfactory Pap test

A Pap is considered "unsatisfactory for evaluation" under any of the following conditions: Paps that cannot be processed because of insufficient labeling, slide breakage, or leakage of liquid specimens, and Paps that are processed and fully evaluated by the laboratory but do not satisfy the minimum criteria for squamous cellularity. This criterion varies depending on whether the Pap is a conventional smear or a LBP test. Although unsatisfactory Paps are unreliable for evaluation, the background elements such as blood or inflammation may provide important information. For example, a cohort of women with unsatisfactory Paps were found to have signifi-

cantly more CIN or cancer on follow-up when compared to patients with satisfactory Paps[121,152] and a retrospective study documented an association between unsatisfactory Paps and development of high grade lesions.[153] Unsatisfactory Paps are common in women with invasive cervical cancer; therefore women with an unsatisfactory Pap should have a repeat Pap within 2–4 months, and clinical correlation may at times suggest the need for additional clinical evaluation such as colposcopy and/or other histologic studies.[121] The only exception to early repeat is in an asymptomatic woman having a Pap that was not necessary in the first place and the background of the Pap is not worrisome for a pathologic process.

18.6 Guidelines for the Management of Women with Abnormal Cervical Cytology

By 2001 a fertile ground for the development of evidence-based management guidelines was established by the availability of extensive new data on abnormal Pap management from the NCI ASCUS/LSIL Triage Study (ALTS) and from other studies, as well as from the new cytologic terminology provided by the Bethesda workshop. In September 2001 evidence-based guidelines for the management of women with cervical cytological abnormalities and cervical cancer precursors were developed at a consensus conference sponsored by the ASCCP.[8] The consensus conference included representatives from 29 participating professional organizations, Federal agencies, and national and international health organizations and included a wide spectrum of experts in cervical screening and management. The following management guidelines were developed at this consensus conference and have become the standard of practice in the United States.

18.6.1 Management of ASC-US

The 1988 Bethesda System placement of cells with changes that lack a clear etiology in a category designated to be abnormal resulted in several management dilemmas.[24] The most important was the substantial increase in Paps reported as abnormal, many not reflecting underlying neoplasia. Also of great significance was marked interobserver variation in the reporting of equivocal cellular changes, which was not resolved with attempts to more specifically define the characteristics of atypical squamous cells.[154] Numerous studies on interobserver variability have shown that the reproducibility of the ASC interpretation is less than 50%, as one cytologist's interpretation of a cellular change as ASCUS may be interpreted by another as reactive and reparative or as squamous intraepithelial lesion (SIL).[155-157] This results in significant variation in the reporting of ASC from one lab to another that may alter the perception of risk and the subsequent clinical response. Additionally, the equivocal nature of many cellular changes and an ever-expanding hunt for safe-refuge from malpractice litigation[158] resulted in ASCUS quickly becoming the most prevalent abnormal Pap interpretation. From 2 to 3 million women per year were now given the Pap interpretation of ASCUS and required some undefined follow-up.[159,160] Although the majority of women with ASCUS are not found to have CIN 2,3 or cancer, the sheer number of women with ASCUS is so large that the overall burden of CIN 2,3 detected in response to an atypical Pap is greater than for any other Pap category.[83] This dichotomy resulted in much confusion over how to best manage women given this Pap interpretation.

The most common response initially was to send all women with ASCUS to colposcopy, but the high prevalence of normal findings led many to conclude that most women with cells interpreted as "of undetermined significance" were normal and consequently that these Paps were not "of significance". However, reports of CIN 2,3 in 10–20% of women with ASCUS and a risk of 1/1000 already having invasive cancer continued to generate a clinical dilemma of how to best find the "needle in the haystack" amongst a majority of women who are normal.[161] The magnitude of this problem generated a major commitment by the National Cancer Institute (NCI) to evaluate the best triage option for ASCUS Paps in ALTS.[162] The findings from ALTS are dramatically changing our understanding not only of the best management strategies for ASCUS and LSIL but also of the natural history of cervical cancer precursor lesions and the parameters of the tests and procedures used to elucidate these lesions.[163] In order to better understand the management issues surrounding an ASC Pap it is important to discuss the risk attendant with this Pap interpretation, the findings of the ALTS trial and of other studies on the initial management of atypical squamous cells, and the findings of these studies during the post-colposcopy management of women evaluated for ASC.

The risk of ASC-US: Atypical cells are often generated in response to events occurring in the vaginal environment that have nothing to do with HPV or with neoplasia. Most of these cellular changes are difficult to interpret reactive and reparative changes secondary to trauma from tampon use, intercourse, bacteria, yeast and other normal "life" events. The epithelial effects of aging and declining estrogen also result in cellular changes whose meaning may be unclear. The other most frequent cause of equivocal

cellular changes is HPV, which depending upon the age of the clinic population screened may account for nearly 70% of the ASCUS (very young) to 30% or less (over the age of 30).[78] Definitive cellular changes due to HPV occur when HPV is actively replicating within infected cells. The classic HPV cellular findings of enlarged, irregular nuclei within cytoplasm that is "ballooned out," or has a perinuclear halo, produce the "koilocyte". Although mimics of koilocytes do occur, when the features are classic they are almost diagnostic of infection with HPV. However, many cellular changes due to HPV are less certain, either because the cellular changes are much less abnormal or the number of abnormal cells is few. When classic, koilocytes designate the Pap interpretation to be LSIL. When less classic, the interpretation is ASCUS.

Even when ASCUS is due to HPV, the majority of patients do not have cervical intraepithelial neoplasia grade 2 or 3 (CIN 2,3) or cancer. However, the detection of HPV from a patient with ASCUS dramatically raises the risk. A review of a number of studies on ASCUS management (Table 18.13) illustrates the point that women with HPV positive ASCUS are 12.5-23 times more likely to be found to have CIN 2,3+ at initial colposcopy than women with HPV negative ASCUS.[24-26] The difference becomes even greater when the cumulative 2-year detection for CIN 2,3 for women referred for HPV positive ASCUS but not initially found to have CIN 2,3 is added in (up from 20.1% at initial colposcopy to 26.9%).[26,163] Although some consider even HPV positive ASCUS to be of minimal risk, most would not consider a risk of high-grade disease of over 1 in 4 to be minimal. In fact, 39% of the total CIN 2,3 reported from a routine screening population was detected following triage of ASCUS and fully 69% was from all equivocal and low-grade Pap diagnoses.[83] Additionally, approximately 1/1000 women with ASCUS already have invasive cervical cancer. While this risk per woman is small, the commonness of ASCUS (2.5 million/year) means that around 2,500 cervical cancers and 222,000 CIN 3s (ALTS rate for CIN 3 of 8.8% × 2.5 million ASCUS) may be found each year following referral of women with this Pap interpretation. It is this risk amongst a majority that is either normal or only have transient low-grade HPV changes that has established ASCUS as a giant clinical headache.[161]

Eliminating ASCUS: Some have proposed that the ASC category be eliminated by relegating atypical cells either into the normal category or into SIL.[164] However, most experts in cytopathology and in the management of women with abnormal Paps believe that it is essential to maintain an equivocal category because this "gray" area is difficult to further define

Table 18.13 Three Studies Indicating the Relative Risk for Initial Detection of CIN 2, 3 for Women Referred for the Evaluation of ASCUS, Depending on HPV Results

Study	Risk for Detection of CIN 2+ at Initial Colposcopy		Total risk for all ASCUS
	ASCUS		
	HPV pos	HPV neg	
Cox*[24] 1995	17% **14/81**	0.74% **1/136**	6.9% **15/217**
Manos**[25] 1999	15% 45/300	1.2% 6/498	6.4% 51/801
Solomon (ALTS)**[26] 2000	20% **195/1087**	1.1% **13/1175**	11.9% **208/2210**

*hc1 (expanded 1st generation Hybrid capture test)

**hc2 (2nd generation Hybrid capture test)

and has a large number of cases with underlying CIN 2 and 3.[165] In a litigious climate such as that in the US, the elimination of an equivocal cytology category might significantly increase risk, given the high expectations for very sensitive cervical cytological screening in this country. The Bethesda 2001 Workshop did recommend the elimination of the subcategory of ASCUS "favor reactive" by placing the interpretation of cells that most likely are reactive and reparative in the normal category, but the equivocal category remained for the other findings interpreted as ASCUS.[164] Eliminating ASCUS "favor reactive" was supported by data showing that women with ASCUS "favor dysplasia" were much more likely to be HPV positive (60%) and to have CIN 2,3 (11.2%), than were women with ASCUS "favor reactive" (24% HPV positive, 2.2% CIN 2,3).[25] One group recently reported on an attempt to eliminate ASCUS by reclassifying each Pap as either negative (within normal limits/benign cellular changes), low-grade SIL (LSIL), or high-grade SIL (HSIL) in a blind retrospective review of Paps originally interpreted as ASCUS, all of which had histologic follow-up.[165] Thirty-nine percent of the women with Paps downgraded to normal had histologic CIN and 17% had CIN 2,3, which reduced the sensitivity for CIN 2,3 of this ASCUS group of Paps from 100% to 41%. The authors concluded that eliminating the ASCUS diagnosis would significantly decrease the sensitivity of the Pap and appears to be no better than chance at predicting a diagnosis of SIL on biopsy, including HSIL.[165]

Clarifying the management of ASCUS—the ALTS trial data: ALTS is the only prospective, randomized clinical trial to evaluate the three primary follow-up options for ASCUS and LSIL Paps: immediate colposcopy, accelerated repeat Pap with liquid-based cytology with ThinPrep Pap®, and testing for the presence of HPV with HC2®.[26,162] ALTS did not formally evaluate other potential candidates for the triage of ASCUS for there was insufficient data on the clinical use of these tests at the time to justify inclusion in the study. Therefore, the potential utility of direct visual inspection (DVI), speculoscopy, cervicography and spectroscopy in the management of equivocal and low-grade Pap interpretations was not evaluated and will await further study. Proponents of immediate colposcopy for all women with ASCUS argue that sending all women with ASCUS to colposcopy would theoretically detect all CIN 2,3 and cancer. However, the positive predictive value of this approach will always be low due to the low (6.4–11.9%) rate of CIN 2,3 among women with ASCUS[24-26] and the cost and anxiety generated are typically high.[166] Repeat cytology requires at least two repeat optimized liquid-based Paps to equal the sensitivity of a single HPV test and is therefore likely to not be cost-competitive with HPV-testing triage due to the high rate of repeat abnormal cytology requiring colposcopic evaluation.[26,66]

Cervical cytology has been a good screening test, but its comparatively low sensitivity (51–83%) and poor reproducibility diminishes its value as a triage test.[37,39,66,157,167] For example, in ALTS out of 1,473 repeat Paps originally read by good clinical center pathologists, only 633 were reread as ASCUS when the interpretation was based upon consensus agreement in a blinded review by an expert panel of cytopathologists.[157] In other words, 840 or 57% were reread as something other than ASCUS. Most were downgraded to normal. In a repeat Pap scenario,

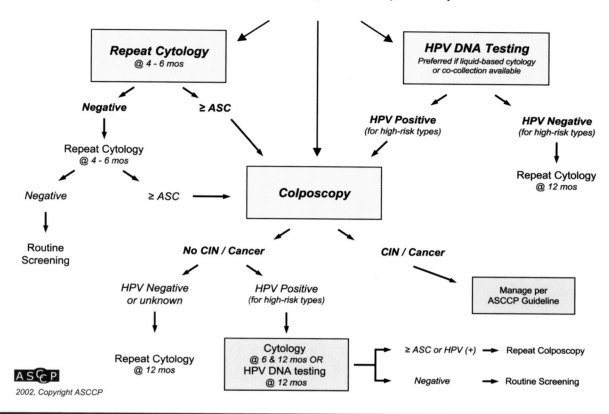

FIGURE 18.2   ASCCP algorithm for the management of women with cervical cytology interpreted as atypical squamous cells of undetermined significance (ASC-US). From: Wright T C Jr, Cox J T, Massad L S, Twiggs L B, Wilkinson E J. 2001 Consensus guidelines for the management of women with cervical cytological abnormalities. *J Low Gen Tract Dis* 2002;6:127–43. With permission.

many of these women would incur the cost and inconvenience of colposcopy. Clearly an objective test that indicates initially which women with ASCUS are at-risk for CIN 2,3 either now or in the future, and which are not, should hold a significant advantage. HPV positive women are clearly at-risk, justifying the anxiety and cost of colposcopic referral, while HPV negative women may be appropriately reassured.

18.6.1.1 Management guidelines for women with ASC-US

A formal evidence-based review of the literature documented that all three options for the management of women with ASCUS are safe and effective.[8] Therefore management by immediate colposcopy, repeat cytology or HPV testing are all acceptable options for the management of ASC-US, but testing for HPV was considered the preferred option when the Pap was obtained on a liquid-based sample or co-collected

(Figure 18.2). This preference was based upon several factors. First, liquid-based Paps have residual cells in the fluid from which a HPV test can be obtained. This eliminates the return visit for the follow-up triage test, whether for repeat Pap or HPV test, that in turn saves clinic and patient time and decreases costs. Second, the ALTS data documented that HPV triage was essentially equivalent to immediate colposcopy in sensitivity for high-grade CIN, while halving colposcopic referrals.[26,167] However, it is important to clarify that data suggest that HPV testing is equally useful for managing ASC-US whether derived from either conventional Pap or from LBP. The problem with HPV triage of ASC-US interpreted from a conventional Pap is the requirement for an added patient office visit to obtain the HPV test, diminishing the cost-effectiveness of this approach.[44] Both the frequency of ASC-US Paps[168] and the rate of HPV detection with ASC-US[169] appear to be comparable for LBPs and conventional smears.

Table 18.14　ASCCP Guidelines for the Management of Women with ASC[8]

- A program of repeat cervical cytology, or colposcopy, or DNA testing for high-risk types of HPV are all acceptable methods for managing women with ASC-US. **(AI)**
- When liquid-based cytology is used, or when co-collection for HPV DNA testing can be done, "reflex" HPV DNA testing is the preferred approach. **(AI)**
- DNA testing for high-risk types of HPV should be performed using a sensitive molecular test and all women who are HPV DNA positive should be referred for colposcopic evaluation. **(AII)**
- Women with ASC-US who are high-risk HPV DNA negative can be followed-up with repeat cytology at 12 months. **(BII)**
- Acceptable management options for women who are positive for high-risk types of HPV, but who do not have biopsy-confirmed CIN, include follow-up with repeat cytology at 6 and 12 months with referral back to colposcopy if a result of ASC-US or greater is obtained, or HPV DNA testing at 12 months with referral back to colposcopy of all HPV DNA positive women. **(BII)**
- When a program of repeat cervical cytology is used, women with ASC-US should undergo repeat cytological testing (either conventional or liquid-based) at 4–6 month intervals until two consecutive "negative for intraepithelial lesion or malignancy" results are obtained. **(AII)**
- Women diagnosed with ASC-US or greater cytological abnormality on the repeat tests should be referred for colposcopy. **(AII)**
- After two "negative for intraepithelial lesion or malignancy" repeat cytology tests are obtained, women can be returned to routine cytological screening programs. **(AII)**
- When immediate colposcopy is used to manage women with ASC-US, women who are referred to colposcopy and not found to have CIN should be followed-up with repeat cytology at 12 months. **(BII)**
- Women with ASC-US who are referred for colposcopy and found to have biopsy-confirmed CIN should be managed according the appropriate Consensus Guideline for the Management of Women with Cervical Histological Abnormalities.[9]
- Because of the potential for overtreatment, diagnostic excisional procedures such as loop electrosurgical excision (i.e., LEEP) should not be routinely used to treat women with ASC in the absence of biopsy-confirmed CIN. **(EII)**

Adapted from: Wright T C Jr, Cox J T, Massad L S, Twiggs L B, Wilkinson E J. Consensus Guidelines for the management of women with cervical cytological abnormalities. *JAMA* 2002;287:2120–2129. With permission.

Comparable sensitivity for detection of CIN 2,3 in ALTS was attained by either a single HPV test or by two repeat liquid-based Paps when the threshold for referral to colposcopy was a positive HPV test or a repeat Pap at ≥ASC-US.[26,167,170] The guidelines recommend that women managed by immediate colposcopy and found to be negative or triaged to observation by a single negative HPV test, should have a follow-up Pap at 12 months.[9] Notice that the guidelines do not state that these women can return directly to routine screening, for in some practice settings "routine screening" is set at 2 or 3 year intervals and some minimal risk for missed CIN 2,3 still exists. For example, 1/83 CIN 2,3s were missed by HPV testing in the Manos et al study, 1/90 in ALTS, and 1/136 in the study by Cox et al.[24-26] Colposcopy did not initially detect 25% of the cumulative high-grade lesions detected over two-year follow-up in ALTS.[167] Therefore to achieve similar sensitivity for CIN 2,3

the guidelines recommend that women managed by repeat cytology have two repeat normal Paps at 4–6 month intervals before returning to routine screening. Some may prefer to repeat the Pap in one year following two repeat negative cervical cytologies similar to the recommendation for follow-up to a negative HPV test. A summary of the management recommendations for women with ASC-US are listed in (Table 18.14).

Because low-risk HPV types are not a cause of CIN 3 or cancer, it is recommended that the HPV test used be a sensitive test and that testing be for high-risk types only.[8] At present the only FDA-approved HPV test is Hybrid Capture 2®, (HC2) [Digene, Gaithersburg, MD] and because this test has available both low- and high-risk HPV panels, it is important for cost-effectiveness to designate to the laboratory that the sample be tested by only the high-risk panel. All women positive for high-risk HPV are to be

Table 18.15   Estimated Triage Test Performance in the ALTS Trial for the Detection of Cumulative CIN 3 Over the 2-years of the Trial.

CIN 3 diagnosis is that given by the ALTS Pathology Quality Control Group. Sensitivity for CIN3 and percent referral to colposcopy is given for the Hybrid Capture 2 HPV test and for repeat liquid-based Pap at one of three potential thresholds for referral to colposcopy: Paps interpreted as HSIL only, LSIL and above or ASCUS and above. One, two and three represents Paps repeated at ASCCP Guideline recommendations of every 4–6 months. Hence "One" is the first Pap usually repeated at 4–6 months, "Two" is the second Pap repeated at 8–12 months, and "Three" would be the third Pap, if three Paps were to be done, repeated at 12–18 months.

	% Sensitivity for CIN 3	% Referral
Enrollment HPV DNA Test	92.4% (88.7–95.2)	53.2% (51.5–54.9)
HSIL Cytology Threshold		
One	35.5% (30.0–41.3)	7.1% (6.2–8.0)
Two	48.3% (38.8–57.7)	10.2% (8.5–12.0)
Three	60.2% (50.8–69.6)	11.7% (9.8–13.6)
LSIL Cytology Threshold		
One	59.3% (53.4–65.0)	25.1% (23.6–26.6)
Two	74.1% (65.8–82.3)	31.7% (29.0–34.4)
Three	82.0% (74.7–89.4)	37.2% (34.4–40.1)
ASCUS Cytology Threshold		
One	83.4% (78.7–87.5)	58.1% (56.4–59.8)
Two	95.4% (91.4–99.3)	67.1% (64.4–69.8)
Three	97.2% (94.1–100)	72.7% (70.1–75.4)

From: ASCUS-LSIL Triage Study (ALTS) Group. Results of a randomized trial on the management of cytology interpretations of atypical squamous cells of undetermined significance. *Am J Obstet Gynecol* 2003;188:1383–92. With Permission.

referred to colposcopy. The sensitivity for CIN 2,3 of the HPV test used in ALTS [Hybrid Capture 2] of 92.4% was matched only by two repeat Paps at a threshold of referral to colposcopy of any repeat abnormal Pap of ≥ASC-US (Table 18.15).[167] Therefore, when repeat cytology is used to triage women with ASC-US, the recommendation is to refer women to colposcopy at the threshold on repeat of any Pap of ≥ASC-US. At this threshold 95% of the CIN 2,3 was detected, but this level of reassurance would only be obtained an average of 8–12 months following nearly identical reassurance provided by the initial HPV test. Additionally, if all women returned as directed for repeat cytology, more women would be referred to colposcopy by repeat abnormal Paps at the ASC-US threshold than would be referred to colposcopy by testing positive for high-risk HPV types. In ALTS 53% tested positive for high-risk HPV and were referred to colposcopy. In contrast, 67% of women managed by repeat Pap had an abnormal Pap on either the first or on the second repeat requiring colposcopy in addition to one or two additional office visits.[167] Reducing

this high rate of referral to colposcopy would require either significant loss to follow-up (which occurs in all practice settings) or increasing the threshold for referral to colposcopy to ≥LSIL on repeat. However, two repeat Paps at a LSIL threshold only detected 74% of the CIN 2,3 and even after 3 repeats only detected 82%.[167] A higher threshold does not provide adequate reassurance and will delay the diagnosis of many significant cervical lesions.

All of these advantages of HPV testing in the triage of women with ASC-US persist when the initial referral ASC-US Pap is a conventional smear except that HPV testing in this setting either requires that the patient return for a repeat office visit to obtain the HPV test, or that a HPV test be co-collected at the time the primary screening Pap is taken. Whether this requirement is cost-effective in comparison to the repeat Pap or immediate colposcopy options depends primarily on the practice setting, including the percent of women in the practice with ASC-US testing positive for HPV, the cost of colposcopy, repeat cytology, HPV test, office visit and follow-up notification system, and on patient related costs such as time away from work, child-care and transportation costs. Co-collection refers to the option of collecting a sample in a standard Digene HC2® HPV test collection kit on all women at the time of their routine Pap and holding all samples until the Pap results are reported.[8] The HPV test samples from women reported to have ASC-US are then sent to the lab for HPV testing and the remaining samples (approximately 95–97% are not reported as ASC-US in most practices) are not tested and are discarded as medical waste. Cost-modeling has reported this approach to be cost-effective.[87]

18.6.1.2 Management of ASC-US in special circumstances

18.6.1.2.1 Management of women with evidence of vaginal atrophy
Management of ASC-US may differ somewhat from the general ASC-US recommendations when the patient is postmenopausal and for the immunosuppressed (Table 18.16). There are no recommended differences in the management of ASC-US in pregnant women.[8] All three management options, immediate colposcopy, repeat Pap or HPV DNA testing are considered acceptable options for the management of postmenopausal women with ASC-US.[8] (Figure 18.3) However, estrogen deficiency is a common cause of ASC-US in postmenopausal women and is responsible for increasing rates of HPV negative ASC-

US in this age group despite continued high sensitivity of HPV testing for CIN 2,3.[78] Therefore treatment with vaginal estrogen cream followed by repeat cytology obtained approximately one week after completing the regimen is also given as an option for postmenopausal women with ASC-US and clinical or cytological evidence of atrophy.[8] The usual recommendation for reversing vaginal atrophy is to have the patient apply 1/2 applicator of estrogen cream in the vagina nightly for 3 weeks. This approach may also be helpful for women with evidence of atrophy who are perimenopausal or are younger and on progestin-only contraception. Women with a result on repeat Pap of ≥ ASC-US should be referred for colposcopy, whereas women with a normal repeat Pap should have a second Pap repeated in four to six months. Repeating the course of vaginal estrogen prior to each Pap repeat may be advantageous when atrophy is likely to persist. Following two repeat normal Paps, the patient can return to routine cytological screening.

18.6.1.2.2 Management of women with immunosuppression
Management of ASC-US in HIV-infected women is particularly problematic, as the rates of ASC-US, HPV detection, and CIN are all two-to-three times those of women not having HIV, and the risk of finding CIN 2,3 is much higher.[171] HPV testing as a triage for ASC-US is not efficient for

---

Table 18.16   ASCCP Guidelines: ASC-US in Special Circumstances[8]

Postmenopausal women:
- Providing a course of intravaginal estrogen followed by a repeat cervical cytology obtained approximately a week after completing the regimen is an acceptable option for women with ASC-US who have clinical or cytological evidence of atrophy and no contraindications to using intravaginal estrogen. **(CIII)**
- If the repeat cervical cytology is "negative for squamous intraepithelial lesion or malignancy", the cervical cytology should be repeated in 4–6 months. If both repeat cytology tests are "negative for squamous intraepithelial lesion or malignancy", the patient can return to routine cytological screening, whereas if either repeat cytology is reported as ASC-US or greater, the patient should be referred for colposcopy. **(BIII)**

Immunosuppressed patients:
- Because of the increased risk for CIN 2,3 in immunosuppressed women and the fact that infection with high-risk types of HPV would be expected to be quite common in HIV-infected women (including all HIV-infected women, irrespective of CD4 count, HIV viral load, or antiretroviral therapy) with ASC-US, referral for colposcopy is recommended for all immunosuppressed patients with ASC-US. **(BIII)**

Pregnant patients:
- It is recommended that pregnant women with ASC-US be managed in an identical manner as non-pregnant women. **(BIII)**

Adapted from: Wright T C Jr, Cox J T, Massad L S, Twiggs L B, Wilkinson E J. Consensus Guidelines for the management of women with cervical cytological abnormalities. *JAMA* 2002;287:2120–2129. With permission.

women who are immunosuppressed, because the majority of ASC-US Paps in these women are HPV-positive. These findings all support the ASCCP recommendation that all immunosuppressed women with ASC-US be referred to colposcopy, irrespective of CD4 count, HIV viral load or anti-retroviral therapy.[8]

18.6.1.2 Logistics of managing ASC

The typical abnormal Pap management system has previously been based exclusively on follow-up by repeat cytology, colposcopy and treatment options. Adding another triage test, i.e. HPV testing, necessarily requires retooling our usual follow-up system. This is not difficult when the laboratory that interprets the liquid-based Pap is also the site that performs the "reflex" HPV test, for this allows the Pap report to be issued as "ASC-US HPV negative" or as "ASC-US HPV positive". However, if the HPV test must be done in a separate reference lab, the Pap report will necessarily come in separate from the HPV report and the clinician will have to collate the two reports before notifying the patient. Because the residual liquid-based sample will need to be sent from the cytopathology laboratory to the reference lab and HPV tests are only run when sufficient quantities are "batched" at the laboratory, there will usually be a delay between receipt of the Pap result and the HPV result. Therefore some mechanism is required that flags the ASC-US report and holds it until receipt of the HPV test result. The same situation occurs when the HPV test sample is "co-collected" with the Pap and is sent to the lab for HPV testing only when the Pap is reported as ASC-US.

"Reflex" HPV testing is the term applied when the lab is instructed to perform a HPV test off the residual liquid-based specimen when the Pap is interpreted as ASC-US.[66] When the practice setting

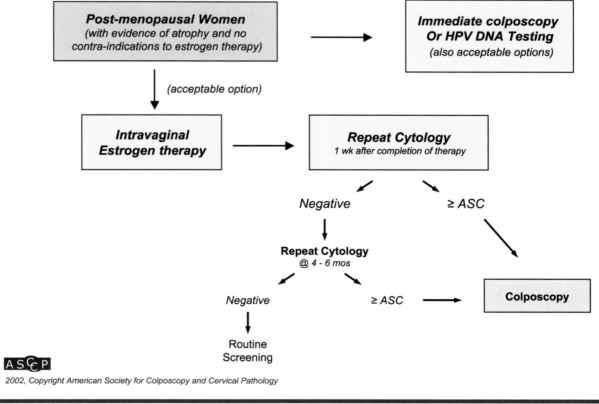

Management of Women with Atypical Squamous Cells of Undetermined Significance (ASC-US) In Special Circumstances

2002, Copyright American Society for Colposcopy and Cervical Pathology

FIGURE 18.3   ASCCP algorithm for the management of women with cervical cytology interpreted as atypical squamous cells of undetermined significance (ASC-US) in special situations. From: Wright T C Jr, Cox J T, Massad L S, Twiggs L B, Wilkinson E J. 2001 Consensus guidelines for the management of women with cervical cytological abnormalities. *J Low Gen Tract Dis* 2002;6:127–43. With permission.

manages all ASC-US except those obtained on immunosuppressed women by "reflex" HPV testing, the lab can be notified to automatically perform the HPV test on all ASC-US without an individual order. However, it must be remembered that a HPV test is a test for a sexually transmitted infection (STI). For that matter, since cervical cancer is caused by HPV, so is a Pap. Therefore, some may want to give all patients a written explanation of the rationale for testing ASC-US Paps for HPV with two check-off options at the bottom indicating whether they would prefer to have HPV testing to clarify their result if it returned as ASC-US, or whether they would prefer one of the other follow-up options. In this scenario the laboratory would need to have a Pap requisition that has a check-off option that designates to the lab whether to do a reflex HPV test if the Pap is ASC-US.

Whenever a new test or procedure is introduced it is also of primary importance that the office staff responsible for completing critical information on the requisition form be adequately trained.[172] This involves knowing when and how to order the test and how to complete insurance information and clinical history on the Pap requisition, including the correct *International Classification of Diseases (ICD-9)* code, to insure that the HPV test is covered by the patient's insurer.

Clinicians using HPV testing must fully understand the usually benign nature of a HPV infection. Reporting a positive HPV test in a manner that does not raise undue concern requires reassuring and non-judgmental communication of the results based upon a broad understanding of the viral natural history, yet fosters responsible follow-up.[161]

18.6.2 Management of ASC-H

Atypical squamous cells "cannot rule out high-grade" (ASC-H) is an uncommon Pap interpretation reported in 0.27%–0.6% of all Paps, or approxi-

mately 1 in 10 Paps read as ASC.[173,174] HPV test and histology results for women in ALTS referred with Paps interpreted as "equivocal low-grade SIL" (ASCUS-L), "equivocal high-grade SIL" (ASCUS-H) and HSIL were compared (Table 18.17).[169] High-risk HPV DNA was detected in 86% of ASCUS-H liquid-based Paps and 69.8% of ASCUS-H conventional smears. CIN 2,3 was found in 40% of ASCUS-H Thin-Preps and in 27.2% of ASCUS-H smears. A three-year retrospective review of ASC-H with follow-up at Johns Hopkins Hospital determined that 49% had no CIN or glandular lesion.[174] Of the 51% with CIN, approximately half were CIN 1 and half were CIN 2,3.

These results indicate that women with ASC-H are clearly more at-risk for CIN 2,3 and therefore should be managed by immediate colposcopy (Figure 18.4). Further management depends on whether CIN is detected. If no CIN is found, the ASCCP Guidelines recommend that the cytology, colposcopy and histology be reviewed and that if there is a change in the diagnosis—for instance if the Pap interpretation is revised to HSIL, then the patient should be managed according to the revised interpretation.[8] In contrast, if there is no change in the diagnosis, then the recommendation is to either follow the patient with repeat cytology at 6 and 12 month intervals or to test for HPV at 12 months. Any repeat abnormal Pap at a threshold of ≥ASC-US or a positive HPV test should prompt repeat colposcopy. ASC-H presents greater risk than ASC-US but less than HSIL, and therefore a surgical excision procedure is not indicated for ASC-H in the absence of documented CIN 2,3.[9] A summary of the management recommendations for ASC-H are listed in (Table 18.18).

18.6.3 Management of LSIL

The 2001 Bethesda System classification defines low-grade squamous intraepithelial lesion (LSIL) as cytological changes associated with cytopathic effects of

Table 18.17 Relative Risk of ASC-H

ALTS data from the Pathology Quality Control cytology interpretations document that the risk for detection of high-risk HPV and CIN 2 and 3 for ASC-H is in-between the risk for ASC-US and the risk for Paps interpreted as HSIL.

Cytology	HPV test results HPV pos	Histology ≥CIN 2	CIN 3
ASC-US	63%	12%	5%
ASC-H	86%	40%	24%
HSIL	99%	59%	38%

From: Sherman M. *AJCP* 2001;116:386–394. With permission.

Management of Women with Atypical Squamous Cells: Cannot Exclude High-grade SIL (ASC - H)

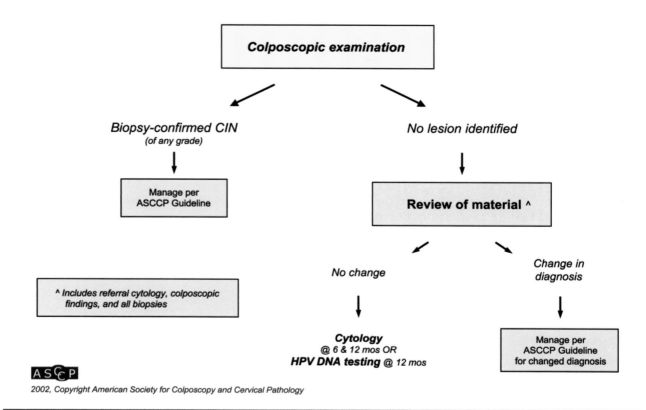

2002, Copyright American Society for Colposcopy and Cervical Pathology

FIGURE 18.4   ASCCP algorithm for the management of women with cervical cytology interpreted as atypical squamous cells "cannot exclude high-grade SIL" (ASC-H). From: Wright T C Jr, Cox J T, Massad L S, Twiggs L B, Wilkinson E J. 2001 Consensus guidelines for the management of women with cervical cytological abnormalities. *J Low Gen Tract Dis* 2002;6:127–43. With permission.

Table 18.18   Management of Women with Atypical Squamous Cells—Cannot Exclude HSIL (ASC-H)[8]

ASCCP Guidelines for the management of women with ASC-H.
• Because of the high prevalence of high-risk types of HPV and of biopsy-confirmed CIN 2,3 among women with ASC-H, the recommended management of women with ASC-H obtained using either conventional or liquid-based cervical cytology is referral for colposcopic evaluation. **(AII)** • When no lesion is identified after colposcopy in women with ASC-H, it is recommended that, when possible, a review of the cytology, colposcopy and histology be performed. **(BIII)** • If the review yields a revised interpretation, management should follow guidelines for the revised interpretation; if a cytological interpretation of ASC-H is upheld, either cytological follow up at 6 and 12 months or HPV DNA testing at 12 months is recommended. **(CIII)**

Adapted from: Wright T C Jr, Cox J T, Massad L S, Twiggs L B, Wilkinson E J. Consensus Guidelines for the management of women with cervical cytological abnormalities. *JAMA* 2002;287:2120–2129. With permission.

Table 18.19 Cumulative Diagnosis* of Two Disease Endpoints (CIN 2, 3 by Clinical Pathology Diagnosis, and CIN 3 by Path QC Consensus Diagnosis) by Referral Pap Interpretations, ASC HPV (+) and LSIL

	HPV + ASCUS (n = 1193)	LSIL (n = 897)
Clinical Center CIN 2 or 3	26.7% (24.2–29.3)	27.6% (24.7–30.7)
Pathology QC Group CIN 3	14.5% (12.6–16.6)	15.9% (13.6–18.5)

*(%) of women diagnosed with the disease endpoints at any time during ALTS enrollment, two-year follow-up, or exit. From: Cox JT, Schiffman M, Solomon D; ASCUS-LSIL Triage Study (ALTS) Group. Prospective follow-up suggests similar risk of subsequent cervical intraepithelial neoplasia grade 2 or 3 among women with cervical intraepithelial neoplasia grade 1 or negative colposcopy and directed biopsy. *Am J Obstet Gynecol.* 2003;188:1406–12. With permission.

HPV known as koilocytotic atypia and mild dysplasia/ CIN 1.[164] LSIL is less common than ASC-US, and in most labs the ASCUS:LSIL ratio will be in the range of 2:1.[8] The 1997 CAP Interlaboratory Comparison Program in Cervicovaginal Cytology (PAP) collected information from participating labs on median Pap rates. The median rate for LSIL was 1.6%, but some laboratories serving young high-risk populations reported rates as high as 7.7%.[175,176]

In 1994 the Interim Guidelines (IG) Subcommittee of the 1991 Bethesda Conference gave two management options for women with a LSIL Pap result; accelerated repeat Paps and return to routine screening once three normal consecutive Paps had been achieved, or referral immediately to colposcopy.[159] Similar options were also endorsed by ACOG in 1993 and by the ASCCP in 2000.[177,178] At the time that the Interim Guidelines document was written, there was little published data on the use of HPV testing in the management of women with abnormal cervical cytology, yet the IG Committee included HPV testing as an option for management of LSIL. At that time it was not clear whether there was a clear advantage to one management option over another. Data was available on the potential of predicting risk for CIN 2,3 for women with LSIL on the basis of social and sexual risk factors and the results were mixed.[155,179–181]

The lack of good clinical data on the best management option for LSIL was clearly an impediment to the provision of verifiable evidence-based guidelines on LSIL and served as the impetus to include the evaluation of LSIL in the randomized ALTS trial. As with women with ASCUS enrolled in the ALTS trial, women with LSIL were initially randomized into one of three arms; immediate colposcopy at the enrollment visit, HPV testing with colposcopy of only those women positive for high-risk HPV types, and follow-up by cytology with colposcopy of only women with HSIL Paps on repeat.[176] However, one year into the trial the HPV testing arm was discontinued because, in these mostly young women with LSIL, high-risk HPV was too commonly detected for HPV testing to be used as a triage test.[176] Hence, just over a year into the trial, randomization for LSIL was narrowed to either immediate colposcopy or to repeat Pap. Patients in all three randomized arms were followed for two years, with treatment reserved for only CIN 2,3.

If cytology perfectly predicted the underlying histologic lesion, repeat cytology would be the clear choice for management of women with LSIL, for most low-grade lesions are transient and long term cytologic follow-up would give time for these lesions to clear.[182] For example, the most comprehensive analysis of all natural history studies between 1952 and 1992 established high rates of regression and low risk of progression for women with CIN 1.[183] Regression of CIN1 averaged 57%, persistence 32%, progression to CIN3 11% and to invasion 1%. Also, the risk that a woman with a LSIL Pap interpretation has an existing invasive cervical cancer is very low.[8] However, extensive data place the risk for detection of CIN 2,3 for women with a LSIL Pap typically between 15–30%, and the recent ALTS data documented the cumulative risk over 2 year follow-up to be 27.6% (Table 18.19).[8,163,184,185] This is the same level of risk associated with HPV positive ASC-US, which is recommended to be sent to colposcopy. Hence new data would appear to indicate that women with LSIL and women with HPV positive ASC-US should be managed similarly by immediate colposcopy.

ALTS confirmed that a Pap interpretation of LSIL, particularly from a young woman, is too accurate a marker for high-risk HPV for HPV testing to be helpful.[176,185] A triage test is only cost-effective if it identifies enough women not needing an expensive follow-up test (i.e., colposcopy) to more than pay for the additional cost of the triage test (HPV test) by savings accrued from decreased referral to the diagnostic procedure.[185–187] Alternatively, the test must identify a significant proportion of patients thought to have disease as being misclassified (false-positive, or overcalled Paps). Both of these requirements are satisfied for the triage of ASC-US, but the 83% rate of high-risk HPV positive women with LSIL indicates that LSIL in young women is rarely misclassified and the high referral to colposcopy does not result in savings that would pay for the cost of the triage test.[185] In contrast, LSIL is decreasingly HPV positive as women age. Only 30–50% of women with LSIL age 40 and over test positive for HPV.[66,188] Because women over this age referred to colposcopy for evaluation of LSIL are also less likely to be found to have CIN that explains the Pap interpretation,[189] it is likely that misclassification of LSIL occurs with increasing frequency as women age, probably secondary to declining estrogen and to the cellular changes associated with aging.[190] Therefore, while HPV testing is not clinically useful for triage of young women with LSIL, it does have utility for older women and has been incorporated in the ASCCP guidelines for the management of postmenopausal women with LSIL.[8]

The two remaining options for the management of LSIL, immediate colposcopy and accelerated repeat cytology, have both had their proponents. The primary advantage of immediate colposcopy is the timely detection of CIN 2,3 or the rare cancer, and reduction in the potential for loss to follow-up. Additionally, this approach reassures women without colposcopic abnormality and permits triage of women with CIN 1 to either observation or to treatment.[191,192] Proponents of repeat Pap stress that low-grade lesions most frequently regress and that repeat Paps provides time for this to occur. However, reduction in cost as a benefit of this approach was not demonstrated in ALTS, as the only threshold for referral to colposcopy that was considered to be safe was ≥ASC. At this threshold, 76% of women followed for LSIL cytology had a first repeat abnormal Pap necessitating colposcopy, a rate not dissimilar to that of HPV testing.[185] Other studies have reported that 53–76% of women with LSIL managed by repeat Pap have been referred to colposcopy on the basis of a single repeat Pap again demonstrating any abnormality.[8,191,192] The costs, both financially and emotionally, of prolonged follow-up that often results in subsequent colposcopic referral may be significantly higher than follow-up brought to quicker closure by immediate referral to colposcopy.[190] Stratifying patients on the basis of social or sexual "risk factors" has been advocated, with referral of "high-risk" patients to colposcopy and "low-risk" patients to Pap follow-up. However, risk-assessment on the basis of these factors has not been shown to reliably predict CIN2,3 or cancer.[181]

A randomized controlled clinical trial from the UK of young women (≤35) with LSIL either managed expectantly for 24 months or having an immediate excisional procedure found that expectant management was not successful without initial colposcopic evaluation.[181] Expectant management of LSIL requires reliable, conscientious accelerated Pap follow-up over a period of two or more years—a level rarely obtained. Because of the high cost of repeating the Pap, yet eventually referring the majority to colposcopy, the perception that this is the most cost-effective triage approach must depend on the high rate of loss-to-follow-up.[190] All studies on Pap follow-up have demonstrated decreased compliance with increasing numbers of follow-up visits.[193] Loss to follow-up has been identified as the most common antecedent to detection of cervical cancers in women followed by repeat cytology for LSIL.[194–196] The largest study in the UK following women with mild dyskaryosis reported that, of 1,781 women with this Pap interpretation followed with repeat cytology, only 35% had obtained two consecutive negative cervical cytology results within 24 months, and 11.5% had biopsy-confirmed CIN 3 or invasive cervical cancer.[194] Twenty-four percent were lost to follow-up. ALTS follow-up of LSIL detected similar rates of CIN 3 over this time frame.[185] Several studies, including ALTS, have demonstrated that repeat Pap with a threshold of LSIL or greater is too insensitive for the detection of CIN 2 or 3, and follow-up at the ASC threshold refers too many women to colposcopy (Table 18.20). Another disadvantage of expectant management of LSIL is that women must accept prolonged uncertainty regarding the nature of their abnormal Pap.[161,190] Therefore, the ASCCP Guidelines recommend that women given the Pap interpretation of LSIL have colposcopic evaluation.[8] (Figure 18.5) Once colposcopy has been performed, subsequent management options depend upon whether a lesion is identified, whether the colposcopy is satisfactory or whether the patient is pregnant, adolescent or post-menopausal (Table 18.21).[8]

Immediate "see and treat" by loop excision of the transformation (LEEP) zone of women with an initial LSIL Pap in the absence of biopsy-confirmed CIN should not be done routinely because CIN is often not identified in the excised specimen, thereby making the risk of excision unacceptable.[8,197,198] Obviously there may occasionally be circumstances that justify this approach, such as when the colposcopic assessment suggests a high-grade lesion and the patient is considered at-risk for non-compliance.

18.6.3.1 LSIL in special circumstances

For adolescent and post-menopausal women with LSIL the ASCCP recommendations vary from those just discussed (Table 18.22).[8]

Table 18.20 Estimated$^{\phi}$ Triage Test Performance

For Detection of Cumulative Histologic Diagnosis of CIN 3* by Pathology Quality Control Group. Initial referral Pap LSIL

	% Sensitivity for CIN 3 +	% Referral
Enrollment HPV DNA Test	95.2% (91.5–97.6)	84.2% (82.2–86.0)
HSIL Cytology Threshold†		
One	36.0% (29.7–42.6)	12.6% (10.9–14.4)
Two	55.1% (44.9–65.2)	16.8% (14.0–19.7)
Three	65.1% (55.1–75.0)	19.5% (16.4–22.6)
LSIL Cytology Threshold†		
One	72.8% (66.5–78.5)	57.4% (54.8–59.9)
Two	86.0% (79.0–93.1)	64.9% (61.3–68.5)
Three	93.0% (87.7–98.3)	68.6% (65.1–72.2)
ASCUS Cytology Threshold†		
One	90.8% (86.3–94.2)	80.8% (78.7–82.8)
Two	98.9% (96.8–100)	87.4% (84.9–90.0)
Three	100.0% (100–100)	88.9% (86.5–91.4)

$^{\phi}$For these estimates, missing test results, missed visits and the timing of visits were ignored, in order to focus on the performance of the tests according to how many were completed.

*CIN 3^{+} includes 5 cases of invasive cancer and 1 case of AIS.

†Each cytology threshold reflects the finding of a cytologic abnormality greater than or equal to the cut point when cytology is performed one, two or three times at approximately 6 month intervals. From: ASCUS-LSIL Triage Study (ALTS) Group. A randomized trial on the management of low-grade squamous intraepithelial lesion cytology interpretations. *Am J Obstet Gynecol.* 2003;188:1393–400. With permission.

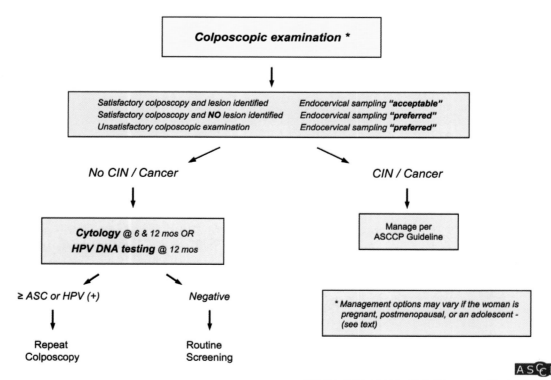

FIGURE 18.5 ASCCP algorithm for the management of women with cervical cytology interpreted as low-grade squamous intraepithelial lesion (LSIL). From: Wright T C Jr, Cox J T, Massad L S, Twiggs L B, Wilkinson E J. 2001 Consensus guidelines for the management of women with cervical cytological abnormalities. *J Low Gen Tract Dis* 2002;6:127–43. With permission.

Table 18.21 ASCCP Recommendations for Managing Women with LSIL[8]

General Management Approaches
- Colposcopy is the preferred management of women with LSIL. **(AII)** Subsequent management options depend on whether a lesion is identified, whether the colposcopic examination is satisfactory, and whether the patient is pregnant.

Satisfactory Colposcopy
- Endocervical sampling is acceptable for non-pregnant women with a satisfactory colposcopy and a lesion identified in the transformation zone **(CII)**
- Endocervical sampling is preferred for non-pregnant women in whom no lesions are identified. **(CII)**
- If biopsy-confirmed CIN is not identified and the colposcopy is satisfactory, acceptable management options include follow up with repeat cytology at 6 and 12 months with a referral to colposcopy if a result of ASC-US or greater is obtained, or HPV DNA testing at 12 months with referral to colposcopy of all HPV DNA positive women. **(BII)**

Unsatisfactory Colposcopy
- Endocervical sampling is preferred for non-pregnant women with an unsatisfactory colposcopy. **(AII)**
- If biopsy-confirmed CIN is not identified and the colposcopy is unsatisfactory, acceptable management options include follow up with repeat cytology at 6 and 12 months, or HPV DNA testing at 12 months. **(BII)**

Management of CIN following LSIL cytology
- Women with LSIL who are found to have biopsy-confirmed CIN should be managed according to the appropriate 2001 Consensus Management Guideline.[9]

ASCCP Guidelines for the management of women with LSIL in special situations. **Adapted from:** Wright T C Jr, Cox J T, Massad L S, Twiggs L B, Wilkinson E J. Consensus Guidelines for the management of women with cervical cytological abnormalities. *JAMA* 2002;287:2120–2129. With permission.

Table 18.22 ASCCP Guidelines: LSIL in Special Circumstances[8]

Adolescents:
- In selected adolescents, follow up without initial colposcopy using a protocol of follow up with repeat cytology at 6 and 12 months with a referral to colposcopy threshold of ≥ASC, or HPV DNA testing at 12 months is an acceptable option. **(CII)**

Postmenopausal women:
- In selected postmenopausal patients, follow up without initial colposcopy using a protocol of follow up with repeat cytology at 6 and 12 months with a referral to colposcopy threshold of ≥ASC, or HPV DNA testing at 12 months is an acceptable option. **(CII)**
- Providing a course of intravaginal estrogen followed by a repeat cervical cytology obtained approximately a week after completing the regimen is an acceptable option for women with LSIL who have clinical or cytological evidence of atrophy and no contraindications to using intravaginal estrogen. **(CIII)**
- If the repeat cervical cytology is "negative for squamous intraepithelial lesion or malignancy", the cervical cytology should be repeated in 4–6 months. If both repeat cytology tests are "negative for squamous intraepithelial lesion or malignancy", the patient can return to routine cytological screening, whereas if either repeat cytology is reported as ASC or greater, the patient should be referred for colposcopy. **(BIII)**

Diagnostic Excisional Procedures in Women with LSIL
- The routine use of diagnostic excisional procedures or ablative procedures is unacceptable for the initial management of patients with LSIL and either a satisfactory or unsatisfactory colposcopy in the absence of a biopsy-confirmed CIN. **(DII)**

ASCCP Guidelines for the management of women with LSIL in special situations. **Adapted from:** Wright T C Jr, Cox J T, Massad L S, Twiggs L B, Wilkinson E J. Consensus Guidelines for the management of women with cervical cytological abnormalities. *JAMA* 2002;287:2120–2129. With permission.

18.6.3.1.1 LSIL in adolescents
Adolescents have high rates of LSIL and high rates of HPV DNA infection, both of which are usually transient.[100] Additionally, cervical cancer at this age is virtually non-existent.[1] These parameters promoted classification of LSIL in adolescents as a special circumstance with expanded management options. Therefore, the ASCCP Guidelines consider the following options to be acceptable; 1). Immediate colposcopy 2). Follow-up without initial colposcopy using a protocol of either repeat cytology at six and twelve months, with referral to colposcopy threshold of ASC or greater or 3). HPV DNA testing at twelve months (Figure 18.6).[8] Expectant management without initial colposcopy provides time for transient lesions to resolve but is considered an option only for adolescents at low risk for loss to follow-up.

18.6.3.1.2 LSIL postmenopausal women
The rate of detection of high-risk HPV amongst postmenopausal women with LSIL is similar to that reported for women with ASCUS, and the sensitivity of HC 2 for CIN 2/3+ is also identical.[167] Therefore, in contrast to the lack of utility of HPV testing in younger women with LSIL, HPV testing of postmenopausal women with LSIL is an option, just as it is for women with ASC-US.[8] The ASCCP guidelines recommend that if initial colposcopy is not selected in the management of postmenopausal women with LSIL that alternative management options for selected women include either a HPV test in 12 months or repeat cytology at 6 and 12 months, with referral to colposcopy at a threshold of ≥ASC, or a positive HPV test (Figure 18.7). Immediate repeat cytology is also an acceptable management option for post-menopausal women with LSIL if the patient has either clinical or cytologic evidence of atrophy and no contraindications to estrogen therapy. In this circumstance, treating the cervix and vagina with a course of intravaginal estrogen therapy and repeating the cytology one week after completion of therapy is acceptable.[8] When repeat

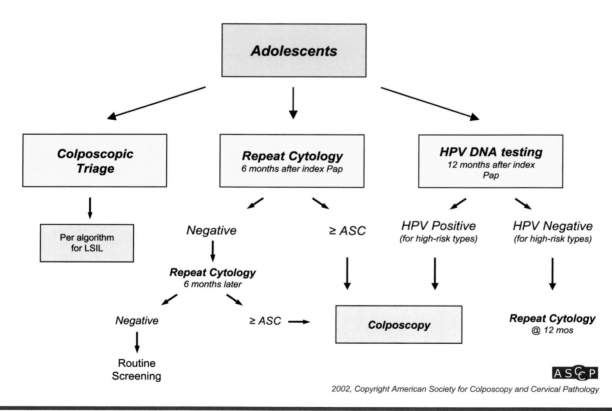

Management of Women with Low-grade Squamous Intraepithelial Lesions In Special Circumstances

2002, Copyright American Society for Colposcopy and Cervical Pathology

FIGURE 18.6   ASCCP algorithm for the management of women with cervical cytology interpreted as low-grade squamous intraepithelial lesion (LSIL) in special situations [adolescents]. From: Wright T C Jr, Cox J T, Massad L S, Twiggs L B, Wilkinson E J. 2001 Consensus guidelines for the management of women with cervical cytological abnormalities. *J Low Gen Tract Dis* 2002;6:127–43. With permission.

cytology is chosen as the option for management of postmenopausal women and the repeat Pap is negative, the Pap should be repeated again in four to six months and if negative the patient may resume routine screening. This management algorithm is the same whether it be in the follow-up of women treated by intravaginal estrogen therapy followed by repeat cytology a week after completion of the estrogen regimen, or in the follow-up of postmenopausal women with LSIL who are not treated with vaginal estrogen due to lack of evidence of atrophy, and who have their Pap repeated six months after the index Pap. Women managed by HPV testing and found to be HPV-negative should return for repeat cytology at 12 months.[8] Although the ASCCP algorithm depicts only the repeat cytology and HPV testing options deemed acceptable for some postmenopausal women with LSIL cytology, immediate colposcopy is also an option for these women as per the primary LSIL man-

agement algorithm for all women and should be the primary option selected for women with any previous history of CIN and for women with inadequate screening histories. Additionally, although the ASCCP algorithm does not give the option of immediate reflex HPV testing of post-menopausal women with LSIL, this option is as valid as it is for the management of women with ASC-US and therefore should be considered.[186]

18.6.4 Management of women with ASC-US or LSIL post-colposcopy

Many clinicians are concerned that women referred for the evaluation of HPV positive ASC-US and not found to have CIN or other manifestations of HPV at colposcopy have a "false positive" HPV test.[186] However, although there are occasional HPV tests that misclassify a low-risk HPV type as high-risk,[68,199] true

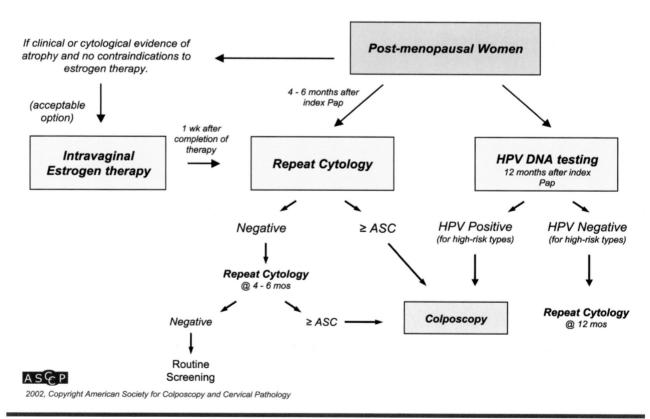

Management of Women with Low-grade Squamous Intraepithelial Lesions In Special Circumstances

2002, Copyright American Society for Colposcopy and Cervical Pathology

FIGURE 18.7   ASCCP algorithm for the management of women with cervical cytology interpreted as low-grade squamous intraepithelial lesion (LSIL) in special situations [post-menopause]. From: Wright T C Jr, Cox J T, Massad L S, Twiggs L B, Wilkinson E J. 2001 Consensus guidelines for the management of women with cervical cytological abnormalities. *J Low Gen Tract Dis* 2002;6:127–43. With permission. ■

"false positive" tests are at most, very rare. The 2–year ALTS longitudinal data provides the best information on what can be expected when a woman referred for HPV positive ASC-US or LSIL is either not found to have CIN at colposcopy or to only have CIN 1 that is subsequently managed expectantly rather than treated.[163] The cumulative risk of CIN 2,3 over the 2 years was equivalent for women referred initially for LSIL (27.6%) and for women referred for HPV positive ASCUS (26.7%). Two-thirds of the CIN 2,3 was detected at initial colposcopy and the remaining one-third during the post-colposcopy 2–year follow-up. The risk for subsequent detection of high-grade CIN was nearly identical for all women not found initially to have CIN 2,3, irrespective of whether CIN 1 was detected at initial colposcopy or whether the colposcopy was initially completely normal or had changes that were biopsied and not found to have CIN (risk for CIN 2,3 was 13.0%, 11.3%, and 11.7% respectively). Hence, all women referred for the evaluation of HPV positive ASC-US or LSIL and not treated for CIN 2,3 require similar diligent follow-up.

Guido et al evaluated the sensitivity of follow-up tests and rates of referral to colposcopy among women in the ALTS longitudinal follow-up (Table 18.23).[170] A single HPV test at 12 months detected 92% of all the CIN 2,3 found over the 24 month follow-up, with 55% testing HPV positive and referred to colposcopy. Repeat ThinPrep cytology at 6 and 12 months referred 63% at a threshold of ≥ASCUS, and sensitivity for CIN 2,3 was slightly less (88.0%). Combining a repeat Pap and with a HPV test did not increase sensitivity but did significantly increase referral to colposcopy. The authors concluded that the most efficient test for identifying women with CIN 2,3 post-colposcopy might be a HPV test alone at 12 months.[170] Further support for this approach can be found in the substantial body of evidence that only persistent HPV progresses to CIN 3[11] and that testing for high-risk HPV detects most CIN 3.[26,167]

These data provided the basis for the ASCCP guidelines for women referred for either HPV positive ASC-US or LSIL and not found to have CIN at initial colposcopy or to only have CIN 1 and managed expectantly.[8,9] In both situations the guidelines

Table 18.23 Follow-up Test Performance for Women not Found to Have CIN 3 at Initial Colposcopy

The performance of both HPV testing and repeat Pap in the 2 year follow-up of women originally referred for the evaluation of ASCUS or LSIL in the ALTS trial and either not found to have CIN at the original colposcopy or found to have CIN 1 and not treated is documented in this table. The sensitivity for CIN 2 or 3 and percent re-referral to colposcopy of HPV testing at 6 and 12 months is compared with that of one, two and three repeat Paps at approximately 6 month intervals.

Management Strategy	Sensitivity of Detection of Subsequent CIN 2 or 3 (95% CI)	% Women That Would Be Positive and Referred to Colposcopy (95% CI)
Follow-up by HPV testing		
At 6 Months HPV DNA Testing	90.9% (85.0–95.1)	62.4% (59.6–65.1)
At 12 Months HPV DNA Testing	92.2% (85.7–96.4)	55.0% (51.9–57.9)
Follow-up by repeat Pap		
Repeat Cytology at LSIL Threshold		
One	49.1% (41.4–56.8)	25.2% (22.9–27.4)
Two	70.5% (63.3–77.7)	34.6% (32.1–37.1)
Three	77.2% (70.4–83.9)	38.3% (35.7–40.9)
Repeat Cytology at ASCUS Threshold		
One	76.7% (70.2–83.2)	51.7% (49.1–54.3)
Two	88.0% (82.9–93.1)	63.6% (61.1–66.1)
Three	95.1% (91.6–98.6)	70.0% (67.5–72.5)

From: Guido R et al. ASCUS LSIL Triage Study (ALTS) Group. Postcolposcopy management strategies for women referred with low-grade squamous intraepithelial lesions or human papillomavirus DNA-positive atypical squamous cells of undetermined significance: a two-year prospective study. Guido R et al. *Am J Obstet Gynecol.* 2003 Jun;188(6):1401–5. With permission.

recommend either HPV testing at twelve months or repeat cytology at 6 and 12 months (see Figure 18.2 and Figure 18.5). Women managed by repeat Pap and having ASC-US or greater on either repeat Pap should be referred back to colposcopy, as should women testing high-risk HPV positive at 12 months. Women not found to have CIN at initial colposcopy and negative on the single HPV test or two repeat Paps are at low-risk of having missed CIN 2,3 or cancer and can return to routine screening, (Figure 18.2) whereas women followed with CIN 1 should have a Pap in 12 months (see Chapter 19). Another option for women with CIN 1 managed expectantly without treatment is repeat cytology and colposcopy at 12 months with annual Paps for women found to have cytological or cytological and colposcopic regression during follow-up.[9]

18.6.5 Management of AGC

The 2001 Bethesda Workshop dropped the term "of undetermined significance" because of clinical confusion generated by the similarity in the terminology of ASCUS and AGUS, thereby shortening AGUS to AGC (atypical glandular cells).[164] The cytologic criteria for interpretation of cells as consistent with adenocarcinoma in-situ (AIS) was considered specific enough to list this as a separate entity.[164] All other glandular cell changes were classified into two groups. The most common subclassification is atypical glandular cells (AGC), which could be further designated endocervical or endometrial if the pathologist considered the cellular characteristics to be well defined, or simply as "glandular cells, not otherwise specified (AGC-NOS)" if not. Far less common are atypical glandular cells (either endocervical or "glandular cells"), favor neoplasia. Grading of atypical endometrial cells has not been successful and therefore, no "favor neoplasia" subcategory exists for this interpretation. AGC is not a common Pap interpretation as the median rate reported in the 1997 College of American Pathologists Interlaboratory Comparison Program in Cervicovaginal Cytology (PAP) was only 0.3%.[175] Other evaluations have placed the AGC rate in the same range as that reported for HSIL cytology (0.13 to 0.8%).[15-18] That many women with AGC Paps are found to be normal reflects the difficulty differentiating reactive and reparative changes, dysplasia, and carcinoma.

AGC is a Pap interpretation that carries great import, for only HSIL Paps have more CIN 2,3 detected in follow-up, and AGC is more likely than other cytologic interpretations to be associated with difficult to detect glandular lesions.[200] Despite this the majority of women with AGC do not have significant lesions. It is this dichotomy that makes atypical glandular cells a Pap interpretation with so much risk for missing significant disease. Complicating management decisions have been uncertainty regarding the natural history of glandular atypia and difficulty detecting these lesions by both cytology and colposcopy.

The most common benign changes found in women with AGC are cellular changes secondary to chronic endocervicitis, to ciliated cell metaplasia of the endocervix, usually seen in women who have IUDs, or to hormonal conditions such as microglandular hyperplasia.[201,202] More efficient capture of endocervical cells secondary to use of the endocervical brush has resulted in Pap smears with a higher concentration of endocervical cells for evaluation, which may also have contributed to finding more atypical benign glandular cell changes as well as more squamous and endocervical neoplastic lesions.[203] Use of the endocervical brush has also been found to increase cell distortion and clumping as well as to induce "toothpick" or "brush" artifact which may falsely inflate the category of AGC.[204] Metaplastic and high-grade squamous cells may also be very difficult to differentiate from abnormal glandular cells.

The CAP Q-Probes Study determined that 40% of women with AGC had CIN, 6% had adenocarcinoma in-situ (AIS) and 6% had invasive carcinoma.[205] In other words, the most common finding in the follow-up of atypical glandular cells was not glandular neoplasia but rather, squamous lesions. Other studies have demonstrated similar proportions of squamous lesions (9–54%), AIS (0–8%) and invasive cancers (<1–9%).[206,207] While adenocarcinomas and adenosquamous carcinomas account for only 10–20% of cervical cancers, they appear to pose an increasing risk for women born since the 1930s, with much of the increase being in women less than 40 years of age.[208] At this time the reason for the increased rate of these glandular cancers is only speculative, but part of the increase may be due to the increasing prevalence of HPV, to the use of oral contraceptives, or to the greater success of cytology in detecting squamous lesions for eradication.[190,209] Because the median age of women having adenocarcinoma of the cervix is lower than that for squamous cancer, it has been suggested that glandular lesions may progress more rapidly.[210] The combination of cancers occurring in young, often adequately screened women results in the increased medicolegal liability associated with glandular lesions.[190]

When AIS is found, it is most commonly detected at the edge of CIN, invasive squamous cell carcinoma or adenocarcinoma.[211] Multifocal AIS may occur that is not adjacent to the squamocolumnar junction or to CIN, but most AIS is situated next to these more obvious landmarks.[212,213] This often makes the finding of AIS on histology unexpected, because adjacent CIN 2,3 easily diverts attention away from the colposcopically less impressive AIS lesion. Often AIS looks similar to a normal ectopy with only slightly accentuated acetowhitening of the columnar villi that may appear similar to the findings of some women on hormonal contraception or during pregnancy.[214] The small size of focal AIS, its frequent location in the cervical canal, and the occasional multifocal nature of many of these lesions, all complicate the detection and correct interpretation of these findings.[211] Approximately 50–66% with AIS or adenocarcinoma will have coexisting squamous lesions.[212]

The Bethesda 2001 Workshop designated the subcategories of AGC as "not otherwise specified" (NOS) and "favor neoplasia" on the basis of data that demonstrated that women with ACG-NOS are at a significantly less risk for having CIN 2,3 and AIS.[164] For example, CIN 2,3 has been detected in 9–41% of women with AGC NOS compared to 27–96% of women with AGC "favor neoplasia".[15–18,205–207,213–217] A Pap interpretation of AIS yields highest risk, for a false positive rate as low as 2% has been reported, with 48–69% having histologic AIS and 38% invasive cervical adenocarcinoma.[217,218]

Data suggest that the traditional management options for the follow-up of abnormal cervical cytology are all less effective in identifying AIS and small invasive cervical adenocarcinomas than similar squamous lesions. However, screening with cervical cytology does detect invasive adenocarcinomas and adenosquamous carcinomas of the cervix at an earlier stage with lower disease-specific mortality than glandular cancers detected only when unscreened women develop symptoms.[218,219] The sensitivity of the Pap for glandular lesions is reported to be from 50–72%, and similar low sensitivities for identifying glandular neoplasia have been reported for both colposcopy and for endocervical sampling.[218,220–224] Therefore, in order to maximize sensitivity for detection of both glandular and squamous lesions, the ASCCP Guidelines incorporate both colposcopy and endocervical sampling in the initial management of all categories of AGC except for atypical endometrial cells. For that diagnosis, endometrial sampling is the initial recommended procedure (Figure 18.8).[8] Follow-up to a non-confirmed AGC "favor neoplasia" or AIS Pap is also more comprehensive than to any other level of Pap abnormality not confirmed at colposcopy other than HSIL, because AIS can look like a normal ectopy or be hidden within the endocervical canal and be easily missed at colposcopy.[212,225,226]

When the AGC rate is higher than normal in a routine screening population, it is increasingly likely that the abnormal glandular cell category is being diluted with minor cellular changes that would be better categorized as normal. This does not change risk, however, for the number of women with significant disease remains the same despite the increase in the number of normal women. The result for AGC, as for dilution of ASC with reactive and reparative changes, is that it results in greater difficulty and higher cost in detecting the women who do have significant disease.[190] That atypical glandular cells may also come from tubal, ovarian, and metastatic lesions in the upper genital tract further complicates the matter.

Were AGC not such an uncommon Pap interpretation, there would likely be extensive data on the use of HPV testing in the management of this Pap abnormality. However, AGC is not common and hence data on management by HPV testing is sparse. There is no question that HPV is as commonly found in glandular lesions as it is in those that are squamous. Several studies have documented HPV DNA in over 95% of AIS and 90% of invasive cervical adenocarcinomas and adenosquamous carcinomas.[227–230] However, the one large study on detection of histologic AIS in the follow-up of glandular cytologic abnormalities documented only 5 cases of AIS in a screening pool of 50,000 women.[206] That all 5 were positive for high-risk HPV is compelling, as was demonstration of poor predictive value of repeat cervical cytology, but these findings were not considered to be numerically sufficient to promote HPV testing in the management of AGC. Additionally, endometrial carcinomas and rare clear cell and mesonephric carcinomas would test negative for HPV DNA. All of these factors highlighted colposcopy as the primary procedure for initial evaluation of women with AGC Paps.

Endometrial cells on the Pap: While endocervical adenocarcinoma is of increasing concern in young women, endometrial cancers predominate as women age beyond 35.[217,231] Normal endometrial cells appearing on the Pap smear are not of significance in premenopausal women but are of some concern when found in women beyond this age, particularly for women not on hormonal replacement therapy. The 1988 Bethesda System recommended that endometrial cells "out of phase" in a menstruating woman be evaluated, for there was concern that cytologically bland endometrial cells shed during the proliferative phase of the menstrual cycle might be associated with endometrial pathology.[29] Lack of confirmation of this perceived risk, however, resulted in dropping this reference in TBS 1991 revisions.[232,233]

In contrast, normal endometrial cells found on Pap in postmenopausal women do identify increased

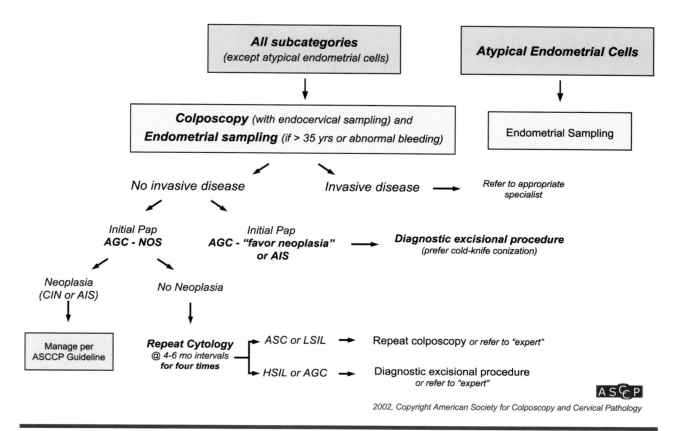

FIGURE 18.8   ASCCP algorithm for the management of women with cervical cytology interpreted as atypical glandular cells (AGC). From: Wright T C Jr, Cox J T, Massad L S, Twiggs L B, Wilkinson E J. 2001 Consensus guidelines for the management of women with cervical cytological abnormalities. *J Low Gen Tract Dis* 2002;6:127–43. With permission.

risk and require further evaluation even though they may only come from vigorous sampling the lower uterine segment.[215] Other causes for normal appearing endometrial cells in a postmenopausal smear include endometrial polyps, endometrial hyperplasia, or endometrial carcinoma. Hence, the presence of normal endometrial cells in a post-menopausal smear requires endometrial sampling.[190] This recommendation may be modified for postmenopausal women on hormonal replacement therapy.

The primary cellular determinant for the definition of "atypical endometrial cells" is increased nuclear size. Approximately one-third of endometrial cancers are detected in follow-up to AGC Paps,[215,234] and cellular changes more definitive for malignancy precede detection of endometrial cancer in another 13–47%.[235–237] Overall, abnormal cytology correctly identifies the endometrium as the primary site in only half.[215] Although the Pap is not intended to be a screen for endometrial disease and most women

with endometrial hyperplasia or cancer are symptomatic with irregular bleeding or increased mucous discharge, any glandular abnormality in women of this age increases concern for endometrial neoplasia. Endometrial hyperplasia and endometrial cancer have been detected in the follow-up of an AGC Pap in only 3% of women under 49 years of age but in 19% of older women.[215] For these reasons, the ASCCP Guidelines recommend endometrial sampling for all women over the age of 35 with atypical glandular cells or AIS.[8] Additionally, unexplained vaginal bleeding at any age requires comprehensive evaluation, particularly when the Pap also returns as AGC.

Because AGC is not a common Pap interpretation, the evidence supporting management options for glandular cell abnormalities was not as robust as it was for other Pap interpretations.[8] However, the guidelines that were developed at the ASCCP conference are based on expert assessment of the existing data (Table 18.24).

Table 18.24   ASCCP Guidelines for the Initial Management of Women with AGC[8]

- Colposcopy with endocervical sampling is recommended for women with all subcategories of AGC, including atypical endocervical cells, with the exception that women with atypical endometrial cells should initially be evaluated with endometrial sampling. **(AII)**
- Endometrial sampling should be performed in conjunction with colposcopy in women over the age of 35 years with AGC and younger women with AGC who have unexplained vaginal bleeding. **(AII)**
- Colposcopy with endocervical sampling is also recommended for women with a cytological result of adenocarcinoma in situ (AIS). The presence of a coexisting squamous abnormality does not change management of women with AGC or AIS. Management of women with an initial AGC or AIS using a program of repeat cervical cytology is unacceptable. **(EII)**
- There is insufficient data to allow an assessment of the use of HPV DNA testing in the management of women with ASC or AIS. **(CII)**

ASCCP Guidelines for the initial management of women with AGC. Adapted from: Wright T C Jr, Cox J T, Massad L S, Twiggs L B, Wilkinson E J. Consensus Guidelines for the management of women with cervical cytological abnormalities. *JAMA* 2002;287:2120–2129. With permission.

Table 18.25   ASCCP Guidelines for the Post-colposcopy Management of Women with AGC[8]

- If invasive disease is not identified during the initial colposcopic workup, it is recommended that women with atypical glandular / endocervical cells "favor neoplastic" or endocervical adenocarcinoma in situ undergo a diagnostic cervical excisional procedure. **(AII)**
- The preferred diagnostic cervical excisional procedure for women with AGC is cold-knife conization. **(BII)**
- If biopsy-confirmed CIN (of any grade) is identified during the initial workup of a woman with atypical glandular / endocervical cells (unqualified), management should be according to the appropriate 2001 Consensus Management Guideline.
- If no neoplasia is identified during the initial workup of a woman with atypical glandular / endocervical cells (unqualified), it is recommended that the woman be followed using a program of repeat cervical cytology at 4 to 6 month intervals until four consecutive "negative for squamous intraepithelial lesion or malignancy" cytology results are obtained. After four negative cervical cytology results are obtained the woman may be returned to routine screening. **(BII)**
- If an ASC or LSIL result is obtained on any of the follow-up Papanicolaou tests, acceptable options include a repeat colposcopic examination or referral to a clinician experienced in the management of complex cytological situations. **(BIII)**
- If an AGC or HSIL result is obtained on any of the follow-up Papanicolaou tests, acceptable options include a diagnostic cervical excisional procedure or referral to a clinician experienced in the management of complex cytological situations. **(BIII)**

ASCCP Guidelines for the post-colposcopy management of women with AGC. Adapted from: Wright T C Jr, Cox J T, Massad L S, Twiggs L B, Wilkinson E J. Consensus Guidelines for the management of women with cervical cytological abnormalities. *JAMA* 2002;287:2120–2129. With permission.

18.6.5.1 Management of women with AGC post-colposcopy

Women with AGC not found to have CIN, AIS or cancer at initial colposcopy continue to be at more risk for missed disease than those with other Pap abnormalities because the sensitivity of colposcopy and endocervical sampling for detecting glandular abnormalities is less than for squamous. A number of cases of AIS and invasive adenocarcinoma were detected following initially negative colposcopy in one large series.[234] Hence, management of women referred for any glandular abnormality on Pap and not found on initial colposcopy to have a lesion that explains the Pap must have follow-up that varies in degree with the subclassification of AGC (e.g., either NOS or "favor neoplasia") (Table 18.25). Women with AGC NOS who have a negative initial work-up are at relatively low risk for having a missed significant lesion. Therefore appropriate follow-up of these women is repeat cytology at 4–6 month intervals. Extrapolating from the known false negative rate of cervical cytology for glandular neoplasia, 3–4 repeat Pap's would appear to be sufficient reassurance that a significant lesion is not present. Although there is only limited clinical information available on the most appropriate response to a repeat cytological abnormality in these women, it is logical that the response be adjusted to the degree of abnormality on the repeat Pap. Women with a repeat cytology interpreted as AGC appear to be at high-risk for significant neoplasia, including endometrial carcinoma,[217] and HSIL cytology is always worrisome, particularly following a non-confirmed AGC Pap. Therefore, women with repeat cytology of AGC or HSIL should have a cervical excisional procedure.

Additionally, the significant risk for women with negative colposcopy, endocervical sampling, and, possibly, endometrial sampling referred for a cytological result of AGC "favor neoplasia" or AIS warrants a cervical excisional procedure rather than by relying on relatively insensitive repeat cervical cytology.[222] Because obscuring of the surgical excisional margins was considered to be more problematic with glandular lesions than with squamous, the ASCCP Guidelines recommended that cold knife conization was preferred over excisional procedures that could result in burned margins. However, the Guidelines also recognize that the choice of procedure is best based on the procedure best performed by the operating clinician. It is important to note that the management of glandular cytological abnormalities can be quite challenging, and it is recommended that women with unexplained glandular cytological findings be referred to a clinician experienced in the management of complex cytological situations.[8]

18.6.6 Management of HSIL

HSIL is not a common Pap interpretation. The 1997 CAP Interlaboratory Comparison Program in Cervicovaginal Cytology found HSIL in only 0.45% of women screened.[175] CIN 2,3 is found at colposcopy in approximately 70–75% of women referred for evaluation of a HSIL Pap and invasive cancer in 1–2%.[83,175] When cytology is suggestive of invasive cervical cancer, the predictive value increases to 78–95%.[238,239] This very high risk associated with HSIL cytology ensures that management of patients with HSIL is non-contentious, for there is no argument that all women with a HSIL Pap must have colposcopy, appropriately directed cervical biopsies and an ECC (Figure 18.9).[8] Management only becomes problematic when no lesion can be found that

explains the finding of high-grade cytologic changes on the Pap. The only alternative to colposcopic biopsy for management of women with HSIL occurs when the colposcopic impression is high-grade, the patient is not pregnant, and it is considered more prudent to proceed directly to immediate excision of the transformation zone using LEEP (i.e., "See and Treat"). This option is taken most often when the patient is considered at-risk for noncompliance.[8] Such an approach is common in the United Kingdom and in some clinical settings in the US, where efficacy and safety have been confirmed in centers with expert colposcopy.[195,198,240]

There are a number of reasons why HSIL cytology may not be confirmed colposcopically. These include: misinterpretation of colposcopic findings, lesion in the canal or endocervix not seen by the colposcopist, and poor biopsy placement.[190] Atrophy due to estrogen deficiency and small CIN 2,3s within a large low-grade lesion or area of complex immature metaplasia may all make identification of the most abnormal area for biopsy difficult. Even when the biopsy specimen correctly contains an area of CIN 2,3, the lesion may not be detected in the lab due to inadequate sectioning of the tissue specimen or misclassification of the histology. For example, one-third of women with persistent SIL on two or more Paps but negative, satisfactory colposcopies, negative biopsies and endocervical sampling were subsequently found to have CIN 2,3 on conization.[190] Increased risk for subsequent detection of CIN 2,3 or microinvasion at conization has also been shown when the discrepancy between cytologic and colposcopic biopsy is of two grades or more.[241]

This risk for missed serious cervical neoplasia in non-correlating HSIL cytology supports the traditional approach of performing a cervical excisional procedure for all high-grade Paps not confirmed at colposcopy of the cervix and vagina.[242] However, interobserver variability even occurs with HSIL cytology and histology, reducing the accuracy of these interpretations.[157,243,244] Such interobserver variability is inversely associated with age.[245] CIN2 is particularly difficult to differentiate from inflammatory changes in immature metaplasia. This results in only 60–80% interobserver agreement on the interpretation of CIN 2 and is probably responsible for the 25% or more HSIL Paps not confirmed in most studies.[167,238,239,246] Reports of safe expectant management of non-confirmed HSIL Paps by periodic repeat cytology and colposcopy likely reflect in part this variability in the accuracy of the cytologic interpretation.[238,242] Additionally, in the ALTS trial a deficit in the cumulative rate of detection of CIN 2, but not of CIN 3, in the Pap management arm

Management of Women with High-grade Squamous Intraepithelial Lesions (HSIL) *

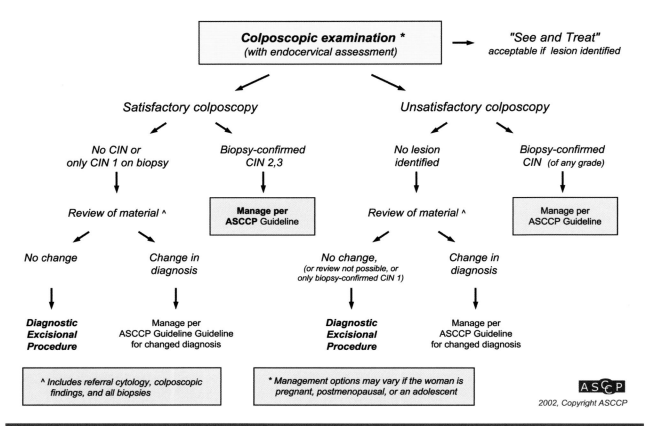

FIGURE 18.9 ASCCP algorithm for the management of women with cervical cytology interpreted as high-grade intraepithelial lesion (HSIL). From: Wright T C Jr, Cox J T, Massad L S, Twiggs L B, Wilkinson E J. 2001 Consensus guidelines for the management of women with cervical cytological abnormalities. *J Low Gen Tract Dis* 2002;6:127–43. With permission.

suggested that regression of CIN 2 lesions might explain some non-correlating HSIL Paps.[167,185] Nasiell also observed complete regression of cytologic CIN 2 to normal in 54% of 894 women with this cytologic interpretation.[247] This may at least partly reflect the finding of low-risk HPV types in CIN 2, arguing that this level of abnormality is not a sufficient surrogate for cancer risk.[248]

Despite the possibility that some women with HSIL cytology do not have significant neoplasia, the non-correlating HSIL Pap requires a comprehensive clinical response that eliminates the risk of missed CIN 2,3 or cancer. Unlike non-confirmed LSIL cytology, which should not have follow-up more aggressive than either repeat accelerated Paps or a HPV test at 12 months, follow-up to non-confirmed HSIL cytology must be much more comprehensive (Table 18.26).[8] The most appropriate course of action may depend upon the age of the patient, the degree of discrepancy, the anxiety level of the patient,

the reliability of the patient for long term follow-up, and the presence of other potentially associated clinical risk factors such as pelvic pain or unexplained bleeding.[190] For most non-pregnant patients with non-correlating HSIL cytology, a cervical excisional procedure will be warranted, but before proceeding to conization, review of the Pap by either the cytopathologist providing the initial interpretation, or a second opinion by another, may be appropriate.[8,190] If such review leads to a revised cytologic interpretation, then management should be according to the new interpretation. However, if the Pap interpretation remains HSIL and no CIN 2,3 or cancer has been found, then cervical conization is recommended even when CIN 1 is documented. This is due to an approximately 35% risk of biopsy-confirmed CIN 2,3 on a subsequent evaluation in this setting.[249,250] Other than pregnancy, the one exception to this approach is in young women with non-confirmed HSIL cytology, satisfactory col-

Table 18.26   ASCCP Guidelines for the Management of Women with HSIL[8]

General Management Approaches

- Colposcopy with endocervical assessment is the recommended management of non-pregnant women with HSIL. **(AII)**
- Subsequent management options depend on whether a lesion is identified, whether the colposcopic examination is satisfactory, and whether the patient is pregnant.

Post-colposcopy management of HSIL when colposcopy is satisfactory

- When no lesion or only biopsy-confirmed CIN 1 is identified after colposcopy in women with HSIL and a satisfactory colposcopy, it is recommended that, when possible, a review of the cytology, colposcopy and histology be performed. **(BIII)**
- If the review yields a revised interpretation, management should follow guidelines for the revised interpretation; if a cytological interpretation of HSIL is upheld or review is not possible, a diagnostic excisional procedure is preferred in non-pregnant patients. **(AII)**
- A colposcopic re-evaluation with endocervical assessment is acceptable in special circumstances (see Table 18.27). **(BIII)**

Post-colposcopy management of HSIL when colposcopy is unsatisfactory

- When no lesion is identified after colposcopy in women with HSIL and an unsatisfactory colposcopy, it is recommended that, when possible, a review of the cytology, colposcopy and histology be performed. **(BIII)**
- If the review yields a revised interpretation, management should follow guidelines for the revised interpretation. If a cytological interpretation of HSIL is upheld, review is not possible, or a biopsy-confirmed CIN 1 is identified, a diagnostic excisional procedure is preferred in non-pregnant patients. **(AII)**
- Ablation is unacceptable. **(AII)**
- Omission of endocervical sampling is acceptable when a diagnostic excisional procedure is planned. In women with HSIL and a colposcopic impression of a high-grade lesion, initial evaluation utilizing a diagnostic excisional procedure is also an acceptable option. **(BI)**
- Triage utilizing either a program of repeat cytology or HPV DNA testing is unacceptable. **(EII)** Women with HSIL who are found to have biopsy-confirmed CIN should be managed according the appropriate 2001 Consensus Management Guideline.[9]

ASCCP Guidelines for the management of women with HSIL. Adapted from: Wright T C Jr, Cox J T, Massad L S, Twiggs L B, Wilkinson E J. Consensus Guidelines for the management of women with cervical cytological abnormalities. *JAMA* 2002;287:2120–2129. With permission.

poscopy, and negative endocervical sampling. Because the risk of missing an invasive cancer in these women is low and CIN 2 may often regress, observation with colposcopy and cytology at 4–6 month intervals for 1 year is considered acceptable.[8]

Management of HSIL cytology in a pregnant woman is more challenging for several reasons. First, overinterpretation of colposcopic findings is common due to accentuation of vascular changes and colposcopic patterns associated with pregnancy. Also, cervical biopsy placement is often less accurate due to accentuation of these changes and biopsy is associated with an increased risk of minor bleeding. However, major bleeding or pregnancy loss has not been reported, whereas cervical cancers have been missed by failure to perform cervical biopsies in pregnant women when criteria for biopsy was restricted to colposcopic evidence of invasion.[8] Therefore cervical biopsy of lesions suspicious for

CIN 2,3 or invasive cancer should be undertaken in pregnant patients by clinicians experienced both in the evaluation of colposcopic changes induced by pregnancy and in managing bleeding from the pregnant cervix after biopsy (Table 18.27).[8] Endocervical sampling is not recommended in pregnancy. Biopsy of lesions that appear to be of lesser grade is acceptable when considered necessary.

18.7 Cervical Screening: Prospects for the Future

The Pap has been very successful in lowering the incidence and mortality from cervical cancer. However, cytology is subjective and has a fairly high false negative rate. The poor sensitivity of the Pap has led to frequent screening, and interobserver variability and misclassification of Pap interpretations drive increased

Table 18.27 ASCCP Guidelines for the Management of Women with HSIL in Special Circumstances[8]

Pregnancy
- It is recommended that the colposcopic evaluation of pregnant women with HSIL be conducted by clinicians who are experienced in the evaluation of colposcopic changes induced by pregnancy. **(BIII)**
- Biopsy of lesions suspicious for high-grade disease or cancer is preferred; biopsy of other lesions is acceptable. **(BIII)**
- Endocervical curettage is unacceptable in pregnant women. **(EIII)**
- Since unsatisfactory colposcopy may become satisfactory as the pregnancy progresses, it is recommended that women with an unsatisfactory colposcopy be followed with repeat colposcopic examination in 6–12 weeks. **(BIII)**
- In the absence of invasive disease, additional colposcopic and cytological examinations are acceptable, with biopsy only if the appearance of the lesion worsens or cytology suggests invasive cancer. Unless invasive cancer is identified, treatment is unacceptable. A diagnostic excisional procedure is recommended only if early invasion is suspected. **(BII)**
- Re-evaluation with cytology and colposcopy is recommended no sooner than 6 weeks postpartum. **(BIII)**

Young Women of Reproductive Age:
- When biopsy-confirmed CIN 2,3 is not identified in a young woman with a HSIL cytology, observation with colposcopy and cytology at 4–6 month intervals for one year is acceptable, provided colposcopy is satisfactory, endocervical sampling is negative, and the patient accepts the risk of occult disease.
- If a lesion appears to progress to a colposcopic high-grade lesion or HSIL cytology persists, a diagnostic excisional procedure is recommended. **(BIII)**

ASCCP Guidelines for the management of women with HSIL in special situations. Adapted from: Wright T C Jr, Cox J T, Massad L S, Twiggs L B, Wilkinson E J. Consensus Guidelines for the management of women with cervical cytological abnormalities. *JAMA* 2002;287:2120–2129. With permission.

cost and anxiety. Testing for high-risk HPV in the management of equivocal cytology and follow-up to non-correlating low-grade Paps and post-treatment surveillance has significantly reduced problems attendant with the misclassification and subjectivity of cytology.[8,9] In addition, the recent approval of HPV testing as an adjunct to the Pap in the primary screening of women 30 and over promises to reduce the false-negative rate to nearly zero, allowing safer extension of the screening interval to 3 years.[19,20] However, it remains impossible to predict which women with confirmed low-grade lesions are at risk for progression and would be most efficiently treated immediately and which are most likely to regress and should be followed. Additionally, many women over 30 found to be HPV-positive and Pap negative are destined to remain normal, while a minority is at-risk for progression. For these reasons, the need for identification of markers that more accurately separate women at-risk for progression from those with benign self-limited HPV infections has never been greater.

Persistent high-risk HPV is presently the only definitive marker for risk of progression to CIN 3 and invasive cancer.[11,14] High HPV viral load has been identified as a marker for CIN 2,3 in some[76] but not all studies.[78] Although high viral loads are linked to cytologic abnormalities, and ultra-low viral loads are associated with microscopic normalcy and with low risk of subsequent precancer or cancer, the prognostic value of increasingly high viral loads is not established.[77,248,251] Individual differences in immunologic responses to HPV play a critical role in determining the fate of HPV infections, but biomarkers identifying individuals most at risk due to a permissive immune response are not yet available despite identification of certain HLA types more commonly found in women with cervical cancer.[248] More specific identification of women at risk for progression will require the documentation of molecular markers known to be more prevalent in invasive than in pre-invasive lesions,[190] such as variants of high-risk HPV types more common in invasive cancer than in CIN3.[252,253] For example, variants of HPV 16 having genomic heterogeneity in areas most responsible for upregulation of the virus and for cellular transformation may be responsible for some women being at highest risk for neoplastic progression, and others infected with HPV 16 having little risk. This could help explain the dichotomy between HPV 16 being the most common high-risk HPV type in women found to be normal and in women with cervical cancer. A clinical test that could identify which women have HPV 16 variants might more specifically distinguish those with increased risk from those without.

Eventually, identification of HLA type or other markers of the immune response, of protein markers elaborated in upregulation of the virus or in cellular dysregulation, of alterations in cellular tumor suppresser genes, or of variations in high-risk HPV types may be valuable markers of risk of progression.[190,254] Cofactors are certainly important in progression of HPV induced neoplasia, but other than age and acquired immunodeficiency, no other cofactors have yet been identified that are important enough to merit separate screening or management protocols.[248] These include a number of cofactors that have been linked to risk in case-control studies of cervical cancer, including smoking, multiparity and long-term oral contraceptive use.[255-257] With the exception of immunodeficiency and age, no cofactor identified to date is important enough to merit separate screening or clinical management protocols.

The rate of change in cervical cancer screening and management protocols has accelerated significantly since the beginning of this new century. The most major change is in the introduction of HPV DNA testing in both primary cervical screening and in management of abnormal cervical cytology, representing a major opportunity to increase screening test sensitivity, help standardize screening, and increase negative predictive value such that screening effectiveness could for the first time approach levels reflecting high public expectations.[258] Management and counseling of women who are HPV positive and cytology negative will continue to be a concern for some time, but should be amenable to education of both the public and providers.

References

1. American Cancer Society, Cancer Facts & Figures 2002.
2. Patsner B. Diagnosis and contemporary management of cervical intraepithelial neoplasia. In: Rock J A, Faro S, Gant N F, Horowitz I R, Murphy A A. *Advances in Obstetrics and Gynecology* 1994;1:261–282.
3. Devesa S S. Descriptive epidemiology of cancer of the uterine cervix. *Obstet Gynecol* 1984;63:605–12.
4. Cox J T. Management of cervical intraepithelial neoplasia. *Lancet* 1999 Mar 13;353:857–9.
5. U. S. Preventative Services Task Force. Guide to clinical preventative services. Washington D.C. US Dept of Health and Human Services, 2003.
6. *Cancer Incidence in Five Continents*, vol. VII. Lyon: International Agency for Research on Cancer; 1997.
7. Walboomers J M, Jacobs M V, Manos M M, et al. Human papillomavirus is a necessary cause of invasive cervical cancer worldwide. *J Pathol* 1999;189:12–19.
8. Wright T C Jr, Cox J T, Massad L S, et al. 2001 Consensus Guidelines for the management of women with cervical cytological abnormalities. *JAMA* 2002;287:2120–29.
9. Wright T C Jr, Cox J T, Massad L S, Carlson J, Twiggs L B, Wilkinson E J; American Society for Colposcopy and Cervical Pathology. 2001 consensus guidelines for the management of women with cervical intraepithelial neoplasia. *Am J Obstet Gynecol* 2003:189:295–304.
10. Wright T C, Schiffman M, Solomon D, Cox J T, Garcia F, Goldie S, et al. Interim guidance on the use of HPV DNA testing as an adjunct to cervical cytology. *Obstet Gynecol* 2004;103:304-9.
11. Nobbenhuis, M, Walboomers, J M, Helmerhorst, T1, Rozendaal, L. Relation of human papillomavirus status to cervical lesions and consequences for cervical-cancer screening: a prospective study. *Lancet* 1999;354:20.
12. Jacobs M V et al. A simplified and reliable HPV testing or archival Papanicolaou-stained cervical smears: Application to cervical smears from cancer. *Br J Cancer* 2000;82:1421–26.
13. Holowaty P, Miller A B, Rohan T, et al. Natural history of dysplasia of the uterine cervix. *J Natl Cancer Inst* 1999;91:252–58.
14. Bosch F X, Lorincz A, Munoz N, Meijer C J, Shah K V. The causal relation between human papillomavirus and cervical cancer. *J Clin Pathol* 2002;55:244–65.
15. Duska L R, Flynn C F, Chen A, et al. Clinical evaluation of atypical glandular cells of undetermined significance on cervical cytology. *Obstet Gynecol* 1998;91:278–82.
16. Goff B A, Atanosoff P, Brown E. et al. Endocervical glandular atypical in Pap smears. *Obstet Gynecol* 1992;79:101–4.
17. Kennedy A W, Salmieri S S, Wirth S L, et al. Results of the clinical evaluation of atypical glandular cells of undetermined significance (AGCUS) detected on cervical cytology screening. *Gynecol Oncol* 1996;63:14–18.
18. Zweizig S, Noller K, Reale F, Collis S, Resseguie L. Neoplasia associated with atypical glandular cells of undetermined significance on cervical cytology. *Gynecol Oncol* 1997;65:314–8.
19. Saslow D, Runowicz C D, Solomon D, Moscicki A B, Smith R A, Eyre H J, Cohen C; American Cancer Society. American Cancer Society guideline for the early detection of cervical neoplasia and cancer. *CA Cancer J Clin* 2002;52:342–62.
20. *ACOG Practice Bulletin*. Cervical cytology screening. Washington, DC. American College of Obstetricians and Gynecologists, 2003.

21. Koss L G, Durfee G R. Unusual patterns of squamous epithelium of the uterine cervix: cytologic and pathologic study of koilocytotic atypia. *Ann NY Acad Sci* 1956;63:1245–61.

22. Meisels A, Fortein R. Condylomatous lesions of the cervix and vagina. I. Cytologic patterns. *Acta Cytol* 1976;20;505–9.

23. Durst M, Gissmann L, Ikenberg H, zur Hausen H. A papillomavirus DNA from a cervical carcinoma and its prevalence in cancer biopsy samples from different geographic regions. *Proc Natl Acad Sci USA* 1983;80:3812–15.

24. Cox J T, Lorincz A T, Schiffman M H, et al. HPV testing by hybrid capture appears to be useful in triaging women with a cytologic diagnosis of ASCUS. *Am J Obstet Gynecol* 1995;172:946–54.

25. Manos M M, Kinney W K, Hurley L B, Sherman M E, Shieh-Ngai J, Kurman R J, Ransley J E, Fetterman B J, Hartinger J S, McIntosh K M, Pawlick G F, Hiatt R A. Identifying women with cervical neoplasia: using human papillomavirus DNA testing for equivocal Papanicolaou results. *JAMA* 1999;281:1605–10.

26. Solomon D, Schiffman M H, Tarone R. Comparison of three management strategies for patients with atypical squamous cells of undetermined significance: baseline results from a randomized trial. *J Natl Cancer Inst* 2001;93:293–9.

27. Papanicolaou G N, Traut H F. *Diagnosis of uterine cancer by the vaginal smear.* New York: Commonwealth Fund, 1943.

28. Clinical laboratory Improvement Amendments of 1988, 42 C.F.R. Part 405. 1992;57:7169.

29. National Cancer Institute Workshop. The 1988 Bethesda System for reporting cervical/vaginal cytologic diagnosis. *JAMA* 1989;262:931–4.

30. The National Breast and Cervical Cancer Early Detection Program, AT-A-GLANCE. 1999.

31. Bogdanich W. *Wall Street Journal,* Nov. 2, 1987: p. 1.

32. Koss L G. The Papanicolaou test for cervical cancer detection: A triumph and a tragedy. *JAMA,* Feb 3, 1989;261:737–43.

33. Braly P, Kinney W, Sheets, E, Walton L, Farber F, Cox J T. Reporting the potential benefits of new technologies for cervical cancer screening. *J Low Gen Tract Dis* 2000;5:73–81.

34. Ries LAG, Kosary C L, Hankey B F, Harras A, Miller B A, Edwards B K (eds). SEER Cancer Statistics Review, 1973–1993: Tables and Graphs, National Cancer Institute. Bethesda, MD, 1996.

35. Ries LAG, Kosary C L, Hankey B F, Miller B A, Clegg L, Edwards B K (eds). SEER Cancer Statistics Review, 1973–1996, National Cancer Institute. Bethesda, MD, 1999.

36. Breen N, Wagener D K, Brown M L, Davis W W, Ballard-Barbash R. Progress in cancer screening over a decade: results of cancer screening from the 1987, 1992, and 1998 National Health Interview Surveys. *J Natl Cancer Inst* 2001;93:1704–13.

37. Evidence Report/Technology Assessment: Number 5, January 1999. Agency for Health Care Policy and Research, Rockville, MD.

38. NIH Consensus Statement Online 1996 April 1–3, cited 1999;43:1–38.

39. Fahey M T, Irwig L, Macaskill P. Meta-analysis of Pap test accuracy. *Am J Epidemiol* 1995;141:680–9.

40. Stoler M H. Advances in cervical screening technology. *Mod Pathol* 2000;13:275–84.

41. Diaz-Rosario L A, Kabawat S E. Performance of a fluid-based, thin-layer Papanicolaou smear method in the clinical setting of an independent laboratory and an outpatient screening population in New England. *Arch Pathol Lab Med* 1999;123:817–21.

42. Hutchinson M L, Zahniser D J, Sherman M E, Herrero R, Alfaro M, Bratti M C, Hildesheim A, Lorincz A T, Greenberg M D, Morales J, Schiffman M. Utility of liquid-based cytology for cervical carcinoma screening: results of a population-based study conducted in a region of Costa Rica with a high incidence of cervical carcinoma. *Cancer* 1999;87:48–55.

43. Ashfaq R, Gibbons D, Vela C, Saboorian M H, Iliya F. ThinPrep Pap Test. Accuracy for glandular disease. *Acta Cytol* 1999;43:81–5.

44. Sherman M E. Chapter 11: Future directions in cervical pathology. *J Natl Cancer Inst Monogr* 2003;31:72–9.

45. Nanda K, McCrory D C, Myers E R, Bastian L A, Hasselblad V, Hickey J D, et al. Accuracy of the Papanicolaou test in screening for and follow-up of cervical cytologic abnormalities: a systematic review. *Ann Intern Med* 2000;132:810–19.

46. Sulik S M, Kroeger K, Schultz J K, Brown J L, Becker L A, Grant W D. Are fluid-based cytologies superior to the conventional Papanicolaou test? A systematic review. *J Fam Pract* 2001;50:1040–6.

47. Lee K R, Ashfaq R, Birdsong G G, et al. Comparison of conventional Papanicolaou smears and a fluid-based thin-layer system for cervical cancer screening. *Obstet Gynecol* 1997;90: 278–84.

48. Obwegeser J H, Brack S. Does liquid-based technology really improve detection of cervical neoplasia? A prospective randomized trial comparing the ThinPrep Pap Test with the conventional Pap Test including follow-up of HSIL cases. *Acta Cytol* 2001;45:709–14.

49. Clavel C, Masure M, Bory J P, et al. Human papillomavirus testing in primary screening for the detection of high-grade cervical lesions: A study of 7932 women. *Br J Cancer* 2001;84:1616–23.

50. Marino J F, Fremont-Smith M. Direct-to-vial experience with AutoCyte PREP in a small New England regional cytology practice. *J Reprod Med* 2001;46:353–58.

51. Belinson J, Qiao Y L, Pretorius R, et al. Shanxi Province Cervical Cancer Screening Study: A cross-sectional comparative trial of multiple techniques to detect cervical neoplasia. *Gynecol Oncol* 2001;83:439–44.

52. Bai H, Sung C J, Steinhoff M M. ThinPrep Pap Test promotes detection of glandular lesions of the endocervix. *Diagn Cytopathol* 2000;23:19–22.

53. Hecht J L, Sheets E E, Lee K R. Atypical glandular cells of undetermined significance in conventional cervical/vaginal smears and thin-layer preparations. *Cancer* 2002;96:1–4.

54. Rosenthal D L. Automation and the endangered future of the Pap test. *J Natl Cancer Inst* 1998;90:738–49.

55. Wilbur D C, Parker E M, Foti J A. Location-guided screening of liquid-based cervical cytology specimens: a potential improvement in accuracy and productivity is demonstrated in a preclinical feasibility trial. *Am J Clin Pathol* 2002;118:399–407.

56. Castle P E, Wacholder S, Lorincz A T, Scott D R, Sherman M E, Glass A G, Rush B B, Schussler J E, Schiffman M. A prospective study of high-grade cervical neoplasia risk among human papillomavirus-infected women. *J Natl Cancer Inst* 2002;94:1406–14.

57. Cuzick J, Beverley E, Ho L, Terry G, Sapper H, Mielzynska I, Lorincz A, Chan W K, Krausz T, Soutter P. HPV testing in primary screening of older women. *Br J Cancer* 1999; 81: 554–8.

58. Cuzick J, for the HART Study Group. Baseline results for the HART multicentre HPV screening study of older women. 19th International Papillomavirus Conference, Florianópolis, Brazil, abstract # P-4, 2001.

59. Franco E L, Ferenczy A. Assessing gains in diagnostic utility when human papillomavirus testing is used as an adjunct to Papanicolaou smear in the triage of women with cervical cytologic abnormalities. *Am J Obstet Gynecol* 1999;181:382–6.

60. Kuhn L, Denny L, Pollack A, Lorincz A, Richart R M, Wright T C. Human papillomavirus DNA testing for cervical cancer screening in low-resource settings. *J Natl Cancer Inst* 2000; 92:818–25.

61. Kulasingam S L, Hughes J P, Kiviat N B, Mao C, Weiss N S, Kuypers J M, Koutsky L A. Evaluation of human papillomavirus testing in primary screening for cervical abnormalities: comparison of sensitivity, specificity, and frequency of referral. *JAMA* 2002;288:1749–57.

62. Macaskill P, Walter S D, Irwig L, Franco E L. Assessing the gain in diagnostic performance when combining two diagnostic tests. *Stat Med* 2002;21:2527–46.

63. Schiffman M, Herrero R, Hildesheim A, Sherman M E, Bratti M, Wacholder S, Alfaro M, Hutchinson M, Morales J, Greenberg M D, Lorincz A T. HPV DNA testing in cervical cancer screening: results from women in a high-risk province of Costa Rica. *JAMA* 2000; 283: 87–93.

64. Sasieni P, Cuzick J. Could HPV testing become the sole primary cervical screening test? *J Med Screen* 2002;9:49–51.

65. Ferris D G, Wright T C Jr, Litaker M S, Richart R M, Lorincz A T, Sun X W, Woodward L. Comparison of two tests for detecting carcinogenic HPV in women with Papanicolaou smear reports of ASCUS and LSIL. *J Fam Pract* 1998;46:136–41.

66. Wright T C, Lorincz A T, Ferris D G, Richart R M, Ferenczy A, Mielzynska I, Borgatta. Reflex human papillomavirus deoxyribonucleic acid testing in women with abnormal Pap smears. *Am J Obstet Gynecol* 1998;178:962–6.

67. Iftner T, Villa L L. Chapter 12: Human papillomavirus technologies. *J Natl Cancer Inst Monogr* 2003;31:80–8.

68. Castle P E, Schiffman M, Burk R D, Wacholder S, Hildesheim A, Herrero R, Bratti M C, Sherman M E, Lorincz A. Restricted cross-reactivity of hybrid capture 2 with nononcogenic human papillomavirus types. *Cancer Epidemiol Biomarkers Prev* 2002;11:1394–9.

69. Peyton C L, Gravitt P E, Hunt W C, Hundley R S, Zhao M, Apple R J, Wheeler C M. Determinants of genital human papillomavirus detection in a US population. *J Infect Dis* 2001;183:1554–64.

70. Kornegay J R, Shepard A P, Hankins C, Franco E, Lapointe N, Richardson H, Coutlee F; Canadian Women's HIV Study Group. Nonisotopic detection of human papillomavirus DNA in clinical specimens using a consensus PCR and a generic probe mix in an enzyme-linked immunosorbent assay format. *J Clin Microbiol* 2001;39:3530–6.

71. Bauer H M, Ting Y, Greer C E, Chambers J C, Tashiro C J, Chimera J, Reingold A, Manos M M. Genital human papillomavirus infection in female university students as determined by a PCR-based method. *JAMA* 1991;265:472–7.

72. Gravitt P E, Peyton C L, Apple R J, Wheeler C M. Genotyping of 27 human papillomavirus types by using L1 consensus PCR products by a single-hybridization, reverse line blot detection method. *J Clin Microbiol* 1998;36:3020–7.

73. Jacobs M V, de Roda Husman A M, van den Brule A J, Snijders P J, Meijer C J, Walboomers J M. Group-specific differentiation between high- and low-risk human papillomavirus genotypes by general primer-mediated PCR and two cocktails of oligonucleotide probes. *J Clin Microbiol* 1995;33:901–5.

74. van den Brule A J, Snijders P J, Gordijn R L, Bleker O P, Meijer C J, Walboomers J M. General primer-mediated polymerase chain reaction permits the detection of sequenced and still unsequenced human papillomavirus genotypes in cervical scrapes and carcinomas. *Int J Cancer* 1990;45:644–9.

75. Kleter B, van Doorn L J, Schrauwen L, Molijn A, Sastrowijoto S, ter Schegget J, Lindeman J, ter Harmsel B, Burger M, Quint W. Development and clinical evaluation of a highly sensitive PCR-reverse hybridization line probe assay for detection and identification of anogenital human papillomavirus. *J Clin Microbiol* 1999;37:2508–17.

76. Ylitalo N, Sorensen P, Josefsson A M, Magnusson P K, Andersen P K, Ponten J et al. Consistent high viral load of human papillomavirus 16 and risk of cervical carcinoma in situ: a nested case-control study. *Lancet* 2000;355:2194–2198.

77. Lorincz A T, Castle P E, Sherman M E, Scott D R, Glass A G, Wacholder S et al. Viral load of human papillomavirus and risk of CIN3 or cervical cancer. *Lancet* 2002;360:228–9.

78. Sherman M E, Schiffman M, Cox J T; Atypical Squamous Cells of Undetermined Significance/Low-Grade Squamous Intraepithelial Lesion Triage Study Group. Effects of age and human papilloma viral load on colposcopy triage: data from the randomized

Atypical Squamous Cells of Undetermined Significance/Low-Grade Squamous Intraepithelial Lesion Triage Study (ALTS). *J Natl Cancer Inst* 2002;94:102–7.

79. van Duin M, Snijders P J, Schrijnemakers H F, Voorhorst F J, Rozendaal L, Nobbenhuis M A, van den Brule A J, Verheijen R H, Helmerhorst T J, Meijer C J. Human papillomavirus 16 load in normal and abnormal cervical scrapes: an indicator of CIN II/III and viral clearance. *Int J Cancer* 2002;98:590–5.

80. Kleter B, van Doorn L J, ter Schegget J, Schrauwen L, van Krimpen K, Burger M, ter Harmsel B, Quint W. Novel short-fragment PCR assay for highly sensitive broad-spectrum detection of anogenital human papillomaviruses. *Am J Pathol* 1998;153:1731–9.

81. Ward J. Population-based mammographic screening: Does 'informed choice' require any less than full disclosure to individuals of benefits, harms, limitations, and consequences? *Aust N Z J Public Health* 1999;23:301–4.

82. Marteau T M, Senior V, Sasieni P. Women's understanding of a "normal smear test result": Experimental questionnaire based study. *Br Med J* 2001;322:526–8.

83. Kinney W K, Manos M M, Hurley L B, Ransley J E. Where's the high grade cervical neoplasia? The importance of the minimally abnormal Papanicolaou diagnoses. *Obstet Gynecol,* Jun 1998; 91:973–6.

84. Frame P S, Frame J S. Determinants of cancer frequency: The example of screening for cervical cancer. *J Am Board Fam Pract,* 1998;11:87–95.

85. Sawaya G F, Brown A D, Washington A E, Garber A M. Clinical practice. Current approaches to cervical-cancer screening. *N Engl J Med* 2001;344:1603–7.

86. Brown A D, Garber A M. Cost-effectiveness of 3 methods to enhance the sensitivity of Papanicolaou testing. *JAMA* 1999;281:347–53.

87. Kim, J J, Wright, T C, and Goldie, S J. 2002. Cost effectiveness of alternative triage strategies for atypical squamous cells of undetermined significance. *JAMA* 287:2382–90.

88. Harlan L C, Bernstein A B, Kessler L G. Cervical cancer screening: who is screened and why? *AM J Pub Hlth* 1991;81:885–90.

89. Burnett C B, Steakley C S, Tefft M C. Barriers to breast and cervical cancer screening in underseved women of the District of Columbia. *Oncol Nurs Forum* 1995;22:1551–7.

90. Katz S J, Hofer T P. Socioeconomic disparities in preventive care persist despite universal coverage. Breast and cervical cancer screening in Ontario and the United States. *JAMA* 1994;272:530–534.

91. Sambamoorthi U, McAlpine D D. Racial, ethnic, socioeconomic, and access disparities in the use of preventive services among women. *Prev Med* 2003;37:475–84.

92. Yu M Y, Seetoo A D, Hong O S, Song L, Raizade R, Weller A L. Cancer screening promotion among medically underserved Asian American women: integration of research and practice. *Res Theory Nurs Pract* 2002;16:237–48.

93. Steinberg A G, Wiggins E A, Barmada C H, Sullivan V J. Deaf women: experiences and perceptions of healthcare system access. *J Womens Health* 2002;11:729–41.

94. Nguyen T T, McPhee S J, Nguyen T, Lam T, Mock J. Predictors of cervical Pap smear screening awareness, intention, and receipt among Vietnamese-American women. *Am J Prev Med* 2002;23:207–14.

95. Fink D J. Change in American Cancer Society Checkup Guidelines for detection of cervical cancer. *CA Cancer J Clin* 1988;38:127–8.

96. Ries L A G, Eisner M P, Kosary C L, et al. (eds). SEER Cancer Statistics Review, 1973–1999. National Cancer Institute. Bethesda, MD, 2002.

97. Gustafsson L, Ponten J, Zack M, Adami H O. International incidence rates of invasive cervical cancer after introduction of cytological screening. *Cancer Causes Control* 1997;8:755–63.

98. Moscicki A B, Shiboski S, Broering J, et al. The natural history of human papillomavirus infection as measured by repeated DNA testing in adolescent and young women. *J Pediatr* 1998;132:277–84.

99. Ho G Y, Bierman R, Beardsley L, et al. Natural history of cervicovaginal papillomavirus infection in young women. *N Engl J Med* 1998;338:423–8.

100. Moscicki A B, Hills N, Shiboski S, Powell K, Jay N, Hanson E, Miller S, Clayton L, Farhat S, Broering J, Darragh T, Palefsky J. Risks for incident human papillomavirus infection and low-grade squamous intraepithelial lesion development in young females. *JAMA* 2001;285:2995–3002.

101. Syrjanen K, Kataja V, Yliskoski M, et al. Natural history of cervical human papillomavirus lesions does not substantiate the biologic relevance of the Bethesda System. *Obstet Gynecol* 1992;79: 675–682.

102. Nasiell K V, Roger V, Nasiell M. Behavior of mild cervical dysplasia during long-term follow-up. *Obstet Gynecol* 1986;67:665–9.

103. Nash J D, Burke T W, Hoskins V J. Biologic course of cervical human papillomavirus infection. *Obstet Gynecol* 1987;69:160–2.

104. Goldie S J, Kim J, Moscicki A B. Alternative policies for the initiation of cervical cancer screening. Plenary presentation at the National Meeting of the Society for Medical Decision Making. San Diego, CA. October 2001.

105. Centers for Disease Control. CDC guideline for immunocompromised women; USPHS/IDSA Guidelines for the prevention of opportunistic infections in persons infected with human immunodeficiency virus: A summary. *Morb Mortal Wkly Rep* 1995;44(RR-8):1–34.

106. Sawaya G F, Grady D, Kerlikowske K, et al. The positive predictive value of cervical smears in previously screened postmenopausal women: The Heart and Estrogen/progestin Replacement Study (HERS). *Ann Intern Med* 2000;133:942–50.

107. Mandelblatt J, Gopaul I, Wistreich M. Gynecological care of elderly women: Another look at Papanicolaou smear testing. *JAMA* 1986;256:367–71.

108. Lawson H W, Lee, N C, Thames S F, et al. Cervical cancer screening among low-income women: Results of a national screening program 1991–1995. *Obstet Gynecol* 1998;92:745–52.

109. Gustafsson L, Sparén P, Gustafsson M, et al. Low efficiency of cytologic screening for cancer in situ of the cervix in older women. *Int J Cancer* 1995;63:804–9.

110. Pearce K F, Haefner H K, Sarwar S F, et al. Cytopathological findings on vaginal Papanicolaou smears after hysterectomy for benign gynecologic disease. *N Engl J Med* 1996;335:1559–62.

111. Videlefsky A, Grossl N, Denniston M, et al. Routine vaginal cuff smear testing in post-hysterectomy patients with benign uterine conditions: When is it indicated? *J Am Board Fam* Pract 2000;13:233–8.

112. Wiener J J, Sweetnam, P M, Jones J M. Long term follow up of women after hysterectomy with a history of pre-invasive cancer of the cervix. *Br J Obstet Gynaecol* 1992;99:907–10.

113. Sigurdsson K. Trends in cervical intra-epithelial neoplasia in Iceland through 1995: Evaluation of targeted age groups and screening intervals. *Acta Obstet Gynecol Scand* 1999;78:486–92.

114. Parazzini F, Negri E, La Vecchia C, et al. Screening practices and invasive cervical cancer risk in different age strata. *Gynecol Oncol* 1990;38:76–80.

115. International Agency for Research on Cancer Working Group on Evaluation of Cervical Cancer Screening Programmes. Screening for squamous cervical cancer: Duration of low risk after negative results of cervical cytology and its implication for screening policies. *Br Med J* 1996;293:659–64.

116. Sato S, Makino H, Yajima A, et al. Cervical cancer screening in Japan. A case-control study. *Acta Cytol* 1997;41:1103–6.

117. Viikki M, Pukkala E, Hakama M. Risk of cervical cancer after a negative Pap smear. *J Med Screen* 1999;6:103–7.

118. Miller M G, Sung H Y, Sawaya G F, Kearney K A, Kinney W, Hiatt R A. Screening interval and risk of invasive squamous cell cervical cancer. *Obstet Gynecol* 2003;101:29–37.

119. Sasieni P D, Cuzick J, Lynch-Farmery E. Estimating the efficacy of screening by auditing smear histories of women with and without cervical cancer. The National Coordinating Network for Cervical Screening Working Group. *Br J Cancer* 1996;73:1001–5.

120. Sawaya G F, Sung H Y, Kinney, et al. Irreducible cervical cancer risk following multiple negative screening Pap smears in long-term members of a prepaid health plan. American Society of Colposcopy & Cervical Pathology March 2002. Oral presentation.

121. Davey D D, Austin R M, Birdsong G, Buck H W, Cox J T, Darragh T M, Elgert P A, Hanson V, Henry M R, Waldman J; American Society for Colposcopy and Cervical Pathology. ASCCP patient management guidelines: Pap test specimen adequacy and quality indicators. *Am J Clin Pathol* 2002;118:714–8.

122. Hutchinson M L, Isenstein L M, Goodman A, et al. Homogeneous sampling accounts for the increased diagnostic accuracy using the ThinPrep Processor. *Am J Clin Pathol* 1994;101:215–19.

123. Joseph M G, Cragg F, Wright V C, et al. Cyto-histological correlates in a colposcopic clinic: A 1-year prospective study. *Diagn Cytopathol* 1991;7:477–81.

124. Kristensen G B, Skyggebjerg K D, Holund B, et al. Analysis of cervical smears obtained within three years of the diagnosis of invasive cervical cancer. *Acta Cytol* 1991;35:47–50.

125. Martin-Hirsch P, Lilford R, Jarvis G, et al. Efficacy of cervical-smear collection devices: a systematic review and meta-analysis. *Lancet* 1999;354:1763–70.

126. Sherman M E, Lorincz A T, Scott D R, Wacholder S, Castle P E, Glass A G, Mielzynska-Lohnas I, Rush B B, Schiffman M. Baseline cytology, human papillomavirus testing, and risk for cervical neoplasia: a 10-year cohort analysis. *J Natl Cancer Inst* 2003;95:46–52.

127. Goldie S J, Kim J J, Wright T C. Decision analytic modeling to inform US national health policy: New guidelines for cervical screening. Oral presentation at the National SMDM Meeting 2002.

128. Clavel C, Masure M, Bory J P, et al. Hybrid Capture II-based human papillomavirus detection, a sensitive test to detect in routine high-grade cervical lesions: A preliminary study on 1518 women. *Br J Cancer* 1999;80:1306–11.

129. Belinson J, Qiao Y, Pretorius R, et al. Prevalence of cervical cancer and feasibility of screening in rural China: A pilot study for the Shanxi Province Cervical Cancer Screening Study. *Int J Gynecol Cancer* 1999;9:411–7.

130. Ratnam S, Franco E L, Ferenczy A. Human papillomavirus testing for primary screening of cervical cancer precursors. *Cancer Epidemiol Biomarkers Prev* 2000;9:945–51.

131. Wright T C Jr, Denny L, Kuhn L, et al. HPV DNA testing of self-collected vaginal samples compared with cytologic screening to detect cervical cancer. *JAMA* 2000;283:81–6.

132. Blumenthal P D, Gaffikin. L, Chirenje Z M, et al. Adjunctive testing for cervical cancer in low resource settings with visual inspection, HPV, and the Pap smear. *Int J Gynaecol Obstet* 2001;72:47–53.

133. Woodman C B, Collins S, Winter H, Bailey A, Ellis J, Prior P, et al. Natural history of cervical human papillomavirus infection in young women: a longitudinal cohort study. *Lancet* 2001;357:1831–6.

134. Ellerbrock, T V, Chiasson, M A, Bush, T J, et al. Incidence of cervical squamous intraepithelial lesions in HIV-infected women. *JAMA* 2000;283:1031–7.

135. Wright, T C, and Schiffman, M. 2003. Adding a test for human papillomavirus DNA to cervical-cancer screening. *New Eng J Med* 2003;348:489–90.

136. Boon M E, de Graaff Guilloud J C, Rietveld W J. Analysis of five sampling methods for the preparation of cervical smears. *Acta Cytol* 1989;33:843–8.

137. Curtis P, Mintzer M, Morrell D, Resnick J C, Hendrix S, Qaqish B F. Characteristics and quality of Papanicolaou smears obtained by primary care clinicians using a single commercial laboratory. *Arch Fam Med* 1999;8:407–13.

138. Germain M, Heaton R, Erickson D, Henry M, Nash J, O'Connor D. A Comparison of the three most common papanicolaou smear collection techniques. *Obstet Gynecol* 1994;84:168–73.

139. Sidawy M K, Tabbara S O, Silverberg S G. Should we report cervical smears lacking endocervical component as unsatisfactory? *Diagn Cytopathol* 1992;8:567–70.

140. Bos A B, van Bellegooijen M, ven den Akker-van Marle M E, et al. Endocervical status is not predictive of the incidence of cervical cancer in the years after negative smears. *Am J Clin Pathol* 2001;115:851–5.

141. Mitchell H. Longitudinal analysis of histologic high grade disease after negative cervical cytology according to endocervical status. *Cancer Cytopathol* 2001;93:237–40.

142. Mitchell H, Medley G. Differences between Papanicolaou smears with correct and incorrect diagnoses. *Cytopathology* 1995;6:368–375.

143. O'Sullivan J P, A'Hern R P, Chapman P A, et al. A case-control study of true-positive versus false-negative cervical smears in women with cervical intraepithelial neoplasia (CIN) III. *Cytopathology* 1998;9:155–161.

144. Fiscella K, Franks P. The adequacy of Papanicolaou smears as performed by family physicians and obstetrician-gynecologists. *J Fam Pract* 1999;48:294–8.

145. Mitchell H, Medley G. Cytological reporting of cervical abnormalities according to endocervical status. *Br J Cancer* 1993;67:585–8.

146. Klinkhamer P J J, Vooijs G P, De-Haan A F. Intraobserver and interobserver variability in the quality assessment of cervical smears. Acta Cytol 1989;33:215–8.

147. Rombach J J, Cranendonk R, Velthuis F J J M. Monitoring laboratory performance by statistical analysis of rescreening cervical smears. *Acta Cytol* 1987;31:887–94.

148. Hamblin J E, Brock C D, Litchfield L, Dias J. Papanicolaou smear adequacy: Effect of different techniques in specific fertility states. *J Fam Pract* 1985;20:257–60.

149. Kost E R, Snyder R R, Schwartz L E, Hankins G D. The "less than optimal" cytology: Importance in obstetric patients and in a routine gynecologic population. *Obstet Gynecol* 1993;81:127–30.

150. Kivlahan C, and Ingram E. Papanicolaou smears without endocervical cells. Are they inadequate? *Acta Cytol* 1986;30:258–60.

151. Bishop J W, Bigner S H, Colgan T J, Husain M, Howell L P, McIntosh K M, Taylor D A, Sadeghi M H. Multicenter masked evaluation of AutoCyte PREP thin layers with matched conventional smears. Including initial biopsy results. *Acta Cytol* 1998;42:189–97.

152. Ransdell J S, Davey D D, Zaleski S. Clinicopathologic correlation of the unsatisfactory Papanicolaou smear. *Cancer Cytopathol* 1997;81:139–43.

153. Sherman M E, Kelly D. High-grade squamous intraepithelial lesions and invasive carcinoma following the report of three negative Papanicolaou smears: screening failures or rapid progression? *Mod Pathol* 1992;5:337–42.

154. Smith A E, Sherman M E, Scott D R, Tabbara S O, Dworkin L, Olson J, et al. Review of the Bethesda System atlas does not improve reproducibility or accuracy in the classification of atypical squamous cells of undetermined significance. *Cancer Cytopathol* 2000;90:201–6.

155. Sherman M, Schiffman M H, Cox J T. The Bethesda System: Biological and Clinical Correlates. *Pathol Case Rev* 1997;2:3–7.

156. Sherman M E, Schiffman M H, Lorincz A T, et al. Towards objective quality assurance in cervical cytopathology: correlation of cytopathologic diagnosis with detection of high risk HPV types. *Am J Clin Pathol* 102;182–7.

157. Stoler M H, Schiffman M. Toward optimal laboratory use. Interobserver reproducibility of cervical cytology and histologic interpretations. Realistic estimates from the ASCUS-LSIL Triage Study. *JAMA* 2001;285:1500–5.

158. Raffle A E, Alden B, MacKenzie E F D. Detection rates for abnormal cervical smears: What are we screening for? *Lancet* 1995;345:1469–73.

159. Kurman R J, Henson D, Herbst A, Noller K, Schiffman M H. Interim guidelines for management of abnormal cervical cytology. *JAMA* 1994;271:1866–9.

160. Ferenczy A. Viral testing for genital human papillomavirus infections: recent progress and clinical potentials. *Int J Gynecol Cancer* 1995;5:321–8.

161. Cox J T. Editorial: Evaluating the role of HPV testing for women with equivocal Papanicolaou test findings. *JAMA* 1999;281:1645–7.

162. Schiffman M, Adrianza M E. ASCUS-LSIL Triage Study. Design, methods and characteristics of trial participants. *Acta Cytol* 2000;44:726–42.

163. Cox J T, Schiffman M, Solomon D; ASCUS-LSIL Triage Study (ALTS) Group. Prospective follow-up suggests similar risk of subsequent cervical intraepithelial neoplasia grade 2 or 3 among women with cervical intraepithelial neoplasia grade 1 or negative colposcopy and directed biopsy. *Am J Obstet Gynecol* 2003;188:1406–12.

164. Solomon D, Davey D, Kurman R, Moriarty A, O'Connor D, Prey M, Raab S, Sherman M, Wilbur D, Wright T C, Young N; The Forum Group Members; The Bethesda 2001 Workshop. The 2001 Bethesda System: terminology for reporting results of cervical cytology. *JAMA* 2002;287:2114–9.

165. Pitman M B, Cibas E S, Powers C N, Renshaw A A, Frable W J. Reducing or eliminating use of the category of atypical squamous cells of undetermined significance decreases the diagnostic accuracy of the Papanicolaou smear. *Cancer* 2002;96:128–34.

166. Jones M H, Singer A, Jenkins D. The mildly abnormal cervical smear: patient awareness and choice of management. *J Roy Soc Med* 1996;89:257.

167. ASCUS-LSIL Triage Study (ALTS) Group. Results of a randomized trial on the management of cytology interpretations of atypical squamous cells of undetermined significance. *Am J Obstet Gynecol* 2003;188:1383–92.

168. Bernstein S J, Sanchez-Ramos L, Ndubisi B. Liquid-based cervical cytologic smear study and conventional Papanicolaou smears: a meta-analysis of prospective studies comparing cytologic diagnosis and sample adequacy. *Am J Obstet Gynecol* 2001;185:308–17.

169. Sherman M E, Solomon D, Schiffman M for the ALTS Group. Qualification of ASCUS. A comparison of equivocal LSIL and equivocal HSIL cervical cytology in the ASCUS LSIL Triage Study. *Am J Clin Pathol* 2001;116:386–94.

170. Guido R, Schiffman M, Solomon D, Burke L; ASCUS LSIL Triage Study (ALTS) Group. Postcolposcopy management strategies for women referred with low-grade squamous intraepithelial lesions or human papillomavirus DNA-positive atypical squamous cells of undetermined significance: a two-year prospective study. *Am J Obstet Gynecol* 2003;188:1401–5.

171. Massad L S, Ahdieh L, Benning L, Minkoff H, Greenblatt R M, Watts H, Miotti P, Anastos K, Moxley M, Muderspach L I, Melnick S. J. Evolution of cervical abnormalities among women with HIV–1: evidence from surveillance cytology in the women's interagency HIV study. *Acquir Immune Defic Syndr* 2001;27:432–42.

172. Lozano R. Successfully integrating human papillomavirus testing into your practice. *Arch Pathol Lab Med* 2003;127:991–4.

173. Selvaggi S M. Reporting of atypical squamous cells, cannot exclude a high-grade squamous intraepithelial lesion (ASC-H) on cervical samples: is it significant? *Diagn Cytopathol* 2003;29:38–41.

174. Alli P M, Ali SZ. Atypical squamous cells of undetermined significance—rule out high-grade squamous intraepithelial lesion: cytopathologic characteristics and clinical correlates. *Diagn Cytopathol* 2003;28:308–12.

175. Jones B A, Davey D D. Quality management in gynecologic cytology using interlaboratory comparison. *Arch Pathol Lab Med* 2000;124:672–81.

176. Human papillomavirus testing for triage of women with cytologic evidence of low-grade squamous intraepithelial lesions: baseline data from a randomized trial. The Atypical Squamous Cells of Undetermined Significance/Low-Grade Squamous Intraepithelial Lesions Triage Study (ALTS) Group. *J. Natl. Cancer Instit* 2000;92:397–402.

177. American College of Obstetricians and Gynecologists. Cervical cytology: Evaluation and management of abnormalities. ACOG Technical Bulletin No. 183. Washington DC. The American College of Obstetricians and Gynecologists, 1993.

178. Cox J T, Massad L S, Lonky N, Tosh R, Waxman A, Wilkinson E. ASSCP Practice Guideline: Management Guidelines for follow-up of low grade squamous intraepithelial lesion (LSIL). *J Low Gen Tract Dis* 2000;4:83–92.

179. Hall S, Wu T C, Soudi N, Sherman M E. Low-grade squamous intraepithelial lesions: Cytologic predictors of biopsy confirmation. *Diagn Cytopathol* 1994;10:3–9.

180. Parrazini F, Sideri M, Restelli S, Schettino F, Chatenoud L, Crosignani P G. Determinants of high-grade dysplasia among women with mild dyskaryosis on cervical smear. *Obstet Gynecol* 1995;86:754–7.

181. Anderson D J, Flannelly G M, Kitchener H C, et al. Mild and moderate dyskaryosis: can women be selected for colposcopy on the basis of social criteria? *BMJ* 1992;305:84–7.

182. Cuzick J. Cervical screening. *Br J Hosp Med* 1988;39:265.

183. Ostor A G. Natural history of CIN: A critical review. *Int J Gynecol Pathol* 1993;12:186–92.

184. Schiffman M, Solomon D. Findings to date from the ASCUS-LSIL Triage Study (ALTS). *Arch Pathol Lab Med* 2003;127:946–9.

185. ASCUS-LSIL Triage Study (ALTS) Group. A randomized trial on the management of low-grade squamous intraepithelial lesion cytology interpretations. *Am J Obstet Gynecol* 2003;188:1393–400.

186. Cox J T. The clinician's view: role of human papillomavirus testing in the American Society for Colposcopy and Cervical Pathology Guidelines for the management of abnormal cervical cytology and cervical cancer precursors. *Arch Pathol Lab Med* 2003;127:950–8.

187. Cox J T. In: Kitchener H, Ed. Human Papillomavirus. Management of atypical squamous cells of undetermined significance and low-grade squamous intra-epithelial lesion by human papillomavirus testing. Harcourt, Publs. London. *Best Pract Res Clin Obstet Gynaecol* 2001;15:715–41.

188. Kaufman R H, Adam E, Icenogle J, et al. Relevance of human papillomavirus screening in management of cervical intraepithelial neoplasia. *Am J Obstet Gynecol* 1997;176:87–92.

189. Giles J A, Deery A, Crow J, Walker P. The accuracy of repeat cytology in women with mildly dyskaryotic smears. *Brit J Obstet Gynecol* 1989;96:1067–70.

190. Cox J T. Evaluation of abnormal cervical cytology. In: Jeanne Carr, Editor. *Clin Lab Med* 2000;20:303–43.

191. Ferris D G, Wright T C, Litaker M S, et al. Triage of women with ASCUS and LSIL Pap smear reports: Management by repeat Pap smear, HPV DNA testing or colposcopy? *J Fam Pract* 1998;46:125–34.

192. Mayeaux E J, Harper M B, Abreo F, et al. A comparison of the reliability of repeat cervical smears and colposcopy in patients with abnormal cervical cytology. *J Fam Prac* 1995;40:57–62.

193. Kirby A J, Spiegelhalter D J, Day N E, et al. Conservative treatment of mild/moderate cervical dyskaryosis: long-term outcome. *Lancet* 1992;339:828–31.

194. Robertson J H, Woodend B E, Crozier E H, Hutchinson J. Risk of cervical cancer associated with mild dyskaryosis. *British Medical Journal* 1988;297:18–21.

195. Bigrigg M A, Codling B W, Pearson P, Read M D, Swingler G R. Colposcopic diagnosis and treatment of cervical dysplasia at a single clinic visit: Experience of low-voltage diathermy loop in 1000 patients. *Lancet* 1990;336:229–31.

196. Luesley D M, Cullimore J, Redman C W E, et al. Loop diathermy excision of the cervical transformation zone in patients with abnormal cervical smears. *British Medical Journal* 1990;300:1690–93.

197. Howells R E, O'Mahony F, Tucker H, Millinship J, Jones P W, Redman C W. How can the incidence of negative specimens resulting from large loop excision of the cervical transformation zone (LLETZ) be reduced? An analysis of negative LLETZ specimens and development of a predictive model. *Br J Obstet Gynecol* 2000;107:1075–82.

198. Denny L A, Soeters R, Dehaeck K, Bloch B. Does colposcopically directed punch biopsy reduce the incidence of negative LLETZ? *Br J Obstet Gynaecol* 1995;102:545–8.

199. Castle P E, Lorincz A T, Scott D R, Sherman M E, Glass A G, Rush B B, Wacholder S, Burk R D, Manos M M, Schussler J E, Macomber P, Schiffman M. Comparison between prototype hybrid capture 3 and hybrid capture 2 human papillomavirus DNA assays for detection of high-grade cervical intraepithelial neoplasia and cancer. *J Clin Microbiol* 2003;41:4022–30.

200. Cox J T (lead author). ASSCP Practice Guideline: Management of glandular abnormalities in the cervical smear. *J Lower Gen Tract Dis* 1997;1:41–45.

201. Bose S, Kannan V, Kline T S. Abnormal endocervical cells: really abnormal? Really endocervical? *Am J Clin Pathol* 1994;101:708–13.

202. Meisels A, Morin C. *Cytopathology of the uterine cervix.* ASCP Press. Chicago. 1990;179–91.

203. Koike N. Efficacy of the cytobrush method in aged patients. *Diagn Cytopathol* 1994;38:310.

204. Chakrabarti. Brush versus spatula for cervical smears. *ACTA Cytol* 1994;38:315.

205. Jones B A, Novis D A. Follow-up of abnormal gynecologic cytology: a college of American pathologists Q-probes study of 16132 cases from 306 laboratories. *Arch Pathol Lab Med* 2000;124:665–71.

206. Ronnett B M, Manos M M, Ransley J E, et al. Atypical glandular cells of undetermined significance (AGUS): cytopathologic features, histopathologic results, and human papillomavirus DNA detection. *Hum Pathol* 1999;30:816–25.

207. Valdini A, Vaccaro C, Pechinsky G, Abernathy V. Incidence and evaluation of an AGUS Papanicolaou smear in primary care. *J Am Board Fam Pract* 2001;14:172–7.

208. Vizcaino A P, Moreno V, Bosch F X, et al. International trends in the incidence of cervical cancer: I. Adenocarcinoma and adenosquamous cell carcinomas. *Int J Cancer* 1998;75:536–45.

209. Sigurdsson K. What is the effect of cervical screening on the incidence of adenocarcinoma? *Int J Cancer* 1993;54:563–5.

210. Jaworski R C. Endocervical glandular dysplasia, adenocarcinoma in situ and early invasive (microinvasive) adenocarcinoma of the uterine cervix. *Semin Diagn Pathol* 1990;7:190–204.

211. Anderson M C. Glandular lesions of the cervix. In: Jones H W, ed. *Cervical Intraepithelial Neoplasia: Baillieres Clinical Obstetrics and Gynecology.* Baillierre Tindall. London 1995;9:105–19.

212. Coppleson M, Atkinson K H, and Dalrymple J C. Cervical squamous and glandular neoplasia: Clinical features and review of management. In Coppleson M (ed.) *Gynecologic Oncology*, pp 571–607. Edinburgh: Churchill Livingston, 1992.

213. Taylor R R, Guerrieri J P, Nash J D, Henry M R, O'Connor D M. Atypical cervical cytology. Colposcopic follow-up using the Bethesda System. *J Reprod Med* 1993;38:443–7.

214. Soofer S B, Sidawy M K. Atypical glandular cells of undetermined significance: clinically significant lesions and means of patient follow-up. *Cancer* 2000;90:207–14.

215. Eddy G L, Wojtowycz M A, Piraino P S, Mazur M T. Papanicolaou smears by the Bethesda system in endometrial malignancy: utility and prognostic importance. *Obstet Gynecol* 1997;90:999–1003.

216. Veljovich D S, Stoler M H, Andersen W A, Covell J L, Rice L W. Atypical glandular cells of undetermined significance: a five-year retrospective histopathologic study. *Am J Obstet Gynecol* 1998;179:382–90.

217. Chhieng D C, Elgert P, Cohen J M, Cangiarella J F. Clinical significance of atypical glandular cells of undetermined significance in postmenopausal women. *Cancer* 2001;93:1–7.

218. Lee K R, Manna E A, St John T. Atypical endocervical glandular cells: accuracy of cytologic diagnosis. *Diagn Cytopathol* 1995;13:202–8.

219. Kinney W, Sawaya G F, Sung H Y, Kearney K A, Miller M, Hiatt R A. Stage at diagnosis and mortality in patients with adenocarcinoma and adenosquamous carcinoma of the uterine cervix diagnosed as a consequence of cytologic screening. *Acta Cytol* 2003;47:167–71.

220. Laverty C R, Farnsworth A, Thurloe J, Bowditch R. The reliability of a cytological prediction of cervical adenocarcinoma in situ. *Aust N Z J Obstet Gynaecol* 1988;28:307–12.

221. Mitchell H, Medley G, Gordon I, Giles G. Cervical cytology reported as negative and risk of adenocarcinoma of the cervix: no strong evidence of benefit. *Br J Cancer* 1995;71:894–7.

222. Kim T J, Kim H S, Park C T, et al. Clinical evaluation of follow-up methods and results of atypical glandular cells of undetermined significance (AGUS) detected on cervicovaginal Pap smears. *Gynecol Oncol* 1999;73:292–8.

223. Lee K R, Minter L J, Granter S R. Papanicolaou smear sensitivity for adenocarcinoma in situ of the cervix. A study of 34 cases. *Am J Clin Pathol* 1997;107:30–5.

224. Krane J F, Granter S R, Trask C E, Hogan C L, Lee K R. Papanicolaou smear sensitivity for the detection of adenocarcinoma of the cervix: a study of 49 cases. *Cancer* 2001;93:8–15.

225. Cullimore J E, Luesley D M, Rollason T P, et al. A prospective study of conization of the cervix in the management of cervical intraepithelial glandular neoplasia (CIGN)—a preliminary report. *Br J Obstet Gynaecol* 1992;99:314–8.

226. Ueki M. *Cervical Adenocarcinoma: A Colposcopic Atlas*. St. Louis: Ishiyaku EuroAmerica, Inc.; 1985.

227. Bosch F X, Manos M M, Munoz N, et al. Prevalence of human papillomavirus in cervical cancer: a worldwide perspective. International biological study on cervical cancer (IBSCC) Study Group. *J Natl Cancer Inst* 1995;87:779–80.

228. Pirog E C, Kleter B, Olgac S, et al. Prevalence of human papillomavirus DNA in different histological subtypes of cervical adenocarcinoma. *Am J Pathol* 2000;157:1055–62.

229. Riethdorf S, Riethdorf L, Milde-Langosch K, Park J W, Loning T. Differences in HPV 16– and HPV 18 E6/E7 oncogene expression between in situ and invasive adenocarcinomas of the cervix uteri. *Virchows Arch* 2000;437:491–500.

230. Madeleine M M, Daling J R, Schwartz S M, et al. Human papillomavirus and long-term oral contraceptive use increase the risk of adenocarcinoma in situ of the cervix. *Cancer Epidemiol Biomarkers Prev* 2001;10:171–7.

231. Obenson K, Abreo F, Grafton W D. Cytohistologic correlation between AGUS and biopsy-detected lesions in postmenopausal women. *Acta Cytol* 2000;44:41–5.

232. The Bethesda System for reporting cervical/vaginal cytologic diagnoses. Report of the 1991 Bethesda Workshop. *Am J Surg Pathol* 1992;16:914–6.

233. Kurman R J, Solomon D. *The Bethesda System for reporting cervical/vaginal cytologic diagnoses. Definitions, criteria, and explanatory notes for terminology and specimen adequacy.* Springer-Verlag, New York, 1993.

234. Eddy G L, Strumpf K B, Wojtowycz M A, et al. Biopsy findings in 531 patients with atypical glandular cells of undetermined significance (AGCUS) as defined by the Bethesda System (TBS). *Am J Obstet Gynecol* 1997;177;1188–95.

235. Demirkiran F, Arvas M, Erkun E, et al. The prognostic significance of cervico-vaginal cytology in endometrial cancer. *Eur J Gynecol Oncol* 1995;16–404–9.

236. Larson, D M, Johnson K K, Reyes C N, Broste S K. Prognostic significance of malignant cervical cytology in patients with endometrial cancer. *Obstet Gynecol* 1994;84:399–403.

237. Cheng R F, Hernandez E, Anderson L L, Heller P B, Shank R. Clinical significance of a cytologic diagnosis of atypical glandular cells of undetermined significance. *J Reprod Med* 1999;44:922–8.

238. Hellberg D, Nilsson S, Valentin J. Positive cervical smear with subsequent normal colposcopy and histology—frequency of CIN in a long-term follow-up. *Gynecol Oncol* 1994;53:148–51.

239. Giles J A, Hudson E, Crow J, Williams D, Walker P. Colposcopic assessment of the accuracy of cervical cytologic screening. *BMJ* 1988;296:1099–1102.

240. Santos C, Galdos R, Alvarez J, et al. One-session management of cervical intraepithelial neoplasia: a solution for developing countries. *Gynecol Oncol* 1996;61:11–15.

241. Ramirez E J, Hernandez E, Miyazawa K. Cervical conization findings in women with dysplastic cervical cytology and normal colposcopy. *J Reprod Med* 1990;35:359–61.

242. Biedermann K, Bannwart F, Staikov D, Schreiner W E. Pathologic Papanicolaou Class IV smear without histologic correlation-What should be done? *Geburtshilfe Frauenheilkd* 1988;48:781–84.

243. Grenko R T, Abendroth C S, Frauenhoffer E E, Ruggiero F M, Zaino R J. Variance in the interpretation of cervical biopsy specimens obtained for atypical squamous cells of undetermined significance. *Am J Clin Pathol* 2000;114:735–40.

244. Joste N E, Rushing L, Granados R, et al. Bethesda classification of cervicovaginal smears: reproducibility and viral correlates. *Hum Pathol* 1996;27:581–5.

245. Kato I, Santamaria M, De Ruiz P A, et al. Interobserver variation in cytological and histological diagnoses of cervical neoplasia and its epidemiologic implication. *J Clin Epidemiol* 1995;48:1167–74.

246. Quantin C, Dusserre L, Montaud A M, et al. A model for quality assessment in cervical cytology used as a screening test. *Qual Assur Health Care* 1992;4:105–13.

247. Nasiell K, Nasiell M, Vaklavinkova V. Behavior of moderate cervical dysplasia during long-term follow-up. *Obstet Gynecol* 1983;61:609–14.

248. Schiffman M, Castle P E. Human papillomavirus: epidemiology and public health. *Arch Pathol Lab Med* 2003;127:930–4.

249. Brown F M, Faquin W C, Sun D, Crum C P, Cibas E S. LSIL biopsies after HSIL smears. Correlation with high-risk HPV and greater risk of HSIL on follow-up. *Am J Clin Pathol* 1999;112:765–8.

250. Chappatte O A, Byrne D L, Raju K S, Nayagam M, Kenney A. Histological differences between colposcopic-directed biopsy and loop excision of the transformation zone (LLETZ): A cause for concern. *Gynecol Oncol* 1991;43:46.

251. Herrero, R, A Hildesheim, and C Bratti. et al. Population-based study of human papillomavirus infection and cervical neoplasia in rural Costa Rica. *J Natl Cancer Inst* 2000;92:464–74.

252. Xi L F, Koutsky L A, Galloway D A, Kuypers J, Hughes J P, Wheeler C M, Holmes K K, Kiviat N B. Genomic variation of human papillomavirus type 16 and risk for high-grade cervical intraepithelial neoplasia. *J Natl Cancer Inst* 1997;89:796–802.

253. Zehbe I, Wilander E, Delius H, Tommassino M. Human papillomavirus 16 E6 variants are more prevalent than the prototype. *Cancer Res* 1998;58:829–33.

254. Larson A A, Liao S-Y, Stanbridge E J, Cavenee W A, Hampton G M. Genetic alterations accumulate during cervical tumorigenesis and indicate a common origin for multifocal lesions. *Cancer Res* 1997;57:4171–6.

255. Munoz, N, S Franceschi, and C Bosetti. et al. Role of parity and human papillomavirus in cervical cancer: the IARC multicentric case-control study. *Lancet* 2002;359:1093–1101.

256. Moreno V, F X Bosch, and N Munoz. et al. Effect of oral contraceptives on risk of cervical cancer in women with human papillomavirus infection: the IARC multicentric case-control study. *Lancet* 2002;359:1085–92.

257. Hildesheim, A, R Herrero, and P E Castle. et al. HPV co-factors related to the development of cervical cancer: results from a population-based study in Costa Rica. *Br J Cancer* 2001;84:1219–26.

258. Austin R M. Human papillomavirus reporting: Minimizing patient and laboratory risk. *Arch Pathol Lab Med* 2003;127:973–7.

Management of Lower Genital Tract Neoplasia

Table of Contents

19.1 Management of Cervical Intraepithelial Neoplasia

19.1.1 Introduction

In 1886, Sir John Williams first described abnormal cell changes that we now know as cervical intraepithelial neoplasia grade 3 (CIN 3, or carcinoma in situ [CIS]) as a case of very early "cervical cancer."[1] In the early decades of the 20th century, it became clear that these cell changes represented a precursor to cervical cancer rather than "early cancer." However, in the United States, it was not until the introduction of widespread cervical screening with the Papanicolaou (Pap) smear in the late 1940s that the ability to detect the precursor lesion to invasive cervical cancer provided the opportunity to develop treatment methods to alter its natural history. Prior to this time, invasive cervical cancer was the second most common cancer among women, but these new capabilities decreased the cervical cancer incidence in the United States from 2nd to 10th among cancers in women.[2,3] The estimated reduction over the last 50 years of 75% in cervical cancer incidence and 74% in mortality is evidence of the success of the cervical cancer screening program and of the modalities developed to treat precursor lesions.[3,4]

Although effective screening programs began to be introduced by the mid-20th century, optimal treatment of precursor lesions was initially limited by lack of knowledge of the natural history of these lesions and by the absence of minimally traumatic procedures for evaluation of women with abnormal Pap test results.[5] Although Koss first described the koilocyte in 1955, the association of the koilocyte with human papillomavirus (HPV) was not reported until the 1976 publication of Meisels and Fortin.[6,7] Even then, the primary role of HPV in the etiology of cervical cancer could not be definitively proclaimed until the 1995 affirmation published by the International Agency for Research on Cancer (IARC).[8]

The modern era of outpatient diagnosis and treatment of precursor lesions began with the popularization of colposcopy and the introduction of cryosurgery in the 1960s. This was followed in the 1970s by carbon dioxide (CO_2) laser therapy and in the early 1990s by loop electrosurgical excision procedure (LEEP). Until recently, CIN 1, CIN 2, and CIN 3 were considered progressive lesions; therefore all were managed by either ablative or excisional procedures. However, recognition that only CIN 3/CIS and some CIN2 are true precancer lesions has fostered an increasing trend to expectantly manage women with CIN 1. This approach was formalized in the Consensus Guidelines Conference for the Management of Women with Cervical Cytological Abnormalities and Cervical Cancer Precursors, sponsored by the American Society for Colposcopy and Cervical Pathology (ASCCP) in September 2001.[9,10] The guidelines developed from this conference were consensus- and evidence-based and serve as a basis for discussion in this chapter of the management of women with CIN.

First, it is important to understand the role that the immune response to human papillomavirus (HPV) plays in the success of any treatment approach.

19.1.2 The role of immunity in successful treatment of CIN

Successful treatment of CIN ultimately depends upon the ability of the host immune response to prevent recurrence. Women with compromised immunity fail to respond adequately to HPV and, therefore, have a very high rate of recurrence following any treatment modality.[11] The primary immune response to tumors and viruses is cellular, although humoral immunity is likely to be important in the initial prevention of HPV infection. This symbiotic relationship between humoral and cellular immunity is demonstrated by the lymphocytic population in the cervix noted in health and in disease. In the normal cervix, the primary function of the lymphocyte population is to serve as a barrier to infection by mounting a B-lymphocyte humoral immune response as the first line of defense against initial infection (Figure 19.1).[12] Therefore, in the normal cervix B-lymphocytes predominate. In contrast, in the presence of CIN 3, B-lymphocytes are a minor part of the population of immune responsive cells, as they are replaced by natural killer cells (NKCs) and cytotoxic T-lymphocytes, the dominant responders of local cellular immunity. In most viral infections, the foreign antigen is recognized quite rapidly, resulting in the activation of antigen-presenting cells and the release of local cytokines within only a day or two. Unfortunately, recognition of the presence of HPV is much slower and extremely variable in timing, resulting in relative delay in the immune response to HPV when compared with the immune response noted with most other viral infections.

Detection of HPV is delayed primarily by the fact that the entire HPV life cycle occurs without the virus ever crossing the basement membrane of the epithelium or being released outside of the protection of the infected host cell. HPV initially infects the basal epithelium by shedding its viral protein coat and injecting its DNA into the cell. HPV resides exclusively in the basal epithelium and does not replicate until a release from a variable period of viral latency results in accelerated HPV DNA production in differentiating keratinocytes above the basal layer (Figure 19.2).[13] These differentiating squamous epithelial cells are inefficient at presenting viral antigens on their surface even after the

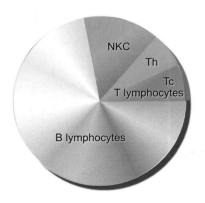

Normal Cervix

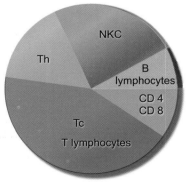

Cervical Intraepithelial
Neoplasia 3

FIGURE 19.1 The lymphocytic population of the cervix changes dramatically in the presence of CIN. B-cells predominate in the normal cervix, whereas women with CIN III have predominantly T-cells and natural killer cells. Modified with permission from Cox J T. In: Lonky N, Ed. Management of women with cervical cancer precursor lesions. *Obstet Gynecol Clin North Am* 2002;29:787–816. ▬

cells contain dozens of HPV genomes.[13] The protein capsule surrounding the HPV genome in infective koilocytes is reassembled in the upper layers of the epithelium as the keratinocytes mature. It is the shedding of these dead or dying cells from the surface epithelium that results in release of the infective unit.[14] Because HPV does not lyse the infected epithelial cells and these cells are not efficient at antigen presentation, the virus remains hidden during its entire life cycle, providing the immune system little opportunity to identify its presence. Several other mechanisms add to the efficiency of HPV in evading immune recognition. Inflammation does not occur because of the absence of release of inflammatory cytokines, such as interleukins and interferon, when immune recognition does not occur. Additionally, HPV genes are expressed at very low levels,[15] and some gene loci have been identified that have the capability to block immune recognition.[16] For example, the HPV genomes E6 and E7 interfere with major histocompatability complex (MHC) class I presentation of antigens and E7 can suppress both the interferon signal and the retinoblastoma gene (pRb) tumor suppressor block.[17,18] HPV E6 also produces a protein that suppresses the other main anti-oncogenic pathway (p53) that is critical in the prevention of the accumulation of mutations that may lead to cancer.[19] Finally, antigen-detecting Langerhans cells are at best sparsely distributed within the epithelium.

An understanding of the capability of HPV to evade host immunity is a critical component of optimal management of HPV-induced lesions. Any treatment that results in lysis of HPV-infected cells increases the opportunity for recognition of the presence of HPV that will initiate a local cellular immune response comprising HPV-specific CD4+ and CD8+ cells (Figure 19.3). Although ablative methods would seem to leave more killed HPV-infected cells behind for exposure to the macrophages and mononuclear cells that initiate immune recognition than that left by excisional methods, clearance rates for both virus and for lesions are similar, indicating this difference is not clinically important.[3,20] Perhaps any modality for treating CIN leaves behind adequate numbers of killed HPV genomes to initiate immune recognition (Figures 19.4a–d). When such recognition does not occur following treatment, recurrence of HPV-induced disease is likely.

Cervical cancer does not occur in the absence of long-term persistence of HPV.[21,22] However, 10% to 20% of patients treated for CIN will have either persistent or recurrent disease, indicating an inability to suppress remaining HPV. It may be that many women in this subset have a diminished immunocompetence to HPV that is genetic, acquired or of unknown etiology.[5]

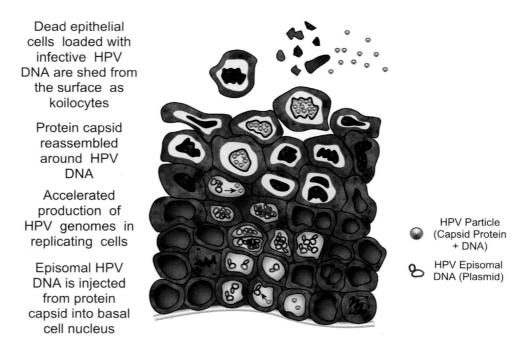

Dead epithelial cells loaded with infective HPV DNA are shed from the surface as koilocytes

Protein capsid reassembled around HPV DNA

Accelerated production of HPV genomes in replicating cells

Episomal HPV DNA is injected from protein capsid into basal cell nucleus

HPV Particle (Capsid Protein + DNA)

HPV Episomal DNA (Plasmid)

Figure 19.2 The life cycle of a HPV infection. During this entire process, HPV remains hidden within the epithelial cells.

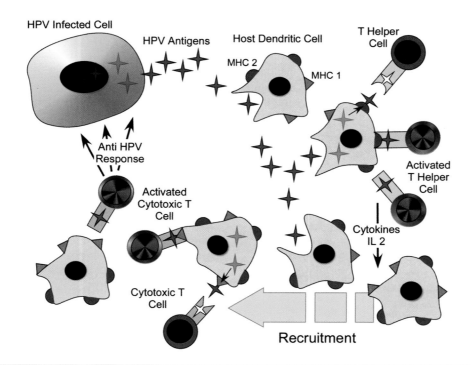

FIGURE 19.3   The sequence of events following immune recognition of the presence of HPV: Dendritic cells engulf HPV antigens and process them into bits of information that can be utilized in initiating an immune response. Dendritic cells may present both MHC Class I and MHC Class II processed antigens on their surface. The major histocompatibility complex, or MHC, is a region of the human chromosome 6 that is responsible for producing glycoproteins that are expressed on the surfaces of most cells. MHC class I processed antigens are presented in the regional lymph nodes to resting cytotoxic T cells, which become activated CD8+ cells. MHC class II processed antigens are presented to resting helper T cells, which become activated CD4+ cells. Activated CD4+ cells produce cytokines such as IL-2, interferon and tumor necrosis factor that further promote recognition of HPV antigens and recruitment of macrophages, monocytes and dendritic cells at the site of infection. Activated CD8+ cells also migrate back to the site of the infection to mount an anti-HPV, anti-tumor response. Modified with permission from Cox J T. In: Lonky N, Ed. Management of women with cervical cancer precursor lesions. *Obstet Gynecol Clin North Am* 2002;29:787–816.

19.1.3 Brief survey of treatment options for CIN

Treatment options for CIN can be grouped into chemically destructive, surgical ablative, and surgical excisional methods. Cryotherapy, laser, and loop electrosurgical methods will be discussed in depth later in this chapter but will be mentioned here as part of the overall survey of modalities.

19.1.3.1 Chemically destructive modalities

Chemical treatments for CIN have neither been adequately evaluated nor achieved widespread use. However, both trichloracetic acid (TCA) and 5-fluorouracil (5-FU) have been proposed for the treatment of CIN and will therefore be mentioned here for completeness. 5-FU is the most commonly used modality for treating actinic keratoses and early skin cancers, and TCA continues to be a mainstay in the treatment of external genital warts.

Trichloracetic Acid   Trichloracetic acid (TCA) is sometimes used by the medical community to treat vaginal low-grade HPV lesions and lesions on the mature squamous epithelium of the cervix in areas not within the transformation zone, and has also been used for this purpose in pregnancy.[23] Consideration of the use of TCA to treat either primary lesions or recurrences post-treatment should be reserved only for those that are low-grade and present on mature squamous epithelium. The use of TCA for the treatment of CIN within active areas of the transformation zone is contraindicated because of concern that topical treatment of surface cells might leave CIN buried in gland ducts at risk for persistence and progression.[24]

5-Fluorouracil   Topical 5-fluorouracil (5-FU) interferes with DNA and RNA synthesis. During the 1980s, 5-FU was widely used to treat both vaginal low- and high-grade intraepithelial neoplasia (VAIN)

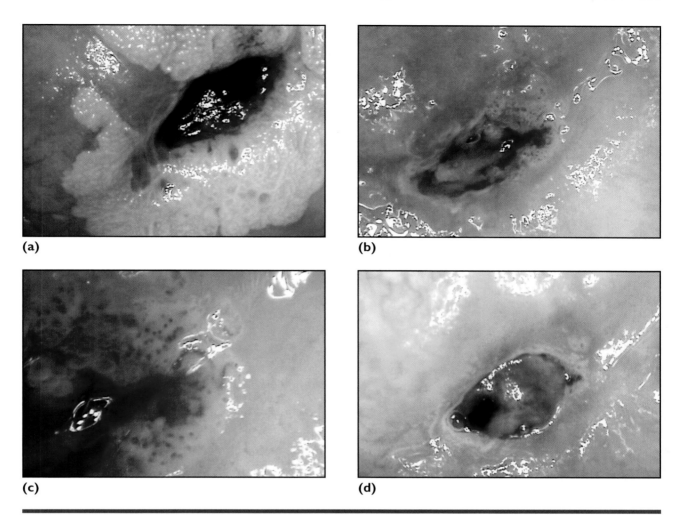

(a)

(b)

(c)

(d)

FIGURES 19.4a–d   **(a)** Extensive recurrent CIN 1 can be seen 4 months following cryotherapy. Expectant management was elected in the expectation that a significant immune response could still occur. **(b)** 4 months later only a very tiny area of mild acetowhite and linear punctation remains, best seen in the magnified view **(c)** HPV test continued to be positive. **(d)** Colposcopy of the cervix was completely normal by nine months post-cryotherapy and the HPV test and Pap were both negative (normal). Modified with permission from Cox J T. In: Lonky N, Ed. Management of women with cervical cancer precursor lesions. *Obstet Gynecol Clin North Am* 2002;29:787–816.

and condylomata.[25] It was also presumed that 5-FU treatment of vaginal HPV lesions would have a secondary advantage of also clearing any low-grade cervical disease present. Although initial reports confirmed that 5-FU did have some efficacy for treating cervical disease,[26] enthusiasm for use in the vagina quickly faded with reports of intractable introital and vaginal ulcers often accompanied by significant acute and chronic introital pain. Not uncommonly, vaginal adenosis developed in areas denuded of vaginal epithelium and at least two cases of clear cell adenocarcinoma were reported to occur in these areas.[27] These problems have eliminated 5-FU from the routine treatment of vaginal HPV-induced disease.

The only arena where 5-FU use in the vagina has been demonstrated to be more helpful than detrimental is in the prevention of recurrence of CIN post-treatment in HIV-positive women. One report indicated that HIV-positive women treated for CIN by standard excisional or ablative procedures and receiving six months of biweekly 2 grams of vaginal 5-FU cream had a significantly prolonged post-treatment disease-free interval compared with women with similar surgical treatment but who were only observed without the application of 5-FU.[28] Also, only 28% recurred in the 5-FU treated group in contrast to 47% in the observation group, and when recurrence occurred, it was more likely to be a lesser grade (8% CIN 2 and 3 in the 5-FU treated group vs. 31% in the observational group). These results have promoted the use of 5-FU in the prophylaxis of individuals at very high risk for post-treatment recurrence secondary to reduced immunocompetence.

19.1.3.2 Cervical ablative procedures

Electrodiathermy CIN is commonly treated in Australia and in Europe by electrocautery with a ball and needle but this procedure is rarely used in the United States. Very high cure rates of 85% to 94% or more have been reported by individuals proficient in electrodiathermy.[29,30] The largest study included 1240 women with CIN 3, with a reported cure rate of 97.5%.[29] Electrodiathermy requires a standard electrical unit capable of generating 40–45 watts, and a needle and ball electrode. Following administration of local or general anesthesia, a radial cut is made with the needle electrode to a depth of 5–7 mm and 2–3 mm beyond the extent of iodine-negative areas. This incision is set as the peripheral margin of the area to be ablated with the ball electrode. The resulting crater should attain a depth of approximately 7 mm. Postoperative instructions and complications are similar to those described for laser later in this chapter. The primary adverse effect of this procedure has been increased scarring within the treated area that has occasionally resulted in prolonging labor.[31]

Cryosurgery Cryosurgery (also called cryotherapy) was the first outpatient procedure for the treatment of CIN to gain wide acceptance. Although it fell out of favor during the late 1980s and early 1990s with the ascendance of laser, and subsequently LEEP, the low cost and high patient safety profile of cryosurgery has resurrected this procedure. As with any ablative procedure, cryosurgery must be performed under stringent patient selection guidelines in order to minimize the failure rate and risk of inappropriately treating occult invasive cancer. When lesions less suitable for treatment by ablation are triaged to excisional procedures, clearance rates for all grades of CIN have varied from 86% to 91.6% following cryosurgery. These rates are comparable to those following both laser and LEEP.[3,32,33] Cryosurgery will destroy the surface 4 to 5 mm of tissue. Safety is ensured by the inability of the destructive temperature to penetrate deeper because of the warmth of the underlying vessels. Comparable clearance rates for women randomized to cryosurgery, laser, and LEEP and paired for gland duct involvement appear to indicate that this depth of cell destruction is adequate even for women with gland duct involvement.[3] As with other treatment methods, the success of cryosurgery is more related to

lesion size than to lesion grade[3,34] and to absence of lesion extension beyond 4 mm to 5 mm into the canal.[35] Other than large lesion size and extension into the canal, treatment failure is most commonly secondary to inadequate freeze caused by poor probe application, insufficient freeze time, and low refrigerant pressure.[36–39]

CO_2 laser During the 1980s, laser vaporization became the treatment of choice for CIN of many gynecologic surgeons. However, the introduction of LEEP to the United States in the early 1990s quickly diminished the laser procedure's popularity. LEEP had many advantages, including being far less costly in both initial investment and in maintenance, as well as being easier to learn. However, very large cervical lesions, high-grade vaginal lesions, and lesions in areas difficult to access are often still best treated by CO_2 laser. Clearance rates for the treatment of CIN by CO_2 laser vaporization are high and comparable to other treatment modalities, with success rates of 90% to 96% reported.[40–44] As with any ablative procedure, selection of patients appropriate for laser ablation should follow strict guidelines similar to those mentioned for cryotherapy. The only exceptions are that laser ablation can successfully treat lesions that extend beyond both the exocervical and the endocervical limits set for cryotherapy. Tissue on the transformation zone of the cervix should be destroyed to a depth of approximately 5 mm to 7 mm. In expert hands, complications are minimal.

19.1.3.3 Cervical excisional procedures

Treatment by cervical biopsy alone Small low-grade lesions may occasionally be completely removed by biopsy with a standard cervical biopsy forceps. Young first described this approach for both diagnosis and treatment of women with abnormal Pap smear results in 1949.[24,45] Because colposcopy was not yet available to better localize abnormal areas, treatment often required multiple biopsies in order to excise by simple punch biopsy the majority of the transformation-zone and squamocolumnar junction (SCJ). Following the introduction of colposcopy, treatment by biopsy could be more focused on the areas of abnormality. Any biopsy may increase the rate of resolution of low-grade CIN, even when the entire lesion is not removed. However, modalities that do not fully treat the transformation zone should be reserved for CIN 1 only or very small post-treatment recurrences, as clearance rates by biopsy alone are significantly less for high-grade lesions (68% for CIN 2 and 46% for CIN 3) than for CIN 1 (82%).[45–47]

Loop electrosurgical excision procedure (LEEP)
The term LEEP (Loop Electrosurgical Excision Procedure) is most commonly used in the United States, whereas LLETZ (Large Loop Excision of Transformation Zone) is the common term in Europe. Both describe the excision of tissue by an electrified wire loop, although LLETZ specifically applies to treatment of the cervix, while the term LEEP encompasses treatment of any area of the lower genital tract or on the skin. The breakthrough in electrical generators that provided renewed interest in this procedure occurred when it became possible to convert 60 Hertz (Hz) low-frequency alternating current into a high frequency AC of 350,000 to 700,000 Hz (or 350 to 700 kHz).[31] The advantage of this frequency is that it cuts by vaporizing tissue rather than by burning it and does not cause muscle twitching or spasm. The result was a significant decrease in thermal damage and an increase in patient comfort. Cartier pioneered small loop biopsy of the cervix.[48,49] The combination of these electrical generator innovations and Cartier's procedural breakthroughs paved the way for the modern development of the larger loops now used.[50]

Although LEEP has been used to excise lesions outside the cervix, many clinicians continue to use LEEP exclusively on the cervix and to treat lesions on the vagina, vulva, and penis with CO_2 laser or other modalities. Because LEEP has several advantages over other procedures, it quickly replaced laser as the procedure of choice for treatment of CIN. The advantages are that the equipment is inexpensive compared to that for laser, the histologic specimen has minimal burn artifact when performed optimally, and the procedure is simple and quick.[51] As with any excisional procedure, treating the cervix while obtaining a histologic specimen virtually eliminates the potential of missing an occult cancer and is therefore ideal when the lesion is large and high grade. Obtaining a specimen is also important when biopsy has not detected CIN 2 or 3 and the referral Pap test is high grade. Recurrent or persistent disease following LEEP has been reported in 5% to 27%,[52–55] which is consistent with rates reported for other treatment modalities. However, widespread overuse during the early to mid-1990s led to reports that 20% to 65% of LEEP specimens were either normal or showed only CIN 1.[56–58] Although some of these were secondary to high-grade lesions having been completely removed by biopsy prior to the LEEP, others reflected cervical excision for noncorrelating misclassified HSIL Paps.[59]

CO_2 laser conization In skilled hands, cervical excision by CO_2 laser can produce a better cone speci-

men with a lower risk of complications than with cold-knife conization.[60,61] The procedure of CO_2 laser conization is more difficult than laser vaporization because of the difficulty in controlling the high-power density generated by the small spot size used to create a cutting instrument. The power density required for excision is greater than 1000 watts/cm² at a spot size of 0.25 to 0.8 mm, whereas the power density for laser ablation is markedly less at the defocused spot size used to vaporize large areas and coagulate blood vessels.[31]

Cold-knife conization Cervical cold-knife (CKC) cone or "cone biopsy" was first described by Martzloff in 1938.[62] Following its introduction, CKC became the mainstay for treatment of high-grade CIN and remained so until the ascent of laser in the 1980s. CKC is not an easy procedure to do well, and the decreased use of this procedure following the introduction of laser, and later LEEP, has greatly reduced the number of clinicians who have the skills required for this procedure. The most common complications with CKC are excessive bleeding and cervical stenosis, complications that are most closely related to the size and shape of the cone and that vary depending on the location of the disease.[31,62] Cervical stenosis can cause dysmenorrhea, inadequate Pap tests, and unsatisfactory colposcopic examinations.

Hysterectomy Hysterectomy is rarely done for CIN alone because of the increased morbidity of the procedure and the likelihood of successful clearance with lesser procedures. However, when CIN occurs in a woman experiencing symptoms of endometriosis, symptomatic leiomyomata, or intractable dysfunctional uterine bleeding, hysterectomy may be a reasonable option. Hysterectomy may be employed when high-grade CIN extends to the endocervical margin of an excised lesion and the woman has completed her family. However, the risk of subsequent detection of cervical cancer in patients with positive cone margins is low enough that most of these women can be followed closely without further treatment, particularly when future childbearing is still a priority.[63]

19.1.4 Principles for managing women with CIN

Promoting a positive attitude While the primary objective in treating women with CIN is to ensure that the cervix returns to normal to minimize the risk for the subsequent development of cervical cancer, it is most important to keep in mind her entire well-being. Anxiety, depression, and other psychological stresses are often manifest following an abnormal Pap test result and subsequent management and their prevention or resolution should be considered a part of any Pap test screening program. Because education is consistently identified as being key to reducing stress related to the management women with abnormal Pap test results,[64,65] providing information about the nature and cause of an abnormal Pap test can be very helpful. When CIN is identified, information on the natural history of HPV-induced lesions and management options should be provided to help the patient understand how common HPV is and how low the risk of cancer is for most infected with HPV. While providing reassurance, however, it must also be emphasized that adherence to management recommendations is imperative. Concern and anxiety over an abnormal Pap test result can be significantly minimized by prior knowledge that the Pap test is primarily a test for cells that may lead to cancer if not detected and treated, and only very rarely identifies cells from an already existing cancer.[66]

Information can be provided in written or verbal form, or optimally by both, since written materials perused at the patient's leisure will often be retained better than verbal communication that may be blurred by the anxiety of the moment. However, verbal communication is important for establishing a relationship of trust between physician and patient and providing the patient an opportunity to ask questions.

Encouraging healthful habits It may also be helpful to encourage good health habits. Perhaps the only definitive evidence that unhealthful habits reduce the immune response to HPV is data related to smoking tobacco. There is little question that smoking depresses the normal immune response. Although a recent analysis did not demonstrate a relationship between smoking and cervical dysplasia after multivariate adjustment,[67] in most studies, the association of smoking with increased risk of cervical cancer and with failure to respond to treatment for CIN is fairly definitive.[68] The mechanism of action of smoking is not proven, but it is likely that a combination of the direct carcinogenic effects of cotinine, nicotine, and nitrosamines and local immunosuppression manifest by decreasing density and function of Langerhans cells are both contributory.[69–71]

Failure to respond to treatment of CIN is significantly more common among smokers than non-smokers, and an increase in persistent HPV infection is seen in heavy smokers.[68] Because of the association of smoking with diminished immune function and cessation of smoking with an increase in cervical Langerhans cells,[71] it is particularly important to advise all women with CIN that smoking increases their risk for cervical cancer and decreases the potential for successful treatment.

Epidemiologic data indicate that there may be an increased risk of cervical cancer in populations with inadequate dietary intake of folic acid, B_6 and B_{12}, beta-carotene, and indole-3-carbinols.[72–74] Although there are no compelling data that diets rich in these substances promote increased regression of CIN,[75–77] recommending a balanced diet is part of good general medical advice and may be beneficial.[78] Other healthy habits that may have a positive impact on general health, or at least not diminish the ability of the immune system to respond, may include avoiding excessive alcohol, drug use, and inadequate sleep. It may be that the most important result of providing common-sense health recommendations is the feeling of empowerment that some women will have when given steps that they can take to gain some control over their disease process.[5] The as-yet unproven health benefits of many of these measures may be far less important than the psychological advantage they foster.[78]

Deciding on active vs. expectant management
Almost all women with high-grade squamous or glandular lesions will be managed actively by either an ablative or an excisional procedure since regression of CIN 2 or 3 is less common than with low-grade CIN and the risk of progression is significantly higher. There are only two exceptions to this rule: pregnant women having a documented high-grade lesion are followed expectantly and a similar option is given to adolescents considered reliable for follow-up who have CIN 2.[10] These options were created because treatment of the pregnant cervix may complicate the pregnancy, and CIN 2 in adolescents often resolves spontaneously. Additionally, once cancer has been ruled out, the risk that a cancer would develop during the pregnancy is small, and the risk of cancer in adolescents is negligible.

In contrast to almost universal active management of CIN 2 or 3, CIN 1 is often managed expectantly without initial treatment in compliant patients because of the high rate of spontaneous regression of low-grade disease. The choice of treatment versus observation is one that ideally should involve the patient after full explanation of the risks and benefits of each approach. Some women will feel treatment brings quicker closure and therefore produces less anxiety than the "wait and see" approach, while others will feel just the opposite. In our mobile society and with the shifting sands of ever-changing insurance plans, continuity of care is often not optimal, increasing the risk that the patient may be lost to follow-up. This is especially the case for indigent or uninsured women, who are both at higher risk for cervical cancer and for problems in accessing follow-up health care. This risk must always be considered when expectant management is elected. It is very important for the patient to understand that if she does not remain in the clinician's care, she must take the responsibility to access appropriate follow-up as directed.

Choosing the procedure for women requiring treatment When treatment is elected the procedure chosen should be one that offers the best cure rate considering the lesion characteristics and the clinician's expertise. Where several options may be equally effective, patient preference should also be taken into consideration. At the present time, the only treatment options are either ablative or excisional, although in the future it is hoped that treatments will become available that more specifically enhance the immune response to HPV or disable regions in the HPV genome that promote viral transcription and transformation. Until that time, the available options are limited to cryosurgery, diathermy, laser ablation or excision, LEEP and cold knife conization. There are numerous comparative advantages and disadvantages for each procedure.[78] Cryosurgery requires minimal skill, is easy to use, has few complications, is reliable, and is very cost-effective. However, the effectiveness of cryosurgery is limited by certain lesion characteristics, including lesion size and extension more than 4 mm to 5 mm into the canal. Additionally, heavy, often odorous, discharge lasting several weeks is a disadvantage. Laser vaporization is more easily tailored to lesion location and size than either cryosurgery or LEEP but requires greater clinical expertise because of the potential for more serious injuries. Also, the initial cost and ongoing expense with maintaining laser equipment has significantly reduced the availability of this modality.

Clearance rates following cryosurgery or laser have not been shown to be statistically different when evaluated in either nonrandomized or randomized trials comparing these two modalities (Table 19.1).[3,38,39,42,79-81] Marked variability in rates of recurrence or persistence of CIN do exist from study to study. For instance, a failure rate of 30% was reported by Kwikkel for laser compared to 14% for cryotherapy,[32] whereas Wright reported that 14% of women treated by cryotherapy and only 3% treated by laser failed to remain clear.[80] Loop excision and laser have also been shown to have similar failure rates in both randomized and in nonrandomized trials.[53,82] Most importantly, the risk of persistent or recurrent disease has been noted in these studies to be associated with three prognostic variables: endocervical gland involvement, lesion size, and lesion grade. In contrast, the largest randomized trial to date in the management of CIN

Table 19.1   Comparison of Failure Rates for Cryo, Laser and LEEP

Study	Year	Total Pts.	Failure Rate(%)*		
Non-randomized			Cryo	Laser	LEEP
Wright	1981	334	14%	3%	NA
Townsend	1983	200	7%	11%	NA
Ferenczy	1985	294	9%	4%	NA
Gunasekera	1990	199	NA	8%	5%
Randomized					
Kirwan	1985	98	17%	11%	NA
Kwikkel	1985	101	14%	30%	NA
Berget	1987	204	9%	10%	NA
Berget	1991	187	4%	8%	NA
Alvarez	1994	375	NA	4%	7%
Mitchell	1998	390	24%	17%	16%

* Persistence and recurrence combined

From Cox J T. In: Lonky N, Ed. Management of women with cervical cancer precursor lesions. Obstet Gynecol Clin North Am 2002;29:790. With permission.

assessed the effectiveness of all three commonly used treatment modalities (cryotherapy, laser, and LEEP) and stratified the patients by prognostic variables that may have accounted for the marked variability in clearance rates noted in previous studies.[3] Cryotherapy had a slightly higher rate of persistent or recurrent disease (24%) when compared with laser (17%) and LEEP (16%) but the difference was not statistically significant. Evaluation of the effect of lesion size, grade, and location, endocervical gland involvement, HPV status, age, and smoking history determined that only the size of the lesion was statistically associated with increased failure rates, regardless of the treatment modality chosen. Lesions involving more than two thirds of the cervical portio were 19 times more likely than smaller lesions to persist following treatment. However, other parameters that more reflect the status of host-immunity or of the infecting virus did appear to be important in determining the patient's risk of recurrence of new disease following a previous negative post-treatment visit. For example, women with any of the following characteristics were more than twice as likely to have recurrent disease: older than 30 years of age, being positive for HPV 16 or 18, or having a history of previous treatment for CIN. These parameters are consistent with the premise that HPV 16 and 18 are higher risk than other high-risk HPV types, and that older women with HPV, or those having failed previous therapy, may have some decreased ability to clear HPV.[78]

Surgical complications were also demonstrated to be reasonably comparable, occurring in only 2% having cryotherapy, 4% having laser, and 8% having LEEP.[3] The difference noted in these rates was almost entirely secondary to an increased rate in postoperative bleeding for LEEP (4.6%) compared with 2.3% for laser, and none with cryotherapy. There was no significant difference in rates of infection or cervical stenosis (less than 1% and 1.5%, respectively, in all groups, (Table 19.2). These data provide reassurance that the efficacy and risks of each of these methods are comparable and are further supported by similar findings in a recent meta-analysis of a much larger number of randomized and quasi-randomized trials evaluating various treatment modalities for CIN.[83]

Colposcopically directed biopsy has been shown to not always detect the most abnormal area.[84] In one study, 47% of women with discordant results have been shown to have a more severe lesion in the excisional specimen than in the previous punch biopsy, and of most concern, was the finding of one microinvasive carcinoma and three cases of AIS.[84] Mac Indoe and colleagues found that 2 of 196 patients with CIN determined to fit the criteria for ablative treatment

Table 19.2	Complication Rates in the Treatment of CIN by Cryotherapy, Laser or LEEP		
	Cryo	Laser	LEEP
Bleeding	0%	2.3%	4.6%
Infection	all < 1.0%		
Cervical stenosis	all < 1.5%		

Data from: Mitchell M F, Tortolero-Luna G, Cook E, Whittaker L, Rhodes-Morris H, Silva E. A randomized clinical trial of cryotherapy, loop electrosurgical excision for treatment of squamous intraepithelial lesions of the cervix. *Obstet Gyneol* 1998;92:737–44.

were subsequently found on laser cone excision to have microinvasive carcinoma and a third had AIS.[85] A review of 15 studies comparing the accuracy of colposcopic biopsy with later excisional treatment found that between 1% and 10% of the women had lesions more severe in the excisional specimen than in the previous biopsy.[86] This included 16 invasive cervical cancers that were missed by the pretreatment colposcopically directed biopsy of 1975 patients. These issues have increased insecurity that direct punch biopsy may be an inadequate endpoint for electing treatment options that do not provide an additional specimen.[84] These reports and those of others showing occult AIS or microinvasive carcinoma in 2% to 3% of biopsy documented high-grade specimens excised by LEEP have convinced many clinicians to not use ablative methods to treat any CIN 2,3.[51,57] However, historical data suggests that ablation may effectively cure microinvasive cancers missed at colposcopy. Ablative techniques for the treatment of CIN continue to be popular and effective if used in strict observance of treatment guidelines that reduce the risk of missed occult disease.

Young women are almost always concerned about the potential for long-term effects of CIN treatment on fertility. Any procedure that destroys or removes a large portion of the cervix theoretically could impair fertility by resulting in decreased cervical mucus, reduced cervical competence, cervical stenosis, or tubal scarring secondary to post-treatment infection.[87,88] An extensive review of the entire literature on the impact of cryotherapy, laser, LEEP, CKC, and electrocoagulation diathermy on fertility provides reassurance that these events are not common with any single treatment with any of the modalities.[89] The only exception was the finding that cold-cone biopsy did result in slightly higher rates of second trimester abortions, pre-term labor, and low birthweight infants. This risk was proportional to the volume and cephalocaudal length of tissue removed Therefore, clinician and patient preference and cost considerations would appear to be more important in the choice of procedure than concern over potential differences in efficacy, complications, or fertility. However, risk of missing the rare occult invasive cancer is highest when the lesion is large and complex or with extension more than 4 mm to 5 mm into the canal.[30] For this reason, guidelines usually suggest ablative procedures only for lesions that do not fit these parameters.[10]

19.1.5 Management guidelines for women with CIN

Evidence-based guidelines on the management of women with CIN were developed at the September 2001 ASCCP consensus workshop and are available at *www.asccp.org*.[10] These guidelines provide the basis for the following discussion of both observational and active treatment management options for CIN.

19.1.5.1 Management of Women with CIN1

Only during the past decade has expectant management of CIN 1 without treatment become a common management option. Prior to the mid-1990s, the prevalent theory was that the various grades of CIN represented a progressive disease continuum and that treatment of all grades was necessary in order to disrupt progression.[90] However, it has become increasingly clear that high-grade lesions represent monoclonal cellular dysfunction independent of CIN 1 and that immunity will usually suppress HPV-induced low-grade lesions.[91-94] Additionally, the accuracy of a histopathological diagnosis of CIN 1 has come under question. For instance, in the ASCUS/LSIL Triage Study (ALTS), an expert review by a pathology quality control panel agreed with only 43% of the original clinical center CIN 1 histologic interpretations.[59] The majority of these discrepancies were downgraded to normal. These observations have promoted a shift to expectant management, which, however, continues to be limited by the present inability to predict the biological potential of a CIN 1 lesion. The risk of detection of CIN 2 and 3 during 2-year follow up of untreated CIN 1 has been shown to be 13%.[95] Although it has traditionally been assumed that women initially referred for LSIL or HPV-positive ASC-US cytology and found to have documented CIN 1 on colposcopic examination were at higher risk for subsequent detection of CIN 2 and 3 than were women with no CIN detected, 2-year follow up has shown the risk to be similar.[95] This similarity in risk promotes similar management.[10,96]

The decision whether to treat CIN 1, or to follow it expectantly, may depend on many factors. One fac-

tor is the impact on the workload of the clinic staff in following large numbers of women with CIN 1 at regular intervals, including an increase in the number of patient notifications, office visits, and treatment for the 11% to 13% that have lesions that progress and another 10% to 20% that will persist as CIN 1.[78,95,96] Sensitive detection of CIN 3 by repeat cytologic testing requires at least two further office visits with a cytologic threshold for repeat colposcopy of ≥ASC-US.[96] Unfortunately, at this threshold, more than two thirds of women with untreated CIN 1 will have a repeat abnormal Pap test, requiring a second referral for colposcopy. Follow-up protocols for the expectant management if CIN 1 have traditionally recommended combining repeat Pap tests with interval colposcopic examinations to decrease the risk of missed CIN 2 or 3, but this approach is costly and increases anxiety.[97] Natural history studies have confirmed that the majority of CIN 1 lesions managed expectantly will spontaneously resolve within 24 months of diagnosis. Although women with CIN 1 persistent at 2 years are not obligated to accept treatment as long as they remain compliant, longer follow-up is less likely to result in spontaneous resolution, and the longer high-risk HPV persists, the greater the risk that CIN 2,3 will develop.[98]

Several other issues related specifically to each individual woman are important determinants in the decision whether to treat or follow CIN 1. The most important of these issues concerns the perceptions and preferences and age of the patient, reliability for compliant follow-up, cost of treatment options in comparison with expectant management, and whether the colposcopy was satisfactory or unsatisfactory.[10,78]

Patient perceptions and preferences For some, the prospect of having a surgical procedure on their cervix is most daunting, while for others, long-term observation only prolongs anxiety secondary to uncertainty over the eventual outcome. The most challenging aspect of any screening test is that a positive result will often make "patients" out of people who otherwise feel well, irrespective of whether a significant lesion is present.[99] Feelings of vulnerability, anger, fear, and mortality in both patient and partner are even stronger once CIN is known to be secondary to a sexually transmitted virus. These feelings, therefore, can threaten sexuality and relationships. Additionally, the level of anxiety does not vary with the level of Pap abnormality or the grade of CIN but can be diminished by appropriate counseling.[64]

Most women have either not heard of HPV or are unaware of its relationship to abnormal Pap test findings, CIN, and cervical cancer.[100] The majority informed of having a HPV infection feel that they had inadequate counseling about the virus. Appropriate counseling about HPV has been shown to diminish psychosocial consequences associated with a positive result on HPV testing,[101] whereas inadequate counseling can have adverse emotional and sexual repercussions.[102] Education via written material, explanatory videos, or individual counseling can all significantly reduce anxiety.[97,103,104]

Patients most anxious about "having a disease" are most likely to elect treatment when given the option, whereas fear of pain and complications, particularly those that might threaten fertility, often drives preference for expectant management.[105] While accurate information can usually allay those fears, many women find the information confusing, and time pressures often make it difficult for clinicians to give the detailed information and reassurance patients need.[106] Despite these challenges, it is imperative that women receive the information they need to feel reassured and to make informed decisions when both conservative treatment and close surveillance are reasonable options.

Reliability for compliant follow-up Safe expectant management requires that the patient be reliable for follow-up and that the clinic have a follow-up reminder system that can dependably aid in such compliance. The most significant challenge with expectant management of CIN 1, as with any aspect of management of abnormal cervical cytologic results, is that achievement of full compliance is never possible and drops significantly with increasing duration of follow-up.[107] A significant proportion of women being observed for CIN 1 at 6-month intervals for a minimum of 2 years will not return for adequate surveillance.[108] A number of factors other than patient fatigue and anxiety can affect adherence to follow-up, including demographic factors, lack of social support and understanding, clinic hours, cost, sensitivity of staff and providers, reliability of the follow-up notification system.[78,109] Robertson et al identified several reasons for loss to follow-up in evaluation of a number of cervical cancers that developed in women with low-grade cervical abnormality who were followed expectantly.[110] These included poorly organized notification systems, transient populations, and a number of psychological and societal barriers. Strategies that have been shown to be successful in improving follow-up include educational programs, telephone counseling, and economic incentives.[109]

Estimation of the reliability for compliance is considered to be a pivotal determinant in the management recommendations for women with CIN 1 made by both the 2001 ASCCP Consensus Confer-

ence and by the 1992 British National Health Service.[10,111] Women with CIN 1 considered to be at-risk for loss to follow-up are best treated. However, since predicting loss to follow-up of individual patients has been shown to be unreliable, clinics with high rates of noncompliance may recommend treatment of CIN 1, although the option of observation should be presented. In order to achieve maximum compliance, patients need to be given a comprehensive explanation of the need for regular follow-up and the risks of not doing so. Additionally, a sound follow-up tracking and notification system needs to be in place.[112] This may not be possible within transient populations.

Cost of observation vs. treatment Cost effectiveness of any management option will vary depending on local factors. One clinical decision analysis comparing expectant management of CIN 1 with treatment demonstrated that the former led to a better outcome for the majority of patients having spontaneous resolution of their disease, but that delay in treatment required more costly surgical procedures for others having progression.[113] However, such cost-comparisons depend on a number of assumptions that cannot cover all variables, such as the lack of a universal approach for expectant management and wide variations in the cost of an office visit, repeat cytologic testing, HPV testing, colposcopic assessment, and treatment options. For example, although expectant management of CIN 1 has traditionally required repeat Pap tests every 6 months, some clinicians also routinely perform colposcopic examinations at one or more follow-up visits, while others refer only patients with repeat abnormal cytologic results for colposcopy. Even then, the threshold for colposcopy referral has been quite variable. Additionally, the recent inclusion of HPV testing as an option for the management of these women is likely to significantly change cost-benefit estimations.

Satisfactory and unsatisfactory colposcopic examinations An unsatisfactory colposcopic examination with CIN 1 extending into the canal beyond visualization may adjoin a higher-grade lesion that has not yet been detected. In contrast, when the examination is satisfactory, the risk of missed disease in the cervical canal is small. One study of women having a cervical excision procedure for CIN 1 in the endocervical curetting and an unsatisfactory colposcopic examination reported that 12% had CIN 2 or 3 detected in the cone specimen.[114] Such data prompted the ASCCP to recommend in its guidelines a surgical excision procedure for women with CIN 1 whose colposcopic examination is unsatisfactory.[10]

19.1.5.1.1 Expectant management of CIN 1   In the ALTS trial, all expectant management strategies with high sensitivity to detect CIN 3 or more severe disease resulted in more than 50% repeat colposcopy referrals.[96] Repeat Pap tests at six and 12 months cumulatively detected 85% of the CIN 3 that occurred in women with ≤CIN 1 at initial colposcopy followed over a two-year period.[96] A single HPV test at 12 months detected 95% of the CIN 3 that developed over the same time period, with slightly less referral back to colposcopy because of a positive result (55% vs. 60%, respectively). The ASCCP Guidelines (Figure 19.5a) incorporated these data along with evidence that only persistent HPV progresses to CIN 3[21] in determining that a single repeat HPV test was a safe alternative to two repeat Pap tests in the expectant management of women with CIN 1 (Table 19.3).[10]

Expectant management is a safe option for women with CIN 1 and is reasonably offered if the patient is deemed compliant and comfortable with this approach, and if the facility responsible for follow-up is equipped to manage the patient long-term and has a reliable follow-up notification system.[10,78] Women who are referred for the evaluation of either LSIL or HPV-positive ASCUS cytologic results but are not found to have CIN on colposcopic examination are at similar risk for the subsequent detection of CIN 2 or 3 as women with biopsy-proven CIN 1. Therefore, the management options are identical for all women with disease severity equivalent to or less than CIN 1 on colposcopic examination, unless initially referred for glandular cell (AGC) or high-grade (HSIL) cytologic abnormality. Management options include either two repeat Pap tests at six-month intervals or a test for high-risk HPV at 12 months. The only observational Pap test management strategy with acceptable sensitivity is referral to colposcopy at the threshold of ≥ASC-US, with return to routine screening for all women with two consecutive negative results on repeat Pap testing. The high sensitivity

Management of Women with Biopsy-confirmed Cervical Intraepithelial Neoplasia - Grade 1 (CIN 1) and Satisfactory Colposcopy

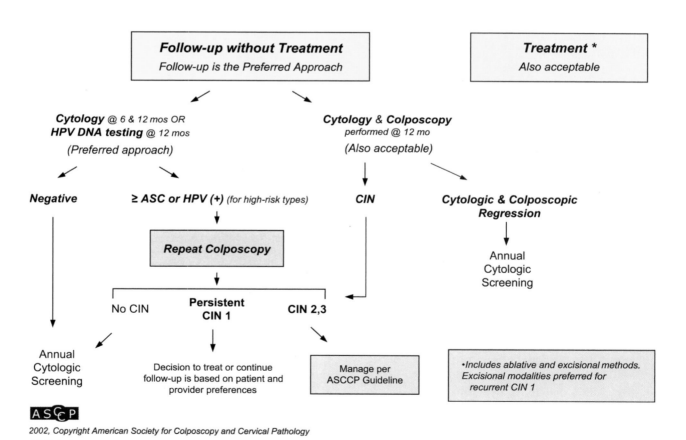

2002, Copyright American Society for Colposcopy and Cervical Pathology

FIGURE 19.5a   ASCCP algorithm for the management of women with biopsy-confirmed CIN1 and a satisfactory colposcopy. With permission from ASCCP.

Table 19.3 ASCCP Recommendations for Managing Women with Biopsy-confirmed CIN 1 and a Satisfactory Colposcopic Examination

Management options for women with biopsy-confirmed CIN 1 include follow-up without treatment or treatment using ablative or excisional modalities.

- Follow-up with a program of either repeat cervical cytology, at 6 and 12 months, or HPV DNA testing for high-risk types of HPV at 12 months, is the preferred management approach for women with biopsy-confirmed CIN 1 and a satisfactory colposcopic examination. **(AI)**
- When follow-up is utilized, referral to colposcopy is preferred if a repeat cytology is reported as ASC or greater or the woman is HPV DNA positive. **(AII)**
- After two negative consecutive cervical cytology tests or a negative DNA test for high-risk types of HPV at 12 months, it is preferred that patients return to annual cytological screening. **(BII)**
- In clinical settings where colposcopy is available, a combination of repeat cytology and colposcopic examination at 12 months is an acceptable approach to follow-up. **(AII)**
- Women found to have cytological or cytological and colposcopic regression during follow-up should be considered high-risk, and it is recommended that they have follow-up with repeat cytology at 12 months. **(BIII)**
- The decision to treat persistent CIN 1 should be based on patient and provider preferences. **(BIII)**

Treatment Options

- Provided the colposcopic examination is satisfactory, the following treatment modalities for biopsy-confirmed CIN 1 are considered acceptable: cryotherapy, electrofulguration, laser ablation, cold coagulation, and loop electrosurgical excision procedures (LEEP). **(AI)**
- If treatment is selected, the choice of treatment should be determined by the judgment of the clinician, and should be guided by experience, resources and clinical value for the specific patient. **(AI)**
- It is recommended that endocervical sampling be performed prior to ablation of CIN 1. **(AII)**
- Excisional modalities are recommended for patients who have recurrent biopsy-confirmed CIN 1 after undergoing previous ablative therapy. **(BII)**

Adapted from: Wright T C, Cox J T, Massad L S, Carlson J, Twiggs L B, and Wilkinson E J for the 2001 Consensus Guidelines for the Management of Women with Cervical Intraepithelial Neoplasia. *Amer J Obstet Gynecol* 2003;189:295–304.

of a single HPV test at 12 months provides similar reassurance. Any woman with a repeat abnormal Pap test result or a positive HPV test result is best referred to colposcopy.

19.1.5.1.2 Active management of CIN 1 The most compelling argument for treating all women with CIN 1 is that limited biopsy sampling of the cervix has been proven to frequently miss CIN 2 and 3 even when the colposcopic examination is satisfactory.[115] When treatment of CIN 1 is elected, the procedure chosen should either ablate or excise not only the entire lesion but also the entire transformation zone. The treatment chosen for women not previously treated can be based upon patient and clinician preference, whether the entire limits of the lesion are visible, and whether the colposcopy is satisfactory or unsatisfactory. Women treated previously may have "skip" lesions within the canal. Therefore, ablative methods are not advised when recurrent or new disease occurs in a woman who has been previously treated.

Whether to perform an endocervical sampling procedure prior to any ablative procedure remains controversial because the sensitivity of endocervical sampling is poor, and it is virtually impossible to miss CIN 2, CIN 3, or cancer in the cervical canal when the colposcopic examination is satisfactory and the canal appears to be normal. However, such estimations depend upon the expertise of the colposcopist, as demonstrated by a number of studies that have shown a higher risk of post-ablation CIN 2, CIN 3, and cervical cancer when pretreatment endocervical sampling has not been done.[116] Despite the low risk, variability in colposcopy expertise dictated that the ASCCP Guidelines recommend endocervical sampling prior to any cervical ablative procedure.[10] Pretreatment endocervical sampling is not mandatory when an excisional procedure is expected, as the canal will be evaluated within the excised portion and an endocervical sample beyond the excisional margin may be obtained at the time of the procedure.[78,115] Endocervical sampling should never be performed during pregnancy. Although the manage-

Management of Women with Biopsy-confirmed Cervical Intraepithelial Neoplasia - Grade 1 (CIN 1) and Unsatisfactory Colposcopy

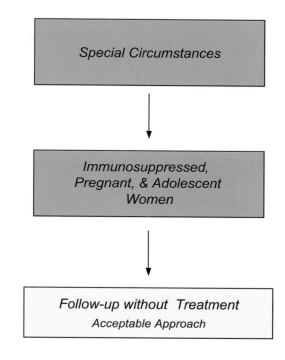

FIGURE 19.5b   ASCCP algorithm for the management of women with biopsy-confirmed CIN1 and an unsatisfactory colposcopy. With permission from ASCCP.

ment options discussed are generally for any woman with CIN 1, they do not apply for women either pregnant or immunosuppressed (see sections below on "Pregnancy" and "Immunosuppressed").

The ASCCP Guidelines recommend that women with CIN 1 and an unsatisfactory colposcopic examination *not* be managed expectantly for the reasons discussed previously (Figure 19.5b). The recommended management is by diagnostic excisional procedure (Table 19.4).

19.1.5.2 Management of women with CIN 2 or 3

In the United States, CIN 2 and 3 are managed similarly primarily because reliable histologic differentiation is only moderate (Figure 19.5c),[59,117] and the progressive potential of CIN 2 is higher than that of CIN 1, although less than that of CIN 3.[118,119]

Women with CIN 2 or 3 and a satisfactory colposcopic examination can be treated equally successfully by either ablative or by excisional methods (Table 19.5),[3] but the risk of missed occult cancer increases with increasing lesion grade and size.[51,119-121] Although numerous studies have failed to demonstrate a significant difference in clearance rates for CIN 2 or 3 treated by either ablative or by excisional methods, concern over the increased risk of missed occult cancer has promoted the use of excisional treatment for large high-grade lesions. The entire transformation zone must be included within the treatment area.[122]

Ablative procedures are contraindicated in the treatment of women with CIN 2 or 3 and an unsatisfactory colposcopic examination.[10] The only exception is when ablation is used peripheral to a central cervical excision procedure in order to eradicate

Table 19.4   ASCCP Guidelines for Managing Women with CIN 1 and an Unsatisfactory Colposcopic Examination

- The recommended treatment for patients with biopsy-confirmed CIN 1 and an unsatisfactory colposcopic examination is a diagnostic excisional procedure. **(AII)**

Unacceptable Treatment Approaches
- Ablative procedures are unacceptable for CIN 1 in patients with an unsatisfactory colposcopic examination. **(EII)**
- Podophyllin or podophyllin related products are unacceptable for use in the vagina or on the cervix. **(EII)**
- Hysterectomy as the primary and principal treatment for biopsy-confirmed CIN 1 is considered unacceptable. **(EII)**

Adapted from: Wright T C, Cox J T, Massad L S, Carlson J, Twiggs LB, and Wilkinson E J for the 2001 Consensus Guidelines for the Management of Women with Cervical Intraepithelial Neoplasia. *Amer J Obstet Gynecol* 2003;189:295–304.

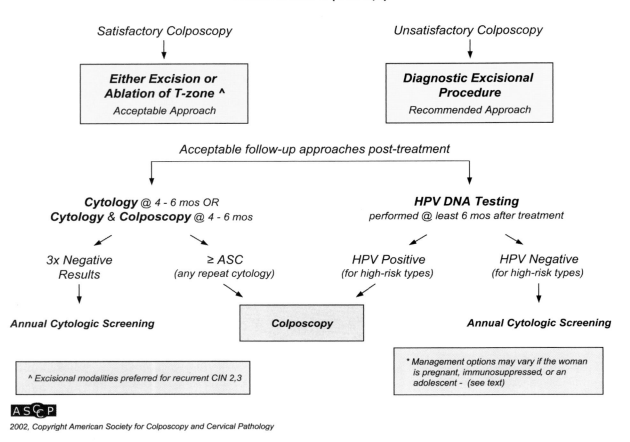

Management of Women with Biopsy-confirmed Cervical Intraepithelial Neoplasia - Grade 2 and 3 (CIN 2,3) *

2002, Copyright American Society for Colposcopy and Cervical Pathology

FIGURE 19.5c   ASCCP algorithm for the management of women with biopsy-confirmed CIN2 or CIN3. With permission from ASCCP.

Table 19.5 ASCCP Guidelines for the Management of Women with CIN 2,3—Initial Management of Biopsy-confirmed CIN 2,3.

- Management decisions in women with biopsy-confirmed CIN 2,3 are determined by whether the colposcopic examination is classified as satisfactory or unsatisfactory. Both excision and ablation of the transformation zone are acceptable for women with biopsy-confirmed CIN 2,3 and a satisfactory colposcopy. **(AI)**
- However, in patients with recurrent CIN 2,3, excisional modalities are preferred. (AII)
- A diagnostic excisional procedure is recommended for women with biopsy-confirmed CIN 2,3 and unsatisfactory colposcopy. **(AI)**
- Observation of CIN 2,3 with sequential cytology and colposcopy is unacceptable except in special circumstances *(see below)*. **(EII)**
- Hysterectomy is unacceptable as primary therapy for CIN 2,3. **(EII)**

Adapted from: Wright T C, Cox J T, Massad L S, Carlson J, Twiggs LB, and Wilkinson E J for the 2001 Consensus Guidelines for the Management of Women with Cervical Intraepithelial Neoplasia. *Amer J Obstet Gynecol* 2003; 189:295–304.

disease outside the area not excised. Acceptable treatment options for women with CIN 2,3 and unsatisfactory colposcopy include cold-knife conization, laser cone, and LEEP. All three options have comparable success rates, but cold-knife conization more frequently results in cervical distortion and an incompetent cervix.[122,123] As discussed previously, hysterectomy is not an acceptable procedure for CIN 2 and 3 unless there are other medical reasons for this procedure.[10]

Women with CIN 2 or 3 should not be managed expectantly with repeat cytologic testing and colposcopic examination unless they are pregnant. The only other exception to this rule is adolescent women with CIN 2 who are considered reliable for follow-up (see discussions below).

19.1.5.2.1 CIN 2 and 3 in pregnancy Cervical treatment for CIN during pregnancy carries unacceptable risks, including excessive bleeding and premature delivery.[124,125] Therefore, high-grade disease occurring in pregnancy is generally followed until the postpartum period (Table 19.6) because of the low risk of progression to invasion and the potential for regression following delivery, which is reported to be up to 69%.[124,126] Follow up of CIN 2 and 3 in pregnancy is by repeat Pap testing and colposcopic examination. Biopsy is warranted when the lesion appears to progress. Conization is indicated only when invasion is suspected. Only invasive cervical cancer is treated during pregnancy and even then, treatment may depend on cancer stage and when in pregnancy the cancer is detected.

19.1.5.2.2 CIN 2 in adolescents CIN 2 in adolescents and very young women is often transient and the risk of cervical cancer is exceedingly small. There-

fore, the ASCCP Guidelines note that observation by means of colposcopic examination and cytologic testing at four- to six-month intervals for one year is acceptable for adolescents with biopsy-confirmed CIN 2, provided the colposcopic examination is satisfactory, endocervical sampling is negative, and the patient accepts the risk of occult disease (Table 19.6).[10] The most important factor is whether the patient is highly likely to be reliable for follow-up. In contrast, except in pregnancy, adolescents with CIN 3 should never be managed expectantly.

19.1.5.2.3 Treatment of the immunosuppressed Management protocols are different for women with CIN 1 who are immunocompromised because of high recurrence rates post-treatment, higher prevalence of HPV, more rapid progression to CIN 2 and 3, and increased incidence of both CIN and cervical cancer.[11,127–132] Clearance rates post-treatment are less than half that seen for immunocompetent women receiving similar treatment, with no difference in rates for HIV-positive women treated with either cryosurgery or LEEP. Additionally, treatment of low-grade lesions does not appear to reduce the risk of progression. Hence, most immunosuppressed women with CIN 1 are followed rather than treated.

Treatment of immunocompromised women with CIN 2 or 3 is also less successful than for immunocompetent women and varies depending on the CD4 cell count and margin status.[131] Half of the women with a negative margin will have recurrence of their CIN. In some studies, recurrence after cold-knife cone is as high as 90%, and up to 100% have recurred following either LEEP or cryosurgery.[130] Because recurrence at the vaginal cuff post-hysterectomy has been reported to be 60%, it would appear that no procedure

Table 19.6 ASCCP Recommendations for Managing Women with CIN 2,3 in Special Circumstances—Pregnancy, Adolescents and the Immunosuppressed

Pregnancy
- The risk of progression of CIN 2,3 to invasive cervical cancer during pregnancy is minimal and the rate of spontaneous regression post-partum is relatively high.
- Excisional procedures performed during pregnancy are associated with complications including significant bleeding and preterm births.
- Excisional procedures performed during pregnancy are frequently non-diagnostic and there is a high rate of recurrent/persistent disease.
- Therefore most authorities recommend that the use of diagnostic excisional procedures during pregnancy be limited to women in whom invasive cancer cannot be ruled out.

Adolescents
- Observation with colposcopy and cytology at 4–6 month intervals for one year is acceptable for adolescents with biopsy-confirmed CIN 2, provided colposcopy is satisfactory, endocervical sampling is negative, and the patient accepts the risk of occult disease. **(BII)**
- Ablation or excision is required for adolescent women with CIN 3. **(BIII)**

Immunosuppressed Patients
- There is a high rate of recurrence/persistence of CIN 2,3 after treatment in women infected with human immunodeficiency virus-1 (HIV) and the level of risk correlates with the level of immunosuppression.
- Even though the efficacy of standard therapies for biopsy-confirmed CIN 2,3 appears to be low in HIV-infected women, the use of multiple excisional procedures appears to be effective in preventing the progression of CIN 2,3 to invasive cervical cancer.
- Use of biweekly topical vaginal 5- fluorouracil (5-FU) maintenance therapy has been shown to significantly reduce the rate of recurrent/persistent CIN after standard therapy.

Adapted from: Wright T C, Cox J T, Massad L S, Carlson J, Twiggs LB, and Wilkinson E J for the 2001 Consensus Guidelines for the Management of Women with Cervical Intraepithelial Neoplasia. *Amer J Obstet Gynecol* 2003; 189:295–304.

is highly effective in eradicating CIN in immunocompromised. Despite this, treatment appears to reduce the risk of progression to invasive cervical cancer.[130]

The inadequacy of treating CIN in the immunosuppressed has promoted the evaluation of vaginal application of 5-fluorouracil (5-FU) following surgical excision of CIN 2 and 3 (Table 19.6).[28] The primary study demonstrated a decrease in the recurrence rate of approximately 50% over 18 months of follow-up when compared with women randomized to the non-5-FU treated observation arm. This success resulted in the addition of 5-FU to many post-treatment CIN 2 and 3 protocols in immunosuppressed patients. Failure rates are also affected significantly by patient compliance with highly active antiretroviral therapy (HAART) administration. Follow-up is to ensure that invasion has not occurred, with hysterectomy the final option for invasion felt to be imminent or detected.

19.1.6 Post-treatment follow-up of women treated for CIN

Although treatment of CIN is highly successful, the long-term risk for cervical cancer remains higher than for women never having had CIN and appears to increase with age.[133–142] The rate of recurrence or persistence of CIN varies from 1% to 21% regardless of the procedure used.[3,133,141,142] Large lesions have the highest treatment failure rate.[3,51,136] Positive cone margins are also indicative of a higher risk of persistent or recurrent disease,[143–148] but margin status is not as predictive in studies that have used multivariate analysis to control for contributing factors.[78,134] Persistent or recurrent disease is more common with both endocervical and ectocervical cone margin involvement than when only one margin is involved.[134] Margins of LEEP specimens are often difficult to interpret,[147,149] and even when margins are

Table 19.7 ASCCP Recommendations for Follow-up after Treatment of Biopsy–confirmed CIN 2,3

- Following treatment of CIN 2,3, follow-up using either cervical cytology or a combination of cervical cytology and colposcopy at four to six month intervals until at least three cytological results are "negative for squamous intraepithelial lesion or malignancy" is acceptable. **(AII)**
- Annual cytological follow-up is recommended thereafter. **(AII)**
- During cytological follow-up the recommended threshold for referral to colposcopy is a result of ASC or greater. **(AII)**
- HPV testing performed at least six months after treatment is acceptable for surveillance. **(B-II)**
- If high-risk types of HPV are identified, colposcopy is recommended. **(B-III)**
- If HPV testing and cytology are negative, triage to annual follow-up is recommended. **(B-III)**
- Repeat conization or hysterectomy based on a single positive HPV test that is not corroborated by other findings (cytology, colposcopy, histology) is unacceptable. **(DIII)**

Management with involved margins or recurrence
- If CIN is identified at the margins of a diagnostic excisional procedure or a post-procedure endocervical assessment contains CIN, the addition of colposcopy and endocervical sampling at the four to six month evaluation is preferred.
- When CIN 2,3 is identified at the endocervical margins, or in the endocervical sampling obtained after the diagnostic excisional procedure, a repeat diagnostic excisional procedure is acceptable. **(AII)**
- Hysterectomy is acceptable in this situation when repeat diagnostic excision is not feasible. **(BII)**
- Hysterectomy is acceptable for treatment of recurrent/persistent biopsy-confirmed CIN 2,3. **(BII)**

Adapted from: Wright T C, Cox J T, Massad L S, Carlson J, Twiggs L B, and Wilkinson E J for the 2001 Consensus Guidelines for the Management of Women with Cervical Intraepithelial Neoplasia. *Amer J Obstet Gynecol* 2003;189:295-304. With permission.

clearly involved, the majority will remain disease-free during follow-up. Therefore, expectant management is reasonable for compliant patients with CIN 3 and positive margins, provided these women have very careful follow up.[10,134,147,148] For large lesions, excision of the central lesion with laser vaporization of the area peripheral to the excised crater-base can reduce the risk of recurrence.[150]

Protocols in the United States for the follow up of women post-treatment range from follow up by Pap tests alone, combinations of Pap tests and colposcopic examinations, and more recently, high-risk HPV DNA testing.[78] Although repeat cytologic testing alone detects up to 90% of recurrent or persistent high-grade lesions,[151,152] the requirement for multiple repeat Pap tests to attain this level of detection depends on diligent patient compliance.[78] Typical repeat Pap test protocols call for repeating the cytology every four to six months for the first year and every six months for the second year, but the threshold for referral back of colposcopy has varied from ≥ASC-US to ≥LSIL. Many clinicians will add colposcopic examination to one or more follow-up visits even though no added benefit has been established when compared with protocols that use only cytology.[152]

Testing for HPV DNA appears to be a very sensitive measure for post-treatment detection of CIN. The majority of women cleared of CIN post-treatment become negative for the type of HPV responsible for the treated lesion within six months post-treatment. In contrast, women with persistent CIN continue to have detectable HPV.[153–159] In one study, 94% of patients successfully treated and positive for HPV pretreatment no longer had detectable high-risk HPV DNA at the 12-month post-treatment visit.[157] Another evaluation of women with negative post-conization margins following treatment for CIN 2 or CIN 3 documented that 100% of women who tested HPV negative post-treatment were completely clear of CIN.[155] The predictive value of persistently detected same-type HPV 16 or 18 six months post-treatment was demonstrated in an increased unadjusted odds ratio (OR) of 8.0 for recurrent disease detected during 5-year follow-up.[159] This high sensitivity and predictive value is likely to establish HPV testing as a standard in post-treatment evaluation.

There are two options in the ASCCP Guidelines for follow up of women post-treatment for CIN 2 or 3 (Table 19.7).[10] The traditional post-treatment management options are to repeat the Pap test either as a stand-alone or to combine repeat cytology with one or more colposcopic exams every four to six months until at least three normal repeat Pap tests are obtained.[78] Once three consecutive "negative for intraepithelial neoplasia or malignancy" Pap test results have been obtained, the patient can resume ongoing annual cytologic follow up. However, any repeat abnormal Pap test result of ≥ASC-US would require a repeat colposcopic examination if not performed at the time the Pap test was obtained. The new approach to following women treated for CIN 2 or 3 is to perform HPV and Pap tests no sooner than six months post-treatment. Women positive for high-risk types of HPV or with abnormal cytology interpreted as AGC, LSIL or HSIL require repeat colposcopic examination, whereas women with normal repeat cytologic test results and a negative HPV test result are at so little risk for missed CIN that the patient may safely resume annual Pap testing. Whether these women can eventually prolong screening intervals to every three years remains to be established, but treated women remain at risk for CIN recurrence and cancer for more than a decade.[135] A positive test for high-risk HPV does not, however, indicate that persistent or recurrent neoplasia is definitively present. Therefore, proceeding to repeat conization or hysterectomy without colposcopic and histologic verification of the indication is not warranted.[10]

A positive margin or a post-procedure positive endocervical sample having CIN usually does not require repeat conization unless endocervical sampling recommended for these women at the 4- to 6-month colposcopic examination is positive.[10] When CIN 2 or 3 is detected during the management of women post-treatment, recommended options are to either repeat the cervical excisional procedure or to do a hysterectomy if childbearing is complete and repeat excision is not feasible.[10]

19.2 Cryotherapy of the Cervix

19.2.1 Introduction

In the past, cervical neoplasia was managed primarily by excisional surgery: either cold-knife conization or hysterectomy. These surgical approaches conveyed a small but significant risk of inadvertent serious harm and morbidity to the patient. A profound reduction of surgical complications was noted following the implementation of cryotherapy to treat premalignant cervical disease.[38] More importantly, treatment failures were no more commonly encountered with the new ablative treatment than when compared with older excisional approaches. Thus, cryotherapy earned a reputation as a safe, similarly efficacious, relatively inexpensive, easy, nonfertility-impairing procedure for treating women with lower genital tract premalignant disease.

19.2.2 Purpose

The purposes of cryotherapy of the cervix are to destroy pathologic tissues of the cervix by cryonecrosis and concomitantly to ablate the entire transformation zone. Cryosurgery involves the freezing of cervical or other lower genital tract tissues using extremely cold gases (nitrous oxide, liquid nitrogen, or carbon dioxide), preferably delivered to the lesion through a closed unit (Figures 19.6a,b). The hypothermic process produces a lethal cold "burn" of premalignant lower genital tract neoplasia and epithelium of the cervical transformation zone. Interchangeable metal probes that are applied to the epithelium convey the thermal damaging effects. Variation in the shape and diameter of probes allows proper selection to match lesion dimension and surface topography. Because cryotherapy is an ablative treatment, no tissues are submitted for histologic analysis. Satisfactory treatment will restore a new, normal transformation zone for the cervix. As with all other cervical therapy, destruction of the entire transformation zone, including "at-risk" epithelium in the distal part of the endocervical canal, is necessary.

19.2.3 Objectives

The objectives of cryotherapy of the cervix are to: (1) expose all cervical intraepithelial neoplasia (CIN) to lethal tissue temperatures; (2) destroy the entire transformation zone; (3) protect surrounding normal lower genital tract tissue from thermal injury; (4) minimize treatment side effects of patient discomfort and complications of cervical stenosis and infertility; and (5) prevent the development of cervical cancer.

19.2.4 Prerequisites, indications, and contraindications

Prior to cryosurgery, the colposcopic triage guidelines for selecting candidates for ablative treatment of the cervical transformation zone must be satisfied (Table 19.8). In review, these consist of: (1) the complete (360°) squamocolumnar junction (SCJ) must be clearly identified; (2) the entire lesion, including both the proximal and distal margins must be seen; (3) the cytologic and colposcopic findings must be no more than one degree of severity worse than histologic findings; (4) the endocervical canal must be free of neoplasia as documented by a negative endocervical curettage, a negative cytobrush endocervical sample, or a normal, satisfactory endocervical colposcopy examination; and (5) the presence of cancer

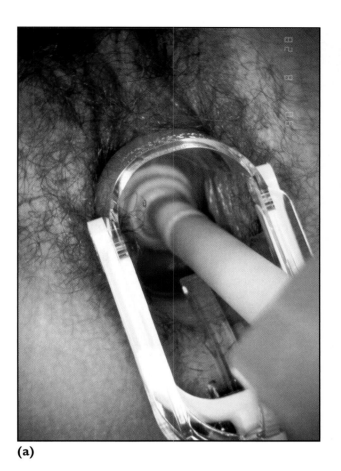
(a)

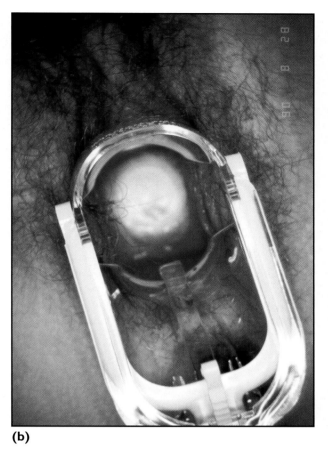
(b)

FIGURES 19.6a,b   Cryotherapy of the cervix. **(a)** The cryoprobe is placed on the cervix and freeze initiated. **(b)** The cervix after the freeze.

Table 19.8   Cervical Ablation Triage Guidelines

Satisfactory colposcopic examination
Pathologic/colposcopic diagnosis agreement
Absence of endocervical canal neoplasia
Cervical cancer presence excluded

Adapted from: Wright T C, Cox J T, Massad L S, Carlson J, Twiggs LB, and Wilkinson E J for the 2001 Consensus Guidelines for the Management of Women with Cervical Intraepithelial Neoplasia. *Amer J Obstet Gynecol* 2003 Jul;189(1):295–304.

must be excluded carefully by means of prior cytologic, colposcopic, and histologic assessment.

The need for proper colposcopic and histologic assessment of the cervix prior to cryosurgery must be re-emphasized. Invasive cervical cancer may present years following a cervical cryosurgical procedure. In many cases, the treatment was performed without a prior careful colposcopic examination and, therefore,

invasive cancer was not excluded.[160] Such an outcome, with inevitable delay in diagnosis, is a tragedy for the patient and is perceived as medicolegally indefensible. If women are to receive cryosurgery for such "soft" indications as "cervicitis" or "ectropion," cytologic and colposcopic assessment is essential prior to the procedure to exclude significant neoplasia. A normal Papanicolaou (Pap) smear is not sufficiently sensitive to guarantee normality.

The indication for cervical cryotherapy is a biopsy-confirmed premalignant cervical lesion (CIN 1 to CIN 3). Women who have a CIN 1 lesion who are compliant and agree to conservative management may be observed by serial cytologic and colposcopic follow up instead of electing immediate treatment. Otherwise, women who have a CIN 1 lesion and are historically noncompliant or simply desire treatment may receive cryotherapy. Many women with small CIN 2 to CIN 3 lesions also may be suitable candidates for cryotherapy. However, most women with CIN 3 are now treated using an excisional method.

The contraindications to cryotherapy (Table 19.9) include: (1) cervical cancer; (2) pregnancy;

Table 19.9 Cervical Cryotherapy Contraindications

Cervical cancer
Prior in-utero DES exposure
Pregnancy
Acute cervicitis
Menstruation
Cryoglobulinemia
Positive endocervical curettage
Unsatisfactory colposcopic examination
Large cervical lesion
Lesions extending into endocervical canal
Lesions with irregular surface contour

(3) in-utero DES exposure because of increased risk for cervical stenosis;[161] (4) acute cervicitis (may potentially precipitate acute salpingitis); (5) menstruating or immediately premenstruating women; (6) cryoglobulinemia; (7) a positive endocervical curettage; or (8) an unsatisfactory colposcopic examination. Other contraindications to cervical cryotherapy include the presence of (1) lesions larger than two cervical quadrants in size; (2) lesions greater than 3 cm in diameter; (3) lesions that extend more than 5 mm into the endocervical canal, and (4) exophytic, nodular, or papillary lesions or obstetrical scars that hinder proper application of the cryoprobe tip to the cervical transformation zone.

19.2.5 Patient preparation

Women are notified of the need for cervical therapy when previously collected cervical biopsies demonstrate premalignant disease that requires treatment. The essence of the biopsy report, concurrence of the colposcopic impression, along with the potential risk for progression, should be reviewed with the patient. Cryotherapy may be one of several options for treatment. Other types of management, including careful observation, electrosurgical loop excision, laser (excision or ablation), conization, or perhaps hysterectomy (provided additional indications exist), should be discussed with the patient. Ideally, the cryotherapy procedure should be described to the patient prior to her actual visit. Written cryotherapy patient education materials may be of benefit prior to and after the procedure. Although the majority of women tolerate cryotherapy reasonably well, some women may wish to have a support person accompany them to the procedure. Cryotherapy is best done immediately following the menses to minimize inadvertent treatment during pregnancy. A pregnancy test should be requested prior to cryotherapy if there is any uncertainty regarding the patient's pregnancy status. Treatment during the early proliferative phase of the menstrual cycle also prevents potential obstruction to menstrual flow, secondary to postoperative edema occluding the endocervical canal that may occur when cryotherapy immediately precedes menstruation.

Explain to the patient that cryotherapy causes a "cold" burn to the skin of the cervix. A large blister develops quickly, the abnormal cells die, and a scab appears eventually sloughing away. New healthy skin will grow back to cover the "burned" area. She may notice mild to moderate menstrual-like cramping pain during the two-step procedure. Use of nonsteroidal antiinflammatory drugs prior to the procedure help minimize discomfort. Following treatment, a very watery, occasionally blood-tinged, malodorous vaginal discharge will be noted. Consequently, the patient will need to use sanitary napkins for two to four weeks. More frequent Pap smears and examinations will be necessary during the first year after therapy to assess therapeutic response. Post-treatment examination compliance must be stressed, as follow-up cytologic and colposcopic assessments are necessary to determine if residual disease lingers or recurrent neoplasia returns.

19.2.6 Equipment and supplies

Several different cryogens (refrigerants or "freezing gases") may be used for cervical cryotherapy. While carbon dioxide and liquid nitrogen units are available, the majority of ambulatory-based cryosurgical units are designed for nitrous oxide. Although it is a relatively "warmer" gas than liquid nitrogen, nitrous oxide units may be kept "closed." This requirement is in contrast with liquid nitrogen systems that must always remain "open" to continually vent gas to the atmosphere whether in use or not. Cryosurgical units, the equipment necessary for nitrous oxide cryotherapy, consist of a gas cylinder, pressure gauge, cryogun, and cryoprobe tips (Figure 19.7).[162] Units are commonly mounted on carts to facilitate mobility between examination rooms.

Gas cylinders store the nitrous oxide used for cryosurgery. A 20-lb. nonsyphon gas cylinder is preferred over a smaller, narrow "E" cylinder, because the 20-lb. cylinder provides a greater volume of available gas (Figure 19.8). The larger gas reservoir provides a less rapid reduction of gas pressure and depletion of available gas; consequently, less frequent cylinder refilling is required. Smaller cryosurgical cylinders carry the distinct disadvantage of failing to maintain adequate pressures to ensure sufficient depth of freeze. The efficacy of cryotherapy is directly dependent on maintaining adequate gas pressure within the gas cylinder. The cylinder contains liquid

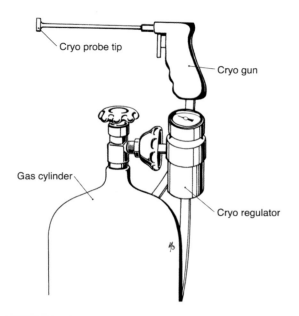

FIGURE 19.7 The cryosurgical unit, consisting of a gas cylinder, pressure gauge, cryogun, and cryoprobe tip. From: Ferris DG, Ho JJ. Cryosurgical Equipment: A critical review. J Fam Pract 1992; 35: 185–93. Reprinted with permission. Dowden Health Media, Inc. ■

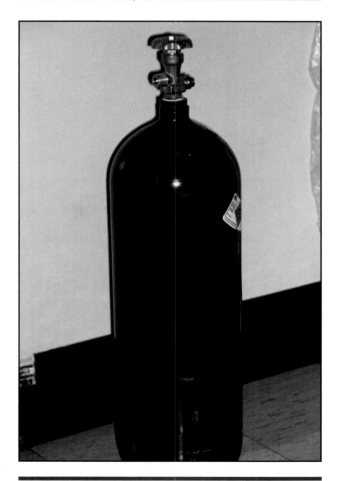

FIGURE 19.8 A 20-lb cylinder used to store nitrous oxide is the most practical for office procedures. ■

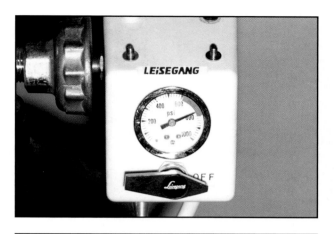

FIGURE 19.9 A pressure gauge indicates the amount of available nitrous oxide gas for cryotherapy. The arrow within the "blue" zone means cryotherapy can be effectively initiated. ■

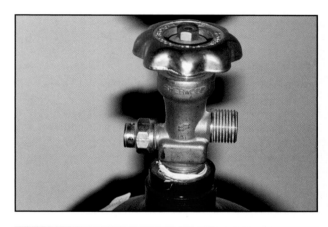

FIGURE 19.10 The "pop off" valve on the left is designed to release before the gas pressure within the cylinder reaches a dangerously high level. ■

nitrous oxide that subsequently produces nitrous oxide gas from the liquid phase. This gas is depleted from the top of the cylinder and transferred through a pressure gauge and tubing to the cryogun and cryoprobe tip during cryosurgery.

The pressure gauge monitors the pressure of nitrous oxide gas within the cylinder and is measured as kg/cm^2 or lbs/in^2 (Figure 19.9). There are three demarcated pressure ranges of concern: high, normal, and low pressure. When the pressure is too high, a potential disaster may be imminent. Rapidly discharging gas venting through the top of the cylinder would render the cylinder a potentially damaging missile. A "pop off" safety valve on the cylinder yoke is designed to prevent this hazardous event from occurring (Figure 19.10). If high pressure is indicated,

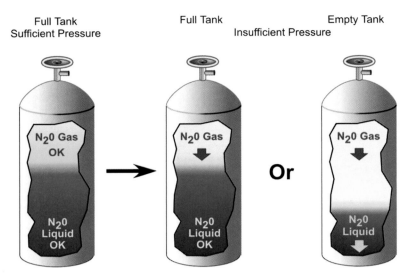

Full Tank
Sufficient Pressure

Full Tank

Insufficient Pressure

Empty Tank

N₂0 Gas
OK

N₂0
Liquid
OK

N₂0 Gas

N₂0
Liquid
OK

N₂0 Gas

N₂0
Liquid

Or

FIGURE 19.11 Two reasons for a low pressure reading on the cryosurgical pressure gauge: sufficient liquid but depleted gas, and insufficient liquid nitrous oxide and, thus, an inadequate supply of gas.

the "closed" cylinder should be taken to an outdoor location and the pressure gauge removed from the cylinder. Cautiously opening the cylinder valve allows excess gas pressure to vent to the atmosphere. Another way to deplete excessive pressure is to activate the cryogun to commence freezing. Otherwise, assistance can be obtained from the cylinder supplier.

When the pressure gauge indicates a normal range, cryotherapy may be performed adequately (Figure 19.9). However, if the pressure gauge indicates a subnormal or low range, cryotherapy should *never* be performed. An inadequately shallow and possibly too-small area of cryonecrosis will result even though a small amount of tissue is visibly frozen. There are two possible explanations for the low pressure indication (Figure 19.11). The first is that the essential gas phase in the top of the cylinder has been depleted to an insufficient pressure level, even though there is still sufficient liquid nitrous oxide remaining in the bottom of the cylinder. This problem can be avoided by allowing ample time for regeneration of gas from the liquid phase to raise the gas pressure once again to the normal range. The time required for gas regeneration may be reduced by placing the cylinder in a warmer environment, either directly in the sun or near a warm radiator/vent. Careful monitoring of the pressure is essential, however, because rapid warming can generate dangerously high gas pressures. A low level pressure indication can also occur when there is an inadequate amount of liquid nitrous oxide in the gas cylinder to generate sufficient nitrous oxide gas. In this case, the cylinder should be replenished with liquid nitrous oxide. It may be difficult to estimate how much usable gas remains in the cylinder, particularly when the pressure gauge indicates normal pressure prior to

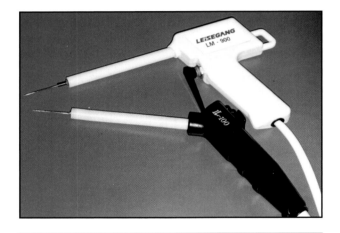

FIGURE 19.12 Two types of cryoguns used for cryosurgery. The top unit has a single trigger, and the bottom one has two buttons—one to initiate the freeze and one to defrost.

freezing. If sufficient pressure cannot be adequately maintained throughout a typical cryotherapy procedure, the cylinder should be refilled. In humid climates, a condensation line demarcating the liquid/gas level may be apparent on the outside of the cylinder. Another way to determine if there is enough gas remains is to simply lift the cylinder. It will be considerably lighter when nearly empty than when full.

The cryogun, a hand-held device resembling a gun with a trigger and barrel, is used to control and direct the procedure (Figure 19.12). Cryoprobe tips, the part that contacts the mucosal or skin surface, attach to the end of the gun barrel on most cryosurgical units. The cryogun is activated by depressing a trigger or by extending a trigger forward in a locked

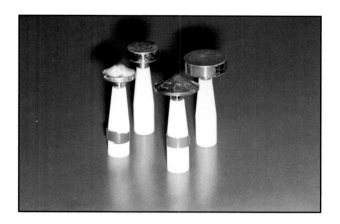

FIGURE 19.13 19-mm and 25-mm diameter flat- and cone-shaped cryoprobe tips used for treating the cervix.

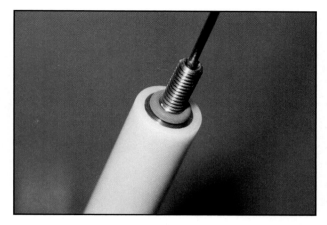

FIGURE 19.14 Rubber "O rings" prevent leakage of gas between the barrel and cryoprobe tip joint.

position (depending on the design of cryosurgery equipment). Conversely, one cryosurgical unit is activated by releasing the trigger and defrosted by depressing the trigger. Some units have an independent on/off switch located on the gunstock or pressure gauge housing. Cryoprobe tips come in different sizes and shapes for cervical cryotherapy (Figure 19.13). The 25-mm and 19-mm diameter probe tips are the most commonly used sizes for treatment of cervical intraepithelial neoplasia. Both a flat and a cone- or nipple-shaped probe tip, with approximately a 5-mm projection, are used. Nipple-shaped probe tips with a central projection longer than 5 mm should never be used on the cervix. Probe tips should conform to the shape of the tissue being treated in order to maximize heat transfer. As a result, the nipple-shaped tips are almost always used during the initial freeze because it adheres to the inner, central curve of the cervix where most neoplasias are located. If the cervical lesion(s) is not completely encompassed within the cryoiceball (frozen tissue) following the first freeze, overlap treatment using a flat probe tip is required for unfrozen lesions that extend toward the periphery of the cervix. Otherwise, if the entire cervical lesion is encompassed within the initial iceball, the same nipple probe tip may be used during the second freeze.

The aim of cryosurgery is to minimize the chance of residual atypia or risk for future development of disease on the ectocervix and in the lower endocervical canal. Failure to destroy the entire transformation zone to adequate depth is the most common cause of cryotherapy failure. Residual or recurrent neoplasia often presents in the distal endocervical canal and escapes detection by residing deeply within gland clefts. This hidden tissue may be at risk for eventually

progressing to invasive cancer. The frequently espoused use of flat cryosurgery probes may predispose to recurrent or residual neoplasia. By using these flat probe tips, the distal 5 mm of the endocervical canal may not be adequately treated. Use of the cone-shaped probe tip, on the other hand, may cause the SCJ to be inaccessible to colposcopic view after treatment. However, a colposcopically inaccessible SCJ after conservative treatment is common and should not cause alarm. It simply mandates adequate endocervical sampling in future screening.

When attaching probe tips to the cryogun barrel, the tip should be fastened tightly. Many models have rubber 0-rings that prevent leakage of gas between the probe and barrel joint (Figure 19.14). An extra supply of 0-rings should be available, since they occasionally dry, crack, and rupture during use, causing an obscuring spray of gas at the joint and rendering the equipment temporarily useless. The long, narrow tube that delivers gas through the barrel, shown in Figure 19.15 as projecting several inches beyond the end of the barrel and located inside of the cryoprobe tip, should always be protected with a secured probe tip to prevent the fragile tube from bending and breaking. Such trauma would require purchase of a new cryogun and tubing. Because nitrous oxide exhaust produced during cryotherapy can accumulate in the treatment room to toxic levels, scavenging tubing must be attached to the cryosurgical unit exhaust port (usually found on the pressure gauge) to vent the gas safely to an external location.

Supplies necessary for cryotherapy include a small amount of water-soluble gel, gloves, a vaginal speculum, vaginal sidewall retractor (when necessary), disinfectants, water at body temperature, syringes and large cotton swabs, and a freeze ball

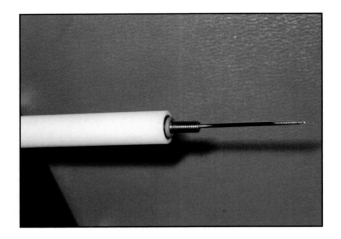

FIGURE 19.15 The fragile narrow tube delivers gas to the cryoprobe tip. It is susceptible to damage if not properly protected. ▬

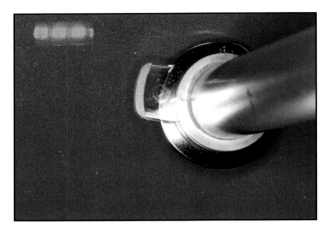

FIGURE 19.16 A freeze-ball scale, which is used to accurately measure the lateral spread of freeze and determine adequate treatment termination. ▬

scale (optional). A thin coating of water-soluble gel is applied to the cryoprobe tip prior to cryotherapy. The gel assists transfer of heat and also permits easy release of the probe tips from the frozen tissue following cryotherapy. A vaginal sidewall retractor, tongue blade, condom, or rubber glove finger tube placed over the vaginal speculum may partially rectify obscuring vaginal sidewall prolapse, when present. A freeze ball scale permits accurate, objective iceball measurements to precisely determine treatment adequacy (Figure 19.16).[163] By observing that the iceball extends to the frosted rim of the freeze ball scale, a therapeutic 5-mm to 7-mm iceball can be objectively assured. The movable scale also helps to retract prolapsing vaginal sidewalls. Following use, probe tips need to be disinfected, using a compatible product as recommended by the unit manufacturer. When disinfecting with liquid agents, such as glutaraldehyde, keep the inside of the probe tip dry. Use of a screw-type plug in the probe tip during cleaning should prevent problems. Body temperature water and syringes are useful to accelerate the defrost phase between the two cryotherapy freezes.

19.2.7 Principles of cryotherapy

19.2.7.1 Heat transfer

An important principle of physics is that heat is transferred between entities, as opposed to cold being added to an entity. As an example, your home refrigerator's condenser removes heat from the refrigerator to lower the temperature inside. During cryotherapy of the cervix, heat is removed from the cervix to the cryoprobe tip at a rate faster than heat can be delivered to the cervix through blood flow from the cervical branches of uterine arteries.

19.2.7.2 Joule-Thomson effect

When gas is passed from a small chamber to a large cavity and expands in volume, the Joule-Thomson effect (adiabatic principle of gas expansion) occurs, resulting in a reduction of gas temperature.[164] During cryotherapy, gas exits the cylinder and travels through the pressure gauge, down the tubing to the cryogun. Gas then travels through the barrel of the gun and exits through a very narrow tube positioned within the hollow cryoprobe tip (Figure 19.15). Gas expands rapidly from the narrow tube into the hollow probe tip, causing a drop in temperature.

19.2.7.3 Cellular injury and cell death

Tissue injury is determined by the final temperature produced and the duration of freeze. Temperatures of less than −20°C are required for tissue necrosis.[165] Tissue frozen transiently at 0°C to −20°C remains viable. The exact reason for cellular injury secondary to thermal damage from cryotherapy is not known specifically. However, it is postulated that intra- and intercellular ice crystals form, producing dehydration in adjoining cells. Later, the cellular membranes are pierced by the ice crystals that form, releasing the intracellular contents and causing vascular thrombosis and microcirculatory failure, anoxia, and ischemia.[166–168] A freeze-thaw-freeze (double-freeze) treatment is more effective than a single-freeze procedure.[169,170]

19.2.7.4 Induction and defrost

A method of rapid freeze and a slow defrost is the most effective means of inducing tissue damage. A slow freeze and rapid defrost technique is less effective. Modern cryosurgical equipment provides for a quick freeze. Defrost can be rapidly accelerated with the cryosurgical unit, accomplished by natural tissue rewarming (lengthy), or greatly facilitated by body temperature water lavage.

19.2.7.5 Relevant cryotherapy temperatures

Liquid nitrous oxide has a boiling point of $-195.8°C$, nitrous oxide $-89.5°C$, and carbon dioxide $-78.5°C$. The temperature of the cryoprobe tip, using a nitrous oxide system, is approximately $-65°C$ to $-75°C$ during cryotherapy. As previously stated, lethal tissue temperatures are generated below $-20°C$. The leading edge of the expanding frozen tissue, or iceball, which represents $0°C$, is the reference parameter for cryotherapy (Figure 19.17). The lateral spread of freeze or the extent of the iceball on the surface of the tissue is defined as the distance from the margin of the cryoprobe edge to the interface of frozen tissue and nonfrozen tissue. The lateral spread of freeze equates to the depth of freeze in an approximately one-to-one ratio.[171] Thereby, a 3-mm lateral spread of freeze equates to a depth of freeze of 3 mm.

During cryotherapy two clinically relevant temperature zones are produced within the iceball (Figure 19.17). The lethal zone is the frozen area located between the cryoprobe tip and $-20°C$ isotherm. Tissue in this area will not survive the freeze. However, a more peripherally located recovery zone is represented by frozen tissue with temperatures between $-20°C$ and $0°C$. Tissue in the recovery zone is temporarily frozen during the procedure but will remain viable after defrosting. The recovery zone equates to frostbite. The recovery zone generated by most cryosurgical units represents the most peripheral 2-mm rim of frozen tissue adjoining the leading margin of the iceball.[162]

19.2.7.6 Determining freeze termination

The termination of cryotherapy may be determined by the measurement of the iceball generated. Based on morphometric data of cervical neoplasia, CIN 3 can extend approximately 5 mm deep into gland clefts within the transformation zone.[172] Therefore, in order to eradicate all possible CIN 3, a lethal zone extending 5 mm beneath the surface of the epithelium is required. However, a recovery zone of 2 mm must be additionally considered in the total iceball measurement. Therefore, during cryotherapy, the lateral spread of freeze, or $0°C$ isotherm (edge of the iceball) ideally should extend 7 mm from the edge of the cryoprobe tip.[173] This distance is very difficult to achieve using nitrous oxide systems. A 7-mm freeze would adequately treat CIN 3 located deeply (5 mm) within gland clefts. In vivo monitoring of cryother-

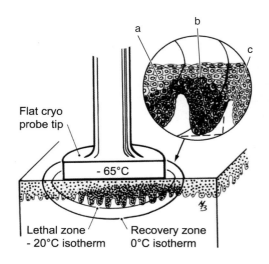

FIGURE 19.17 A cryo iceball on squamous epithelium with CIN 2, demonstrating the visible ice-tissue interface or 0°C isotherm, the −20°C isotherm, and the temperature at the cryoprobe tip (−65°C). The lethal zone (insert A) represents the iceball volume between the cryoprobe tip and the −20°C isotherm. The recovery zone (insert B) represents the iceball area between the −20°C isotherm and the 0°C isotherm. Cells located in the lethal zone (insert A) will not remain viable, but cells located in the recovery zone (insert B) will be temporarily frozen but viable. Cells lateral to the 0°C isotherm (insert C) are not frozen and, thus, not altered by the procedure. From: Ferris DG, Ho JJ. Cryosurgical Equipment: A critical review. J Fam Pract 1992; 35: 185–93. Reprinted with permission. Dowden Health Media, Inc. ▄▄▄

apy using a thermocouple needle positioned in cervical tissue 5 mm from the cryoprobe tip demonstrated that after 6.5 minutes of freezing, a 4.2-mm lethal zone was produced.[163] Such treatment would result in a theoretical cryotherapy failure rate of 12.5% for CIN 3.[163] This theoretically calculated failure rate is quite similar to the aggregate 15.7% clinical cryotherapy failure rate for CIN 3 reported by multiple investigators.[173] The outcomes of nitrous oxide cryotherapy are limited by several principles of thermal physics. Heat transfer eventually reaches equilibrium or steady state during cryotherapy as the amount of heat removed by the cryogen equals the amount of heat delivered by the cervical arteries. Furthermore, the expanding, thick iceball creates ice insulation (much like an igloo) that inhibits heat transfer. Thus, clinicians *cannot* excessively freeze the cervix using nitrous oxide. Freezing until the iceball lateral spread of freeze is 5 mm to 7 mm from the cryoprobe tip or until the iceball margin fails to advance further defines the clinical parameters for freeze termination. A commercially available gauge that permits accurate measurement of the iceball during cryosurgery (Figure 19.16) may reduce the frequent tendency for iceball measurement overestimation and premature cessation of the freeze. Use of the gauge may improve outcomes by limiting the premature termination of freeze.[163] All of the cervical lesion must be encompassed within an iceball. Additional overlapping freezes may be necessary to adequately treat large lesions that occupy an expansive surface area of the cervix. It is critically important to realize that the termination of cryosurgery should never be determined by a specific duration of time. Watches are not essential equipment for cervical cryotherapy. Several researchers have demonstrated that cervical cryotherapy produces a potentially inadequate iceball after only a 5-minute freeze.[173,174] Early cryotherapy researchers indicated that a 7-minute freeze was necessary even during the era when timing cryotherapy was once considered standard care for determining freeze termination.[35]

19.2.7.7 Cryoprobe tips

Cryoprobe tips are hollow and made of a metal that conducts heat well (Figure 19.13). The shape of the cryoprobe tip determines the shape of the cryoiceball within the tissue. A flat cryoprobe tip produces a relatively flat square iceball, and a rounded cryoprobe tip produces a rounded area of cryonecrosis and rounded iceball. Poor contact between the cryoprobe surface and the cervical epithelium may lead to treatment failure. A flat cryoprobe tip does not conform to the relief contour of the cervix and, thus, is less efficacious than a nipple-shaped probe tip.[175] Yet, use of the nipple- or cone-shaped probe tip may be more likely to cause the SCJ to reposition within the endocervical canal following treatment, primarily because a greater extent of ectocervical tissue surrounding the endocervical canal is affected. This may make direct colposcopic visualization of the canal following cryotherapy more difficult, but the endocervical canal can still be assessed subsequently by cytologic sampling. However, for the sake of maximizing patient cure, a nipple-shaped probe tip, with no more than a 5-mm nipple extension should be used for most initial freezes.

19.2.7.8 Cryonecrosis stages

Cervical tissue responds to the thermal insult in a characteristic fashion after cryotherapy. Erythema and hyperemia are noted at and surrounding the treatment site immediately following cryotherapy. Within the next 24 to 48 hours, bullae or local edema associated with vesicular formation develops. Thereafter, an eschar (scab) covers the treated site, followed by a re-epithelialization and neovascularization. During the healing stages, epithelial tissue, stroma, and blood vessels grow horizontally from the periphery and crater base of the wound to fill the tissue void. Loop capillaries extend vertically from the horizontal vessels to the epithelium. When viewed colposcopically from above, a fine linear or radial punctation pattern of neovascularization, extending from the periphery toward the os (much like spokes of a bicycle wheel) may be noted. This is a normal finding and can be confirmed by the lack of associated acetowhite epithelium or other colposcopic signs of neoplasia (excluding leukoplakia). Reepithelialization is complete for nearly 50% of patients at six weeks posttreatment. Reparative and inflammatory cytologic changes may be observed for three to four months after therapy.

19.2.7.9 Immunologic response

The direct thermal effects of cryotherapy determine eventual treatment success. Neoplasia within the lethal zone is readily destroyed by cryonecrosis. However, adjoining tissue temporarily frozen in the recovery zone and more peripherally positioned nonfrozen residual minor neoplasia may regress following cryotherapy through the actions of the immune system. After cryotherapy debulks a large, central viral (HPV) load, the immune system may be better able to eradicate a limited amount of surrounding low-grade residual disease. This assumption is based on anecdotal evidence noted by many clinicians. The specifics of the immune response in relation to cryotherapy, however, are poorly understood. The potential adjunctive effect of the immune system on cryotherapy outcomes is further elucidated by evidence that patients who are immunosuppressed (i.e., have AIDS) have very poor outcomes when treated by cryotherapy, in contrast to better cure rates experienced by immunocompetent patients. Moreover, immunosuppressed women who are treated by excisional methods, such as electrosurgical loop excision, have significantly better cure rates than do women treated by cryotherapy. This difference is probably related to the greater amount of pathologic tissue removed by excision.

19.2.8 Cryotherapy procedure

Prior to initiating cryotherapy, one must review and satisfy the treatment triage guidelines for ablative therapy. Informed consent may be obtained once the colposcopist has fully informed the patient of the procedural details, risks, and potential complications. Prophylactic treatment with short-acting nonsteroidal anti-inflammatory drugs approximately 60 minutes prior to treatment may help block prostaglandin-mediated tissue effects and, hence, reduce cramping associated with treatment. Cryotherapy should not be performed on patients who are pregnant or menstruating. To ensure the procedure is performed when neither of these conditions exists, cryotherapy should be scheduled immediately following the patient's normal menstrual period. A routine, pretherapeutic pregnancy test may be reasonable for assurance purposes. Some clinicians also screen women for occult cervicitis (*Chlamydia trachomatis* and *Neiserria gonorrhea*) prior to initiating treatment.

Before initiating cryotherapy, sufficient gas pressure must be available within the nitrous oxide cylinder, as indicated by the pressure gauge. Cryotherapy should never be attempted when the pressure gauge indicates insufficient pressure. Following the application of acetic acid to the cervix, the cervical lesion should be visualized with the colposcope to determine size and disease distribution. Cryotherapy is best performed when the cervical mucosa is moistened. Next, an appropriate, warm, cervix-conforming cryoprobe tip should be selected to cover the lesion and abnormal transformation zone. If the lesion is not completely covered, a second overlap treatment using a flat cryoprobe tip will be required to encompass the lesion and transformation zone. Lesions that are laterally positioned or located more than 3 mm to 5 mm from the cryoprobe tip within the endocervical canal will not be ablated by cryotherapy.[176] A thin layer of water-soluble gel should be applied to the cryoprobe tip before the tip is applied to the cervix. A colposcope is not necessary to assist cryotherapy. In fact, use of a colposcope tends to cause overestimation of the lateral spread of freeze distance and, thus, premature treatment termination.[163]

Cryotherapy is initiated by activating a trigger or switch on the cryogun, provided the probe is carefully visualized to be clear of the vaginal walls. Placement of the nipple projection into the cervical os will help prevent probe tip displacement during the activation of freeze. The cryoprobe position should be steadily maintained on the cervix. Once the freeze is activated, the cryoprobe tip will adhere to the cervix. When necessary, gentle retraction or forward pressure on the cervix may straighten prolapsing vaginal sidewalls to improve visualization. If the vaginal walls come in contact with the probe, gently rotate or twist the cryogun, or push the adhering vaginal wall off the edge of the cryoprobe tip with a cotton-tipped swab. If these steps are unsuccessful, the cervix should be allowed to thaw completely and the freeze subsequently reinitiated.

Cryotherapy should continue until a 5-mm to 7-mm lateral spread of iceball freeze from the margin of the cryoprobe tip is accomplished (Figures 19.18a,b). In other words, a 5-mm to 7-mm rim or band of frozen tissue should circumferentially surround the probe-tip prior to terminating the freeze. The lateral spread of freeze of the cryoiceball on the tissue surface equates to the approximate depth of the iceball. A 5-mm to 7-mm distance is best determined by the use of a freeze-ball scale (Figure 19.16). Because many external variables may affect cryotherapy, it is neither necessary nor advisable to time the procedure. For instance, with a borderline low gas pressure, more time is required to produce an iceball of adequate proportion. Patients who are vasodilated may also require a longer duration of freeze. Conversely, women who are vasoconstricted may need a shorter freeze compared with the freeze time for a "normal" patient. The probe should be defrosted completely before the tip can be removed freely from the frozen cervix. Defrost is initiated by quickly squeezing then releasing ("flashing") the cryogun trigger several times. Using this technique, all nitrous oxide cryotherapy probe tips should defrost within six seconds.[162] Because cryotherapy causes tissue dehydration, the probe tip will be depressed slightly within the frozen cervical tissue (Figure 19.18c). Remove the probe by gently prying up on one side of the probe from the frozen base (Figure 19.18d). A water lavage may also facilitate the release of the probe tip from the epithelium.

Once the probe is removed, the cervix should then be reinspected to ensure that the cryoiceball is positioned in the desired location or intended area of treatment. A frozen depression of the cervix will be transiently noted (Figure 19.18d). Prior to initiating a second freeze, the temporary depression should return to a normal contour and the icy-white tissue should return to a normal pink color. Cervical defrosting may be hastened by bathing the cervix in 5 cc to 10 cc of body-temperature water. Once the tissue is defrosted and prior to initiating the second freeze, this water should be removed from the posterior fornix. Otherwise, the cervix will defrost naturally over a 10- to 15-minute time span. The cryoprobe also may be activated in a defrost mode to help thaw the frozen tissue; however, this procedure wastes a considerable amount of cryogen.

Cryotherapy should then be repeated a second time as necessary to completely cover lesions and ablate the entire transformation zone. A freeze-thaw-freeze, or double-freeze, technique is recommended for cervical cryotherapy. Researchers have demonstrated a reduced failure rate (19% from 49%) when a double-freeze method is utilized.[169] Following the first freeze, the cervix should be defrosted prior to attempting the second freeze. Cryoprobe adherence is not possible for the second freeze until the probe

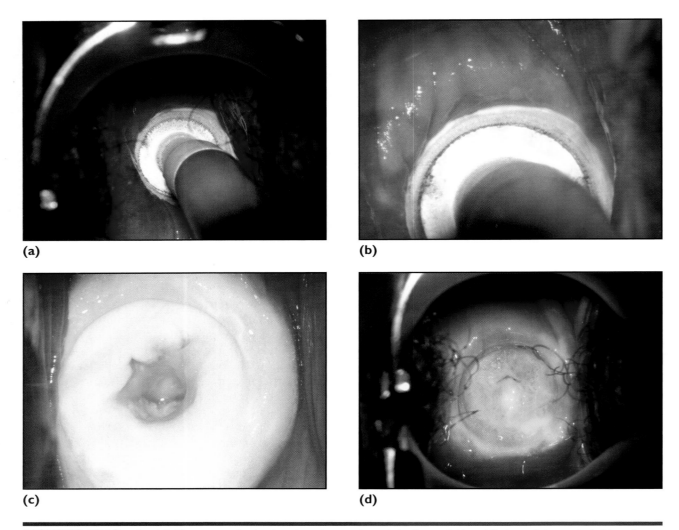

(a)

(b)

(c)

(d)

FIGURES 19.18a–d **(a)** The cryoprobe is placed on the cervix and the freeze initiated if clear of the vaginal sidewalls; **(b)** a 1-mm iceball is seen shortly after beginning the freeze; **(c)** the cervix immediately following cryotherapy (notice a frozen depressed area caused by the dehydration of cryotherapy; a wide 5-mm to 7-mm iceball extends peripheral to the central depressed area formerly occupied by the cryoprobe tip; **(d)** with partial thawing, the cervix begins to resemble its baseline appearance.

and superficial epithelium defrost. Because the cervical epithelium and stroma are still very cold (but not frozen), the second freeze should occur much more quickly. With large lesions or large transformation zones, multiple overlapping freeze applications may be required to ensure complete coverage (Figures 19.19a–c). Optional cryodebridement of the devitalized tissue 48 hours postoperatively will minimize the odor but will not diminish the hydrorrhea or watery discharge associated with cryotherapy.[177] The procedure is painless and takes only minutes in the office. Ring forceps can be used to remove the necrotic tissue, followed by gentle further debridement with gauze as needed. Cryodebridement, however, does not appear to be a clinically useful or cost-

effective technique and is of little benefit to the patient. A patent cervical os may be documented by passing a cotton swab into the canal, although such a maneuver at this early stage may not predict or prevent cervical stenosis.

19.2.9 Patient education

Patients should be instructed that a very watery, malodorous, slightly blood-tinged vaginal discharge will be noted for the subsequent 3 to 4 weeks.[177] Patients should be instructed to wear pads rather than tampons to absorb this discharge, and pelvic rest should be encouraged during this healing phase. Nonsteroidal antiinflammatory drugs may minimize

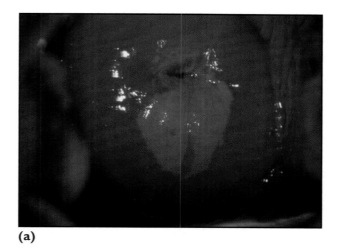

(a)

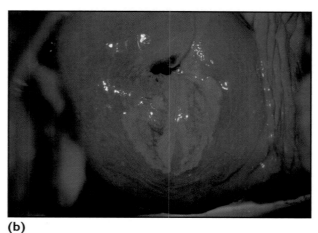

(b)

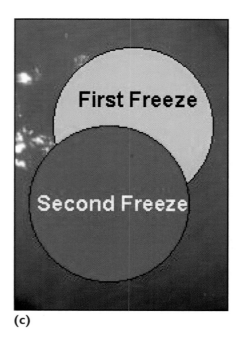

(c)

FIGURES 19.19a–c **(a,b)** Cervix with large neoplasia extending to the distal ectocervix; **(c)** schematic of overlapping freezes (1 and 2) to treat the entire transformation zone and lesion.

immediate postoperative discomfort. If present, uterine cramping usually resolves within 24 to 48 hours. Acidification of the vagina with agents such as Aminocerv® may help alleviate odor and promote healing, but the efficacy of this product has not been proven scientifically. The patient should be instructed to return within 48 hours if optional cryodebridement is desired, but if fever, unusual bleeding or severe pelvic pain develops, she should notify the cryotherapist immediately. Cryotherapy may precipitate acute salpingitis in women previously infected with potential pathogens. In this case, women usually develop symptoms within one week of cryotherapy. Finally, the patient should clearly understand that 5% to 15% of women treated by cryotherapy will have residual disease. Therefore, follow-up visits for cervical cytologic and colposcopic assessment are mandatory to determine therapeutic cure.

19.2.10 Follow-up

Post-treatment follow-up is critically important to establish therapeutic cure. Several serial Pap smears should be performed during the postoperative period. Pap smears obtained before the four-month interval may demonstrate reparative changes, inflammation, and/or atypia. Colposcopy may be performed during the post-treatment phase (at four and/or 12 months). Not all clinicians perform postoperative colposcopic assessment, but follow-up cytologic testing is mandatory. Evidence of three negative or normal cytologic smears and a normal colposcopic examination are usually considered standard for defining therapeutic cure. A Pap test report of low-grade squamous intraepithelial lesion is not uncommon for women previously treated for CIN, as residual disease may remain on the cervix. Recurrent disease also may suddenly appear, or vaginal HPV disease may actually be the source for the mildly abnormal smear when the cervix appears free of disease following colposcopic examination (Figures 19.20a–d). Postoperative use of HPV DNA tests, which have a negative predictive value of 99%, may be beneficial to confirm normalcy.

19.2.11 Side effects and complications

All women undergoing cryotherapy of the cervix experience some side effects, including a profuse, occasionally malodorous, blood-tinged hydrorrhea (watery vaginal discharge) lasting three to four weeks.[177] The volume of hydrorrhea can exceed more than 100 cc per day for some women. Many women notice menstrual-like, crampy uterine pain during cryotherapy, but it usually resolves within 24 to 48 hours.

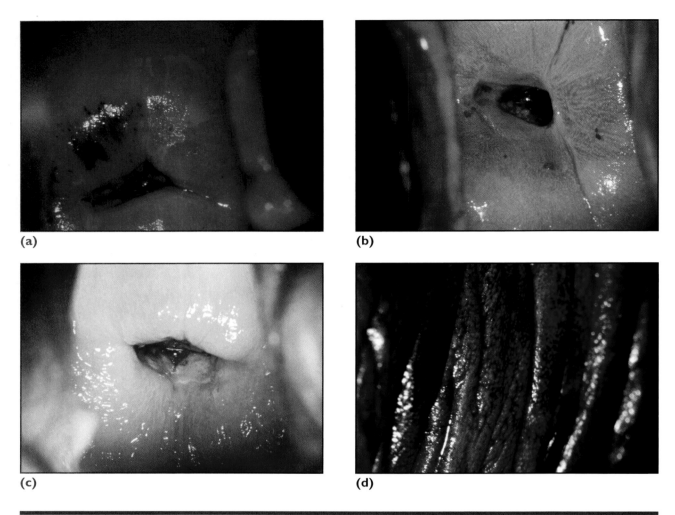

(a)

(b)

(c)

(d)

FIGURES 19.20 a–d **(a–c)** Recurrent and residual disease of the cervix is seen following cryotherapy; acetowhite areas of CIN 1 can be seen on the cervix after treatment. VAIN **(d)** may be the source for an abnormal Pap smear following cryotherapy when the cervix is entirely normal. A diffusely iodine-negative area of the vagina can be seen in this woman following cryotherapy. Her biopsy diagnosis of VAIN 1 correlates with her LSIL Pap smear and normal cervical colposcopic findings.

Premedication with nonsteroidal antiinflammatory drugs may minimize the prostaglandin-mediated discomfort. Paracervical block has been advocated for use prior to cervical cryotherapy, but the effectiveness of this block is clinically questionable and thus, is used by few clinicians.[178]

Severe complications secondary to cryotherapy are quite unusual. The main complication is inadvertent injury or freezing of the proximal vagina, which can be avoided by careful visualization, selection of a smaller (19 mm) cryoprobe tip, use of a freeze-ball scale, placement of a vaginal sidewall retraction device, steady positioning, and discontinuation of cryotherapy, if adhering vaginal side walls cannot be

freed from the cryoprobe tip. Heavy bleeding is a very unusual postoperative complication, but mild spotting may be noted approximately 10 days following treatment as the eschar sloughs from the cervix. Some blood-tinged hydrorrhea is also not uncommon. Although postoperative infections are rare, acute salpingitis may be precipitated in women who have occult or acute cervicitis. In order to prevent salpingitis, women who are found to have acute cervicitis should be first treated with an appropriate antibiotic and cured prior to initiating cryotherapy.[179] Women discovered to have bacterial vaginosis prior to treatment should also receive treatment prior to cryotherapy (Figure 19.21). Moderate or clinically sig-

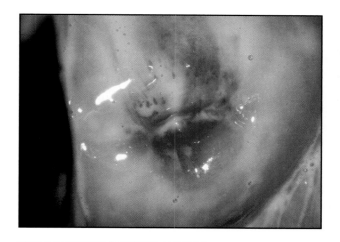

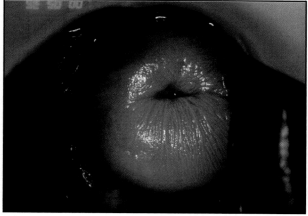

(a)

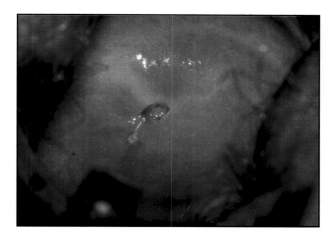

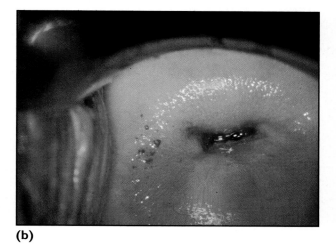

(b)

FIGURE 19.21 Bacterial vaginosis is a relative contraindication to cryotherapy because of an increased risk for postoperative infection. A thin adherent off-white discharge is seen covering the cervix. Her vaginal pH was 5.0 (elevated), clue cells were detected on microscopic examination, and a positive sniff test was noted.

FIGURES 19.23a,b Parakeratosis seen following cryotherapy of the cervix is a normal finding and may also be observed in an accompanying Pap smear. The surface appears granular and not smooth.

FIGURE 19.22 Mild cervical stenosis following cryotherapy.

nificant cervical stenosis is rare[180] but may occur in approximately 5% or less of women (Figure 19.22). Severe or complete stenosis requiring dilation is uncommon but possible. Women exposed to DES in utero are especially at an increased risk for cervical stenosis.[181] Cervical incompetence would be an extremely rare complication of cryotherapy. Although limited data are available, there is no evidence to support impaired fertility following cryotherapy.[181] Unsatisfactory colposcopy examinations will be encountered in a minority of women following cryotherapy. Occasionally, the SCJ cannot

be seen following cryotherapy, not unlike other cervical procedures, because it has relocated within the endocervical canal. This is not particularly problematic because representative sampling of the new transformation zone within the endocervical canal using a brush device will provide sufficient cytologic information during follow-up examinations. Postoperative Pap smears and colposcopic examinations may detect parakeratosis, one type of leukoplakia (Figures 19.23 a,b). In this case, the ectocervix is not completely smooth but has a fine granular texture. Some individuals experience transient vasomotor or vagal symptomatology with flushing, lightheadedness, bradycardia and rarely, tonic-clonic activity. It may be prudent to have women remain in a sitting or lying position for a brief period of time following cryotherapy to prevent syncope. A simple assessment of pulse rate may help to predict this occurrence. Finally, clinicians have a tendency to overestimate the lateral spread of freeze measurement during cryotherapy, particularly when viewing the procedure through colposcopic magnification.[171] Such error results in premature termination of cryotherapy, thereby potentially increasing the risk of inadequate treatment, the ultimate complication.

19.2.12 Outcomes

The efficacy of cryosurgery in the treatment of CIN has been studied extensively. Just as with any other form of therapy, treatment failures occur with cryotherapy. Average cure rates in relation to severity of cervical dysplasia have been reported, 94% cure rate for CIN 1, 93% for CIN 2, and 84% for CIN 3/CIS.[163] Following second or third additional treatments, the cure rate surpasses 95% for immunocompetent women. Immunodeficient women suffer from very poor cryotherapy cure rates. It should be understood that the cryotherapy cure rates for CIN 1 and CIN 2 are equivalent to cure rates expected using other treatment modalities. The cure rate for CIN 3 using cryotherapy may be lower than those rates expected for other ablative or excisional therapies. Satisfactory cryotherapy outcomes correlate better with lesion size and not necessarily severity of disease, although these two parameters are proportionally related.[182] High-grade cervical lesions tend to be morphometrically larger in size and extend more deeply into gland clefts.[171] Therefore, some high-grade lesions may be more effectively treated by an excisional method to ensure adequate therapeutic depth, as documented by histologic analysis.

To minimize the risk for poor outcomes, certain specific indications for cervical cryotherapy must be recognized. For best results, the lesion should measure less than 3 cm in diameter, occupy two or less quadrants of the cervix, and extend no more than 5 mm into the endocervical canal. Lesion parameters greater than previously described require excisional therapy. CIN 3 and CIS lesions described as deeply occupying gland clefts may be best treated by contemporary excisional techniques. Treatment failure also tends to arise in patients presenting with scarred, misshaped cervices from previous pregnancies, exophytic or nodular cervical lesions (poor probe/tissue adherence), or, more commonly, lesions extending close to or within the endocervical canal. Cryonecrosis is limited to no more than the distal 5 mm of the endocervical canal. Greater treatment failure rates have been noted for cervical lesions located at the 3 o'clock and 9 o'clock positions where the cervical branches of the uterine artery are located.[175] These areas of the cervix are relatively warmer and more resistant to cryotherapy effects than are lesions in the cooler 12 o'clock and 6 o'clock positions. Although a long-term analysis of 2839 patients treated by cryotherapy demonstrated a negligible risk for residual disease,[183] cervical cancer has been reported in women following cryotherapy of CIN.[184] Moderately abnormal cytologic findings after cryosurgery are worrisome, particularly when the endocervix is constricted and the SCJ is inaccessible. At this point, the full advantage of local destructive therapy may be lost. When recurrent or residual CIN is identified, a conservative, excisional approach to retreatment is advisable, following proper preliminary colposcopic examination with histologic sampling.

19.2.13 Documentation

The specifics of the cryotherapy procedure should be fully documented. A standardized paper form or computer-based format may be helpful, so that necessary notations can be comprehensively recorded. The procedural report should include pertinent history, cytologic, colposcopic, and histologic findings; type of cryotherapy; dimension of iceball(s), or more importantly, the lateral spread of freeze measurements; complications, and follow-up plans. A patient management tracking log should be maintained to ensure appropriate post-treatment care and follow-up screening.

19.2.14 Procedural and diagnostic codes

Correct documentation of cryotherapy is essential for financial purposes as well. Use proper CPT codes to minimize audit difficulties. The CPT code for cryotherapy of the cervix is 57511. Several ICD-9 diagnostic codes for cryotherapy-related purposes are condyloma acuminata 078.1, cervical dysplasia 622.1, and CIN 3/CIS 233.1.

19.2.15 Consent

It may be advisable to obtain informed consent prior to performing cryotherapy. As with all informed consent, the nature of the disease, the procedure to be performed, reasonable risks and complications involved, the prognosis with and without treatment, possible alternative procedures, and the opportunity to ask questions must be acknowledged in writing by the patient following explanation by the clinician. A witness and clinician should also sign and date the informed consent. A small effort to ensure appropriate notification of potential adverse but accidental outcomes should be considered a wise and necessary obligation.

19.3 Treatment of External Genital Warts

19.3.1 Introduction

Genital warts, caused by various types of HPV, are seen primarily in young, sexually active people. In many cases, these warts are quite small and, because of their anatomical location, remain unnoticed. These lesions frequently regress without therapeutic intervention in immunocompetent patients. However, in some cases, condylomas multiply in number and expand in size so that they produce symptoms of itching, irritation, bleeding and a mass effect that can interfere with hygiene, function, and sexual activity (Figure 19.24). Emotional awareness causes potentially crippling psychological sequelae that arise from typical concerns about sexually transmitted infection. Evaluation and therapy are usually sought once individuals become symptomatic.

Although prophylactic and therapeutic HPV vaccine trials are in progress, currently no effective way exists to prevent genital warts or cure HPV. Instead, clinicians have a wide variety of unique treatment options available that allow therapy to be tailored for each patient. A rational and selective treatment plan will maximize optimal outcomes and may minimize side effects even though cure rates are quite similar for the different approaches. This section describes the various methods for treating genital warts. Specifically, the composition and mechanism of action, indications and contraindications, application or delivery techniques, advantages and disadvantages, and effectiveness of each option will be discussed.

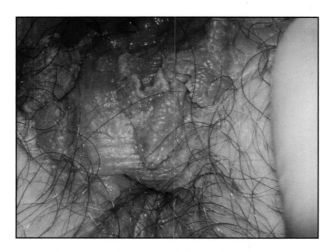

FIGURE 19.24   These perineal condyloma caused itching followed by a self-inspection that detected a growth.

19.3.2 Purpose and objectives

Patients want genital warts treated for many reasons. However, one must remember that observation may be a very reasonable alternative. Because genital warts pose few serious risks, treatment should be considered elective in most cases. The main purpose for treating genital warts is to eliminate the lesion(s) and allow the restoration of healthy epithelium. Until therapeutic HPV vaccines become available, it is important to note that the expression of HPV (condyloma) is treated and not the actual virus. Successful treatment currently means that the active expression of HPV is removed, but latent HPV may persist in adjoining tissues thereafter. Consequently, all forms of treatment are associated with a certain risk for recurrent disease.

The objectives of genital wart management are to: (1) destroy clinically evident genital warts, when desired, (2) preserve the integrity of normal adjoining tissue, (3) reduce the potential for infectious transmission to sexual partners or infants, (4) prevent the development of high grade cancer precursors or cancer (a relatively rare event), (5) minimize the chance of disease recurrence, (6) address psychologically related concerns, and (7) provide appropriate patient education.

19.3.3 Prerequisites

Prior to treating patients with genital warts, certain considerations must be entertained. First, clinicians should be confident of their diagnosis. What appear to be condylomas may not always be. Potentially serious complications can result from mistakenly treating condyloma mimics as simply condylomas. The differential diagnosis includes molluscum contagiosum, verrucous carcinoma, Buschke-Loewenstein tumor, condyloma lata (syphilis), micropapillomatosis labialis, or pearly penile papules, and other papular or plaque-like dermatologic conditions. Condylomas that do not respond to conventional therapy, present in the elderly or are pigmented, hard or ulcerated demand additional appraisal. Therefore, pretreatment evaluation may include histologic sampling or serologic testing, if necessary.

The distribution and site of disease must be considered. Diffuse anogenital condylomas may present different implications for therapy when compared with unifocal disease (Figures 19.25a-d). Likewise, choice of treatment may be influenced whether disease is located on mucosal or keratinized epithelium. External genital lesions may extend internally within the vagina, urethra, minor vestibular glands, or rectum necessitating two or more different treatment approaches. Condylomas involving "sensitive" areas,

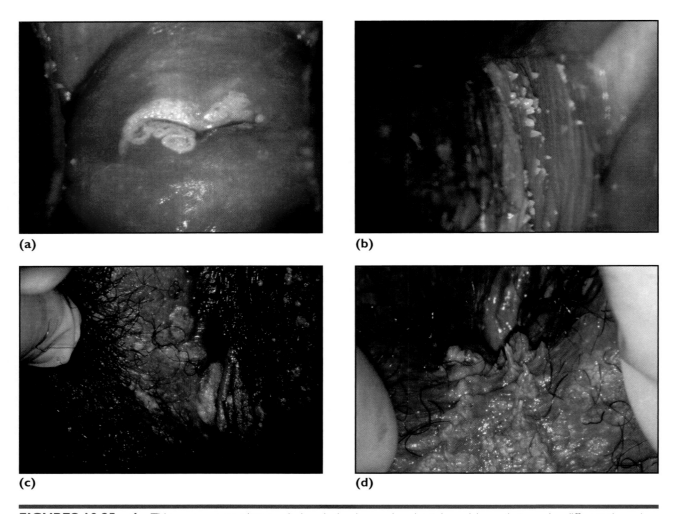

(a)

(b)

(c)

(d)

FIGURES 19.25a–d   This young woman has cervical, vaginal, vulvar, and perirectal condyloma that require different therapies.

such as the clitoris or glans penis, require tissue-sparing therapy that avoids excessive treatment of normal epithelium and prevents postoperative discomfort. Cervical condylomas are treated along with the underlying transformation zone, much of which may appear entirely normal. Management is also influenced by the number, size, and shape of the condylomas. For instance, simple excision may be preferred for treating large, solitary, pedunculated warts, while topical application or vaporization may be more appropriate for multiple small sessile or papular warts. Irregularly shaped warts are not conducive to treatment using flat or rounded cryotherapy probe tips.

Clinicians must also consider the patient's age, immune status, use of tobacco, other associated medical conditions, history of response to past therapy, drug allergies, and pregnancy status (Figure 19.26). Some patients may prefer to treat themselves inconspicuously at home, while others may insist on clinician-directed treatment. Others may

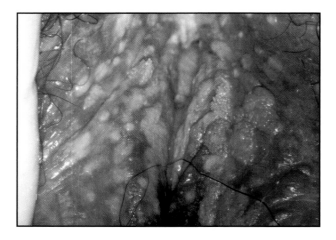

FIGURE 19.26   Several vulvar condyloma were noted on this pregnant woman. Podophyllin and 5-FU would be contraindicated for use.

wish to forego any therapy. Because each type of treatment is associated with potentially bothersome side effects, full patient disclosure of the anticipated cure rate, average length of treatment, potential adverse reactions and cost is necessary prior to initiating therapy.

19.3.4 Chemical agents

19.3.4.1 Podophyllin

Podophyllin resin is derived from the root of the "may apple plant," podophyllin peltatum. The solution is commonly formulated as a 25% concentration in tincture of benzoin, although the actual concentration may vary considerably. Podophyllin arrests cellular replication of warts by inhibiting mitosis. This effect is noted particularly in rapidly growing tissue.

Podophyllin is used infrequently because newer, and perhaps more effective, forms of treatment are now available. However, podophyllin is indicated for use on small anogenital condyloma that cover a limited area and reside primarily on keratinized epithelium. Podophyllin is absorbed quite readily through mucosal epithelium. Therefore, care should be exercised to prevent potential drug-induced toxicity by limiting the extent of condyloma treatment involving this tissue. Because podophyllin is a teratogen, its use is contraindicated in pregnant women.

The solution containing podophyllin can be applied directly to condyloma using a cotton tip applicator (Figure 19.27). Approximately four to eight hours following application, patients may wash the treated area with soap and water even though the tincture of benzoin is water insoluble. Although

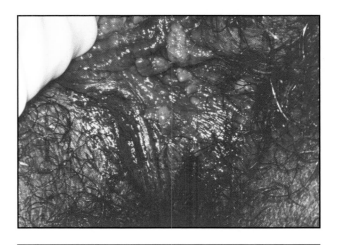

FIGURE 19.27 Podophyllin applied to external genital condyloma.

latent HPV can be found in the normal appearing epithelium surrounding warts, care should be exercised to treat only the warts and not the normal adjoining tissues. Therefore, some advocate covering the adjoining normal epithelium with a protective barrier of petrolatum before applying podophyllin to the wart. However, in our experience, this simply prolongs the time required for treatment, and frequently leads to ineffectual treatment after petrolatum is inadvertently applied to the condyloma. Treated areas should be allowed to air dry following podophyllin application. Podophyllin can be reapplied weekly for four to six weeks or until wart resolution. If warts do not respond within this interval, biopsy confirmation of the original diagnosis and/or treatment with another modality is advised.

Because podophyllin is fairly inexpensive, it has been an attractive therapeutic option. Furthermore, some patients prefer its painless application. In our experience, however, podophyllin acts rather slowly and many patients require multiple clinician-applied treatments. Consequently, it may not be the best treatment for impatient or noncompliant patients. If a condyloma must be biopsied following recent unsuccessful podophyllin use, clinicians should disclose this important information to the pathologist. By promoting mitotic cells, podophyllin may produce histopathologic changes that mimic epithelial atypia. Podophyllin should not be used to treat warts located within the urethra, vagina, or rectum. Excessive exposure and absorption may cause hepatotoxicity, neurotoxicity, or even death. Podophyllin can precipitate skin erythema, ulceration, and pain.

Wart cure rates reported for podophyllin vary between 20% to 80%, depending on the clinical trial.[185–187] Because some study endpoints for cure were defined at six treatments, greater cure rates may be expected with longer treatment. Unfortunately, 25% to 70% of patients have a recurrence of condylomas following use of podophyllin.

19.3.4.2 Podophyllotoxin

Podophyllotoxin is simply a purified form of podophyllin (Figure 19.28). Podophyllotoxin works in the same fashion as podophyllin by arresting cellular division in mitosis. Both solution and gel forms of the drug are commercially available. The indications and contraindications for podophyllotoxin are the same as that for podophyllin.

In contrast with podophyllin, podophyllotoxin is a patient-applied product. Patients apply podophyllotoxin to warts twice a day for three successive days followed by a rest period of four days. This sequence is repeated on a weekly basis for as long as four weeks or until wart resolution occurs.

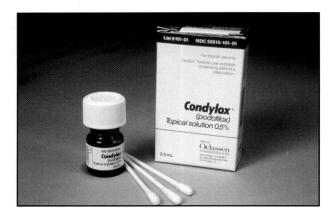

FIGURE 19.28 Commercially available podophyllotoxin used to treat external genital condyloma. ▬▬▬

Podophyllotoxin has two main advantages when compared with podophyllin. First, it is a patient-applied form of treatment, which allows easy home application in a confidential setting. Furthermore, it is a purified form of podophyllin that is prepared at a standardized concentration. The main disadvantages are similar to those mentioned for podophyllin. However, since podophyllotoxin is self-applied, improper application risks treatment failure. Epidermal erythema, ulceration, irritation, and pain may accompany its use.

The cure rates expected with podophyllotoxin vary between 45% and 80%.[185,188,189] Recurrences have been reported in 0% to 90% of the patients. Depending upon the spectrum of disease, a four- to six-week course of treatment may be necessary to completely eradicate the condyloma.

19.3.4.3 Di- or tri-chloroacetic acid (DCA, TCA)

Di- and tri-chloroacetic acid are potent caustic solutions used to treat external genital condyloma. Although not advocated by all experts, these acids can be applied to condyloma within the vagina or those on the ectocervix if located outside the transformation zone. However, care must be taken when using these products to treat internal condyloma because depth of tissue destruction may be difficult to control. Patients who have a limited number of condylomas are ideal candidates for DCA/TCA. Multiple, diffusely distributed condylomas may be better treated using other agents. Di- and tri-chloroacetic acid can be used safely to treat external genital condylomas in pregnant women.

When treating small solitary condylomas, DCA and TCA are best applied using a small-caliber wood stick or the end of a wooden-shaft, cotton-tipped

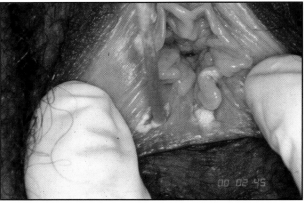

(a)

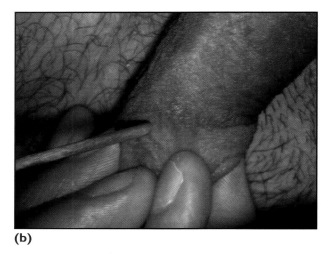

(b)

FIGURES 19.29a,b Use of a wood stick to apply DCA/TCA to external genital condyloma on the vulva **(a)** and penis **(b)**. ▬▬▬

applicator (Figures 19.29a,b). Larger lesions may be treated using a cotton-tip applicator soaked in TCA. The surface of the condyloma will assume a stark white color following proper application (Figures 19.30a,b). Patients do not need to rinse the treated areas following treatment. Several days later, the affected desicated tissues will slough, sometimes leaving slight erosion. Care must be exercised to keep the wooden application device perpendicular to the surface of the epithelium so as to treat only the warts. Wooden-shaft applicators have inherent capillary action that tends to draw solutions up the shaft from the immersed tip. If the wet applicator is held parallel and touches the surface of the skin, some linear trauma to normal adjoining tissue is possible. Some advocate applying petrolatum to the normal epithelium surrounding condylomas prior to using DCA/TCA. However, in our experience, this additional effort is not usually necessary if the DCA/TCA

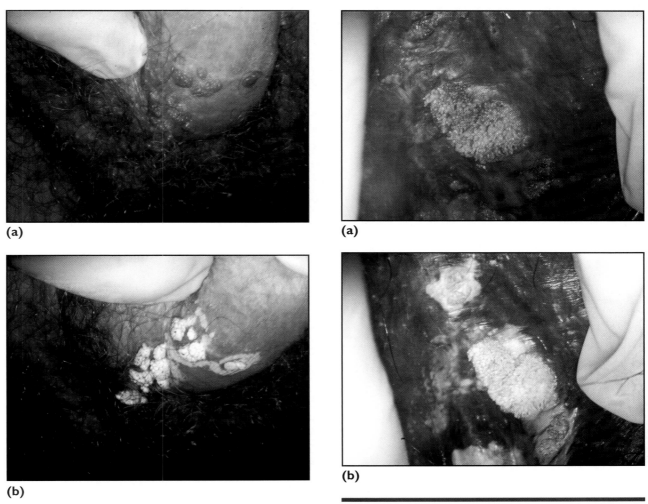

(a)

(b)

FIGURES 19.30a,b Penile condyloma before **(a)** and after **(b)** application of TCA. Note the immediate white discoloration of treated epithelium. ▬

(a)

(b)

FIGURES 19.31a,b Vulvar condyloma before **(a)** and following **(b)** treatment. Notice some runoff of the TCA onto normal surrounding epithelium. ▬

is applied cautiously only to the wart. Because of its low viscosity, large drops of DCA/TCA tend to flow easily off warts and onto surrounding tissue. Therefore, before removing the wooden shaft applicator from the vial of DCA/TCA, tap the drop that usually adheres at the end of the stick against the container to dislodge it prior to wart application. This simple "flick" prevents acid runoff (Figures 19.31a,b). TCA/DCA is considered a clinician-applied form of treatment for condylomas. Potentially extensive and deep burns may occur if the product is applied improperly. Sodium bicarbonate can be used to neutralize TCA/DCA, if necessary.

DCA/TCA works quite effectively for most patients. It is comparatively inexpensive and reasonable outcomes can be expected. The solutions may cause an immediate mild-to-moderate burning sen-

sation if normal epithelium is treated accidentally. Usually this discomfort resolves within five to ten minutes. When present, a post-treatment erosion may also cause some pain for several days (Figure 19.32). Deeper ulcerations can occur following aggressive treatment. In this case, healed tissue may be depigmented if the melanocytes are permanently damaged. Small warts usually resolve following a single application. Particularly large or heavily keratinized condyloma may be reduced in size or in some cases completely eradicated following a single application (Figure 19.33). Multiple applications may be necessary. Patients are usually treated on a bimonthly basis to allow interval healing. Therapeutic response depends on the host immune status, size of the lesions, viral load, type of epithelium and spectrum of HPV disease.

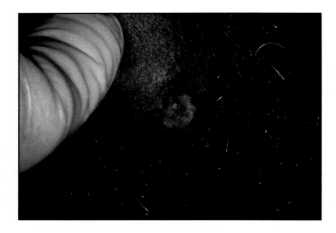

FIGURE 19.32   Healing ulceration on base of penis 2 weeks after treating a condyloma with TCA.

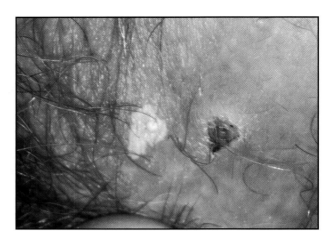

FIGURE 19.34   Healing penile site after condyloma treatment with TCA. Notice a new condyloma has become apparent since the past treatment.

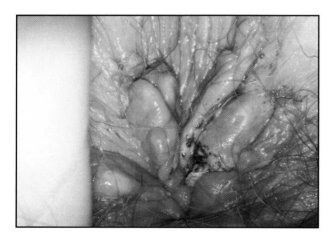

FIGURE 19.33   Residual perianal warts after a prolonged course of treatment. Notice the smooth contour of these incompletely eradicated warts.

Cure rates of between 50% and 100% may be expected with the use of DCA/TCA.[185,190] Low cure rates may reflect inappropriate selection of DCA/TCA as the agent of choice. Condyloma recurrence rates vary between 5% and 50% (Figure 19.34).

19.3.4.4 5-Fluorouracil (5-FU)

5-fluorouracil is an agent that inhibits DNA synthesis. This drug acts by causing a chemically induced inflammation and denuding of squamous epithelium. It is used primarily as an antimetabolite for treating certain epithelial pre-cancers and cancers. 5-FU is available as a 5% cream, 1% solution, and injectable gel combined with epinephrine.

Currently, 5-fluorouracil is rarely used for treating external genital condylomas. It is contraindicated

for use during pregnancy and in individuals with a history of hypersensitivity to the product. Therefore, contraceptives must be utilized when treating women of childbearing age.

5-FU cream or solution is applied directly to the involved areas and the gel is injected beneath the condyloma. If used prior to bedtime, the area should be washed with soap and water the next morning. When used previously for treating vaginal condyloma, it was applied using various treatment strategies. One method consisted of a once weekly intravaginal application of 5-FU cream (1/2 of a 5-gm vaginal applicator) for up to 10 weeks.[191] Patients were examined monthly and were told to report any significant irritation or pain. Any reported discomfort precipitated an immediate follow-up examination and probable drug discontinuation. A petrolatum or zinc oxide barrier may help protect normal surrounding epithelium before using 5-FU.

When used carefully, in a reliable and compliant patient, 5-FU performed as well as other forms of treatment for intravaginal and intraurethral condyloma. However, 5-FU cream may cause a local irritation along with burning, itching, or pain. When used in treating vaginal condylomas, erythema, vaginal adenosis, ulcerations, and vaginal and labial coaptation have occurred. Because of these significant adverse effects, 5-FU is no longer considered standard of care for treating vaginal condylomas.

There have been very few clinical trials evaluating the effectiveness of 5-FU cream. However, cure rates between 10% and 50% have been reported.[185] Little is known about recurrence rates following 5–FU use. One study reported a condyloma recurrence rate of 10% up to nine months following treatment.

19.3.4.5 Interferon

Interferon alpha, beta, and gamma are derived from components of the immune system (i.e. lymphocytes, fibroblasts, and macrophages). In particular, alpha interferon has been used to treat external genital warts. Interferon is an immunomodulatory protein that has antiproliferative properties.

Interferon has been used primarily as an adjuvant or tertiary agent for treating condyloma. The benefit of interferon, when used as an adjuvant, however, remains suspect. Although used infrequently, interferon may be of value in the treatment of recalcitrant condyloma. Interferon is contraindicated in patients with a known hypersensitivity to this product. Interferon cannot be used in immunocompromised patients, patients under 18 years of age, or people with allergies to egg or neomycin.

When used to treat external genital condyloma, interferon is delivered as an intralesional injection. The typical intralesional dose is 1 million units injected directly into the wart. As many as three warts can be injected per visit (maximum allowed dose per patient visit = 3 million units). Injections can be given three times per week for as long as two weeks, then if response is noted, once a week for up to a total of six weeks. Systemic therapy is no longer condoned.[185]

Interferon use is considered tertiary, and therefore it may be advantageous in patients who have failed other primary forms of treatment. Unfortunately, many patients do not tolerate the somewhat severe potential side effects: flu like systems, headache, fever, chills, myalgia, vomiting, nausea, dizziness and backpain. Elevated liver function studies, leukopenia and thrombocytopenia have been reported following interferon use. When injected into a condyloma, patients may notice pain, burning, itching and irritation. The limited dose per visit precludes its effective use in patients with multiple condyloma. The high cost of interferon restricts its use to very select cases.

Intralesional interferon has been shown to produce cure rates in approximately 40% to 60% of patients.[192–194] Recurrence rates have been reported in the range of 20% to 50%.

19.3.4.6 Imiquimod

Imiquimod is an immune response modifying agent with properties that induce alfa interferon, tumor necrosis factor, interleukin-6 and other cytokines. The exact mechanism of action is unknown. However, the resulting immune response has been shown to decrease the amount of HPV DNA in affected tissues. It is commercially formulated as a 5% cream (Figure 19.35).

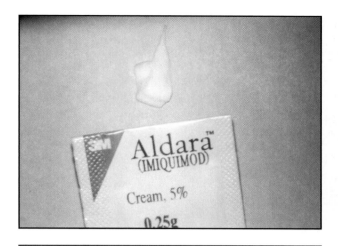

FIGURE 19.35 Commercially available imiquimod cream used to treat external genital condyloma. Imiquimod is an immune-response modifying agent.

Imiquimod is the newest primary form of treatment for external genital condylomas. Patients with diffusely located condylomas are ideal candidates. This scenario is very conducive to a regional cream application, instead of a precise site-specific application. However, patients with focal or solitary condyloma can also be treated with imiquimod. Because imiquimod is a self-applied product, patients should be comfortable to participate in their own care. Women need to understand that imiquimod is contraindicated for use during pregnancy. Even though off-label use of this drug occurs, imiquimod should not be used to treat condylomas of the cervix, vagina, urethra or rectum.

Imiquimod cream is applied to condylomas three times a week (i.e., Monday, Wednesday, Friday). The cream is washed off after each application eight hours later. Although complete cure may be achieved in a much shorter interval, application for up to sixteen weeks may be necessary to clear some condyloma.

There are several therapeutic advantages observed with imiquimod. As opposed to most of the other agents listed previously, imiquimod works by boosting the local immune system. Therefore, some regional antiviral effect may be noted. As a consequence, very small adjoining condyloma, not even apparent to casual inspection, may also be unknowingly treated. Furthermore, imiquimod is intended to be used as a self-application product so that patients may treat themselves at home. This is particularly appealing to embarrassed individuals or those otherwise inconvenienced by multiple health care appointments. Not unlike other products mentioned previously, imiquimod use may precipitate erythema, ulceration, and discomfort at the treatment site.

Between 40% to 80% of patients treated with imiquimod are cured following treatment (Figures 19.36a,b).[195] Condylomas in women may respond more favorably than those in men,[196] although cure rates in men may actually be equivalent.[197] Because of its mechanism of action, imiquimod is no more effective than placebo when treating HIV-infected patients.[198] In the general population, recurrence rates are low and vary between 10% to 20%. The low recurrence rates may be explained by the regional effect on the immune system.

19.3.5 Surgical approaches
19.3.5.1 Cryotherapy

Nitrous oxide, liquid nitrogen, and carbon dioxide cryogens can be used to treat condylomas. Each cryogen generates tissue temperatures below –20°C that are sufficient to cause cell death. Initially, cryother-

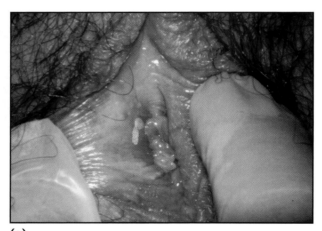

(a)

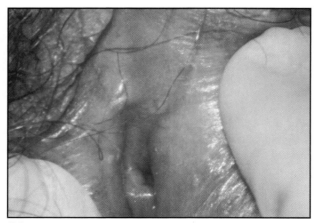

(b)

FIGURES 19.36a,b A small vulvar condyloma **(a)** cleared following one application of topical imiquimod **(b)**.

apy produces an intracellular dehydration. Thereafter, ice crystals pierce the cell membranes, releasing vasoactive substances that cause small vessel thrombosis, leading to anoxia and ischemia.

Cryotherapy is an ablative method used to treat selected external genital warts. Each cryogen may be better suited to treat certain warts based on their size and shape, and cryogen delivery method (i.e. spray, probe, etc). Liquid nitrogen can be used to treat all types of warts. Nitrous oxide systems use a probe that should conform to the shape of the wart. Consequently, these latter systems may be of limited utility in treating large, irregularly shaped exophytic warts. However, nitrous oxide systems are probably preferred for treating condylomas arising within the transformation zone of the cervix. Because of the difficulty controlling depth of freeze, vaginal condyloma are not usually treated by cryotherapy. Similarly, because of a limited depth of freeze, genital cancers are not treated by cryotherapy. Cryotherapy is contraindicated in patients with cryoglobulinemia. Cryotherapy is also contraindicated for treating cervical condyloma in pregnant women. However, pregnant women with external genital warts may be treated using cryotherapy.

There are three ways that liquid nitrogen may be used to treat external condylomas. The cryogen may be applied directly to the wart using large or small cotton-tip applicators that have been dipped in liquid nitrogen. Liquid nitrogen may also be applied by a device that directs a focal spray onto the wart. Finally, a metal probe that contains liquid nitrogen can be placed against condylomas to complete a freeze. Hollow cryoprobe tips of various sizes and shapes are also used when nitrous oxide cryotherapy is conducted. A thin film of water-soluble lubricant gel is first applied to the probe tip and then the tip is applied to the condyloma. Freezing is initiated by depressing a trigger located on a cryogun. Once the condyloma is completely frozen, including a surrounding 1-mm to 2-mm rim of normal tissue, the freeze may be discontinued for any cryotherapy method. Care should be taken not to freeze neurovascular tissue that may lie directly beneath condyloma. To prevent this from occurring, once the cryoprobe tip adheres to the wart, the wart should be gently retracted away from deeper structures. A double freeze (freeze, thaw, repeat freeze) technique may improve cryotherapy efficacy.

Cryotherapy is a clinician-directed treatment that causes minimal to moderate operative discomfort. Patients with solitary or a limited number of condyloma are perhaps the best candidates. Aggressive treatment may cause postoperative ulceration, pain, and depigmentation. Many patients respond to a single treatment provided the condyloma are of a smaller size and adequately frozen.

Cryotherapy successfully treats condylomas in 60% to nearly 100% of cases.[185] Treatment technique greatly determines outcome. Many clinicians have a tendency to undertreat using an abbreviated approach. Recurrence rates vary between 20% to 80%.

19.3.5.2 Laser vaporization

Carbon dioxide laser is the preferred way to ablate warts. The depth and extent of vaporization is determined by the power of the laser, diameter of the beam, duration of laser activation, and skill of the surgeon.

Laser vaporization is best indicated for widely distributed, recalcitrant, or heavily keratinized condylomas. Laser vaporization is also an effective form of treatment for condylomas found in anatomical locations that are difficult to reach. These sites include the rectum and the vagina. In contrast with some of the previously mentioned types of therapy, laser effectively treats neoplasia that may coexist with condylomas. It is contraindicated to use laser vaporization in patients who are fully anticoagulated or have a hemorrhagic diathesis. Laser vaporization is not contraindicated for treating external genital warts in pregnant women.

The surgeon guides the laser beam with either a handpiece instrument or a joy stick mounted on a colposcope. Following either local or general anesthesia, the laser beam is directed at the condyloma using a small laser beam spot size. The small beam size (high-power density) minimizes thermal injury to surrounding normal tissue. The treatment continues until the entire condyloma is vaporized. Caution must be taken to not treat too deeply or ineffectively. Such aggressive treatment may cause prolonged healing and increased scar formation.

Patients with condylomas that are numerous and spread diffusely or recalcitrant to prior therapy are best managed by laser vaporization. Because of the high cost and moderate postoperative morbidity, laser vaporization is generally reserved for select cases. Furthermore, laser requires surgical expertise and, for many clinicians, this means patient referral. Even properly performed laser vaporization may be associated with significant postoperative discomfort and pain, scar formation, and postoperative bleeding.

Condyloma cure rates using laser vaporization vary between 60% to 100%.[185,199] Furthermore, recurrence rates vary between 0% and 80%. These figures may reflect the more difficult cases reserved for laser vaporization.

19.3.5.3 Excisional procedures

Although not commonly done, a simple excision procedure may easily remove raised or pedunculated condyloma. Excision can be accomplished using scissors, electrosurgical loop, or scalpel, with few complications, limited to pain, infection, scar formation, and bleeding. Preoperative local anesthesia is usually necessary unless a pedunculated wart's stalk is quite narrow or general anesthesia is given. Surgical excision is best reserved for patients with a solitary or a limited number of condyloma. Lesions are excised to or just above the level of the papillary dermis. Surgical excision cure and recurrence rates vary between 10% and 35%.[185]

19.3.6 Therapeutic vaccines

Therapeutic HPV vaccines are currently undergoing clinical trials. Several different viral antigens are being evaluated. The ability of these antigens to produce effective neutralizing antibodies in the genital tract is unknown.[200] Therefore, at this point in time, it is premature to speculate on the potential efficacy of these vaccines. However, if shown to be effective, this approach could become a standard of care in the near future.

19.4 Cold Coagulation of the Cervix

19.4.1 Introduction

Cervical intraepithelial neoplasia (CIN) may be managed effectively by excisional or ablative procedures. Most providers recognize cryotherapy and laser vaporization as two of the more frequently performed types of ablation of the cervical transformation zone. Each technique is based on a distinct thermal or spectral energy, which is sufficient to produce cell death or tissue destruction. Because these therapeutic approaches do not allow for histologic examination of treated tissue, they are done less frequently than excisional methods. Another ablative procedure, referred to as cold coagulation, is also used by some clinicians to treat women with CIN. Although not widely utilized in North America, this relatively simple approach expands the therapeutic options available to women.

19.4.2 Purpose

Cold coagulation is a surgical method used to treat premalignant cervical neoplasia and the encompassing cervical transformation zone.[201] Since the procedure is ablative, no tissue is submitted for histologic interpretation. Therefore, it is preferable that only patients with histologically confirmed CIN involving the ectocervix receive cold coagulation. Proper treatment should eradicate disease and allow the regeneration of normal healthy epithelium.

19.4.3 Objectives

The objectives of cold coagulation are to (1) expose all CIN to lethal tissue temperatures; (2) eradicate the complete transformation zone; (3) minimize injury to normal tissue and post-treatment complications; and, most importantly, (4) prevent cervical cancer.

19.4.4 Prerequisites, indications, and contraindications

Because cold coagulation is an ablative type of therapy, specific pretreatment conditions must be met prior to initiating the procedure. These include visualizing the entire squamocolumnar junction (SCJ) and full extent of any cervical lesion; documenting cytologic, colposcopic, and histologic concordance; ensuring an endocervical canal free of neoplasia; and excluding the presence of cervical cancer by prior clinical examination and laboratory tests. Patients who do not satisfy these triage principles are better managed by conization.

The primary indication for cold coagulation is the presence of CIN, even though some benign conditions may be treated in the same manner. Cold coagulation is contraindicated in women with an unsatisfactory colposcopic examination; evidence of glandular neoplasia or cervical cancer; or discordant colposcopic and laboratory diagnoses.

19.4.5 Patient preparation

Prior to undergoing cold coagulation, women should be informed of their condition, treatment options, pretreatment preparation, expected reaction during therapy and post-treatment care. Patient education pamphlets are generally well accepted and serve as a printed source of information that may be reviewed at a later date. Premenopausal women are best scheduled immediately following menstruation. A urine pregnancy test may be necessary should any uncertainties arise concerning their current risk for pregnancy. An informed consent document pertaining to cold coagulation should be read and signed by the patient before surgery is initiated. Women may benefit by taking a nonsteroidal anti-inflammatory drug several hours prior to cold coagulation to minimize potential procedure-induced uterine cramping.

19.4.6 Equipment and supplies

A coagulator (Semm) is a medical device able to generate temperatures of 100° C in order to effectively destroy tissue.[202] "Cold coagulation" is a misnomer of sorts, as this device should not be confused with a cryosurgical unit that destroys tissue with freezing temperatures. The "cold" term implies coagulation by relatively cooler temperatures than those generated by electrocoagulation/electrocautery. The electrical device heats thermosounds (probes) to the selected temperature that is sufficient to produce tissue desiccation. The probes are similar in shape to cryotherapy probes, some are flat and others are rounded at the tip so as to achieve maximum tissue/probe adherence. These reusable probes are coated with Teflon to make post-treatment cleaning easier. No other equipment is required than optional anesthetics.[201] It is important to note from the cost-incurred standpoint, no disposable equipment is used.

19.4.7 Principles of cold coagulation

Cold coagulation causes tissue desiccation sufficient to destroy the epithelium and stroma to a depth of 3 mm to 4 mm.[201] The extent of desiccation depends on the temperature selected and the duration of application. In practical terms, the cold coagulator cooks tissue by invoking a rapid dehydration. Because of the extremely high temperatures, relatively brief application times are required. Excessively prolonged application causes increased scar formation and delayed healing.

19.4.8 Cold coagulation procedure

Cold coagulation is perhaps the easiest of all cervical surgeries to perform. After properly preparing the patient and visualizing the cervical transformation zone, the coagulator is activated. Once the probe reaches 100°C, the rounded tip is placed into the vagina and onto the ectocervix, centrally positioned at the external os for approximately 20 seconds. Care must be taken to not inadvertently touch the vulva or vagina while introducing the hot probe. Therefore, lateral sidewall retractors may be necessary to protect women with prolapsing vaginal walls. Once the probe is placed on the cervix, the clinician may hear soft crackling or snapping noises as the tissue is treated. Next, a flat probe is used to treat each quadrant of the ectocervix for 20 seconds. Four overlapping treatments usually ablate the entire transformation zone since the probe usually covers just one quadrant of the cervix.[201] However, a small cervical transformation may need only two or three treatments. Total treatment time, therefore, should not exceed two minutes. Local anesthesia or paracervical blocks are not always necessary; however, it is probably safer to administer anesthetic, particularly for women with very large transformation zones.

19.4.9 Patient education and follow-up

Patients may take nonsteroidal anti-inflammatory medication for any postoperative uterine cramping or pelvic pain. Women are free to resume sexual intercourse immediately. Because postoperative vaginal discharge or bleeding is minimal, tampon use is not essential. A follow-up appointment should be scheduled before the patient is discharged from the treatment visit.

19.4.10 Side effects and complications

Few side effects and complications are experienced with cold coagulation. Women may notice mild uterine cramping, although a significant number experience no side effects either during or following the treatment.[203] Mild vaginal discharge, spotting, and pelvic pain may be noted for a brief duration after the procedure.[204] Since endocervical canal lesions are not treated by cold coagulation, cervical stenosis is a rare postoperative complication. Cold coagulation appears to have no adverse effect on future fertility, although most studies are limited by inclusion of small numbers of women.

Outcomes Excellent cure rates can be expected with cold coagulation. In one study, a single treatment cured 93% of women with CIN 3 based on cytologic follow-up.[205] Similar cure rates of 90% to 97% for treatment of CIN 2 and 3 have been reported by other investigators.[203,206] These cure rates compare favorably with those experienced after loop excision, laser and cryotherapy. Cure rates for CIN 1 (97%) and CIN 2 (97%) have also been documented, based on a "see and treat" approach.[207] An excisional technique is recommended for any primary treatment failures because of a relatively unacceptable cure rate (19%) following a repeat cold coagulation.[205]

19.4.11 Documentation

The surgical procedure should be fully documented in writing. Temperature, duration, application number, probe shape, and complications, if applicable, can be noted in the operative note. Appropriate follow-up should be mentioned.

19.5 Carbon Dioxide Laser Surgery for the Cervix: Indications, Operative Methods, Complications, and Results

19.5.1 Introduction

Carbon dioxide laser surgery permits precise and complete tissue eradication. However, the success of laser surgery depends upon removing all obviously diseased and potentially involved tissue. Many gynecologists have adopted laser surgery and incorporated it into routine practice in offices and operating rooms. Still, in some settings, laser surgery remains the method of choice for first intervention in many cervical and lower genital tract diseases.

19.5.2 Characteristics of laser energy

Various substances in different physical states have been used to produce laser action. Lasers produce nonionizing electromagnetic radiation in the optical and infrared portions of the spectrum. Laser radiation is coherent (all waves are in phase in both space and time), collimated (all rays are virtually parallel), and essentially monochromatic (all waves have the same wavelength, frequency, and color). These characteristics account for the unique directionality of laser light, the predictable and uniform effect the light will have on a particular target, and the enormous intensity of the light, which is achieved by focusing the beam and, thus, concentrating the energy in a small area.

The wavelength or its reverse, the frequency determines the effect a laser beam will have on biological tissue. CO_2 laser energy, which is absorbed on the surfaces of tissues with a high water content, vaporizes the tissue, producing steam and scattered carbonized particles. Tissue necrosis, caused by thermal denaturing of proteins, occurs within $50\ \mu m$ to $100\ \mu m$ of the crater with limited exposure time (Figure 19.37).

The development of high energy per pulse lasers permits a high maximum power output for very short periods of time. Since thermal damage is time related, even less thermal damage is seen since the high energy per pulse noted with such lasers reduces the opportunity for heat conduction. The inherent hemostatic effect is the result of heat sealing smaller blood vessels in the zone of thermal necrosis. A wider zone of injury, caused by elevated temperature, surrounds the zone of necrosis, but the tissue will recover.

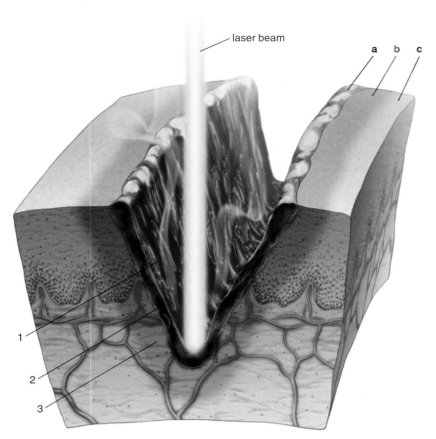

laser beam

a b c

FIGURE 19.37 The three zones of laser thermal injury:
Zone 1—zone of vaporization
Zone 2—tissue necrosis usually less than 100 μm
Zone 3—further tissue necrosis, which can delay healing

1
2
3

19.5.3 Lasers in cervical surgery

The laser most commonly used for treating diseases of the lower female genital tract is the CO_2 laser. For best control of laser energy, the laser is coupled to a colposcope or an operating microscope (Figure 19.38) rather than to a pen-like handpiece. The laser beam is delivered to the microscope in one of two ways: either the laser head is attached to the scope directly or an articulated arm containing mirrors connects the laser head to the microscope (colposcope). The scope and laser lenses are parfocal and coaxial, so that the surgical beam is in focus when the microscope is in focus with a matched lens system. The beam is controlled by the surgeon using a gimbaled mirror attached by a joystick (Figure 19.38). The surgical field is unobstructed, and surgery can be performed without touching the target.[208–210]

19.5.4 Rationale for employing the carbon dioxide laser

The advantages of laser surgery, when properly performed, over other modalities include the following: (1) microsurgical precision; (2) complete removal of diseased tissue to any depth or breadth required;

(3) no-touch surgery with an unobstructed operating field; (4) minimal effect on adjacent normal tissue and rapid healing to normal or near-normal volume with a new squamocolumnar junction (SCJ) located most often at the level of the external os; (5) quick, virtually painless treatment performed in the vast majority of cases in an office or clinic with little discharge, minimal complications, and no apparent effect on subsequent fertility or cervical incompetence; (6) in most cases, concomitant hemostasis; (7) a high rate of success after one treatment; (8) early identification of persistent disease; and (9) easy retreatment, usually in the office or clinic.[60,208,211]

19.5.5 Disease distribution

The laser surgical procedures on the cervix are based on the following disease parameters.

19.5.5.1 Area of susceptibility

Tissue susceptible to developing squamous cell intraepithelial neoplasia lies between the original SCJ and the histological os. The transformation zone (the area between the original and new SCJs) is usually transformed into normal squamous epithelium during the phases of metaplasia. Once normal squa-

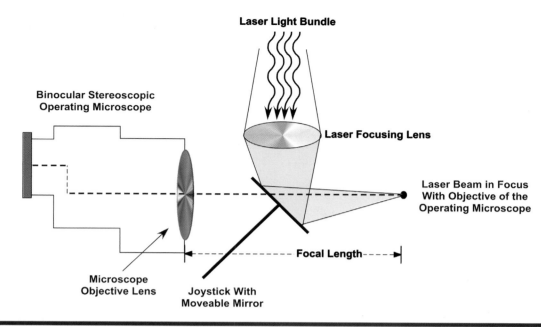

FIGURE 19.38 Basic instrumentation for the laser for microsurgery. The laser is coupled with the optical system of the colposcope or operating microscope. Adapted from Wright V C. Laser surgery for cervical intraepithelial neoplasia. In: Wright V C, Lickrish G M, Shier R M (eds). *Basic and Advanced Colposcopy (2nd Ed): A Practical Handbook for Treatment.* Houston: Biomedical Communications, 1995;21:1.

mous tissue is formed, it appears to be resistant to the development of squamous intraepithelial neoplasia and ultimately carcinoma. The area of susceptibility diminishes as columnar epithelium is replaced by normal squamous epithelium and as the new SCJ moves toward and later into the cervical canal. During the dynamic phases of metaplasia, however, atypical metaplastic squamous epithelium can develop in the transformation zone, creating a field of neoplastic potential.

Squamous lesions begin at the caudal part of the remaining area of susceptibility and then extend cephalad, becoming histologically more severe in the process.

19.5.5.2 Cervical intraepithelial lesions (CIN) involving cervical crypts

CIN can extend into the underlying cervical crypts. Higher-grade lesions (severe dysplasia and carcinoma in situ [CIS]) extend into cervical crypts up to 5.2 mm, but in most cases, crypt depth varies between 1.24 mm and 1.6 mm.[172,212,213] In CIN 3 lesions (severe dysplasia/CIS) 85% to 95% will have some crypt extension.[208] However, 96% of these cases have depth of disease extension of less than 2.9 mm. It has been hypothesized that destruction of lesions to a depth of 3.8 mm will eradicate all involved crypts in 99.7% of patients.[212]

19.5.5.3 Radial linear length

The radial linear length of CIN can vary between 2 mm and 22 mm, but the usual linear length varies between 6 mm and 10 mm.[172,213-216] CIN lesions do not extend more than 22 mm up the endocervical canal when measured from the lowermost border of the lesions.[215] Therefore, when planning tissue destruction or removal for a particular patient, the surgeon must consider that the more exposed the columnar epithelium appears, the less likely it is that disease is located high within the endocervical canal. The more endocervical the columnar epithelium, the more likely there is involvement high in the canal. This is very important and helps to determine the correct procedure to remove the CIN.

19.5.5.4 Disease location

The transformation zone recedes into and up the endocervical canal with age.[217] In women of reproductive age, CIN lesions do not extend above the level of the internal os.

19.5.5.5 Location of cancer

Invasive squamous cell cancer appears on the canal side. That is, the worst disease is located centrally,[218] indicating that for ectocervical CIN, sampling the innermost margin provides the most severe histological information. To exclude invasive cancer for lesions in the canal, the upper margin must be carefully assessed regardless of the histology of the more caudal component.

19.5.6 The geometry of cervical intraepithelial neoplasia as a guide to its removal

Accepting the known dimensions of CIN, one can conceptualize the three-dimensional geometry of disease bearing tissue in a given patient and apply appropriate operative techniques to remove or destroy it.[60,172,208–219] It is obvious that a defect resembling a cylinder best represents the solid geometry of disease regardless of its location.[60,211,214,219,220] Figure 19.39 compares volumes of tissue removed with the cylindrical approach and with the cone-shaped method when all potentially involved tissue is incorporated in the specimen and when cure, not just diagnosis, is anticipated.[219] Figure 19.39a depicts ectocervical CIN. The vertical "5 mm" arrows indicate the maximum potential depth of involvement in crypts and the heavier horizontal "1.9 cm" arrow indicates diameter of the lesion. To surround the arrows, a cone-shaped specimen would be deeper and wider and would include much more normal tissue, but a domed cylinder would match the diseased tissue and incorporate a smaller volume.

When an excision is required, the specimen must also be cylindrical in shape to incorporate lateral crypt involvement (horizontal 5-mm arrows) and the lesion along the surface of the endocervical canal (vertical 1.6-cm arrow). Figure 19.39b illustrates that a cylindrical approach removes half the volume of tissue required by a cone-shaped specimen when diagnosis as well as cure is intended.

Approximately 18% of CIN cases have lesions with a long length and occupy the ectocervix and extend into the endocervical canal. The principles of colposcopy dictate that the disease in the canal must be excised to rule out invasive cancer since the worst histologic evidence is located centrally. Figure 19.39c

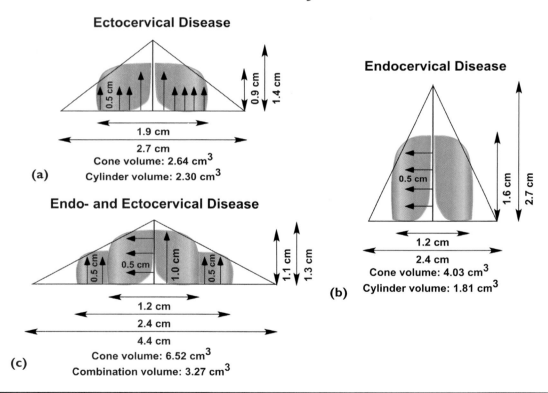

The Geometry of CIN

Ectocervical Disease

0.5 cm
0.9 cm
1.4 cm
1.9 cm
2.7 cm
Cone volume: 2.64 cm³
(a) Cylinder volume: 2.30 cm³

Endocervical Disease

0.5 cm
1.6 cm
2.7 cm
1.2 cm
2.4 cm
Cone volume: 4.03 cm³
(b) Cylinder volume: 1.81 cm³

Endo- and Ectocervical Disease

0.5 cm
0.5 cm
1.0 cm
0.5 cm
1.1 cm
1.3 cm
1.2 cm
2.4 cm
4.4 cm
Cone volume: 6.52 cm³
(c) Combination volume: 3.27 cm³

FIGURES 19.39a–c The measurements of crypt involvement and linear length provide therapeutic guidelines for eradication of CIN. Successful eradication of disease is based upon a cylindrical defect, whether vaporized or excised. The destroyed or removal volume of tissue is less than that with the conical approach. Adapted from Wright V C. Laser surgery for cervical intraepithelial neoplasia. In: Wright V C, Lickrish G M, Shier R M (eds). *Basic and Advanced Colposcopy (2nd Ed): A Practical Handbook for Treatment.* Houston: Biomedical Communications, 1995;19:1–7.

illustrates a logical approach to these lesions, that is, a central cylinder excision plus peripheral vaporization that removes disease, establishes a diagnosis, and requires half the volume of tissue excised by a cone-shaped specimen.[60,211,219]

From these concepts, three surgical procedures account for the distribution of CIN.[60,211,219] These procedures include a shallow, dome-shaped cylinder for ectocervical CIN, a tall cylinder for canal disease, and a moderately tall central cylinder surrounded by a donut or inner tube configuration (similar in shape to a cowboy hat) for disease occupying the endocervical canal and extending beyond a radius of 8 mm onto the cervix.

19.5.7.1 The laser vaporization procedure for ectocervical CIN

The following criteria must be fulfilled for laser ablation: (1) cytologic, colposcopic, and histologic information must be correlated to establish an accurate cervical tissue diagnosis; (2) the entire transformation zone must be colposcopically defined; (3) the colposcopist must be certain from the qualitative assessment of the transformation zone that no cancer or adenocarcinoma in situ (AIS) is present; (4) the CIN must occupy the ectocervix at or below the level of the external os with no extension into the endocervical canal (Figure 19.40).

19.5.7.1 Basic setup and instrumentation

The patient is comfortably placed in stirrups and the cervix is exposed by using the largest bivalve speculum possible. The cervix is infiltrated with local anes-

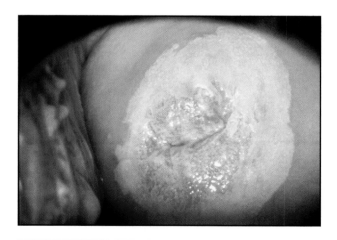

FIGURE 19.40 A colpophotograph of ectocervical CIN 2 which meets the criteria for laser ablation. Figure 19.40 reprinted with permission from Wright V C: Color Atlas of Colposcopy—Cervix, Vagina and Vulva. Houston: Biomedical Communications, 2000. ■

thetic, or a paracervical block can be used. Local infiltration of 1% lidocaine (Xylocaine) with 1:100,000 dilution of epinephrine (pH 4.05) produces a stinging sensation most likely related to its acid pH. The pain can be decreased by adding sodium bicarbonate (1 mEq/mL) at a dilution of 10:1. For example, 5 mL of 1% lidocaine with epinephrine is mixed in the same syringe with 0.5 mL of sodium bicarbonate. This results in a pH of 7.37 (alkaline). Alternately, vasopressin (the total dose not exceeding one pressor unit) can be mixed with the 1% lidocaine (pH 6.49) for local anesthesia. The purpose of using a vasoconstricting agent is to decrease the diameter of the blood vessels so that the laser beam's heat will seal them and minimize bleeding. Table 19.10 illustrates the pH of commercial local anesthetics and those modified. The author recommends local infiltration into the posterior cervical lip first, then lateral infiltration, with injection of the anterior lip last, because the anterior cervical lip appears to be more sensitive than the posterior lip.

A smoke evacuation system is necessary to remove the vapor plume. A handheld suction tip can be positioned in the vagina by an assistant or the suction device can be attached to the upper blade of the speculum. Custom speculae with suction device attachments are commercially available. A trap is placed between the speculum and the filter to permit suction of both plume and blood should bleeding occur.

The CO_2 laser is attached to a colposcope or operating microscope employing a magnification of 2.5× to 3.5×. This gives an adequate diameter of view of 57 mm to 80 mm. Although higher magnification offers the advantage of permitting more colposcopic detail, low magnifications allow an operator to see the entire operative field during surgery. The working distance should be 300 mm, which reflects the focal length of the microscope's main objective lens. A matched 300-mm focal lens system is used in the laser system. Thus, when the microscope is in focus,

Table 19.10 pH of 1% Lidocaine + Epinephrine and Sodium Bicarbonate

Solution	pH
Lidocaine + commercial epinephrine	4.05
Lidocaine	6.49
Lidocaine + added epinephrine	6.39
Normal saline	6.85
Lidocaine + epinephrine + sodium bicarbonate	7.37
Lidocaine + sodium bicarbonate	7.38

the laser beam will be in focus at the focal plane (in this case, the cervix). The main objective lens of the microscope should be at the same level as the target (cervix). A small beam diameter (0.5 mm) is effective for cutting but will produce potholes and furrowing if used for vaporization. The recommended effective laser beam diameter for laser vaporization is a minimum of 2 mm to 2.5 mm; this is obtained with the variable-spot-size mechanism. The laser power setting is between 25 and 40 watts. A 2-mm effective laser beam diameter and 25 watts results in a power density (PD) of 625 watts/cm^2 (PD = 100 × W divided by d^2 where d is the effective laser beam diameter and W is the watts of power chosen by the surgeon). Larger beam diameters can be used, but the watts of power have to be increased accordingly to produce the appropriate power density. Alternately using high energy per pulse 200 millijoules of energy per pulse and an average power between 25 and 40 watts can be used.

The lesion on the cervix is redefined by colposcopy. The entire transformation zone including the CIN lesion is outlined with a 2-mm laser beam. This marking must be 2 mm to 3 mm beyond the lesion border. Most cases of CIN do not have a linear length greater than 8 mm. The entire transformation zone, including the area of pathology, is then vaporized to a minimum depth of 6 mm to 8 mm, with the surgeon beginning at the 6 o'clock position and never leaving an area until proper depth is achieved. Centrally, a further vaporization of 4 mm to 8 mm is recommended, creating the dome-shaped defect (Figures 19.39a and 19.41). The latter step takes into account the topographical anatomy of the cervix and removes part of the

remaining area of susceptibility in order to prevent new disease from developing in the future. This procedure usually takes 1 to 5 minutes to perform in an office or clinic setting. The detailed operative techniques for this procedure have been previously published.[60,208,211,220]

When CIN occupies the ectocervix and has a radial linear length exceeding 8 mm, a central cylindrical dome-shaped is vaporized. CIN peripheral to the 8-mm radial length is then vaporized to a depth of 4 mm to 6 mm. This results in a cowboy-hat type of configuration. These ablative methods help to preserve the cervix. Should disease extend onto the vagina, laser vaporization can be extended to encompass the disease, but vaporization depth should not exceed 1.5 mm.

19.5.7.2 Pitfalls in vaporization management in CIN

Persistent disease occurs as a result of any of three vaporization procedure errors: the initial outline of the intended defect did not include a 2-mm to 3-mm normal tissue border, a minimum vaporization depth of at least 6 mm was not uniformly achieved along the cervical surface, or activation of latent virus (not a procedure error) occurred. Proper depth is relatively easy to obtain at the defect's margin but harder to achieve at the external os where there is no tissue by which to judge depth. It is essential for the defect to be dome-shaped and to match the anatomical topography of the cervix and assure adequate depth at the external os (Figure 19.41)

Vaporization of larger CIN lesions (those longer than 8 mm) creating the standard dome-shaped defect can result in central or complete loss of the cervix and can produce a large central ectopy of columnar epithelium when healed. Both situations are undesirable, the first for obvious reasons and the second because the columnar epithelium is exposed to any potential carcinogenic agent(s) contained within the vaginal environment. To remedy these problems, the standard procedure should be modified as described.

19.5.8 Cylindrical laser excision for endocervical lesions

This procedure is indicated when discrepancies exist between cytology, colposcopy, and histology; when lesions and the transformation zone are located in the endocervical canal and require tissue for histological evaluation (Figure 19.42); when either cytologic or colposcopic results suggest possible invasive carcinoma that is not clinically visible and has not been proven by colposcopically directed biopsy;

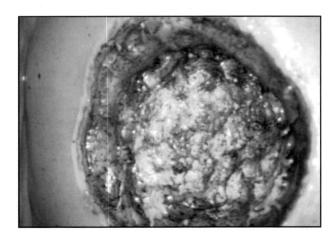

FIGURE 19.41 A colpophotograph of the laser ablation procedure using the continuous mode of the laser. ▬▬

when there is a positive ECC or to differentiate adenocarcinoma in situ from adenocarcinoma.

Figure 19.39b illustrates the geometry of endocervical disease. In this case, the disease extends to a maximum depth of 5 mm into the underlying cervical crypts and involves the endocervical canal to a height of 1.6 cm. By removing a cylinder rather than a cone, the surgeon excises half as much tissue. This procedure is performed under anesthesia as day surgery in a hospital or surgery center. The operating requirements include a CO_2 laser attached to an operating microscope, an effective laser beam diameter of 0.5 mm, a working distance of 300 mm, and a power density greater than 1500 watts/cm^2 (usually between 1500 and 18,000 watts/cm^2). To ensure a virtually bloodless operating field, hemostatic sutures are placed at the 3 o'clock and 9 o'clock positions, then a vasopressin solution (not exceeding one pressor unit and mixed in 10 cc of normal saline) is injected into the cervical stroma. A cylindrical rather than a cone-shaped specimen is removed for histological interpretation (Figures 19.39b and 19.43). The specimen height varies from 1.5 mm to 1.8 cm in a reproductive woman. To proceed, the upper pole is cut with a scalpel or a tonsil snare, followed by flashing (quickly moving the beam over the apex with a 2-mm diameter laser beam to seal the blood vessels). The only thermal damaged tissue is located at the outer margin (less than 100 μm). This procedure takes less than 6 minutes when properly performed. The step-by-step details of this procedure have been published elsewhere.[60,220]

19.5.8.1 Pitfalls in management of endocervical CIN

Persistent disease occurs for several reasons: because initial marking of the defect's periphery by the laser beam did not incorporate at least 6 mm of lateral radius; because adequate depth was not achieved, leaving disease in the canal; when the shape of the defect resembled a cone, with sloping sides cutting across glands and leaving disease in place; or if latent human papillomavirus becomes activated, producing condyloma or low grade CIN during the healing process.

19.5.8.2 Reasons for an inadequate specimen

Specimens are inadequate for many reasons. Mostly they are the following: inadequate power density prolonged the procedure; the specimen was excised by repeated encircling of the cervix with the beam, causing excessive thermal damage; it is better to achieve the desired height in one location before moving onward; the apex of the specimen was "coned in" and severed by the laser beam, producing a thermal effect at the upper margin and making histological interpretation difficult (vaporization of a coned-shaped defect to correct the final defect's shape and create a cylindrical defect may destroy evidence of invasion).

19.5.8.3 Reason for poor healing

The reason for poor healing is that the specimen's radius was excessive and a large central core was removed that was not restored during healing resulting in a large central ectopy with the new SCJ located widely on the ectocervix—an undesirable situation

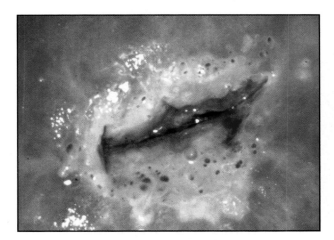

FIGURE 19.42 CIN 3 around the external os and extending into the endocervical canal. A candidate for laser cylindrical excision. Figure 19.40 reprinted with permission from Wright V C: *Color Atlas of Colposcopy—Cervix, Vagina and Vulva.* Houston: Biomedical Communications, 2000.

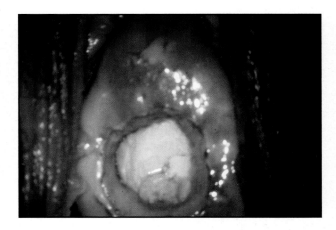

FIGURE 19.43 A colposcopic photo of the cervix after the cylindrical excisional procedure performed using a high energy per pulse laser.

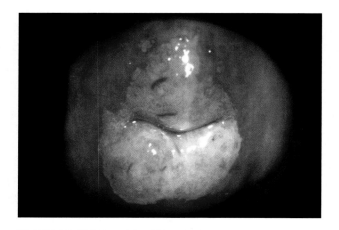

FIGURE 19.44 Ectocervical and endocervical disease. A typical candidate for the combination procedure (central excision and peripheral ablation). Figure 19.44 reprinted with permission from Wright V C: *Color Atlas of Colposcopy—Cervix, Vagina and Vulva.* Houston: Biomedical Communications, 2000.

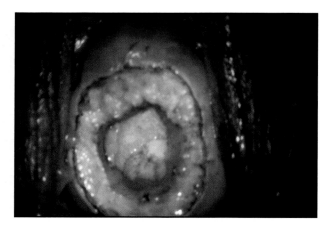

FIGURE 19.45 A colpophotograph after the combination procedure using a high energy per pulse laser. Note the absence of carbonization. Figure 19.45 reprinted with permission from Wright V C: *Color Atlas of Colposcopy—Cervix, Vagina and Vulva.* Houston: Biomedical Communications, 2000.

because the area is then exposed to the carcinogenic agent(s) and therefore capable of promoting new disease. The typical cervix after a properly performed procedure reveals the new SCJ to be located at the level of the external os or slightly within the endocervical canal.

19.5.9 Laser excision and vaporization (the combination procedure)

In approximately 18% of cases, extensive disease occupies the transformation zone on the ectocervix but extends beyond colposcopic view into the endocervical canal (Figures 19.39c and 19.44). Although cytologic and colposcopic examinations indicate CIN disease, histological examination of the endocervical tissue is necessary to completely evaluate this area. A suitable defect incorporating the ectocervix and lower endocervical canal can effectively eliminate the distribution of this disease. The combination procedure is used when the ectocervical component has a radius greater than 8 mm.

With the patient under anesthesia, the central cylinder is removed first for histological evaluation, as above. Specimen heights usually range from 1.0 cm to 1.5 cm. This part of surgery is similar to the laser cylindrical excision. Then, using a 2-mm CO_2 laser beam, the remaining outer disease and transformation zone are vaporized to a depth of 6 mm. This results in a cowboy-hat configuration (Figure 19.45). By removing a central cylinder with

peripheral vaporization, the surgeon removes half as much tissue than if the entire disease had been included within a cone-shaped specimen (Figure 19.39c). The entire procedure takes less than 8 minutes. The step-by-step operative details of this procedure have been published elsewhere.[220]

19.5.10 Cervix cases: discharge instructions, post-operative complications, healing, and follow-up

Patients are advised to refrain from douching, having intercourse, or using tampons for 3 weeks following laser surgery. They should be instructed to notify the physician's office immediately if brisk, red bleeding develops and to expect some spotting during the first 10 days after treatment. Most problems can be managed in the office or clinic setting more easily than if the patient comes into the hospital emergency room. Patients should be advised to return to the clinic or office for their first complete follow-up examination 4–6 months following surgery. The examination includes cytology or cytology and colposcopy or HPV DNA testing at 6 months after treatment with biopsy if necessary. At this time, metaplastic cellular changes are few and a satisfactory Pap smear can be obtained. The second visit is scheduled 4–6 months afterward and the third after another 4–6 months. Usually, any persistent disease is discovered at the first or second visit. Yearly cytologic examination is recommended after 3 satisfactory, normal follow-ups.

19.5.11 Delayed bleeding

Troublesome bleeding requiring medical intervention is rarely a problem following laser ablation. It is slightly more common following laser excision (about 5% to 10% of cases). Surgical intervention is also not commonly required to control postoperative bleeding. Examination of the cervix with the colposcope will usually identify a small area of ooze or heavier bleeding. These conditions can be controlled by one or a combination of the following measures: application of Monsel's paste; placing a pack against the cervix and removing it 24 hours later; focal electrosurgical coagulation (very effective); laser coagulation (defocused laser beam while sucking the blood out of the operative site); suturing; arterial embolization; or if all fails, hysterectomy.

The last two would be unusual methods to stop the bleeding. Further, it is important not to soak a pack in Monsel's paste and leave it in the cervix for any period of time, since considerable sloughing of cervical tissue could result. If an inflammatory process is present, appropriate cultures should be taken and appropriate antibiotics prescribed. The maximum probability of encountering bleeding, hence the greatest chance of difficulty, occurs between the 6th and 10th postoperative day.

19.5.12 Infection

Infection is virtually non-existent, probably because of the sterilized wound, the absence of necrotic debris, and the sealing of lymphatics and blood vessels. Antibiotics, therefore, are unnecessary except as prophylaxis, for example, in patients with previous pelvic inflammatory disease.

19.5.13 Healing

Healing patterns are well documented. Some sloughing of necrotic tissue and carbon residue occurs during the first 2 days. If taken, cytologic samples reveal the presence of acute inflammatory cells. By day 3, squamous epithelium begins to proliferate in the defect, and specks of carbonized debris on the crater surface can be seen through the colposcope and within the new epithelium as it begins to fill the cavity. Soon the inflammatory reaction subsides. When the cervical procedure is appropriately planned, the original or near-original mass of cervical tissue is usually restored by day 21 with normal topography. Mature epithelium with normal tensile strength has been documented cytologically, histologically, and by scanning electron microscopy.[221,222]

19.5.14 Stenosis

Cervical stenosis after excisional procedures on the cervix is not common. While some narrowing of the cervix after these procedures is frequently seen, symptomatic cervical stenosis only occasionally presents as a problem in management. When stenosis occurs, it usually involves only the cervical os but does not exceed 2 mm. In most cases, a small membrane of tissue covers the external os. Regardless, prevention is better than cure. Cervical stenosis can occur in the following circumstances: women of reproductive age group with oligomenorrhea or amenorrhea; women on low dose birth control pills who have oligomenorrhea or amenorrhea; women who are postpartum and lactating; postmenopausal women who are not on hormone replacement therapy; women who are on estrogen and progesterone therapy with amenorrhea; women using progestin-only contraception.

Cyclic systemic estrogen and progesterone at doses that cause menstruation will likely prevent stenosis in the hormonal deficiency group. This should occur before, during, and after the excisional procedure and can be achieved by prescribing conjugated estrogen 1.25 mg daily and progestin 10 mg per day for days 1 to 12 of each month for 3 or 4 cycles. In lactating women, topical vaginal estrogen can be prescribed before, during, and after the procedure. Alternately, the procedure may be postponed, provided there is no concern about cancer, until breastfeeding is discontinued and menstrual periods resume. For medroxyprogesterone patients, it is best to stop the drug and let the cycles return or use vaginal estrogen twice daily for 14 days before the procedure and until healing is achieved.

High-risk patients should be examined every 2 weeks for at least 6 to 8 weeks following excision, and their endocervical canals should be probed. Stenosis cannot be completely prevented, but the incidence can be reduced.[223]

19.5.15 Results of laser surgery

In one series, a single operator treated 2327 patients with CIN by the CO_2 laser (1,454 by laser vaporization and 873 by cylindrical excision or the combination procedure).[208] Vaporization produced cure rates of 94.8% and the excisional and/or the combination procedure 95.1% after one surgery. Pregnancy outcome in 195 patients within the whole group (142 laser vaporizations and 53 laser excisions) indicated no increase in the premature delivery rate or cesarean rate.[208,224,225] Similar cure rates have been published elsewhere.[226–231] The first follow-up examination performed at the 3-month anniversary, including colposcopic and cytologic exams, was very accurate in predicting any persistent disease. That is, 90% of all patients who were shown to have persistent disease were identified at the first follow-up visit, with the remaining noted at the second visit, except for one case, whose persistence was not identified until the third visit (9 months post-procedure). After laser surgery, the new SCJ formed at the external os in 90% of cases, and in all cases, the cervix appeared to regenerate to its original or near-original organ mass.[208]

19.6 Loop-and-Needle Electrosurgical Procedures for Treatment of Cervical Intraepithelial Neoplasia

19.6.1 Introduction

Electrosurgery was first introduced in the late 1920s by William Bovie and Harvey Cushing. They invented the first electrosurgical generator (ESG) that produced high-frequency energy for surgical cutting and coagulation of biological tissue. Since that time, safer and more flexible equipment has been developed, and electrosurgery has become popular in a variety of disciplines.[50,232–238]

19.6.2 Definition of electrosurgery

Electrosurgery can be defined as the use of radio frequency current to cut tissue or achieve hemostasis. The primary rules of electricity pertain to the following: 1) electricity flows to ground; 2) electricity follows the path of least resistance; 3) impedance to electric current produces heat.

19.6.3 Basic electrical terms

For best therapeutic results, the colposcopist should understand four basic electrical terms and appreciate how they relate to clinical electrosurgery: current, volts, resistance and power.

19.6.3.1 Current

An electric current is a stream of charged electrons flowing through a conducting body (e.g., a wire). The amount of electric current can be defined as the amount of charge (q) that passes a given point per unit of time (t), usually a second. That is, I (current) = q (charge transported) / t (time required to transport the charge) measured in amperes or coulombs per second, since the unit of charge is the coulomb. That is, 1 ampere = 1 coulomb/sec (1A = 1 C/S). A coulomb is the amount of charge on 6.25×10^{18} electrons. This means that 6.25×10^{18} electrons are passing a given point per second ($I = q/t$).

19.6.3.2 Volt

A definite amount of energy is required to move each unit of charge from one place to another. The volt is a measure of electromagnetic force. When applied to a resistance of one ohm, one volt will produce a current of one amp. That is $V = IR$, where V = volts, I = current (amperes) and R = electrical resistance of a conductor.

19.6.3.3 Impedance (resistance)— how much current will be inhibited

A conductor permits the flow of electronic charge. However, the electrons collide with one of the atoms of the conductor, slowing them down. This results in a loss of energy to the atoms, and the energy appears as heat. In electrosurgery, impedance to current flow is principally related to the dimensions of the tissue electrodes, the resistivity of conductors, inductance, capacitance (electrosurgical generators), and the impedance related to the type of human tissue.

A capacitor (condenser) is an electrical component that stores electric charges. It consists of two plates, which are inductors separated by an insulator, called a dielectric. Capacitors store electric energy in the dilectric. Capacitance is the amount of electric charge stored in the dilectric, measured in Farads (F). The greater the capacitance, the greater and more intense is the flow of the alternating current. The higher the frequency of the electrosurgical generator, the more the current flows.

Inductance (energy stored in a magnetic field) provides high resistance to current flow to alternating current. Capacitance, frequency, and inductance vary between electrosurgical generators.

19.6.3.4 Watts and power

A watt is the rate of work represented by a current of one ampere with a force of one volt; that is, watts = volts × amps. The rate at which energy or work is performed (or transformed, such as electricity into heat or light) is termed *power*. In the International System of Units (ISU), the unit of power is the watt (W), and, it is expressed as 1 watt (W) = 1 joule/second.

Power is expressed as $P=IV$, where I = current and V = volts. From Ohm's law ($V=IR$ or $I =V/R$); thus, power can also be expressed as $P = I^2R$ and $P = V^2/R$.

In electrosurgery, human tissue resists the flow of current. This impedance creates the heat required for tissue cutting or coagulation. The amount of tissue heated is proportional to the square of the current, the resistance (P= I²R), and the current density. Current density (j) is current divided by area (j=I/area). The power setting on any ESG is representative of the power (volts × amps) the particular unit is capable of delivering into a fixed load (e.g., tissue type with its characteristic impedance). Many generators are designed for an impedance load of approximately 500 ohms, which accounts for the impedance of most human tissues. The power in watts displayed on the panel of the ESG reflects the maximum power that can be obtained at that setting. The actual power delivered in watts to tissue varies with changes in tissue impedance in conventional generators. For some high impedance in tissue, the ESG may not have the capacity to deliver sufficient current to match the power settings. The amount of power to do the procedure depends in part upon the physical characteristics of the ESG (keeping the tissue electrodes and operative techniques constant). This varying power is related to the differences in frequency, waveforms, capacitance, inductance, etc., which are peculiar to different manufacturers' products. Thus, the setting in watts of power as a base to perform certain procedures will not be the same for all generators, and the operator cannot expect the same ESG settings to produce the same tissue response. Individuals without electrosurgical experience who are using the conventional ESG for a procedure should set the generator, which varies the voltage to maintain a constant current flow, at a low setting and slowly increase the power until the desired effect is obtained.

Electrosurgery requires high voltage, high frequency, and low current density, as opposed to low voltage, low frequency, and high current provided by the standard power sources (e.g., household electricity). The use of a step-up transformer within the ESG increases the typical 60 Hz household current to greater than 300,000 Hz (300 kHz). The frequencies employed in electrosurgery are within the frequencies of AM radio. Hence, electrosurgery is at times referred to as radiofrequency surgery. Frequencies below 100 kHz can stimulate muscles and nerves (Faradic effect). Should this occur, surgery must be discontinued and the cause of the low frequency investigated.

19.6.4 Stages of thermal destruction

The utilization of thermal energy permits the physician to perform electrosurgical cutting (flash boiling or vaporization) and electrosurgical dehydration of tissue termed coagulation (desiccation and fulguration). Table 19.11 illustrates the stages of thermal destruction in tissue.

19.6.5 Waveforms produced by electrosurgical generators

The basic waveforms employed in electrosurgery are: pure sine waves (Figure 19.46), damped sine waves (Figure 19.47), and modulated sine waves (Figure 19.48).

19.6.6 Monopolar electrosurgical cutting

Unless the voltage is kept constant, the alternating current flows from the ESG under a variable voltage to the active tissue electrode and through the patient to a return electrode, termed the *dispersive plate* or *electrode*. The dispersive plate provides an electrical contact over a very large area on the patient. The current density at the dispersive plate is small in comparison to the current density at the active tissue electrode. In modern ESGs, an isolation transformer inside the unit isolates the therapeutic current from ground (isolated electrosurgical generator, which protects against current division); hence, the generator, not the

Table 19.11 Stages of Thermal Destruction*

Temperature	Effect
Up to approximately 40° C	No significant effect
Above approximately 40° C	Reversible cell damage depending upon duration of exposure
Above 40° C	Irreversible cell damage (denaturing of protein occurs)
Above approximately 70° C	Coagulation. Collagen is converted to glucose
At 100° C	Flash boiling, vaporization
Above 100° C	Desiccation occurs
Above approximately 200° C	Carbonization occurs

*The most severe thermal effects in electrosurgery pertain to coagulation. Electrosurgical cutting produces the least thermal effect.

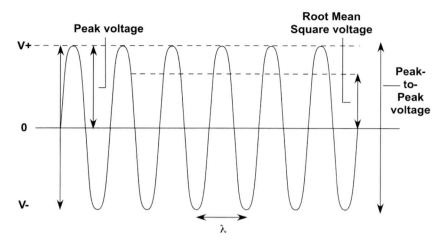

FIGURE 19.46 A pure sine wave. (Image provided courtesy of Dr. V. Cecil Wright: *Understanding Electrosurgery.* Houston: Biomedical Communications, 1995.)

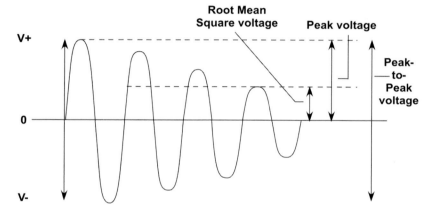

FIGURE 19.47 A damped sine wave (Image provided courtesy of Dr. V. Cecil Wright: *Understanding Electrosurgery.* Houston: Biomedical Communications, 1995.)

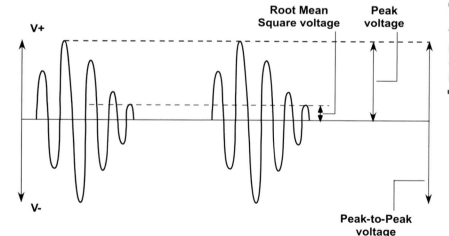

FIGURE 19.48 A modulated sine wave (RMS = root mean square). (Image provided courtesy of Dr. V. Cecil Wright: *Understanding Electrosurgery.* Houston: Biomedical Communications, 1995.)

ground, completes the circuit (Figure 19.49a). Return electrode monitoring systems (REM) help reduce the incidence of burns at the site of the dispersive plate (Figure 19.49b). In order to cut tissue, electric arcs must be produced and sparking to tissue must occur. The following parameters appear to be of surgical importance: a voltage greater than 200 peak volts is required to produce the electric spark between a metal tissue electrode and biological tissue; with a voltage greater than 200 peak volts, electric sparks increase in length and strength in proportion to the voltage; the radial extent of coagulation along the cut increases with voltage and with the length and intensity of the electric spark; at more than 500 peak volts,

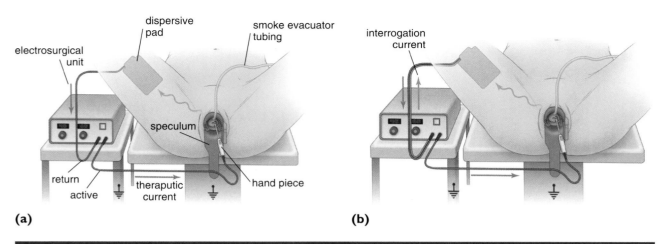

(a)

(b)

FIGURES 19.49a,b   **(a)** The flow of alternating current in an isolated electrosurgical unit. Such a unit prevents current division and alternate site burns (except at the potential site of the dispersive plate if improperly attached). **(b)** The return electrode monitoring system (REM). The REM circuitry recognizes the quality of the return electrode's pats; that is, any reduction of surface area contact between patient and dispersive plate (increased current concentration) or lack of conductivity between patient's skin and the dispersive plate surface deactivates the generator.

carbonization occurs; control of thermal damage and carbonization is maximized when the voltage in the active tissue electrode is between 200 and 500 peak volts, irrespective of tissue impedance while employing a pure sine wave (Figure 19.46).

Many commercial ESGs used for general surgery greatly exceed 1000 peak volts in the cut mode. In some instances, these units are also used for cervical procedures, but they are less than ideal.

19.6.6.1 The pure sine wave

If the voltage output of an ESG is plotted over time, a pure cut waveform is representative of a continuous sine wave alternating from positive to negative at the frequency of the generator (Figure 19.46). The amplitude of the waveform is the voltage (Figure 19.46). The peak voltage is the highest voltage when measured from zero, and the peak-to-peak voltage represents the voltage to the highest positive voltage, the RMS (root mean square) being the mathematical average of the waveform (Figure 19.46). The ratio of peak voltage to RMS voltage (average voltage) of a periodic waveform is termed the *Crest Factor*.

Clinically, the Crest Factor is a method of indicating the potential degree of thermal effect (providing hemostasis) in an electrosurgical waveform. The lower the Crest Factor, the less is the thermal effect. Hence, pure sine waves have the lowest Crest Factor (approximately 1.4). Crest factors for the individual settings (like cut, blend 1, COAG) are different from one generator to the other.

19.6.6.2 The blended cut

Blend is cutting waveform with more hemostatic effect than a pure sine wave (has a higher Crest Factor than a pure sine wave). Basically, this is achieved by employing a damped (Figure 19.47) or a modulated waveform (Figure 19.48). The latter consists of on and off periods producing a duty cycle (e.g. 80% on and 20% off). The duty cycle is the ratio of the duration of output bursts to the time between the initiation of the bursts. For example, a pure sine wave has a duty cycle of 100%. A modulated waveform is less than 100%.

19.6.6.3 Increasing the voltage and maintaining a pure sine wave (constant voltage™, ERBE)

A pure sine wave is employed (Crest Factor 1.4) for all tissue mode settings (Figure 19.46). The voltage can be selected between 200 and 500 peak volts and is kept relatively constant during the cutting process regardless of the variations in tissue impedance. Increasing the voltage while maintaining a pure sine wave will uniformly increase the thermal effect. The sparking to tissue increases in direct proportion to the voltage. This is the principle of constant voltage technology (Figure 19.50).

19.6.6.4 Instant Response™ electrosurgical generators

Tissue impedance is not uniform. In the Instant Response System™ (Valleylab), a computer-controlled feedback system is incorporated so that

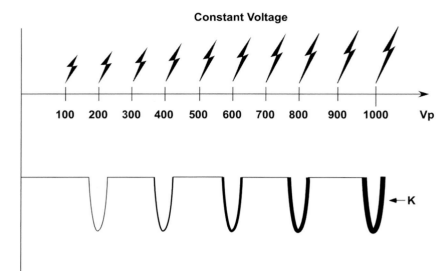

Constant Voltage

FIGURE 19.50 In constant voltage technology the increased thermal effect (K) occurs due to increasing the peak voltage (Vp). (Image provided courtesy of Dr. V. Cecil Wright: *Understanding Electrosurgery.* Houston: Biomedical Communications, 1995.)

the unit can respond to changing tissue impedances while maintaining a constant power and controlling the current density. The current density around the tissue electrode varies by the formula $j = I/\text{Area}$, where j = current density and I = current. In electrosurgery, tissue electrodes are used to deliver current to the body. Tissue electrodes vary in length and diameter: they are usually in the configuration of a wire loop, a needle or spatula, and ball electrode. Since current density varies directly with the amount of current and inversely with the cross-sectional area, or in the case of the ball electrode, the surface area, it follows that current density varies with the configuration of the tissue electrode. Watts being constant, thin wires have more than thick ones, long wires less than shorter ones, and big balls less than smaller ones.

19.6.6.5 Core concepts for electrosurgical cutting

1. The active tissue electrode must be in contact with the tissue.
2. There is sparking to tissue.
3. The tissue is cut by moving the electrode through tissue.
4. Low-amplitude continuous sinusoidal waveforms produce the least thermal effect (lowest Crest Factor).
5. To provide better hemostasis and minimal thermal effect to the tissue, a blend (mixed mode), damped, or modulated waveform is used. This is accomplished by adjusting the amplitude and degree of modulation of the high-frequency voltage. The degree of this alteration is reflected in the Crest Factor.
6. The higher the Crest Factor, the greater the tissue coagulation.
7. The Crest Factor is not equal for the same setting on different generators.
8. A duty cycle is expressed as a ratio of the burst duration of the sine wave to the time between the initiation of the bursts.

19.6.7 Monopolar electrosurgical coagulation

A coagulation (COAG) waveform consists of short bursts (microseconds) of radiofrequency sine waves (Figures 19.47 and 19.48). The COAG waveform has a considerably greater peak-to-peak voltage (higher Crest Factor) than the cut waveform. The energy (heat per second) is less because the COAG is turned off most of the time. Figures 19.51 and 19.52 indicate that COAG waveforms vary in frequency and duration between different electrosurgical generators. Therefore, the tissue effect per unit of time will not be the same for similar power settings.

The three methods used surgically to produce coagulation are desiccation, fulguration, and puncture coagulation.

19.6.7.1 Monopolar electrosurgical desiccation

Desiccation occurs with the active tissue electrode (ball electrode) in contact with the tissue. Heat is generated in the tissue as a result of current moving

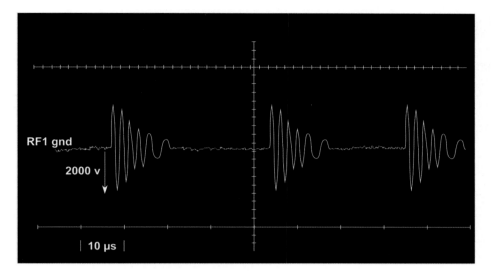

FIGURE 19.51 An oscilloscope tracing of a COAG waveform of a conventional electrosurgical generator (Image provided courtesy of Dr. V. Cecil Wright: *Understanding Electrosurgery.* Houston: Biomedical Communications, 1995.) ▬▬

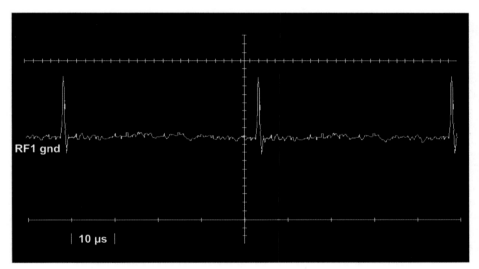

FIGURE 19.52 An oscilloscope tracing of a COAG waveform from a constant voltage generator. This varies considerably from the one shown in Figure 19.51. (Image provided courtesy of Dr. V. Cecil Wright: *Understanding Electrosurgery.* Houston: Biomedical Communications, 1995.) ▬▬

against tissue impedance. Steam forms as the tissue evaporates, resulting in dehydration and increased tissue impedance to current flow. If the voltage is sufficient (greater than 200 peak volts), electric sparking will occur to the nearest moist tissue.

Desiccation can be accomplished in any waveform. The amount of sparking lateral to the site of desiccation that occurs depends on the peak voltage of the waveform.

Soft coagulation (no spark coagulation) is the term applied when no sparking is produced between the coagulating electrode and tissue during the coagulation process. This is achieved by employing a pure sine wave; however, the voltage must be less than 200 peak volts. Forced coagulation occurs when the spark is intentionally generated between the coagulation electrode and the tissue. Intense sparking is produced when the peak voltage is the highest (COAG waveform, highest Crest Factor).

19.6.7.2 Core concepts of monopolar desiccation

1. For desiccation to occur, the tissue electrode is held in contact with the tissue.
2. Tissue desiccation can occur in any waveform.
3. Dehydration of tissue occurs, followed by sparking to the nearest moist tissue, if the voltage is greater than 200 peak volts. The sparks are finer than those produced by fulguration (non-contact coagulation).
4. The intensity of the sparking to the adjacent moist tissue increases proportionally with increase in voltage; thus, the greatest sparking is observed when desiccating in the COAG waveform.
5. The power density (PD) varies inversely with the contact surface area of the coagulating electrode, i.e., PD = watts (volts × amps)/ contact surface area.

6. The larger the electrode contact area, the more current is required to produce the same effective current density.

7. The higher the power setting (watts), the greater the amount of current delivered and the quicker the desiccation.

19.6.7.3 Monopolar electrosurgical fulguration (spraying)

Fulguration is non-tissue contact by the tissue electrode. High voltage is required (COAG waveform). If the peak voltage is insufficient, the operator will touch the tissue electrode to the tissue, which defeats the purpose of fulguration. The sparks produced cause superficial tissue necrosis. Excessive fulguration can char tissue and cause excessive damage once the tissue has become dehydrated. The sparks produced by each cycle of voltage have a high current density. The greater the frequency of the ESG, the more frequent is the sparking to tissue.

19.6.7.4 Core concepts of fulguration

1. In fulguration, the tissue electrode is not in contact with the tissue.

2. There is long sparking to tissue across the electrode-tissue gap.

3. Fulguration occurs with relatively high voltage and low amperage current.

4. Superficial dehydration of tissue results.

5. With fulguration, in contrast to desiccation, only one fifth of the amount of current enters the tissue.

6. High voltage (COAG waveform) with sparking to tissue raises the possibility of neuromuscular stimulation resulting from production of low frequency waveforms.

19.6.7.5 Monopolar puncture coagulation

Puncture coagulation consists of plunging the tissue electrode needle into the tissue—frequently the center of the lesion—resulting in high current density inside the lesion. Puncture coagulation must be used with extreme caution since the high current density must leave the lesion and return through the patient to the dispersive plate. For example, puncture coagulation of a large condyloma attached by a small pedicle causes excessive current density to occur in its base with resulting excessive depth of thermal burn to the underlying dermis.

19.6.8 Bipolar electrosurgery

Bipolar electrosurgery can be used for tissue cutting and desiccation. Both require two similar active tissue electrodes. This bipolar (two-pole) tissue electrode provides one tip as the active electrode and the other as the return electrode; therefore, no separate dispersive plate is required. The current flows from the bipolar connection port to one of the tips of the bipolar forceps, through the grasped tissue between the forceps tips and returns back to the electrosurgical generator via the other tip. A high frequency, low voltage unmodulated waveform (sine wave) is employed (Figure 19.46). The high frequency flows through the tissue (between electrode tips) within a well-defined area; lateral spread of tissue coagulation does not occur. The amount of tissue desiccation depends on the volume of tissue grasped.

19.6.8.1 Core concepts of bipolar electrosurgery

1. Bipolar electrodes are combined with a bipolar instrument.

2. The high-frequency, low-voltage current (sine waveform) flows through the tissue within a well-defined area between two similar electrodes. Thus, lateral spread of thermal damage does not occur.

3. Because of low voltage, there is less risk of interference with the electronic circuits simultaneously connected to the patient.

4. Bipolar desiccation potentially eliminates sparking, lowering the risk of inadvertent burning to adjacent tissue.

5. Because there is no dispersive plate, alternate site burns, as seen in monopolar electrosurgery, do not occur.

6. The reduction of generator power reduces the potential of nerve and muscle stimulation.

7. Bipolar instruments can be used in a normal saline bathing solution (a urological advantage).

19.6.9 Electrosurgery vs. electrocautery

The term *electrocautery* is often confused with the term *electrosurgery*. The reader is advised to know the difference and, when recording the procedure, to use correct terminology. The following list the considerable differences. In electrocautery:

1. No current is passed to the patient.

2. Tissue effects are caused by heat transference.

3. High amperage and low voltage are used.

4. The electrocautery tip is a resistance wire similar to that used in an electric stove or toaster.

5. The wire is a platinum alloy, rather than tungsten or stainless steel, as used in electrosurgery.
6. Impedance to current flow determines the temperature of the tip.
7. There is no radiofrequency current.
8. The low voltage is created by a step-down transformer (taking 120 volts to 6 volts).

19.6.10 Electrosurgical systems

There are three basic components to all electrosurgical systems: the electrosurgical generator, the patient return electrode (dispersive plate), and the active tissue electrode. As previously discussed, the isolated ESG (Figure 19.49a) has replaced the grounded unit (Bovie ESG). The addition of return electrode monitoring (REM) circuitry has helped eliminate burns at the site of the dispersive plate. This mechanism monitors the quality of the electrical contact between the return electrode (dispersive plate) and the patient during electrosurgery. Specifically, it measures the electro-patient impedance. Any imbalance or poor dispersive plate contact signals an alarm system and shuts down the generator (Figure 19.49b).

19.6.11 Electrosurgical safety

Most electrosurgical injuries relate to the following:

1. Not using an isolated, return electrode monitoring system
2. Accidental burns caused by improper use of the dispersive plate
3. Accidental burns resulting from the following:
   a. High-frequency current leakage
   b. Unintentional activation of the high-frequency generator
   c. Accidental touching of an organ (body part) by hot electrodes
   d. Use of unsuitable and or defective accessories
   e. Ignition of flammable liquids, gases, and or vapors
   f. Stimulation of muscles and nerves (Faradic effect)
   g. Interference with electrical equipment (e.g., pacemakers)

19.6.12 Preventative maintenance program

Policies and procedures for the maintenance and safe use of the ESG should be written by the biomedical engineering department staff or safety committee. The material should be readily available and reviewed annually within the office or institution. Factors that should be considered include:

1. Testing new equipment before employing it surgically.
2. Frequently testing equipment.
3. Establishing authority, responsibility, and accountability for the proper use of the ESG.
4. Accurately recording mishaps, equipment maintenance, and repairs.
5. Providing in-service education for personnel.
6. Appointing a safety officer to oversee safety aspects, such as having fire equipment available, checking electrical accessories (intact cords, secure connections, wire breakage, fraying, etc.) making maintenance checks and repairs, and being familiar with the manufacturer's operating manual.

19.6.13 Electrosurgical approaches to remove cervical intraepithelial neoplasia

Electrosurgical excision is the newest modality being used to treat cervical intraepithelial neoplasia (CIN). With electrosurgery, a straight-needle electrode or a curved- or square-loop electrode is used to excise the abnormal transformation zone, with a ball electrode (3 mm or 5 mm in diameter) for coagulation purposes.

Loop excision is sometimes referred to as large loop excision of the transformation zone, or LLETZ, a term coined in England by investigators who first studied the techniques.[50,52,239] In North America, the same procedure is referred to as loop electrosurgical excision procedure.[240]

19.6.13.1 Rationale for excision of CIN

Electrosurgical techniques produce one or more specimens of cervical tissue for histological interpretation. These procedures reduce the chance of potential diagnostic errors by minimizing the possibility of missing an invasive squamous cell cancer, adenocarcinoma in situ, or an adenocarcinoma. They are used to confirm the complete removal of diseased tissue. Ideally, these electrosurgical procedures could replace other excisional methods, such as scalpel and CO_2 laser conization and many ablative procedures.

Each specimen is examined in the same manner as a traditional cone specimen. Reported studies demonstrate that loop specimens are adequate for thorough evaluation of cervical dysplasia.[241–243] In evaluating and reporting on these specimens, the pathologist needs to report both margin status and severity of disease. However, in reality, specimens are far from ideal. In some cases, the pathological interpretation is insufficient for adequately grading the lesion, excluding malignancy, or predicting persistent disease because of excessive thermal effects or having to report on multiple bits of excised tissue.[149,244–248] In reviewing LLETZ specimens, Ioffe et al[244] found that the presence of tissue artifacts interfering with interpretation was only rarely mentioned within the original pathology report. Furthermore, the status of margins was a better predictor of abnormal follow up in cold knife conization than in the LLETZ specimens. The worst thermal effect occurs at the upper margin (base of specimen or apex of defect), where the worst disease potentially exists. Significant injuries to adjacent normal anatomical structures such as bladder and bowel have also occurred.[247]

19.6.13.2 Evaluating the patient prior to electrosurgery

A colposcopic evaluation of the cervix and vagina is necessary before any excisional procedure. This evaluation, in part, determines the location and size of the lesion and its potential grade. It further helps the practitioner decide which electrode should be chosen and what electrosurgical technique should be used to encompass the lesion.[240] Two options exist for management of women with lesions.

19.6.13.3 One- or two-visit appointment to remove the lesion

The electrosurgical method has been used for both diagnosis and treatment at the same visit.[249] This approach is termed *see and treat*. The colposcopic examination is performed based on abnormal cytologic results and colposcopic identification of an ectocervical lesion. Because the loop procedure supplies a specimen for pathological interpretation, no preliminary biopsies or endocervical curettage are necessary. This quick approach is considered appropriate in the presence of HSIL and a colposcopic lesion without prior biopsy. It is inappropriate in other circumstances because there are mimics of significant CIN lesions, such as low-grade squamous intraepithelial lesions and squamous metaplasia and repair. This approach does seem to be a reasonable treatment for patients with significant lesions who are expected to be noncompliant.[250]

Alternately, a more traditional approach, consisting of standard colposcopic examination, directed biopsies and ECC, can be used. This approach relies on subsequent correlation of the three diagnoses—cytologic, colposcopic, and histologic—followed by treatment at the next patient visit or further investigation, if warranted. Thus, the strategy of patient management is influenced by the grade of the cytologic specimen, the reliability of the patient, the location of the lesion, the colposcopic impression, and the confidence of the colposcopist.

19.6.13.4 Contraindications for the loop procedure

Regardless of the number of visits, there are contraindications for the loop procedure, including the presence of a cervical inflammatory process, bleeding disorders, an obvious cancer, the need to differentiate between microinvasive cancer on biopsy and advanced disease, disease high within the endocervical canal, suspected glandular disease, pregnancy, and DES abnormality and states of amenorrhea (e.g., patients in the postpartum period or menopause, and patients who are breast feeding or using medroxyprogesterone). In the amenorrhea group, the absence of menstruation can lead to stenosis unless remedied.

19.6.14 Surgical approaches

Various surgical approaches have been previously described in detail.[50,61,251] These procedures are designed to deal with ectocervical disease (large and small), endocervical canal disease, and ectocervical disease with endocervical canal extension. The operator chooses the desired loop or needle electrode with intention to remove all lesional tissue while at the same time sparing as much normal tissue as possible. In doing so, the linear length of disease, the location of disease, and the potential for crypt involvement must be considered. The specimen removed must be cylindrical rather than conical in configuration. The resulting defect must spare peripheral cervical stroma to minimize cervical volume loss during the healing and regenerative process.

Properly insulated instrumentation as well as a smoke evacuation system are required, preferably with a blood trap in the line to suck out blood so desiccation can be achieved. Local anesthesia is usually appropriate in combination with a vasoconstricting agent (epinephrine or vasopressin). The manufacturer usually suggests power settings appropriate to specific conventional ESGs and electrode sizes. With the constant voltage generator (Figure 19.50), the operator chooses the tissue effect setting and the watts of power are automatically selected by the unit in response to the differences in tissue impedance while employing a pure sine wave (Figure 19.46). In the conventional ESG, a modulated sine wave (also called blended waveform) is preferred over the pure cut (Figure 19.48) for better hemostasis. The coagulation mode (COAG waveform) is chosen for coagulation of any bleeding sites (Figures 19.47, 19.51 and 19.52). Fulguration is preferred over desiccation to any remaining bleeding points because fulguration involves only superficial thermal injury to the remaining cervix and less current enters the remaining cervix. Unfortunately, it is impossible to fulgurate through blood, particularly the blood pool that accumulates in the cavity of the posterior cervix. In many cases, the operator pushes the ball electrode into the blood mass to create the coagulation process, which results in desiccation. A blood trap in the smoke evacuation system and use of a plastic suction device handles both smoke and blood simultaneously. The removal of blood from the operative sites permits fulguration. The plastic suction device can also serve as an insulated retractor.

19.6.14.1 Removal of ectocervical tissue with one pass of the loop electrode

In the presence of an ectocervical lesion not encroaching the endocervical canal the operator selects an appropriate loop electrode, which should be larger in width than the largest lesion diameter and greater than 5 mm but not exceeding 8 mm in height from crossbar to the wire's upper arc. The cervix is exposed with the insulated bivalve speculum with appropriate suction apparatus. It is important to have the cervix in the mid-position. If not, a large swab or dental cylindrical cottonoid (a long string attached for removal and reminder purposes) can be put in place to relocate its position.

The cervix is anesthetized, and the peripheral component of the lesion is identified by applying a solution, either iodine or acetic acid. Some operators prefer to monitor the surgical procedure while looking through the colposcope. Others find this awkward and use the colposcope as a light source. The handpiece to be employed can be activated by switches ("cut" or "coag") or by a footswitch. Some generators come with both activation sources, others with only a footswitch. Activating the current just before tissue contact (termed *open circuit voltage*), the operator positions the upper arc of the semicircular loop just outside the outer boundary of the lesion, which is identified by staining, and then directs it straight ahead into the cervical stroma up to the crossbar. Most operators have the entrance point at 3 o'clock and the exit point at 9 o'clock or the reverse. Others find a beginning point of 6 o'clock and exiting point at 12 o'clock to be technically good. However, when beginning at the 12 o'clock position and approaching the 6 o'clock exit point, the partially excised specimen falls forward as the cutting process continues and can drape over the exit point, obscuring the procedure. This may require stopping the procedure until the situation is remedied. After reaching the desired depth in the stroma and using the same

smooth, continuous motion, the operator moves the handpiece to the opposite lesion border, keeping the same depth throughout the cut by touching or almost touching the surface of the cervix with the crossbar as it moves over the lesion. A backstop (insulated or cylindrical cottonoid) can be placed to protect the exit side in the vagina for extra protection should the upper electrode's wire arc come in contact with the vaginal wall during removal of the loop from the cervical tissue. This is helpful because resistance against motion at that point drops dramatically. When the crossbar is at the exit point, the operator pulls the handpiece straight out, continuing in the same smooth motion, and when the upper arc cuts through the tissue surface, the current is shut off. Frequently the specimen remains in place and needs to be removed with forceps and placed in fixative. Any bleeding sites are fulgurated using a ball electrode in the COAG waveform. Monsel's paste is applied to the crater bed to complete the procedure. Figures 19.53a–c illustrate the removal of tissue with one pass of the tissue electrode.

19.6.14.2 Problems encountered during the procedure

The cutting process may be halted because of sudden poor exposure, painful stimuli requiring more local anesthetic, or tissue impedance exceeding the output power of the generator. When these situations are remedied, the procedure is best restarted from the stop point. However, with some ESGs, the restart process will not occur at the stop point and the operator must begin at the initial start point and follow the initial incision. This can lead to further tissue damage. Thus, it is suggested to start at the exit point and end at the initial cut stop point. Another mistake is losing concentration and activating the COAG mode instead of the cut mode when cutting. If this happens, very little cutting will occur, the wire loop will drag, and likely the wire will fracture because of the high voltage and the physical properties of the COAG waveform. These problems can lead to excessive thermal damage and difficulties in pathological interpretation.

19.6.14.3 Removal of ectocervical CIN with multiple passes of the loop electrode

Approximately 10% of cases will require more than one pass of the loop electrode because of the extent of disease. Multiple passes using one or two different loops can excise the diseased tissue. This approach produces two or more specimens, each of which must be pathologically evaluated. The central portion of the lesion, which potentially has the worst disease, is usually removed first. Further passes are made to remove the remaining disease (Figures 19.54a–e). This

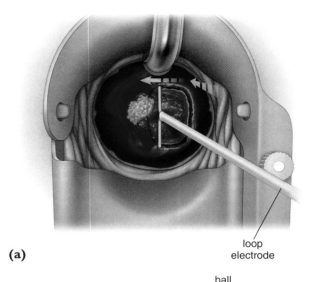

(a)

loop
electrode

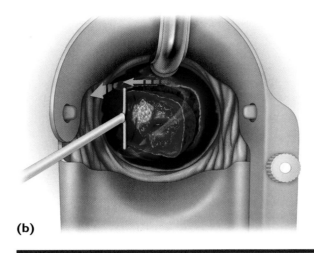

(b)

ball
electrode

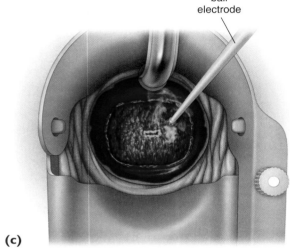

(c)

FIGURES 19.53a–c Tissue removal with one pass of the tissue electrode. **(a)** For a one pass loop excision, the activated loop tissue electrode is pushed into the cervical stroma at the 3 o'clock position up to the level of its crossbar. **(b)** With current continuing to flow through it, the loop electrode is slowly and deliberately moved laterally, keeping the crossbar at or just slightly above the surface as it moves towards the 9 o'clock exit position. There it is pulled straight out and afterwards the cylindrical severed specimen is removed with forceps. **(c)** Any bleeding sites are fulgurated using a ball electrode held above the surface of the defect. In this step the sparks which impact the tissue produce heat to coagulate the vessels and control bleeding. Then Monsel's paste is applied to the crater to provide residual coagulation.

method of excision is similar to that for the single-pass approach already described. After each pass, the specimen is picked up with forceps, and placed in containers with fixative for pathological interpretation.

19.6.14.4 Excision of endocervical CIN

Disease confined to the endocervical canal can potentially extend as far as 22 mm from its lowermost border, but 86% of CIN 3 lesions have a length of 10 mm or less. Because of this, most endocervical lesions can be entirely removed with one pass of the loop electrode using the same technique as described for ectocervical disease. Longer lesions or those that extend beyond the limits of view require more than one pass or cylindrical excision using the needle elec-

trode. Older patients and those with higher grades of CIN are more likely to require this procedure. If two specimens are taken from the canal, it is important for pathological identification that the upper margin of the second specimen be marked (e.g., using India ink) to define final margin status.

19.6.14.5 Needle excision of endocervical CIN

Needle excision can be performed on an outpatient basis by working through a bivalve speculum, although it is probably better performed under local or general anesthesia in an operating room (Figures 19.55a–c).[251,252] A weighted speculum is placed along the posterior vaginal wall and an insulated

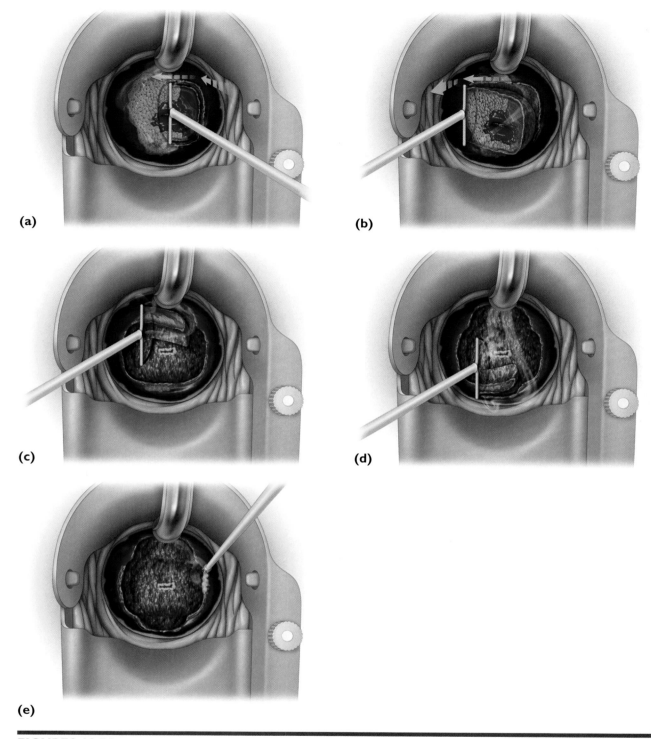

FIGURES 19.54a–e Excision of disease requiring more than one pass of the tissue electrode. **(a)** When more than one pass is required to remove ectocervical disease the central portion is first removed by beginning at the 3 o'clock position. **(b)** The loop exists at the 9 o'clock position; after the central disease is removed, residual disease can be seen peripheral to the excision defect. **(c)** The anterior residual disease is removed. **(d)** The posterior disease is removed. Each specimen is placed in fixative in different marked containers. **(e)** The procedure is completed by fulguration to any bleeding areas.

tenaculum grasps the anterior cervix outside the tissue to be excised. The tenaculum can be used to position the cervix so that the canal is parallel to the needle electrode angle. A vasopressin solution (the total dose not exceeding one pressor unit) is infiltrated into the cervix to decrease blood flow to the surgical site. Viewing directly or through the colposcope (operating microscope), the operator positions the long needle electrode and activates it in the blend mode (conventional ESG) just before the needle tip comes into contact with the tissue. A circle with a radius not exceeding 8 mm is marked on the cervix. If disease extends beyond this radius on the ectocervix, the combination procedure (to be described next) is recommended which would remove any remaining transformations zone. Insulated forceps are positioned within the developing specimen, pulling inward from the incision being developed by the needle tip. The incision will be made to a height (depth) of approximately 15 mm, or deeper if necessary. When the circular incision is completed to the anticipated height, the cylindrical specimen is severed transversely at the apex using a scalpel or a ton-

sil snare. This provides a specimen with an upper nonthermal edge for accurate histological reporting of diseased margins. An ECC can follow the procedure. Alternately, colposcopy can be performed to identify persistent disease as acetowhite rather than pink epithelium. If desired, more tissue can be removed and identified for pathological examination accordingly. Following this, the defect's base is fulgurated with the ball electrode in the COAG mode.

19.6.14.6 The combination procedure for ectocervical and endocervical CIN

Approximately 18% of CIN lesions are found widely on the ectocervix with canal extension. The ectocervical portion usually can be excised by one pass of a large loop (Figures 19.56a–c). The remaining disease in the canal is excised with a smaller loop (Figure 19.56d) or using the technique of long needle excision as described (Figures 19.55a–c). It is important to mark the upper margin of the second specimen for pathological orientation. Figures 19.56e and 19.57 demonstrate the cervical defect following

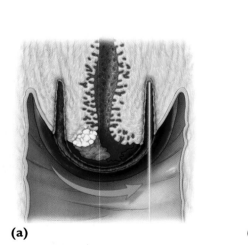

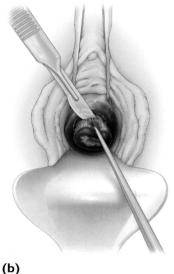

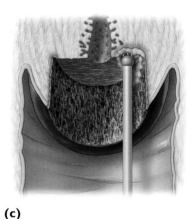

(a)   **(b)**   **(c)**

FIGURES 19.55a–c Operative schematics for endocervical disease. **(a)** When disease is confined to the endocervical canal needle electrode excision is performed similar to the laser cylindrical excision procedure. The circular incision is developed around the os using forceps for traction as the line of incision is developed parallel to the canal. **(b)** After sufficient depth is achieved, the specimen is severed at the apex with a scalpel or tonsil snare, producing a cylinder of tissue which is removed by forceps and fixed. **(c)** The base of the defect is fulgurated using a ball electrode for hemostasis.

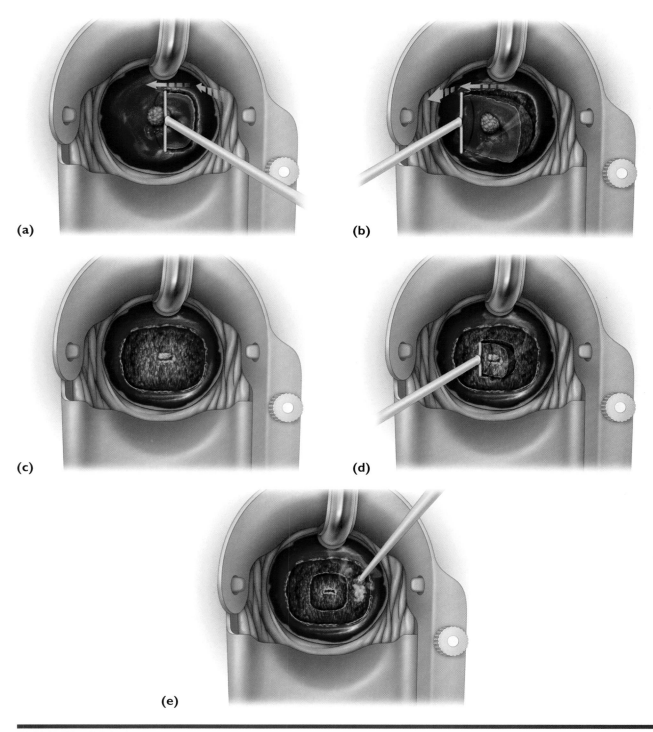

FIGURES 19.56a–e The combination procedure for extensive ectocervical disease involvement with canal extension. **(a)** When a combination procedure is required to deal with ectocervical disease as well as endocervical disease, the ectocervical disease is first removed using the same approach as for the simple ectocervical disease starting at 3 o'clock. **(b)** The loop electrode exits the ectocervical tissue at the 9 o'clock position. **(c)** The defect in the cervix appears after the specimen is removed with forceps. **(d)** Using a smaller loop, the endocervical canal component is removed. **(e)** The final two-tiered defect appears after the smaller specimen is removed. Any bleeding or ooze is controlled by fulguration with the ball electrode followed by the application of Monsel's paste.

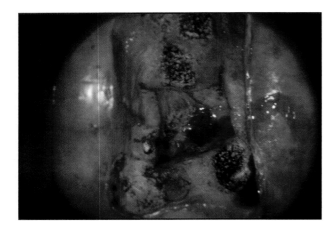

FIGURE 19.57   A colpophotograph of the cervix after the combination procedure.

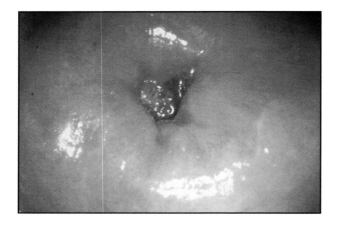

FIGURE 19.58   The cervix as shown in Figure 17 nicely healed with good restoration of volume and an appropriately located squamocolumnar junction.

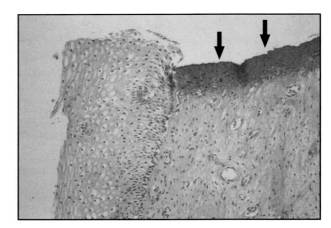

FIGURE 19.59   The histopathology employing a constant open circuit voltage of 250 peak volts. There is no cellular distortion or epithelial stripping. Carbonization is minimal and the zone of thermal necrosis (eosinophilic zone, See arrows) is uniform, measuring 200 μm. In: Wright, VC, Lickrish, GM, Shier, RM: *Basic and Advanced Colposcopy—A Practical Handbook for Diagnosis* (2nd ed.). Houston Biomendical Communications, 1995.

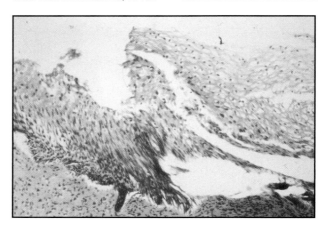

FIGURE 19.60   With open circuit voltage greater than 1200 peak volts, epithelial stripping and considerable cellular distortion occurs. In: Wright, VC, Lickrish, GM, Shier, RM: *Basic and Advanced Colposcopy—A Practical Handbook for Diagnosis* (2nd ed.). Houston Biomendical Communications, 1995.

the combination procedure and Figure 19.58 the healed cervix with good restoration of cervical tissue margin.

19.6.15 The pathological specimen

The excised specimen is usually placed in a 10% neutral buffered formalin, and the usual radial sections are processed for conventional microscopy. The pathologist should study three zones: the attachment of squamous epithelium to the underlying stroma; the lateral (deep) thermal cut; and the base of the excised specimen. The degree of thermal

artifact is studied further according to the (1) degree of detachment of the epithelium or denudation and stripping of the squamous epithelium; (2) degree of cellular distortion; (3) degree of charring; (4) and amount of coagulation necrosis (eosinophilia of the connective tissue stroma). Figures 19.59 to 19.62 illustrate some classical undesirable features of loop histology.

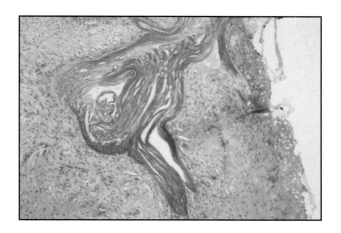

FIGURE 19.61   Electric current has completely destroyed the cellular structure of an endocervical gland. (Image provided courtesy of Dr. V. Cecil Wright)

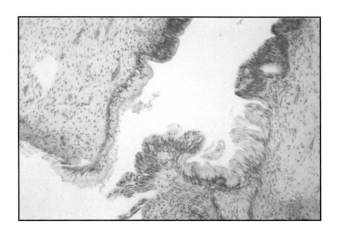

FIGURE 19.62   Adenocarcinoma in situ involves the upper part of the cervical crypt. The epithelium below the disease shows distortion and pseudostratification making pathological assessment difficult. (Image provided courtesy of Dr. V. Cecil Wright.)

19.6.16 Postoperative instructions

Patient management after treatment is similar to that after laser surgery. The methods for management for loop procedures are identical to those for bleeding management in laser surgery, which have been previously described. Patients are evaluated by cytology at 4–6 months or cytology and colposcopy at 4–6 months or with HPV DNA testing at least 6 months after treatment. Persistent disease is usually discovered at one of these intervals (usually the first). After three normal and satisfactory examinations, the patient can have annual cytological surveillance.

19.6.17 Therapeutic effectiveness

In general, loop specimens using the one-pass technique are smaller than the traditional cold knife conization specimens. Some authors state that both procedures are equally effective. The main difference is the nonthermal effect and the better histological interpretation in the cold knife group.[130,142,253,254]

Studies indicate that the overall disease eradication rate after a single treatment ranges from 63% to 95%. The most common complication is bleeding (peri- and post-operative) in 4% to 6% of patients. Most patients with bleeding are managed on an outpatient basis with 2% requiring hospitalization.[50–52,56,130,239,252]

19.7 Cold-Knife Conization of the Cervix

19.7.1 Introduction

Traditionally cold knife conization (CKC) was used for investigation of abnormal cytology and for definitive management of carcinoma in situ (CIS).[255–258] The CKC procedure was usually performed on an inpatient basis (average 3 to 6 days) rather than as day surgery. Because of complications—mostly bleeding—outpatient procedures were recommended under anesthesia only when an operating room was immediately accessible and there was an adequate blood replacement service on site.[259]

19.7.2 Basic operative technique

Whether the patients were inpatients or outpatients, in the past general anesthesia was most often used. A vasoconstricting agent was injected into the cervical stroma, and an iodine-staining solution was applied to the cervix. The margins of the excision were planned according to lesion topography. The identification of normal-appearing columnar epithelium above the lesion was proof that no tissue abnormality existed above that point; therefore, tissue removal above that point was unnecessary. The procedure was radical enough to remove the lesion "completely," but the cone dimensions varied considerably. A shallow cone was done for ectocervical disease (wide base, short height) but with canal involvement, an increase in excisional height with a corresponding decrease in base was planned. In each case, the incision line was slanted inward toward the internal os and some endocervical canal was removed. Later, using colposcopy, clinicians improved in their ability to predict the location and dimensions of the lesions, which enabled them to design the surgical approach to remove all lesional tissue and also to spare as much normal tissue as possible.[257,259] Bleeding was controlled by electrosurgical coagulation, sutures, (including Sturmdorf type, and packing).[260] To prevent infection, prophylactic antibiotics were prescribed.[216,257]

Early on, CKC was often followed by a dilatation and curettage (D&C). Later, studies indicated that this step was probably unnecessary for evaluating abnormal squamous cytology. D&C still follows conization in the peri- or post-menopausal patient when there is a reason to sample the endometrium, when there is a suspicion of glandular abnormalities, or in the presence of abnormal glandular cells. Eliminating the routine dilatation and curettage was found to be a cost-saving step.[261,262]

19.7.3 Changing the trend

Early publications correlating cytopathology, colposcopy, and histopathology and demonstrating success in predicting the ultimate diagnosis brought to a close the era of mandatory conization for abnormal cytology of cervical dysplasia in most cases.[80,263–266] However, there are still valid indications for the CKC. The operative technique is described in any modern operative gynecological textbook.

19.7.4 Current indications for conization

The following are indications for conization: 1) lack of correlation between cytology, colposcopy, and histology; 2) a positive ECC; 3) when any portion of a lesion is located within the endocervical canal requiring tissue to be submitted for histological evaluation; 4) when cytologic or colposcopic findings suggest invasive carcinoma that has not been proven by colposcopically directed biopsy; 5) when colposcopic biopsy or cytologic findings indicate adenocarcinoma in situ (AIS) since colposcopic and cytologic examinations cannot differentiate between AIS and adenocarcinoma; 6) when colposcopic biopsy indicates microinvasive squamous cell carcinoma; and 7) when colposcopy is unsatisfactory for any reason, particularly in the presence of high-grade cytologic findings.

Some practitioners prefer excision for CIN 3 lesions confirmed on histologic examination, regardless of patient age or disease location, to exclude malignancy, but this opinion is fading.

19.7.5 Results of cold knife conization

The older literature must be reviewed to appreciate the results of this procedure, since it was historically performed for both diagnostic and therapeutic purposes, mostly for carcinoma in situ (CIS) lesions. Publications between 1956 and 1995 reported that residual disease was found at subsequent hysterectomy or repeat CKC in 12% to 47% (average 23.8%) of women undergoing CKC. The most common positive margin was apical because of coning inward toward the internal os; hence, the high persistent disease rate.[216,256,259,267–276] Performing colposcopy before the procedure decreased the persistent disease rate somewhat.[257,277] More recent studies indicate that 2.8% to 7.7% of CIN 3 cases will have squamous cell carcinoma, half of which will be microinvasive.[273,278–280] Therefore, CIN 3 patients with postcone-positive apical margins are at risk of harboring more advanced disease.

It is difficult to predict residual disease after CKC. There are no consistent predictive factors.[144,273,281,282] Some studies indicate margin status failed to predict residual neoplasia in the excised uterus.[144,273,281,282] Negative endocervical margins are associated with a 32% residual disease rate, which is similar for positive margins.[281] However, the cancers were found in the positive margin (CIN 3) cases, not negative margin ones. Some authors indicate that the only predictors of residual dysplasia are increased age and severity of disease in the cone specimen.[281] Other investigators disagree.[144] In one study of HIV-positive women, cervical conization was not shown to be an effective method for eradication of CIN. Disease recurred in most HIV patients despite complete excision of the dysplasia. Surgical margin status, ECC status, and CD4 count had no effect on the recurrence rate.[144] The contribution of conization is to prevent progression to invasive cancer.[144]

Despite this conservative approach, invasive squamous cell cancer develops in the cervix in 0.9% and recurrent CIS in 2.3% of patients,[258] while after hysterectomy 1.2% of women develop CIS and 2.1% invasive cancer in the vaginal vault. Women who had CIS of the cervix are at risk for recurrence and malignancy whether treated conservatively or more radically.[258]

19.7.6 Complications

Cold knife conization is a major operative procedure associated with complications that are significant in both incidence and morbidity.[269] There does not appear to be any appreciable correlation between the technique of CKC and the incidence of complications.[275,283]

The most major and immediate complications are perioperative and postoperative bleeding. The blood supply to the cervix is predominantly from the uterine artery (a branch of the internal iliac artery). The overall blood supply to the cervix involves anastomotic pelvic and extrapelvic sources (Figure 19.63). The intrapelvic anastomotic vessels include the vaginal artery, the middle hemorrhoidal artery and internal pudendal artery (which are all branches of the anterior division of the internal iliac artery). Extrapelvic sources include the ovarian artery, which arises from the aorta and anastomoses with the ascending branch of the uterine artery; the superior hemorrhoidal artery (the terminal branch of the inferior mesenteric artery arising from the aorta), which anastomoses with the middle and inferior hemorrhoidal vessels; the middle sacral artery which arises at the aortic bifurcation and anastomoses with the lateral sacral vessels, a branch of the posterior division; and the anastomosis of the lumbar artery (a branch of the aorta) and the iliolumbar (a branch of the posterior division of the interior iliac). Hemorrhage, defined as blood loss greater than 100 cc or heavy bleeding requiring suturing, packing, or other procedures, varied between 9.3% and 15% of all CKCs.[256,259,270,271,275,284]

The hospital readmission rate for supervision and bleeding control is 2.2%.[268,269] The transfusion rate in those who bled varied between 10.0% and 78.5%.[256,259,266,269,275] In older studies, when transfusion was necessary, so was hysterectomy as a lifesaving procedure in 14.3% to 18.3% of these cases.[269,275]

Symptomatic cervical stenosis occurs in 1.0% to 3.2% of CKC cases[259,270] and uterine perforation in 0.4% to 1.9%.[259,268-270,276] Measurement of the cone dimensions showed that the factor most responsible for these complications was the length of the cone biopsy (specimen height > 25 mm) rather than the overall volume of tissue removed.[256,257,267,275]

19.7.7. Modifying the procedure to account for disease distribution

The CKC has advantages over the loop excision in that there are no thermal effects. This can be critical in managing patients with one of three indications

for excision: these are to differentiate microinvasive squamous carcinoma from more advanced disease, to differentiate AIS from adenocarcinoma, and to sort out the abnormal glandular smear. In these three situations, a cylindrical specimen as described accounts best for the distribution of disease. In squamous disease, any peripheral CIN can be managed by loop excision or laser ablation. If the excised specimen (which includes the entire transformation zone) demonstrates cancer, the patient is staged and treated accordingly. If the histology of the central disease is CIN, the patient is routinely followed as with any patient treated for CIN.

Excisions in glandular disease should also use the cylindrical configuration. Its dimensions vary according to the distribution of disease similar to squamous. The loop procedure should not be employed in these situations for two reasons: the high probability of thermal injury and the pathologist being unable to grade the lesion and exclude malignancy.[244] As with squamous, the worst disease potentially lies centrally (apically, Figure 19.64). Figure 19.65 illustrates the anatomical location of CIN as a function of age. Figures 19.39 and 19.66 illustrates that a single cylinder or a combination of cylinders compared with a conical defect removes far less tissue but still encompasses the distribution of disease.[60,219] The processing is illustrated in Figure 19.67.

19.8 Hysterectomy for Cervical Intraepithelial Neoplasia

19.8.1 Introduction

Before 1970, hysterectomy was the definitive method for the management of cervical carcinoma in situ (CIS).

19.8.2 Indications for hysterectomy

Hysterectomy is employed only in special circumstances, including the following:[230,257,258,269,272,275,282,285]

1. Persistent or recurrent CIN lesions for which excision treatment has failed. Hysterectomy will certainly eradicate the cervical disease.
2. Extensive disease occupying the cervix with vaginal extension for which conservative management may be difficult. Vaginal extension occurs in 4% of cases.[258] In this situation, the involved vagina is removed as a cuff attached to the hysterectomy specimen. Alternately, laser ablation of the vaginal

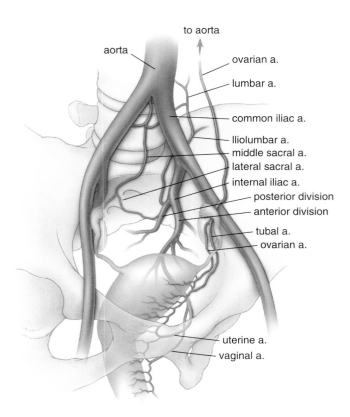

FIGURE 19.63 The pelvic superfluous blood supply to the cervix.

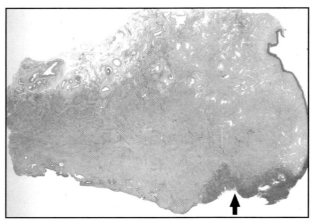

FIGURE 19.64 Cervical histology specimen demonstrating CIN 3 lesion peripherally and invasive cancer centrally (See arrow) in the endocervical canal. Reprinted with permission from Wright V C: Loop electrosurgical excisional procedures for treatment of cervical intraepithelial neoplasia. In: Wright V C, Lickrish G M, Shier R M: *Basic and Advanced Colposcopy—A Practical Handbook for Diagnosis (2nd ed.).* Houston: Biomedical Communications, 1995.

involvement plus hysterectomy may be appropriate.

3. The presence of coexisting gynecological conditions necessitating hysterectomy, such as large fibroids, uterine prolapse, endometriosis, or intractable menorrhagia. Because of advances in endoscopic surgery, some of these cases could be managed by hysteroscopic and laparoscopic methods. Each case must be considered on an individual basis.

4. Technical difficulties (exposure problems) for conservative management. An example of this circumstance is a nulliparous, postmenopausal, never-estrogenized woman. It may be easier to remove the cervix and its lesion (usually in the canal) by hysterectomy rather than risking major complications, such as uncontrolled hemorrhage and injury to adjacent organs.

5. Unresolved stenosis after conservative treatment, particularly when a positive upper margin exists. This circumstance inhibits long-term post-treatment assessment and detection of postmenopausal bleeding, induced by either malignancy or hormones.

6. Definitive management for adenocarcinoma in situ (AIS) when fertility is no longer an issue.

7. To control hemorrhage postconization.

8. Cancer phobia.

19.8.3 Operative methods

A Class I hysterectomy (extrafacial) is advised to ensure removal of all cervical tissue.[286] Reflection and retraction of the ureters laterally without actual dissection from the ureteral bed allows clamping of the adjacent paracervical tissue without cutting the side of the cervical tissue. This procedure is recommended primarily for CIS, true microinvasive carcinoma, and AIS.

The various options for operative approach are: vaginal hysterectomy, laparoscopically assisted vaginal hysterectomy, total abdominal hysterectomy with or without salpingoophorectomy, and total abdominal hysterectomy plus vaginal cuff if there is vaginal extension. A more modified radical hysterectomy will be required for extensive vaginal involvement since the ureters must be isolated to ensure safe excision of the upper third of the vagina (Class II hysterectomy without pelvic lymphadenectomy.[287] The approach must be chosen on an individual case basis, taking into consideration other associated disease states and medical conditions.

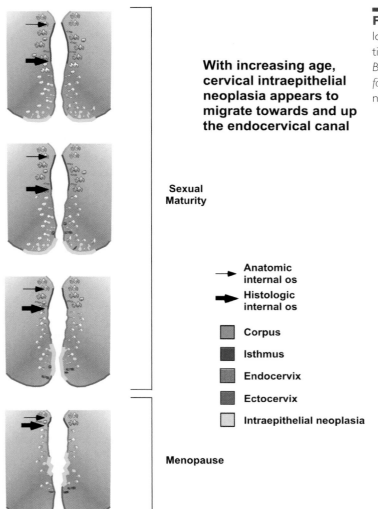

With increasing age, cervical intraepithelial neoplasia appears to migrate towards and up the endocervical canal

FIGURE 19.65   Schematics of the anatomical location of cervical intraepithelial neoplasia as a function of age. (In: Wright, VC, Lickrish, GM, Shier, RM. *Basic and Advanced Colposcopy—A Practical Handbook for Diagnosis* (2nd ed.), Houston: Biomedical Communications, 1995.)

Sexual Maturity

→ Anatomic internal os

➡ Histologic internal os

▢ Corpus

▢ Isthmus

▢ Endocervix

▢ Ectocervix

▢ Intraepithelial neoplasia

Menopause

19.8.4 Post-hysterectomy assessments

Hysterectomy offers no assurance that the patient will be free from disease. Vaginal intraepithelial neoplasia (VAIN) seen at the vaginal vault immediately post-hysterectomy indicates that there was unrecognized disease at the time of the hysterectomy. Prior to a hysterectomy, vaginal colposcopy should always be carried out using iodine staining in the estrogenized patient. Disease noted at the vaginal vault suture line may reflect buried disease (hidden disease), which requires a more complicated plan of management.

VAIN that develops many years after hysterectomy likely represents inadequate screening or new disease (Figures 19.68 and 19.69). Kolstad and Valborg[258] found CIS of the vaginal vault developing later in 1.2% of patients and invasive carcinoma in

2.1%. Creasman and Parker[288] reported recurrent CIS in 1.5% and invasive disease in 0.5%, and Boyes et al[289] noted recurrent CIS in 0.7% and cancer in 0.1%. Because of these findings, all women undergoing hysterectomy for CIN require initial surveillance with Pap tests from the vaginal vault and upper third of the vagina since these are the frequent sites of recurrence/persistence (Figures 19.68 and 19.69).

The American Cancer Society[290] recommends for women with CIN 2/3 treated as the primary indication by hysterectomy have follow-up cytology every 4 to 6 months. Three documented, consecutive, technically satisfactory normal/negative vaginal cytology tests and no abnormal/positive cytology tests should be achieved within an 18- to 24-month period following hysterectomy before discontinuing cytology screening. These recommendations suggest that

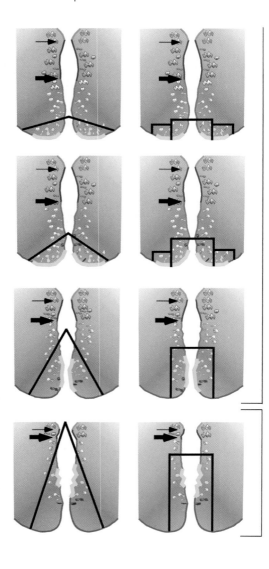

Sexual Maturity

→ **Anatomic internal os**

⟹ **Histologic internal os**

▨ **Corpus**

▨ **Isthmus**

▨ **Endocervix**

▨ **Ectocervix**

☐ **Intraepithelial neoplasia**

Menopause

FIGURE 19.66   Schematics of a cone-shaped specimen vs. a cylindrical configuration. The cylindrical excisional method removes less tissue when accounting for the distribution of disease (linear length and crypt involvement). Reprinted with permission from Wright V C: The Geometry of Cervical Intraepithelial Neoplasia: An applied guide to its removal. In: Wright V C, Lickrish G M, Shier RM: *Basic and Advanced Colposcopy—A Practical Handbook for Diagnosis (2nd ed.).* Houston: Biomedical Communications, 1995. ■

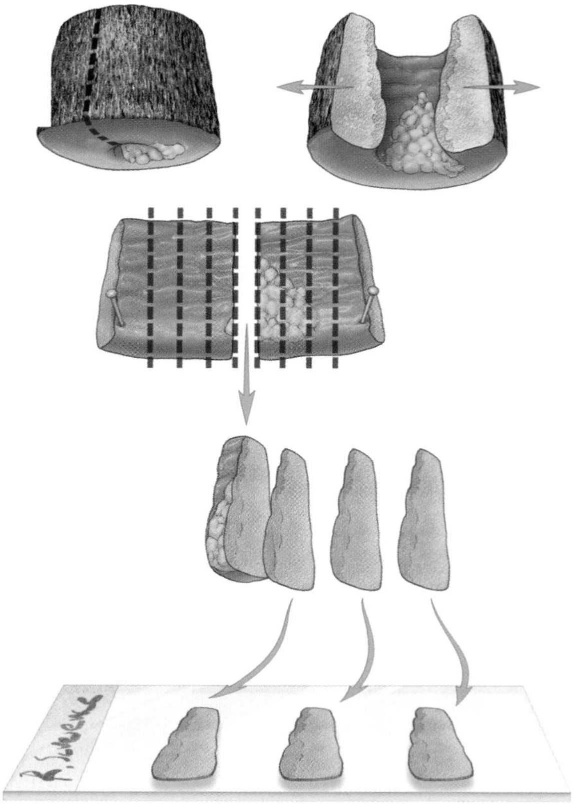

FIGURE 19.67   The cylindrical specimen is opened and pinned with the stromal side down. The larger tissue pieces are cut into smaller serial cross-sections—termed bread loafing. Single 5 micron sections from each slice are placed on a glass slide for histological diagnosis and to establish whether or not the margins are free of disease. ■

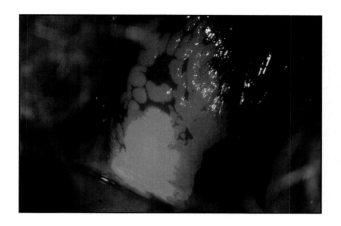

FIGURE 19.68   VAIN 3 of the vaginal vault after Lugol's staining of the estrogenized epithelium. The lesion is multifocal and the diseased areas fail to retain the iodine solution because of a lack of glucose in the intraepithelial lesion. A previous hysterectomy for CIN 3 was done 5 years earlier. From: Wright, V.C.: *Color Atlas of Colposcopy—Vervix, Vagina and Vulva.* Houston: Biomedical Communications, 2000.

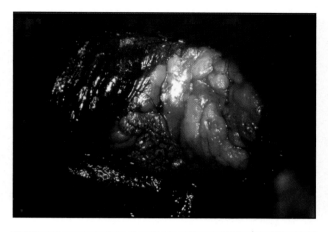

FIGURE 19.69   Four years post-hysterectomy, VAIN 3 disease of the left upper third of the lateral vaginal wall is identified by a positive Lugol's iodine test. From: Wright, V.C.: *Color Atlas of Colposcopy—Vervix, Vagina and Vulva.* Houston: Biomedical Communications, 2000.

lesions found years later are related to initial inadequate screening post-hysterectomy.

Occasionally, the pathologist will report invasive cancer in the extirpated specimen. If it is microinvasive by standard definition and all margins are clear, surgery is sufficient. If advanced disease is reported, a referral to an appropriate cancer specialist is necessary.

References

1. Williams J. Cancer of the uterus. *Harveian Lectures for 1886.* London: HK Lewis.
2. Cox J T. Answer to: "How long will screening myths survive?" *Lancet.* 2000
3. Mitchell M F, Tartorlaro-Luna G, Cook E, Whittaker L, Rhodes-Morris H, Silva E. A randomized clinical trial of cryotherapy, loop electrosurgical excision, and laser for treatment of squamous intraepithelial lesions of the cervix. *Obstet Gynecol* 1998;92:737–44.
4. Krone K R, Kiviat N B, Koutsky L A. The epidemiology of cervical neoplasms. In: Luesley D, Jordan J, Richart R M, Eds. *Intraepithelial neoplasia of the lower genital tract.* Churchill Livingston, Edinburgh. 1995, pp. 49–60.
5. Cox J T. In: Lonky N, Ed. Management of precursor lesions of cervical carcinoma: history, host defense, and a survey of modalities. *Obstet Gynecol Clin North Am* 2002;29:751–85.
6. Koss L G, Durfee G R. Unusual patterns of squamous epithelium of the uterine cervix.: cytologic and pathologic study of koilocytotic atypia. *Ann NY Acad Sci* 1956;63:1245–61.
7. Meisels A, Fortein R. Condylomatous lesions of the cervix and vagina. I. Cytologic patterns. *Acta Cytol* 1976;20;505–9.
8. Bosch F X, Manos M M, Munoz N et al. Prevalence of human papillomavirus in cervical cancer: a worldwide perspective. *J Natl Cancer Inst* 1995;87:796–802.
9. Wright T C, Cox J T, L. Massad L S, Twiggs L B, Wilkinson E J for the 2001 ASCCP-sponsored Consensus Workshop. 2001 Consensus Guidelines for the Management of Women with Cervical Cytological Abnormalities and Cervical Cancer Precursors—Part I: Cytological Abnormalities. *JAMA* 2002;287:2120–9.
10. Wright T C Jr, Cox J T, Massad L S, Carlson J, Twiggs L B, Wilkinson E J; American Society for Colposcopy and Cervical Pathology. 2001 consensus guidelines for the management of women with cervical intraepithelial neoplasia. *Am J Obstet Gynecol.* 2003;189:295–304.
11. Tate D R, Anderson R J. Recurrence of cervical dysplasia in the human immunodeficiency virus-seropositive patient. *Obstet Gynecol* 2001;97(Suppl 1):S60.

12. Crowley-Nowick P A, Bell M, Edwards R P, McCallister D, Gore H, Kanbour-Shakir A, Mestecky J, Partridge E E. Normal uterine cervix: characterization of isolated lymphocyte phenotypes and immunoglobulin secretion. *Am J Reprod Immunol* 1995;34:241–7

13. Chow L T, Broker T R. Papillomavirus DNA replication. *Intervirology* 1994;37:150–8.

14. Cheng S, Schmidt-Grimminger D-C, Murant T, et al. Differentiation-dependent up-regulation of the human papillomavirus gene reactivates cellular DNA replication in suprabasal differentiated keratinocytes. *Genes Dev* 1995;9:2335–49.

15. Dollard S C, Wilson J L, Demeter L M, et al. Production of human papillomavirus and modulation of the infectious program in epithelial raft cultures. *Genes Dev* 1992;6:1131–42.

16. Flores E R, Lambert P F. Evidence for a switch in the mode of human papillomavirus type 16 DNA replication during the viral life cycle. *J Virol* 1997;71:7167–79.

17. Jian Y, Schmidt-Grimminger D-C, Chien W-M, et al. Post-transcriptional induction of p21cip 1 protein by human papillomavirus E7 inhibits unscheduled DNA synthesis reactivated in differentiated keratinocytes. *Oncogene* 1998;17:2027–38.

18. Dyson N, Howley P M, Munger K, et al. The human papillomavirus-16 E7 oncoprotein is able to bind to the retinoblastoma gene product. *Science* 1989;243:934–6.

19. Werness B A, Levine A J, Howley P M. Association of human papillomavirus types 16 and 18 E6 proteins with p53. *Science* 1990;248:76–9.

20. Nuovo G J, Banbury R, & Calayag P T. Human papillomavirus types and recurrent cervical warts in immunocompromised women. *Mod Pathol* 1991;4:632–5.

21. Nobbenhuis, M., Walboomers, J. M., Helmerhorst, T.1., Rozendaal, L. Relation of human papillomavirus status to cervical lesions and consequences for cervical-cancer screening: a prospective study. *Lancet* 1999;354,20–5.

22. Hopman E H, Rozendaal L, Voorhorst F J, Walboomers J M, Kenemans P, Helmerhorst T J. High risk human papillomavirus in women with normal cervical cytology prior to the development of abnormal cytology and colposcopy. *BJOG* 2000;107:600–4.

23. Bergeron C. Management of infection caused by HPV in pregnancy. *J Gynecol Obstet Biol Reprod* (Paris). 1989;18:895–8.

24. Burke L. Evolution of therapeutic approaches to cervical intraepithelial neoplasia. *J Lower Genital Tract Dis* 1997;1:267–73.

25. Pride G, Chuprevich T W. Topical 5-fluorouracil treatment of the transformation zone intraepithelial neoplasia of cervix and vagina. *Obstet Gynecol* 1982;60:467–72.

26. Barten G. Local treatment of cervical intraepithelial neoplasia with a 5 percent fluorouracil ointment. *Zentralbl Gynakol* 1987;109:1510–6.

27. Goodman A, Zukerberg L R, Nikrui N, Scully R E. Vaginal adenosis and clear cell carcinomas after 5-fluorouracil treatment for condylomas. *Cancer* 1991;68:1628–32.

28. Maiman M, Watts D H, Andersen J, Clax P, Merino M, Kendall M. Vaginal 5-fluorouracil for high-grade cervical dysplasia in human immunodeficiency virus infection: a randomized trial. *Obstet Gynecol* 1999;94:954–61.

29. Chanen W, Rome R M. Electrocoagulation diathermy for cervical dysplasia and carcinoma-in-situ: A 15-year survey. *Obstet Gynecol* 1983;67:673–9.

30. Giles J A, Walker P C, Chalk P A. The treatment of CIN by radical electrocoagulation diathermy: five years' experience. *Br J Obstet Gynaecol* 1987;94:1089–93.

31. Singer A, Monaghan J M, Quek S C. *Lower Genital Tract Precancer: colposcopy, pathology and treatment. 2nd edition.* Blackwell Science Ltd. 2000.

32. Kwikkel H J, Helmerhorst T J M, Bezemer P D, Quaak M J, Stolk J G. Laser or cryotherapy for cervical intraepithelial neoplasia: A randomized study to compare efficacy and side effects. *Gynecol Oncol* 1985;22:23–31.

33. Ostergard D R. Cryosurgical treatment of cervical intraepithelial neoplasia. *Obstet Gynecol* 1980;56:231–3.

34. Morrow C P, Townsend D E. *Synopsis of Gynecologic Oncology, 3rd Ed.* John Wiley and Sons, Publ., New York, 1987, pp. 17–28.

35. Stuart G C E, Anderson R J, Corlett B M A, et al. Assessment of failures of cryosurgical treatment in cervical intraepithelial neoplasia. *Am Obstet Gynecol* 1982;142:658–63.

36. Hatch K D, Shingleton H M, Austin J M, Soong S-J, Bradley D H. Cryosurgery of cervical intraepithelial neoplasia. *Obstet Gynecol* 1981;57:692–8.

37. Savage E W, Matlock D L, Salem F A, Charmes E H. The effect of endocervical gland involvement on the cure rates of patients with cervical intraepithelial neoplasia undergoing cryosurgery. *Gynecol Oncol* 1982;14:194–8.

38. Townsend D E, Richart R M. Cryotherapy and carbon dioxide laser management of cervical intraepithelial neoplasia: A controlled comparison. *Obstet Gynecol* 1983;61:75–8.

39. Ferenczy A. Comparison of and carbon dioxide laser therapy for cervical intraepithelial neoplasia. *Obstet Gynecol* 1985;66:793–8.

40. Burke L. The use of carbon dioxide laser in the treatment of intraepithelial neoplasia. *Colposc Gynecol Lasers Surg* 1986;2:77–81.

41. Tsukamoto N. Treatment of cervical intraepithelial neoplasia with carbon dioxide laser. *Gynecol Oncol* 1985;21:331–6.

42. Berget A, Andreasson B, Bock J E, Bastofte E, Hebjorn S, Isager-Sally L, et al. Outpatient treatment of cervical intraepithelial neoplasia: The CO_2 laser versus cryosurgery, a randomized clinical trial. *Acta Obstet Gynecol Scand* 1987;66:531–6.

43. Benedet J L, Miller D M, Nickerson K C. Results of conservative management of cervical intraepithelial neoplasia. *Obstet Gynecol* 1992;79:105.

44. Paraskevaidis E, Jandial L, Mann E M, Fisher P M, Kitchener H C. Patterns of treatment failure following laser for cervical intraepithelial neoplasia; implication for follow-up protocol. *Obstet Gynecol* 1991;78:80–3.

45. Younge P A, Hertig A, Armstrong D. A study of carcinoma in situ of the cervix—135 cases. *Am J Obstet Gynecol* 1949;58:867–95.

46. Tronstadt S E, Kirschner K. Treatment of cervical intraepithelial neoplasia with local excision biopsy and cryosurgery. *Acta Obstet Gynecol Scand* 1980;59:349–53.

47. Younge P A. Pre-malignant lesions of the cervix: clinical management. *Clin Obstet Gynecol* 1962;5:1137–47.

48. Cartier, R. Therapeutic choices in treatment. In: Cartier, R. (ed.) *Practical Colposcopy*, 1984 p. 162. Laboratoire Cartier, Paris.

49. Cartier I, Richart R M, Wright T C. The evolution of loop diathermy in cervical disease. In Prendeville W. (Ed) *Large Loop Excision of the Transformation Zone: A Practical Guide to LLETZ.* Pp. 93–7. London: Chapman and Hall Medical.

50. Prendiville W, Cullimore J, Norman S. Large loop excision of the transformation zone (LLETZ: A new method of management for women with intraepithelial neoplasia. *Br J Obstet Gynecol* 1989;96:1054–60.

51. Wright T C, Gagnon S, Richart R M, Ferenczy A. Treatment of cervical intraepithelial neoplasia using the loop electrosurgical excision procedure. *Obstet Gynecol* 1992;79:173–8.

52. Luesley D M, Cullimore J, Lawton F G, et al. Loop diathermy excision of the cervical transformation zone in patients with abnormal cervical smears. *Br J Med* 1990;330:1690–3.

53. Gunasekera P C, Phipps J H, Lewis B V. Large-loop excision of the transformation zone (LLETZ) compared to carbon dioxide laser in the treatment of CIN: A superior mode of treatment. *Br J Obstet Gynaecol* 1990;97:995–8.

54. Whitely P F, Olah K S. Treatment of cervical intraepithelial neoplasia: Experience with low-voltage diathermy loop. *Am J Obstet Gynecol* 1990;162:1272–7.

55. Minucci D, Cinel A, Insacco E. Diathermic loop treatment for CIN and HPV lesions. *Eur J Gynaecol Oncol* 1991;12:385–93.

56. Bigrigg M A, Codling B W, Pearson P, et al. Colposcopic diagnosis and treatment for cervical dysplasia at a single clinic visit. *Lancet* 1990;336:229–31.

57. Ferenczy A, Choukroun D, Arseneau J. Loop electrosurgical excision procedure for squamous intraepithelial lesions of the cervix: Advantages and potential pitfalls. *Obstet Gynecol* 1996;87:332–7.

58. Wiser-Estin M, Niloff J, Burke L. Is loop excision over-utilized in the management of high grade squamous intraepithelial lesions of the cervix? *Cervix Lower Female Genital Tract* 1995;13:41–5.

59. Stoler M H, Schiffman M. Interobserver reproducibility of cervical cytologic and histologic interpretations: realistic estimates from the ASCUS-LSIL Triage Study. *JAMA.* 2001;285:1500–5.

60. Wright V C, Davies E, Riopelle M A. Laser cylindrical excision to replace conization. *Am J Obstet Gynecol* 1984;150:704–9.

61. Baggish M S, Dorsey J H. Carbon dioxide laser for combination excisional-vaporization conization. *Am J Obstet Gynecol* 1985;151:23–7.

62. Martzloff K H. Cancer of the cervix uteri: recognition of early manifestations. *JAMA* 1938;111:1921–24.

63. Coppleson, M, Atkinson, K H, & Dalrymple J C. Cervical squamous and glandularintraepithelial neoplasia; clinical features and review of management. In: Coppleson, M. (ed.) *Gynaecological Oncology,* Vol. 1, 2nd ed. Edinburgh: Churchill Livingstone, 1992.

64. Bjork S, Hagstrom H G. Of what significance is abnormal result of smear test? Anxiety because of insufficient information in connection with abnormal result of cervical smear test. *Lakartidningen* 2001;98:2796–800.

65. Jones M H, Singer A, Jenkins D. The mildly abnormal cervical smear: patient anxiety and choice of management. *J R Soc Med* 1996;89:257–60.

66. Wilkinson C, Jones J M, McBridge J. Anxiety caused by abnormal result of a cervical smear test: a controlled trial. *Br Med J* 1990;300:440.

67. Moore T O, Moore A Y, Carrasco D, Vander Straten M, Arany I, Au W, Tyring S K. Human papillomavirus, smoking, and cancer. *J Cutan Med Surg* 2001;5:323–8.

68. Acladious N N, Sutton C, Mandal D, Hopkins R, Zaklama M, Kitchener H. Persistent human papillomavirus infection and smoking increase risk of failure of treatment of cervical intraepithelial neoplasia (CIN). *Int J Cancer* 2002;98:435–9.

69. Schiffman M H, Haley N J, Felton J S, Andrews A W, Kaslow R A, Lancaster W D, Kurman R J, Brinton L A, Lannom L B, Hoffmann D. Biochemical epidemiology of cervical neoplasia: measuring cigarette smoke constituents in the cervix. *Cancer Res* 1987;47:3886–8.

70. Hellberg D, Nilsson S, Haley N J, Hoffman D, Wynder E. Smoking and cervical intraepithelial neoplasia: nicotine and cotinine in serum and cervical mucus in smokers and nonsmokers. *Am J Obstet Gynecol* 1988;158:910–3.

71. Szarewski A, Maddox P, Royston P, Jarvis M, Anderson M, Guillebaud J, Cuzick J. The effect of stopping smoking on cervical Langerhans' cells and lymphocytes. *BJOG* 2001;10:295–303.

72. Alberg A J, Selhub J, Shah K V, Viscidi R P, Comstock G W, Helzlsouer K J. The risk of cervical cancer in relation to serum concentrations of folate, vitamin B12, and homocysteine. *Cancer Epidemiol Biomarkers Prev.* 2000;9:761–4.

73. Thomson S W, Heimburger D C, Cornwell P E, Turner M E, Sauberlich H E, Fox L M, Butterworth C E. Effect of total plasma homocysteine on cervical dysplasia risk. Nutr *Cancer* 2000;37:128–33.

74. Weinstein S J, Ziegler R G, Frongillo E A Jr, Colman N, Sauberlich H E, Brinton L A, Hamman R F, Levine R S, Mallin K, Stolley P D, Bisogni C A. Low serum and red blood cell folate are moderately, but nonsignificantly associated with increased risk of invasive cervical cancer in U.S. women. *J Nutr* 2001;131:2040–8.

75. Palan P R, Chang C J, Mikhail M S, Ho G Y, Basu J, Romney S L. Plasma concentrations of micronutrients during a nine-month clinical trial of beta-carotene in women with precursor cervical cancer lesions. *Nutr Cancer* 1998;30:46–52.

76. Bell M C, Crowley-Nowick P, Bradlow H L, Sepkovic D W, Schmidt-Grimminger D, Howell P, Mayeaux E J, Tucker A, Turbat-Herrera E A, Mathis J M. Placebo-controlled trial of indole-3-carbinol in the treatment of CIN. *Gynecol Oncol* 2000;78:123–9.

77. Comerci J T Jr, Runowicz C D, Fields A L, Romney S L, Palan P R, Kadish A S, Goldberg G L. Induction of transforming growth factor beta-1 in cervical intraepithelial neoplasia in vivo after treatment with beta-carotene. Clin Cancer Res 1997;3:157–60.

78. Cox J T. In: Lonky N, Ed. Management of women with cervical cancer precursor lesions. *Obstet Gynecol Clin North Am* 2002;29:787–816.

79. Kirwan P H, Smith I R, Naftalin N J. A study of cryosurgery and the CO₂ laser in treatment of carcinoma in situ (CIN III) of the uterine cervix. *Gynecol Oncol* 1985;22:195–200.

80. Wright V C, Davies E M. The conservative management of cervical intraepithelial neoplasia: the use of cryosurgery and the carbon dioxide laser. *Br J Obstet Gynaecol.* 1981;88:663–8.

81. Berget A, Andreasson B, Bock J E. Laser and cryosurgery for cervical intraepithelial neoplasia: A randomized trial and long-term follow-up. *Acta Obstet Gynecol Scand.* 1991;70:231–5.

82. Alvarez R D, Helm C W, Edwards R P, Naumann R W, Partridge E E, Shingleton H M, et al. Prospective randomized trial of LLETZ versus laser ablation in patients with cervical intraepithelial neoplasia. *Gynecol Oncol* 1994;52:175–9.

83. Martin-Hirsch P L, Paraskevaidis E, Kitchener H. Surgery for cervical intraepithelial neoplasia. *Cochrane Database Syst Rev* 2000;2:13–18.

84. Buxton E J, Luesley D M, Shafi M I & Rollason M. Colposcopically directed punch biopsy; a potentially misleading investigation. *Br J Obstet Gynaecol* 1991;98:1273–6.

85. McIndoe A, Robson M, Tidy J, Mason P, Anderson M. Laser excision rather than vaporization: the treatment of choice for cervical intraepithelial neoplasia. *Obstet Gynecol* 1989;74:165–8.

86. Sze E, Rosenzweig B, Birenbaum D et al. Excisional conization of the cervix-uteri. *J Gynecol Surg. 1989;* 5:325–31.

87. Cox J T. Management of cervical intraepithelial neoplasia. *Lancet* 1999 Mar 13;353(9156):857–9.

88. Hammond R H, Edmonds D K. Does treatment for cervical intraepithelial neoplasia affect fertility and pregnancy? Little to worry about. *Br Med J.* 1990;301:1344–5.

89. Montz F J. Impact of therapy for cervical intraepithelial neoplasia on fertility. *Am J Obstet Gynecol* 1996;175:1129–36.

90. Richart R M, Barron B A. A follow-up study of patients cervical dysplasia. *Am J Obstet Gynecol* 1969;105:386–92.

91. Shafi M I, Luesley D M, Jordan J A, Dunn J A, Rollason T P, Yates M. Randomized trial of immediate versus deferred treatment strategies for the management of minor cervical cytological abnormalities. *Br J Obstet Gynaecol* 1997;104:590–4.

92. Ostor A G. Natural history of CIN: A critical review. *Int J Gynecol Pathol* 1993;12:186–92.

93. Nasiell K, Roger V, Nasiell M. Behavior of mild cervical dysplasia during long-term follow-up. *Obstet. Gynecol.* 1986;67:665–9.

94. Nasiell K, Nasiell M, Vaclavinkova V: Behavior of moderate cervical dysplasia during long-term follow-up. *Obstet Gynecol* 1983; 61:609–14.

95. Cox J T, Schiffman M, Solomon D; ASCUS-LSIL Triage Study (ALTS) Group. Prospective follow-up suggests similar risk of subsequent cervical intraepithelial neoplasia grade 2 or 3 among women with cervical intraepithelial neoplasia grade 1 or negative colposcopy and directed biopsy. *Am J Obstet Gynecol* 2003;188:1406–12.

96. Guido R, Schiffman M, Solomon D, Burke L, for the ASCUS LSIL Triage Study (ALTS) Group Post-Colposcopy Management Strategies for Patients Referred with LSIL or HPV DNA Positive ASCUS: A Two-Year Prospective Study. *Am J Obstet Gynecol* 2003;188:1401–5.

97. Freeman-Wang T, Walker P, Linehan J, Coffey C, Glasser B, Sherr L. Anxiety levels in women attending colposcopy clinics for treatment for cervical intraepithelial neoplasia: a randomized trial of written and video information. *BJOG* 2001;108:482–4.

98. Holowaty P, Miller A B, Rohan T, To T. Natural history of dysplasia of the uterine cervix. *J Natl Cancer Inst* 1999;91:252–8.

99. Doherty I E, Richardson P H. Psychological ascpects of the investigation and treatment of abnormalities of the cervix. [Luesley D, Jordan J, Richart R, eds.] *Intraepithelial Neoplasia of the Lower Genital Tract* London: Livingston Ltd, Publs, 1995:241–250.

100. Ramirez J E, Ramos D M, Clayton L, Kanowitz S, Moscicki A B. Genital human papillomavirus infections: knowledge, perception of risk, and actual risk in a nonclinic population of young women. *J Womens Health* 1997;6:113–21.

101. Reed B D, Ruffin M T, Gorenflo D W, Zazove P. The psychosexual impact of human papillomavirus cervical infections. *J Fam Pract* 1999;48:110–6.

102. Clarke P, Ebel C, Catotti D N, Stewart S. The psychosocial impact of human papillomavirus infection: implications for health care providers. *Int J STD AIDS* 1996;7:197–200.

103. Nugent L S, Tamlyn-Leaman K, Isa N, Reardon E, Crumley J. Anxiety and the colposcopy experience. *Clin Nurs Res* 1993;2:267–77.

104. Stewart D E, Lickrish G M, Sierra S, Parkin H. The effect of educational brochures on knowledge and emotional distress in women with abnormal Papanicolaou smears. *Obstet Gynecol* 1993;81:280–2.

105. Meana M, Stewart D E, Lickrish G M, Murphy J, Rosen B. Patient preference for the management of mildly abnormal Papanicolaou smears. *J Womens Health Gend Based Med* 1999;8:941–7.

106. Kavanagh A M, Broom D H. Women's understanding of abnormal cervical smear test results: a qualitative interview study. *BMJ* 1997;314:1388–91.

107. Jones B A, Novis D A. Follow-up of abnormal cervical cytology: a College of American Pathologists Q-Probes Study of 16,132 cases from 306 laboratories. *Arch Pathol Lab Med* 2000;124:672–81.

108. Hartz L E, Fenaughty A M. Management choice and adherence to follow-up after colposcopy in women with cervical intraepithelial neoplasia. *Obstet Gynecol* 2001;98:674–8.

109. Abercrombie P D. Improving adherence to abnormal Pap smear follow-up. *J Obstet Gynecol Neonatal Nurs* 2001;30:80–8.

110. Robertson J H, Woodend B E, Crozier E H, Hutchinson J. Risk of cervical cancer associated with mild dyskaryosis. *Brit Med J* 1988;297:18–21.

111. Duncan I D. NHS Cervical Screening Programme: *Guidelines for Clinical Practice and Programme Management.* Oxford: National Coordinating Network, 1992.

112. Cox J T (lead author). ASSCP Practice Guideline: Management of an abnormal Pap follow-up system. *J Lower Gen Tract Dis* 1997;1:167–70.

113. Hamm R M, Loemker V, Reilly K L, Johnson G, Dubois P, Staveley-O'Carroll K, Brand J, Owens T, Smith K. A clinical decision analysis of cryotherapy compared with expectant management for cervical dysplasia. *J Fam Pract* 1998;47:193–201.

114. Spitzer M, Chernys A E, Shifrin A, Ryskin M. Indications for cone biopsy: pathologic correlation. *Am J Obstet Gynecol* 1998;178:74–9.

115. Kobak W H, Roman L D, Felix J C, Muderspach L I, Schlaerth J B, Morrow C P. The role of endocervical curettage at cervical conization for high-grade dysplasia. *Obstet. Gynecol* 1995;85:197–201.

116. Fine B A, Feinstein G I, Sabella V. The pre- and postoperative value of endocervical curettage in the detection of cervical intraepithelial neoplasia and invasive cervical cancer. *Gynecol Oncol* 1998;71:46–9.

117. Ismail S M, Colelough A B, Dinnen J S, et al. Observer variation in histopathological diagnosis and grading of cervical intraepithelial neoplasia. *BMJ* 1989;298:707–10.

118. Nuovo J, Melnikow J, Willan A R, Chan B K. Treatment outcomes for squamous intraepithelial lesions. *Int J Gynaecol Obstet* 2000;68:25–33.

119. Tidbury P, Singer A, Jenkins D. CIN 3: the role of lesion size in invasion. *Br J Obstet Gynaecol* 1992;99:583–6.

120. Andersen E S, Nielsen K, Pedersen B. The reliability of preconization diagnostic evaluation in patients with cervical intraepithelial neoplasia and microinvasive carcinoma. *Gynecol Oncol* 1995;59:143–7.

121. Burke L, Covell L, Antonioli D. Carbon dioxide laser therapy of cervical intraepithelial neoplasia: factors determining success rate. *Lasers Surg Med* 1980;1:113–22.

122. Duggan B D, Felix J C, Muderspach L I, et al. Cold-knife conization versus conization by the loop electrosurgical excision procedure: a randomized, prospective study. *Am J Obstet Gynecol* 1999;180:276–82.

123. Naumann R W, Bell M C, Alvarez R D, et al. LLETZ is an acceptable alternative to diagnostic cold-knife conization. *Gynecol Oncol* 1994;55:224–8.

124. Connor J P. Noninvasive cervical cancer complicating pregnancy. *Obstet Gynecol Clin North Am* 1998;25:331–42.

125. Robinson W R, Webb S, Tirpack J, Degefu S, O'Quinn A G. Management of cervical intraepithelial neoplasia during pregnancy with LOOP excision. *Gynecol Oncol* 1997;64:153–5.

126. Economos K, Perez Veridiano N, Delke I, Collado M L, Tancer M L. Abnormal cervical cytology in pregnancy: a 17-year experience. *Obstet Gynecol* 1993;81:915–8.

127. Wright T C, Ellerbrock T V, Chiasson M A, Van De Vanter N, Sun X W. Cervical intraepithelial neoplasia in women infected with human immunodeficiency virus: prevalence, risk factors, and validity of Papanicolaou smears. New York Cervical Disease Study. *Obstet Gynecol* 1994;84:591–97.

128. Sun X W, Kuhn L, Ellerbrock T V, Chiasson M A, Bush T J, Wright T C Jr. Human papillomavirus infection in women infected with the human immunodeficiency virus. *N Engl J Med* 1997;337:1343–9.

129. Palefsky J M, Minkoff H, Kalish L A, et al. Cervicovaginal human papillomavirus infection in human immunodeficiency virus-1 (HIV)-positive and high-risk HIV-negative women. *J Natl Cancer Inst* 1999;91:226–36.

130. Holcomb K, Matthews R P, Chapman J E, et al. The efficacy of cervical conization in the treatment of cervical intraepithelial neoplasia in HIV-positive women. *Gynecol Oncol* 1999;74:428–31.

131. Ellerbrock TV, Chiasson MA, Bush TJ, Sun XW, Sawo D, Brudney K, Wright TC Jr. Incidence of cervical squamous intraepithelial lesions in HIV-infected women. *JAMA* 2000;283:1031–7.

132. Massad LS, Ahdieh L, Benning L, Minkoff H, Greenblatt RM, Watts H, Miotti P, Anastos K, Moxley M, Muderspach LI, Melnick S. Evolution of cervical abnormalities among women with HIV-1: evidence from surveillance cytology in the women's interagency HIV study. *J Acquir Immune Defic Syndr* 2001;27(5):432–42.

133. Reich O, Pickel H, Lahousen M, Tamussino K, Winter R. Cervical intraepithelial neoplasia III: long-term outcome after cold-knife conization with clear margins. *Obstet Gynecol* 2001;97:428–30.

134. Reich O, Lahousen M, Pickel H, Tamussino K, Winter R. Cervical intraepithelial neoplasia III: long-term follow-up after cold-knife conization with involved margins. *Obstet Gynecol* 2002;99:193–6.

135. Soutter WP, de Barros Lopes A, Fletcher A, et al. Invasive cervical cancer after conservative therapy for cervical intraepithelial neoplasia. *Lancet* 1997;349:978–80.

136. Kolstad P, Klem V. Long-term follow-up of 1121 cases of carcinoma in situ. *Obstet Gynecol* 1976;48:125–9.

137. Anderson MC. Invasive carcinoma of the cervix following local destructive treatment for cervical intraepithelial neoplasia. *Br J Obstet Gynaecol* 1993;100:657–63.

138. Brown JV, Peters WA, Corwin DJ. Invasive carcinoma after cone biopsy for cervical intraepithelial neoplasia. *Gynecol Oncol* 1991;40:25–28.

139. Gornall RJ, Boyd IE, Manolitsas T, Herbert A. Interval cervical cancer following treatment for cervical intraepithelial neoplasia. *Int J Gynecol Cancer* 2000;10:198–202

140. Flannelly G, Bolger B, Fawzi H, De Lopes AB, Monaghan JM. Follow up after LLETZ: could schedules be modified according to risk of recurrence? *BJOG* 2001;108:1025–30.

141. Gardeil F, Barry-Walsh C, Prendiville W, Clinch J, Turner MJ. Persistent intraepithelial neoplasia after excision for cervical intraepithelial neoplasia grade III. *Obstet Gynecol* 1997;89:419–22.

142. Giacalone PL, Laffargue F, Aligier N, Roger P, Combecal J, Daures JP. Randomized study comparing two techniques of conization: cold knife versus loop excision. *Gynecol Oncol* 1999;75:356–60

143. Chan KS, Yu KM, Lok YH, Sin SY, Tang LC. Conservative management of patients with histological incomplete excision of cervical intraepithelial neoplasia after large loop excision of transformation zone. *Chin Med J (Engl)* 1997;110:617–9.

144. Narducci F, Occelli B, Boman F, Vinatier D, Leroy JL. Positive margins after conization and risk of persistent lesion. *Gynecol Oncol* 2000;76:311–4.

145. Felix JC, Muderspach LI, Duggan BD, Roman LD. The significance of positive margins in loop electrosurgical cone biopsies. *Obstet Gynecol* 1994;84:996–1000.

146. Zaitoun AM, McKee G, Coppen MJ, Thomas SM, Wilson PO. Completeness of excision and follow up cytology in patients treated with loop excision biopsy. *J Clin Pathol* 2000;53:191–6.

147. Murdoch JB, Morgan PR, Lopes A, Monaghan JM. Histological incomplete excision of CIN after large loop excision of the transformation zone (LLETZ) merits careful follow up, not retreatment. *Br J Obstet Gynaecol* 1992;99:990–3.

148. Lapaquette TK, Dinh TV, Hannigan EV, Doherty MG, Yandell RB, Buchanan VS. Management of patients with positive margins after cervical conization. *Obstet Gynecol* 1993;82:440–3.

149. Mathevet P, Dargent D, Roy M, Beau G. A randomized prospective study comparing three techniques of conization: cold knife, laser, and LEEP. *Gynecol Oncol* 1994;54:175–9.

150. Bar-Am A, Daniel Y, Ron IG, Niv J, Kupferminc MJ, Bornstein J, Lessing JB. Combined colposcopy, loop conization, and laser vaporization reduces recurrent abnormal cytology and residual disease in cervical dysplasia. *Gynecol Oncol* 2000;78:47–51.

151. Paraskevaidis E, Lolis ED, Koliopoulos G, Alamanos Y, Fotiou S, Kitchener HC. Cervical intraepithelial neoplasia outcomes after large loop excision with clear margins. *Obstet Gynecol* 2000;95:828–31.

152. Lopes A, Mor-Yosef S, Pearson S, Ireland D, Monaghan JM. Is routine colposcopic assessment necessary following laser ablation of cervical intraepithelial neoplasia? *Br J Obstet Gynecol* 1990;97:175–7.

153. Paraskevaidis E, Koliopoulos G, Alamanos Y, Malamou-Mitsi V, Lolis ED, Kitchener HC. Human papillomavirus testing and the outcome of treatment for cervical intraepithelial neoplasia. *Obstet Gynecol* 2001;98:833–6.

154. Strand A, Wilander E, Zehbe I, Rylander E. High risk HPV persists after treatment of genital papillomavirus infection but not after treatment of cervical intraepithelial neoplasia. *Acta Obstet Gynecol Scand* 1997;76:140–4.

155. Jain S, Tseng CJ, Horng SG, Soong YK, Pao CC. Negative predictive value of human papillomavirus test following conization of the cervix uteri. *Gynecol Oncol* 2001;82:177–80.

156. Lin CT, Tseng CJ, Lai CH, et al. Value of human papillomavirus deoxyribonucleic acid testing after conization in the prediction of residual disease in the subsequent hysterectomy specimen. *Am J Obstet Gynecol* 2001;184:940–5.

157. Kucera E, Sliutz G, Czerwenka K, Breitenecker G, Leodolter S, Reinthaller A. Is high-risk human papillomavirus infection associated with cervical intraepithelial neoplasia eliminated after conization by large-loop excision of the transformation zone? *Eur J Obstet Gynecol Reprod Biol* 2000;100:72–6.

158. Kjellberg L, Wadell G, Bergman F, Isaksson M, Angstrom T, Dillner J. Regular disappearance of the human papillomavirus genome after conization of cervical dysplasia by carbon dioxide laser. *Am J Obstet Gynecol* 2000;183:1238–42.

159. Cruikshank M E, Sharp L, Chambers G, Smart L, Murray G. Persistent infection with human papillomavirus following the successful treatment of high-grade cervical intraepithelial neoplasia. *BJOG* 2002;109:579–81.

160. Schmidt C, Pretorius R G, Bonin M, Hanson L, Semrad N, Watring W. Invasive cervical cancer following cryotherapy for cervical intraepithelial neoplasia or human papillomavirus infection. *Obstet Gynecol* 1992:180:797–800.

161. Kalstone C. Cervical stenosis in pregnancy: a complication of cryotherapy in diethylstilbestrol-exposed women. *Am J Obstet Gynecol* 1992;166:502–3.

162. Ferris D G, Ho J J. Cryosurgical equipment: A critical review. *J Fam Pract* 1992;35:185–93.

163. Ferris D G, Crawley G R, Baxley E G, Line R, Ellis K E, Wagner P. Cryotherapy precision: Clinician's estimate of cryosurgical iceball lateral spread of freeze. *Arch Fam Med* 1993;2:269–75.

164. Garamy G. Engineering aspects of cryosurgery. In: Rand R W, Rinfret A P, von Leden H, eds. *Cryosurgery.* Springfield, IL: Charles C. Thomas, 1968:92–132.

165. Gage A A. What temperature is lethal for cells? *J Dermatol Surg Oncol* 1979;5:459–64.

166. Cooper I S. Cryogenic surgery. *NEJM* 1963;268:743–9.

167. Daniels F. Some of the cryobiology behind cryosurgery. *Cutis* 1975;16:421–4.

168. Rubinsky B, Lee C Y, Bastacky J, Onik G. The process of freezing and the mechanism of damage during hepatic cryosurgery. *Cryobiology* 1990;27:85–97.

169. Creasman W T, Weed J C Jr, Curry S L, Johnston W W, Parker R T. Efficacy of cryosurgical treatment of severe cervical intraepithelial neoplasia. *Obstet Gynecol* 1973;4:501–6.

170. Schantz A, Thormann L. Cryosurgery for dysplasia of the uterine ectocervix: a randomized study of the efficacy of the single- and double-freeze techniques. *Acta Obstet Gynecol Scand* 1984;63:417–20.

171. Torre D. Understanding the relationship between lateral spread of freeze and depth of freeze. *J Dermatol Surg Oncol* 1979;5:51–3.

172. Abdul-Karim F H, Fu Y S, Reagan J W, Wentz W B. Morphometric study of intraepithelial neoplasia of the uterine cervix. *Obstet Gynecol* 1982;60:210–4.

173. Ferris D G. Lethal tissue temperature during cervical cryotherapy with a small flat cryoprobe. *J Fam Pract* 1994;38:153–6.

174. Kashimura M. Reparative process of benign erosion of the uterine cervix following cryosurgery. *Gynecol Oncol* 1980;9:334–50.

175. Boonstra H, Koudstaal J, Oosterhuis J W, Wymenga H A, Aalders J G, Janssens J. Analysis of cryolesions in the uterine cervix: application techniques, extension and failures. *Obstet Gynecol* 1990;75:232–9.

176. Rothenborg H W, Fraser J. "Third generation" cryotherapy. *J Dermatol Surg Oncol* 1977;3:408–13.

177. Harper D M, , Mayeaux E J, Daaleman T, Woodward L D, Ferris D G, Johnson C A. The natural history of cervical cryosurgical healing. *J Fam Pract* 2000;49:694–700.

178. Harper D M. Paracervical block diminishes cramping associated with cryosurgery. *J Fam Pract* 1997;44:71–5.

179. Hillard P A, Biro F M, Wildey L. Complications of cervical cryotherapy in adolescents. *J Reprod Med* 1991;36:711–6.

180. Ostergard D R, Townsend D E, Hirose F M. The long-term effects of cryosurgery of the uterine cervix. *J Cryosurgery* 1969;2:17–22.

181. Weed J C, Curry S L, Duncan I D, Parker R T, Creasman W T. Fertility after cryosurgery of the cervix. *Obstet Gynecol* 1978;52:245–6.

182. Townsend D E. Cryosurgery for CIN. *Obstet Gynecol Surv* 1979;34:828.

183. Richart R M, Townsend D E, Crisp W, et al. An analysis of "long-term" follow-up results in patients with cervical intraepithelial neoplasia treated by cryotherapy. *Am J Obstet Gynecol* 1980;137:823–6.

184. Sevin B U, Ford J H, Girtanner R D, Hoskins W J, Ng A B P, Nordqvist S R B, et al. Invasive cancer of the cervix after cryosurgery: pitfalls of conservative management. *Obstet Gynecol* 1979;53:465–71.

185. Beutner K R, Wiley D J, Douglas J M, Tyring S K, Fife K, Trofatter K, et al. Genital warts and their treatment. *Clin Inf Dis* 1999;28:S37–56.

186. von Krogh G, Lacey C J N, Gross G, Barrasso R, Schneider A. European course on HPV associated pathology: Guidelines for primary care physicians for the diagnosis and management of anogenital warts. *Sex Transm Inf* 2000;76:162–8.

187. Simmons P D. Podophyllin 10 percent and 25 percent in the treatment of anogenital warts: A comparative double-blind study. *Br J Vener Dis* 1981;57:208–9.

188. Greenberg M D, Rutledge L H, Reid R, Berman N R, Precop S L, Elswick R K. A double-blind, randomized trial of 0.5% podofilox and placebo for the treatment of genital warts in women. *Obstet Gynecol* 1991; 77: 735–9.

189. Beutner K R, Friedman-Kien A E, Artman N N, Conant M A, Illeman M, Thisted R A, et al. Patient-applied podofilox for treatment of genital warts. *Lancet* 1989;1:831–4.

190. Abdullah A N, Walzman M, Wade A. Treatment of external genital warts comparing cryotherapy (liquid nitrogen) and trichloroacetic acid. *Sex Transm Dis* 1993;30:544–5.

191. Krebs H B. Treatment of vaginal condyloma by weekly topical application of 5-fluororuracil. *Obstet Gynecol* 1987;70:68–71.

192. Welander C E, Homesley H D, Smiles K A, Peets E A. Intralesional interferon alfa-2b for the treatment of genital warts. *Am J Obstet Gynecol* 1990;162:348–54.

193. Eron L J, Judson F, Tucker S, Prawer S, Mills J, Murphy K, et al. Interferon therapy for condylomata acuminata. *N Engl J Med* 1986;315:1059–64.

194. Reichman R C, Oakes D, Bonnez W, Greisberger C, Tyring S, Miller L, et al. Treatment of condyloma acuminatum with three different interferons administered intralesionally. *Ann Intern Med* 1988;108:675–9.

195. Fife K H, Ferenczy A, Douglas J M Jr, Brown D R, Smith M, Owens M L. Treatment of external genital warts in men using 5% imiquimod cream applied three times a week, once daily, twice daily or three times a day. *Sex Transm Dis* 2001;28:226–31.

196. Edwards L, Ferenczy A, Eron L, Baker D, Owens M L, Fox T L, et al. Self-administered topical 5% imiquimod cream for external genital warts. *Arch Dermatol* 1998;134:25–30.

197. Gollnick H, Barrasso R, Jappe U, Ward K, Evl A, Carey-Yard M, et al. Safety and efficacy of imiquimod 5% cream in the treatment of penile genital warts in uncircumcised men when applied three times weekly or once per day. *Int J STD AIDS* 2001;12:22–8.

198. Gilson R J, Shupack J L, Friedman-Kien A E, Conant M A, Weber J N, Nayagam A T, et al. A randomized, controlled, safety study using imiquimod for the topical treatment of anogenital warts in HIV-infected patients. *AIDS* 1999;13:2397–404.

199. Baggish M S. Improved laser techniques for the elimination of genital and extragenital warts. *Am J Obstet Gynecol* 1985;153:545–50.

200. Fife K H. Human papillomavirus vaccine development. *Australas J Dermatol* 1998;39:S8–10.

201. Duncan I D. Cold coagulation. *Baillieres' Clinical Obstetrics and Gynecology* 1995;9:145–55.

202. Semm K. New apparatus for the "cold coagulation" of benign cervical lesions. *Am J Obstet Gynecol* 1966;95:963–6.

203. Staland B. Treatment of premalignant lesions of uterine cervix by means of moderate heat thermosurgery using the Semm coagulator. *Ann Chir Gynecol* 1978;67:112–6.

204. Duncan I D. The Semm cold coagulator in the management of cervical intraepithelial neoplasia. *Clin Obstet Gynecol* 1983;26:996–1006.

205. Gordon H K, Duncan I D. Effective destruction of cervical intraepithelial neoplasia (CIN) 3 at 100° C using the Semm cold coagulator: 14 years experience. *Br J Obstet Gynecol* 1991;98:14–20.

206. Smart G E, Livingstone J R B, Gordon A, et al. Randomized trial to compare laser with cold coagulation therapy in the treatment of CIN II and III. *Colposcopy and Gynecologic Laser Surgery* 1987;3:47.

207. Loobuyck H A, Duncan I D. Destruction of CIN 1 and 2 with Semm cold coagulator: 13 years' experience with a see-and-treat policy. *Br J Obstet Gynecol* 1993;100:465–8.

208. Wright V C. Carbon dioxide laser surgery for the cervix and vagina: indications, complications, and results. *Comprehensive Therapy* 1988;14:54–64.

209. Wright V C, Riopelle M A. Laser physics for surgeons. *Acta Obstet Gynecol Scand Suppl* 1984;125:5–15.

210. Fisher J C. Qualitative and quantitative tissue effects of light from important surgical lasers: optimal surgical principles. In: Wright V C, Fisher J C (eds): *Laser Surgery in Gynecology.* Philadelphia: W B Saunders Company, 1993:73–8.

211. Wright V C, Davies E, Riopelle M A. Laser surgery for cervical intraepithelial neoplasia: principles, and results. *Am J Obstet Gynecol* 1983;145:181–4.

212. Anderson M C, Hartley R B. Cervical crypt involvement by intraepithelial neoplasia. *Am J Obstet Gynecol* 1980;55:546–9.

213. Boonstra H, Aalders J G, Koudstaal J et al. Minimum extension and appropriate topographic position of tissue destruction for treatment of cervical intraepithelial neoplasia. *Obstet Gynecol* 1990;75:227–31.

214. Reagan J W, Patten S F Jr. Dysplasia: A basic reaction to injury in the uterine cervix. *Ann NY Acad Sci* 1962;97:662–7.

215. Przybora L A, Plutowa A. Histological topography of carcinoma in situ of the uterine cervix. *Cancer* 1959;12:268–73.

216. Scott R B, Reagan J W. Diagnostic cervical biopsy technique for the study of early cancer. Value of the cold-knife conization procedure. *JAMA* 1956;160:343–8.

217. Hamperl H, Kaufmann C. The cervix uteri at various stages. *Obstet Gynecol* 1959;14:621–5.

218. Holzer E. Localization of dysplastic epithelium. In: Burghardt E, Holzer E, Jordan J A. *Cervical Pathology and Colposcopy.* Massachusetts, PSG Publishing Company, 1978.

219. Wright V C, Riopelle M A. The geometry of cervical intraepithelial neoplasia as a guide to its eradication. *Cervix* 1986;4:21–38.

220. Wright V C. CO_2 laser surgery for cervical intraepithelial neoplasia. In: Wright V C, Fisher J C. *Laser Surgery in Gynecology: A Clinical Guide.* Philadelphia: WB Saunders Company,1993.

221. Holmquist N D, Bellina J H, Danol M L. Vaginal and cervical cytologic changes following laser treatment. *Acta Cytol* 1976;20:290–4.

222. Bellina J H, Seto Y J. Pathological and physiological investigations into CO_2 laser-tissue interactions with specific emphasis on cervical intraepithelial neoplasia. *Lasers Surg Med* 1980;1:47–55.

223. Lickrish G M. Colposcopy in the management of cervical intraepithelial neoplasia: Problems and solutions. *J Soc Obstet Gynaecol Can* 2000;22:429–34.

224. Larsson G, Grundell H, Gullberg H, et al. Outcome of pregnancy after conization. *Surg Gynecol Obstet* 1982;54:59–61.

225. Anderson M C, Howell D H, Broby Z. Outcome of pregnancy after laser vaporization conization. *Colpos Gynecol Laser Surg* 1984;1:35–9.

226. Baggish M S. High-power density carbon dioxide laser therapy for early cervical dysplasia. *Am J Obstet Gynecol* 1980;136:117–21.

227. Baggish M S. Management of cervical intraepithelial neoplasia by carbon dioxide laser. *Obstet Gynecol* 1982;60:379–83.

228. Dorsey J H, Diggs E S. Microsurgical conization of the cervix by carbon dioxide laser. *Obstet Gynecol* 1979;54:565–70.

229. Bertelsen B, Tande T, Sandvei R, et al. Laser conization of cervical intraepithelial neoplasia grade 3: free resection margins indicative of lesion survival. *Acta Obstet Gynecol Scand* 1999;78:54–9.

230. Hagen B, Skjeldestad F E, Tingulstad S, et al. CO_2 laser conization for cervical intraepithelial neoplasia grade II – III: complications and efficacy. *Acta Obstet Gynecol* 1998;77:558–63.

231. Fevalli G, Lomini M, Schreiber C, et al. The use of carbon-dioxide laser surgery in the treatment of intraepithelial neoplasia of the uterine cervix. *Przegl Lek* 1999;56:58–64.

232. Pearce J A. *Electrosurgery*. London: Chapman & Hall, 1986.

233. Soderstrom R. Principles of electrosurgery as applied to gynecology. In: Rock J A, Thompson J D (eds.). *Te Linde's Operative Gynecology* (8th ed.). Philadelphia: Lippincott-Raven, 1997:321–36.

234. Ferris D G, Saxena S, Hainer B L, et al. Gynecologic and dermatologic electrosurgical units. *J Fam Pract* 1994;39:160–6.

235. Health Devices. ESU electrode contact quality monitors. *ECRI* 1985;14:115–20.

236. Sebben J E. Electrosurgical principles. Cutting current and cutaneous surgery—Part I. *J Dermatol Surg Oncol* 1988;14:29–35.

237. Tucker R D, Schmitt O H, Sievert C E, et al. Demodulated low frequency currents from electrosurgical procedures. *Surg Gynecol Obstet* 1984;159:39–42.

238. Wright V C. *Understanding Electrosurgery*. Houston: Biomedical Communications, 1995.

239. Murdoch J B, Grimshaw R N, Monaghan J M. Loop diathermy excision of the abnormal transformation zone. *Int J Gynecol Cancer* 1991;1:105–9.

240. Wright T C, Richart R M, Ferenczy A. *Electrosurgery for HPV related diseases of the anogenital tract*. New York, Arthur Vision, 1992.

241. Huang L-W, Huang J-L. A comparison between loop electrosurgical excision procedure and cold knife conization for the treatment of cervical dysplasia: residual disease in a subsequent hysterectomy specimen. *Gynecol Oncol* 1999;73:12–5.

242. Baggish M S, Barash F, Noel Y, et al. Comparison of thermal injury zone in loop electrical and laser excisional conization. *Am J Obstet Gynecol* 1992;166:545–8.

243. Wright T C, Richart R M, Ferenczy A, et al. Comparison of specimens removed by CO_2 laser conization and loop electrosurgical procedures. *Obstet Gynecol* 1991;79:147–53.

244. Ioffe O B, Brooks S E, De Rezende R B, et al. Artifact in cervical LLETZ specimens: correlation with follow-up. *Int J Gynecol Pathol* 1999;18:115–21.

245. Messing M J, Otken L, King L A, et al. Larger loop excision of the transformation zone (LLETZ): a pathological evaluation. *Gynecol Oncol* 1994;52:207–11.

246. Montz F J, Holschneider C H, Thompson L D R. Large-loop excision of the transformation zone: effect on the pathological interpretation of resection margins. *Obstet Gynecol* 1993;81:976–82.

247. Krebs H, Pastor L, Helmkamp B F. Loop electrosurgical procedures for dysplasia. Experience in a community hospital. *Am J Obstet Gynecol* 1993;169:289–95.

248. Thomas P A, Zaleski M S, Ohlhausen W W, et al. Cytomorphologic characteristics of thermal injury related to endocervical brushing following loop electrosurgical procedure. *Diag Cytopathol* 1996;14:212–5.

249. Darwish A, Gadallah H. One step management of cervical lesions. *Int J Gynaecol Obstet* 1998;61:261–7.

250. Spitzer M, Chernys A E, Seltzer V L. The use of large loop excision of the transformation zone in an inner city population. *Obstet Gynecol* 1993;82:731–5.

251. Wright V C. Loop electrosurgical procedures for treatment of cervical intraepithelial neoplasia: Principles and results. In: Wright V C, Lickrish G M, Shier R M (eds.). *Basic and Advanced Colposcopy—Part Two: A Practical Handbook for Treatment (2nd ed.)*. Houston: Biomedical Communications, 1995:, 20/1–20/31.

252. Sadek A L. Needle excision of the transformation zone: a new method for treatment of cervical intraepithelial neoplasia. *Am J Obstet Gynecol* 2000;182:866–71.

253. Takac I, Gorisek B. Cold knife conization and loop excision for cervical intraepithelial neoplasia. *Tumori* 1999;85:243–6.

254. Simmons J R, Anderson L, Hernadez E, et al. Evaluating cervical neoplasia. LEEP as an alternative to cold knife conization. *J Reprod Med* 1998;43:1007–13.

255. Kreiger J S, McCormack L J. The indications for conservative therapy for carcinoma in situ of the cervix. *Am J Obstet Gynecol* 1963;76:312–20.

256. Bjerre B, Eliasson G, Linell F. Conization as only treatment of carcinoma in situ of the uterine cervix. *Am J Obstet Gynecol* 1976;125:143–52.

257. Jordan J A. Symposium on cervical dysplasia I. Excisional methods. *Colpo Gynecol Laser Surg* 1984;4:271–4.

258. Kolstad P, Valborg K. Long term follow-up of 1121 cases of carcinoma in situ. *Obstet Gynecol* 1976;48125–9.

259. Berkus M, Daly J W. Cone biopsy: An outpatient procedure. *Am J Obstet Gynecol* 1980;137:953–8.

260. Sturmdorf A. Tracheloplastic methods and results. *Surg Gynecol Obstet* 1916;22:93–103.

261. Helmkamp B F, Denslow B L, Bonfiglio T A et al. Cervical conization: when is uterine dilatation and curettage also indicated. *Am J Obstet Gynecol* 1983;146:893–4.

262. Rubin S, Battistini M. Endometrial curettage at the time of cervical conization. *Obstet Gynecol* 1986;67:663–4.

263. Thompson B H, Woodruff J D, Davis H J et al. Cytopathology, histopathology, and colposcopy in the management of cervical neoplasia. *Am J Obstet Gynecol* 1872;114:329–34.

264. Hovadhanakul P, Mehra U, Terragno A, et al. Comparison of colposcopy directed biopsies and cold knife conization in patients with abnormal cytology. *Surg Gynecol Obstet* 1976;142:333–6.

265. Townsend D E, Ostergard D R. Cryocauterization for preinvasive cervical dysplasia. *J Reprod Med* 1971;6:171–3.

266. Creasman W T, Weed J C, Jr. Conservative management of cervical intraepithelial neoplasia. *Clin Obstet Gynecol* 1980;43:281–5.

267. Larsson G, Alm P, Grundell H. Laser conization verses cold knife conization. *Surg Gynecol Obstet* 1982;154:59–61.

268. McCann S, Mickal A, Crapazano J T. Sharp conization of the cervix. *Obstet Gynecol* 1969;33:470–5.

269. Van Nagell J R, Parker J C, Hicks L P, et al. Diagnostic and therapeutic efficacy of cervical conization. *Am J Obstet Gynecol* 1976;124:134–9.

270. Hester L L, Read R A. An evaluation of cervical conization. *Am J Obstet Gynecol* 1960;80:715–21.

271. Bostofte E, Berget A, Larsen J F, et al. Conization by carbon dioxide laser or cold knife in the treatment of cervical intraepithelial neoplasia. *Acta Obstet Gynecol Scand* 1986;65:199–202.

272. Burghardt E, Holzer E. Treatment of carcinoma in situ. Evaluation of 1609 cases. *Am J Obstet Gynecol* 1980;55:539–45.

273. Ostegard D R. Prediction of clearance of cervical intraepithelial neoplasia by conization. *Obstet Gynecol* 1980;56:77–80.

274. Adelman H C, Hajdee S I. Role of conization in the treatment of cervical carcinoma in situ. *Am J Obstet Gynecol* 1967;56:173–9.

275. Villasanta U, Durkan J P. Indications and complications of cold conization of the cervix. Observation on 200 consecutive cases. *Obstet Gynecol* 1965;27:717–23.

276. Davis R M, Cooke J K, Kirk R F. Cervical conization—an experience with 400 patients. *Obstet Gynecol* 1972;40:23–7.

277. Holdt D G, Jacobs A J, Scott J et al. Diagnostic significance and sequelae of cone biopsy. *Am J Obstet Gynecol* 1982;143:312–5.

278. Killackey M A, Jones W B, Lewis J, Jr. Diagnostic conization of the cervix: Review of 460 consecutive cases. *Obstet Gynecol* 1986;67:766–70.

279. Jafari K, Ravindranaths S: Role of endocervical curettage in colposcopy. *Am J Obstet Gynecol* 1978;131:83–87.

280. Benedet J L, Anderson G H, Boyes D A. Colposcopic accuracy in the diagnosis of microinvasive and occult invasive carcinoma of the cervix. *Obstet Gynecol* 1985;65:551–61.

281. Moore B C, Higgins R V, Laurent S L, et. al. Predictive factors from cold knife conization for residual intraepithelial neoplasia in subsequent hysterectomy. *Am J Obstet Gynecol* 1995;173:361–8.

282. Murta E F, Resende A V, Adad S J, et al. Importance of surgical margins in conization for cervical intraepithelial neoplasia grade III. *Arch Gynecol Obstet* 1999;263:42–4.

283. Claman A D, Lee N. Factors that relate to complications of cone biopsy. *Am J Obstet Gynecol* 1974;120:124–8.

284. Larsen G. Conization for cervical dysplasia and carcinoma in situ: long term follow-up of 1013 women. *Annales Chirugiae et Gynaecologiae* 1981;70:79–85.

285. Lickrish G M. Hysterectomy for cervical intraepithelial neoplasia. In: Wright V C, Lickrish G M, Shier R M. *Basic and Advanced Colposcopy—A Practical Handbook for Treatment (2nd ed.)*. Houston: Biomedical Communications, 1995:23-1 to 23-4.

286. Piver M S, Rutledge F N, Smith P J. Five classes of hysterectomy of extended hysterectomy of women with cervical cancer. *Obstet Gynecol* 1974;44:265–9.

287. Way S, Hennigan M, Wright V C. Some experiences with preinvasive and microinvasive carcinoma of the cervix. *J Obstet Gynaecol Br Commwlth* 1968;75:593–8.

288. Creasman W T, Parker R T. Management of early cervical neoplasia. *Clin Obstet Gynecol* 1975;18:233–8.

289. Boyes D A, Worth J, Fidler H K. The results of treatment of 4389 cases of pre-clinical cervical squamous carcinoma. *J Obstet Gynaecol Br Commwlth* 1979;77:769–73.

290. Saslow D, Runowicz C D, Solomon D, et al. American Cancer Society Guidelines for the early detection of cervical neoplasia and cancer. *J Lower Gen Tract Dis* 2003;7:67–79.

Potential Mistakes That Can Be Made during Colposcopy and Management of Lower Genital Tract Neoplasia

Table of Contents

20.1 Introduction

Performing colposcopy requires unique knowledge and sophisticated skills. Because the processes involved in colposcopy demand more complex cognitive skills than psychomotor skills, a greater risk for assessment and management errors exists. Technical and procedural complications can also occur. Structured training, ample experience, reasonable dexterity, problem-solving capabilities, and sufficient knowledge collectively determine a colposcopist's procedural proficiency.[1] Mastery of all of these areas is required to perform colposcopy effectively and determine an appropriate plan for patient care. Proficiency with a series of four colposcopic steps must be achieved and maintained: *visualization*, which involves identifying normal anatomical landmarks and lower genital tract neoplasia; *assessment*, which involves assessing the extent of disease and selection of biopsy site(s); *sampling*, which involves removing a representative portion of the most severe disease present, as well as tissue from other areas with high potential for containing neoplasia; and *correlation*, which involves correlating the cytologic, colposcopic, and histologic findings to determine an accurate diagnosis and proper patient management.

Colposcopic errors result from ignorance, carelessness, misinterpretation, deviation, or omission of any component of these basic colposcopic processes. By adhering to these 4 colposcopic steps, with the acronym (VASC), untoward outcomes can be minimized. Intentional errors almost always evolve from educational deficiencies, whether in initial training or in continuing education. Judgment errors, whether related to diagnosis or management, occur most commonly. Neglecting the therapeutic triage guidelines increases the chance that improper care will occur. Learning from others' mistakes or recognizing possible traps may minimize problems. This chapter provides insight into potential colposcopic and management errors, and suggests ways to avoid making these mistakes.

20.2 Errors Occurring Prior to the Colposcopy Examination

Many errors, primarily decisional, are actually committed prior to the patient's colposcopic examination. In most cases, abnormal cytology is the reason women are referred for colposcopy. The inherent deficiencies in the Papanicolaou (Pap) smear system of screening are well known.[2] Interpretive errors and lack of consensus are particularly frequent with cervical cytology, especially in cases of minimal abnormality (e.g., atypical squamous cells or ASC).[3]

Cytologic results may either over or under represent the true state of cervical epithelial change (Figure 20.1). False negative Pap smears are particularly troublesome when a high grade squamous intraepithelial lesion (HSIL) or cancer is missed (Figure 20.2). Simple awareness of the difficulty in reaching cytologic agreement among pathologists should prompt the colposcopist to seek further cytopathologic consultation when the preliminary result determined by cytology reports does not agree with relevant clinical findings. This may consist of requesting the initial pathologist to review their findings or consulting with another gynecologic pathologist. The advice or second opinion of pathology experts, when

necessary, may provide a more accurate understanding of difficult, perplexing cases. Colposcopists should never assume that the Pap smear report is always accurate. The Pap smear is an imperfect screening test, the results of which may not agree precisely with the histologic and colposcopic diagnosis. Total dependence on the validity of normal findings from a Pap smear, especially when clinical findings raise suspicion of lower genital tract neoplasia, will invariably lead to negative patient outcomes. Furthermore, when unsatisfactory results are obtained on a Pap smear, the test must be repeated and not ignored. The reason for the unsatisfactory result (obscuring inflammatory cells, lack of endocervical cells, etc.) should be addressed by the clinician. In the case of lack of endocervical cells, a deeper more vigorous sampling of the endocervix or cervical dilation when stenosis is present, will help to increase the yield of endocervical cells with subsequent sampling.

Guidelines have been developed to help clinicians appropriately manage abnormal cervical cytologic findings in women.[4-6] However, guidelines are not always readily adhered to nor easily understood by clinicians.[7] Clearly, clinicians do fail at times to respond appropriately concerning abnormal Pap smear results.[8] Most errant clinicians suffer few repercussions, especially when the underlying cytologic abnormality is minor. Because cervical neoplasia usually progresses at a rather slow rate, cases involving negligence on the part of a provider will likely be discovered before serious abnormalities have evolved if the patient is compliant with normal recommen-

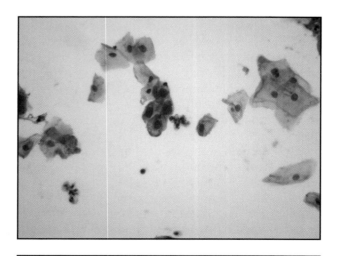

FIGURE 20.1 Cervical cytology revealing ASC-US that was initially diagnosed as normal (Papanicolaou stain, high power magnification). ■

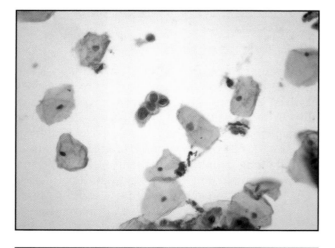

FIGURE 20.2 Findings on cervical cytology that were originally interpreted as negative, but upon review were diagnosed as HSIL (Papanicolaou stain, high power magnification). ■

dations for screening. In contrast, an error of *omission*, such as not evaluating a patient colposcopically after a severe cytologic abnormality has been detected on screening tests may result in significant problems. All clinicians must be able to recognize the absolute cytologic indications for colposcopy; such as a series of Pap smear results indicating atypical squamous cells of undetermined significance (ASC-US), atypical squamous cells, cannot exclude a high grade squamous intraepithelial lesion (ASC-H) or more severe squamous neoplasia, adenocarcinoma in situ, or severe glandular neoplasia. Performing colposcopy when not indicated may lead to overdiagnosis of mimics as neoplasia, with morbidity from overtreatment. Conversely, underdiagnosis may result in missed cancer. In addition to poor triage judgment, lapses in patient tracking (appropriate patient scheduling, recall, follow up, etc) sometimes occur. A patient's failure to return for necessary evaluation or treatment when indicated places her at risk for developing more severe disease (Figure 20.3). When used conscientiously, commercially available computer-based tracking systems for colposcopy (e.g., EasyTrack, DenVu, Tucson, Arizona) minimize unintentional noncompliance.

A failure to appreciate the non-cytologic indications for colposcopic examination also can lead to a multitude of problems. Any cervical or vaginal mass, or persistent ulceration, seen or palpated during a routine gynecologic examination should be evaluated by colposcopy or biopsied (Figures 20.4 and 20.5). Any patient, but especially an older woman, with chronic cervical or vaginal bleeding

that cannot be readily explained, should be referred for colposcopy to rule out the possibility of a lower genital tract malignancy. Unexplained vaginal bleeding during pregnancy also demands colposcopic evaluation after more common pregnancy-associated causes such as abruption and placenta previa have been excluded. Women with vulvar condylomas and vulvar neoplasia are at increased risk for having a coexisting cervical or vaginal neoplasia. Although subject to debate, these women may benefit from a colposcopic examination (Figures 20.6a,b). However, some clinicians consider cervical cytology a sufficient, appropriate alternative. Other indications for conducting colposcopy include obtaining a positive Cervigram or a DNA test result indicating a patient

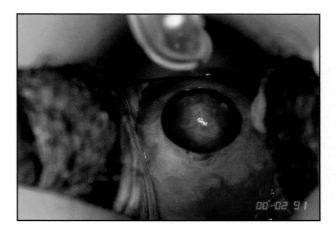

FIGURE 20.4 A cervical mass discovered by palpation and subsequently examined by colposcopy. The mass was a prolapsed uterine fibroid tumor that was soon passed by the patient.

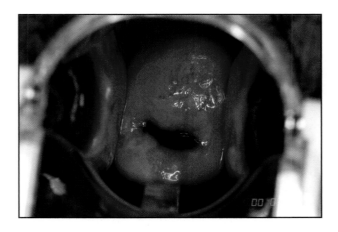

FIGURE 20.3 This 35-year-old woman failed to return for treatment of her cervix after a cervical biopsy indicated the presence of CIN 3. She presented 3 years later with cervical cancer, which can be seen here on the anterior lip of the cervix at the 2 o'clock position.

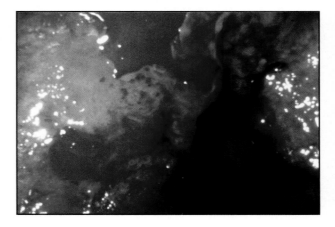

FIGURE 20.5 A cervical ulceration associated with an occult cancer.

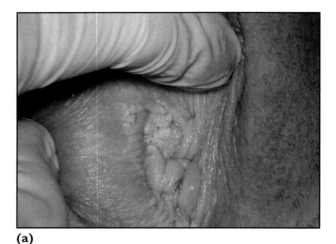

(a)

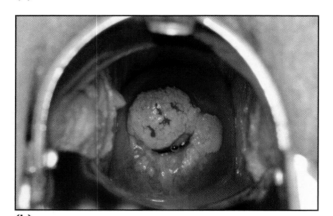

(b)

FIGURES 20.6a,b During a routine annual examination, condylomas were noted on this young woman's vulva **(a)**. Her Pap smear was interpreted as satisfactory and within normal limits. However, a colposcopic examination done later because of a palpable cervical mass revealed this very large cervical lesion **(b)**.

has high-risk human papillomavirus (HPV).[9] The positive HPV test result may merely indicate the patient has a lower genital tract infection, which is likely to resolve spontaneously without intervention or formation of an invasive cancer. However, HPV tests are extremely effective at identifying women with cancer or cancer precursors. Failure to respond by ordering a colposcopic examination could potentially lead to disastrous consequences. Even though most women exposed to DES in utero have already been identified, and at a minimal age of 30 years are likely to have fully mature transformation zones, colposcopic examination remains the foundation for appropriate assessment of these patients, along with conducting a pelvic examination and serial cervico-vaginal cytology.

20.3 Errors during the Colposcopy Examination

20.3.1 Visualization errors

20.3.1.1 Causes of poor visualization

The initial step in conducting a colposcopic examination is establishing proper visualization of the pertinent anatomy of the lower genital tract. The effectiveness of the remainder of the examination is ultimately contingent upon this important step. That which is not seen cannot be diagnosed. Diagnostic errors can occur when blood, debris, mucus, discharge, or chemicals obscure cervical or vaginal lesions or when other parts of the anatomy obstruct the colposcopist's view. Consequently, the lesions are not identified, visually inspected, or biopsied. Therefore, attempts must be made to remove, reposition, modify, or otherwise control anything that may cause the colposcopist's view to be obstructed.

Bleeding Traumatic bleeding points, occurring de novo or induced inadvertently by minor trauma, may be controlled by applying firm pressure with a cotton swab. Hemostasis may be more difficult to achieve in women with acute cervicitis or advanced cancer. Care must be exercised when using hemostatic agents (Monsel's paste and silver nitrate sticks) that can obscure proper visualization of surrounding features. Yet, when used carefully following biopsy, these agents curtail hemorrhage that may obscure other areas of colposcopic interest. Moistening cotton swabs before using them to maneuver the cervix can prevent bleeding (Figure 20.7). Using cotton balls or swabs to apply acetic acid to the cervix also minimizes trauma. Avoid using gauze pads, which can be abrasive. Using a scouring or rotary motion with a dry cotton swab against columnar epithelium can cause bleeding and also should be avoided.

Mucus, debris, and discharge Cervical mucus can be thin and watery or thick and cloudy depending on the phase of the patient's menstrual cycle. The latter type of mucus may especially hinder visualization. Thick, opaque mucus can be removed, pushed to the side, or positioned deeper within the endocervical canal using a very small cotton swab. Endocervical mucus can also be removed using a cytobrush®; however, this frequently causes bleeding. Debris or discharge can be gently removed with a large cotton swab.

Prolapsing vaginal walls In pregnant, elderly, or obese patients, laxity of vaginal tissue may cause the sidewalls to protrude laterally between the speculum

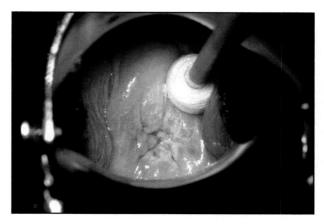

FIGURE 20.7 Large moistened cotton swab used to atraumatically maneuver the cervix.

blades. Prolapsing vaginal sidewalls can be retracted using a vaginal speculum covered by a condom or the finger from a latex glove (Figures 20.8a,b). A lateral sidewall retractor also works well, but should be used cautiously to prevent pinching from occurring if the sidewall prolapses between the retractor and speculum blades. Small cotton swabs, tongue blades, or forceps also can be used to retract the vaginal walls. A tenaculum is not an instrument typically used during colposcopy because its use traumatizes tissue and may cause bleeding, which would obscure inspection.

Often, gentle manipulation of the vaginal speculum will enhance visualization. For instance, applying a downward pressure against the anterior cervix with the anterior vaginal speculum blade can align an anteriorly oriented ectocervix so that it is perpendicular to the colposcopist's line of sight. In addition, proper illumination from the colposcope's light source is essential for identifying necessary anatomy and disease. Adjusting the light rheostat to maximum, directing the light beam down toward the central axis of the vagina, and opening the yoke of the vaginal speculum as wide as the patient can tolerate are ways of maximizing proper illumination and visibility. Using the colposcope at a low power magnification setting provides greater illumination, depth of field, and field of view than using a high power magnification setting. The external genitalia are also best examined with the colposcope set at low magnification so subtle lesions are not missed. Accumulation of dust and dirt on the colposcope can impair visualization as well. Covering the colposcope when it is not in use and routinely cleaning it will help to maintain dust free lenses and eyepieces.

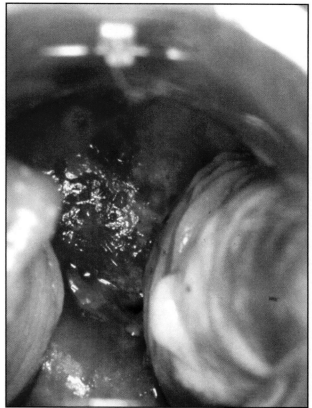

(a)

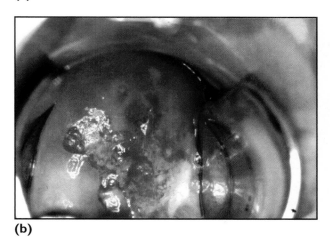

(b)

FIGURES 20.8a,b Prolapsed vaginal sidewalls hinder proper colposcopic evaluation of this woman's cervix. Colposcopists should not curtail their inspection if this occurs. Vaginal sidewall retractors help reveal the source (seen at the 3 o'clock position) of her abnormal cytology report.

20.3.1.2 Inadequate visualization of the squamocolumnar junction

A potentially lethal error of colposcopy is to assume the entire squamocolumnar junction has been examined when only a portion has been observed (Figures 20.9 and 20.10). If a woman was referred for colposcopy because of an abnormal result on a Pap smear, but during colposcopy no visible abnormality is found, and the entire squamocolumnar junction (SCJ) cannot be seen, then the source of neoplasia may very well be located within that unvisualized SCJ segment. Every effort must be taken to identify the elusive SCJ section. By opening the vaginal speculum

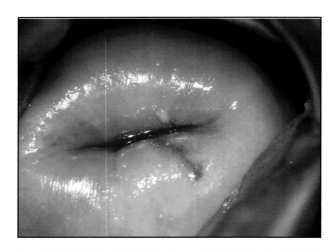

FIGURE 20.9 Examining only the area visible here would result in an unsatisfactory colposcopy examination because the entire squamocolumnar junction cannot be seen. ▬

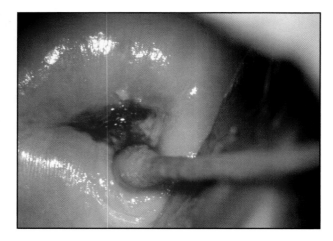

FIGURE 20.10 The same patient in Figure 20.9. Now the entire squamocolumnar junction is seen along with the previously undetected high-grade neoplasia located at the 3 o'clock position. ▬

blades in both planes as widely as the patient can tolerate, the resulting cervical eversion should allow the hidden areas of the SCJ to be inspected. If this step does not permit adequate visualization of the SCJ, the vagina may be gently forced open by applying pressure to the vaginal fornices or directly on the ectocervix in opposing directions using moistened cotton swabs. As a last resort, a closed endocervical speculum or forceps can be placed gently within the canal, then carefully opened to permit viewing. These instruments should be used cautiously since the thin, fragile columnar epithelium can be easily sheared, resulting in bleeding, which will obscure visibility.

Endocervical canal bleeding significantly compromises inspection of an area that is already difficult to examine. As described above in the section on bleeding, tamponade with a cotton swab moistened with a 5% acetic acid solution will sometimes help if the etiology of the bleeding is only minor trauma. When acute cervicitis or menstruation is the source of the bleeding, it is often necessary to treat and then reschedule the examination. Pregnant women with unsatisfactory colposcopic examinations during the first trimester should be reexamined after 20 weeks gestation when cervical eversion and os dilation facilitate identification of the SCJ.

20.3.1.3 Inadequate visualization of the proximal margin of a lesion

Colposcopists may be unable initially to identify the proximal margin of a lesion that extends deeply within the endocervical canal (Figures 20.11a,b). The same visualization maneuvers described in the previous section can be used to identify the proximal margin of endocervical neoplasia. *Never* assume the entire SCJ or the proximal margin of a lesion can be seen when, in fact, it cannot! By definition, such an evaluation qualifies as an unsatisfactory colposcopic examination. If the woman is elderly and/or estrogen deficient, a 2- to 3-week course of estrogen replacement therapy may make it possible to conduct a satisfactory colposcopic examination about 1 month later. If the woman has sufficient estrogen, and the exact reason for being unable to visualize the proximal margin of a lesion cannot be determined, then the colposcopic examination should be rescheduled for another day or the colposcopist should have a colleague examine the patient.

20.3.1.4 Special situations in which comprehensive colposcopic visualization of the vagina and vulva is necessary

When no lesions can be seen on the cervix of a patient who had an abnormal result on a cytologic smear, the entire vagina must be carefully inspected. Frequently in these circumstances, an occult lesion is found in the proximal vagina near the cervix (Figures 20.12a,b). Vaginal neoplasia may also be the cause of abnormal cytology in women who have an unsatisfactory colposcopy examination (Figures 20.13a,b). Both cervical and vaginal sites must be assessed to determine the location of the disease. The disease may involve only the cervix or vagina, or both locations. The cervix must be gently manipulated towards the opposite side to view the entire vaginal fornix. In most cases of vaginal neoplasia, disease is located in the proximal vagina near the cervix. Use of an acetic acid solution, and

more importantly, dilute Lugol's iodine solution, is necessary for adequately identifying most vaginal neoplasias. Confluent iodine-negative yellow areas represent potential sites of vaginal neoplasia and contrast well with the surrounding mahogany-brown staining of healthy vaginal squamous epithelium.

Visualizing some vulvar lesions may be difficult because of their anatomic position. Identifying vulvar neoplasias and condylomas may be challenging when these are hidden within the urethra, beneath the clitoral hood, protruding from minor vestibular glands, or behind hymenal redundant tissue. Applying a 5% acetic acid solution directly to these areas and using low power colposcopic magnification to inspect them may be helpful. Regular cursory examinations of the external genitalia at the conclusion of

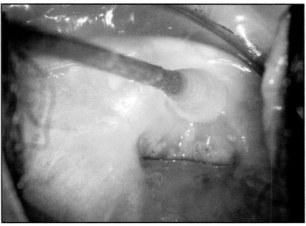

(a)

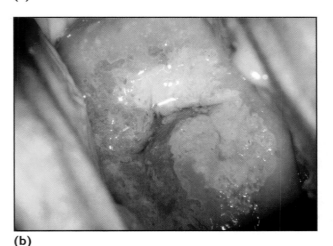

(b)

FIGURES 20.11a,b   A small CIN 1 lesion is seen on the anterior lip of the cervix **(a)**. The lesion extends into the endocervical canal beyond colposcopic view. The patient may have a more severe lesion along the SCJ. In **(b)**, a large 2-quadrant lesion is seen. This examination would also be considered unsatisfactory because the lesion extends within the endocervical canal beyond view. ▬▬▬

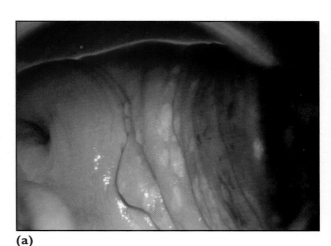

(a)

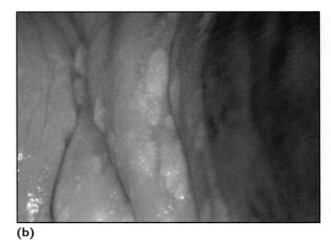

(b)

FIGURES 20.12a,b   The results on this woman's Pap smear indicated LSIL. Although her cervical examination by colposcopy was normal, acetowhite lesions were found on the left proximal vaginal wall **(a,b)**. A vaginal biopsy revealed VAIN 1. ▬▬▬

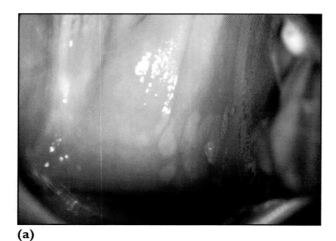

(a)

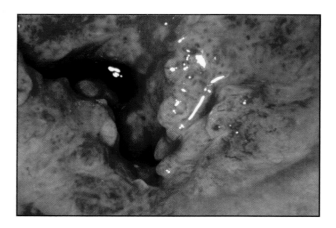

FIGURE 20.14 An occult cervical cancer not readily detected.

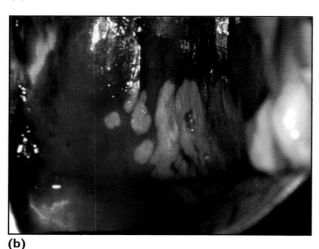

(b)

FIGURES 20.13a,b This woman also had a normal cervical examination by colposcopy. Acetowhite **(a)** and corresponding iodine negative lesions **(b)** can be seen on the left vaginal wall. This biopsy was interpreted as VAIN 2.

cervicovaginal colposcopy may prevent overlooking vulvar neoplasia in these areas. However, casual inspection alone may miss occult disease. Therefore, a comprehensive colposcopic examination of the epithelium of the entire lower genital tract is recommended for minimizing visualization errors.

20.3.2 Assessment errors

20.3.2.1 Developing colposcopic assessment skills

Once proper visualization of the lower genital tract has been achieved the colposcopist must critically assess each area. The process of visualization involves primarily psychomotor skills that are readily learned by most novice colposcopists. In contrast, colpo-

scopic assessment demands cognitive skills that must be learned and then continuously refined through years of experience. Perfection in assessing cervical or vaginal neoplasia is never achieved, but skills can be improved by comparing the final colposcopic impression of a patient with the cytologic and histologic findings from biopsies taken. Only by critical feedback can these important assessment skills be maintained and improved. Routine use of a colposcopic index with standardized assessment categories provides objective criteria for deriving an accurate colposcopic impression. Innately derived colposcopic impressions are more prone to diagnostic error, particularly those formed by beginning colposcopists.

20.3.2.2 Failing to recognize cervical cancer

The most detrimental assessment error is failing to recognize cervical cancer when it is present (Figure 20.14).[10] Such an error may harm the patient if it results in a significant delay in diagnosis. In a retrospective study, Shumsky et al. evaluated the outcomes of women who developed invasive cervical cancer following treatment of cervical intraepithelial neoplasia (CIN). The mean interval between treatment and the diagnosis of cancer was approximately 24 months. Most of the cancers were detected at an early stage. In 13% of these cases, however, Shumsky and his colleagues concluded that the invasive disease may have been present prior to ablative therapy, but simply had not been detected. Potentially disastrous medicolegal consequences obviously await the errant colposcopist who fails to identify cervical cancer that is readily apparent.

Certainly, cancers residing within the endocervical canal can be missed even by experts. However,

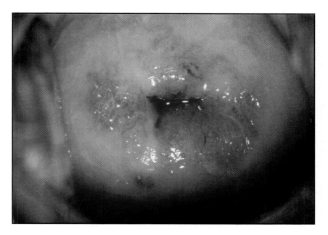

FIGURE 20.15 This atypical blood vessel in a field of normal immature metaplasia is benign but mimics atypical blood vessels of invasive cancer. Cervical biopsy is usually warranted to define the status of the epithelium.

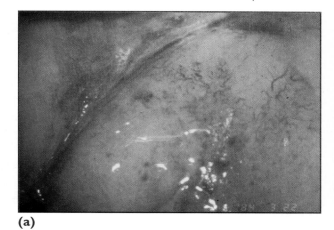

(a)

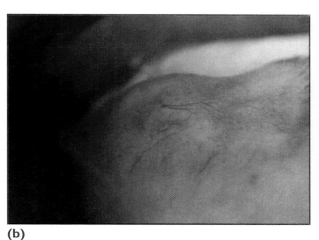

(b)

FIGURES 20.16a,b Atypical blood vessels noted in this elderly woman following radiation therapy for cervical cancer. These vessels are benign and induced by her therapy **(a,b)**. However, discrimination from recurrent disease can be exceedingly difficult.

colposcopists should always look for the warning signs of cervical cancer, even in women who were referred for colposcopy simply because minor cytologic abnormalities were found. Colposcopists fail to diagnose microinvasive and invasive cancer at significant rates of 15.9% and 10.4%, respectively.[11] These errors arise from inexperience, inadequate training, insufficient patient volume, and failure to consult with experts.[11]

As stated previously, the site of the cancer also influences the colposcopist's success in detecting it. Even the most novice colposcopist is expected to recognize atypical blood vessels and to biopsy the involved tissue. However, if the atypical blood vessels are located in an area of very immature squamous metaplasia or are present in a patient who has undergone radiation therapy, even an experienced colposcopist may mistakenly assume the involved tissues are benign (Figures 20.15 and 20.16 a,b). The latter case presents a difficult challenge for all colposcopists. Are the atypical vessels the result of successful radiation therapy or, in fact, could the vessels represent a recurrent cancer? Maintaining a low threshold for biopsying any atypical vessels minimizes errors committed in diagnosing new or recurring cancers.

Similarly, ulcerations thought to be iatrogenic, viral, or bacterial in etiology actually may result from a malignancy. Large vaginal ulcerations caused by a retained tampon can mimic a cancer because of the associated necrosis, discharge, and inflammation. Biopsy, especially when ulcers are of a chronic nature, or careful observation and mandatory reexamination at a later date are reasonable management options for ulcers. However, when they are accompa-

nied by warning signs of cancer, or adjoin intact acetowhite or non-iodine-staining epithelium, a less conservative approach to management should be selected (Figure 20.17).

Both microglandular hyperplasia, which is associated with the use of progestins in oral contraceptives, and decidual tissue, which is seen in women during pregnancy, can be mistaken for a malignancy. In both cases, the women affected are young and the risk for cancer is low. Yet, if in doubt, a biopsy should be taken to eliminate cancer as the etiology for the noted change. Even experienced colposcopists can overlook small high-grade lesions or occult areas of microinvasive cancer positioned within larger low-grade lesions. Establishing a regimen of checking for internal margins will help to reduce the probability of this error occurring.

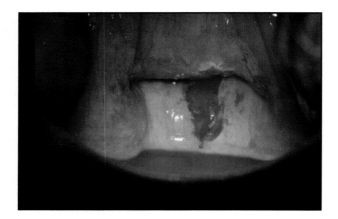

FIGURE 20.17 A large vaginal ulceration and opaque thickened acetowhite epithelium are seen raising the suspicion of vaginal cancer. A biopsy of the area was interpreted as VAIN 3.

One of the most difficult lesions to discriminate from cancer is a large, 4-quadrant, exophytic cervical condyloma (Figures 20.18a,b and 20.19). Generally, condylomas will be symmetrical and papillary in contour. The presence of ulcerations, yellow necrotic epithelium, irregular surface contour, and atypical vessels would indicate cancer. Fine central capillary vessels may be observed within the papillary projections of condylomas when viewed colposcopically at high magnification. Obtaining a representative biopsy for histologic analysis is always necessary to establish the true etiology since the discrimination of condylomas from cancer can be very challenging, even for an expert colposcopist. Discriminating between cancer and benign impostors during colposcopy is even more difficult when the patient has a history of abnormal cervical cytology results.

Insufficient and infrequent application of 5% acetic acid solution to the cervix during the examination will adversely affect the colposcopist's ability to assess disease. Lesions will either not be detected or, if seen, appear to be less significant levels of neoplasia than they actually are (Figures 20.20 and 20.21). The color and opacity of the lesion(s) are important features to note when attempting to correctly identify and classify cervical neoplasia. The use of contrast agents greatly facilitates the colposcopic examination; however, they may also hinder assessment. For example, use of Lugol's iodine solution may help in discriminating between neoplasia and benign tissue changes; however, if it is applied prematurely, the resulting brown and yellow staining may obscure important colposcopic features. Applying topical benzocaine gel or a solution of 10% sodium hypochlorite to the area can reverse unintentional

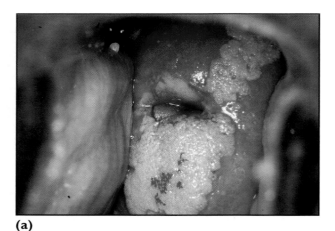

(a)

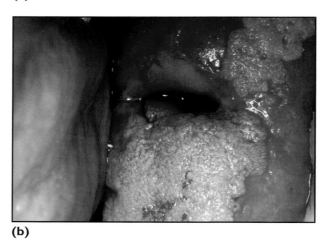

(b)

FIGURES 20.18a,b A large exophytic cervical condyloma that mimics an invasive lesion is seen **(a,b)**. The irregular surface contour is apparent.

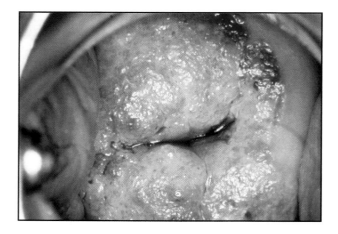

FIGURE 20.19 A cervical cancer that appears strikingly similar to the large condyloma seen in Figures 20.18a,b. Photo courtesy of Dr. Vesna Kesic.

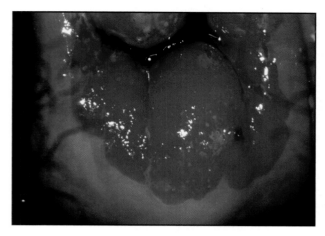

FIGURE 20.20 The cervix of a woman with a HSIL Pap smear report seen with insufficient 5% acetic acid application. Her lesion is not easily apparent.

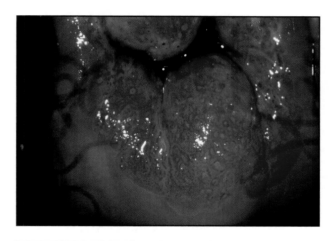

FIGURE 20.21 The same cervix seen in Figure 20.20 after sufficient acetic acid application. Now a high grade lesion can be readily appreciated.

iodine uptake by glycogen-containing epithelium. The green filter accentuates vessel appearance and aids with vessel recognition, particularly by the novice colposcopist. However, the green filter may modify the appearance of the epithelium by darkening the field of view.

Failure to evaluate the true caliber of blood vessels prior to applying an acetic acid solution or as the acetic acid effect is diminishing also may lead to incorrect assessment. In this case, the acetic acid, which exerts a vasoconstrictive effect, narrows the caliber of the vessels, sometimes causing the colposcopist to underestimate the presence of disease. This error can be prevented by applying a saline solution to the area prior to applying the 5% acetic acid solution, or by simply not rushing the colposcopic assessment.

20.3.2.3 Failing to form a colposcopic impression

Finally, the primary goal of the assessment process is to formulate a colposcopic impression. An objectively derived colposcopic impression should be formulated at the completion of each colposcopic examination. Only in this way can a good colposcopist compare their colposcopic impressions with the findings from cytologic and histologic tests. Furthermore, disease may not be properly managed if the colposcopist overlooks the important step of making a clinical or presumptive diagnosis. Many novice colposcopists are uncomfortable initially with their ability to form an accurate colposcopic impression. Yet, failure to derive a clinical diagnosis prevents the colposcopist from determining whether important clinical findings and the overall colposcopic impression correlate with laboratory findings and with histologic and cytologic diagnoses.

Colposcopists should realize that pathologists commonly fail to reach a consensus among themselves with regard to their findings on cytologic smears and, more importantly, their findings on histologic specimens.[12,13] In other words, cytologic and histologic interpretation suffer from subjectivity and human error just as colposcopic interpretation does. Nevertheless, when findings from histology and colposcopy are considered collectively, diagnostic error is minimized. Making the "casual" error of failing to state a colposcopic impression potentially threatens patient management.

20.3.3 Sampling errors

An obligatory component of colposcopy is retrieving representative histologic specimens from lesions following assessment of the most severe areas of change. Procedurally speaking, this phase primarily involves psychomotor skills that can be quickly learned with moderate practice. Biopsying inanimate materials that simulate cervical anatomy and neoplasia may allow the novice colposcopist to gain confidence and become more competent prior to performing a biopsy on a patient.[14] In addition to developing proper technique, proper sampling equipment should be selected and carefully maintained. Biopsy instruments must be kept sharp to minimize the amount of crushing artifact resulting from a biopsy and to insure retrieval of an adequate specimen. Moreover, dull biopsy instruments are probably the main cause of patient discomfort.[15]

It is impossible to collect too deep of a cervical biopsy when using commercially available instruments intended for that purpose (Figure 20.22). However, timid, superficial sampling may result in a

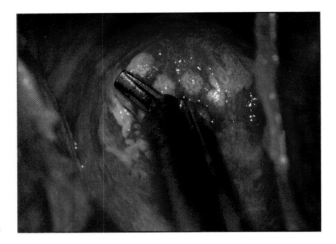

FIGURE 20.22 An adequate cervical biopsy is necessary to properly determine a histologic diagnosis. It is impossible to take too deep or too large of a cervical biopsy using modern biopsy forceps. The risk is from taking too small or too shallow a sample. ▬▬▬

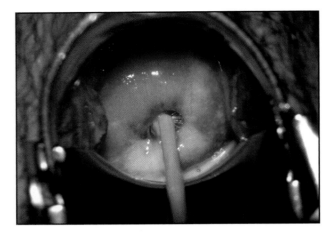

FIGURE 20.23 A Cytobrush® can effectively remove cellular contents of the endocervical canal following endocervical curettage. ▬▬▬

biopsy of inadequate depth and because the basement membrane of the tissue was not captured in the specimen, may prevent a pathologist from properly assessing whether an invasive process exists. Such biopsies are infrequent and usually result from inexperience. A biopsy forceps with small jaws (baby Tischler) may also be more apt to produce an inadequate specimen. A shallow biopsy also can result when the colposcopist samples a lesion located on a flat epithelial surface such as the cervix or, more likely, the vagina. A satisfactory biopsy is more easily obtained when the speculum blades are released slightly, which reduces the tautness of sidewalls and increases tissue folding, allowing the colposcopist to insert the biopsy instrument into the tissue with little resistance. Dull instruments are more likely to obtain a thin, superficial specimen. The specimen may also exhibit "crush" artifact. When dull, the jaws tend to slip from the surface before procuring an adequate specimen. Opening the sharp jaws of a biopsy instrument widely and pushing the cervix backwards until the cardinal ligaments prevent further cephalad motion will prevent the biopsy instrument from slipping.

Occasionally, biopsy specimens will be "lost" immediately after sampling the tissue. Sometimes when the biopsy is taken aggressively, the movable upper jaw of the instrument will force the specimen through the bottom jaw and the specimen retention grid of the forceps. A search of the posterior, proximal vaginal fornix or posterior speculum blade will usually locate the missing specimen. Tissue may also

fall out of the jaws when the closed jaws are accidentally opened prior to placing the tissue into formalin. Using biopsy forceps that have a locking device, which is easily activated by turning a thumbscrew, limits the possibility of losing a specimen.

Retrieving an insufficient amount of tissue from the cervix following endocervical curettage is a more common sampling problem. Using a sharp curette and applying firm pressure when scraping the tissue of the endocervical canal and assuring that all of the contents of the canal resulting from the curettage (i.e., blood, mucus, and cellular material) are evacuated are crucial for obtaining sufficient tissue. It may not be readily apparent upon clinical inspection whether an ample specimen has been obtained because of the large volume of blood and mucus collected. Using a Cytobrush® to evacuate the contents of the endocervical canal after metal curettage may help to increase the number of endocervical cells included in the specimen (Figure 20.23).

Even more important is recognizing when collection of an endocervical specimen is necessary to reach an accurate diagnosis. Experienced colposcopists may forego endocervical sampling when the complete squamocolumnar junction and the entire cervical lesion are visible. However, inexperienced colposcopists should always perform endocervical sampling unless doing so is otherwise contraindicated. Although recent guidelines suggest that endocervical curettage should not be performed universally, colposcopists should still perform some type of sampling procedure on the endocervical canal because this anatomical site cannot be assessed visually.[16] Certainly, if the patient has cytologic evidence of cervical neoplasia, an endocervical curettage must

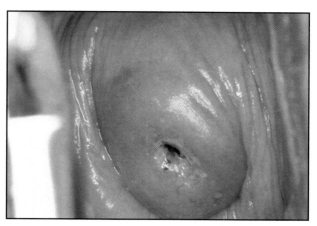

FIGURE 20.24 The colposcopic examination is clearly unsatisfactory in this woman with a HSIL Pap smear report. The squamocolumnar junction is not visualized. Provided that the vagina is free of disease, the source of the cytologic abnormality resides hidden within the canal.

be performed, even if the findings from the colposcopic examination are normal. Moreover, when the colposcopic examination is unsatisfactory because the squamocolumnar junction is positioned within the endocervical canal, endocervical sampling is necessary (Figure 20.24).

Failing to perform endocervical curettage is a common reason for failing to diagnose cervical cancer.[17,18] Cytologic and histologic evaluation of the products of an endocervical curettage (ECC) is very likely to detect cervical cancer if it is present. In one study in which colposcopic biopsy and ECC were performed in 2,304 women, neoplastic epithelium was found in the ECC specimens of 15 of the women, but not found in the colposcopic biopsies from these same women.[19] However, in another study of 763 women with suspected cervical neoplasia, the rate of undetected cancer was not increased by omitting ECC.[20] Nor did failure to perform ECC reduce the accuracy of the colposcopic impression. Nevertheless, glandular neoplasias, even of the ectocervix, are exceedingly difficult to detect colposcopically. Failure to perform an ECC also increases the chance that subtle adenocarcinoma in situ or adenocarcinoma will not be detected clinically (Figures 20.25a–d). Although they are very rare and found primarily in women with a history of prior cervical treatment, when present, skip lesions of the endocervical canal are more likely to be detected by ECC. These separate, usually occult, endocervical lesions are separated from a more readily apparent ectocervical lesion by normal epithelium. The ectocervical lesion may explain the previous abnormal

cytology result. However, the skip lesion may be more severe histologically. All women with a history of prior surgical treatment of the cervix and abnormal cytologic results on a recent test probably should have an endocervical specimen collected. No colposcopist will ever be criticized for performing an ECC, except when contraindicated during pregnancy. It may be prudent to make ECC or endocervical sampling with a Cytobrush® a routine part of the colposcopic evaluation unless the colposcopist is completely sure that the endocervical canal is entirely normal. Samples obtained using a Cytobrush® are more sensitive for detecting neoplasia, while samples obtained using a curette are more specific. Thus, the Cytobrush® may be more useful for collecting specimens for screening purposes and the curette ideal for collecting specimens for diagnostic testing.

Errors made in sampling sometimes result in submitting non-representative specimens for cytologic and histologic evaluation. Preventing such errors depends on the cervix being properly assessed and the site of most severe disease being accurately determined, particularly when a large complex lesion is present. In general, the most severe lesions are usually those located along or closest to the SCJ. Recognition of this principle can help guide biopsy site selection particularly if a large, seemingly homogeneous lesion is present. Therefore, the ideal location for obtaining the biopsy is along the SCJ and usually within the center of uniformly appearing lesions. Routine use of colposcopic indices (e.g., Reid Colposcopic Index or RCI) should help to minimize errors in identifying and assessing lesions. When normal immature metaplasia and cervical neoplasia coexist, frequently the larger benign tissue is mistakenly biopsied because it is more visible. (Figures 20.26 a–c). Failing to biopsy the most severe disease present is perhaps the most critical error that can be made during colposcopy. Occasionally, during the biopsy, the jaws of the forceps will slip from the intended sampling site. Quickly examining the site using the colposcope immediately following the biopsy, before bleeding obscures visualization, will allow the colposcopist to determine whether the desired specimen was obtained. If the site was missed, another biopsy should be performed to assure that the tissue most likely to be diseased is sampled. Mucus, debris, or blood may obscure an area of severe disease. Excessive bleeding also may be encountered when performing biopsies in pregnant women or women with acute cervicitis or cancer. A potential for hemorrhage should not preclude a biopsy when indicated since a rapid hemostatic reaction will curtail bleeding. By anticipating possible complications and having hemostatic agents readily available to control the

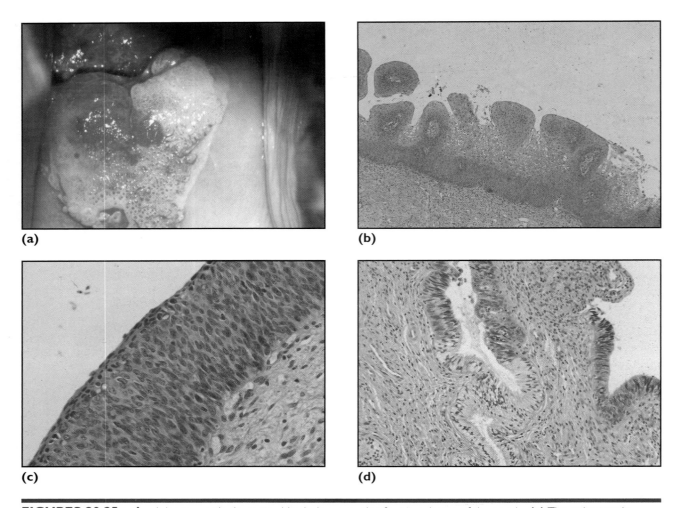

FIGURES 20.25a–d A large exophytic acetowhite lesion occupies four quadrants of the cervix. **(a)** The colposcopic examination was unsatisfactory. Cervical biopsies demonstrate **(b)** condyloma (Hematoxylin-eosin stain; medium power magnification) and **(c)** CIN 3 (Hematoxylin-eosin stain; high power magnification). A loop conization **(d)** also detected occult adenocarcinoma in situ in the endocervical canal (Hematoxylin-eosin stain; medium power magnification).

bleeding, excessive blood loss is unlikely. Occasionally a suture will need to be placed. Limiting the number of biopsies performed because of misplaced concern about the patient's discomfort or over the amount of time required to identify the best sites to sample is not a wise approach colposcopically. Large lesions or multiple distinct lesions may require several biopsies to insure that tissue representative of the disease is obtained. Even aggressive use of biopsy forceps will never remove as much tissue as is removed during cervical conization. Obtaining deep or wedge-shaped biopsies is indicated when cancer is suspected.

Unintentional trauma inflicted while inserting or removing biopsy instruments can also jeopardize care. For example, while using the endocervical curette, an ectocervical lesion located on the external os could be "nicked" accidentally (Figure 20.27). If

the lesion was subsequently sampled, the pathologist would diagnose an endocervical neoplasia when it really represented ectocervical tissue collected with an endocervical sampling device. When a specimen obtained by ECC is found to contain abnormal cells, cervical conization should be performed to properly diagnose (and possibly treat) endocervical neoplasia. Some colposcopists argue that if properly documented, a conization would be unnecessary under this "accidental" circumstance. However, such an assumption probably cannot be substantiated. Sound colposcopy practice dictates that a positive ECC is always reason for concern and dictates further histologic evaluation no matter what the circumstances were in which it was obtained.

Passing the Cytobrush® or curette through a protective straw or tube-like device placed in the cervical

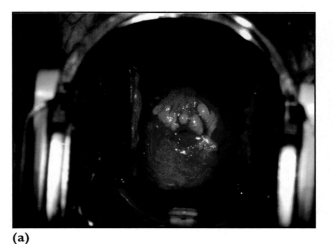

(a)

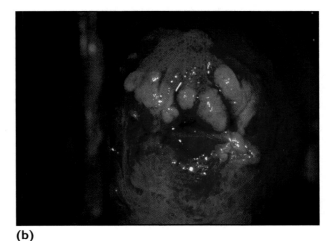

(b)

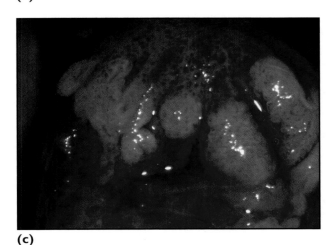

(c)

FIGURES 20.26a–c   Acetowhite epithelium is noted on the anterior and posterior lips of the cervix **(a)**. The cervical biopsy of the posterior lip revealed normal immature metaplasia. A second biopsy of the anterior lip detected her CIN 3. An internal margin demarcating the more proximally positioned CIN 3 from the less severe, peripherally located CIN is clearly seen **(b,c)**. Hence, three different acetowhite areas of different densities are observed.

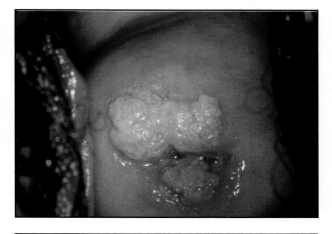

FIGURE 20.27   A cervical neoplasia extending within the endocervical canal that could be easily sampled accidentally by a careless ECC.

os can prevent the colposcopist from accidentally scraping the vagina or ectocervix and contaminating the instrument. Otherwise, endocervical sampling should be carefully performed under direct visualization through the colposcope, and the curette should be withdrawn with the cutting edge turned away from any observed lesions to limit the possibility of contaminating the instrument being used to acquire the sample.

Colposcopy has resulted in a reduction in the number of cervical conizations performed during the past 30 years. However, cervical conization should always be performed when the procedure is clearly indicated to insure a comprehensive evaluation of the lower genital tract. Conization provides an adequately deep specimen for thorough pathologic analysis of the endocervical canal, including the detection of cancer (Figure 20.28). Cervical conization is indicated in the following circumstances: (1) when preliminary histology, cytology, or colposcopy results indicated the possible presence of microinvasion or invasive cancer; (2) when adenocarcinoma in situ has been diagnosed cytologically; (3) when significant cervical neoplasia was identified by preliminary cytologic tests, but during colposcopic examination no ectocervical disease or vaginal lesions were noted that would explain the cytologic abnormality; or (4) when an endocervical tissue sample obtained during a previous examination contained neoplastic cells. As discussed thus far, some sampling errors are caused by inadequate visualization or poor assessment skills; however, the majority of mistakes are the direct result of poor colposcopic technique.

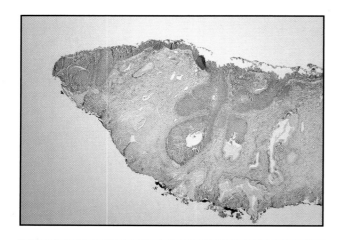

FIGURE 20.28 A histologic section from a cervical conization demonstrating CIN 3 (Hematoxylin-eosin stain; low power magnification). The conization was necessary because of a colposcopic and cytologic discordance. ▬

20.4 Errors after the Colposcopy Examination

20.4.1 Correlation errors

Following careful visualization, critical assessment, and precise, comprehensive sampling, the colposcopist must collectively consider the results from the cytologic smear and histologic specimen(s), along with the colposcopic impression. Ideally, these clinical and laboratory results should "make sense" at this point by being equivalent or very similar in terms of the level of neoplasia or the degree of normalcy found. One level of difference (i.e., CIN 2 and CIN 3, or normal and CIN 1) among the results is acceptable because of the somewhat subjective nature of both pathology and colposcopy. Concordance among these findings either confirms normalcy or confirms the presence of disease. Hence, the optimal management plan may then be pursued with reasonable confidence.

Lack of agreement within one degree of severity (i.e., CIN 1 and CIN 3 or normal and cancer) among cytologic, histologic, and colposcopic results does occur and should not necessarily be considered the fault of the colposcopist, clinician, or pathologist (Figures 20.29a–c). When their findings concerning neoplasia do not correlate within one degree of severity, the colposcopist must determine why discrepancy exists. Imprecise selection of the biopsy site, misinterpretation of pathology results, patient identification errors, or faulty reasoning in formulating the colposcopic impression may lead to diagnostic

disagreement. When this occurs, colposcopy may need to be repeated. Consultation should be sought concerning the cytologic and histologic findings. Initially, the colposcopist should request that the primary pathologist(s) reevaluate the specimens in question. If a second evaluation does not resolve the disagreement, then a second opinion should be obtained from an expert gynecologic pathologist.

In the face of continued disagreement with colleagues regarding findings, clinicians may be tempted to disregard their colposcopic impression. However, the merit of the colposcopic impression, especially if arrived at using a valid colposcopic index, should not be underestimated or quickly dismissed. In fact, doing so might jeopardize a satisfactory patient outcome. Nevertheless, errors may be made in formulating a colposcopic impression. Of particular concern are cases in which the colposcopic impression is that more severe disease exists than is indicated (Figures 20.30a–c). In those cases, the colposcopist should consider reexamining the patient or referring the woman to an expert colposcopist for a second opinion. Many times, reevaluation by another colposcopist and further histologic sampling will help to resolve discordance. As a last resort, the colposcopist should consider conization, since laboratory findings from the deeper layers of tissue obtained by conization might provide an explanation for the diagnostic discrepancy.

Subjecting a patient to therapy prior to establishing clinical and pathologic agreement on a diagnosis risks improperly managing the disease, which will ultimately result in patient morbidity. This is particularly true when only one of several findings suggests the presence of microinvasive or invasive cancer, so the contradictory finding is ignored (Figure 20.31). A pathology report that suggests even the "possibility of cancer" should always be considered seriously and follow-up testing should be diligently pursued, regardless of what the colposcopic impression was.

Likewise, disregarding an unsatisfactory colposcopic examination may eventually lead to horrendous problems for both the patient and clinician. The risk of undetected neoplasia, either premalignant or cancerous, is great, especially when even minor (ASC) cervical cytologic abnormalities are detected. This scenario is common in older women, estrogen deficient women, and women who have had prior ablative or excisional cervical therapy. Women who have previously received cervical radiation treatment present the added challenge of delineating the SCJ and transformation zone. Consequently, the results of the colposcopic examination will frequently remain unsatisfactory and cytology and histology alone must be used to

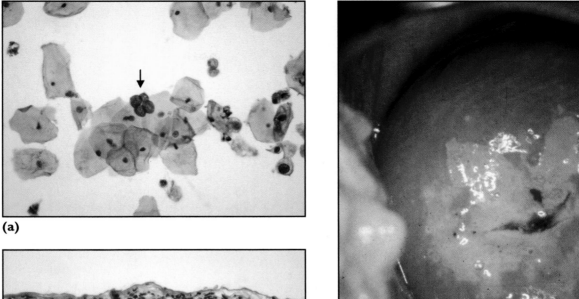

(a)

(b)

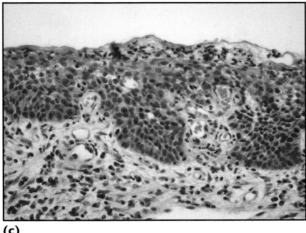

(c)

FIGURES 20.29a–c   Lack of agreement of cytology, histology and colposcopic impression. The cytology **(a)** indicates CIN 3 (Papanicolaou stain, high power magnification), the colposcopy **(b)** was normal but unsatisfactory, and the histology **(c)** was reported as immature metaplasia. (Hematoxylin-eosin stain; medium power magnification). Further evaluation is necessary to determine proper management.

determine appropriate management. However, if ecto-cervical or vaginal disease is observed during colposcopy, additional assessment is imperative. Invariably, women with colposcopic or histologic evidence of neoplasia located deep within the endocervical canal should undergo cervical conization. In such cases, further colposcopic evaluation or histologic testing of specimens from endocervical curettage will not provide a more accurate or specific diagnosis. When evidence of significant endocervical disease is present, the diagnosis ultimately resides in the hands of the pathologist. Management is then usually directed by the histologic results from the diagnostic conization. Because the area biopsied often includes the entire site of diseased tissue, conization is sometimes considered a therapeutic as well as a diagnostic procedure.

20.4.2 Management errors

As stated previously, the procedure of colposcopy consists of 4 unique and sequential steps: visualization, assessment, sampling, and correlation (VASC). From the last step of correlating the cervical cytology and histology results with the colposcopic impression, patient management evolves. The patient's characteristics, relevant history, and personal desires also influence the decision-making process regarding therapy. These factors collectively form the basis on which a proper strategy for patient management of cervical neoplasia is built.

Determining a plan for optimum patient care is usually straight forward and relatively easy; however, it can be intimidating if uncertainties regarding your

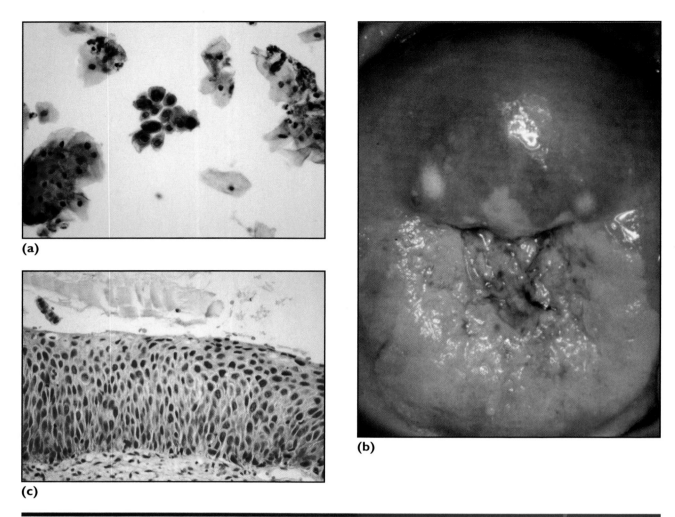

(a)

(b)

(c)

FIGURES 20.30a–c Discordance of the **(a)** Pap smear (Papanicolaou stain, High power magnification), biopsy report and colposcopic impression. A colposcopically visible cervical cancer appears present **(b)**, but the Pap smear was interpreted as reactive vs. ASC-US and the biopsy **(c)** as CIN 2 (Hematoxylin-eosin stain; Medium power magnification). Repeat sampling (wedge biopsy or conization) should help resolve the disagreement. Colposcopic photograph courtesy of Dr. Vesna Kesic. ▬

patient exist, conflicting or confusing data are presented, extraneous influences arise, seemingly equivalent therapeutic techniques are considered, or dilemmas concerning balance of risk emerge. Tailoring management plans to suit the patient when multiple therapeutic options are available requires an extensive understanding of the disease process and of the likely scenarios associated with each treatment option. Furthermore, patient management is frequently a dynamic process since unexpected events may alter the original treatment plans. Consequently, the process of selecting an appropriate management plan may sometimes seem extremely complex. A structured and systematic approach that considers all relevant information optimizes the likelihood of achieving satisfactory patient outcomes.

Prior to embarking upon any cervical treatment, a comprehensive colposcopy examination should

be performed. Normal, large cervical ectropions have been confused by clinicians as representing cervical pathology. Some clinicians consider the beefy red color to represent significant pathology. In the past, a clinician would often diagnose a copious, clear vaginal discharge as "cervicitis" or a cervical "erosion" and perform an ablative procedure without first conducting a colposcopic examination, only to later discover that the patient actually had invasive cancer.[17] Cervical friability may be a sign of acute cervicitis in most cases, but this same inflammatory, necrotic tissue could be caused by invasive cancer (Figure 20.32). A careful colposcopist will biopsy every large cervical wart and review the pathology report prior to making a definitive decision on treatment to eliminate the possibility that a benign-looking finding is actually a malignant imposter.

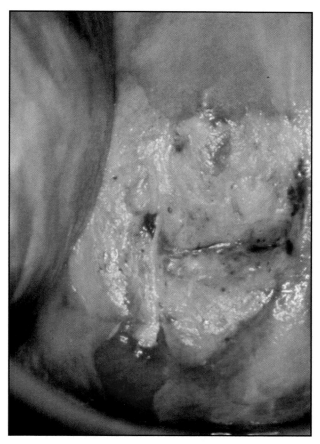

FIGURE 20.31 Regardless of cytology or histology results, a colposcopic diagnostic conization is mandatory for this woman with colposcopic suspicion of microinvasion. The cone specimen revealed less than 4 mm of invasion. Photo courtesy of Dr. Vesna Kesic.

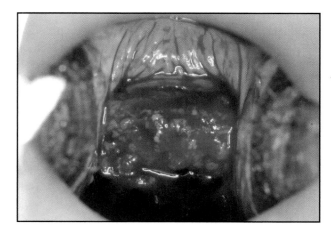

FIGURE 20.32 The cervical friability and bleeding seen on this patient's cervix can be diagnosed erroneously as cervicitis. Instead, this woman was found to have cervical cancer.

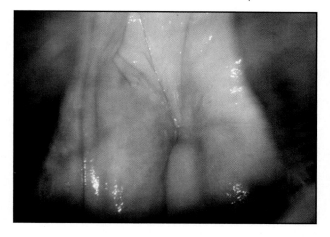

FIGURE 20.33 Complete cervical stenosis following electrosurgical loop conization in a young woman treated for CIN 3. She required further surgery to open the canal to allow menstrual flow and follow-up cytologic sampling.

All colposcopists should be able to properly evaluate at least 90% of patients seen in normal practice. However, a greater level of colposcopic expertise may be necessary to evaluate patients with more challenging conditions. As colposcopic expertise increases, the spectrum of diseases and challenging cases that the colposcopist can effectively manage will also increase. However, during the early learning phase, questions concerning colposcopic technique or management will arise and consultation should be obtained. Pregnant patients, particularly those in the late second and third trimesters of pregnancy, are extremely difficult to evaluate because of normal, hormonally mediated lower genital tract responses to pregnancy (Chapter 12). Many of these physiologic changes can make proper visualization of the cervix difficult. Normal cervical changes during pregnancy, such as the development of decidual tissue and dilated vessels, may have an appearance that mimics that of severe cervical neoplasia. Immunosuppressed patients also present unique challenges, particularly in regard to choosing effective treatment and managing neoplasia, which is notoriously persistent in these patients. Patients who have received prior cervical treatment may have grossly deformed cervices or cervical stenosis, which make performing an adequate evaluation almost impossible (Figure 20.33). Postmenopausal women or women who are estrogen deficient can be challenging to evaluate because of the resulting epithelial changes and anatomical modifications. Women with cytologic evidence of glandular disease are extremely difficult to evaluate colposcopically because of the anatomical location of the neoplasia within the endocervical canal.

Furthermore, glandular neoplasia may be very subtle and difficult to recognize because it does not have the same colposcopic signs as those seen with squamous disease (Chapter 11). Finally, women afflicted with cancer deserve the expertise of a gynecologic oncologist to ensure their care is properly managed.

The triage guidelines for determining ablative versus excisional therapy of the cervix also must be considered prior to embarking on definitive treatment. In review, the guidelines for ablative treatment are: (1) no cytologic, colposcopic or histologic evidence of cancer; (2) satisfactory findings from a thorough colposcopic examination that included full visualization of the SCJ and transformation zone, as well as evaluation of any cervical lesions; and (3) a normal or negative test result on an endocervical sample (obtained by Cytobrush® or curette, when necessary). If these guidelines are met, an ablative therapy (cryotherapy, laser ablation, etc) may be performed. Otherwise, excisional treatment or further diagnostic assessment by cervical conization must be done. Failing to perform conization in patients who have a positive test result from a specimen obtained by ECC risks failing to diagnose cancer.[18,19] Ablation performed for the wrong indication risks providing only partial treatment, or in the case of cancer, improper therapy. Thus, invasive cancer must be ruled out during the preliminary colposcopic evaluation and prior to performing any definitive treatment.

Recent studies have clearly demonstrated that women who underwent only conservative cytologic follow-up after receiving a Pap smear report indicating ASC-US or low grade squamous intraepithelial lesions (LSIL), and who later have a follow-up Pap smear result that again indicates ASC-US or more severe disease, should be examined by colposcopy (Figure 20.34).[21] A triage threshold that dictated only those women in whom LSIL or more severe disease was identified by a repeat Pap smear should undergo colposcopy would miss a significant number of women with CIN 2 or 3. Therefore, if a clinician wishes to initially monitor these women cytologically instead of performing colposcopy, then a low threshold of cytologic abnormality (ASC) should be established for referral to more comprehensive colposcopic examination.

Cervical biopsy allows the colposcopist to obtain a tissue diagnosis prior to initiating therapy. In an evaluation of the treatment histories of patients discovered to have cervical cancer following therapy, a frequent error that was identified was treating the cervix based only on the results of cytology and the findings from a colposcopic examination.[17] Essentially, the purpose of performing a cervical biopsy and the subsequent histology is to define the severity of disease and determine the presence of cancer whenever possible. As stated earlier, using ablative

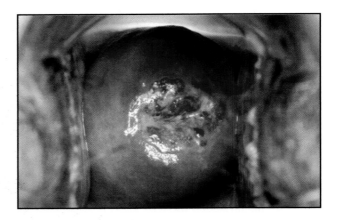

FIGURE 20.34 The cervix of a 24-year-old woman who had an initial ASC-US Pap smear report and repeat cytologic sampling 6 months later that also indicated ASC-US. Adherence to the ASC-US triage threshold prevented her clinician from overlooking this subtle high grade cervical lesion.

therapy to treat cervical disease without first obtaining biopsies and a histology report is contraindicated. Some suggest that the biopsy and treatment can be performed in a single visit if a high suspicion of severe preinvasive disease exists. However, this "see and treat" approach to the management of cervical neoplasia risks administering inappropriate treatment. Most of the studies that have evaluated outcomes in women who have undergone electrosurgical loop excision procedures have found that occult microinvasive or invasive cancer is later diagnosed in 1% to 2% of the patients.[22,23] Conversely, as many as 35% to 40% of these women are subsequently found to have normal histology, further suggesting that a "see and treat" approach is not in the patient's best interest. Most of these cases occur when a woman with a mildly abnormal Pap smear is referred to a colposcopist who, upon examination of the patient, subsequently interprets normal immature squamous metaplasia as significant neoplasia (Figure 20.35). When a biopsy of what appears to be a high-grade lesion is performed during a colposcopic examination of a woman who previously received cytologic results indicating high-grade disease, in most cases the cytologic results will confirm that the lesion contains high-grade disease. Given this scenario, only 5% of the patients who fall victim to the "see and treat" approach will be diagnosed as normal. Certainly, there may be advantages to diagnosing and treating the patient in one visit, but potentially serious errors can result. This approach to treatment might be appropriate if conducted by an expert colposcopist and if patient noncompliance, excessive costs, or limited medical access are signifi-

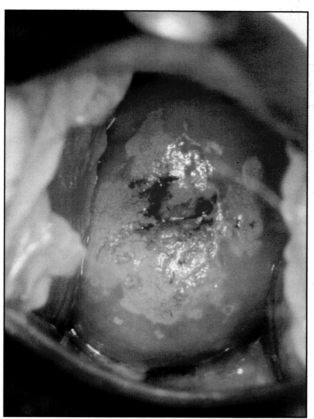

FIGURE 20.35   Colpophotograph of a woman's cervix that was managed by the "see and treat" approach. The histologic diagnosis of normal immature metaplasia means this woman was treated inappropriately. ▬

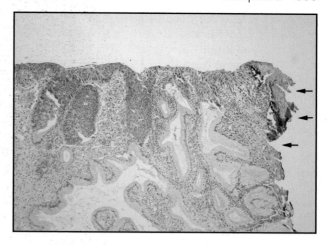

FIGURE 20.36   A positive endocervical margin is noted in this conization specimen (Hematoxylin-eosin stain; medium power magnification. The patient should have serial endocervical sampling postoperatively to identify residual disease that occurs in 15% to 20% of these cases. ▬

cant enough issues to justify combining therapy with a single colposcopic evaluation.

Similarly, a hysterectomy should not be performed prior to conducting a preliminary evaluation. Among 148 women who underwent a simple hysterectomy in the presence of undiagnosed invasive cervical cancer, in 21%, a previously obtained abnormal Pap smear or cervical biopsy result had been inadequately evaluated, in 11%, a grossly apparent cancer had been overlooked, and in 2%, a gross cervical lesion had not been biopsied.[24] Preoperative colposcopy would have prevented the majority of these errors.

Several other treatment errors are more common than most colposcopists believe. During any cervical treatment, the entire abnormal transformation zone must be treated and not just the cervical lesion(s). In addition to the observed lesion(s), the surrounding normal-appearing tissue must be removed or ablated to assure that all of the cancerous and precancerous cells are destroyed. Then new, healthy tissue can replace the diseased epithelium. Incomplete treatment of the abnormal transformation zone risks leav-

ing residual disease that may later give rise to neoplasia. Of equal importance, the treatment should penetrate to a depth that is sufficient to eliminate all neoplasia located on the surface tissue of the endocervical canal or positioned deeply within gland clefts. Because gland clefts are located radially around the endocervical canal, the width of the excision must be sufficient (a minimum of 10 mm) as well. Performing a narrow conization risks leaving behind a "positive" margin and residual disease (Figure 20.36).

Women with CIN 1 may be managed in a variety of ways including by observation of findings from serial cytologic sampling, by periodic colposcopic examination, and by treatment. However, CIN 2/3 has a real risk of progressing to cervical cancer; thus, women with this stage of disease require immediate treatment. There is always a risk that residual disease is present following ablative treatment of the cervix. Disease may remain in the periphery of the treated area or, more commonly, deep within gland clefts because the ablation was not sufficiently deep. If cytologic, histologic, and colposcopic evidence of significant cervical neoplasia is found in a woman who has undergone ablative therapy, an excisional approach to treatment should then be used to clearly define the extent and nature of disease (Figures 20.37a,b). In such cases, the risk of occult cancer is real; therefore, further treatment must be performed to rule out the presence of a malignancy and provide information concerning the margins of excision.

Comprehensive patient follow-up is almost as important as the primary treatment of disease. No form of cervical treatment, including hysterectomy, guarantees a 100% cure rate for lower genital tract neoplasia. Therefore, postoperative cytology and colposcopy are obligatory to detect residual disease, which is present in an average of 5% to 15% of women following treatment of CIN. This rate is even greater among women with immunodeficiency disease and those who smoke tobacco products.[22] Obviously, postoperative follow-up is also mandatory for women with cervical cancer since lower cure rates would be expected, depending on the stage to which the disease had progressed before detection. Patient noncompliance challenges the effectiveness of otherwise rational follow-up strategies. Therefore, the importance of careful follow-up must be effectively communicated to women prior to leaving the clinic following therapy. Even if recurrent disease is not detected in a patient after an intensive, long-term

follow-up period, annual screening with Pap smears will still be necessary for the remainder of her life. Her risk of developing other neoplasias in the lower genital tract is greater than that for women in the general population. Tracking systems help to monitor and limit the frequency of subsequent "no shows" (Figures 20.38a,b). Whether cytology alone is a sufficient means of screening during the immediate follow-up period is subject to debate. Most colposcopists consider at least one posttreatment colposcopic examination in addition to more frequent cytologic smears to be essential for providing adequate care.

Errors occur in colposcopy and the management of women with lower genital tract neoplasia. The wise clinician must be aware of these potential pitfalls so poor outcomes may be minimized.

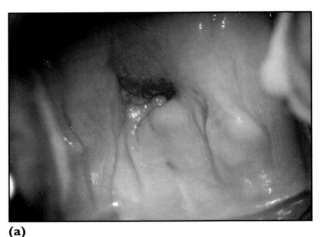

(a)

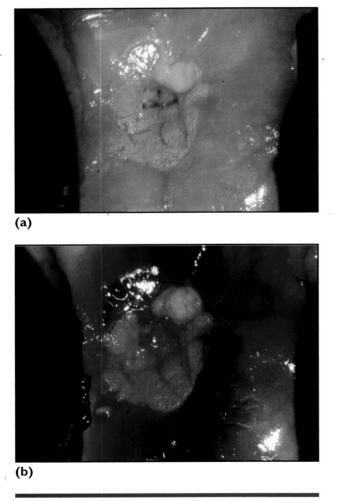

(a)

(b)

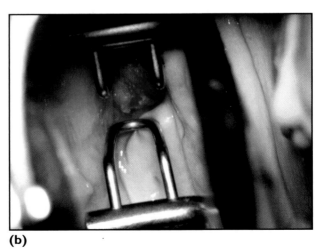

(b)

FIGURES 20.37a,b   Residual CIN 2 identified 8 months following cryotherapy **(a,b)**. An excisional treatment modality would be preferred for this circumstance.

FIGURES 20.38a,b   Woman lost to follow up for 2 years following cervical treatment by electrosurgical loop excision. A high grade cervical lesion within the endocervical canal can be seen using the endocervical speculum **(a,b)**.

References

1. Ferris D G, Miller N M. Colposcopic accuracy in a residency program: Defining competency and proficiency. *J Fam Pract* 1993;36:515–20.

2. Koss L G. The Papanicolaou test for cervical cancer detection. *JAMA* 1989;261:737–43.

3. Sherman M E, Schiffman M H, Lorincz A T, et al. Toward objective quality assurance in cervical cytopathology: Correlation of cytopathologic diagnosis with detection of high risk Human papillomavirus types. *Am J Clin Pathol* 1994;102:182–7.

4. Kurman R J, Henson D E, Herbst A L, Noller K L, Schiffman M H. Interim guidelines for management of abnormal cervical cytology. *JAMA* 1994;271:1866–9.

5. Wright T C, Cox J T, Massad L S, Carlson J, Twiggs L B, Wilkinson E J. 2001 Consensus guidelines for the management of women with cervical intraepithelial neoplasia. *J Lower Genital Tract Dis* 2003;7:154–67.

6. Wright T C, Cox J T, Massad L S, Twiggs L B, Wilkinson E J. 2001 Consensus guidelines for the management of women with cervical cytologic abnormalities. *JAMA* 2002;287:2120–9.

7. Titus K. Abnormal Pap smears, ASCUS still ob/gyn puzzle. *JAMA* 1996;276:1014–6.

8. Ferris D G, Miller M D, Wagner P, Walaitis E, Lawler F H. Clinical decision making following abnormal Papanicolaou smear reports. *Fam Pract Res J* 1993;13:343–53.

9. Ferris D G, Payne P, Frisch L E. Cervicography: An intermediate triage test for the evaluation of cervical atypia. *J Fam Pract* 1993;37:463–8.

10. Shumsky A G, Stuart G C E, Nation J. Carcinoma of the cervix following conservative management of cervical intraepithelial neoplasia. *Gynecol Oncol* 1994;53:50–4.

11. Benedet J L, Anderson G H, Boyes D A. Colposcopic accuracy in the diagnosis of microinvasive and occult invasive carcinoma of the cervix. *Obstet Gynecol* 1985;65:557–62.

12. Stoler M H, Schiffman M. Interobserver reproducibility of cervical cytologic and histologic interpretations: realistic estimates from the ASCUS-LSIL triage study. *JAMA* 2001;285:1500–5.

13. Ismail S M, Colclough A B, Dinnen J S, et al. Observer variation in histopathological diagnosis and grading of cervical intraepithelial neoplasia. *BMJ* 1989;298:707–10.

14. Ferris D G, Waxman A G, Miller N M. Colposcopy and cervical biopsy educational training models. *Fam Med* 1994;26:30–5.

15. Ferris D G, Harper D M, Callahan B, et al. The efficacy of topical benzocaine gel in providing anesthesia prior to cervical biopsy and endocervical curettage. *J Low Gen Tract Dis* 1997;1:221–6.

16. Cox J T. ASCCP Practice Guidelines: Endocervical curettage. *J Low Gen Tract Dis* 1997;1:251–6.

17. Townsend D E, Richart R M. Diagnostic errors in colposcopy. *Gynecol Oncol* 1981;12:S259–S264.

18. Townsend D E, Richart R M, Marks E, Nielsen J. Invasive cancer following outpatient evaluation and therapy for cervical disease. *Obstet Gynecol* 1981;57:145–9.

19. Hatch K D, Shingleton H M, Orr J W, Gore H. Soong S J. Role of endocervical curettage in colposcopy. *Obstet Gynecol* 1985;65:403–8.

20. Swan R W. Evaluation of colposcopic accuracy without endocervical curettage. *Obstet Gynecol* 1979;53:680–4.

21. Ferris D G, Wright T C, Litaker M S. Triage of women with ASCUS and LSIL on Pap smear reports: Management by repeat Pap smear, HPV DNA testing, or colposcopy? *J Fam Pract* 1998;46:125–34.

22. Ferris D G, Hainer B L, Pfenninger J L, Zuber T J, DeWitt D E, Line R L. Electrosurgical loop excision of the cervical transformation zone: The experience of family physicians. *J Fam Pract* 1995;41:337–44.

23. Spitzer M, Chernys A E, Seltzer V L. The use of large-loop excision of the transformation zone in an inner-city population. *Am J Obstet Gynecol* 1993;82:731–5.

24. Roman L D, Morris M, Eifel P J, Burke T W, Gershenson D M, Wharton J T. Reasons for inappropriate simple hysterectomy in the presence of invasive cancer of the cervix. *Obstet Gynecol* 1992;79:485–9.

Glossary

Ablation (laser ablation): A surgical procedure that removes tissue by vaporization. No tissue specimen is submitted for histological review. Cryotherapy is also an ablative-type surgery.

Acantholysis: Abrupt separation of the epidermal cells, which results in a bullous lesion (blister).

Acanthosis: Thickening of the vulvar epidermis, specifically due to lengthening and broadening of the rete pegs.

Acetic acid: A 3% to 5% acidic solution (e.g., vinegar) that enhances the detection of anogenital neoplasia during colposcopy.

Adenocarcinoma: Cancer of the glandular (columnar) cells. In the cervix, adenocarcinomas arise in the endocervical canal, but can represent cancers of the endometrium, fallopian tube, or ovary metastatic to the cervix. Endocervical adenocarcinomas can be multifocal and can originate anywhere along the endocervical canal.

Adenocarcinoma in situ (AIS): An abnormal glandular neoplasia (severe dysplasia of columnar epithelium) characterized by architecturally normal glands with cells that are cytologically abnormal. The basement membrane is intact. The majority of AIS is confined to the transformation zone. However, up to 20% of these lesions will be multifocal.

Adenosis: The presence of glandular cells in the vagina. This process is most often seen in connection with in-utero diethylstilbestrol (DES) exposure but also occurs in the normal vagina, often after ablative or topical (5-FU) therapy.

Atrophy: A condition whereby the number of squamous cell layers is decreased and immature squamous cells predominate. Usually seen in women with decreased levels of the hormone estrogen (postmenopausal state).

Atypical cells: Cells that have an altered appearance from normal. *Atypical squamous cells of undetermined significance (ASC-US, previously ASCUS)* are squamous cells that have altered morphologic features resulting in an unclear impression as to how they might behave, although, in most cases, they are equivalent to a low-grade squamous intraepithelial lesion. *Atypical squamous cells, cannot exclude a high-grade squamous intraepithelial lesion (ASC-H)* are altered immature squamous cells that have features suggesting a high-grade dysplasia. *Atypical glandular cells* (AGC, previously AGUS) are altered glandular cells with morphologic features that suggest a glandular cell abnormality such as adenocarcinoma in situ.

Atypical Squamous Cells of Undetermined Significance/Low-Grade Squamous Intraepithelial Lesion Triage Study (ALTS): A large National Cancer Institute-sponsored, multisite study designed to determine the best way to triage women with minimally abnormal cytologic results.

Basement membrane: The barrier that separates the surface epithelial cells from the underlying stroma or connective tissue.

Carcinoma in situ: The traditional term for a premalignant lesion defined by a replacement of the entire surface epithelium by dysplastic cells. The basement membrane remains intact. In squamous lesions, carcinoma in situ is the equivalent of a cervical intraepithelial neoplasia 3 or, using cytology terminology, a high-grade squamous intraepithelial lesion.

Cervical incompetence: Congenital or iatrogenically-induced injury to the cervix resulting in abortion or premature delivery.

Cervical Intraepithelial Neoplasia (CIN):
Evidence of abnormal squamous epithelial cell growth; a histologic grading system for cervical dysplasia. CIN is graded depending on the amount of abnormal proliferation. CIN 1 is equivalent to mild dysplasia; CIN 2 is equivalent to moderate dysplasia; and, CIN 3 incorporates severe dysplasia and carcinoma in situ.

Cervical stenosis: A narrowed cervical os (< 3 mm) usually secondary to a previous surgical procedure. In some cases, obstruction may be complete. Increased depth of surgery and lack of estrogen are risk factors.

Cervicitis: Inflammation of the cervix, usually chronic in nature, and most often seen in the region of the transformation zone. Although usually nonspecific, certain types may be associated with particular organisms (follicular cervicitis and Chlamydia trachomatis).

Cervix: The inferior extension of the uterus, which is divided into two portions: the lower portion (portio or vaginal cervix) that can be visualized after speculum placement, and the upper or supravaginal cervix that extends from the vaginal attachment to the lower uterine segment.

Clinical Laboratory Improvement Amendments (CLIA): Federal regulations that govern how pathology laboratories examine Pap test specimens. The last major revision was in 1988, which now limits the number of slides a technologist can review in a day, and requires that a certain percentage of normal slides be reexamined by another technologist before issuing a final report.

Cold knife conization: The removal of a cervical conical or cylindrical specimen using a scalpel under anesthesia.

Colposcope: An optical instrument or microscope that permits illuminated and magnified examination of the lower genital tract.

Colposcopy: The procedure during which the cervix is inspected using a special type of microscope (i.e., the colposcope) after the application of a dilute solution of acetic acid.

Condylomata acuminata: Also known as genital condylomas or genital warts. These are sexually transmitted lesions found on the surface of the lower genital tract in men and women. They are commonly raised papillae, but can be flat, and are indicative of human papillomavirus infection.

Conization (see cold knife conization): A deep surgical excision of the transformation zone and portions of the endocervical canal using electrosurgery, knife or laser.

Cryotherapy (cryosurgery): An ablative procedure of the abnormal transformation zone using very cold temperatures provided by nitrous oxide, carbon dioxide or liquid nitrogen.

Cytokeratins: Intermediate filament cytoskeleton proteins unique to epithelial cells.

Cytopathology (Cytology): The subspecialty area of pathology that involves examination of individual cell preparations (such as Pap tests) by an individual (cytotechnologist or cytopathologist) with expertise in this area. Individuals undergo postgraduate training and sit for a written examination to obtain special qualification in this area.

Dermis: The underlying connective tissue in the vulva.

Diethylstilbestrol (DES): Estrogen-like compound given to pregnant women from 1940 to 1970 to prevent miscarriage. Since 1970 numerous reports have shown that females with early in-utero exposure to this drug have increased risk for cervicovaginal dysplasias and cancers.

Dyskeratosis: Keratin production within individual immature squamous cells.

Dysplasia: Abnormal growth or proliferation of the surface epithelial cells. The basement membrane, however, remains intact. Dysplasia is graded based on the number or amount of surface cells that are transformed from normal to abnormal. This transformation usually starts in the cells at the base, or basal cells. *Mild dysplasia* implies that the lower one-third of the cells are abnormal; *moderate dysplasia* implies that one-half to two-thirds of the cells are abnormal; and, *severe dysplasia* implies that two-thirds or more of the surface cells are abnormal.

Dystrophy: A term used in the past to identify various vulvar skin conditions. Dystrophy means abnormal nutrition.

Ectocervix (or Exocervix): The area of cervix extending from the external os to the vaginal fornix (recessed cervicovaginal junction), which is usually covered by squamous epithelial cells.

Ectropion: Eversion of columnar epithelium onto the ectocervix.

Endocervical curettage (ECC): A form of histologic sampling performed to evaluate non-visualized areas of the endocervical canal for squamous or glandular neoplasia, and other abnormalities beyond colposcopic view.

Endocervical polyp: Raised growth, usually benign, arising in the endocervical canal from glandular epithelium.

Endocervix: The area of cervix extending from the external to the internal cervical os, which is usually covered by columnar (glandular) epithelial cells.

Epidermis: The layer of keratinized squamous epithelium, usually applied to the vulvar skin. The epidermis is divided into different layers or *strata* (*corneum, granulosum, spinosum, basalis, malpighii*) that reflect different levels of maturity or keratin production.

Epithelium: Cells that line a surface. *Squamous cells* are highly cohesive flattened cells with excellent protective qualities. They are commonly found in exposed areas such as the ectocervix and vagina. Squamous cells are subdivided into different layers (superficial, intermediate, parabasal, basal) based on levels of maturity. *Glandular cells* (columnar cells) are tall, thin, and less cohesive cells found in closed areas. These cells are usually involved in production of sugars and mucoproteins that act as nutritional materials, transport systems, and barriers to bacteria.

Exocytosis: Inflammatory cells in the epidermal layer.

False negative Papanicolaou (Pap) Test: A cytology specimen that is interpreted as negative in a woman who is subsequently found to have a cervicovaginal abnormality.

Hart's Line: The interface between the skin and mucosal surfaces within the vulvar vestibule, located slightly lateral to the vaginal introitus. Hart's line represents the embryologic junction between the ectoderm and endoderm (urogenital sinus).

Histopathology: Also known as *surgical pathology.* The division of the pathology laboratory that processes (performed by histotechnologists) and examines (completed by the surgical pathologist) tissue specimens. Of note is the fact that cytology specimens (Papanicolaou or Pap tests) and histology specimens (colposcopically directed biopsies or loop excision specimens) may not be examined by the same laboratory.

Human papillomavirus (HPV): A sexually transmitted DNA virus that is found in most women with invasive cervical cancer and high-grade cervical cancer precursors. There are over 100 types of HPV, only a few of which cause significant cervical lesions.

Hyperkeratosis: Excessive production of keratin along the skin surface. On mucosal surfaces, the presence of any surface keratin.

Inflammation: A pathophysiologic reaction to injury irritation, or infection, which results in vascular proliferation and an influx of leukocytes.

Introitus: Round entrance to the vagina, bordered by the hymeneal ring.

Invasive carcinoma: Extension of abnormally proliferating (malignant) cells into the underlying connective tissue due to loss of basement membrane integrity. These malignant cells can also have the potential to spread to remote sites distant from the initial invasion. Squamous cell carcinoma represents invasion of malignant squamous cells. Invasive adenocarcinoma consists of malignant glandular cells.

Keratin: An insoluble protein produced by epithelial cells that forms a protective layer over the skin surface. Also an element in hair and nails.

Keratinocytes: Keratinized stratified squamous epithelial cells (e.g., surface cells of the vulva).

Koilocyte: Cell that reflects marked degeneration of a mature squamous cell with a nucleus filled with particles of HPV. *Koilocytosis* is the process of transforming a squamous cell into a koilocyte. *Koilocytotic atypia* or *condylomatous atypia* indicates the presence of the characteristic pathologic features of a koilocyte.

Large loop electrosurgical excision of the transformation zone (LLETZ): Electrosurgical loop excision using a large loop electrode to excise the transformation zone.

Lentigenous or Lentigo: An increase in melanocytes (specialized cells in the epidermal base that produce melanin pigment) that results in a pigmented skin lesion.

Leukoplakia: A white, thickened area of epithelium that is visible before the application of acetic acid. Note: In January 2003, the International Federation for Cervical Pathology and Colposcopy (IFCPC) Terminology introduced the term "keratosis" for "leukoplakia."

Lichenoid: A plaque-like skin lesion that contains a dermal band-like inflammatory infiltrate.

Liquid-based cytology: A cervical cancer screening process in which the cells that are removed from the cervix are transferred to a container of liquid-fixative rather than spread on a glass slide.

Loop electrosurgical excision procedure (LEEP): The removal of tissue by a tungsten or stainless steel loop electrode employing the principles of electrosurgery.

Metaplasia: The transformation from one mature cell type to a different type of mature cell. In the uterine cervix, metaplasia usually involves conversion from a columnar cell to a stratified squamous cell, although conversion from one glandular cell type to another also occurs.

Microglandular hyperplasia: A form of benign gland proliferation that results in sheets of endocervical cells that coalesce to form individual cell spaces and small gland-like structures.

Mosaic (mosaicism):   The term referring to a vascular pattern produced when capillaries in stromal papillae are arranged parallel to the epithelial surface and form a basket-like structure around blocks or pegs of epithelium. Mosaic vasculature appears colposcopically as a red, tile-like, polygonal grid viewed within an area of acetowhite epithelium.

Original (or native) squamocolumnar junction: The point at which cervical columnar and squamous cells meet during fetal life. Following metaplasia-induced migration, it will be known as the new squamocolumnar junction.

Os (internal cervical os):   The opening into the uterine cervix at the upper end of the endocervical canal.

Papanicolaou (Pap) Test: Traditionally known as a *Pap smear*. A screening procedure named after George Papanicolaou, one of the first investigators to describe the removal of cellular material from the cervix and vagina for microscopic examination.

Papillary dermis: Superficial rounded extensions of the dermal connective tissue into the epidermis. The papillary dermis is bordered laterally by the rete pegs.

Papillomatosis: Extension of the papillary dermis, which results in raised epidermal spikes with central fibrovascular cores (papillae).

Parakeratosis: The presence of nuclei in the keratin surface.

Pilosebaceous line: The junction between the hair bearing and non hair bearing vulvar skin, usually located near the interlabial sulcus.

Portio: The segment of cervix that extends into the vagina. The cervix area that is accessible to colposcopy.

Punctation: The term referring to the appearance of single-looped terminal capillaries within stromal papillae of either the original squamous epithelium or the transformation zone. Punctation appears as tiny red dots of variable dimensions usually present within an area of acetowhite epithelium.

Reactive changes: The process of cell change similar to reparative changes (see below). Nuclei of the affected glandular cells are enlarged and multinucleation can occur; nuclear membranes are smooth.

Reflex HPV DNA testing: Approach in which either the residual fluid left over after a liquid-based Papanicolaou test is prepared or a second specimen that is co-collected at the time of cervical cancer screening is tested for HPV when a cervical cytology is diagnosed as ASC-US.

Reparative changes: The healing process of immature metaplastic squamous cells quickly replacing the squamous or glandular epithelia. These cells have larger nuclei than the usual metaplastic cell, with nuclear chromatin being more dense and nucleoli more prominent.

Reserve cells: A single layer of undifferential cells that form beneath exposed columnar cells. Reserve cells represent the initial step in the process of squamous metaplasia.

Rete pegs: Rounded extensions of the basal portion of the vulvar epidermis.

Rugae: Small transverse ridges covering the surface of the vagina, not apparent after childbirth and during the postmenopausal period.

Satisfactory colposcopy: Defined as when the entire transformation zone (360° of columnar epithelium, squamous epithelium, and the current SCJ) can be visualized. Additionally, if a cervical lesion is present, the entire lesion to include the distal and proximal margins, must be visualized.

Schiller's stain: The iodine test for nongylcogen-containing areas of the vagina and cervix, which may be the site of early carcinoma. Very similar to Lugol's iodine solution now more commonly used during colposcopy.

Spongiosis: Epidermal edema, characterized by separation of individual keratocytes.

Squamocolumnar junction (SCJ) (see also original squamocolumnar junction): The area where the stratified squamous and columnar cells meet. An area of squamous metaplasia is located at this cellular interface.

Squamous Intraepithelial Lesion (SIL): A cytopathology term used (as part of The Bethesda System) to describe dysplasia. *Low Grade Squamous Intraepithelial Lesions (LSIL)* encompass mild dysplasias and Cervical Intraepithelial Neoplasia 1; this entity is felt to represent evidence of human papillomavirus infection only. *High Grade Squamous Intraepithelial Lesions (HSIL)* include moderate and severe dysplasias, Cervical Intraepithelial Neoplasias 2 and 3, and Carcinoma in Situ. This entity is felt to represent an abnormal transformation of a high risk papillomavirus DNA in the cervical cell.

The Bethesda System (TBS): A NIH-organized standardized terminology for reporting cervicovaginal cytologic abnormalities. The first Bethesda conference occurred in 1988, subsequent conferences occurred in 1991 and 2001.

Transformation zone: The area bordered by the original or native SCJ and the new SCJ; it reflects the presence of endocervical gland elements (Nabothian follicles and gland openings) adjacent to or beneath squamous epithelium.

Vagina: A mucosa-lined tube that extends from the vulva to the cervix and separates the bladder neck and urethra from the rectum and anus.

Vaginal Intraepithelial Neoplasia (VAIN): The term used to refer to biopsy-confirmed vaginal cancer precursors. The precursors are divided into low-grade forms called VAIN 1 and high-grade forms referred to as VAIN 2 and VAIN 3.

Vestibule: The area of the vulva bordered laterally by the labia minora and medially by the introitus, and bordered anteriorly by the clitoris and posteriorly by the labial convergence (posterior fourchette). Structures found with the vestibule include the urethral opening, Skene's glands, the hymeneal ring, the major (Bartholin's) and minor vestibular glands.

Vulva: The area of the female external genital tract that extends from the symphysis pubis anteriorly to the anus posteriorly and lateral to the inguinal-gluteal folds.

Vulvar Intraepithelial Neoplasia (VIN): The term used to refer to biopsy-confirmed vulvar cancer precursors. The precursors are divided into low grade forms called VIN 1 and high grade forms referred to as VIN 2 and VIN 3.

Vulvar noninvasive neoplastic abnormalities: A category of vulvar neoplastic growths with varying degrees of premalignant potential. The general category is subdivided into squamous abnormalities (vulvar intraepithelial neoplasias) and non-squamous abnormalities (Paget's disease or adenocarcinoma in situ, and superficial melanocytic lesions).

Vulvar nonneoplastic abnormalities: Also known as dermatoses, these are skin abnormalities with little or no premalignant potential, and include lichen sclerosis, squamous hyperplasia, and other dermatosis such as psoriasis and lichen planus.

Abbreviated Index

Page numbers in italics indicate tables, figures, and photographs

A

Abnormal cervical epithelium. *See* Colposcopic signs

Abnormal Pap management guidelines, 6–9, *6–9*, 540–69
  ASC-US or LSIL post-colposcopy, 559–61, *560*
  atypical glandular cells (AGC), 561–65, *563–64*
    endometrial cells on the Pap, 562–63, *564*
    post-colposcopy, 564–65, *564*
  atypical squamous cells-high grade (ASC-H), 552, *552–53*
  atypical squamous cells of unidentified significance (ASC-US), 544–52, *547–50*, *547–49*
  with a Pap lacking an endocervical/transformation zone (EC/TZ) component, 542–43, *543*
  with a Pap that has partially obscuring blood, inflammation, other partial obscuring factors or partial air-drying, 543–44, *543*
  with an unsatisfactory Pap test, *543*, 544
    ALTS trial data, 546–47, *549*
    eliminating the category, 545–46
    immunosuppression, 550–51, *550*
    logistics of, 551–52
    risk of, 545, *546*
    in special circumstances, 550–51, *550–51*
    vaginal atrophy, 550, *550*
  high-grade squamous intraepithelial lesion (HSIL), 565–67, *566–68*
  low-grade squamous intraepithelial lesion (LSIL), 552, 554–59, *554*
    in special circumstances, 555, *557–59*, *558–59*
  specimen adequacy guidelines, 542–44, *543*
  see also Cervical screening

Abortion, cervical neoplasia and, 387–88
Acantholysis, 451
Acanthosis, 451
Acetic acid solution, 138–39
  application of, 152–53, *153–54*
    abnormal cervix and, 245–48, *245–48*
    epithelial color and, 194–201, *195–201*
    naked-eye test, 509–11, *510–11*
Acetowhitening, 454–56, *455–56*
American Cancer Society (ACS)
  cervical screening recommendations, *535–536*
  HPV test with the Pap in primary screening, *540*
  screening after hysterectomy, *536*
  screening intervals, *538*
American College of Obstetricians and Gynecologists (ACOG)
  cervical screening recommendations, *535–536*
  HPV testing with the Pap in primary screening, *540*
  screening after hysterectomy, *537*
  screening intervals, *538*
American Society for Colposcopy and Cervical Pathology (ASCCP)
ASCCP Consensus Conference, 542
ASCCP Consenses Guidelines, 540–594
  guidelines for biopsy-confirmed CIN, 2, 3, *595*
  guidelines for biopsy-confirmed CIN 2, 3, special circumstances, *596*
  guidelines for biopsy-confirmed CIN 2, 3 follow-up treatment, *597*
  guidelines for management of LSIL, *556–59*
  guidelines for the management of AGC, *563–64*
  guidelines for the management of ASC, *548*, *550*
  guidelines for the management of ASC-H, *553*
  guidelines for the management of HSIL, *566–68*

recommendations for biopsy-confirmed CIN 1–satisfactory colposcopy, *591–92*
recommendations for biopsy-confirmed CIN 1–unsatisfactory colposcopy, *593–94*
specimen adequacy guidelines, *543*
Actinomyces, *55*
Active vs. expectant management, 586–87
Adenocarcinoma in situ and adenocarcinoma, 329–49
  atypical vessels, 341–47, *342–47*
  columnar epithelium, 329–30, *330*
    fate of, 330
    neoplastic transformation of, 330, *331*
  confirming the diagnosis, 346–47
    management of the patient who desires fertility, 347
    significance of negative margins in the excised specimen, 347
    significance of positive margins in the excised specimen, 347
  invasive, 48–49, *48*
  morphologic spectrum of glandular intraepithelial lesions, 332
  problems detecting, 332–34
    buried disease, *331*, 333
    colposcopic inexperience, 332–33
    cytologic difficulties, 332
    lesion size and location, 333
    mixed disease, 333–34, *333–34*
    skip (multifocal) lesions, 333
  stimulus of disease development, 330–32, *331*
  surface patterns
    elevated lesions, 335, 337, *337*
    epithelial budding, 340, *340–41*
    lesions with a patchy (variegated) red and white surface, 341–2, *341–42*
    lesions with large crypt openings, 337, *337*
    papillary lesions, 337–38, *337–40*
  three colposcopic presentations, 334, *334–35*
  vaginal, 441–42
  vulvar, 483